W9-CNE-547

For Reference

Not to be taken from this room

SALEM HEALTH

MAGILL'S MEDICAL GUIDE

SALEM HEALTH

MAGILL'S MEDICAL GUIDE

Sixth Edition

Volume IV

Kinesiology — Parasitic diseases

Medical Editors

Brandon P. Brown, M.D.
Indiana University School of Medicine

H. Bradford Hawley, M.D.
Wright State University

Margaret Trexler Hessen, M.D.
Drexel University College of Medicine

Clair Kaplan, A.P.R.N./M.S.N.
Yale University School of Nursing

Paul Moglia, Ph.D.
South Nassau Communities Hospital

Judy Mouchawar, M.D., M.S.P.H.
University of Colorado Health Sciences Center

Nancy A. Piotrowski, Ph.D.
Capella University and
University of California, Berkeley

Claire L. Standen, Ph.D.
University of Massachusetts Medical School

SALEM PRESS
Pasadena, California   Hackensack, New Jersey

Editor in Chief: Dawn P. Dawson
Editorial Director: Christina J. Moose
Project Editor: Tracy Irons-Georges
Copy Editors: Desiree Dreeuws, Connie Pollock
Editorial Assistant: Brett S. Weisberg

Photo Editor: Cynthia Breslin Beres
Production Editor: Andrea E. Miller
Acquisitions Editor: Mark Rehn
Page Design and Layout: James Hutson
Additional Layout: William Zimmerman

Illustrations: Hans & Cassidy, Inc., Westerville, Ohio

Magill's Medical Guide: Health and Illness, 1995
Supplement, 1996
Magill's Medical Guide, revised edition, 1998
Second revised edition, 2002
Third revised edition, 2005
Fourth revised edition, 2008
Sixth edition, 2011

∞ The paper used in these volumes conforms to the American National Standard for Permanence of Paper for Printed Library Materials, Z39.48-1992 (R1997).

Note to Readers

The material presented in *Magill's Medical Guide* is intended for broad informational and educational purposes. Readers who suspect that they suffer from any of the physical or psychological disorders, diseases, or conditions described in this set should contact a physician without delay; this work should not be used as a substitute for professional medical diagnosis or treatment. This set is not to be considered definitive on the covered topics, and readers should remember that the field of health care is characterized by a diversity of medical opinions and constant expansion in knowledge and understanding.

Library of Congress Cataloging-in-Publication Data

Magill's medical guide / Brandon P. Brown ... [et al.]. — 6th ed.
    p. cm. — (Salem health)
    Includes bibliographical references and index.
    ISBN 978-1-58765-677-4 (set : alk. paper) — ISBN 978-1-58765-681-1 (v. 4 : alk. paper) —
1. Medicine—Encyclopedias. I. Brown, Brandon P. II. Title: Medical guide.
    RC41.M34 2011
    610.3—dc22

                                                                                    2010031862

First Printing

CONTENTS

COMPLETE LIST OF CONTENTS

VOLUME 1

VOLUME 2

Volume 3

Contents lxxiii
Complete List of Contents lxxvii

VOLUME 4

VOLUME 5

VOLUME 6

Contents clvii
Complete List of Contents clxi

SALEM HEALTH

MAGILL'S MEDICAL GUIDE

KINESIOLOGY
SPECIALTY

ANATOMY OR SYSTEM AFFECTED: Brain, cells, circulatory system, heart, lungs, muscles, musculoskeletal system, nervous system, psychic-emotional system, respiratory system, spine

SPECIALTIES AND RELATED FIELDS: Cardiology, exercise physiology, orthopedics, physical therapy, psychology, sports medicine

DEFINITION: The applied science of human movement, which combines the general areas of anatomy (the study of structure) and physiology (the study of function).

SCIENCE AND PROFESSION

In 1989, the American Academy of Physical Education endorsed the term "kinesiology" to describe the entire field traditionally known as physical education, which includes the following subdisciplines: exercise physiology, biomechanics, motor control and learning, sports nutrition, sports psychology, sports sociology, athletic training programs, pedagogy, adapted physical education, cardiac rehabilitation, and physical therapy.

Exercise physiology describes the body's muscular, cardiovascular, and respiratory functioning during both short-term and long-term exercise. Research has focused on muscle fiber typing, oxygen uptake assessment, lactic acid metabolism, thermoregulation, body composition, and muscle hypertrophy. Biomechanics applies Isaac Newton's laws of physics to improve the mechanical efficiency of muscle movement patterns; using high-speed video and computer analysis, flaws in joint and limb dynamics can be assessed and changed to optimize performance. Motor control and learning pinpoint the areas of the brain and spinal cord that are responsible for the acquisition and retention of motor skills. Understanding the neurological basis of reflex and voluntary muscle movements helps to refine teaching strategies and describe the mechanisms of fatigue.

Sports nutrition describes how the body stores, circulates, and converts nutrients for aerobic and anaerobic energy production through carbohydrate loading and other strategies. Sports psychology explores the workings of the mind before, during, and after exercise and competition. Sports sociology examines aspects such as cultural, ethnic, and gender differences; dynamics in small and large groups; and the role of sports in ethical and moral development. Athletic trainers work with sports physicians and surgeons to prevent and rehabilitate injuries caused by overuse, trauma, or disease.

Physical therapists use clinical exercise therapy and other modalities in a variety of rehabilitation settings.

Allied health areas under the kinesiology umbrella include pedagogy (teaching progressions for movement skills), adapted physical education (activities for the physically and mentally challenged), and cardiac rehabilitation (recovery stages for those disabled by heart disease). Professional organizations in the field of kinesiology include the American College of Sports Medicine, the American Physical Therapy Association, the National Athletic Trainers Association, the National Strength and Conditioning Association, and the American Alliance for Health, Physical Education, Recreation, and Dance.

—Daniel G. Graetzer, Ph.D.

See also Allied health; Anatomy; Cardiac rehabilitation; Dyskinesia; Exercise physiology; Muscles; Nervous system; Neurology; Physical rehabilitation; Physiology; Respiration; Sports medicine.

FOR FURTHER INFORMATION:

Brooks, George A., and Thomas D. Fahey. *Fundamentals of Human Performance.* Mountain View, Calif.: Mayfield, 2000.

McArdle, William, Frank I. Katch, and Victor L. Katch. *Exercise Physiology: Energy, Nutrition, and Human Performance.* 7th ed. Boston: Lippincott Williams & Wilkins, 2010.

Oatis, Carol A. *Kinesiology: The Mechanics and Pathomechanics of Human Movement.* 2d ed. Philadelphia: Lippincott Williams & Wilkins, 2009.

Plowman, Sharon A., and Denise L. Smith. *Exercise Physiology for Health, Fitness, and Performance.* New York: Wolters Kluwer/Lippincott Williams & Wilkins, 2008.

Powers, Scott K., and Edward T. Howley. *Exercise Physiology: Theory and Application to Fitness and Performance.* 7th ed. New York: McGraw-Hill, 2009.

Sharkey, Brian J. *Fitness and Health.* 6th ed. Champaign, Ill.: Human Kinetics, 2007.

KLINEFELTER SYNDROME
DISEASE/DISORDER

ANATOMY OR SYSTEM AFFECTED: Breasts, endocrine system, genitals, hair, psychic-emotional system, reproductive system

SPECIALTIES AND RELATED FIELDS: Embryology, endocrinology, genetics, psychology

DEFINITION: A male chromosomal disorder causing infertility and significant femaleness.

CAUSES AND SYMPTOMS

Klinefelter syndrome is caused by a variation in the number of sex chromosomes. Normal males possess one X and one Y chromosome, while females have two X chromosomes. When an embryo has two X chromosomes and one Y chromosome (XXY), normal development and reproductive function are hampered and the boy shows the symptoms of Klinefelter syndrome. These symptoms include breast development, incomplete maleness, and school or social difficulties. The major symptom is sterility or very reduced fertility. The testes remain small after puberty and produce few, if any, sperm.

In adolescence, breast tissue develops significantly in about 50 percent of all cases. In addition, normal facial and pubic hair may not develop in these boys. Although their average height is six feet, young men with Klinefelter syndrome are often unathletic and less physically strong or coordinated than their peers. Some affected individuals exhibit some degree of subnormal intelligence. Others appear passive and without self-confidence or experience difficulties learning language and speech.

TREATMENT AND THERAPY

Klinefelter syndrome is diagnosed using a karyotype, an analysis of the chromosomes from blood or cheek cells. It can determine the presence of forty-seven chromosomes, including one Y and two X. Although Klinefelter syndrome is genetic and cannot be cured, treatment in the form of a monthly injection of testosterone can be administered to supplement the usually insufficient amount produced by the boy's own testes. This therapy should enhance male physical development by increasing the size of the penis and causing pubic and facial hair growth and greater muscle bulk.

Hormone therapy cannot increase the size of the testes, however, nor can it cure sterility. It cannot reverse breast tissue development, which can only be treated by surgical removal. It may, however, increase self-esteem and a sense of maleness, thereby easing social interactions.

PERSPECTIVE AND PROSPECTS

Found in one or two of every thousand males born, Klinefelter syndrome is the most common human chromosomal variation. Described by Harry Klinefelter in 1942, its cause was discovered by Patricia Jacobs and John Strong in 1959. Affected males have normal erections and may suffer no major effects other than those mentioned above.

—*Grace D. Matzen*

See also Genetic diseases; Genetics and inheritance; Gynecomastia; Hermaphroditism and pseudohermaphroditism; Hormone therapy; Puberty and adolescence; Reproductive system; Sexual differentiation.

FOR FURTHER INFORMATION:

Bandmann, H.-J., and R. Breit, eds. *Klinefelter's Syndrome*. New York: Springer, 1984.

Klinefelter Syndrome and Associates. http://www.genetic.org.

Kronenberg, Henry M., et al., eds. *Williams Textbook of Endocrinology*. 11th ed. Philadelphia: Saunders/Elsevier, 2008.

Martin, Richard J., Avroy A. Fanaroff, and Michele C. Walsh, eds. *Fanaroff and Martin's Neonatal-Perinatal Medicine: Diseases of the Fetus and Infant*. 2 vols. 8th ed. Philadelphia: Mosby/Elsevier, 2006.

Milunsky, Aubrey, ed. *Genetic Disorders of the Fetus: Diagnosis, Prevention, and Treatment*. 6th ed. Hoboken, N.J.: Wiley-Blackwell, 2009.

Morales, Ralph, Jr. *Out of the Darkness: An Autobiography of Living with Klinefelter Syndrome*. Louisville, Ky.: Chicago Spectrum Press, 2002.

Parker, James N., and Philip M. Parker, eds. *The Official Parent's Sourcebook on Klinefelter Syndrome*. San Diego, Calif.: Icon Health, 2002.

Sørensen, Kurt. *Klinefelter's Syndrome in Childhood, Adolescence, and Youth: A Genetic, Clinical, Developmental, Psychiatric, and Psychological Study*. Park Ridge, N.J.: Parthenon, 1988.

KLIPPEL-TRENAUNAY SYNDROME
DISEASE/DISORDER

ALSO KNOWN AS: Angio-osteohypertrophy, nevus vasculosus osteohypertrophicus syndrome, hemangiectasia hypertrophicans, Klippel-Trenaunay-Weber syndrome

---

INFORMATION ON KLINEFELTER SYNDROME

CAUSES: Genetic chromosomal disorder
SYMPTOMS: Infertility, breast development, small testes that produce few, if any, sperm
DURATION: Lifelong
TREATMENTS: None; hormonal therapy for symptoms

ANATOMY OR SYSTEM AFFECTED: Blood vessels, circulatory system, gastrointestinal system, joints, lymphatic system

SPECIALTIES AND RELATED FIELDS: Genetics, internal medicine, pediatrics, vascular medicine

DEFINITION: A rare congenital syndrome characterized by hemangiomas of the vascular system that can affect bone or soft tissue throughout the body.

CAUSES AND SYMPTOMS

Klippel-Trenaunay syndrome was first described in 1900 in patients exhibiting a combination of varicose veins, multiple vascular nevi (birthmarks on the skin sometimes called port-wine stains), and excessive growth or development (hypertrophy) of limbs or soft tissue. Increased vascularity is common. At birth, a large vein may be observed running from the lower leg into the upper thigh, referred to as the Klippel-Trenaunay vein.

The molecular basis for the disease is unclear, as most cases appear as simply random occurrences. Among those few cases which appear to be heritable, it is believed that an autosomal dominant gene may be at fault, possibly linked to chromosome numbers 5 or 11. Evidence suggests that, at the molecular level, deregulation of deoxyribonucleic acid (DNA) methylation of imprinted genes may play a role.

Whichever gene may be at fault, it is believed the mutation occurs early in embryonic development. The result is that the defect appears randomly among cells as they migrate and differentiate early during embryonic stages, resulting in the seemingly haphazard distribution of the trait as the fetus develops.

Diagnosis is based upon the triad of vascular or soft tissue defects, with venous or capillary malformations leading to localized, and often extensive, tumors. Preliminary diagnosis can be based upon any two of the characteristics. Another symptom may be excessive bleeding, especially from the rectum or detected in the urine.

TREATMENT AND THERAPY

If the disorder becomes apparent during the prenatal period, then the prognosis is generally poor. Treatment in the adult is generally symptomatic, although the possibility of internal organ involvement, as well as pulmonary embolisms, leaves the patient at risk even in the absence of symptoms.

Since varicose veins are generally apparent, the pa-

INFORMATION ON KLIPPEL-TRENAUNAY SYNDROME

CAUSES: Unknown, possibly genetic

SYMPTOMS: Varicose veins, port-wine stains, limb or soft tissue hypertrophy, noticeable large vein running from lower leg into upper thigh, localized tumors, excessive bleeding

DURATION: Lifelong

TREATMENTS: Alleviation of symptoms, such as compression garments and leg elevation for varicose veins, surgery for limb hypertrophy, anticoagulants

---

tient may wear compression garments, elevating the legs at intervals. Surgery may be necessary to correct limb hypertrophy. Because the formation of embolisms is a risk, the patient may utilize anticoagulants prophylactically, particularly prior to surgery. Corticosteroid use may help limit swelling in some cases. In the absence of significant malformations, the patient should simply be monitored on an annual basis.

PERSPECTIVE AND PROSPECTS

The rare and sporadic nature of the disorder complicates routine screening. At best, proper prenatal care during pregnancy may result in diagnosis if the disorder does appear. Research into the molecular basis of the disorder may eventually determine its origins.

—*Richard Adler, Ph.D.*

See also Birthmarks; Blood vessels; Congenital disorders; Hypertrophy; Skin; Skin disorders; Varicose veins; Vascular medicine; Vascular system.

FOR FURTHER INFORMATION:

Baskerville, P. A., et al. "The Etiology of the Klippel-Trenaunay Syndrome." *Annals of Surgery* 202 (November, 1985): 624-627.

Evans, Jeff. "Klippel-Trenaunay Stains Predict Complications." *Skin and Allergy News* 34, no. 2 (February 1, 2003): 40.

Mulliken, John B., and Anthony E. Young, eds. *Vascular Birthmarks: Hemangiomas and Malformations.* Philadelphia: W. B. Saunders, 1988.

Telander, R. L., et al. "Prognosis and Management of Lesions of the Trunk in Children with Klippel-Trenaunay Syndrome." *Journal of Pediatric Surgery* 19 (1984): 417-422.

KLUVER-BUCY SYNDROME

DISEASE/DISORDER

ANATOMY OR SYSTEM AFFECTED: Brain, eyes, genitals

SPECIALTIES AND RELATED FIELDS: Family medicine, ophthalmology, pediatrics, psychiatry, psychology

DEFINITION: A behavioral disorder characterized by lack of emotional activity or responses similar to that often observed in patients with Alzheimer's disease.

KEY TERMS:

agnosia: inability to recognize common objects

amygdala: the front portion of the temporal lobe of the brain

hyperorality: use of the mouth for the examination of objects

lobotomy: the severance of nerve fibers in the frontal lobe of brain

temporal lobes: lateral portions of the cerebrum of the brain

---

> ### INFORMATION ON KLUVER-BUCY SYNDROME
>
> **CAUSES:** Malfunction in communication between left and right temporal lobes or damage to amygdala
> **SYMPTOMS:** Unusual fear response, use of mouth for examining objects, inability to recognize objects
> **DURATION:** Lifelong
> **TREATMENTS:** Symptomatic

CAUSES AND SYMPTOMS

Kluver-Bucy syndrome was first observed in 1937 when German neuroanatomist Heinrich Kluver, working with American neuropathologist Paul Bucy at Northwestern University, observed that the removal of the temporal lobes, including the amygdala, of a rhesus monkey resulted in significant behavioral changes in the animal. More specifically, the monkey displayed visual agnosia, the inability to recognize objects while at the same time displaying excessive responses to visual stimulation (hypermetamorphosis). The animals also demonstrated a significantly increased tendency to orally examine objects (hyperorality) and heightened sexual responses.

The syndrome was first described in humans in 1955 by Sergio Dalle Ore and a colleague following a temporal lobectomy in a male being treated for epilepsy. Symptoms largely followed those previously observed by Kluver and Bucy in monkeys and are still considered valid for the diagnosis of the illness. Specific characteristics of the syndrome in humans include auditory, tactile, or visual agnosia; the inability to recognize familiar objects including other persons (psychic blindness); hyperorality; the examination of objects orally rather than visually; docility; complete lack of aggressiveness sometimes termed as placidity; and changes in diet that can include either overeating or the eating of inappropriate objects (hyperphasia). Hyperphasia has been reported to take the form of not only placing in the mouth unusual foods but also placing in the mouth dangerous objects such as cigarettes, razors, and nails or even excrement. Altered sexuality, attempting to achieve sexual satisfaction not through intercourse or masturbation but through comments or touching, has also been observed in persons diagnosed with Kluver-Bucy syndrome. Humans generally do not exhibit all the characteristics of the syndrome, with diagnosis based upon manifestation of three or more of these symptoms.

The underlying physiological basis for the syndrome remains unclear. Kluver-Bucy syndrome may be triggered by damage either to the temporal lobes or within the amygdala, the frontal portion of the temporal lobes. The function of the cells that constitute the amygdala includes production of a variety of neurotransmitters; the initial studies carried out by Kluver and Bucy that resulted in the description of the condition had involved investigation of the effect of mescaline on this region of the brain. Kluver-Bucy syndrome has been triggered by pathological conditions associated with, or secondary to, more than fifty different conditions, including encephalitis, strokes, tumors, and dementias such as Alzheimer's or Pick's diseases.

Specific diagnosis beyond the appearance of behavioral changes has been difficult and controversial. Radioimaging studies as well as positron emission tomography (PET) scans have shown the presence of damage to neural connections within the amygdala as well as other regions in the temporal lobes. The issue has been controversial, however, since not all patients diagnosed with the syndrome exhibit such changes or the presence of lesions.

TREATMENT AND THERAPY

Few effective treatments have been described. However, the use of anti-cholinergics, drugs that inhibit the activity of the neurotransmitter acetylcholine, have shown some success in causing regression of the syndrome. Several studies have reported that treatment of patients with carbamazepine, an anticonvulsant and analgesic prescribed for treatment of seizures that have their origin in the trigeminal ganglia region, has had some success, particularly in adults.

Treatments have also been directed toward the functioning of the amygdala directly. The region is associated with cognitive recognition and social behaviors, the result of its interconnections with other regions of the cortex of the brain. The amygdala is characterized by neural interactions involving the neurotransmitter serotonin. Inhibitors of serotonin uptake have shown some success in addressing the syndrome. This class of drugs has been categorized as selective serotonin reuptake inhibitors (SSRI) and includes at least eight major categories of drugs. SSRIs are frequently prescribed as antidepressants, and they function to increase serotonin levels within the nerve synapse, with the result that neurotransmitter action on nerves is increased.

PERSPECTIVE AND PROSPECTS

No cure for Kluver-Bucy syndrome currently exists; fortunately, the syndrome is a relatively rare disorder with no more than several hundred cases being reported since it was first described in humans in 1955. Furthermore, Kluver-Bucy syndrome manifests itself in behavior difficulties rather than in life-threatening conditions. Therefore, management of the problem is the primary means of dealing with the condition. Since the syndrome most commonly manifests itself in the aftermath of other diseases or difficulties, prevention of the condition is indirect, reflecting the elimination or prevention of other underlying causes. They include recognition and rapid treatment of the causes of encephalitis or intervention during birth to address conditions that may result in oxygen deprivation (hypoxia).

Rare cases may evolve into Korsakow syndrome, a brain disorder characterized by significant encephalopathy. Korsakow syndrome is generally observed only among alcoholics.

—*Richard Adler, Ph.D.*

See also Alzheimer's disease; Brain; Brain damage; Brain disorders; Dementias; Encephalitis; Frontotemporal dementia (FTP); Neurology; Pick's disease; Psychiatric disorders; Psychiatry.

FOR FURTHER INFORMATION:

Goscinski, I., et al. "The Kluver-Bucy Syndrome." *Journal of Neurosurgical Sciences* 41, no. 3 (1997): 269.

Jha, Sanjeev, et al. "Cerebral Birth Anoxia, Seizures and Kluver-Bucy Syndrome: Some Observations." *Journal of Pediatric Neurology* 3, no. 4 (2005): 227.

Kalat, James. *Biological Psychology.* Belmont, Calif.: Wadsworth, 2008.

Malloy, Paul, and Jeffrey Cummings. *The Neuropsychiatry of Limbic and Subcortical Disorders.* Washington, D.C.: American Psychiatric Press, 1997.

Salim, Ali, et al. "Kluver-Bucy Syndrome as a Result of Minor Head Trauma." *Southern Medical Journal* 95, no. 8 (August 1, 2002): 929.

KNEECAP REMOVAL
PROCEDURE

ALSO KNOWN AS: Patellectomy

ANATOMY OR SYSTEM AFFECTED: Bones, joints, knees, legs, muscloskeletal system, tendons

SPECIALTIES AND RELATED FIELDS: General surgery, orthopedics

DEFINITION: The surgical removal of the kneecap.

INDICATIONS AND PROCEDURES

The kneecap, or patella, is the triangular bone at the front of the knee. It is held in position by the lower end of the quadriceps muscle, which surrounds the patella and is attached to the upper part of the tibia by the patellar tendon. The role of the kneecap is to protect the knee.

Kneecap removal surgery, or patellectomy, is performed as a result of fracture, frequent dislocation, or painful arthritis in the kneecap. Fracture is usually caused by a direct or sharp blow to the knee. Dislocation of the patella is often linked to a congenital abnormality, such as the underdevelopment of the lower end of the femur or excessive laxity of the ligaments that support the knee. Painful degenerative arthritic conditions, such as retropatellar arthritis and chondromalacia patellae, inflame and roughen the undersurface of the kneecap. Arthritic pain often worsens with the climbing of stairs or bending of the knee.

Before surgery begins, a clinical examination is conducted including blood and urine studies, and X rays of both knees. The knee is thoroughly cleansed with antiseptic soap. Anesthesia is administered either by local injection or spinal injection or by inhalation and injection (general anesthesia).

Surgery begins with an incision made around the

kneecap. The skin is pulled back, exposing the muscle-covered kneecap. Surrounding muscle and connecting tendons attached to the kneecap are cut, and the kneecap is carefully removed. The remaining muscle is then sewn back together with strong suture material. Surgery is completed with the closing of the skin with sutures or clips. Full recovery takes about six weeks.

USES AND COMPLICATIONS

Following surgery, a scar will form along the incision. As the incision heals, the scar will recede gradually. Pain from the incision can be alleviated with heating pads. The affected leg should be elevated with pillows. Frequent movement of legs while resting in bed will decrease the likelihood of deep vein blood clots. General activity and returning to work is encouraged as soon as possible. Standing for prolonged periods of time, however, is not recommended during recovery. Following the approximate six-week recovery time, physical therapy is often used to restore strength to the knee.

Possible complications associated with kneecap removal include excessive bleeding and surgical wound infection. Additional complications can occur during recovery if general postoperative guidelines are not followed. Some loss of function can be expected.

—*Jason Georges*

See also Arthritis; Bones and the skeleton; Fracture and dislocation; Joints; Lower extremities; Orthopedic surgery; Orthopedics; Orthopedics, pediatric; Physical rehabilitation.

FOR FURTHER INFORMATION:

Doherty, Gerard M., and Lawrence W. Way, eds. *Current Surgical Diagnosis and Treatment.* 12th ed. New York: Lange Medical Books/McGraw-Hill, 2006.

Halpern, Brian. *The Knee Crisis Handbook: Understanding Pain, Preventing Trauma, Recovering from Knee Injury, and Building Healthy Knees for Life.* Emmaus, Pa.: Rodale Books, 2003.

Mulholland, Michael W., et al., eds. *Greenfield's Surgery: Scientific Principles and Practice.* 4th ed. Philadelphia: Lippincott Williams & Wilkins, 2006.

Tapley, Donald F., et al., eds. *The Columbia University College of Physicians and Surgeons Complete Home Medical Guide.* Rev. 3d ed. New York: Crown, 1995.

Tierney, Lawrence M., Stephen J. McPhee, and Maxine A. Papadakis, eds. *Current Medical Diagnosis and Treatment 2007.* New York: McGraw-Hill Medical, 2006.

KNOCK-KNEES
DISEASE/DISORDER

ALSO KNOWN AS: Genu valgum

ANATOMY OR SYSTEM AFFECTED: Bones, feet, hips, joints, knees, legs, ligaments, muscles

SPECIALTIES AND RELATED FIELDS: Orthopedics, pediatrics, physical therapy

DEFINITION: A deformity in which the knees are positioned close together or turn toward each other and the tibias and ankles are apart when the feet are placed in a normal standing position.

CAUSES AND SYMPTOMS

Knock-knees, affecting both knees or occasionally only one, are a normal condition as children mature. Infants' leg bones are slightly rotated because of uterine positioning. As toddlers' legs straighten after having bowlegs, their tibias and knees often temporarily rotate toward the body's axis, causing the feet to be several inches apart. When knock-knees are not representative of normal physical development, they occur because of health conditions such as infections, obesity, or fractured legs that disrupt knee growth. Knock-knees are sometimes a symptom of other conditions.

Mobility may be affected with knock-knees. Patients sometimes adjust leg and foot movement to compensate for altered knee positioning and imbalanced centers of gravity. Usually, children walk with their toes turned in for balance when they have knock-knees. Knock-kneed adults sometimes develop arthritis because of the strain on knee joints and ligaments. Knock-knees can also place stress on patients' backs and hips.

TREATMENT AND THERAPY

Medical professionals do not treat most knock-knees unless specific cases seem abnormal, cause pain, or

---

INFORMATION ON KNOCK-KNEES

CAUSES: Normal condition in infants; infections, obesity, or fractures in older individuals

SYMPTOMS: Altered knee positioning, imbalanced center of gravity, sometimes arthritis

DURATION: Usually temporary

TREATMENTS: None, unless pain develops or movement is impeded; may include stretching, shoe inserts, physical therapy, orthopedic braces, surgery

impede movement. Growth usually corrects knee positioning. Physicians measure legs and the distance between ankles to assess the progress of natural correction. X rays are useful to detect bone problems that may exacerbate knock-knees. Photographs can document leg alignment.

Stretching the leg muscles can aid the natural resolution of knock-knees. Shoes designed with inserts can mitigate the stress on feet and manipulate patients to walk straight. Physical therapy can alleviate cartilage and joint pain associated with knock-knees.

If young patients do not outgrow knock-knees, ankle distances increase to 4 inches or more, or the condition worsens, particularly in one knee, then medical intervention often becomes necessary to ensure that patients are capable of normal movement. Physicians sometimes advise patients to wear a brace. If such efforts are unsuccessful, then the patient may undergo surgery to adjust leg bones and growth plates.

Treatment is essential for diseases or conditions in which knock-knees is a symptom. Some patients seek medical correction for aesthetic reasons.

PERSPECTIVE AND PROSPECTS

Beginning in the late nineteenth century, physicians routinely recommended therapeutic braces to treat knock-knees. During the 1950's, Soviet doctor Gavril Abramovich Ilizarov devised a fixator that encircles legs and uses tension to correct rotation problems associated with knock-knees. Italian doctor Antonio Bianchi-Maiocchi first used this device in Western countries in 1981. James Aronson brought the method to the United States in the 1980's. In that decade, Ukrainian doctor Veklich Vitaliy adapted Ilizarov's fixator for a procedure that is often used to correct severe knock-knees.

By the late twentieth century, however, physicians discouraged the use of braces to treat normal cases of knock-knees. Most advised patients to permit natural correction to occur, emphasizing that devices would not quicken that process.

—*Elizabeth D. Schafer, Ph.D.*

See also Bones and the skeleton; Growth; Joints; Lower extremities; Orthopedics; Orthopedics, pediatric.

FOR FURTHER INFORMATION:

Bianci-Maiocchi, Antonio, and James Aronson, eds. *Operative Principles of Ilizarov: Fracture Treatment, Nonunion, Osteomyelitis, Lengthening, Deformity Correction*. Baltimore: Williams & Wilkins, 1991.

England, Stephen P., ed. *Common Orthopedic Problems*. Philadelphia: W. B. Saunders, 1996.

Halpern, Brian. *The Knee Crisis Handbook: Understanding Pain, Preventing Trauma, Recovering from Knee Injury, and Building Healthy Knees for Life*. Emmaus, Pa.: Rodale Books, 2003.

Herring, John A., ed. *Tachdjian's Pediatric Orthopaedics*. 4th ed. 3 vols. Philadelphia: Saunders/Elsevier, 2008.

KWASHIORKOR
DISEASE/DISORDER

ALSO KNOWN AS: Malignant malnutrition, protein malnutrition, protein-calorie malnutrition, Mehl hrschaden

ANATOMY OR SYSTEM AFFECTED: Gastrointestinal system, muscles, skin

SPECIALTIES AND RELATED FIELDS: Family medicine, nutrition, pediatrics

DEFINITION: A form of malnutrition caused by inadequate protein intake.

CAUSES AND SYMPTOMS

Kwashiorkor occurs most commonly in areas of famine, limited food supply, and low levels of education, which can lead to inadequate knowledge of diet and appropriate dietary intakes. Early symptoms are general and include fatigue, irritability, and lethargy. As protein deprivation continues, symptoms include failure to gain weight and linear growth. Other progressed symp-

---

INFORMATION ON KWASHIORKOR

CAUSES: Protein deprivation

SYMPTOMS: Fatigue, irritability, lethargy, poor growth, apathy, edema, decreased muscle mass, large belly, diarrhea, dermatitis, loss of skin pigmentation, changes in color and texture of hair, infections; may progress to shock, coma, and death

DURATION: Progressive if untreated

TREATMENTS: Depends on degree of malnutrition; may include treatment for shock and increased calorie intake (first as carbohydrates, simple sugars, and fats, then proteins)

toms include apathy, decreased muscle mass, edema, a large protuberant belly (resulting from decreased albumin in the blood), diarrhea, and dermatitis. Skin may lose pigment where it has peeled away or darken where it has been irritated or traumatized. Hair may become thin and brittle and may change color, becoming lighter or reddish. As a result of immune system damage, patients may suffer from increased numbers of infections and increased severity of what normally might be mild infections. In the final stages, shock and/or coma usually precede death.

TREATMENT AND THERAPY

A physical examination may show an enlarged liver and generalized edema. Treatment varies depending on the degree of malnutrition. Patients in shock will require immediate treatment. Often, calories are given first in the form of carbohydrates, simple sugars, and fats. Proteins are started after other caloric sources have provided increased energy. Vitamin and mineral supplements are essential. Many children will have developed intolerance to milk lactose (sugar intolerance) and will need to be supplemented with lactase (an enzyme) if they are to benefit from milk products. Adequate diet with appropriate amounts of carbohydrates, fat, and protein will prevent kwashiorkor.

PERSPECTIVE AND PROSPECTS

Kwashiorkor means "deposed child" in one African dialect, referring to a child "deposed" from the mother's breast by a newborn sibling. Kwashiorkor is found largely in tropical and subtropical regions where the diet is high in starch (such as cereal grains or plantains) and low in protein. The incidence of kwashiorkor in children in the United States is extremely low, and only rare, isolated cases are seen. Treatment early in the course of kwashiorkor generally produces positive results. Treatment in later stages will improve a child's general health, but the child may be left with permanent physical ailments and mental disabilities. With delayed or no treatment, the condition is fatal.

—*Jason A. Hubbart, M.S.*

See also Dietary reference intakes (DRIs); Edema; Food biochemistry; Malnutrition; Nutrition; Protein.

FOR FURTHER INFORMATION:

Champakam, S., S. G. Srikantia, and C. Gopalan. "Kwashiorkor and Mental Development." *American Journal of Clinical Nutrition* 21 (1968): 844.

Golden, M. H. N. "Severe Malnutrition." In *Oxford Textbook of Medicine*, edited by D. J. Weatherall, J. G. G. Ledingham, and D. A. Warrell. 3d ed. New York: Oxford University Press, 1996.

Kleinman, Ronald E., ed. *Pediatric Nutrition Handbook*. 5th ed. Elk Grove Village, Ill.: American Academy of Pediatrics, 2004.

KYPHOSIS

DISEASE/DISORDER

ALSO KNOWN AS: Dowager's hump

ANATOMY OR SYSTEM AFFECTED: Back, bones

SPECIALTIES AND RELATED FIELDS: Orthopedics

DEFINITION: A marked increase of the normal curvature of the thoracic vertebrae or upper back, sometimes referred to as dowager's hump because of its prevalence in elderly women.

CAUSES AND SYMPTOMS

Patients with kyphosis appear to be looking down with their shoulders markedly bent forward. They are unable to straighten their backs, their body height is reduced, and their arms therefore appear to be disproportionately long. The increased curvature of the thoracic vertebrae tilts the head forward, and the patient has to raise her head and hyperextend her neck in order to look forward. This posture increases the strain on the neck muscles and leads to discomfort in the neck, shoulders, and upper back. It limits the field of vision and increases the patient's chances of tripping over an object not directly in the line of vision. It also shifts forward the body's center of gravity and increases the chances of falling.

In severe cases, kyphosis limits chest expansion during breathing. As a result, less air gets into the lungs, which become underventilated and prone to infections. Pneumonia is a common cause of death in these patients. In very severe cases, the curvature of the thoracic vertebrae is so pronounced that the lower ribs lie over the pelvic cavity. Patients with severe kyphosis are not able to lie flat on their backs, and many spend most of their time sitting up in a chair or in bed, propped by a number of pillows. Unless the patient changes positions frequently, the pressure exerted by the vertebrae on the skin and subcutaneous tissue may precipitate pressure sores (bed sores) on the upper back. Pressure sores may also develop on the buttocks. The sores often become infected, and the infection may spread to the blood, leading to septicemia and death.

INFORMATION ON KYPHOSIS

CAUSES: Osteoporosis, tumors, infection

SYMPTOMS: Inability to straighten one's back, reduced body height, appearance of disproportionately long arms, strain on neck muscles leading to discomfort, pain

DURATION: Chronic

TREATMENTS: Hormone therapy, drug therapy (e.g., Fosamax, teriparatide)

The most common cause of kyphosis is osteoporosis, a disease in which the bone mass is reduced. As a result, the bones become mechanically weak and are unable to sustain the pressure of the body weight. The vertebrae gradually become wedged and partially collapsed, more so in the front (anteriorly) than in the back (posteriorly), thus increasing the forward curvature of the thoracic vertebrae. Sometimes, the compression of a vertebra is associated with sudden, very severe, and incapacitating pain that is usually relieved spontaneously after about four weeks. In most cases, however, the compression is a gradual process associated with slowly worsening back discomfort. The discomfort is caused by the strain imposed on the muscles on either side of the vertebrae. In rare instances, the nerves exiting the spinal cord become trapped by the wedged or collapsed vertebrae, and the patient experiences severe pain that tends to radiate to the area supplied by the entrapped nerve.

Less common causes of kyphosis include the compression of a vertebra as a result of tumors or infections. In these cases, the angulation of the thoracic curvature is very prominent.

TREATMENT AND THERAPY

The availability of medications to treat and prevent osteoporosis should reduce significantly the prevalence of both that disease and kyphosis.

—*Ronald C. Hamdy, M.D.*

See also Aging; Back pain; Bone disorders; Bones and the skeleton; Braces, orthopedic; Orthopedic surgery; Orthopedics; Orthopedics, pediatric; Osteoporosis; Pneumonia; Safety issues for the elderly; Spinal cord disorders; Spine, vertebrae, and disks.

FOR FURTHER INFORMATION:

Byyny, Richard L., and Leonard Speroff. *A Clinical Guide for the Care of Older Women.* 2d ed. Baltimore: Williams & Wilkins, 1996.

Currey, John D. *Bones: Structures and Mechanics.* Princeton, N.J.: Princeton University Press, 2002.

Heaney, Robert P. "Osteoporosis." In *Nutrition in Women's Health*, edited by Debra A. Krummel and Penny M. Kris-Etherton. Gaithersburg, Md.: Aspen, 1996.

Hodgson, Stephen F., ed. *Mayo Clinic on Osteoporosis: Keeping Bones Healthy and Strong and Reducing the Risk of Fractures.* Rochester, Minn.: Mayo Clinic, 2003.

Meredith, C. M. "Exercise in the Prevention of Osteoporosis." In *Nutrition of the Elderly*, edited by Hamish Munro and Gunter Schlierf. Nestle's Nutrition Workshop Series 29. New York: Raven Press, 1992.

Nelson, Miriam E., and Sarah Wernick. *Strong Women, Strong Bones: Everything You Need to Know to Prevent, Treat, and Beat Osteoporosis.* Rev. ed. New York: Berkley Books, 2006.

Van De Graaff, Kent M. *Human Anatomy.* 6th ed. New York: McGraw-Hill, 2002.

LABORATORY TESTS

PROCEDURES

ANATOMY OR SYSTEM AFFECTED: Blood, cells

SPECIALTIES AND RELATED FIELDS: Bacteriology, cytology, endocrinology, epidemiology, forensic medicine, genetics, hematology, histology, immunology, microbiology, oncology, pathology, pharmacology, serology, toxicology, virology

DEFINITION: The collection and analysis of body fluids such as blood and urine to establish a diagnosis or to monitor a treatment regimen.

KEY TERMS:

antibody: a protein produced in the body by the immune system that recognizes and binds selectively to foreign material (antigens) to facilitate their elimination; antibodies can be cultivated in animals or by artificial means in the laboratory and chemically altered for use as reagents in immunoassays

clinical chemistry: a chemistry specialty that deals with an analysis of the chemical components of body fluids

clinical laboratory: a general term for those areas of a medical facility where analyses of body fluids are performed

clinical microbiology: the scientific discipline involving the study of microscopic organisms (such as bacteria, fungi, and viruses) that cause disease

coagulation: the process of blood clotting, a very complicated process that can be affected by many disease states; the clotting process is inhibited for specimen collection purposes using substances called anticoagulants

hematology: the medical specialty dealing with the detection and diagnosis of blood-related diseases

immunoassay: the use of antibody-antigen recognition as the basis of a medically useful method of detecting and measuring a substance in body fluids

pathology: the medical specialty that deals with the structural and biochemical changes that are produced by disease

INDICATIONS AND PROCEDURES

Clinical laboratory testing is a vital element in diagnosis. After physical examination and the taking of the patient's medical history, the physician will often request that specific tests be performed on blood, urine, or other body fluids. Appropriate specimens are collected and forwarded to the laboratory for specimen processing.

Blood is the most common specimen submitted for testing in the clinical laboratory. In a hospital or large referral laboratory, there may be special personnel, called phlebotomists, employed to collect blood. In a small office laboratory, blood may be collected by the attending physician or nurse. Blood is collected in a syringe or in special tubes that may contain anticoagulants.

Urine is the next most common laboratory specimen and is collected as a result of a single void (random urine specimen) or for a time period of twenty-four hours or more. In the latter case, the collection container may also contain substances that act as a preservative. If a long-term urine specimen is necessary, it is very important for the patient to follow the directions regarding collection. Failure to follow these directions can lead to erroneous laboratory results.

Less commonly collected specimens include cerebrospinal fluid, gastric (stomach) fluid, and amniotic fluid. Cerebrospinal fluid is usually collected by a physician by direct sampling with a needle (lumbar puncture, or spinal tap). Gastric fluid is obtained by the insertion of a gastric collection tube. Amniotic fluid is collected by an obstetrician in the process called amniocentesis, in which a sample of the fluid surrounding the fetus is removed by the insertion of a needle through the mother's abdomen. Frequently, laboratory tests are also ordered on infectious material associated with a wound or surgical incision.

A major aspect of specimen collection is ensuring that the sample is correctly labeled and that no mix-up of specimens has occurred. Part of this process may involve checking identification armbands or asking patients or nursing staff to confirm identification. While this procedure may be exasperating to the patient or nursing personnel, it is a necessary part of detecting errors.

Immediately after the specimen is received in the laboratory, documentation of time of receipt and the tests requested is made, which is referred to as logging in the specimen. Each sample receives a special code called an accession number. The test performance and results are tracked with this number, since multiple specimens can be received on a single patient in a given day. This process is usually computerized and may utilize bar code labeling in a process very similar to that used for automatic cash-register pricing of grocery items.

In large hospital or referral laboratories, the processing center is responsible for distributing the sample to the laboratory sections, where various tests are performed. Since each test requires a specific amount of sample, specimen processing also involves determining that the correct amount of fluid has been collected and reserved for proper performance of the test.

For blood specimens, many laboratory determinations are made regarding plasma, or serum, which is the liquid component of blood that contains no cells. The whole blood specimen is separated into cellular and liquid components by centrifugation. The sample is spun rapidly so that the force of the spin sediments the cells, with the serum or plasma layer on top.

Once the specimen is distributed to the pertinent laboratory sections, testing is done using a variety of analytical techniques. The testing methodology is almost as varied as the types of analyses requested. A few general statements, however, are applicable. Automation is the guiding force behind laboratory test methodology development. Routinely ordered tests are done with instruments specifically designed to perform a group or panel of tests, rather than each test being performed individually by a technologist using manual chemistry methods. Automation coupled with computerization has greatly increased laboratory efficiency, decreased turnaround time (the time required for a test to be performed and results to be reported to the physician), eliminated human errors, and allowed more tests to be performed on smaller sample material. The latter advantage is particularly important for pediatric specimens, in which sample size is usually an important consideration. Automation also eliminates much of the technologist's contact with the specimen, considerably reducing the risk of spreading infectious diseases.

Each section of the laboratory is responsible for a specific set of tests. The chemistry section performs chemical analyses of body fluids. Panels of tests related to kidney, heart, and liver function are also done. In addition, tests to measure amounts of therapeutic drugs, hormones, blood proteins, and cancer-related proteins are accomplished with immunoassay techniques. The development of antibody-related techniques has revolutionized testing in all areas of the clinical laboratory. The ability to customize antibody production and adapt it to specific analytical requirements has allowed the continual development of new tests and methodologies.

The hematology section is responsible for monitoring the levels of blood cells and clotting factors. Other specialized tests to diagnose cancer of the blood cells

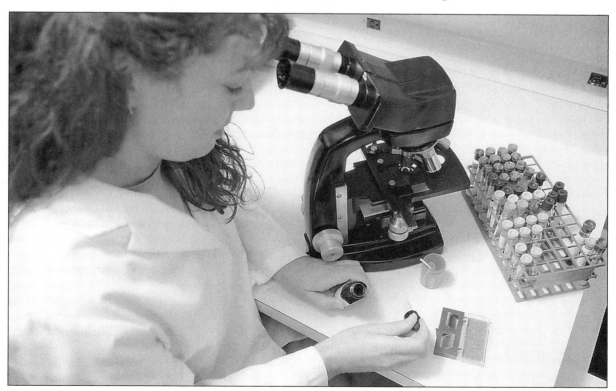

Laboratory tests are vital in the diagnosis of disease. A scientist examines samples with a microscope. (PhotoDisc)

may also be done. Blood typing and donor testing are technically hematology-related tests, but they are usually reserved for a separate section designated as blood bank or transfusion services. Transfusion service is a specialty in its own right and is almost always reserved for hospital-associated laboratories.

Microbiology is the section where body fluids are checked for infectious microorganisms. Once an organism is identified, the section can also determine which antibiotics may be useful for treatment by performing antibiotic susceptibility tests.

As the laboratory tests are performed, the results are recorded and reported to the physician. Computerization has permitted the transfer of patient results directly from the instrument performing the test to the patient's file, eliminating many tedious and error-prone clerical functions.

For hospital and reference laboratories, a laboratory director—either a physician (usually a pathologist) who specialized in laboratory medicine or a scientist with doctoral level training in a laboratory specialty—monitors the performance of the laboratory, helps physicians with the interpretation of ambiguous or complex laboratory results, and provides guidance on the introduction of new tests or instrumentation. Most laboratories also have a section supervisor or administrator who is an experienced medical technologist to oversee the daily laboratory routine.

In the United States, hospital and reference laboratories are inspected periodically by federal and state government agencies as well as professional medical societies to check the quality of the work performed. The most commonly used proficiency testing program is that administered by the College of American Pathology (CAP), which also sponsors a program of peer inspection of laboratories. Many state and federal agencies will accept CAP approval of a laboratory as a substitute for its own detailed inspection.

USES AND COMPLICATIONS

Because of the variety of laboratory testing, it is impractical to cover its applications in depth in a brief review. Instead, a few illustrative tests that are performed often or are associated with familiar disorders will be presented. The most frequently ordered laboratory tests are serum glucose tests, serum electrolyte (salt) level measurements, and complete blood count (CBC) tests.

The maintenance of blood glucose (sugar) levels is essential for body activity and brain function. The laboratory measurement of blood glucose is one of the oldest known procedures performed in the clinical laboratory. It is part of the diagnostic procedures used to monitor and test for diabetes mellitus. Glucose and electrolyte testing are performed in the chemistry section of the laboratory, while a CBC takes place in hematology. Certain levels of electrolytes—sodium, chloride, potassium, and calcium—are needed for proper cardiac function. An abnormal level of these salts could also indicate possible hormonal or kidney malfunction. The CBC is a measure of the cell populations that carry oxygen (red blood cells), fight infection or invasion by foreign substances (white blood cells), and activate the blood-clotting mechanism (platelets). The white cell population is elevated in infections but also in cases of leukemia (malignant growth of a white cell population). More specialized testing is needed when leukemia is suspected. An instrument called a flow cytometer can be used to count and detect subtypes of white cells. These data, along with a pathologist's microscopic examination of a blood smear and the results of clinical examination, are used to arrive at a diagnosis of the specific type of leukemia present. The identification of the cell population causing the cancer is important for determining treatment and prognosis.

A deficiency of red cells or their oxygen-carrying hemoglobin molecule is called anemia. It can be caused by iron deficiency and other impairments of red cell production, chronic bleeding, or accelerated red cell destruction (hemolysis). Each of the causes must be either confirmed or ruled out through additional testing or by clinical examination.

Platelet deficiency is a major cause of clotting disorders, although many other causes of bleeding disorders exist. The specific defect can be determined by measuring the clotting time and by using special immunoassays to measure clotting substances in the blood.

Many hormonal (endocrine) disorders can be diagnosed through laboratory testing. For example, the thyroid, the regulator gland for body metabolism, can produce a variety of symptoms when it is not functioning properly. Thyroid testing is the most common endocrine-related laboratory procedure requested by physicians. The blood levels of thyroid hormone and of the pituitary factor that stimulates the thyroid gland are measured in the laboratory using immunoassay methods. These types of assays can also be used to monitor other hormones involved in fertility, growth, and the function of the adrenal gland (the gland that helps maintain sugar metabolism and electrolyte balance).

IN THE NEWS: IN-HOME MEDICAL TESTING

In-home health testing has become increasingly popular as a result of its convenience, privacy, and affordability. Home tests can enable the consumer to determine the potential risk for developing a health problem even when no immediate signs or symptoms exist, or they can enable the consumer to follow a specific medical condition more accurately. Several home tests are available for over-the-counter purchase, including those that test for cholesterol levels, drugs of abuse, fecal occult blood, glucose levels, hepatitis C, human immunodeficiency virus (HIV), ovulation timing, pregnancy, prothrombin time screening, and vaginal pH. Home test kits should not be used as stand-alone measures to determine one's health care, but rather the results should be used in conjunction with proper medical advice in order to confirm the test results.

Most reports state that the test kits approved by the Food and Drug Administration (FDA) are either "about as accurate" or "fairly accurate," when compared to those that a doctor would use, provided that the instructions are carefully followed. The consumer should understand that no test is 100 percent accurate; test accuracy is improved when the consumer can read, understand, and follow the directions for test administration carefully. A home test kit will require accurate timing, specific collection materials, and typically a body fluid sample. Failure to comply with any of these factors could result in an inaccurate reading. If a product is not approved by the FDA, then the test's safety and efficacy is in question. Internet shopping for diagnostic test kits can be particularly misleading, since not all test kits available for purchase in this fashion are FDA-approved and some are illegal to sell over the Internet.

A search of the Clinical Laboratory Improvement Amendments (CLIA) database will inform the consumer if a home test has FDA approval. To use this search engine, the consumer must know if the test is considered a "test kit" (a consumer takes a sample, performs the test, and analyzes it, all on one's own) or a "collection kit" (a consumer takes a sample but sends it out to a laboratory for analysis). Collection kits are not currently listed on the CLIA database, although one can contact the FDA directly to find out if a kit is FDA-approved. The FDA maintains another database called Manufacturer and User Facility Device Experience (MAUDE), which lists reports on problems with kits and testing devices. *Consumer Reports* magazine and its Web site can also provide the consumer with additional product comparison information for a handful of home tests.

—*Bonita L. Marks, Ph.D.*

Immunoassay methodology has also permitted the routine laboratory testing of therapeutic drugs as well as of drugs of abuse. In the past, the technology for analyzing drugs in biological fluids involved expensive, labor-intensive techniques that were impractical for routine laboratory use. With the introduction of immunologically based testing for drugs, however, it became possible to monitor patients on antibiotics, immunosuppressive agents, cardiac drugs, and antiseizure medication. Testing has been automated so that these drug levels can be performed as routine laboratory procedures. Assay results can be used to establish an individual dosage schedule so that dosage is maintained in the therapeutic range and does not exceed the concentration threshold, leading to toxic effects, or decline to values too low to achieve adequate treatment (subtherapeutic levels).

A continuing research effort is directed toward developing specific diagnostic cancer tests. These tests could be used to screen patients for tumors in order to detect them early, when therapy would be most effective. Substances that appear in body fluids coincident with the growth of tumors are referred to as tumor markers. The ideal tumor marker would appear only in patients afflicted with a specific type of cancer. Its concentration would reflect the size of the tumor as well as the presence of metastasis, in which tumor cells migrate from the initial cancer site to other sites in the body.

The ideal tumor marker has not yet been discovered. Most have not been specific or sensitive enough to use as a screening tool for detecting tumors, although they have been useful for monitoring the effects of therapy. One example of a useful marker is prostate-specific antigen (PSA). The level of this protein in serum is very low when the prostate gland is normal. When prostate cancer is present, however, the serum level, as measured by immunoassay, is elevated. The test can also be used for screening, provided that any positive result is confirmed by clinical examination. It is also used following prostate surgery or radiation therapy in order to determine the completeness of tumor removal. Continually high or rising levels of PSA in the serum following treatment indicate that residual tumor is still present.

In the microbiology department, the culturing of body fluids and antibiotic susceptibility studies allow the selection of the most appropriate antibiotic for treatment. The course and duration of treatment can then be followed in the chemistry laboratory using the therapeutic drug monitoring techniques discussed above. When an infection is suspected, body fluids are cultured or incubated with media selected to grow only specific microorganisms. Antibiotic susceptibility studies are performed by culturing the organism with various antibiotics until growth is arrested. Many strains of bacteria and other microorganisms will become resistant to an antibiotic that had proven effective previously, and patients who are allergic to some antibiotics may need to be treated with an alternative regimen.

The detection and identification of viruses has become a subspecialty in microbiology with distinctly different culturing techniques. Newer immunoassay methods and other biotechnologically based methods have made virus diagnosis easier. Acquired immunodeficiency syndrome (AIDS) testing is a prime example of the application of immunoassay techniques to virology testing. A detection technique that required growth of the human immunodeficiency virus (HIV) in the laboratory would be extraordinarily difficult and tedious. It would also be prohibitively expensive and time-consuming to screen large populations such as blood donors and high-risk groups. Instead, laboratory screening for HIV utilizes an automated immunoassay technique based on the detection of patient antibodies to virus-specific antigens. Although this test is very specific, the possibility of false positives is greatly minimized by confirming all positive screening results with another antibody test called a Western blot. In this test, a serum sample from a suspected HIV-positive patient is applied to a membrane impregnated with virus proteins. The virus proteins are localized at a characteristic position determined by their migration rate when the membrane coated with virus proteins is subjected to an electric field in a process called protein electrophoresis. After the membrane has been treated with patient serum and color development reagents, the presence in the patient sample of an antibody to one or more of these proteins is revealed as a colored stripe on the membrane. A combination of the two tests is a cost-efficient and extremely accurate procedure to confirm a suspected diagnosis of HIV infection.

PERSPECTIVE AND PROSPECTS

According to a 2002 study of the history of the clinical laboratory by J. Büttner, the concept of the modern hospital laboratory was first documented in 1791 when French physician and chemist Antoine-François de Fourcroy wrote that in hospitals "a chemical laboratory should be set up not far away from a ward having twenty or thirty beds." Büttner asserts that the two suppositions necessary for the creation of these laboratories were the idea that the results of laboratory examinations can be used as "chemical signs" in medical diagnosis and a new concept of disease that was the result of the "birth of the clinic" at the end of the eighteenth century.

During this phase of laboratory development, investigations were performed at patients' bedsides by physicians themselves. In the period from 1840 to 1855, clinical laboratories were established as operations distinct from hospitals and clinics. Most of these laboratories were developed in German-speaking countries and staffed by scientists who performed tests for the hospitals and taught medical students physiological chemistry. From 1855 onward, the concept of the clinical laboratory spread rapidly, with clinicians assuming directorship roles. The laboratory ultimately serving as a model for clinical laboratories in the United States was established by the renowned pathologist Rudolf Virchow at Berlin University. As the chair for pathological anatomy, he set up a "chemical department" within the institute for pathology in 1856. This laboratory represented a center of clinical chemistry research and established the clinical laboratory as integral to pathology.

Laboratories have evolved as essential but distinctly separate specialties of medical services. Although there is little or no participation in the analytical process by the physicians ordering the tests, a major part of a physician's diagnostic skill is knowing which tests to order as a supplement to examination and medical history. Laboratory tests cost money and time, and they may be useless in the diagnostic process if not ordered in a judicious fashion. The old medical admonishment to "treat the patient, not the laboratory result" is still an appropriate consideration. Moreover, responsibility for the correct interpretation of the results lies with the attending physician, who has access to all the pertinent patient data.

Laboratory results are usually interpreted with the help of a reference range. Reference ranges ideally represent laboratory values characteristic of a sample population that is free of known disease. If the results lie within this range, however, the laboratory result cannot always be assumed to rule out a specific diagnosis. Since considerable biological variation exists for most laboratory values, diseased individuals can sometimes yield test values in the normal range and, conversely, healthy individuals can occasionally have low or elevated values.

To verify a diagnosis, all laboratory results and clinical impressions should complement one another. The detection of blood-clotting deficiencies by the hematology department could be related to a poorly functioning liver, which will also be reflected in changes in enzymes and blood proteins measured in the chemistry laboratory. Cardiac disorders are diagnosed not only by examining an electrocardiograph (EKG or ECG) but also by measuring the levels of specific cardiac-related enzymes that rise to abnormally high levels when cardiac blood supply is diminished (such as with myocardial infarction, or heart attack). In summary, the clinical laboratory provides a valuable tool for physicians, but it should never displace clinical examination and medical history as methods of determining the final diagnosis.

—*David J. Wells, Jr., Ph.D.*

See also Amniocentesis; Bacteriology; Biopsy; Blood and blood disorders; Blood testing; Breast biopsy; Cells; Cytology; Cytopathology; Diagnosis; DNA and RNA; Endometrial biopsy; Forensic pathology; Genetic engineering; Genetics and inheritance; Gram staining; Hematology; Hematology, pediatric; Histology; Hormones; Karyotyping; Lymph; Microbiology; Microscopy; Pathology; Screening; Serology; Toxicology; Urinalysis.

FOR FURTHER INFORMATION:

Bennington, James L., ed. *Saunders Dictionary and Encyclopedia of Laboratory Medicine and Technology.* Philadelphia: W. B. Saunders, 1984. An excellent reference to laboratory vocabulary and terminology. Gives detailed information about complicated procedures and topics, rather than simple dictionary definitions.

Cavanaugh, Bonita Morrow. *Nurse's Manual of Laboratory and Diagnostic Tests.* 4th ed. Philadelphia: F. A. Davis, 2003. Provides information on hundreds of laboratory and diagnostic tests, with each test presented in two distinct, cross-referenced sections: "Background Information" sections provide a complete description of each test and its purposes; "Clinical Application Data" sections focus on the information nurses most commonly need while caring for clients.

Griffith, H. Winter. *Complete Guide to Symptoms, Illness, and Surgery.* Revised and updated by Stephen Moore and Kenneth Yoder. 5th ed. New York: Perigee, 2006. Covers more than five hundred diseases and disorders and includes information about causes and risk factors, preventive techniques, and diagnostic tests.

McPherson, Richard A., and Matthew R. Pincus, eds. *Henry's Clinical Diagnosis and Management by Laboratory Methods.* 21st ed. Philadelphia: Saunders/ Elsevier, 2007. The classic text on the clinical laboratory. Multiple authors cover all aspects of laboratory operations, including management and administration. The most recent edition should be consulted.

Pagana, Kathleen Deska, and Timothy J. Pagana. *Mosby's Diagnostic and Laboratory Test Reference.* 9th ed. St. Louis, Mo.: Mosby/Elsevier, 2009. A clinical handbook that gives alphabetically organized laboratory and diagnostic tests for easy reference. Each listing includes such things as alternate or abbreviated test names, type of test, normal findings, possible critical values, test explanation and related physiology, and potential complications.

Price, Christopher P., and David J. Newman, eds. *Principles and Practice of Immunoassay.* 2d ed. New York: Stockton Press, 1997. This work covers all aspects of immunoassays, including assay development, laboratory quality assurance, and test methodology.

Wu, Alan H. B., ed. *Tietz Clinical Guide to Laboratory Tests.* 4th ed. St. Louis, Mo.: Saunders/Elsevier, 2006. A paperback condensation of the vital information needed for the interpretation of clinical laboratory tests. Tests are arranged alphabetically in tabular form for easy reference.

LACERATION REPAIR

PROCEDURE

ANATOMY OR SYSTEM AFFECTED: Skin
SPECIALTIES AND RELATED FIELDS: Emergency medicine, general surgery, plastic surgery
DEFINITION: The closure of an irregular skin wound.

INDICATIONS AND PROCEDURES

A laceration is a jagged, torn, mangled, or ragged wound. This type of wound is most commonly encountered in the skin, although any tissue may be lacerated. Lacerations are caused by sharp objects such as a piece of metal, glass, or a stick, or they may occur in accidents involving machinery or animals.

The first priority in laceration repair is to stop bleeding, thereby minimizing blood loss. This is usually accomplished by pressure either directly on the wound or on the injured blood vessel nearest the injury site.

The second priority with a laceration is to clean the wound, which involves the removal of any foreign material or debris. With penetrating injuries, this cleaning must be done carefully lest the removal of the object initiate bleeding. Tissue that has been destroyed beyond the body's ability to repair it must also be removed; this process is called debridement. Devitalized tissue is removed to prevent infection. The wound site is then cleaned through irrigation with saline and a disinfectant, usually a mild soap or a chemical.

Lacerations may then be treated for bacterial or other pathogenic contamination. Aqueous solutions containing an antibiotic are used with most wounds. If contamination with other pathogens is suspected, appropriate agents are used to rinse the wound. Antibiotic powders may be employed in field conditions, although this form of treatment is unusual in a hospital setting. Other than soap and water, there is no special treatment for viral contamination.

Closure of the wound is then completed. The edges are brought together and may be held in place with forceps. Sutures, or stitches, are inserted to hold the edges together while the tissue heals. On skin surfaces, these sutures are usually nonabsorbable and are later removed. The amount of time that sutures are kept in place varies with the location of the wound and the age of the patient: Mucous membranes heal more quickly than the palm, for example, and children's skin heals more rapidly than that of adults. Removable sutures are made of nylon or a similar material. Sutures that are used beneath the skin cannot be removed and are made of material that will break down within the body. Wound closure may also be accomplished with wire, staples, or adhesive tape. These materials have some advantages—durability (wire), ease of placement (staples), and minimal pain (tape)—and disadvantages—potential contamination (wire) and premature, accidental removal (tape). Lacerations should be rechecked by a physician when sutures or other means of wound closure are removed.

USES AND COMPLICATIONS

The techniques of laceration repair are used on all parts of the body where such wounds occur. Plastic surgery may be required to improve the appearance of the repaired tissue and to reduce scars when the patient believes that cosmetic results are an issue. In addition to scarring, other complications that may be associated with the repair of lacerations include infection and tetanus. All these problems can be minimized through good surgical techniques, the use of antibiotics, and careful postoperative care. The repair of lacerations to

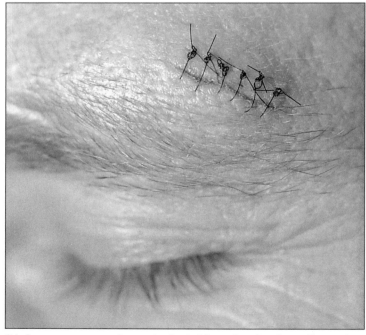

Stitches or sutures may be required to hold together the edges of lacerations that are large, deep, or ragged. (PhotoDisc)

exposed facial skin is especially important. Careful technique minimizes scarring, as do some new methods of wound closure.

—*L. Fleming Fallon, Jr., M.D., Ph.D., M.P.H.*

See also Bleeding; Bruises; Emergency medicine; Grafts and grafting; Healing; Plastic surgery; Skin; Wounds.

FOR FURTHER INFORMATION:

American Academy of Orthopaedic Surgeons. *Emergency Care and Transportation of the Sick and Injured.* Edited by Benjamin Gulli, Les Chatelain, and Chris Stratford. 9th ed. Sudbury, Mass.: Jones and Bartlett, 2005.

Handal, Kathleen A. *The American Red Cross First Aid and Safety Handbook.* Boston: Little, Brown, 1992.

Mulholland, Michael W., et al., eds. *Greenfield's Surgery: Scientific Principles and Practice.* 4th ed. Philadelphia: Lippincott Williams & Wilkins, 2006.

Thygerson, Alton L. *First Aid and Emergency Care Workbook.* Boston: Jones and Bartlett, 1987.

Weedon, David. *Skin Pathology.* 3d ed. New York: Churchill Livingstone/Elsevier, 2010.

LACTOSE INTOLERANCE

DISEASE/DISORDER

ANATOMY OR SYSTEM AFFECTED: Gastrointestinal system, intestines, stomach

SPECIALTIES AND RELATED FIELDS: Gastroenterology, nutrition

DEFINITION: Lactose intolerance is an inability to break down and absorb milk sugar, known as lactose, resulting in stomach pain, gas, and diarrhea if lactose is consumed.

CAUSES AND SYMPTOMS

Lactose is a complex sugar commonly found in dairy products. It is composed of two simple sugars, glucose and galactose. In babies and young children, a gene produces an enzyme called lactase that breaks down lactose into its two component sugars, which are then absorbed into the bloodstream through the intestinal wall. In many people, sometime after early childhood, the lactase gene is "turned off." It no longer synthesizes lactase, which prevents the digestion and absorption of lactose.

Normal bacterial inhabitants of the intestines synthesize lactase and break down the lactose molecules, producing large quantities of gas as a by-product. This can lead to cramping for the lactose-intolerant individ-

---

> **INFORMATION ON LACTOSE INTOLERANCE**
>
> **CAUSES:** Insufficient lactase production
> **SYMPTOMS:** Gas, cramping, and diarrhea after consumption of lactose-containing food or drink
> **DURATION:** One to two days
> **TREATMENTS:** Avoidance of dairy products, lactase pills

ual. The presence of lactose in the large intestine causes excessive amounts of water to move into the intestine, which can lead to diarrhea. Symptoms subside one to two days after the last lactose-containing food has been consumed.

TREATMENT AND THERAPY

Lactose intolerance can often be misdiagnosed as a host of gastrointestinal disorders, largely as a result of the commonness of its major symptoms, cramps and diarrhea. Typically, a dietary history must be kept. Patients with lactose intolerance will note an association between their symptoms and the consumption of milk products containing lactose. After elimination of these products from the diet, symptoms should not recur.

There is no cure for lactose intolerance; prevention of symptoms is the general course of action. Avoidance of foods that contain lactose—including milk, ice cream, and cheese—is usually the best recourse. For those who wish to indulge in these products, over-the-counter lactase pills are available; their use usually prevents symptoms of the disorder.

PERSPECTIVE AND PROSPECTS

The vast majority of the world's population is lactose intolerant, yet this disorder was not recognized in the United States until the latter third of the twentieth century. Today, lactase supplements are available to help prevent symptoms for lactose-intolerant people who choose to consume dairy products. Alternatively, more and more dairy products are being manufactured as lactose-free; they can be consumed safely by the lactose-intolerant population.

—*Karen E. Kalumuck, Ph.D.*

See also Acid reflux disease; Diarrhea and dysentery; Digestion; Enzymes; Gastroenterology; Gastroenterology, pediatric; Gastrointestinal disorders;

Gastrointestinal system; Gluten intolerance; Irritable bowel syndrome (IBS); Metabolic disorders; Nutrition.

FOR FURTHER INFORMATION:

Dobler, Merri Lou. *Lactose Intolerance Nutrition Guide*. Chicago: American Dietetic Association, 2002.

Gracey, Michael, ed. *Diarrhea*. Boca Raton, Fla.: CRC Press, 1991.

Greenberger, Norton J. *Gastrointestinal Disorders: A Pathophysiologic Approach*. 4th ed. Chicago: Year Book Medical, 1989.

Icon Health. *Lactose Intolerance: A Medical Dictionary, Bibliography, and Annotated Research Guide to Internet References*. San Diego, Calif.: Author, 2004.

Janowitz, Henry D. *Your Gut Feelings: A Complete Guide to Living Better with Intestinal Problems*. Rev. ed. New York: Oxford University Press, 1995.

National Digestive Diseases Information Clearinghouse. National Institute of Diabetes and Digestive and Kidney Diseases. National Institutes of Health. "Lactose Intolerance." http://digestive.niddk.nih.gov/ddiseases/pubs/lactoseintolerance.

Peikin, Steven R. *Gastrointestinal Health*. Rev. ed. New York: Quill, 2001.

LAMINECTOMY AND SPINAL FUSION
PROCEDURES

ANATOMY OR SYSTEM AFFECTED: Back, bones, spine

SPECIALTIES AND RELATED FIELDS: General surgery, orthopedics

DEFINITION: Surgical procedures that join two or more vertebrae, the arching bones that make up the spine.

INDICATIONS AND PROCEDURES

Laminectomies, which are designed to relieve pressure on the spinal cord, are often performed as the initial surgery in cases of extreme back pain caused by the compression of the spinal canal. An incision is made in the patient's back to expose the laminae, the flattened portions of the vertebral arch, and one or more adjacent laminae are chipped away. On occasion, several laminae are excised.

In such cases, spinal fusion, which involves the immobilization of the spine with steel rods or bone grafts, is indicated. Spinal fusion, like laminectomy a major surgery done under general anesthesia, is performed if

X rays reveal unusual motion between adjacent vertebrae.

The causes of the severe back pain that usually precedes laminectomy or spinal fusion may be related to three conditions: osteoarthritis, which causes deterioration of the spinal joints; scoliosis caused by an injury or tumor that is destroying vertebrae; or spondylolisthesis, the dislocation of facet joints. In spinal fusion, when the damaged vertebrae are exposed, joint fusion is sometimes performed by using bone chips from the patient's pelvis. Following surgery, the vertebrae are held in place with plates or screws.

USES AND COMPLICATIONS

Both laminectomy and spinal fusion usually relieve the persistent back pain that has caused patients to seek treatment. Such surgery involves distinct risks, inasmuch as the spinal cord is exposed and there is often considerable blood loss. In the hands of a seasoned orthopedic surgeon, however, the risk is minimized.

Recovery from the surgery can be slow and often involves up to six weeks of confinement in bed. After this confinement, patients are usually required to wear a plaster cast until final vertebral fusion has occurred. This process can take half a year.

Fusion sometimes places an additional burden on the rest of the spinal column. In some cases, this pressure results in renewed back pain in other areas of the spine. Additional surgery may be indicated to control this pain.

—*R. Baird Shuman, Ph.D.*

See also Back pain; Bone grafting; Bones and the skeleton; Disk removal; Fracture and dislocation; Grafts and grafting; Orthopedic surgery; Orthopedics; Orthopedics, pediatric; Osteoarthritis; Scoliosis; Spinal cord disorders; Spine, vertebrae, and disks.

FOR FURTHER INFORMATION:

Boden, Scott D., ed. *Spinal Fusion*. Philadelphia: W. B. Saunders, 1998.

Devlin, Vincent J., ed. *Spine Secrets*. Philadelphia: Hanley & Belfus, 2003.

Frymoyer, John W., and Sam W. Wiesel, eds. *The Adult and Pediatric Spine: Principles, Practice, and Surgery*. 3d ed. Philadelphia: Lippincott Williams & Wilkins, 2004.

Hitchon, Patrick W., Setti Rengachary, and Vincent C. Traynelis, eds. *Techniques in Spinal Fusion and Stabilization*. New York: Thieme Medical, 1995.

Lewandrowski, Kai-Uwe, et al., eds. *Advances in Spi-*

nal Fusion: Molecular Science, Biomechanics, and Clinical Management. New York: Marcel Dekker, 2004.

Nakamura, K., Y. Toyama, and Y. Hoshino, eds. Cervical Laminoplasty. New York: Springer, 2003.

Wetzel, F. Todd, and Edward Nathaniel Hanley, Jr. Spine Surgery: A Practical Atlas. New York: McGraw-Hill, 2002.

LAPAROSCOPY

PROCEDURE

ANATOMY OR SYSTEM AFFECTED: Abdomen, gallbladder, gastrointestinal system, intestines, kidneys, reproductive system, urinary system, uterus

SPECIALTIES AND RELATED FIELDS: Endocrinology, gastroenterology, general surgery, gynecology

DEFINITION: The examination of the abdominal organs with a laparoscope, a fiber-optic tube that can also be used to perform surgery to correct several disease conditions.

KEY TERMS:

abdomen: the area of the body between the diaphragm and the pelvis; it contains the visceral organs

cholecystectomy: the surgical removal of the gallbladder

ectopic pregnancy: the development of a fertilized egg in a Fallopian tube instead of the uterus; can be fatal to the mother unless it is corrected surgically

endometriosis: a female reproductive disease in which cells from the uterine lining (the endometrium) grow outside the uterus, causing severe pain and infertility and sometimes the need for hysterectomy

Fallopian tubes: the two tubes through which eggs pass on the way from the ovaries to the uterus

general anesthesia: anesthesia that induces unconsciousness

implant: a section of endometrial tissue found outside the uterus

local anesthesia: anesthesia that numbs the feeling in a body part, administered by injection or direct application to the skin

INDICATIONS AND PROCEDURES

Laparoscopy is a surgical technique for examining the abdominal organs and for treating surgically many diseases of these organs. The instrument used is called a laparoscope. It is a flexible tube that contains fiber optics for visualization purposes and a channel through which physicians can pass special surgical instruments into the abdominal cavity.

Upon insertion of a laparoscope into the abdomen through a small surgical incision (usually near the navel), physicians can observe the liver, kidneys, gallbladder, pancreas, spleen, and exterior aspects of the intestines in both sexes. Hence the technique is useful for detecting cirrhosis of the liver, the presence of stones and tumors, and many other diseases of the abdominal organs. The female reproductive organs can also be examined in this manner.

Before laparoscopy can be carried out, the patient must fast for at least twelve hours. The patient is given a local or general anesthetic, depending on the purpose of the procedure. In exploratory abdominal examinations, the instrument is inserted into the abdomen through a small incision in the abdominal wall after local anesthesia has numbed it. Often, especially when extensive surgery is anticipated, the procedure begins after general anesthesia produces unconsciousness. Upon the completion of exploration or surgery, the laparoscope is withdrawn and the incision is closed.

Laparoscopic abdominal examination is often used to detect endometriosis, the presence of endometrial cells outside the uterus. This procedure begins with the

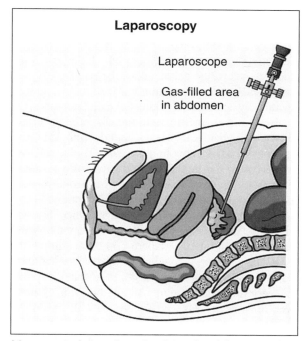

Laparoscopy

Laparoscope —

Gas-filled area in abdomen

Many surgical procedures involving the abdomen, such as appendectomy or the removal of eggs from the ovaries for in vitro fertilization, can be performed using laparoscopy. Gas is pumped into the abdominal cavity, and a fiber-optic scope and instruments are inserted through a small hole in the skin.

administration of local anesthesia when only exploration or biopsy is planned. General anesthesia is used when the removal of implants (endometrial tissue) is anticipated. The entry incision is made near the navel, and the laparoscope is inserted. The fiber-optics system is used to search the abdominal organs for implants. Visibility of the abdominal organs is usually enhanced by pumping in a harmless gas, such as carbon dioxide, to distend the abdomen. After the confirmation of endometriosis, surgical implant removal is carried out immediately, unless the decision is made to institute drug therapy instead. Full recovery from this surgery requires only a day of postoperative bed rest and a week of curtailing activities.

Laparoscopy can also be employed for female sterilization. The patient is given a general anesthetic. After laparoscopic visualization of the Fallopian tubes in the gas-distended abdomen is achieved, surgical instruments for tube cauterization or cutting are introduced and the sterilization is carried out. The entire procedure often requires only thirty minutes, which is one reason for its popularity. In addition, patients can go home in a few hours and have fully recovered after a day or two of bed rest and seven to ten days of curtailing activities.

USES AND COMPLICATIONS

Common laparoscopic surgeries are cholecystectomy (the removal of the gallbladder), the removal of gallstones and kidney stones, tumor resection, female sterilization by cutting or blocking the Fallopian tubes, the treatment of endometriosis through the removal of implants from abdominal organs, and the removal of biopsy samples from abdominal organs. Traditional uses of laparoscopy in female reproductive surgery are to identify and correct pelvic pain resulting from endometriosis, ectopic pregnancy, and pelvic tumors.

Laparoscopy has several advantages. There is rarely a need for patients on chronic drug therapy to discontinue medication before laparoscopy. In addition, the use of laparoscopy dramatically lowers surgical incision size, surgical trauma, length of hospital stay, and recovery time. Laparoscopy should be avoided, however, in cases of advanced abdominal wall cancer, severe respiratory or cardiovascular disease, or tuberculosis. Extreme obesity does not disqualify a patient from undergoing laparoscopy but makes the procedure much more difficult to perform.

As laparoscopic surgery has increased in scope, more procedures yield surgical tissues that are larger in size than the laparoscope channel (for example, the removal of gallbladders, gallstones, and ovaries). In many cases these organs and structures are cut into small pieces for removal. If potentially dangerous items are involved—such as malignancies that can spread on dissection—larger, more conventional incisions are often combined with laparoscopy.

PERSPECTIVE AND PROSPECTS

Since the 1970's, the uses of laparoscopy have constantly expanded. Once confined to the exploratory examination of the abdomen, the methodology has been applied to a large number of different types of surgery in addition to those already mentioned. Such versatility is attributable to the development of better laparoscopes, advanced instrumentation for diverse surgeries, and improved fiber-optic and video technologies.

As a consequence of these advances, many surgeons predict that most future abdominal surgery will be laparoscopic. The driving force for such innovation includes the public demand for quicker recovery times. In the United States, this desire is intensified by the requirements of insurance companies, employers, and the federal government for shorter hospital stays. Both changes are made possible by decreased severity of surgical trauma in laparoscopy when compared to traditional surgery, a result of the smaller incisions. The dramatic trend toward laparoscopy can be seen with cholecystectomies: Of those done in 1992, 70 percent were laparoscopic, compared to less than 1 percent in 1989.

—*Sanford S. Singer, Ph.D.*

See also Abdomen; Abdominal disorders; Appendectomy; Appendicitis; Biopsy; Cholecystectomy; Ectopic pregnancy; Endometriosis; Endoscopy; Gynecology; Internal medicine; Sterilization; Stone removal; Stones; Tubal ligation; Tumor removal; Tumors.

FOR FURTHER INFORMATION:

Graber, John N., et al., eds. *Laparoscopic Abdominal Surgery*. New York: McGraw-Hill, 1993. A text for surgery residents and practicing surgeons wishing to gain an understanding of the theory and technique of laparoscopic surgery, written by experts in each area who were instrumental in the development of laparoscopic approaches. Abundantly illustrated with clear, detailed line drawings and color photographs.

Henderson, Lorraine, and Ros Wood. *Explaining Endometriosis*. 2d ed. St. Leonards, N.S.W.: Allen and Unwin, 2000. Details possible causes, diagnosis, surgeries, and current treatment options for endometriosis.

Kapadia, Cyrus R., James M. Crawford, and Caroline Taylor. *An Atlas of Gastroenterology: A Guide to Diagnosis and Differential Diagnosis.* Boca Raton, Fla.: Pantheon, 2003. Provides a fully illustrated, nonspecialist understanding of myriad gastrointestinal diseases, including heartburn, dyspepsia, diarrhea, irritable bowel syndrome, and pancreatitis. Includes bibliographic references and an index.

Reddick, Eddie Joe, ed. *An Atlas of Laparoscopic Surgery.* New York: Raven Press, 1993. Discusses such topics as cholecystectomy and peritoneoscopy. Includes an index.

Zollinger, Robert M., Jr., and Robert M. Zollinger, Sr. *Zollinger's Atlas of Surgical Operations.* 8th ed. New York: McGraw-Hill, 2003. A comprehensive examination of surgery. Covers basic surgical anatomy and vascular, gynecologic, gastrointestinal, and miscellaneous abdominal procedures.

Zucker, Karl A., ed. *Surgical Laparoscopy.* 2d ed. Philadelphia: Lippincott Williams & Wilkins, 2001. Discusses the gastrointestinal system, peritoneoscopy, and the methods of biliary tract surgery and endoscopic surgery.

LARYNGECTOMY

PROCEDURE

ANATOMY OR SYSTEM AFFECTED: Respiratory system, throat

SPECIALTIES AND RELATED FIELDS: General surgery, oncology, otorhinolaryngology

DEFINITION: The removal of all or part of the voice box, or larynx.

INDICATIONS AND PROCEDURES

Continued hoarseness and coughing can indicate laryngeal disorders. Polyps, which may be caused by excessive smoking or drinking, can form on the larynx. Children sometimes develop warts on it. Although these polyps and warts are generally benign, they should be removed and subjected to biopsy to preclude the presence of cancer.

Polyps, warts, and tumors are all detected quite easily with a laryngoscopic examination carried out by an otorhinolaryngologist with a mirror, an endoscope (a flexible fiber-optic tube), or a combination of the two. Such an examination, in addition to determining whether a growth is benign or cancerous, can detect signs of cancer in the lining of the larynx.

If cancer is detected early enough, radiation can usually control it. If the disease has advanced significantly, however, a laryngectomy may be necessary. In this surgical procedure, performed under general anesthesia, an incision is made in the neck and the larynx is removed. The windpipe directly below the larynx is then sewn to the skin around the surgical opening to form a permanent opening, or stoma, through which the patient breathes.

USES AND COMPLICATIONS

This surgery is used when cancer is sufficiently advanced that radiation therapy cannot destroy it. The major complication is that the patient's air supply is now taken through the stoma, meaning that swimming is precluded and that bathing must be undertaken with considerable caution.

A more apparent complication is that, with the loss of the larynx, one cannot speak. Through an extensive and painstaking course of speech therapy, however, esophageal speech can be achieved. This involves swallowing air and expelling it in such a way that it can be shaped by the palate, lips, and tongue into understandable words and sentences. An electronic larynx is also available. It makes a buzzing sound that the patient can convert into words when the device is pressed against the top of the throat.

—*R. Baird Shuman, Ph.D.*

See also Cancer; Endoscopy; Esophagus; Head and neck disorders; Mouth and throat cancer; Otorhinolaryngology; Polyps; Speech disorders; Tumors; Voice and vocal cord disorders; Warts.

FOR FURTHER INFORMATION:

Blom, Eric D., Mark I. Singer, and Ronald C. Hamaker, eds. *Tracheoesophageal Voice Restoration Following Total Laryngectomy.* San Diego, Calif.: Singular, 1998.

Casper, Janina K., and Raymond H. Colton. *Clinical Manual for Laryngectomy and Head/Neck Cancer Rehabilitation.* 2d ed. San Diego, Calif.: Singular, 1998.

Edels, Yvonne, ed. *Laryngectomy: Diagnosis to Rehabilitation.* Rockville, Md.: Aspen Systems, 1983.

Ferrari, Mario. *PDxMD Ear, Nose, and Throat Disorders.* Philadelphia: PDxMD, 2003.

Griffith, H. Winter. *Complete Guide to Symptoms, Illness, and Surgery.* Revised and updated by Stephen Moore and Kenneth Yoder. 5th ed. New York: Perigee, 2006.

Montgomery, William W., ed. *Surgery of the Larynx, Trachea, Esophagus, and Neck.* Philadelphia: W. B. Saunders, 2002.

Zollinger, Robert M., Jr., and Robert M. Zollinger, Sr. *Zollinger's Atlas of Surgical Operations.* 8th ed. New York: McGraw-Hill, 2003.

LARYNGITIS

DISEASE/DISORDER

ANATOMY OR SYSTEM AFFECTED: Throat

SPECIALTIES AND RELATED FIELDS: Otorhinolaryngology, speech pathology

DEFINITION: Inflammation of the larynx (voice box), often associated with common colds, bacterial infection, or straining the voice. The throat is dry, swallowing becomes difficult, and speech is a hoarse whisper.

CAUSES AND SYMPTOMS

The larynx, located directly above the windpipe (trachea), is the short, hollow tube containing the vocal cords, two heavily lined slits in a mucous membrane. Voiced sounds, such as vowels, result when air from the lungs induces vocal fold vibration. Laryngitis occurs when the folds are obstructed or do not vibrate properly; depending on the cause, laryngitis is classified as simple, chronic, diphtheritic, tuberculous, or syphilitic.

Simple laryngitis may be caused by bacterial infection (common cold, typhoid fever), a virus (influenza), or nonbacterial irritants (chemical fumes, dust, or tobacco smoke). The primary infection site is the mucous membrane lining the larynx. It becomes red and swollen, secreting a viscous discharge that impedes vocal fold vibration. In severe cases of viral infection, the larynx may become completely obstructed, causing suffocation.

Chronic laryngitis often results from excessive smoking, alcoholism, or consistent strain or abuse of the voice. It is an occupational hazard of auctioneers, orators, singers, and those who frequently shout for long periods, such as cheerleaders. Nondisease-induced chronic laryngitis may also be instigated by hysteria, allergic reaction, remote disease of the nerves serving the voice, strong external pressure against the larynx, or irritation caused by tubes inserted down the throat to sustain breathing.

Diphtheritic laryngitis occurs when diphtheria afflicting the upper throat spreads to the larynx. The result may be a membrane of diseased cells infiltrating the mucous membrane and obstructing the vocal cords.

Tuberculous laryngitis is a secondary infection spread from the lungs. Tubular nodulelike growths are formed in larynx tissue, leaving ulcers on the surface. Starting at the vocal cords, this infection may spread over the entire larynx and eventually destroy the epiglottis and laryngeal cartilage.

Syphilitic laryngitis is one of the many complications of syphilis. Sores or mucous patches form in the larynx, eventually producing tissue destruction and scar formation. The mucous membrane becomes dry and covered with polyps (small bumps of tissue that project from the surface). These polyps distort the larynx, shorten the vocal cords, and produce persistent hoarseness.

TREATMENT AND THERAPY

Simple laryngitis is best treated by resting the voice. When it is absolutely necessary to speak, it should be with a soft, breathy voice, not a whisper. The throat should be kept well lubricated by frequent drinks of water and not cleared. Relative humidity in the recovery room should be maintained at 40 to 50 percent, and alcohol, tobacco, and decongestants should be avoided.

Complete recovery usually occurs within several days.

A persistent hoarseness indicates a bacterial infection (usually curable by antibiotics) or polyps, cysts, or other fibrous growths on the vocal cords. These growths may become ulcerated and require surgical intervention. Although cancer of the larynx is not uncommon (2 percent of malignancies), it is usually completely curable if detected sufficiently early.

Systemic diseases not localized in the larynx, such as tuberculosis and syphilis, are best treated by antibiotics.

—*George R. Plitnik, Ph.D.*

INFORMATION ON LARYNGITIS

CAUSES: Bacterial infection (common cold, typhoid fever, diphtheria, syphilis), viral infection (influenza), irritants (chemical fumes, dust, smoke, alcohol), consistent strain or abuse of voice

SYMPTOMS: Red and swollen larynx; discharge; obstruction that can cause suffocation if severe; polyps, cysts, or other fibrous growths on vocal cords

DURATION: Acute or chronic

TREATMENTS: Depends on cause; may include resting the voice, antibiotics, or surgery

See also Common cold; Laryngectomy; Multiple chemical sensitivity syndrome; Nasopharyngeal disorders; Otorhinolaryngology; Pharyngitis; Pharynx; Polyps; Sore throat; Strep throat; Tonsillectomy and adenoid removal; Tonsillitis; Voice and vocal cord disorders.

FOR FURTHER INFORMATION:

Bellenir, Karen, and Peter D. Dresser, eds. *Contagious and Noncontagious Infectious Diseases Sourcebook.* Detroit, Mich.: Omnigraphics, 1996.

Colton, Raymond H., Janina K. Casper, and Rebecca Leonard. *Understanding Voice Problems: A Physiological Perspective for Diagnosis and Treatment.* 3d ed. Philadelphia: Lippincott Williams & Wilkins, 2006.

Icon Health. *Laryngitis: A Medical Dictionary, Bibliography, and Annotated Research Guide to Internet References.* San Diego, Calif.: Author, 2004.

Ossoff, Robert H., et al., eds. *The Larynx.* Philadelphia: Lippincott Williams & Wilkins, 2003.

Sataloff, Robert T., ed. *Reflux Laryngitis and Related Disorders.* 3d ed. San Diego, Calif.: Plural, 2006.

Swartzberg, John Edward. *Wellness Self-Care Handbook: The Everyday Guide to Prevention and Home Remedies to Over 150 Common Ailments.* New York: Times Books, 1999.

LASER USE IN SURGERY
PROCEDURE

ANATOMY OR SYSTEM AFFECTED: Eyes, skin

SPECIALTIES AND RELATED FIELDS: Dermatology, oncology, ophthalmology, urology

DEFINITION: The application of laser technology to surgical procedures, such as the vaporization of blood clots or arterial plaque, the breaking up of kidney stones into small fragments, the removal of birthmarks, and the stoppage of hemorrhaging in the retina of the eye.

KEY TERMS:

ionization: a process in which a neutral atom loses one or more of its orbital electrons because of light, heat, or electrical collisions

laser: an acronym for light amplification by stimulated emission of radiation; a laser produces a very-high-intensity light beam at a single wavelength

optical fiber: a very thin thread made of high-purity glass, plastic, or quartz; used to transmit light from a laser into the body

photon: a particle of light whose energy depends on its wavelength (that is, its color); many billions of individual photons make up a light beam

pulsed laser: a laser technique used to deliver a light beam of high power for a very short time in order to localize the heating effect without damaging surrounding tissue

shock wave: a miniature explosion caused by intense local heating with a laser beam; used to fragment stones in the kidney or gallbladder

stimulated emission of radiation: the process in a laser whereby an avalanche of photons is created, all of which are synchronized in wavelength and direction of travel

wavelength: a property used to measure colors in the spectrum of light from infrared to ultraviolet; usually expressed in units of microns (one micron is equal to one-millionth of a meter)

THE FUNDAMENTALS OF LASER TECHNOLOGY

The first successful laser was built in 1960 by Theodore H. Maiman at the Hughes Aircraft Research Laboratory in Palo Alto, California. Since then, many applications have been developed for lasers. These include the compact disc player, telephone systems with fiber optics, guidance systems for military weapons, supermarket checkout scanners, quality control in industry, entertainment with laser light shows, and numerous medical applications.

Ordinary light sources such as flashlights, flames, and the sun do not emit laser light. The individual atoms emit their light waves in a random, uncoordinated manner, in the same way that water waves spread out at random when a handful of pebbles is thrown into a pool. In contrast, a laser beam consists of light waves that are all synchronized; they all have the same wavelength and remain in step as they travel in the same direction. Synchronizing the light emission from billions of atoms in a light source is the chief difficulty in building a laser.

The key idea for solving this problem had been proposed in an article on the general theory of light absorption and emission by atoms written by the famous physicist Albert Einstein in the 1920's. When an atom absorbs a burst of light energy (a photon), an electron in the atom is raised from a lower energy level to a higher one. A short time later, the electron spontaneously falls back down to the lower energy level, emitting a photon of light in the process. Einstein's contribution was to suggest a third mechanism in addition to ordinary absorption and emission. Based on theoretical arguments of symmetry and the conservation of energy, he proposed a new process called "stimulated emission of radiation." (The word "laser" is an acronym for light amplification by stimulated emission of radiation.)

To understand stimulated emission, consider an atom whose electron has been raised to a higher energy level, called an "excited state." This state is unstable, and the electron ordinarily will fall back down to the lower energy level in a short time. Suppose, however, that a photon of precisely the right energy strikes the atom while the electron is still in its temporary excited state. This photon cannot be absorbed because the electron is already in its excited state. Einstein reasoned that the incoming photon would cause the excited electron to fall to the lower energy level. A photon would then be emitted from the atom and would join the incoming photon. The two photons would be exactly synchronized in wavelength and direction.

If there were many atoms whose electrons had previously been raised to excited states, the process of stimulated emission would continue. The two photons could strike two other excited atoms and stimulate them to emit light energy, making a total of four photons. These four would trigger four more atoms, making eight photons, and so forth. Eventually, a so-called photon avalanche consisting of a huge number of synchronized light waves would be generated, which is the desired laser beam.

To make a successful laser, some additional requirements must be met. For one thing, a source of energy must be provided to raise most of the electrons to their excited states. For a gas laser, this energy is normally supplied by a high voltage. Examples of gas lasers are those using carbon dioxide, argon, or a mixture of helium and neon. A solid crystal, such as a clear ruby rod, would be excited by a bright burst of light from a device similar to a camera flash attachment. A solid-state diode laser is energized by a flow of electric current across a diode junction. In each case, it is necessary to "pump" the laser so that many atoms are in their excited state, ready and waiting to be triggered by an incoming photon to release their energy.

Another requirement for a successful laser is that the electrons must remain in their excited state for a longer-than-normal time. The problem with most materials is that electrons fall spontaneously to their lower energy level almost instantaneously, in less than one-millionth of a second. The photon avalanche effect requires that a substantial majority of the atoms be in their excited state. For very short-lived excited states, it is not possible to maintain this condition. Experimenters have no way to control the lifetime of excited states, so they must search for those atoms and molecules that already have the appropriate longer lifetime supplied by nature. It has not been possible to build a laser using hydrogen gas, for example, because hydrogen does not have any long-lived excited states. The spontaneous emission of light takes place so quickly that there is no time for a photon avalanche to develop.

Another condition for laser action is to have two parallel mirrors at the ends of the laser material. The laser beam bounces back and forth many times between the mirrors at the speed of light, gaining or maintaining its energy from the excited atoms of the laser material. One of the mirrors is made slightly less than 100 percent reflecting, so that a small portion of the laser energy is allowed to exit in a narrow beam. For most medical applications, a thin optical fiber is joined directly to the end of the laser in order to transmit the beam to the desired location in the body.

Much research has been done to develop good optical fibers. The fiber should transmit a laser beam with very little loss of energy along the way. The technology of drawing thin glass fibers with few impurities or imperfections has become quite sophisticated. A fiber must be thin and uniform so that the laser beam will be forced to travel down its center, thus avoiding the loss of light energy through the walls.

For an ultraviolet laser, glass fibers cannot be used because of absorption. (The sun's ultraviolet radiation is absorbed by ordinary eyeglasses.) Special quartz fibers with low absorption have been developed for lasers in the ultraviolet region of the spectrum. In the infrared region of the spectrum, new optical materials are still under continuing investigation.

The wavelength (color) of a laser is determined entirely by the energy levels of the atoms or molecules being used. For example, a carbon dioxide laser always has a wavelength of 10.6 microns, which is infrared. The helium-neon gas laser always produces visible red light at a wavelength of 0.63 microns. A wide range of laser wavelengths has become available as a result of extensive research efforts by physicists and optical engineers. Since 1960, lasers have become much more rugged and dependable in construction. Some lasers operate with a continuous beam, while others produce very short pulses, depending on the desired application. Also, lasers can be designed to operate at a low power level for diagnostic purposes or a high power level for surgery.

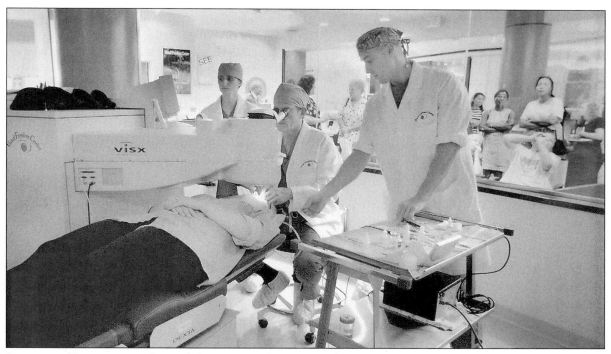

Lasers are taking a more prominent role in many procedures, especially eye surgery. Some worry that the popularity of laser vision correction—here a patient is treated at a shopping mall as spectators look on—has compromised safety. (AP/Wide World Photos)

Safety precautions must be followed when working with a laser. Not only the patient but also the surgical team must be protected from possible harmful radiation. The eyes must be protected from laser beam reflections from a shiny surface. Ultraviolet light is a special hazard because its high-energy photons can cause cell damage and genetic mutations. The great benefits of laser surgery can be negated by an inexperienced or careless surgeon.

USES AND COMPLICATIONS

The first medical use of a laser beam was for surgery on the retina of the eye, in 1963. Diabetic patients in particular frequently develop excessive blood vessels in the retina that give their eyes a typically reddish color. In advanced cases, the blood vessels can hemorrhage and eventually cause blindness. The green light of an argon laser will pass through the clear cornea and lens of the eye, but when it hits the dark brown melanin pigment of the retina, it will be absorbed and cause a tiny hot spot. The physician uses a series of laser pulses, carefully focused on affected areas of the retina, to burn away the extra blood vessels. The remarkable property of the laser beam in this procedure is that its energy penetrates to the rear of the eye, leaving the clear fluid unaffected.

In a greenhouse, light from the sun comes in through the glass but infrared radiation cannot get back out. This example illustrates that some materials, such as glass, are transparent for visible light but opaque for infrared light. Similarly, the front of the eye is transparent for visible light but absorbs infrared light. Therefore, an infrared laser such as the YAG (yttrium-aluminum-garnet) laser can be used for surgery near the front of the eye because its light energy is selectively absorbed there.

A particular problem following cataract surgery is that a secondary cataract may develop on the membrane behind the implanted artificial lens. About one-third of patients with such a lens implant require a second surgery to remove the secondary cataract. A YAG laser beam will pass through the cornea and artificial lens but can be focused to produce a hot spot at the site of the secondary cataract to destroy it. More than 200,000 such procedures are performed each year in the United States, and the result is a dramatic, almost instantaneous improvement of vision.

A third form of laser eye surgery, laser-assisted in

situ keratomileusis (LASIK), became quite popular at the end of the twentieth century; it has, in fact, become the most commonly performed surgery in the country. In LASIK surgery, the cornea of the eyeball is reshaped to help patients overcome myopia (nearsightedness), hyperopia (farsightedness), or astigmatism. The procedure is done with a cool beam laser that can be used to remove thin layers of tissue from selected sites on the cornea to change its curvature. Success rates for the surgery are high: 90 to 95 percent of the patients get 20/ 40 vision, and 65 to 75 percent of the patients get 20/20 vision or better. The surgery is not without its problems, however. Because of its popularity and the large fee charged for a quick and fairly simple procedure, unqualified or less experienced physicians are oftentimes performing the delicate procedure; approximately 5 percent of patients receiving LASIK surgery receive less-than-satisfactory results. Two other corrective procedures for eyesight involving lasers are the use of Kera-Vision Intacs (intrastomal corneal rings), which involves placing a lens in the cornea, and PRK (photorefractive keratectomy), in which the cornea is scraped without actual incision into the cornea.

Another dramatic medical application of the laser is the breaking up of stones in the kidney, ureter, or gallbladder. Such calcified, hard deposits previously could be removed only by surgery. It is now possible, for example, to insert an optical fiber of less than half a millimeter in diameter through the urethra and then transmit the laser beam to the site of the stone. High-power light pulses of very short duration (less than one-billionth of a second) create a shock wave that breaks the stone into small fragments that the body can eliminate.

Another promising application of laser surgery that has received much publicity is laser angioplasty, which is used to open up a blood vessel near the heart that is partially or wholly blocked by a deposit of plaque. The hope is that the laser procedure may be able to replace heart bypass surgery, but the results are still preliminary.

Laser angioplasty involves inserting a catheter that contains a fiberscope, an inflation cuff, and an optical fiber into the artery of the arm and advancing it into the coronary artery. The fiberscope enables the physician to see the blockage, the cuff is used to stop the blood flow temporarily, and the optical fiber transmits the laser energy that vaporizes the plaque. Sometimes, the laser method is used only to open up a small channel, after which balloon angioplasty is used to stretch the walls of the blood vessel.

The main risk in using the laser beam is that the alignment of the optical fiber inside the artery may be deflected and cause a puncture of the blood vessel wall. Improvements in the imaging system are needed. Also, further work must be done to see which light wavelengths are most effective in removing plaque and preventing recurrence of the obstruction.

The heating effect of a laser beam has been used by surgeons to control bleeding. For example, bleeding ulcers in the stomach, intestine, and colon have been successfully cauterized with laser light transmitted through an optical fiber. A similar procedure has been used to treat emphysema patients. An optical fiber is inserted through the wall of the chest, and the laser's heat is used to shrink the small blisters that are present on the surface of the lungs. Also, the heat from a laser has been used during internal surgery to seal the surrounding capillaries that contribute to bleeding.

For the preceding procedures, a carbon dioxide gas laser that emits infrared light is normally used. The reason is that water molecules in the tissue absorb the infrared wavelengths most efficiently. The optical fibers used to transmit infrared light are not as efficient and reliable as those used for visible or ultraviolet light, however, so further research on fiber materials is in progress.

One notable success of laser surgery has been the removal of birthmarks. Because of their typically reddish-purple coloration, birthmarks are commonly called port-wine stains. They can be quite unsightly, especially when located on the face of a person with an otherwise light complexion. To remove such a birthmark, the laser beam has to burn out the network of extra blood vessels under the skin. A similar procedure can be used to remove unwanted tattoos.

The color of the laser must be chosen so that its wavelength will be absorbed efficiently by the dark purple stain. What would happen if a purple laser beam were used? Its light would be reflected rather than absorbed by a purple object, and it would not produce the desired heating. Yellow or orange is most effectively absorbed by a purple object. The surgeon must be careful that the laser light is absorbed primarily by the purple birthmark without harming the normal, healthy tissue around it.

Experimental work is being done to determine whether laser surgery can be applied to cancer. Small malignant tumors in the lungs, bladder, and trachea have been treated with a technique called photodynamic therapy. The patient is injected with a colored dye that is preferentially absorbed in the tumor. Porphyrin, the reddish-brown pigment in blood, is one substance that has been known for many years to become concentrated in malignant tissue. The suspected site is irradiated with ultraviolet light from a krypton laser, causing it to glow like fluorescent paint, which allows the surgeon to determine the outline of the tumor. To perform the surgery, an intense red laser is focused on the tumor to kill the malignant tissue. Two separate optical fibers must be used for this procedure, one for the ultraviolet diagnosis and one for the red laser therapy.

The three traditional cancer treatments of surgery, chemotherapy, and radiation therapy all seek to limit damage to healthy tissue surrounding a tumor. Photodynamic surgery by laser must develop its methodology further to accomplish the same goal.

Much has already been accomplished in applying laser surgery to various body organs. Future developments are likely to emphasize microsurgery on smaller structures, such as individual cells or even genetic material in DNA molecules.

PERSPECTIVE AND PROSPECTS

Some inventions, such as the printing press, the steam engine, and the electric lightbulb, were made by innovators who were trying to solve a particular practical problem of their time. Other inventions, such as the microscope, radio waves, and low-temperature superconductivity, initially were scientific curiosities arising from basic research, and their later applications were not at all anticipated. The laser belongs to this second category.

The first successful laser, built by Theodore Maiman, consisted of a small cylindrical ruby rod with shiny mirrored ends and a bright flash lamp to excite the atoms in the rod. Maiman's goal was to determine whether the separately excited atoms could be made to release their absorbed energy almost simultaneously in one coordinated burst of monochromatic (single-wavelength) light.

No one could have foreseen the wide range of technological applications that resulted from Maiman's experiment. It is important to appreciate that he did not set out to improve telephone communication or eye surgery; those developments came about after the laser became available.

It is worthwhile here to summarize some of the general uses for lasers in modern technology. The tremendous advances in medical applications could not have happened without the concurrent development of new types of lasers, with a variety of wavelengths and power levels, needed for other industrial products.

Among laser applications are the following: the compact disc (CD) player, in which the laser beam replaces the LP record needle; optical fibers that can carry several thousand simultaneous telephone calls; supermarket checkout scanners, in which a laser beam reads the universal product code on each item; three-dimensional pictures, called holograms, that are displayed at many art museums; military applications, such as guided weapons and Star Wars technology; surveying, bridge building, and tunneling projects in which exact alignment is critical; and nuclear fusion research, in which high-power lasers can produce nuclear reactions that may become a future source of energy as coal and oil resources are depleted. Sophisticated advances in using lasers to control specific chemical reactions and to predict earthquakes are under development.

Laser technology in medicine will continue to advance as biologists, electrical and optical engineers, physicians, biophysicists, and people from related disciplines share this common interest.

—Hans G. Graetzer, Ph.D.;
updated by Cassandra Kircher, Ph.D.

See also Angioplasty; Astigmatism; Bionics and biotechnology; Birthmarks; Bleeding; Blood vessels; Blurred vision; Cataract surgery; Cataracts; Cervical procedures; Dermatology; Electrocauterization; Eye surgery; Eyes; Melanoma; Myopia; Neurosurgery; Ophthalmology; Plaque, arterial; Plastic surgery; Refractive eye surgery; Skin; Skin disorders; Skin lesion removal; Stone removal; Stones; Tattoo removal; Ulcer surgery; Ulcers; Vision.

FOR FURTHER INFORMATION:

Alster, Tina S., and Lydia Preston. *Skin Savvy: The Essential Guide to Cosmetic Laser Surgery.* New York: Cadogan, 2002. A guide that provides an overview of current laser procedures in cosmetic surgery, information on the variety of lasers used for different procedures, and practical advice on whether or not certain surgeries would be right for specific conditions.

American Society for Laser Surgery and Medicine. http://www.aslms.org. Site offers a database for referral to a laser practitioner, as well as links to the journal *Lasers in Surgery and Medicine.*

Azar, Dimitri T., and Douglas D. Koch, eds. *LASIK: Fundamentals, Surgical Techniques, and Complica-*

tions. New York: Marcel Dekker, 2003. A description of LASIK eye surgery and potential complications.

Buettner, Helmut, ed. *Mayo Clinic on Vision and Eye Health: Practical Answers on Glaucoma, Cataracts, Macular Degeneration, and Other Conditions.* Rochester, Minn.: Mayo Foundation for Medical Education and Research, 2002. A helpful handbook on all the medical, social, and emotional facets of vision impairment and the treatments available.

Goldman, Mitchel P., ed. *Cutaneous and Cosmetic Laser Surgery.* Philadelphia: Mosby/Elsevier, 2006. Discusses methods of cosmetic surgery using lasers. Includes bibliographical references and an index.

IEEE Journal of Quantum Electronics 26, no. 12 (December, 1990). A special issue on lasers in biology and medicine. This journal is the professional publication of the Institute of Electrical and Electronic Engineers. The articles require some technical background on the part of the reader.

Narins, Rhoda S., and Paul Jarrod Frank. *Turn Back the Clock Without Losing Time: Everything You Need to Know About Simple Cosmetic Procedures.* New York: Three Rivers Press, 2002. A user-friendly guide to procedures that covers laser resurfacing and includes a "frequently asked questions" section for each treatment.

Sutton, Amy L., ed. *Eye Care Sourcebook: Basic Consumer Health Information About Eye Care and Eye Disorders.* 3d ed. Detroit, Mich.: Omnigraphics, 2008. A complete guide to eye care that includes such topics as eye anatomy, preventive vision care, refractive disorders and eye diseases, current research and clinical trials, and a list of organizations.

Victor, Steven, and Ina Yalof. *Ageless Beauty: A Dermatologist's Secrets for Looking Younger Without Surgery.* New York: Crown, 2003. Details several innovative approaches to skin care, including laser surgery.

LAW AND MEDICINE
ETHICS

DEFINITION: The use of medicine in legal contexts—to determine whether a person has been injured by the act of another, the extent of such an injury and its treatment, and whether a defendant was physically or emotionally capable of committing a crime or tort—and in related ethical and philosophical contexts—to determine when life begins (in the abortion debate) or how one evaluates "quality of life" (the euthanasia debate).

KEY TERMS:

compensable injury: an injury for which damages may be awarded

competency: the capacity to understand and act reasonably under given circumstances

diminished capacity: partial insanity; a legal determination that a defendant does not have the ability to achieve the state of mind required to commit a crime

DNA testing: a technique for identifying a person based on matching unique gene-bearing proteins (deoxyribonucleic acid, or DNA) from an organic sample taken from that person (such as hair, blood, or tissue) with another organic sample

emotional distress: damage to a plaintiff's emotional state caused by fear, anger, anxiety, stress, depression, or other negative emotions; such damage may be judged compensable

euthanasia: the act of putting a person or other living being to death in order to end incurable pain or disease; popularly called mercy killing

forensic: having to do with a court of justice; forensic medicine and its various subspecialties apply medical science to the purposes of the law

insanity: a mental disease or defect that renders a person incapable of appreciating the wrongfulness of certain acts or of conforming to the requirements of the law

tort: a wrongful act for which civil courts, rather than criminal courts, are empowered to render justice

MEDICINE IN LEGAL AND ETHICAL DEBATES

Medicine as it relates to law is referred to as forensic medicine. Forensic medicine plays a part in three basic areas of the law. The first two involve the practical application of medicine in civil law and in criminal law. The third area involves the use of medical science to help in defining philosophical or ethical issues, such as when life begins and ends. Ethics in medicine, also called bioethics, refers to a set of moral standards and a code for behavior that govern people's interactions with one another and with society. Bioethics deals with moral issues and problems that have arisen as a result of modern medicine and research. Bioethical principles focus on autonomy (self-determination), beneficence (doing good), nonmaleficence (avoiding evil), and justice (the fair distribution of scarce resources).

In a civil case, a private party, the plaintiff, files a complaint in court against another party, the defendant, requesting that a judge or a jury settle a dispute between the two parties. A party to a civil suit can be an individual, a corporation, an association, a government organization, or any other group. A civil suit differs from a criminal case in that neither party is claiming that a crime (such as theft, kidnapping, or murder) was committed and that someone should be put in jail. Instead, the plaintiff in a civil suit is asking that the defendant pay some amount of money to the plaintiff to compensate for damages that the plaintiff has suffered because of something the defendant did.

In a criminal case, however, the government, on behalf of "the people," files a complaint with the court claiming that the defendant committed a crime, and the government seeks to have a judge or a jury determine the guilt or innocence of that defendant. If the defendant is determined to be guilty, the judge has the authority to punish the defendant, usually by imposing a fine, by requiring community service, by setting a jail sentence, or ultimately, in some states, by having the defendant put to death.

In both civil and criminal cases, medical science is called upon to provide evidence that can be used to prove or disprove a party's case. In a civil case, the parties will often resort to medical experts to determine the extent of a plaintiff's mental and physical injuries. These experts act as witnesses in their areas of expertise and testify in a court of law. For example, a plaintiff in a civil suit might claim that he or she was born with birth defects as a result of drugs that the mother had taken during pregnancy and may present evidence of that injury and its cause in the form of testimony of doctors and medical research experts specializing in those related areas of medicine. Such testimony would be presented to the jury to show that the plaintiff's claim of birth defects being caused by such a drug is supported by medical research.

As medical science reveals more about the causes of disease, injuries, and the workings of the body, more distinct specialties have been created. This trend is reflected in the increasing number of expert witnesses: At the beginning of the twentieth century, a general practitioner was considered qualified to testify on most areas of medicine; today, the courts require expert witnesses to be specifically qualified in the area of medicine about which they testify.

The practice of using highly qualified and specialized doctors as expert witnesses has long been accepted by courts as an effective way to educate a jury regarding the extent, cause, and treatment of the injury in question, but there are some limitations on the use of such testimony. In order for the court to allow a medical ex-

pert to testify as to specific facts from which conclusions are to be drawn, the facts must be outside what is considered to be the general or common knowledge of a lay jury. For example, a court may not allow a party to use a medical expert to explain sprained ankles. The court would, however, allow a medical expert to explain toxic shock syndrome, because the existence, causes, and effects of that impairment are not common knowledge. The reasoning behind this limitation is that the jury members are supposed to form their own opinions when such opinions do not involve or require specialized knowledge. Only when it is necessary or helpful to the jury to be educated in a specialized area of knowledge is expert testimony usually allowed. In contrast to a lay witness, an expert witness is permitted to testify about the ultimate issue in the case. The medical expert in an accident case, for example, may testify about causation: whether the accident caused the injury that is the subject of plaintiff's lawsuit. Lay witnesses are not permitted to testify along these lines because they do not have the expertise to do so.

The court also recognizes a distinction between testimony from a medical expert and testimony from the plaintiff's treating doctor. Whereas the former educates the jury regarding an area of medicine that is relevant to the case, the latter does not. Instead, the treating doctor is called to testify to actual events or facts of the case that the doctor personally witnessed: that the plaintiff was examined on a certain date, the extent of his or her injuries, and so on. Thus, although an expert witness may not be allowed by the court to educate the jury on the subject of a sprained ankle or other topic of common knowledge, the fact that the plaintiff sustained a sprained ankle and was treated for it may be testified to by the treating doctor.

In a civil suit, the plaintiff must prove that he or she was injured by some act of the defendant. That injury can be economic (the loss of property or money), physical (such as a torn muscle or broken leg), or mental (stress or anxiety). Over the years, more and more types of injuries have become recognized as compensable injuries in civil cases. The term "pain and suffering" has been used to describe physical and emotional symptoms that a plaintiff may claim were caused by the defendant. Medical facts can help determine the existence and extent of all these types of injury.

Sometimes the expert will testify only hypothetically. In the hypothetical question, the expert may be asked to render an opinion based on certain assumptions concerning a hypothetical case that closely resembles the case at bar. The hypothetical question provides an opportunity for counsel to summarize his or her client's position. Sometimes, however, a medical expert will need to examine a plaintiff. It is not unusual for such examinations to take place years after the injury occurred, and the doctor will have to determine whether the injury exists, the extent of the injury, the cause of the injury, what (if any) limitations are caused by the injury, the treatment that is indicated, and the probable duration of the injury (perhaps based on the average rate of recovery for such an injury).

In the criminal justice system, medical experts may testify on a variety of scientific and medical issues. In the case of a murder, for example, it may be necessary to identify blood, tissue, bone, or some other human remains and to determine the source of those remains— namely, whether the remains belong to the alleged victim or perpetrator of the crime. Doctors who specialize in forensic medicine are often called upon to conduct special tests, such as DNA testing, to identify whose blood or tissue was found at the scene of a crime or on a murder weapon. Forensic experts can also determine the approximate time and cause of death. Testimony on these issues helps a jury determine the guilt or innocence of the accused.

Criminal cases occasionally also require the testimony of a forensic psychiatrist, who is an expert in mental and emotional disorders as they relate to legal principles. Testimony from such an expert assists in determining whether the defendant is "insane." According to section 4.01 of the Model Penal Code, a person is insane if he or she "lacks substantial capacity either to appreciate the criminality [wrongfulness] of his conduct or to conform his conduct to the requirements of the law." Not every state follows the Model Penal Code. Other variations of the insanity defense exist that deal with a person's ability to distinguish right from wrong. Psychiatric evaluations of the accused are performed to determine whether the defendant fit this definition at the time the crime was committed. Testimony regarding the defendant's insanity would significantly affect the case's outcome and sentencing.

A separate issue, unrelated to the defendant's mental condition at the time of the crime, is the defendant's "competency" to stand trial. According to *Black's Law Dictionary* (9th ed., 2008), a defendant is competent to stand trial if he or she has "the capacity to understand the proceedings, to consult meaningfully with counsel, and to assist in the defense." The law ensures that an accused person's rights are protected by requiring that the defendant be capable of understanding these proceedings and their implications before he or she is allowed to stand trial. If either of the attorneys, or the judge, asserts that the defendant is not competent to stand trial, the court will hold a competency hearing to decide whether the defendant is "competent." In determining the competency of the defendant, the court will hear the testimony of psychiatric experts. If the defendant is determined to be incompetent at the time of the trial, the defendant will not be tried but may instead be sent to a mental institution until such time as he or she is competent to stand trial.

In addition to being used in civil cases and criminal cases, medical science is used to provide scientific information to support or disprove wholly nonscientific determinations. Such philosophical and ethical issues include abortion and euthanasia. In the long-running debate over the legality of abortion, for example, many issues and circumstances come into play, including rape and the possibility that pregnancy may endanger the woman's life. One central and hotly contested question, however, is "When does life begin?" This question may also involve an equally difficult and controversial one: "What is life?" The courts and various state legislatures have turned to medical science to address these profound, and possibly unanswerable, questions. Medical science has identified two key concepts to answer these questions: the concept of "viability" (that is, the ability of the fetus to survive outside the womb) and the distinction between the first, second, and third trimesters of a pregnancy. The distinction of trimesters was originally based on the concept of viability: A fetus generally could not survive outside the womb during the first trimester (that is, was not viable), while a fetus was generally considered viable during the third trimester. Thus, the courts and legislature would often use the concept of trimesters in determining a cutoff date after which an abortion could not be performed.

These concepts have been used as the basis for legislation to regulate and authorize abortions. Medical science is, however, a rapidly evolving field. Because it is now possible for a human egg, once fertilized, to become viable outside the womb, the legal foundation upon which abortions are based is becoming more unstable.

Another important area that has emerged from late twentieth and early twenty-first century technology concerns the use of human embryonic stem cells. Widely acknowledged as extremely valuable in assisting scientists in understanding basic mechanisms of embryo development and gene regulation, stem cell research holds the promise of enabling scientists to direct stem cells to grow into replacement organs and tissues to treat a wide variety of diseases. Embryos are valued in research for their ability to produce stem cells, which can be harvested to grow a variety of tissues for use in transplantation to treat serious illnesses such as cancer, heart disease, and diabetes.

THE APPLICATIONS OF MEDICAL TESTIMONY

Medical experts in almost every field of medicine have played a part in civil cases, criminal cases, and controversies involving philosophical and ethical issues. Sometimes, the interaction between medicine and the law has spawned new medical or legal subspecialties. In fact, medical expert testimony has become a field and an occupation in itself, supporting an entire group of medical professionals to the exclusion of actual medical practice. This phenomenon has occurred in large part in response to the greater acceptance by the courts of medical expert testimony and the increased reliability of recent medical testing.

Personal injury cases afford a good example of all the different types of testimony that come into play in civil suits. A physical injury case, as the name suggests, is based on a physical (or mental) injury, as opposed to a purely financial injury, suffered by the plaintiff. A physical injury case may involve an automobile accident and its resulting injuries. In such a case, doctors who are experts in the field of muscle damage, neurology (for head and nerve injuries), orthopedic surgery, and countless other areas could be called as experts, depending on the extent of the injuries.

Another type of case, called a product liability case, will often use expert medical testimony. A product liability case is one in which a person has been injured by a specific product on the market and sues the manufacturer, and often the seller, claiming that the product was defective. Famous examples of product liability cases include claims filed against manufacturers of asbestos products, certain tampons (for causing toxic shock syndrome), contraceptive devices such as the Dalkon Shield, and some generic or prescription drugs, such as thalidomide and Halcion. All these cases required medical experts in recently developed fields of medicine. Prior to the product liability suits filed against some tampon manufacturers, few people had heard of toxic shock syndrome. The testimony of medical experts was required to prove a link between an allegedly defective product and the resulting injury that was claimed.

Without expert medical testimony in these cases, it would be impossible to prove that the defective products caused the injuries of which the defendants complained.

Another example of the medical profession developing to suit the law is in the area of workers' compensation. The California legislature, like the legislatures of many states, has established by statute (Labor Code section 3600 and following) a method by which to compensate any employee who has suffered a job-related injury. An employer is required by law to carry workers' compensation insurance, which will compensate an injured employee. If an employee is injured on the job in any manner, that employee is supposed to file a claim notifying his or her employer of the injury. The claim is then submitted to the workers' compensation insurance carrier. If the employer and the carrier accept liability, necessary treatment is provided to the employee. If the carrier denies further treatment or denies that an employee is disabled, the employee may file a claim with the Workers' Compensation Appeal Board. Once such a claim is filed, a judge will review all the medical reports of the injured worker. Additional medical evidence and testimony may be introduced to prove or disprove the employee's claim of injury or disability. The award of the Workers' Compensation Appeal Board is determined by the medical condition of the person claiming the injury. The growing popularity of workers' compensation has spawned an entire field of medicine, that of work-related injuries.

California courts routinely allow damages for "mental distress" in almost every type of tort action. Accordingly, psychiatrists and psychologists are routinely called upon to testify regarding whether a plaintiff has suffered such an injury. Emotional distress is not a specific medical condition, but rather a general emotional state, which may include anger, fear, frustration, anxiety, depression, and similar symptoms. Although psychiatric or psychological testimony is not required by the court for the plaintiff to recover damages for mental distress, it can be very effective in explaining to the jury the extent of the injuries and the effect of those injuries on the plaintiff's future life.

If a jury determines that the plaintiff suffered a physical or mental injury caused by the defendant, then, based on the medical testimony—of either the medical witness or the treating doctor—the jury may award any medical fees incurred, as well as anticipated medical fees and costs and compensation for the pain and suffering of the defendant. The jury may also award further damages not related to the medical condition of the plaintiff, if the case warrants such damages.

In a criminal case, particularly a case of homicide, forensic medicine often provides the key and fundamental evidence upon which the entire case is based. During the investigations of the assassination of President John F. Kennedy in the 1960's, the forensic evidence played a vital, although controversial, role. The testimony presented by the doctors who examined the president's body was used to reconstruct the crime. Forensic science was used to interpret the angle of entry of the bullets that killed Kennedy and thereby to extrapolate the source of the shots. Furthermore, forensic science was called upon to demonstrate how many shots were fired and the paths of the bullets upon entering the bodies of the president and Governor John Connally. Using medical evidence, along with other evidence, the Warren Commission concluded that the bullets all came from the book depository building behind the presidential caravan. Also using medical evidence and experts, critics of the Warren Commission's findings have alleged that the injuries suffered by the president could have been caused only by a bullet entering from the front of the president's neck and exiting the rear of the skull.

In another case, forensic evidence was able to reach a conclusive determination that certain bones were those of the Nazi war criminal Josef Mengele, known as the Angel of Death. In 1992, forensics experts discovered, using a method known as DNA testing, that some bones retrieved from a grave in Brazil were those of Mengele. To make this determination, doctors compared the DNA found in the blood of Mengele's son with DNA from the bones found in the grave. They found that the DNA from both sources matched. Because DNA constitutes a "genetic fingerprint" that remains the same from parent to offspring, the doctors were able to conclude that the remains found in Brazil were those of Mengele.

DNA testing is now also commonly used in suits to determine the father of an infant. According to the Genetics Institute, DNA testing is at least 99.8 percent accurate. Medical science has so refined its ability to chart DNA "fingerprints" that the chance of coming upon two identical DNA patterns is approximately one in six billion. Prior to DNA testing, a blood testing method called human leukocyte antigen (HLA) typing was used to determine paternity, but this typing was only 95 percent accurate.

Some medical or scientific tests, while accepted by the courts, remain subject to much controversy. The Breathalyzer test, used to determine blood alcohol levels, is one such test. While the courts regularly accept the results of such tests to determine whether a suspect was intoxicated, the test is based on several assumptions and averages. Based on the alcohol content in the suspect's breath, the test extrapolates a probable amount of alcohol in the suspect's blood. The reliability of this test depends on the correct calibration of the equipment and the care of the person taking the readings. Since the tests are taken by nonmedical or nonscientific personnel in the field, mistaken readings are not uncommon. Furthermore, if the suspect used a spray breath freshener just before the test, the readings may be skewed, since such breath fresheners are usually alcohol-based.

Perspective and Prospects

Medicine has always played some role in the outcome of court cases, but this relationship did not come into full flower until relatively recently. In the early twentieth century, courts placed strict limitations on the type and amount of medical testimony allowed into evidence. Often, certain types of medical evidence were not admissible because the science was not deemed reliable—there was too much room for error. The polygraph (lie detector), for example, could not be relied upon to reveal consistently whether a person was telling the truth, since it simply measured galvanic skin response, respiration rate, and other factors that only tend to be correlated with the subject's feelings of guilt. Most other evidence presented by medical experts concerned the likelihood of events or outcomes and therefore usually constituted opinion, rather than fact.

With the advent of new technologies in the later part of the twentieth century, medical science began to present "hard" (more precise) data that became more frequently accepted by the courts as reliable and relevant evidence. Even so, it took some time before medical scientists were able to present enough data to persuade the courts that the evidence of such methods as DNA "fingerprinting" was truly reliable. The acceptance of DNA testing, for example, was a long and hard-fought battle among legions of medical experts on both sides of the issue. Finally, DNA testing was accepted by the courts as a reliable source of evidence. As forensic medicine advances, no doubt its contribution to the law will also advance. The ability of the medical and other scientific professions to determine reliable conclusions relating to court cases is progressing rapidly with increases in scientific knowledge, methods, and technology.

In an ironic twist, however, this progress has clouded other areas of the law. In the early twentieth century, for example, no one could have dreamed of the technology that makes life support possible. With the advent of kidney dialysis machines, pacemakers, respirators, and other life-support devices, medical science has achieved the ability to prolong an individual's bodily functioning. Whether this functioning alone is sufficient to define "life," however, remains a question that cannot be addressed by medical science alone but must be considered in the light of philosophical, ethical, and other values. Medicine is therefore becoming an area with which the law must contend. Issues that have challenged existing laws include abortion and the point at which life begins, euthanasia, the individual's right not to have life extended by extraordinary means if there is no hope of recovery, the right to reveal an individual's genetic predisposition toward disease, egg implantation, and genetic engineering. Medical science has propagated these dilemmas but may also be called upon to solve them.

—Larry M. Roberts, J.D.;
updated by Marcia J. Weiss, M.A., J.D.

See also Abortion; Animal rights vs. research; Assisted reproductive technologies; Autopsy; Blood testing; Cloning; Environmental health; Ethics; Euthanasia; Forensic pathology; Genetic engineering; In vitro fertilization; Living will; Malpractice; Occupational health; Screening.

FOR FURTHER INFORMATION:

Boumil, Marcia M., Clifford E. Elias, and Diane Bissonnette Moes. *Medical Liability in a Nutshell.* 2d ed. St. Paul, Minn.: Thomson/West, 2003. Succinctly discusses salient topics in medical liability: medical negligence, standard of care, intentional torts, informed consent and the right to refuse treatment, the duty of disclosure, causation and damages, and various defenses to liability.

Fremgen, Bonnie F. *Medical Law and Ethics.* 2d ed. Upper Saddle River, N.J.: Pearson/Prentice Hall, 2006. Essential legal and ethical principles for the health care provider. Contains case studies and legal citations.

Furrow, Barry R., et al. *Health Law: Cases, Materials, and Problems.* 6th ed. St. Paul, Minn.: Thomson/West, 2008. Covers a range of issues related to health and the law, including cost control, prospective payment, health care antitrust, and federal and state regulation of health care delivery; legal and ethical issues created by reproductive technology and by the dilemmas of death and dying; and the core topics of professional liability and the physician-patient relationship.

Garner, Bryan A., ed. *Black's Law Dictionary.* 9th ed. St. Paul, Minn.: Thomson/West, 2008. The fundamental legal dictionary, containing definitions and examples of how terms have been interpreted by courts.

James, Stuart H., and Jon J. Nordby, eds. *Forensic Science: An Introduction to Scientific and Investigative Techniques.* 2d ed. Boca Raton, Fla.: CRC Press, 2005. An introductory text that covers a range of topics, including trace evidence, forensic toxicology, DNA analysis, crime scene investigation, fingerprints, traumatic death, forensic anthropology, bloodstain patterns, and criminal profiling, among many others.

Jonsen, Albert R., Mark Siegler, and William J. Winslade. *Clinical Ethics: A Practical Approach to Ethical Decisions in Clinical Medicine.* 6th ed. New York: McGraw-Hill, 2006. Discusses the whole range of medical ethics, including legal issues, confidentiality, care of the dying patient, and euthanasia and assisted suicide.

Lewis, Marcia A., and Carol D. Tamparo. *Medical Law, Ethics, and Bioethics for Ambulatory Care.* 6th ed. Philadelphia: F. A. Davis, 2007. Directed to the general health care provider, the book covers practical topics such as management, guidelines and regulations for medical and allied health professionals, public duties, medical records, collection, allocation of scarce resources, genetic engineering, abortion, and life-and-death issues from the legal and ethical perspectives.

Munson, Ronald, comp. *Intervention and Reflection: Basic Issues in Medical Ethics.* 7th ed. Belmont, Calif.: Thomson/Wadsworth, 2004. An undergraduate text that combines social context, case studies, readings, and decision scenarios for topics that include abortion, advances in gene therapy, genetic discrimination, and health care rights.

Pence, Gregory E. *Classic Cases in Medical Ethics: Accounts of Cases That Have Shaped Medical Ethics, with Philosophical, Legal, and Historical Backgrounds.* 4th ed. Boston: McGraw-Hill, 2004. Surveys important cases that have defined and shaped the field of medical ethics. Each case is accompanied by careful discussion of pertinent philosophical theories and legal and ethical issues.

LEAD POISONING

DISEASE/DISORDER

ALSO KNOWN AS: Saturnism, plumbism, painter's colic

ANATOMY OR SYSTEM AFFECTED: Brain, circulatory system, endocrine system, musculoskeletal system, nervous system, reproductive system

SPECIALTIES AND RELATED FIELDS: Environmental health, pediatrics, preventive medicine, toxicology

DEFINITION: A condition caused by high levels of lead in the blood. This major preventable environmental health problem is found in both children and adults, but more frequently in children.

KEY TERMS:

arthralgia: severe joint pain, especially when inflammation is not present

chelation: the taking up or release of a metallic ion by an organic molecule

encephalopathy: any disease of the brain

lead: a limited naturally occurring element widely distributed throughout the environment by industrial uses and pollution

paresis: partial paralysis

paresthesia: an abnormal sensation, such as burning, tingling, tickling, or pricking

CAUSES AND SYMPTOMS

Lead poisoning is a major, preventable environmental health problem. Elevated lead levels in adults can increase blood pressure and cause fertility problems, nerve disorders, arthalgia, and problems with memory and concentration. Children under the age of six are at high risk for harm because their brains and nervous systems are still maturing. Blood lead levels as low as 10 micrograms per deciliter are associated with harmful effects on children's ability to learn. Very high blood lead levels of 70 micrograms per deciliter can cause devastating health consequences, including seizures and other neurological symptoms, abdominal pain, developmental delays, attention deficit, hyperactivity, behavior disorders, hearing loss, anemia, coma, and death.

Children can be exposed to lead in many ways. Sources of exposure include automobile exhaust, lead-based paint, and environmental contaminants released by industrial processes that use or produce lead-containing materials. Contributors to childhood lead exposure also include lead-contaminated containers, food, dust, soil, air, and water; toys contaminated with lead paint; lead-containing ceramics and hobby sup-plies; substance abuse such as gasoline sniffing; parental transfer from lead-rich occupational environments; and traditional medicines such as azarcon and greta. Deteriorating lead-based paint in older homes is the most important source of lead exposure in children. Swallowing lead-based paint dust through normal hand-to-mouth activity and chewing directly on painted surfaces are major methods of lead ingestion. Children are often attracted to lead paint because of its sweet taste. Lead exposure in adults is usually a result of jobs in house painting, welding and smelting, the manufacturing of car batteries, and other occupations involving lead.

Upon entering the human body, inorganic lead is not metabolized but is directly absorbed, distributed, and excreted. The rate at which lead is absorbed depends on its chemical and physical form and on the physiologic characteristics of the exposed person. Once in the blood, lead is distributed among three compartments: the blood; soft tissue zones such as the kidneys, bone marrow, liver, and brain; and mineralizing tissues such as bones and teeth. For lead poisoning to take place, major acute exposures to lead need not occur. The body accumulates lead and releases it slowly; therefore, even small doses over time can be toxic. It is the total body accumulation of lead that is related to the risk of adverse effects. Whether lead enters the body through inhalation or ingestion, the biologic effects are the same—interference with normal cell function and with certain physiologic processes.

By and large, children show a greater sensitivity to the effects of lead than do adults. Parents working in lead-related industries not only may inhale lead dust and lead oxide fumes but also may eat, drink, and smoke in or near contaminated areas, increasing the probability of lead ingestion and subsequent transfer to their children. Since lead readily crosses the placenta, the fetus is at risk. Fetal exposure can cause potentially

---

INFORMATION ON LEAD POISONING

CAUSES: Environmental exposure

SYMPTOMS: Vary; can include abdominal discomfort, fatigue, muscle pain, tremor, difficulty concentrating, headache, vomiting, weight loss, constipation, hearing loss, changes in consciousness

DURATION: Can be short-term or chronic

TREATMENTS: Chelation drug therapy

adverse neurological effects in utero and during post-natal development. The incomplete development of the blood-brain barrier in very young children, up to thirty-six months of age, increases the risk of the entry of lead into the developing nervous system, which can result in prolonged neurobehavioral disorders. Children absorb and retain more lead in proportion to their weight than do adults. Young children also show a greater preva-lence of iron deficiency, a condition that can increase the gastrointestinal absorption of lead.

Symptoms of lead poisoning and lead intoxication vary because of differences in individual susceptibility, and the severity of symptoms increases with increased exposure. Symptoms of mild lead toxicity include ab-dominal discomfort, fatigue, muscle pain, or pares-thesia. Moderate toxicity is indicated by arthralgia, tremor, fatigue, difficulty concentrating, headache, ab-dominal pain, vomiting, weight loss, and constipation. Severe toxicity symptoms include paresis or paralysis, encephalopathy, seizures, severe abdominal cramps, hearing loss, changes in consciousness, and coma.

TREATMENT AND THERAPY

If a child is suspected of having lead poisoning, labora-tory tests are necessary to evaluate lead intoxication levels. Laboratory techniques defining lead toxicity include blood lead level screening, erythrocyte proto-porphyrin (EP) and zinc protoporphyrin (ZPP) screen-ing, creatinine, urinalysis, and hematocrit and hemo-globin tests with peripheral smear.

The physical examination for suspected lead poison-ing cases includes special attention to hematologic, cardiovascular, gastrointestinal, and renal systems. Any neurological or behavioral changes are considered significant indicators. In addition, severe and pro-longed lead poisoning may be indicated by a purplish line on the gums. A complete interview and medical evaluation of a suspected lead poisoning patient in-cludes a full workup and medical history. Clues to po-tential exposure vectors can be obtained by discussing family and occupational history, use of traditional med-icines, remodeling activities, hobbies, table and cook-ware, drinking water source, nutrition, proximity to in-dustry or waste sites, and the physical condition and age of the patient's residence, school, and/or day care facility.

The treatment and management of lead poisoning first involves the separation of the patient from the source of lead. After a diagnosis of lead poisoning is made, local environmental health officials should be contacted to determine the lead source and what remediation action is necessary for its control. A diet high in calcium and iron may help to decrease the ab-sorption of lead.

The Centers for Disease Control and Prevention rec-ommends that children with blood lead levels of 45 mi-crograms per deciliter or greater should be referred for chelation therapy immediately. Several drugs are capa-ble of binding or chelating lead, depleting both soft and hard (skeletal) tissues of lead and reducing its acute toxicity. All these drugs have potential side effects and must be used with caution. The most commonly used chelating agent is calcium disodium edetic acid, but several other agents are available.

—Randall L. Milstein, Ph.D.; updated by Sharon W. Stark, R.N., A.P.R.N., D.N.Sc.

See also Developmental disorders; Environmental diseases; Environmental health; Learning disabilities; Mental retardation; Occupational health; Poisoning; Safety issues for children; Screening; Toxicology.

FOR FURTHER INFORMATION:

Centers for Disease Control and Prevention. "Lead: Topic Home." http://www.cdc.gov/lead. This Web site provides a variety of information and sources re-lated to lead, lead poisoning, statistics, treatments, and prevention.

Environmental Protection Agency. http://www.epa .gov/oppt/lead. A comprehensive site, providing in-formation on lead and lead poisoning, details on where one can find lead in and near the home, and family protection.

Goldstein, Inge F., and Martin Goldstein. *How Much Risk? A Guide to Understanding Environmental Health Hazards*. New York: Oxford University Press, 2002. A critical analysis of environmental health hazards and their threat to the public. Includes discussions of radiation from nuclear testing, radon in the home, the connection between electromag-netic fields and cancer, environmental factors and asthma, and pesticides and breast cancer.

Kessel, Irene, and John T. O'Connor. *Getting the Lead Out: The Complete Resource on How to Prevent and Cope with Lead Poisoning*. Rev. ed. Cambridge, Mass.: Perseus, 2001. A comprehensive resource for parents and homeowners describing the major sources of lead in the home and environment, as well as medical concerns, prevention strategies, and tech-niques for controlling lead hazards.

Morgan, Monroe T. *Environmental Health*. 3d ed.

Belmont, Calif.: Thomson/Wadsworth, 2003. Examines the links between environmental sciences and human population, focusing on the practices that support human life as well as the need to control factors that are harmful to human life.

National Safety Council. "Lead Poisoning." http://www.nsc.org/safety_home/resources. This Web site provides an overview of lead poisoning and its sources, its effects on health, and treatments and prevention.

Warren, Christian. *Brush with Death: A Social History of Lead Poisoning.* Baltimore: Johns Hopkins University Press, 2001. Traces the history of lead poisoning from paint and gasoline in the United States. Examines occupational, pediatric, and environmental exposure and the regulatory mechanisms, medical technologies, and epidemiological tools that arose in response to lead poisoning.

LEARNING DISABILITIES

DISEASE/DISORDER

ANATOMY OR SYSTEM AFFECTED: Brain, nervous system, psychic-emotional system

SPECIALTIES AND RELATED FIELDS: Neurology, pediatrics, psychology

DEFINITION: A variety of disorders involving the failure to learn an academic skill despite normal levels of intelligence, maturation, and cultural and educational opportunity; estimates of the prevalence of learning disabilities in the general population range between 2 and 20 percent.

KEY TERMS:

achievement test: a measure of an individual's degree of learning in an academic subject, such as reading, mathematics, and written language

dyslexia: difficulty in reading, with an implied neurological cause

intelligence test: a psychological test designed to measure an individual's ability to think logically, act purposefully, and react successfully to the environment; yields intelligence quotient (IQ) scores

neurological dysfunction: problems associated with the way in which different sections and structures of the brain perform tasks, such as verbal and spatial reasoning and language production

neurology: the study of the central nervous system, which is composed of the brain and spinal cord

perceptual deficits: problems in processing information from the environment, which may involve distractibility, impulsivity, and figure-ground distor-

tions (difficulty distinguishing foreground from background)

standardized test: an instrument used to assess skill development in comparison to others of the same age or grade

CAUSES AND SYMPTOMS

An understanding of learning disabilities must begin with the knowledge that the definition, diagnosis, and treatment of these disorders have historically generated considerable disagreement and controversy. This is primarily attributable to the fact that people with learning disabilities are a highly diverse group of individuals with a wide variety of characteristics. Consequently, differences of opinion among professionals remain to such an extent that presenting a single universally accepted definition of learning disabilities is not possible. Definitional differences most frequently center on the relative emphases that alternative groups place on characteristics of these disorders. For example, experts in medical fields typically describe these disorders from a disease model and view them primarily as neurological dysfunctions. Conversely, educators usually place more emphasis on the academic problems that result from learning disabilities. Despite these differences, the most commonly accepted definitions, those developed by the United States Office of Education in 1977, the Board of the Association for Children and Adults with Learning Disabilities in 1985, and the National Joint Committee for Learning Disabilities in 1981, do include some areas of commonality.

Difficulty in academic functioning is included in the three definitions, and virtually all descriptions of learning disabilities include this characteristic. Academic deficits may be in one or more formal scholastic subjects, such as reading or mathematics. Often the deficits will involve a component skill of the academic area, such as problems with comprehension or word knowledge in reading or difficulty in calculating or applying arithmetical reasoning in mathematics. The academic difficulty may also be associated with more basic skills of learning that influence functioning across academic areas; these may involve deficits in listening, speaking, and thinking. Dyslexia, a term for reading problems, is the most common academic problem associated with learning disabilities. Because reading skills are required in most academic activities to some degree, many view dyslexia as the most serious form of learning disability.

The presumption of a neurological dysfunction as

the cause of these disorders is included, either directly or indirectly, in each of the three definitions. Despite this presumption, unless an individual has a known history of brain trauma, the neurological basis for learning disabilities will not be identified in most cases because current assessment technology does not allow for such precise diagnoses. Rather, at least minimal neurological dysfunction is simply assumed to be present in anyone who exhibits characteristics of a learning disorder.

The three definitions all state that individuals with learning disabilities experience learning problems despite possessing normal intelligence. This condition is referred to as a discrepancy between achievement and ability or potential.

Finally, each of the three definitions incorporates the idea that learning disabilities cannot be attributed to another handicapping condition such as mental retardation, vision or hearing problems, emotional or psychiatric disturbance, or social, cultural, or educational disadvantage. Consequently, these conditions must be excluded as primary contributors to academic difficulties.

Reports on the prevalence of learning disabilities differ according to the definitions and identification methods employed. Consequently, statistics on prevalence range between 2 and 20 percent of the population. Many of the higher reported percentages are actually estimates of prevalence that include individuals who are presumed to have a learning disorder but who have not been formally diagnosed. Males are believed to constitute the majority of individuals with learning disabilities, and estimated sex ratios range from 6:1 to 8:1. Some experts believe that this difference in incidence may reveal one of the causes of these disorders.

A number of causes of learning disabilities have been proposed, with none being universally accepted. Some of the most plausible causal theories include neurological deficits, genetic and hereditary influences, and exposure to toxins during fetal gestation or early childhood.

Evidence to support the assumption of a link between neurological dysfunction and learning disabilities has been provided by studies using sophisticated brain imaging techniques such as positron emission tomography (PET) and computed tomography (CT) scanning and magnetic resonance imaging (MRI). Studies using these techniques have, among other findings, indicated subtle abnormalities in the structure and electrical activity in the brains of individuals with learning disabilities. The use of such techniques has

---

INFORMATION ON LEARNING DISABILITIES

CAUSES: Unclear; possibly neurological deficits, genetic and hereditary influences, exposure to toxins during pregnancy or early childhood

SYMPTOMS: Difficulty in academic functioning (including deficits in listening, speaking, and thinking)

DURATION: Often chronic

TREATMENTS: Medication, patterning, teaching of specific reading skills and repeated language drills (imprinting)

---

typically been confined to research; however, the continuing advancement of brain imaging technology holds promise not only in contributing greater understanding of the nature and causes of learning disabilities but also in treating the disorder.

Genetic and hereditary influences also have been proposed as causes. Supportive evidence comes from research indicating that identical twins are more likely to be concordant for learning disabilities than fraternal twins and that these disorders are more common in certain families.

A genetic cause of learning disabilities may be associated with extra X or Y chromosomes in certain individuals. The type and degree of impairment associated with these conditions vary according to many genetic and environmental factors, but they can involve problems with language development, visual perception, memory, and problem solving. Despite evidence to link chromosome abnormalities to those with learning disabilities, most experts agree that such genetic conditions account for only a portion of these individuals.

Exposure to toxins or poisons during fetal gestation and early childhood can also cause learning disabilities. During pregnancy nearly all substances the mother takes in are transferred to the fetus. Research has shown that mothers who smoke, drink alcohol, or use certain drugs or medications during pregnancy are more likely to have children with developmental problems, including learning disabilities. Yet not all children exposed to toxins during gestation will have such problems, and the consequences of exposure will vary according to the period when it occurred, the amount of toxin introduced, and the general health and nutrition of the mother and fetus.

Though not precisely involving toxins, two other conditions associated with gestation and childbirth have been linked to learning disabilities. The first, anoxia, or oxygen deprivation, occurring for a critical period of time during the birthing process has been tied to both mental retardation and learning disabilities. The second, and more speculative, involves exposure of the fetus to an abnormally large amount of testosterone during gestation. Differences in brain development are proposed to result from the exposure, causing learning disorders and other abnormalities. Known as the embryological theory, it may account for the large number of males with these disabilities, since they have greater amounts of testosterone than females.

The exposure of the immature brain during early childhood to insecticides, household cleaning fluids, alcohol, narcotics, and carbon monoxide, among other toxic substances, may also cause learning disabilities. Lead poisoning resulting from ingesting lead from paint, plaster, and other sources has been found in epidemic numbers in some sections of the country. Lead poisoning can damage the brain and cause learning disabilities, as well as a number of other serious problems.

The number and variety of proposed causes not only reflect differences in experts' training and consequent perspectives but also suggest the likelihood that these disorders can be caused by multiple conditions. This diversity of views also carries to methods for assessing and providing treatment and services to individuals with learning disabilities.

TREATMENT AND THERAPY

In 1975, the U.S. Congress adopted the Education for All Handicapped Children Act, which, along with other requirements, mandated that students with disabilities, including those with learning disabilities, be identified and provided appropriate educational services. Since that time, much effort has been devoted to developing adequate assessment practices for diagnosis and effective treatment strategies.

In the school setting, assessment of students suspected of having learning disabilities is conducted by a variety of professionals, including teachers specially trained in assessing learning disabilities, school nurses, classroom teachers, school psychologists, and school administrators. Collectively, these professionals are known as a multidisciplinary team. An additional requirement of this educational legislation is that parents must be given the opportunity to participate in the assessment process. Professionals outside the school setting, such as clinical psychologists and independent educational specialists, also conduct assessments to identify learning disabilities.

Because the definition of learning disabilities in the 1975 act includes a discrepancy between achievement and ability as a characteristic of the disorder, students suspected of having learning disabilities are usually administered a variety of formal and informal tests. Standardized tests of intelligence, such as the third edition of the Wechsler Intelligence Scale for Children, are administered to determine ability. Standardized tests of academic achievement, such as the Woodcock-Johnson Psychoeducational Battery and the Wide Range Achievement Test, also are administered to determine levels of academic skill.

Whether a discrepancy between ability and achievement exists to such a degree as to warrant diagnosis of a learning disability is determined by various formulas comparing the scores derived from the intelligence and achievement tests. The precise methods and criteria used to determine a discrepancy vary according to differences among state regulations and school district practices. Consequently, a student diagnosed with a learning disability in one part of the United States may not be viewed as such in another area using different diagnostic criteria. This possibility has been raised in criticism of the use of the discrepancy criteria to identify these disorders. Other criticisms of the method include the use of intelligence quotient (IQ) scores (which are not as stable or accurate as many assume), the inconsistency of students' scores when using alternative achievement tests, and the lack of correspondence between what students are taught and what is tested on achievement tests.

In partial consequence of these and other problems with standardized tests, alternative informal assessment methods have been developed. One such method that is frequently employed is termed curriculum-based assessment (CBA). The CBA method uses materials and tasks taken directly from students' classroom curriculum. For example, in reading, CBA might involve determining the rate of words read per minute from a student's textbook. CBA has been demonstrated to be effective in distinguishing among some students with learning disabilities, those with other academic difficulties, and those without learning problems. Nevertheless, many professionals remain skeptical of CBA as a valid alternative to traditional standardized tests.

Other assessment techniques include vision and hearing tests, measures of language development, and tests examining motor coordination and sensory perception and processing. Observations and analyses of the classroom environment may also be conducted to determine how instructional practices and a student's behavior contribute to learning difficulties.

Based on the information gathered by the multidisciplinary team, a decision is made regarding the diagnosis of a learning disability. If a student is identified with one of these disorders, the team then develops an individual education plan to address identified educational needs. An important guideline in developing the plan is that students with these disorders should be educated to the greatest extent possible with their nonhandicapped peers, while still being provided with appropriate services. Considerable debate has occurred regarding how best to adhere to this guideline.

Programs for students with learning disabilities typically are implemented in self-contained classrooms, resource rooms, or regular classrooms. Self-contained classrooms usually contain ten to twenty students and one or more teachers specially trained to work with these disorders. Typically, these classrooms focus on teaching fundamental skills in basic academic subjects such as reading, writing, and mathematics. Depending on the teacher's training, efforts may also be directed toward developing perceptual, language, or social skills. Students in these programs usually spend some portion of their day with their peers in regular education meetings, but the majority of the day is spent in the self-contained classroom.

The popularity of self-contained classrooms has decreased significantly since the 1960's, when they were the primary setting in which students with learning disabilities were educated. This decrease is largely attributable to the stigmatizing effects of placing students in special settings and the lack of clear evidence to support the effectiveness of this approach.

Students receiving services in resource rooms typically spend a portion of their day in a class where they receive instruction and assistance from specially trained teachers. Students often spend one or two periods in the resource room with a small group of other students who may have similar learning problems or function at a comparable academic level. In the elementary grades, resource rooms usually focus on developing basic academic skills, whereas at the secondary level time is more typically spent in assisting students with their assignments from regular education classes.

Resource room programs are viewed as less restrictive than self-contained classrooms; however, they too have been criticized for segregating children with learning problems. Other criticisms center on scheduling difficulties inherent in the program and the potential for inconsistent instructional approaches and confusion over teaching responsibilities between the regular classroom and resource room teachers. Research on the effectiveness of resource room programs also has been mixed; nevertheless, they are found in most public schools across the United States.

Increasing numbers of students with learning disabilities have their individual education plans implemented exclusively in a regular classroom. In most schools where such programs exist, teachers are given assistance by a consulting teacher with expertise in learning disabilities. Supporters of this approach point to the lack of stigma associated with segregating students and the absence of definitive research supporting other service models. Detractors are concerned about the potential for inadequate support for the classroom teacher, resulting in students receiving poor quality or insufficient services. The movement to provide services to educationally handicapped students in regular education settings, termed the Regular Education Initiative, has stirred much debate among professionals and parents. Resolution of the debate will greatly affect how individuals with learning disabilities are provided services.

No one specific method of teaching these students has been demonstrated to be superior to others. A variety of strategies have been developed, including perceptual training, multisensory teaching, modality matching, and direct instruction. Advocates of perceptual training believe that academic problems stem from underlying deficits in perceptual skills. They use various techniques aimed at developing perceptual abilities before trying to remedy or teach specific academic skills. Multisensory teaching involves presenting information to students through several senses. Instruction using this method may be conducted using tactile, auditory, visual, and kinesthetic exercises. Instruction involving modality matching begins with identifying the best learning style for a student, such as visual or auditory processing. Learning tasks are then presented via that mode. Direct instruction is based on the principles of behavioral psychology. The method involves developing precise educational goals, focusing on teaching the exact skill of concern, and providing frequent opportunities to perform the skill until it is mastered.

With the exception of direct instruction, research has generally failed to demonstrate that these strategies are uniquely effective with students with learning disabilities. Direct instruction, on the other hand, has been demonstrated to be effective but has also been criticized for focusing on isolated skills without dealing with the broader processing problems associated with these disorders. More promisingly, students with learning disabilities appear to benefit from teaching approaches that have been found effective with students without learning problems when instruction is geared to ability level and rate of learning.

PERSPECTIVE AND PROSPECTS

Interest in disorders of learning can be identified throughout the history of medicine. The specific study of learning disabilities, however, can be traced to the efforts of a number of physicians working in the first quarter of the twentieth century who studied the brain and its associated pathology. One such researcher, Kurt Goldstein, identified a number of unusual characteristics, collectively termed perceptual deficits, that were associated with head injury.

Goldstein's work influenced a number of researchers affiliated with the Wayne County Training School, including Alfred Strauss, Laura Lehtinen, Newell Kephart, and William Cruickshank. These individuals worked with children with learning problems who exhibited many of the characteristics of brain injury identified by Goldstein. Consequently, they presumed that neurological dysfunction, whether it could specifically be identified or not, caused the learning difficulties. They also developed a set of instructional practices involving reduced environmental stimuli and exercises to develop perceptual skills. The work and writings of these individuals through the 1940's, 1950's, and 1960's were highly influential, and many programs for students with learning disabilities were based on their theoretical and instructional principles.

Samuel Orton, working in the 1920's and 1930's, also was influenced by research into brain injury in his conceptualization of children with reading problems. He observed that many of these children were left-handed or ambidextrous, reversed letters or words when reading or writing, and had coordination problems. Consequently, he proposed that reading disabilities resulted from abnormal brain development and an associated mixing of brain functions. Based on the work of Orton and his students, including Anna Gilmore and Bessie Stillman, a variety of teaching strategies were developed that focused on teaching phonics and using multisensory aids. In the 1960's, Elizabeth Slingerland applied Orton's concepts in the classroom setting, and they have been included in many programs for students with learning disabilities.

A number of other researchers have developed theories for the cause and treatment of learning disabilities. Some of the most influential include Helmer Mykelbust and Samuel Kirk, who emphasized gearing instruction to a student's strongest learning modality, and Norris Haring, Ogden Lindsley, and Joseph Jenkins, who applied principles of behavioral psychology to teaching.

The work of these and other researchers and educators raised professional and public awareness of learning disabilities and the special needs of individuals with the disorder. Consequently, the number of special education classrooms and programs increased dramatically in public schools across the United States in the 1960's and 1970's. Legislation on both state and federal levels, primarily resulting from litigation by parents to establish the educational rights of their children, also has had a profound impact on the availability of services for those with learning disabilities. The passage of the Education for All Handicapped Children Act in 1975 not only mandated appropriate educational services for students with learning disabilities but also generated funding, interest, and research in the field. The Regular Education Initiative has since prompted increased efforts to identify more effective assessment and treatment strategies and generated debates among professionals and the consumers of these services. Decisions resulting from these continuing debates will have a significant impact on future services for individuals with learning disabilities.

—Paul F. Bell, Ph.D.

See also Aphasia and dysphasia; Asperger's syndrome; Attention-deficit disorder; Autism; Brain; Brain disorders; Developmental disorders; Down syndrome; Dyslexia; Mental retardation; Neuralgia, neuritis, and neuropathy; Neurology; Neurology, pediatric; Psychiatry; Psychiatry, child and adolescent; Speech disorders.

FOR FURTHER INFORMATION:

Bender, William N. *Learning Disabilities: Characteristics, Identification, and Teaching Strategies.* 6th ed. Boston: Pearson/Allyn & Bacon, 2006. A text with a pedagogical slant that examines the controversial issues of the changing definition of learning disabilities, theories, and medical aspects to assessment, placement, and instructional approaches.

Hallahan, Daniel P., et al. *Learning Disabilities: Foundations, Characteristics, and Effective Teaching.* 3d ed. Boston: Allyn & Bacon, 2005. This text addresses different learning disabilities and the education of the learning disabled. Includes a bibliography and indexes.

Jordan, Dale R. *Overcoming Dyslexia in Children, Adolescents, and Adults.* Austin, Tex.: Pro-Ed, 2002. Examines the role of genetics and brain development in relation to learning disabilities, and explains the perceptual and emotional nature of dyslexia. Eight "success stories," strategies for improving academic performance and social skills, and assessment checklists are included.

Learning Disabilities Association of America. http://www.ldanatl.org. Information, publications, and referral service concerning learning disabilities. State and local groups provide services to families, including camps and recreation programs.

Levinson, Harold N. *Smart but Feeling Dumb: The Challenging New Research on Dyslexia—and How It May Help You.* Rev. ed. New York: Warner Books, 2003. Argues that the basis of dyslexia and other disorders is an inner ear dysfunction that can be cured with judicious application of the correct medications. Also discusses adults and families with dyslexia, speech disorders, and attention deficit disorders.

Lovitt, Thomas. *Introduction to Learning Disabilities.* Needham Heights, Mass.: Allyn & Bacon, 1989. This book is exceptionally well written and comprehensive in its review of topics associated with learning disabilities, including assessment and treatment issues, the history of these disorders, and recommendations for future efforts in the field.

Rief, Sandra F. *The ADHD Book of Lists: A Practical Guide for Helping Children and Teens with Attention Deficit Disorders.* San Francisco: Jossey-Bass, 2003. Designed for school personnel and parents, this resource book details recent research and strategies, supports, and interventions that help minimize the problems and optimize the success of children and teens with ADHD.

Swanson, H. Lee, Karen R. Harris, and Steve Graham, eds. *Handbook of Learning Disabilities.* New York: Guilford Press, 2006. A thorough text that synthesizes current understanding on the nature of learning disabilities, their causes, and how students with these difficulties can be identified and helped to succeed.

LEGIONNAIRES' DISEASE
DISEASE/DISORDER

ANATOMY OR SYSTEM AFFECTED: Chest, lungs, respiratory system

SPECIALTIES AND RELATED FIELDS: Bacteriology, environmental health, epidemiology, internal medicine, public health

DEFINITION: A rapidly progressing bacterial pneumonia caused by infection with an organism of the genus *Legionella* and characterized by influenza-like illness, with high fever, chills, headache, and muscle aches.

KEY TERMS:

alveolus: an outpouching of lung tissue in which gas exchange takes place between air in the lungs and blood capillaries

legionellosis: another name for any infection caused by a member of the genus *Legionella*; generally denotes Legionnaires' disease

macrophage: any of a variety of phagocytic cells; macrophages are found in highest numbers in tissue; alveolar macrophages are found in lungs and function to remove respiratory pathogens

phagocytes: white cells capable of ingesting and digesting microbes, a process referred to as phagocytosis; primarily refers to neutrophils and macrophages

Pontiac fever: a self-limiting, nonpneumonic disease caused by *Legionella* bacteria; clinically and epidemiologically distinct from Legionnaires' disease

virulence factor: a bacterial factor that enhances the pathogenic potential of the organism; includes products such as toxins and capsules

CAUSES AND SYMPTOMS

Legionnaires' disease, or legionellosis, is an acute bacterial pneumonia that was unknown prior to 1976. In July and August of that year, an outbreak of pneumonia occurred among persons who had either attended an American Legion convention in Philadelphia or had been in the vicinity of the Bellevue-Stratford Hotel in the downtown area. The likely source of the epidemic was a contaminated air-conditioning unit in the hotel. Though speculation among the media and general public suggested all sorts of causes for the epidemic, the specific etiological agent was isolated by January, 1977. It turned out to be a somewhat common bacterium, which was subsequently given the genus and species names *Legionella pneumophila*; the genus name reflected the first known victims, while the species name meant "lung-loving."

Within several years, additional strains of *Legionella* bacteria were isolated from patients suffering from bacterial pneumonia. Through 2005, forty-one species have been identified, of which eighteen have been associated with human disease. Most cases of Legionnaires' disease have been linked to infection by *L. pneumophila* or, to a lesser degree, *L. micdadei*.

Genetic evidence confirmed that *Legionella* was indeed a newly isolated bacterium. Several factors contributed to its previous invisibility. First, Legionnaires' disease is similar in its characteristics to other forms of nonbacterial pneumonia, such as that caused by viruses. Since no bacteria were readily isolated, there was no immediate reason to suspect a bacterium as the infectious agent. The second reason related to the initial difficulty of growing *Legionella* bacteria in the laboratory. Aspirates from pneumonia victims were inoculated onto routine laboratory media; most common bacteria grow quite readily on such media. No growth was observed, however, in the case of *Legionella*. Many nutrient supplements were tried. *Legionella* bacteria grew only on media that were supplemented with iron and the amino acid cysteine. Since the early 1980's, the medium of choice has been agar containing buffered charcoal yeast extract (BCYE). Nutrients such as amino acids, vitamins, and iron are included in the medium while the charcoal removes potentially toxic materials.

Legionellosis actually constitutes two separate clinical entities: Legionnaires' disease and Pontiac fever. Legionnaires' disease is potentially the more serious of the two. The victim is initially infected through a respiratory route. In general, the source of the infection is an aerosol generated by contaminated water supplies such as those found in the cooling units of building air-conditioning systems. Rarely, if at all, does the disease pass from person to person. Most infections are unapparent, with either mild disease or none at all. The estimate is that less than 5 percent of exposed individuals actually contract Legionnaires' disease. Certain factors seem to increase the chances that the infection will progress toward pneumonia. Often, the lungs of the victim have suffered from previous trauma, such as that caused by emphysema or smoking. The person is generally, though not always, middle-aged or older. These observations suggest that, in most instances, the person's immune system is quite capable of handling the infection.

The disease begins with a dry cough, muscle aches, and rising fever—symptoms that resemble the flu. The person may also suffer from vomiting and diarrhea. In serious cases, the disease becomes progressively more severe over the next three to six days. The alveoli, or air sacs, of the lung become necrotized, increasing the difficulty in breathing. Small abscesses may also form in the lungs, as phagocytes infiltrate the area. The mortality rate has ranged from 15 to 60 percent in various outbreaks, although with early treatment, these numbers can be significantly lowered. Patients with other underlying lung problems, or who may be immunosuppressed, are at particular risk.

Pontiac fever is a much less serious form of disease. Named for the Michigan city in which a 1968 outbreak occurred in the Public Health Department building, the disease is self-limiting, nonpneumonic, and not life-threatening. Pontiac fever also seems to follow the inhalation of the etiological agent. Though the attack rate in exposed individuals appears to approach 100 percent, there is no infiltration of lung tissue and no abscess formation. A febrile period occurs one to two days following infection, with the individual progressing to recovery after several days. The difference between the two forms of disease remains obscure. There appears to be no obvious difference between the organisms associated with the two diseases, though strains associated with Pontiac fever may not replicate as readily inside human cells.

The mechanism by which infection by *Legionella* bacteria results in pneumonia is not altogether clear. Research into this area has centered on forms of virulence factors produced by the organism and their relationships to disease. Following their infiltration into the lung, *Legionella* bacteria are phagocytized by alveolar macrophages or other leukocytes (white blood cells). Unlike other ingested microbes, however, *Legionella* bacteria often survive the process and begin a process of intracellular replication. In this intracellular state, *Legionella* bacteria are shielded from many of the host's immune defenses.

Certain questions lend themselves to understanding this approach in elucidating the mechanisms of Le-

---

INFORMATION ON LEGIONNAIRES' DISEASE

CAUSES: Bacterial infection
SYMPTOMS: Dry cough, muscle aches, rising fever, possible vomiting and diarrhea
DURATION: Acute
TREATMENTS: Antibiotics (erythromycin, rifampin)

gionnaires' disease. First, are intracellular survival and multiplication necessary factors in the development of the disease? Second, if these factors are indeed relevant, exactly how does the organism manage to evade the killing mechanisms that exist inside the cell?

The first question has been dealt with by various animal studies. Guinea pigs were exposed to a *Legionella* aerosol, and lung aspirates were prepared after forty-eight hours. Large numbers of viable organisms were found inside alveolar macrophages. Few live *Legionella* bacteria, however, were observed outside cells. In addition, mutant *Legionella* bacteria that were incapable of intracellular growth showed reduced virulence in guinea pigs. Therefore, initial intracellular infection and multiplication does appear to be necessary to initiate the disease process.

The mechanism of intracellular survival is less clear. Macrophages are phagocytes that have a wide variety of means for killing ingested microorganisms. These mechanisms range from the production of reactive oxygen molecules to the synthesis of oxidizing agents such as peroxides. In addition, after a foreign microbe has been phagocytized within the membrane-bound vessel called a phagosome, a cell organelle, the lysosome, will fuse with the phagosome. Contained within the lysosome are large numbers of digestive enzymes that proceed to digest the target. Under normal circumstances, foreign microbes are ingested and digested, eliminating the threat of infection.

Somehow, *Legionella* bacteria evade these defense mechanisms. Different strains of *Legionella* bacteria appear to have evolved a variety of mechanisms for survival. In particular, there are two types of molecules, a phosphatase and a cytotoxin, whose presence is correlated with intracellular survival. Both appear to act by preventing the phagocytes from producing potentially lethal oxidation molecules such as hydrogen peroxide.

Another virulence factor that appears to be important for infectivity is a surface protein known as the macrophage infectivity potentiator, or MIP. The MIP proteins are apparently unique to *Legionella* bacteria; mutants that lack the MIP gene are significantly less virulent than wild-type strains. The MIP protein appears to be necessary for the internalization of *Legionella* bacteria by the macrophage, and for survival against the array of bacteriocidal activities.

A variety of other mechanisms may also exist that allow *Legionella* bacteria to escape the killing mechanisms of the macrophage. For example, in addition to the phosphatase, which removes phosphate molecules from host proteins or lipids, *Legionella* bacteria also produce protein kinases, which can add phosphate molecules to host cell proteins. In this manner, *Legionella* bacteria can potentially regulate the metabolism of the cells in which they find themselves by adding or subtracting phosphates from various sites or metabolic pathways.

Though a precise sequence of events that leads to the development of Legionnaires' disease remains to be worked out, certain steps appear to be necessary. Following the inhalation of a *Legionella* aerosol, probably from a contaminated water source, the organism lodges in the alveoli of the lung. Resident macrophages phagocytize the microbe, resulting in its internalization. Through a variety of virulence factors, *Legionella* survives, and multiplies within the macrophage. Death of the host cells along with the concomitant infiltration of other white cells results in the inflammation and lung damage recognized as Legionnaires' disease.

Treatment and Therapy

Despite the hysteria associated with the Philadelphia outbreak of Legionnaires' disease and the difficulty associated with the initial isolation of the etiological agent, there is nothing particularly unusual about the organism. The *Legionella* bacterium is a small, thin microbe some 2 to 10 micrometers in length, about the size of most average bacteria. Because of its characteristic staining pattern, it is classified as a gram-negative organism. This results from the molecular nature of its cell wall, which has a high lipopolysaccharide (LPS) content.

Since legionellosis can resemble other forms of pneumonia, improper diagnosis can be a problem. Though the prognosis of the disease is generally favorable with early intervention, improper or delayed treatment can prove fatal. In general, legionellosis is suspected in a patient with a progressive pneumonia for which other organisms do not appear to be a factor.

Legionnaires' disease pneumonia may be diagnosed microbiologically in a number of ways. The simplest, most rapid, and least costly test is the urinary antigen. The test is available only for *L. pneumophila* serogroup 1, but this organism is responsible for 80 percent of pneumonia cases. The antigen is detectable in the urine three days after symptoms begin and persists for several weeks. Expectorated sputum or secretions obtained through bronchoscopy may be stained and cultured. A special stain to visualize the bacteria through the microscope, called direct fluorescent antibody

(DFA), is very specific but not very sensitive, because it requires large numbers of bacteria to be positive and such number are usually present only in the most severe cases. The definitive diagnostic method is culture using BCYE media. The bacteria grow slowly and colonies become visible only after three to five days of incubation. Lastly, blood (sera) may be collected as acute and convalescent specimens. A fourfold rise in the antibody titer is considered diagnostic. A single specimen of high titer (1:128 dilution or higher) is considered presumptive, but not definitive, evidence of infection. In the case of Pontiac fever, serologic testing is the usual method for diagnosis.

There are several aspects of the clinical significance of the gram-negative character of the organism, one of which is that this type of bacteria responds poorly to penicillin or penicillin derivatives. This serves to limit the type of antimicrobial therapy available for treatment of severe cases of legionellosis. Other antibiotics exist, of course, that exhibit antibacterial characteristics similar to those of penicillin—for example, the cephalosporins. And, indeed, penicillin derivatives have been used to treat at least some types of gram-negative infections. Legionellosis patients did not respond well, however, to treatment with any of these agents. It was subsequently found that the basis for the resistance by *Legionella* bacteria to these antibiotics lay in a type of extracellular enzyme produced by these bacteria—a beta-lactamase.

The lack of pharmacologic activity associated with the penicillins, the cephalosporins, and certain other antibiotics is thus easy to explain. The activity of these antibiotics is associated with the presence of a structure in the molecule called a beta-lactam ring. The beta-lactamase produced by the *Legionella* bacterium causes a break in the ring, rendering the antibiotic harmless to the microbe, and thus useless as a form of treatment. Such resistance has become increasingly common among bacteria, since the genes encoding the beta-lactamase are passed from organism to organism.

Fortunately, other antibiotics did prove to be useful in the treatment of legionellosis. To a certain extent, the determination of the antibiotics of choice was fortuitous. During the Philadelphia outbreak, the nature of the illness was unknown. The primary assumption was that an infectious agent was at fault, but determination of the nature of that agent lay months beyond the extent of the epidemic. Therefore, as would be true in the treatment of any illness of unknown origin, various treatments were carried out. Two antibiotics in particular proved to be useful: erythromycin and rifampin. Erythromycin, which specifically inhibits bacterial protein synthesis, has continued to be useful. Though long-term use can result in liver damage and some individuals are hypersensitive to the drug, the intravenous administration of erythromycin remains the treatment of choice for legionellosis. Rifampin is used on occasion in association with other methods of treatment, but the high frequency of bacterial resistance to the drug precludes its use as a treatment of first choice.

Since the virulent properties of the *Legionella* bacterium depend on its intracellular presence in the macrophage, those antimicrobial agents that exhibit intracellular penetration would be expected to be most effective. Erythromycin fits this requirement, as do a number of other antibiotics. Newer antibiotics with intracellular activity have replaced erythromycin and rifampin as first choices for treatment of Legionnaires' disease pneumonia. Azithromycin, a macrolide antibiotic similar to erythromycin, yields higher intracellular levels than erythromycin and has proven to be more effective. Alternative monotherapy can be employed using one of the new respiratory fluoroquinolones such as levofloxacin or moxifloxacin. The quinolones are used for those who have undergone transplantation, as they do not interfere with the immunosuppressive drugs used in these patients.

Other aspects of treatment center on maintaining the comfort of the individual. This may include the use of analgesics for relief of pain. Pontiac fever is a self-limiting disease and requires only such symptomatic therapy.

Prevention of the disease is obviously preferable to dealing with the sequelae of infection. Epidemiological studies have demonstrated that the *Legionella* bacterium is a common soil organism that is often found in bodies of water contaminated by soil. The organism has been found in lakes and pond water, and it can survive for long periods in unchlorinated tap water. In fact, contaminated water appears to have been the source of infection for most outbreaks of the illness. Problems have often been associated with cooling towers, evaporative condensers, and other water supplies found with air-conditioning units of buildings. Infectious aerosols may be generated from these units, allowing for a respiratory route of infection. Though the disease is thus spread in an airborne manner, there is no evidence that it can be passed from person to person.

The epidemiological evidence for the disease supports an airborne hypothesis. Most outbreaks have occurred in regions of soil disruption, such as that occurring during construction. Subsequent isolation of *Legionella* bacteria from the cooling towers confirmed such contamination. Though the air-conditioning unit of the Bellevue-Stratford Hotel in Philadelphia was replaced prior to isolation of the organism, the assumption is that the unit was contaminated. The outbreaks of the disease during the summer, when air-conditioning use has peaked, are consistent with the role of air-conditioning units in the spread of *Legionella* bacteria.

The method by which the *Legionella* bacterium survives in the environment has not been completely determined. The organism is somewhat resistant both to chlorine treatment and to heat as high as 65 degrees Celsius. It appears to grow best in the presence of biological factors secreted by other microflora in the environment; growth stimulation may also be enhanced by the presence of physical factors such as sediment, silicone, and rubber compounds. Its ability to survive, and indeed be transmitted, may also be related to its tendency to penetrate and multiply intracellularly within environmental protozoa or amoeba.

Prevention of disease transmission must take into account these problems. Contamination of water supplies must be minimized. The resistance of the *Legionella* bacterium to standard methods of decontamination has made the process more difficult, and methods of choice remain controversial. Chlorination at relatively high levels remains the preferred method, with subsequent treatment at lower concentrations over the long term. The disadvantages of this method include the cost of constant treatment and the eventual corrosion of the units. Continuous or intermittent heating of the water has also proved effective in decontamination.

PERSPECTIVE AND PROSPECTS

Prior to August, 1976, Legionnaires' disease was unknown. From July 21 to 24 of that year, however, the Pennsylvania branch of the American Legion held its annual convention at the Bellevue-Stratford Hotel in Philadelphia. Some 4,000 delegates and their families attended the festivities. Following the convention, as delegates returned to their homes, a mysterious illness began to appear among the attendees. A total of 149 conventioneers and 72 others became ill. Characterized by a severe respiratory infection that progressed into pneumonia, and high fever, the illness proved fatal to 34 of the victims.

By August, it became clear to the Pennsylvania Department of Health that an epidemic was at hand. The cause of the outbreak was not clear, and rumors began to circulate. At various times, the news media explained the outbreak as a Communist plot against former military men, a Central Intelligence Agency test gone awry, and even an infectious agent arriving from space. The truth was less dramatic. By the beginning of 1977, David Fraser, Joseph McDade, and their colleagues from the Centers for Disease Control isolated the etiological agent: a bacterium subsequently named *Legionella pneumophila*.

With the isolation and identification of the organism, it became possible to explain earlier outbreaks of unusual illness. For example, during July and August of 1965, an outbreak of pneumonia at a chronic-care facility at St. Elizabeth's Hospital in Washington, D.C., resulted in 81 cases and 14 deaths. An outbreak among personnel at the Oakland County Health Department in Pontiac, Michigan, during July and August of 1968 of a disease that was subsequently called Pontiac fever was also traced to the same organism. In this case, however, though 144 persons were affected, none died. In fact, illness associated with the *Legionella* bacterium has been traced as far back as 1947. The 1976 outbreak was not new; it was merely the first time that medical personnel were able to isolate the organism that caused the disease.

The precise prevalence of the *Legionella* bacterium remains murky, but it is clearly more common than was at first realized. Despite the public's fear of the disease, in most instances it probably remains a mild respiratory infection, resembling nothing worse than a bad cold. Most cases remain undetected. A study of hospitalized community-acquired pneumonia patients conducted in Ohio showed that about 3 percent of cases were caused by *Legionella*. Estimates have suggested that as many as 25,000 persons in the United States develop infection. Based on seroconversions—the production of anti-*Legionella* antibody in the sera of persons—it has been estimated that more than 20 percent of the population of Michigan has been exposed to the organism. There is no reason to doubt that the same situation exists in many other states. In addition to sporadic cases, outbreaks continue to occur around the world. The most recent large outbreak was in Toronto. A colonized air-conditioning cooling tower atop the Seven Oaks Home for the Aged caused illness in 127 residents and workers, and 20 of the residents died.

The basis for the difference in severity between Legionnaires' disease and Pontiac fever is also unclear. There is no obvious difference between the two diseases that accounts for the differences in virulence. It also remains to be seen whether *Legionella* bacteria are associated with other illnesses.

The final lesson of Legionnaires' disease is as subtle as its initial appearance. Humans exist in an environment replete with infectious agents. Despite the battery of modern methods of treatment for illness, there always remains the potential for new outbreaks of previously unknown disease.

—*Richard Adler, Ph.D.;*
updated by H. Bradford Hawley, M.D.

See also Antibiotics; Bacterial infections; Epidemics and pandemics; Epidemiology; Lungs; Pneumonia; Pulmonary diseases; Pulmonary medicine; Pulmonary medicine, pediatric; Respiration.

FOR FURTHER INFORMATION:

Brock, Thomas D., ed. *Microorganisms: From Smallpox to Lyme Disease.* New York: W. H. Freeman, 1990. A collection of readings from *Scientific American.* The book includes a collection of accounts of the history of major infectious diseases. Divided into sections dealing with medical histories, methods of prevention, and means of transmission.

Dowling, John N., Asish K. Saha, and Robert H. Glew. "Virulence Factors of the Family *Legionellaceae*." *Microbiological Reviews* 56 (March 1, 1992): 32. A thorough discussion of the roles played by various virulence factors related to intracellular survival of the bacterium. A review article for which basic knowledge of microbiology would be helpful. Nevertheless, the article contains a wealth of information on the subject.

Frank, Steven A. *Immunology and Evolution of Infectious Disease.* Princeton, N.J.: Princeton University Press, 2002. Blends research from molecular biology, immunology, pathogen biology, and population dynamics to discuss how and why parasites vary to escape recognition by the immune system, vaccine design, and the control of epidemics.

Gorbach, Sherwood L., John G. Bartlett, and Neil R. Blacklow, eds. *Infectious Diseases.* 3d ed. Philadelphia: W. B. Saunders, 2004. A thorough discussion of infectious diseases. Included is a brief history, an account of the mechanisms of disease and immunity, and a concise discussion of a broad range of infectious agents.

Hoebe, Christian J. P. A., and Jacob L. Kool. "Control of *Legionella* in Drinking-Water Systems." *The Lancet* 355, no. 9221 (June 17, 2000): 2093-2094. This article discusses the process of copper-silver ionization for the control of *Legionella.* This process has reduced *Legionella* counts when used simultaneously with continuous chlorine injection.

Kasper, Dennis L., et al., eds. *Harrison's Principles of Internal Medicine.* 16th ed. New York: McGraw-Hill, 2005. The standard textbook of internal medicine with an excellent chapter on Legionnaires' disease.

Ryan, Kenneth J., and C. George Ray, eds. *Sherris Medical Microbiology: An Introduction to Infectious Diseases.* 4th ed. New York: McGraw-Hill, 2004. A textbook dealing with major pathogenic organisms. The section on *Legionella* is a concise outline of what is known about the disease.

Springston, John. "*Legionella* Bacteria in Building Environments." *Occupational Hazards* 61, no. 8 (August, 1999): 51-56. *Legionella* bacteria tend to be unwanted occupants of the building environment. Their ability to contaminate domestic water systems, coupled with their potential to cause severe health complications, presents a very real concern to building owners and managers.

LEISHMANIASIS
DISEASE/DISORDER
ALSO KNOWN AS: Kala-azar
ANATOMY OR SYSTEM AFFECTED: Bones, immune system, lymphatic system, skin
SPECIALTIES AND RELATED FIELDS: Family medicine, public health
DEFINITION: A complex of diseases caused by protozoan parasites of the genus *Leishmania.*

CAUSES AND SYMPTOMS

Leishmaniasis, also known as kala-azar in its visceral form, is a parasitic disease that strikes nearly 2 million persons each year. At least 350 million persons, from eighty-eight subtropical and tropical countries around the world, are at risk of contracting the disease. Leishmaniasis has received more attention among United States' medical authorities because of the risk of contracting the disease faced by U.S. military personnel in Southwest Asia, including Iraq, and Central Asia, including Afghanistan. Leishmaniasis may be a contributor to the complex of illnesses called Gulf War syndrome reported from veterans of the first Persian Gulf War in 1991.

Leishmaniasis is caused by any of more than twenty species of the protozoan parasite *Leishmania.* They are

INFORMATION ON LEISHMANIASIS

CAUSES: Transmission of protozoa through sandflies
SYMPTOMS: Skin infection and ulcers; vomiting, fever, abdominal discomfort, diarrhea, weight loss, and cough in children; also fatigue, weakness, and appetite loss in adults; darkening, dry, and flaky skin; thinning hair; enlargement of spleen, liver, and lymph nodes
DURATION: Often chronic
TREATMENTS: Medications containing the mineral antimony (meglumine antimonite, stibogluconate) and sometimes amphotericin B, pentamidine, flagyl, and allopurinol; plastic surgery to correct disfigurement; removal of spleen

transmitted by the bites of sandflies, small bloodsucking insects in the subfamily Phlebotominae. The parasite may also be transmitted by blood transfusion, sharing of needles by intravenous drug abusers, and other modes not requiring the bite of a sandfly. Humans are one of many mammalian hosts of these parasites. Infection can cause skin disease, called cutaneous leishmaniasis. *Leishmania* can also affect the mucous membranes, frequently resulting in ulcers, or cause systemic disease called visceral leishmaniasis, which is often fatal. Infection in children is usually sudden, with symptoms including vomiting, fever, abdominal discomfort, diarrhea, weight loss, and cough. Adults suffer from similar symptoms, but they may be accompanied by nonspecific symptoms such as fatigue, weakness, and loss of appetite. The skin may become darker, dry, and flaky, and the hair may begin to thin. Other signs include an enlarged spleen, liver, and lymph nodes.

Diagnosis is based on demonstration of the organism in spleen pulp, lymph nodes, liver, or peripheral blood. Species of *Leishmania* cannot be differentiated morphologically. They are distinguished on the basis of the disease produced, the host and its immune response, and geographical distribution.

TREATMENT AND THERAPY

Compounds containing the mineral antimony are the principal medications used to treat leishmaniasis. These compounds include meglumine antimonite and sodium stibogluconate. When these drugs are ineffective, other antiprotozoan medications may be utilized, including amphotericin B, pentamidine, flagyl, and

allopurinol. With mucocutaneous leishmaniasis, plastic surgery may be needed to correct the disfigurement caused by destructive facial lesions. Removal of the spleen may be required in drug-resistant cases of visceral leishmaniasis. Relapse may occur and infection may persist despite treatment.

PERSPECTIVE AND PROSPECTS

Cases of infection by *Leishmania* have been reported on all the continents except Australia. In the Americas, *Leishmania* can be found from southern Mexico into the South American continent. The disease is widespread in the tropics. In the United States, cases have been reported in dogs, cats, and humans in Texas, Ohio, and Oklahoma.

The prognosis for leishmaniasis is quite variable and depends on the specific strain of infecting protozoan, as well as on the individual patient's immune system response to infection. Cure rates are high with antimony compounds. There are no preventive vaccines. Preventing sandfly bites is the most immediate form of protection. Insect repellent, appropriate clothing, screening of windows, and fine mesh netting will reduce exposure.

—Jason A. Hubbart, M.S.;
updated by David M. Lawrence
See also Bites and stings; Insect-borne diseases; Parasitic diseases; Protozoan diseases; Tropical medicine; Ulcers.

FOR FURTHER INFORMATION:

Chang, K.-P., and R. S. Bray, eds. *Leishmaniasis.* New York: Elsevier, 1985.

Hide, G., et al. *Trypanosomiasis and Leishmaniasis: Biology and Control.* Wallingford, Oxon, England: CAB International, 1997.

Lane, R. P. "Sandflies (Phlebotominae)." In *Medical Insects and Arachnids*, edited by Richard P. Lane and Roger W. Crosskey. New York: Chapman & Hall, 1993.

Raghunath, D., and R. Nayak, eds. *Trends and Research in Leishmaniasis: With Particular Reference to Kala Azar.* New York: Tata/McGraw-Hill, 2005.

Ryan, Kenneth J., and C. George Ray, eds. *Sherris Medical Microbiology: An Introduction to Infectious Diseases.* 4th ed. New York: McGraw-Hill, 2004.

Leprosy

Disease/disorder

Also known as: Hansen's disease

Anatomy or system affected: Immune system, nerves, nervous system, skin

Specialties and related fields: Bacteriology, epidemiology, immunology, internal medicine, public health

Definition: A bacterial infection that affects skin and nerves, causing symptoms ranging from mild numbness to gross disfiguration.

Key terms:

acid-fast: the ability of a bacterium to retain a pink stain in the presence of a mixture of acid and alcohol

antibody: a protein found in the blood and produced by the immune system in response to bodily contact with an antigen

antigen: a foreign substance (such as a bacterium, toxin, or virus) to which the body makes an immune response

Bacillus Calmette-Guérin (BCG): a vaccine for tuberculosis made from a harmless strain of *Mycobacterium bovis*

bacterium: microscopic single-celled organism that multiplies by simple division; bacteria are found everywhere; most are beneficial, but a few species cause disease

cellular immune response: the reaction of the body that produces active white blood cells that can destroy antigens associated with other body cells

humoral immune response: the reaction of the body that produces antibodies that can destroy antigens present in body fluids

hypersensitivity: an overreaction by the immune system to the presence of certain antigens; this overreaction often results in some damage to the person as well as the antigen

immune response: the working of the body's immune system to prevent or combat an infectious disease

Causes and Symptoms

Leprosy, also known as Hansen's disease, is caused by the bacterium *Mycobacterium leprae (M. leprae)*. Humans are the only natural host for this bacterium; it can be found only in leprosy victims. Most people who are exposed to this bacterium are unaffected by it; in the remainder, the bacterium grows inside skin and nerve cells, causing a wide range of symptoms that depend upon the person's immune response to the growth of the bacteria.

M. leprae is an obligate intracellular parasite, which means that it can grow only inside other cells. *M. leprae* has a unique waxy coating that helps to protect it while it is growing inside human skin and nerve cells. The bacterium grows very slowly, dividing once every twelve days, whereas the average bacterium will divide every twenty to sixty minutes. *M. leprae* grows best at temperatures slightly below body temperature (37 degrees Celsius). The leprosy bacterium is the only bacterium known to destroy peripheral nerve tissue (nerves that are not a part of the central nervous system) and will also destroy skin and mucous membranes. This bacterium is closely related to the bacterium that causes tuberculosis: *Mycobacterium tuberculosis.*

Leprosy is not very contagious. Several attempts to infect human volunteers with the bacteria have been unsuccessful. It is believed that acquiring leprosy from an infected person requires prolonged intimate contact with that person, such as living in the same house for a long time. Although the precise mode of transmission of *M. leprae* bacteria is unclear, it is highly probable that the bacteria are transferred from the nasal or respiratory secretions of the victim to the nasal passages or a skin wound of the recipient.

Once inside a person, *M. leprae* will grow and reproduce inside skin and nerve cells and destroy tissue. The exact mechanism of tissue destruction is not understood, but it probably results from a combination of nerve damage, massive accumulation of bacteria, and immunological reactions. Because the bacteria grow so slowly, the length of time from infection to appearance of the symptoms (the incubation period) is quite long. The average incubation period is two to seven years, but incubation can range from three months to forty years. Since the bacteria prefer temperatures slightly lower than normal body temperature, symptoms appear first in the cooler parts of the body, such as the hands, fingers, feet, face, nose, and earlobes. In severe cases, symptoms also appear in the eyes and the respiratory tract.

The symptoms associated with leprosy can range from very mild to quite severe, and the symptoms that a person gets depend heavily on that person's ability to mount a cellular immune response against the bacteria. In a normal infection, the human body is capable of defending itself through two processes of the immune system; the humoral immune response and the cellular immune response. The humoral response produces chemicals called antibodies that can attack and destroy infectious agents that are present in body fluids such as the blood. The cellular response produces white blood

INFORMATION ON LEPROSY

CAUSES: Bacterial infection
SYMPTOMS: Skin lesions, numbness, disfiguration
DURATION: Lifelong
TREATMENTS: Antibiotics

cells that can destroy infectious agents that are associated with cells. Since *M. leprae* hides and grows inside human cells, a cellular response is the only type of immune response that can be of any help in fighting the infection. The ability to generate a cellular immune response against *M. leprae* is dependent upon the genetic makeup and overall health of the victim, as well as the number of infecting bacteria and their ability to invade the body and cause disease. A quick and strong cellular response by a person infected with *M. leprae* will result in no symptoms or in the mild form of the disease: tuberculoid leprosy. A slow or weak cellular response by a person exposed to leprosy may result in the more severe form of the disease: lepromatous leprosy.

Only one in two hundred people exposed to leprosy will get some form of the disease. The earliest symptom is a slightly bleached, flat lesion several centimeters in diameter that is usually found on the upper body or on the arms or legs. About three-fourths of all patients with an early solitary lesion heal spontaneously; the rest progress to tuberculoid or lepromatous leprosy or to one of the many forms that fall between these two extremes.

Tuberculoid leprosy is characterized by flat skin lesions 5 to 20 centimeters in diameter. The lesions are lighter in color than the surrounding skin and are sometimes surrounded by nodules (lumps). The lesions contain only a few bacteria, and they, along with the surrounding tissue, are numb. These lesions are caused by a hypersensitive cellular immune response to the bacteria in the nerves and skin. In an attempt to destroy the bacteria, the immune system overreacts, and some of the surrounding nerve and skin tissue is damaged while the bacteria are being killed. This causes the areas of the skin to lose pigment as well as sensation. Often, tuberculoid leprosy patients can experience more extensive physical damage if the numbness around the lesions leads to accidental loss of digits, skin, and so forth. Leprosy victims may burn and cut themselves unknowingly, since they have no feeling in certain areas of their bodies.

In lepromatous leprosy, the bacteria grow unchecked because of the weak cellular immune response. Often, there are more than 100 million bacterial cells present per square centimeter of tissue. These bacteria cause the formation of tumorlike growths called lepromas as well as tissue destruction of the skin and mucous membranes. Also, the presence of so many bacteria causes large numbers of antibacterial antibodies to be produced, but these antibodies are of no benefit in fighting off the infection. Instead, they can contribute to the formation of lesions and tissue damage both internally and on the skin through a process called immune complex hypersensitivity. This is a process whereby the large number of antibodies bind to the large number of bacteria in the body and form immune complexes. These complexes can be deposited in various parts of the body and trigger a chemical reaction that destroys the surrounding tissue. The large number of bacteria puts pressure on the nerves and destroys nerve tissue, which causes loss of sensation and tissue death.

The initial symptoms of lepromatous leprosy are skin lesions that can be spread out or nodular and are found on the cooler parts of the body, such as the inside of the nose, the front part of the eye, the face, the earlobes, the hands, and the feet. Often, the victim loses all facial features because the nodules enlarge the face, and the eyebrows and nose deteriorate, giving the victim a characteristic lionlike appearance. Severe lepromatous leprosy erodes bones; thus, fingers and toes become needlelike, pits form in the skull, nasal bones are destroyed, and teeth fall out. Also, the limbs become twisted and the hands become clawed. The destruction of the nerves leads to the inability to move the hands or feet, deformity of the feet, and chronic ulceration of the limbs. In addition, as is the case with tuberculoid leprosy, destruction of the small peripheral nerves leads to self-inflicted trauma and secondary infection (infection by another bacterium or virus). As the disease progresses, the growth of bacteria in the respiratory tract causes larynx problems and difficult breathing. Deterioration of the optic nerve leads to blindness. Bacteria can invade the bloodstream and spread infection throughout the whole body except the central nervous system. Death associated with leprosy usually results from respiratory obstruction, kidney failure, or secondary infection.

TREATMENT AND THERAPY

A physician can tell whether a person has leprosy by looking for characteristic symptoms (light-colored and numb lesions, nodules, and so forth) and by determining whether the patient may have been exposed to someone with leprosy. In addition, samples of scrapings from skin lesions, nasal secretions, fluid from nodules, or other tissue secretions can be examined for the presence of *M. leprae*. Samples are treated with a procedure called the acid-fast technique. Because of *M. leprae*'s waxy coating, these bacteria retain a pink stain after being washed in an acid-alcohol mixture, whereas all other bacteria lose the pink stain. Therefore, pink, rod-shaped bacteria observed in samples treated with the acid-fast technique indicate the presence of *M. leprae*. It is easy to find the acid-fast *M. leprae* in lepromatous leprosy patients because they have so many bacteria in their lesions, but the bacteria are more difficult to find in the lesions of tuberculoid leprosy patients.

The lepromin test was originally developed to be used as a diagnostic tool for leprosy, in the same way that the tuberculin test is used as a diagnostic tool for tuberculosis. Lepromin, which is heat-killed *M. leprae* taken from nodules, is injected under the skin in the lepromin test. Two reactions are possible: an early reaction that appears twenty-four to forty-eight hours later and a late reaction that appears three to four weeks later. In both reactions, a hard red lump at the injection site indicates a positive lepromin test. This test is not specific for leprosy, however, because a person who has been exposed to *M. leprae*, *M. tuberculosis*, or the tuberculosis vaccine, Bacillus Calmette-Guérin (BCG), will show a positive early reaction. Even though this test is not useful as a diagnostic tool, it is useful in determining whether a patient has a strong or a weak cellular immune response to *M. leprae*. Tuberculoid leprosy patients show both the early and late reactions, while lepromatous leprosy patients show no reaction at all.

Leprosy can be treated with antibiotics. The antibiotic dapsone began to be used on a wide scale in the treatment of leprosy in 1950. Since that time, however, many dapsone-resistant strains of *M. leprae* have appeared. This means that, for some victims, this drug is no longer helpful in fighting the disease. In 1981, in response to the problem of dapsone-resistant strains, the World Health Organization (WHO) rec-

ommended a multidrug regimen for leprosy victims. For lepromatous leprosy patients, dapsone, rifampin, and clofazimine are recommended, whereas tuberculoid leprosy patients need take only dapsone and rifampin. For patients who are intolerant of one or more of the standard antibiotics or who suffer from infections unresponsive to these medications, doxycycline and moxifloxacin are additional antibiotics that have been found to be effective. Treatment is expected to continue until skin smears are free from acid-fast bacteria, which can last from two years up to the lifetime of the patient. Since 1989, the U.S. recommendations for tuberculoid leprosy are six months of rifampin and dapsone daily, then dapsone alone for three years. For lepromatous leprosy, the recommendation is to use rifampin and dapsone daily for three years, then dapsone only for the rest of the person's life.

Often, antibiotics are given to family members of leprosy patients to prevent them from contracting the disease. Antibiotic therapy can make a leprosy victim noncontagious, stop the progress of the disease, and in some cases cause a reversal of some of the symptoms.

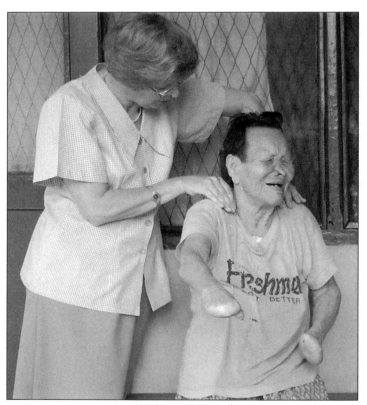

A man with leprosy receives a massage from a health care worker at a rehabilitation center in Thailand. (AP/Wide World Photos)

Until treatment is complete, however, it is recommended that patients sleep in separate bedrooms, use their own linens and utensils, and not live in a house with children. Thus, leprosy victims can lead nearly normal lives without fear of infecting others in the community.

The best ways to keep from getting leprosy are to avoid exposure to leprosy bacteria and to receive antibiotic therapy following exposure. It should be possible to control and, eventually, eliminate leprosy. If every case of leprosy were treated, the disease could not spread and the bacteria would die out with the last leprosy victim. Progress in this direction is slow, however, because of ignorance, superstition, poverty, and overpopulation in areas with many leprosy cases. The first strategy in controlling leprosy is to treat all leprosy cases with antibiotics. As of 1991, about 50 percent of all leprosy victims were not receiving drug therapy. Second, the early detection and rigid isolation of lepromatous leprosy patients are important, as is preventive antibiotic therapy for individuals in close contact with those patients. Finally, even in the early twenty-first century, too many countries lack adequate basic health resources, and too many patients disabled by leprosy are not receiving adequate care. The development of a vaccine for leprosy would aid control efforts.

A global effort for the production of a vaccine for leprosy is being made under the auspices of WHO. The first problem with vaccine development is that, until recently, it was not possible to grow *M. leprae* bacteria outside a leprosy victim; therefore, not much is known about the nature of the bacteria. Even though this bacterium was the first to be associated with a disease, it cannot be grown on an artificial laboratory medium, whereas nearly all other bacteria known can be grown artificially. It was not until 1960 that scientists at the Centers for Disease Control (CDC) discovered that the bacterium could be grown in the footpads of mice. Finally, in 1969, scientists at the National Hansen's Disease Center in Carville, Louisiana, found that the bacteria would grow in the tissues of the nine-banded armadillo. Several potential vaccines for leprosy have been tested since that time. One vaccine being tested is BCG, a live bacterial vaccine of the bacteria *Mycobacterium bovis*, which is a close relative of *M. leprae*. In four major trials with BCG, a range of 20 to 80 percent protection from leprosy was obtained. It is not known why there was such a wide variation in results. Recent strategies for vaccine development include making a modified BCG that contains *M. leprae* cell wall antigens. It is more advantageous to use BCG than *M. leprae* in a vaccine because BCG is much easier to grow. In addition, scientists are trying to find a way to grow *M. leprae* artificially so that larger quantities will be available to be used for a vaccine. In 1999, WHO set up a strategic plan titled "The Final Push Toward Leprosy Elimination: 2000-2005" and the Global Alliance for the Elimination of Leprosy was launched.

PERSPECTIVE AND PROSPECTS

Leprosy is one of the oldest known diseases. References to leprosy are contained in Indian writings that are more than three thousand years old. The Bible refers to leprosy and the isolation of lepers, although the term refers to other skin diseases as well. The examination of ancient skeletons has provided insights into how leprosy spread in past centuries. Early evidence suggests that the disease was highly contagious and that leprosy was widespread in Europe during the Middle Ages. Leprosy was so prevalent, in fact, that both governments and churches moved to deal with the problem. At that time, the cause of leprosy was unknown, and the disease was generally believed to be a punishment for some personal sin. Lepers were treated as outcasts and required to shout "unclean." They were required to wear gloves and distinctive clothes and carry a bell or clapper to warn people of their approach. They were forbidden to drink from public fountains, speak loudly, eat with healthy people, or attend church. Some lepers were even pronounced legally dead, burned at the stake, or buried alive. Later, they were isolated in asylums called leprosaria, and at one time about nineteen thousand leprosaria existed—mostly in France.

There was a sharp decrease in the number of leprosy cases in the sixteenth century. Several factors may have contributed to this decline, including the isolation of lepers, a better diet, warmer clothes, the plague epidemic, and the increase in tuberculosis, which may have provided resistance to leprosy. Leprosy is no longer as deadly or contagious as it once was, yet the stigma attached to this disease has remained. In an effort to alleviate the social stigma, the Fifth International Congress on Leprosy in 1948 banned the use of the word "leper" and encouraged the use of the term "Hansen's disease" instead of leprosy. *M. leprae*, the causative agent of leprosy, was first identified in the tissues of leprosy patients by the Norwegian physician Gerhard Armauer Hansen in 1873—hence the alternate name, Hansen's disease. Today, victims of leprosy are referred to as Hansenites or Hansenotic.

From the 1960's to the 1980's, estimates of the number of cases of leprosy worldwide ranged from 10 to 12 million. In 2001, at the Fifty-fourth World Health Assembly, it was announced that the global prevalence of leprosy had fallen to below 1 case per 10,000 by the end of 2000 and health experts believed that eliminating leprosy in all countries was an attainable goal by the year 2005. More than 600,000 new cases of leprosy were reported globally in 2002. A new combination of drugs known as multidrug therapy has been used to treat and completely cure patients. The drugs are donated free through foundations, and since these donations began in 2000, millions of the "blister packs," each of which provides one month's treatment to one patient, have been shipped. By 2008, some countries had achieved elimination, but leprosy remained endemic in others.

Leprosy is prevalent in tropical areas such as Africa, Southeast Asia, and South America. In the United States, most cases occur in Hawaii and small parts of Texas, California, Louisiana, and Florida. The number of new cases in the United States annually—mostly from foreign-born immigrants from leprosy-prone areas—has been very low in the last several decades.

—*Vicki J. Isola, Ph.D.*

See also Antibiotics; Bacterial infections; Immune system; Immunology; Necrosis; Nervous system; Numbness and tingling; Thalidomide; Tropical medicine; Tuberculosis; World Health Organization.

For Further Information:

Biddle, Wayne. *A Field Guide to Germs*. 2d ed. New York: Anchor Books, 2002. This comprehensive book is easily accessible to the nonspecialist and includes a discussion of nearly every virus, bacterium, and fungus known to cause human and nonhuman animal disease. Includes the history of the microbe and the treatment of diseases.

Bloom, B. R. "Learning from Leprosy: A Perspective on Immunology and the Third World." *Journal of Immunology* 137 (July, 1986): i-x. This article discusses leprosy as a disease, the immune response to leprosy, possible leprosy vaccines, and the problems of administering vaccines in the developing world.

Donnelly, Karen J. *Leprosy (Hansen's Disease)*. New York: Rosen, 2002. Traces the history of leprosy and discusses current and future directions in research. Written especially for young adults.

Frank, Steven A. *Immunology and Evolution of Infectious Disease*. Princeton, N.J.: Princeton University Press, 2002. Blends research from molecular biology, immunology, pathogen biology, and population dynamics to discuss how and why parasites vary to escape recognition by the immune system, vaccine design, and the control of epidemics.

Hastings, Robert C., ed. *Leprosy*. 2d ed. New York: Churchill Livingstone, 1994. This book contains a series of articles describing all aspects of leprosy, from the characteristics of the organism to the disease process to treatment.

Joklik, Wolfgang K., et al., eds. *Zinsser Microbiology*. 20th ed. Norwalk, Conn.: Appleton and Lange, 1997. An excellent textbook describing all infectious diseases. The information presented is thorough and logical, and it is supplemented by interesting diagrams, photographs, and charts. Discusses all diseases caused by species of mycobacteria, including leprosy and tuberculosis.

Mandell, Gerald L., John E. Bennett, and Raphael Dolin, eds. *Mandell, Douglas, and Bennett's Principles and Practice of Infectious Diseases*. 7th ed. New York: Churchill Livingstone/Elsevier, 2010. Describes leprosy, discussing the organism, epidemiology, symptoms, complications, and diagnosis; an expanded section on therapy is included.

Sehgal, Alfica. *Leprosy*. Philadelphia: Chelsea House, 2006. A book intended for young adults. Includes a historical overview and a scientific description.

Weedon, David. *Skin Pathology*. 3d ed. New York: Churchill Livingstone/Elsevier, 2010. Text with extensive photographs, covering tissue reaction patterns; the epidermis, dermis and subcutis; the skin in systemic and miscellaneous diseases; infections and infestations; and tumors, among other topics.

Leptin

Biology

Anatomy or system affected: All

Specialties and related fields: Biochemistry, cardiology, endocrinology, genetics, gynecology, nutrition

Definition: A protein hormone involved in regulation of food intake and obesity, with secondary effects on immunity, reproduction, and heart disease.

Structure and Functions

Leptin (from the Greek *leptos*, meaning "thin") is a protein hormone with important effects in regulating body weight, metabolism, and reproductive function. It is the product of the obese (*ob*) gene occurring on chromosome 7 in the human. Leptin is produced primarily by adipocytes (white fat cells). It is also produced by cells of the epithelium of the stomach and in the placenta. It appears that as adipocytes increase in size because of accumulation of triglycerides (fat molecules), they synthesize more and more leptin. However, the mechanism by which leptin production is controlled is largely unknown. It is likely that a number of hormones modulate leptin output, including corticosteroids and insulin.

Disorders and Diseases

At first leptin was assumed to be simply a signaling molecule involved in limiting food intake and increasing energy expenditure. Studies published as early as 1994 showed a remarkable difference in weight gain in mice deficient in leptin (mice with a nonfunctional ob gene). Daily injections of leptin into these animals resulted in a reduction of food intake within a few days and a 50 percent decrease in body weight within a month.

More recent studies in the human have not been as promising. It appears that leptin's effects on body weight are mediated through effects on hypothalamic (brain) centers that control feeding behavior and hunger, body temperature, and energy expenditure. If leptin levels are low, appetite is stimulated and use of energy limited. If leptin levels are high, appetite is reduced and energy use stimulated. The most likely target of leptin in the hypothalamus is inhibition of neuropeptide Y, a potent stimulator of food intake. However, this inhibition alone could not account for the effects seen, and studies looking at other hormones are under way.

Leptin also affects reproductive function in humans. It has long been known that very low body fat in human females is associated with cessation of menstrual cycles, and the onset of puberty is known to correlate with body composition (fat levels) as well as age. Several studies have suggested that leptin stimulates hypothalamic output of gonadotropin-releasing hormone, which in turn causes increases of luteinizing and follicle-stimulating hormones from the anterior pituitary gland. These hormones stimulate the onset of puberty. Prepubertal mice treated with leptin become thin and reach reproductive maturity earlier than control mice. One report has also indicated that humans with mutations in the ob gene that prevent them from producing leptin not only become obese but also fail to achieve puberty.

Leptin has been identified in placental tissues; newborn babies show higher levels than those found in their mothers. Leptin has also been found in human breast milk. Together, these findings suggest that leptin aids in intrauterine and neonatal growth and development, as well as in regulation of neonatal food intake.

Finally, leptin appears to have a role in immune system function. Studies have suggested a role for leptin in production of white blood cells and in the control of macrophage function. Mice that lack leptin have depressed immune systems, but the mechanisms for this remain unclear.

Perspective and Prospects

Although early reports claimed that leptin could be useful in treating human obesity, clinical reports to date have not looked promising. It appears that deficiencies in leptin production are a rare cause of human obesity. However, since most obese individuals have plenty of leptin available, additional leptin will have no effect. In those individuals with a genetic deficiency of leptin, clinical use would require either daily injections of leptin or gene therapy. At this point neither of these options looks particularly promising.

—*Kerry L. Cheesman, Ph.D.*

See also Appetite loss; Endocrinology; Endocrinology, pediatric; Hormones; Immune system; Obesity; Obesity, childhood; Puberty and adolescence; Reproductive system; Weight loss and gain.

For Further Information:

Barinaga, Marcia. "Obesity: Leptin Receptor Weighs In." *Science* 271 (January 5, 1996): 29. This article presents a summary of leptin receptor research accessible to the nonspecialist, as well as prospects for obesity drug research.

Castracane, V. Daniel, and Michael C. Henson, eds. *Leptin*. New York: Springer, 2006. Describes the discovery, history, roles, and regulation of leptin in all the major areas of physiology.

Goodman, H. Maurice. *Basic Medical Endocrinology*. 4th ed. Boston: Academic Press/Elsevier, 2009. Focuses on research advances in the understanding of hormones involved in regulating most aspects of bodily functions. Includes in-depth coverage of individual glands and regulatory principles.

Henry, Helen L., and Anthony W. Norman, eds. *Encyclopedia of Hormones*. 3 vols. San Diego, Calif.: Academic Press, 2003. A comprehensive overview of the role of hormones, the major physiological systems in which they operate, and the biological consequences of an excess or deficiency of a particular hormone.

Holt, Richard I. G., and Neil A. Hanley. *Essential Endocrinology and Diabetes.* 5th ed. Malden, Mass.: Blackwell, 2007. This text addresses the field of endocrinology, describing the physiology of the endocrine glands and the hormones that they produce. Includes an index.

Rink, Timothy J. "In Search of a Satiety Factor." *Nature* 372 (December 1, 1994): 372-373. A history of the research into weight regulation and how leptin supports prior theories is presented in a general news format. References are provided for further reading.

LESIONS

DISEASE/DISORDER

ANATOMY OR SYSTEM AFFECTED: All

SPECIALTIES AND RELATED FIELDS: Cardiology, dermatology, gastroenterology, general surgery, gynecology, internal medicine, nephrology, neurology, oncology, ophthalmology, otorhinolaryngology, podiatry, pulmonary medicine, urology, vascular medicine

DEFINITION: Any tissue damaged by injury or disease.

CAUSES AND SYMPTOMS

"Lesion" is the general term describing any damage to tissue. It results from some insult to the body and may take many forms: physical injury from an accident; intentional surgical incisions to treat a disorder; bacterial, parasitic, or viral disease, such as ringworm or syphilis; stomach ulcers caused by excess acid production; an autoimmune reaction, such as arthritis; heart muscle damage during a heart attack; malformations in the circulatory system; or brain tissue harmed by a stroke.

Because of this great variety, lesions are often classified by location and by whether they develop on their own (primary) or are related to another lesion (secondary). Primary skin lesions, for example, include cuts and scrapes, pustules, birthmarks, hives, and cancers—anything that changes the color and texture of the skin. Secondary lesions include such things as scabs,

---

INFORMATION ON LESIONS

CAUSES: Disease, physical trauma, cancer, autoimmune action, genetic abnormality
SYMPTOMS: Pain, reduced function
DURATION: Various
TREATMENTS: Medication, surgery

---

scratches from itching hives, or scars from removing or picking at a primary lesion. Most of these examples are benign, or at least more annoying than harmful. Skin cancers, on the other hand, can be deadly if left untreated.

Likewise, internal lesions vary from benign to deadly. Ulcers of the stomach or duodenum may heal on their own, but some worsen and can penetrate the bowel wall, leaking digestive fluid into the body cavity. In addition to cancerous lesions, some types are progressively dangerous, such as the scarring left by tuberculosis or the plaques of multiple sclerosis. Yet others require immediate medical attention, such as an aneurysm in the brain or a puncture of a lung.

TREATMENT AND THERAPY

Therapy depends on the type of lesion. Topical ointments or creams, such a cortisol cream, soothe the effects of many skin lesions. Lesions caused by a specific disease clear up with the appropriate medication for the disease. Likewise, medications can clear up some internal lesions, such as the antacids or H_2-receptor antagonists that reduce stomach acid production in an attempt to treat gastric ulcers.

Surgery, heat therapy, ultrasound, cautery, chemotherapy, radiation, and laser surgery are used to remove lesions or destroy damaged tissue. Classic examples include removal of a polyp in the colon with a cauterizing snare, radiation to destroy cancer cells and shrink a tumor, surgery to cut out a melanoma, and the suturing of a wound.

—*Roger Smith, Ph.D.*

See also Aneurysms; Birthmarks; Cancer; Dermatology; Dermatopathology; Disease; Electrocauterization; Grafts and grafting; Heart attack; Hives; Melanoma; Multiple sclerosis; Plastic surgery; Skin; Skin cancer; Skin disorders; Skin lesion removal; Strokes; Tuberculosis; Ulcers; Wounds.

FOR FURTHER INFORMATION:

Anderson, Robin L. *Sources in the History of Medicine: The Impact of Disease and Trauma.* Upper Saddle River, N.J.: Pearson/Prentice Hall, 2006.

Beers, Mark H. *The Merck Manual of Medical Information.* New York: Pocket Books, 2003.

Feliciano, David, Kenneth Mattox, and Ernest Moore. *Trauma.* 6th ed. New York: McGraw-Hill Medical, 2008.

Sompayrac, Lauren. *How Cancer Works.* Sudbury, Mass.: Jones and Bartlett, 2004.

LEUKEMIA

DISEASE/DISORDER

ANATOMY OR SYSTEM AFFECTED: Blood

SPECIALTIES AND RELATED FIELDS: Hematology, internal medicine, serology, toxicology

DEFINITION: A family of cancers that affect the blood, characterized by an increase in the number of white blood cells.

KEY TERMS:

blast cell: an immature dividing cell

bone marrow: the tissue within bones that produces blood cells; in children, all bones have active marrow, but in adults, blood cell production occurs only in the trunk

bone marrow transplant: the removal of bone marrow from an immunologically matched individual for infusion into a patient whose bone marrow has been destroyed

chemotherapy: the use of drugs to kill rapidly growing cancer cells; this treatment will also kill some normal cells, producing undesirable side effects

granulocytes: white blood cells that generally help to fight bacterial infection; these cells are capable of passing from the blood capillaries into damaged tissues

hematopoiesis: the process by which blood cells develop in the bone marrow; this maturation is regulated by specific molecules called growth factors

immune system: the cells and organs of the body that fight infection; destruction of these cells leaves the body vulnerable to numerous diseases

lymphocytes: white blood cells that specifically target a foreign organism for destruction; the two classes of lymphocytes are B cells, which produce antibodies, and T cells, which kill infected cells

oncogenes: genes found in every cell that are capable of causing cancer if activated or mutated

CAUSES AND SYMPTOMS

The blood is essential for all the physiological processes of the body. It is composed of red cells called erythrocytes, white cells called leukocytes, and platelets, each of which has distinct functions. Erythrocytes, which contain hemoglobin, are essential for the transport of oxygen from the lungs to all the cells and organs of the body. Leukocytes are important for protecting the body against infection by bacteria, viruses, and other parasites. Platelets play a role in the formation of blood clots; therefore, these cells are critical in the process of wound healing. Blood cell development, or

---

INFORMATION ON LEUKEMIA

CAUSES: Unclear; possibly environmental and genetic factors

SYMPTOMS: Mild cold symptoms; fever; enlargement of lymph nodes, spleen, and liver; fatigue; paleness; weight loss; repeated infections; increased susceptibility to bleeding and bruising

DURATION: Acute or chronic with recurrent episodes

TREATMENTS: Chemotherapy, bone marrow transplantation

---

hematopoiesis, begins in the bone marrow with immature stem cells that can produce all three types of blood cells. Under the influence of special molecules called growth factors, these stem cells divide rapidly and form blast cells that become one of the three blood cell types. After several further divisions, these blast cells ultimately mature into fully functional erythrocytes, leukocytes, and platelets. In a healthy individual, the number of each type of blood cell remains relatively constant. Thus, the rate of new cell production is approximately equivalent to the rate of old cell destruction and removal.

Mature leukocytes are the key players in defending the body against infection. There are three types of leukocytes: monocytes, granulocytes, and lymphocytes. In leukemia, leukocytes multiply at an increased rate, resulting in an abnormally high number of white cells, a significant proportion of which are immature cells. All forms of leukemia are characterized by this abnormally regulated growth; therefore, leukemia is a cancer, even though tumor masses do not form. The cancerous cells live longer than the normal leukocytes and accumulate first in the bone marrow and then in the blood. Since these abnormal cells crowd the bone marrow, normal hematopoiesis cannot be maintained in a person with leukemia. The patient will usually become weak as a result of the lack of oxygen-carrying red cells and susceptible to bleeding because of a lack of platelets. The abnormal leukocytes do not function effectively in defending the body against infection, and they prevent normal leukocytes from developing; therefore, the patient is immunologically compromised. In addition, once the abnormal cells accumulate in the blood, they may hinder the functioning of other organs, such as the liver, kidney, lungs, and spleen.

It has become clear that leukemia, which was first recognized in 1845, is actually a pathology that comprises more than one disease. Leukemia has been divided into four main types, based on the type of leukocyte that is affected and the maturity of the leukocytes observed in the blood and the bone marrow. Both lymphocytes and granulocytes can be affected. When the cells are mainly immature blasts, the leukemia is termed acute, and when the cells are mostly mature, the leukemia is termed chronic. Therefore, the four types of leukemia are acute lymphocytic (ALL), acute granulocytic (AGL), chronic lymphocytic (CLL), and chronic granulocytic (CGL). The granulocytic leukemias are also known as myologenous leukemias (AML, CML) or nonlymphoid leukemias (ANLL, CNLL). These are the main types of leukemia, although there are additional rarer forms. These four forms of leukemia account for 5 percent of the cancer cases in the United States. The incidence of acute and chronic forms is approximately equivalent, but specific forms are more common at different stages of life. The major form in children is ALL; after puberty, there is a higher incidence of AGL. The chronic forms of leukemia occur in the adult population after the fourth or fifth decade of life, and men are twice as likely to be affected as women.

The causes of leukemia are still not completely understood, but scientists have put together many pieces of the puzzle. It is known that several environmental factors increase the risk of developing leukemia. Among these are exposure to radiation, chemicals such as chloramphenicol and benzene, and possibly viruses. In addition, there is a significant genetic component to this disease. Siblings of patients with leukemia have a higher risk of developing the disease, and chromosomal changes have been found in the cells of most patients, although they disappear when the patient is in remission. For example, the genetic basis of certain forms of CML is an exchange of information (translocation) between chromosome 22 and chromosome 9; the shortened chromosome 22 is referred to as the Philadelphia chromosome. These different "causes" can be linked by understanding how oncogenes function. Every person, as part of his or her genetic makeup, has several oncogenes that are capable of causing cancer. In the healthy person, these oncogenes function in a carefully regulated manner to control cell growth. After exposure to an environmental or genetic influence that causes chromosome abnormalities, however, these oncogenes may become activated or deregulated so that

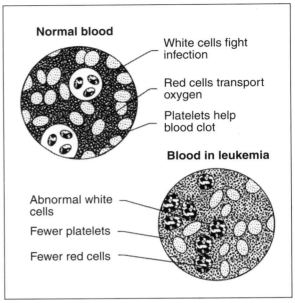

Leukemia is characterized by a high number of white blood cells and a reduced number of red blood cells and platelets; also, abnormal cells may be visible.

uncontrolled cell growth occurs, resulting in the abnormally high number of cells seen in leukemia. The translocation associated with the Philadelphia chromosome results in abnormal expression of an oncogene encoding an enzyme that regulates cell division.

Leukemia is often difficult to diagnose in the early stages because the symptoms are similar to more common or less serious diseases. "Flulike" symptoms, sometimes accompanied by fever, may be the earliest evidence of acute leukemia; in children, the first symptoms may be less pronounced. The symptoms quickly become more pronounced as white cells accumulate in the lymph nodes, spleen, and liver, causing these organs to become enlarged. Fatigue, paleness, weight loss, repeated infections, and an increased susceptibility to bleeding and bruising are associated with leukemia. As the disease progresses, the fatigue and bleeding increase, various skin disorders develop, and the joints become painfully swollen. If untreated, the afflicted individual will die within a few months. Chronic leukemia has a more gradual progression and may be present for years before symptoms develop. When symptoms are present, they may be vague feelings of fatigue, fever, or loss of energy. There may be enlarged lymph nodes in the neck and armpits and a feeling of fullness in the abdomen because of an increase in the size of the spleen as much as tenfold. Loss of appetite and sweating at night may be initial symptoms. Often, chronic leukemia eventually leads to a syndrome resembling acute leukemia, which is ultimately fatal.

If these symptoms are present, a doctor will diagnose the presence of leukemia in two stages. First, blood will be drawn and a blood smear will be analyzed microscopically. This may indicate that there are fewer erythrocytes, leukocytes, and platelets than normal, and abnormal cells may be visible. A blood smear, however, may show only slight abnormalities, and the number of leukemic cells in the blood may not correspond to the extent of the disease in the bone marrow. This requires that the bone marrow itself be examined by means of a bone marrow biopsy. Bone marrow tissue can be obtained by inserting a needle into a bone such as the hip and aspirating a small sample of cells. This bone marrow biopsy, which is done under local anesthetic on an outpatient basis, is the definitive test for leukemia. Visual examination of the marrow usually reveals the presence of many abnormal cells, and this finding is often confirmed with biochemical and immunological tests. After a positive diagnosis, a doctor will also examine the cerebrospinal fluid to see if leukemic cells have invaded the central nervous system.

Treatment and Therapy

The treatment and life expectancy for leukemic patients varies significantly for each of the four types of leukemia. Treatment is designed to destroy all the abnormal cells and produce a complete remission, which is defined as the phase of recovery when the symptoms of the disease disappear and no abnormal cells can be observed in the blood or bone marrow. Unfortunately, a complete remission may be only temporary, since a small number of abnormal cells may still exist even though they are not observed under the microscope. These can, with time, multiply and repopulate the marrow, causing a relapse of the disease. With repeated relapses, the response to therapy becomes poorer and the durations of the remissions that follow become shorter. It is generally believed, however, that a remission that lasts five years in ALL, eight years in AGL, or twelve years in CGL may be permanent. Therefore, the goal of leukemia research is to develop ways to prolong remission.

By the time acute leukemia has been diagnosed, abnormal cells have often spread throughout the bone marrow and into several organs; therefore, surgery and radiation are usually not effective. Treatment programs include chemotherapy or bone marrow transplants or both.

Chemotherapy is usually divided into several phases. In the first, or induction, phase, combinations of drugs are given to destroy all detectable abnormal cells and therefore induce a clinical remission. Vincristine, methotrexate, 6-mercaptopurine, L-asparaginase, daunorubicin, prednisone, and cytosine arabinoside are among the drugs that are used. Combinations that selectively kill more leukemic cells than they do normal cells are available for the treatment of ALL; however, in AGL no selective agents are available, resulting in the destruction of equal numbers of diseased and healthy cells. An alternative strategy does not rely on destroying the abnormal cells but instead seeks to induce immature leukemic cells to develop further. Once the cells are mature, they will no longer divide and will eventually die in the same way that a normal leukocyte does. Drugs such as cytarabine and retinoic acid have been tested, but the results are inconclusive.

Although the induction phase achieves clinical remission in more than 80 percent of patients, a second phase, called consolidation therapy, is essential to prevent relapse. Different combinations of anticancer drugs are used to kill any remaining cancer cells that were resistant to the drugs in the induction phase. Once the patient is in remission, higher doses of chemotherapy can be tolerated, and sometimes additional intensive treatments are given to reduce further the number of leukemic cells so that they will be unable to repopulate the tissues. During these phases of treatment, patients must be hospitalized. The destruction of their normal leukocytes along with the leukemic cells makes them very susceptible to infection. Their low numbers of surviving erythrocytes and platelets increase the probability of internal bleeding, and transfusions are often necessary. The dosages of chemotherapeutic agents must be carefully calculated to kill as many leukemic cells as possible without destroying so many normal cells that they cannot repopulate the marrow. In general, children handle intensive chemotherapy better than adults.

Following the induction and consolidation phases, maintenance therapy is sometimes used. In ALL, maintenance therapy is given for two to three years; however, its benefit in other forms of leukemia is a matter of controversy.

A second form of therapy is sometimes indicated for patients who have not responded to chemotherapy or are likely to relapse. Bone marrow transplantation has been increasingly used in leukemic patients to replace diseased marrow with normally functioning stem cells. In this procedure, the patient is treated with intensive chemotherapy and whole-body irradiation to destroy all leukemic and normal cells. Then a small amount of marrow from a normal donor is infused. The donor can be the patient himself, if the marrow was removed during a previous remission, or an immunologically matched donor, who is usually a sibling. If a sibling is not available, it may be possible to find a matched donor from the National Marrow Donor Program, which has on file approximately 350,000 people who have consented to be donors. Marrow is removed from the donor, broken up into small pieces, and given to the patient intravenously. The stem cells from the transplanted marrow circulate in the blood, enter the bones, and multiply. The first signs that the transplant is functioning normally occur in two to four weeks as the numbers of circulating granulocytes and platelets in the patient's blood increase. Eventually, in a successful transplant, the bone marrow cavity will be repopulated with normal cells.

Bone marrow transplantation is a dangerous procedure that requires highly trained caregivers. During this process, the patient is completely vulnerable to infection, since there is no functional immune system. The patient is placed in an isolation unit with special food-handling procedures. There is little chance that the patient will reject the transplanted marrow, because the immune system of the patient is suppressed. A larger problem remains, however, because it is possible for immune cells that existed in the donor's marrow to reject the tissues and organs of the patient. This graft-versus-host disease (GVHD) affects between 50 and 70 percent of bone marrow transplant patients. Even though the donor is immunologically matched, the match is not perfect, and the recently transplanted cells regard the cells in their new host as a "foreign" threat. Twenty percent of the patients who develop GVHD will die; therefore, drugs such as cyclophosphamide and cyclosporine, which suppress the immune system, are usually given to minimize this response. GVHD is not a problem if the donor is the patient. Since the availability of matching bone marrow cells is exceeded by the need, recent studies have involved the testing of hematopoietic umbilical cord cells from unrelated donors. The incidence of relapse as well as GVHD was similar to that when using matched bone marrow cells, suggesting that cord blood cells have the potential to serve as an alternative to conventional transplants.

Aggressive chemotherapy and bone marrow transplantation have dramatically increased the number of long-lasting remissions. For those who survive the therapy, it appears that, in ALL, approximately 60 percent of children and 35 percent of adults may be cured of the leukemia. The outlook for permanent remission is 10 to 20 percent in AGL and 65 percent for CGL patients. Statistics for chronic lymphocytic leukemia have been difficult to predict, because individual cases that have been similarly treated have had very different outcomes. The average lifespan after a diagnosis of CLL is three to four years; however, some patients live longer than fifteen years.

Perspective and Prospects

As the number of deaths from infectious disease has decreased, cancer has become the second most common cause of disease-related death. It is estimated that one of three people in the United States will develop a form of cancer and that the disease will kill one of five people. The search for causes and treatments of various cancers is perhaps the most active area of biological research today. Multiple lines of experimentation are being pursued, and significant advances have been made.

Leukemia is one of the cancers that scientists understand fairly well, but many unanswered questions remain. Leukemia research can be divided into two broad approaches. In the first, the researcher seeks to modify and improve the current methods for treatment: chemotherapy and bone marrow transplantation. In the second, an effort is being made to understand more about the disease itself, with the hope that completely different strategies for treatment might present themselves.

The risks involved in current therapy for leukemia have been discussed in the previous section. Treatment schedules, individually designed for each patient, will add to the understanding of how other physiological characteristics affect treatment outcome. Significant advances in reducing the risk of GVHD are likely to come quickly. In marrow transplants in which the donor is the patient, research is in progress to improve ways to screen out abnormal cells, even if they are present at very low levels, before they are infused back into the patient. In addition, for transplants in which the donor is not the patient, techniques that remove the harmful components of the bone marrow are being developed. Bone marrow cells can be partially purified, resulting in an enriched population of stem cells. Administering these to the leukemic patient should greatly reduce the risk of GVHD. Since bone marrow can be stored easily, the day may come when healthy people will store a bone marrow stem cell sample in case they contract a disease that would require a transplant.

Basic research in leukemia focuses on a simple question, "Why are leukemic cells different from normal cells?" This question is asked from a variety of perspectives in the fields of immunology, cell biology, and genetics. Immunologists are looking for markers on the surfaces of leukemic cells that would distinguish them from their normal counterparts. If such markers are found, it should be possible to target leukemic cells for destruction by using monoclonal antibodies attached to drugs. These "smart drugs" would be able to home in on the diseased cells, leaving normal cells untouched or only slightly affected. This would be a great advance for leukemia treatment, since much of the risk for the leukemic patient following chemotherapy or bone marrow transplant involves susceptibility to infection because the normal immune cells have been destroyed. Similarly, it may be possible to "teach" the patient's immune system to destroy abnormal cells that it had previously ignored. Similar forms of immunotherapy have shown promise in treating forms of cancer such as melanoma.

Cell biologists are seeking to understand the normal hematopoietic process so that they can determine which steps of the process go awry in leukemia. Some of the growth factors involved in hematopoiesis have been identified, but it appears that the process is quite complex, and as yet scientists do not have a clear picture of normal hematopoiesis. When the understanding of the normal process becomes more complete, it may be possible to localize the defect in a leukemic patient and provide the missing growth factors. This might allow abnormal immature cells to complete the developmental process and relieve the symptoms of disease.

Geneticists are studying the chromosomal changes that underlie the onset of leukemia. As the oncogenes that are involved are identified, the reasons for their activation will also be determined. Once the effects of these genetic abnormalities are understood, it may be possible to intervene by genetically engineering stem cells so that they can develop normally.

These areas of research will likely converge to provide the leukemia treatments of the future. Leukemia is a cancer for which there is already a significant cure rate. It is not unreasonable to expect that this rate will approach 100 percent in the near future.

—Katherine B. Frederich, Ph.D.;
updated by Richard Adler, Ph.D.

See also Blood and blood disorders; Bone marrow transplantation; Cancer; Carcinogens; Chemotherapy; Malignancy and metastasis; Oncology; Radiation sickness; Stem cells.

FOR FURTHER INFORMATION:

Bellenir, Karen, ed. *Cancer Sourcebook: Basic Consumer Health Information About Major Forms and Stages of Cancer.* 5th ed. Detroit, Mich.: Omnigraphics, 2007. This well-written volume provides the reader with a background against which to understand leukemia. Describes each of the four main types of leukemia in a straightforward and practical manner.

Dollinger, Malin, et al. *Everyone's Guide to Cancer Therapy.* 5th ed. Kansas City, Mo.: Andrews McMeel, 2008. An excellent source of medical information about cancer, written for the general public. Describes various cancer sites in the body, and one essay focuses on sarcomas of the bone. Includes a helpful glossary of medical terminology.

Eyre, Harmon J., Dianne Partie Lange, and Lois B. Morris. *Informed Decisions: The Complete Book of Cancer Diagnosis, Treatment, and Recovery.* 2d ed. Atlanta: American Cancer Society, 2002. This text from the American Cancer Society is intended for the layperson. It is exemplary in its discussion of cancer.

Goldman, John, and Junia Melo. "Chronic Myeloid Leukemia: Advances in Biology and New Approaches to Treatment." *New England Journal of Medicine* 349, no. 15 (October 9, 2003): 1451-1464. Review of the causes and treatment for one form of leukemia, comparable to the research in general in that field.

Keene, Nancy. *Childhood Leukemia: A Guide for Families, Friends and Caregivers.* 4th ed. Sebastopol, Calif.: O'Reilly, 2010. Keene uses the story of her daughter's battle with leukemia as a vehicle to explore the physical and emotional impacts of the disease. Offers guidance on coping with procedures, hospitalizations, school, and associated social, emotional, and financial problems.

Kimball, Chad T. *Childhood Diseases and Disorders Sourcebook: Basic Consumer Health Information About Medical Problems Often Encountered in Preadolescent Children.* Detroit, Mich.: Omnigraphics, 2003. Offers basic facts about cancer, sickle cell disease, diabetes, and other chronic conditions in children and discusses frequently used diagnostic tests, surgeries, and medications. Long-term care for seriously ill children is also presented.

Leukemia and Lymphoma Society of America. http://www.leukemia.org. A group dedicated to funding blood cancer research, education, and patient services for patients with leukemia and other lymphatic diseases.

Rennie, Ed. *Beginning of the End of My Life*. Philadelphia: Xlibris, 2005. Diagnosed with leukemia, the author describes the impact on himself as well as his family. Presents the nature of his treatment.

Westcott, Patsy. *Living with Leukemia*. Austin, Tex.: Raintree-Steck-Vaughn, 1999. Designed for students in grades three through five, this book discusses the condition or disease through the stories of children experiencing it. Includes clear and easy-to-understand diagrams and full-color photographs.

LEUKODYSTROPHY

DISEASE/DISORDER

ANATOMY OR SYSTEM AFFECTED: Brain, ears, eyes, muscles, nerves

SPECIALTIES AND RELATED FIELDS: Biochemistry, family medicine, genetics, neurology, nutrition, occupational health, pediatrics, physical therapy

DEFINITION: A group of genetic disorders characterized by progressive deterioration of the white matter (myelin sheath) of the brain.

CAUSES AND SYMPTOMS

Leukodystrophy is caused by a breakdown in the enzyme systems that metabolize fats (lipids) in the nerve cells. As a result, the body can no longer break down very long chain fatty acids (VLCFA), which then accumulate. This causes the substance around nerve fibers, known as the myelin sheath, to degenerate. The myelin sheath protects and insulates the axons of nerve cells, allowing them to transmit impulses between the nerve cells in the brain and other parts of the body. Loss of the myelin sheath around nerve cells short-circuits nerve impulses. As a result, the victim can experience uncontrolled muscle stiffness, paralysis, speech difficulties, memory failures, personality changes, impaired reasoning, urinary incontinence, loss of vision, and loss of hearing. These symptoms may be difficult to recognize during the early stages of the disease. Leukodystrophy usually begins in the back of the brain, eventually spreading throughout the white matter of the cerebral hemispheres and often into the spinal cord. Leukodys-

---

INFORMATION ON LEUKODYSTROPHY

CAUSES: Enzyme defect resulting in degeneration of the myelin sheath

SYMPTOMS: Uncontrolled muscle stiffness, paralysis, speech difficulties, memory failures, personality changes, impaired reasoning, urinary incontinence, vision loss, hearing loss

DURATION: Lifelong

TREATMENTS: Medications (Lorenzo's oil or Lovastatin), dietary supplements, exercise, and occupational and speech therapy

---

trophy is typically diagnosed with a blood test that is used to determine the amount of VLCFA in the body.

The myelin sheath is a complex chemical substance made from a variety of lipids. Different types of leukodystrophy affect one of the particular constituents of myelin. Specific leukodystrophies include adrenoleukodystrophy (ALD), metachromatic leukodystrophy (MLD), Zellweger's syndrome, and Alexander's disease. Having one type of leukodystrophy does not increase the risk of having another type.

TREATMENT AND THERAPY

The effects of leukodystrophy may be tempered through the use of various medications, dietary supplements, exercise programs, and occupational and speech therapies. For ALD, the most common form of leukodystrophy, Lorenzo's oil helps the body bring VLCFA levels back to normal. To be effective, Lorenzo's oil should be coupled with a very-low-fat diet. Lovastatin, an anticholesterol drug, does the same thing as Lorenzo's oil without the patient needing to be on a low-fat diet.

For some types of leukodystrophy, particularly MLD, bone marrow transplants have shown promise in slowing down the disease. Gene therapy is being investigated. The hope is to deliver genes to the patient that will stimulate the oligodendrocyte cells in the brain to produce myelin once again.

PERSPECTIVE AND PROSPECTS

Leukodystrophy is genetically inherited. Most types show up in early childhood, although there are some late childhood forms. Public awareness of the disease was greatly enhanced by the 1992 film *Lorenzo's Oil*, the true story of Augusto and Michaela Odone seeking a cure for ALD for their five-year-old son Lorenzo.

They founded the Myelin Project, a research effort that continues to seek ways for victims of leukodystrophy to produce myelin that will insulate their nerve cells.

—Alvin K. Benson, Ph.D.

See also Adrenoleukodystrophy; Brain; Brain damage; Brain disorders; Multiple sclerosis; Nervous system; Neuralgia, neuritis, and neuropathy; Neuroimaging; Neurology; Neurology, pediatric.

FOR FURTHER INFORMATION:

Icon Health. *Leukodystrophy: A Medical Dictionary, Bibliography, and Annotated Research Guide to Internet References*. San Diego, Calif.: Author, 2004.

Kimball, Chad T. *Childhood Diseases and Disorders Sourcebook: Basic Consumer Health Information About Medical Problems Often Encountered in Preadolescent Children*. Detroit, Mich.: Omnigraphics, 2003.

Lazzarini, Robert A. *Myelin Biology and Disorders*. San Diego, Calif.: Academic Press/Elsevier, 2004.

Salvati, S., ed. *A Multidisciplinary Approach to Myelin Diseases II*. New York: Plenum Press, 1994.

LICE, MITES, AND TICKS
DISEASE/DISORDER

ANATOMY OR SYSTEM AFFECTED: Ears, genitals, hair, skin

SPECIALTIES AND RELATED FIELDS: Dermatology, pediatrics, public health

DEFINITION: Parasites that live on the human body, causing severe itching, skin rashes, and sometimes more serious diseases.

KEY TERMS:

louse (pl. lice): a wingless insect that sucks blood and that can be involved in transmitting diseases

mite: a very small spider that is parasitic to humans and can carry disease

molt: to shed all or part of the skin or outer covering

parasite: an organism that lives off of another organism while contributing nothing to the survival of the host

tick: a wingless insect that sucks blood and can spread disease

CAUSES AND SYMPTOMS

Lice, mites, and ticks are parasites that live on human beings. Two species of lice survive on human blood: body lice and crab lice. Body lice are divided into two subspecies, the head louse (*Pediculus humanus capitis*) and the body louse (*Pediculus humanus corporis*). Head lice live on the scalp among the hairs of the head.

Body lice actually live in and on clothing. They move off clothes and attach themselves to human skin to feed on blood frequently during the day. It is very difficult to tell the difference between these types of lice. They are both flat, wingless, grayish in color, and very small. The body louse is about .08 to .16 inch long, slightly larger than the head louse, which measures only .04 to .08 inch. Body lice are a slightly lighter shade of gray than are head lice.

Both subspecies of body lice live by sucking blood from their victims. These insects of the order *Anoplura* have three pointed tubes on their bodies called stylets that can jab into the skin and draw out blood. When not in use, the stylets are tucked away in a pouch. Body lice begin their lives as eggs dropped into the folds of clothing by mature adult females. Head lice eggs are glued to the base of a strand of hair on top of the head. The eggs, called nits, are about one-fourth the size of a mature female. After about seven to ten days, the nits hatch into young nymphs. Because hair grows about 0.3 millimeter a day, the nits hatch about 3 millimeters away from the scalp. After the nymph emerges, it leaves behind an empty egg shell still tightly cemented to the hair. Nymphs begin sucking blood as soon as they hatch. Within nine days, the nymph molts three times before a full adult louse is formed. Adults then live about two weeks, with females laying about ten eggs every day.

Lice are passed from head to head only by direct contact. This usually happens at school, often on the playground or in the gym. Head lice have different effects on different people. Some experience only slight itching, while others are terribly irritated and develop a swollen and inflamed scalp. An itching scalp is the most obvious symptom of head lice. Nits are visible upon inspection of hair near the scalp. On girls, they are usually found behind the ears, while on boys, they are most likely to be found attached near the top of the head. Parents should be very careful in treating head

---

INFORMATION ON LICE, MITES, AND TICKS

CAUSES: Bites or exposure to diseases through parasites

SYMPTOMS: Severe itching, rashes, development of diseases

DURATION: Acute to chronic

TREATMENTS: Insecticidal shampoos, medications, lotions

lice; they too can be infected. Head lice can be the transmitters of several dangerous infectious diseases, such as epidemic typhus, relapsing fever, and trench fever.

Body lice are less often found on children than are head lice. They thrive in clothing and bodies that are unclean for long periods of time. Body lice are especially troublesome and numerous on homeless people, prisoners of war, and others living in dirty conditions. (Cleanliness, however, is not a factor with head lice; they can thrive in clean or dirty hair.) Body lice have helped spread a number of contagious diseases, the most deadly of which is typhus. This disease starts with flu-like symptoms, followed by a high fever and rash. During World War II, more than three million Russian prisoners of war died from louse-spread typhus. In recent years, however, typhus has been rare.

Crab lice (*Phthirus pubis*) are usually found living in pubic hair and are most likely to infect adults. Like all lice, they are very small, .083 inch in length when fully grown, but they cause great discomfort. As adults, they firmly grab pubic hair with their crablike legs (six per louse), insert their barbed tongue into the skin, and suck blood. The female lays its eggs about .08 inch from the skin. When the eggs hatch, the nymphs begin to feed and stop only while molting. Feeding causes intense itching and a rash. Rarely, but occasionally, the lice spread to the chest, eyebrows, or armpits. They can be passed on only by human carriers through direct contact. Crab lice cannot live on any other species except humans, and about 3 percent of people have them. Crab lice do not carry sexually transmitted diseases but are often associated with them.

Ticks are members of a blood-sucking family of insects called Ixodidae. Several different species suck blood from warm-blooded vertebrates, such as human beings, cows, and dogs. Common species in the United States and Canada include hard ticks and the American dog tick. Ticks have a hard, shieldlike plate on their backs called a scutum that makes them very difficult to crush. A female tick can swell up to the size of a pea when ingesting blood and can lay from four thousand to six thousand eggs within four to ten days.

The eggs hatch after about a month, and six-legged larvae, called seed ticks, emerge. A seed tick waits on

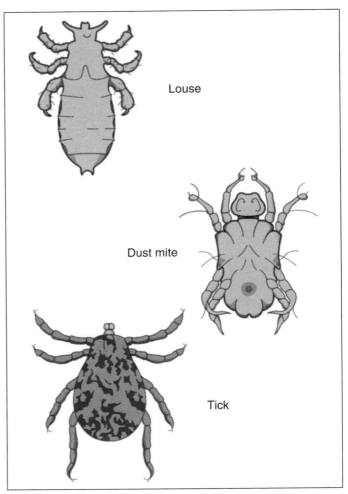

Magnified representations of a louse, a mite (normally microscopic), and a tick.

the tip of a leaf of grass or other low-growing plant until a suitable animal walks by. The seed tick grabs onto its meal and, after sucking enough blood, molts into its next stage, an eight-legged nymph called a yearling tick. It finds another host, sucks more blood, and then molts one more time into an adult. After another week of feeding, adults mate, the female produces its eggs, and the three-stage cycle begins all over again.

Ticks are very good survivors: Eight-legged nymphs can live more than a year without food, while adults can go without a meal of blood for more than two years. Ticks carry many dangerous diseases, including Rocky Mountain spotted fever, Colorado tick fever, tularemia, anaplasmosis, and Lyme disease.

Mites are actually related to spiders, rather than insects. Dust mites (*Dermatophagiodes pteronyssinus*), the chief living forms found in house dust, are among the most numerous inhabitants of human environments. One study of 150 houses in Holland found mites in every one of them. Dust mites measure about .01 inch in diameter. They have eight legs, like all spiders, and are closely related to ear mites found in dogs and cats and scab mites found in sheep. House dust mites spend all of their life stages, from birth to death, in dust. There can be as many as five hundred mites in every gram of house dust. This measures out to about fourteen thousand mites per ounce of dust. They survive by eating human skin that is shed daily, scabs that fall off, and dandruff, which is about 10 percent fat and which they digest with the help of a fungus also found in house dust. Dust mites are responsible for some allergies and asthma attacks. They can also invade the skin and cause allergic reactions such as dermatitis. Although dust mites cannot penetrate the surface of the skin, they can live in ulcers, fungal infections, scabs, and other skin openings.

The scabies mite (*Sarcoptes scabei*) does burrow into the skin in search of its preferred food, skin cells and intestinal fluids. Female scabies mites are about .016 inch long, while males are only about half as big. The female lays its eggs only a few hours after mating and can lay two to three eggs a day for up to four weeks. The eggs hatch after only three to four days. The larvae often move about on the skin surface until they find a suitable space, usually between the fingers or at the bend in the knee, elbow, or wrist. The underarms, breasts, and genitals can also be invaded by these travelers. Frequently, they travel all the way down to the ankles or between the toes. Sometimes it takes up to six weeks before the pests are noticed by the person acting as their host.

Children are especially sensitive to the feces and eggs of scabies mites, which can cause an agonizing itch that is particularly irritating at night. Scabies mites are most active in the fall and winter, but they are transmissible at any time. They can be spread by shaking hands, by touching the infected areas of another person, and even by having contact with the clothes or bedsheets of the infected individual. Scabies mites do not carry any major diseases, but they do cause a good deal of itching and discomfort.

TREATMENT AND THERAPY

Treatments for lice, mites, and ticks vary according to the type and severity of infestation. The only way to protect a child against head lice is through regular inspection of the head. The hair should be combed and brushed every night; this will injure the lice, which will not be able to survive. Treatment involves an insecticidal shampoo such as Proderm, which contains malathion, or Kwell, which contains lindane or gamma benzene hexachlorine. These shampoos kill both the lice and the nits. Removing lice by hand or crushing them is a difficult and usually impossible task. The force required to remove a nit from a hair is greater than most parents can provide. Crushing a louse requires direct pressure of about five hundred thousand times the weight of a louse. The crushed body of a louse can also cause infection. The best treatment for body lice is washing clothes and infected areas with soap. Soap and hot water usually kill body lice. If an infection of either head or body lice is discovered, all members of a family should be checked, and a doctor should be consulted. If a child has head lice, his or her school should always be notified. If crab lice are discovered, a physician should be contacted immediately. Pubic lice can be treated with insecticides such as pyrethrin pediculicide. Pyrethrins are available over the counter in drugstores. Stronger treatments require a prescription. Crab lice can be controlled by washing clothing and bedding and drying them in a very hot dryer.

Ticks are very difficult to remove from the body. A tick should not be pulled or yanked out because its head, filled with jagged teeth, can remain in the wound and cause an infection. Ticks have to be removed so that their mouthparts do not break off. Unattached ticks can be brushed off with a hand, but an attached tick should not be removed with bare fingers. To remove a tick, the hands should be covered with a tissue or gloves. Then, the tick is grabbed with a pair of tweezers as close to its head as possible. Gentle, steady pressure is applied until the tick comes out. The tick should not be twisted or crushed until it is fully out. Body fluids from the tick can carry Lyme disease organisms, which

VIRAL DISEASES SPREAD BY TICKS	
Disease	*Principal Vector*
Colorado tick fever	*Dermacentor andersoni*
Encephalitis, Far East Russian	*Ixodes persulcatus*
Louping ill	*Isodes ricinus*

can enter the body through broken skin. The safest way to kill the tick is to drown it in soapy water or crush it with the tweezers, avoiding contact with the hands. The site of the bite should be washed and checked carefully to see if any part of the head is still embedded. Anything that remains should be removed with tweezers, which will help prevent infection. If all parts cannot be removed, the spot should be rubbed with an antiseptic. A doctor should be consulted if the site becomes inflamed or filled with pus.

Scabies mites can be controlled by insecticidal lotions containing lindane or sulfur. The pesticide lindane is the one most commonly used for scabies mites, but it has been linked to cancer in some tests. Sulfur is preferred by most physicians because it is safer and more widely available. Sulfur requires three applications over three days, however, and frequently leaves stains on bedding and clothes. The fastest-acting miticide is permethrim. It usually requires only one application to be effective, but it is more toxic than sulfur. Scabies mites can be controlled by washing the clothing, bedding, and towels used by the infected person. If scabies mites are found, other people with whom the child has had contact should be told so that they can seek treatment, even though they might not have started to itch. Scabies mites cannot live long if detached from their hosts, usually no more than two to three days. Sealing infected clothes in a plastic bag for a week or so will also kill most of the mites.

Dust mites can be controlled by reducing their sources of food. This can be accomplished by covering mattresses in plastic, keeping pets away from beds and sleeping areas, reducing humidity in the house, and vacuuming once a week. Killing dust mites requires vacuuming with a water vacuum or one with special dust filters, washing sheets and pillowcases in hot soapy water, freezing or heating blankets, or using pesticides such as mosquito repellents containing diethyl-m-toluamide (DEET) or products containing boric acid.

PERSPECTIVE AND PROSPECTS

New chemicals have proven very effective in the treatment of diseases spread by lice, mites, and ticks. Louse-spread typhus, once responsible for millions of deaths, is no longer a great danger. Improved standards of cleanliness have done much to eliminate the problem of body lice in all but the poorest populations in the United States. Unfortunately, head lice cannot be controlled

BACTERIAL AND RICKETTSIAL DISEASES SPREAD BY LICE, MITES, AND TICKS

Disease	Disease Agent	Principal Vectors
Boutonneuse fever	*Rickettsia conori*	Ticks: *Rhipicephalus sanguineus, R. secundus*, and species of *Haemaphysalis, Hyalomma, Amblyomma, Boophilis, Dermacentor*, and *Ixodes*
Q fever	*Coxiella burneti*	Ixodid ticks
Relapsing fever	*Borrelia*	*Ornithodoros* ticks
Rickettsialpox	*Rickettsia akari*	Mite: *Liponyssoides sanguineus*
Rocky Mountain spotted fever	*Rickettsia rickettsi*	Ticks: *Dermacentor andersoni, D. variabilis, Amblyomma americanus, Haemaphysalis leporispalustris* (rabbit-to-rabbit transmission)
Trench fever	*Rickettsia quintana*	Human body louse *Pediculus humanus humanus*
Tularemia	*Francisella tularensis*	Deer flies and ticks
Typhus, louse-borne	*Rickettsia prowazekii*	Human body louse *Pediculus humanus humanus*
Typhus, murine	*Rickettsia mooseri*	The rat louse *Polyplax spinulosa* and the tropical rat mite *Ornthonssus bacoti* are zoonotic vectors
Typhus, scrub	*Rickettsia tsutsugamushi*	Mites: *Leptotrombidium akamushi* and *L. deliensis*

simply by keeping things clean, so they continue to cause itching and scratching when contracted even by the cleanest children. Lice, mites, and ticks will always be with humans, but the diseases that these parasites spread, with a few exceptions such as Rocky Mountain spotted fever and Lyme disease, are now much less deadly because of new medicines and drug treatments.

—*Leslie V. Tischauser, Ph.D.*

See also Allergies; Asthma; Babesiosis; Bites and stings; Dermatitis; Dermatology; Dermatology, pediatric; Ehrlichiosis; Insect-borne diseases; Itching; Lyme disease; Parasitic diseases; Rashes; Rocky Mountain spotted fever; Scabies; Skin; Skin disorders; Typhus.

FOR FURTHER INFORMATION:

Ashford, R. W., and W. Crewe. *The Parasites of "Homo sapiens": An Annotated Checklist of the Protozoa, Helminths, and Arthropods for Which We Are Home.* 2d ed. New York: Taylor & Francis, 2003. A comprehensive checklist of all the animals naturally parasitic in or on the human body. Each parasite includes a complete summary of characteristics.

Berenbaum, May R. *Ninety-nine Gnats, Nits, and Nibblers.* Urbana: University of Illinois Press, 1989. A scientist describes how insects affect human lives. Offers an informative description of the life cycles and habits of lice, mites, ticks, and other troublemakers.

Goddard, Jerome. *Physician's Guide to Arthropods of Medical Importance.* 4th ed. Boca Raton, Fla.: CRC Press, 2003. Nontechnical description of a wide variety of arthropods and conditions related to their stings or bites. Topics include allergy to venoms and the signs and symptoms of arthropod-borne diseases.

Olkowski, William, Sheila Daar, and Helga Olkowski. *Common-Sense Pest Control.* Newton, Conn.: Taunton Press, 1996. A very useful book by a biologist that describes the best methods of dealing with all kinds of insect problems, including lice, mites, and ticks. Offers detailed descriptions of how to remove these pests from your children and the environment safely.

Robinson, William H. *Urban Entomology: Insect and Mite Pests in the Human Environment.* London: Chapman & Hall, 1996. Discusses household pests in urban areas, including how to control them. Provides a bibliography and an index.

Service, M. W., ed. *Encyclopedia of Arthropod-Transmitted Infections of Man and Domesticated Animals.* New York: CAB International, 2001. Offers basic information related to the transmission, symptoms, treatment, and control of infections transmitted by biting midges, ticks, lice, and related organisms.

Sheorey, Harsha, John Walker, and Beverley-Ann Biggs. *Clinical Parasitology.* Melbourne, Vic.: University of Melbourne Press, 2003. Reviews global parasitic diseases and includes information regarding classification and geographical distribution of parasites, details of diagnostic tests, availability and treatment regimens of drugs, and means of obtaining uncommon drugs.

Vanderhoof-Forschner, Karen. *Everything You Need to Know About Lyme Disease and Other Tick-Borne Disorders.* 2d ed. Hoboken, N.J.: John Wiley & Sons, 2003. A consumer guide that aims to provide basic knowledge and useful insights into the prevention and management of disease.

Weedon, David. *Skin Pathology.* 3d ed. New York: Churchill Livingstone/Elsevier, 2010. Text with extensive photographs, covering tissue reaction patterns; the epidermis, dermis and subcutis; the skin in systemic and miscellaneous diseases; infections and infestations; and tumors, among other topics.

LIGAMENTS

ANATOMY

ALSO KNOWN AS: Connective tissue

ANATOMY OR SYSTEM AFFECTED: Joints, musculoskeletal system, reproductive system

SPECIALTIES AND RELATED FIELDS: Exercise physiology, orthopedics, osteopathic medicine, pathology, physical therapy, rheumatology, sports medicine

DEFINITION: White fibrous connective tissue that has a supportive role by attaching to the ends of bones to form movable joints. Ligaments also provide support for internal organs such as the kidneys and the spleen.

KEY TERMS:

articular joint: a freely moving joint consisting of the joining of two bony surfaces covered by cartilage

collagen: a protein arranged in bundles to form the fibers of tendons and ligaments

elastin: a protein that forms the main substance of yellow elastic fibers within connective tissue such as ligaments

fibroblast: a cell in connective tissue that gives rise to other cells which form binding and supportive tissue of the body

osteoarthritis: a degenerative process where components of the joints undergo thinning, resulting in loss of motion, pain, and often inflammation in the later stages

synovium: a transparent fluid secreted by the synovial membrane acting as a lubricant for many joints

STRUCTURE AND FUNCTIONS

Structurally, ligaments appear to be straplike bands or round cords. They are strong yet somewhat pliable. In terms of the musculoskeletal system, they serve to stabilize the adjoining bones making up what is referred to as an articulating joint. Ligaments consist of a cellular component called fibroblasts, making up 20 percent of their total tissue volume. The remaining 80 percent of the tissue volume is outside the fibroblast cells and consists of collagen and elastin. The relative proportion of collagen to elastin varies among ligaments. The degree of stabilization also varies and depends on each particular joint, such as shoulder and ankle joint ligaments. This degree of stabilization may be one which limits the amount of movement or prevents certain movements entirely. Some ligaments surround an entire joint filled with a lubricating fluid called synovium and are termed capsular ligaments. Ligaments located outside this joint capsule are called extracapsular and provide joint stability, while ligaments located inside the capsular ligament are called intracapsular and permit much more movement of the joint.

Other locations outside the musculoskeletal system that consist of ligaments for supporting structures include the broad ligament for the uterus and Fallopian tubes, which attaches these organs to the pelvic wall. Suspensory ligaments are also found in the body supporting a variety of organs, including the eyeball and breasts.

DISORDERS AND DISEASES

Ligaments are elastic, and they gradually lengthen when under tension. The term "sprain" describes an injury to a ligament caused by forces that stretch some or all of the ligament's fibers beyond their limit. This type of ligament injury can result in some degree of rupture of some or all of the fibers. In some instances, the ligament injury includes the possibility of pulling attachments from the bones. The classification for grading ligament injuries is based on two factors, the numbers of fibers ruptured and the resulting instability of the joint involved. Ligament injuries are also classified clinically as first-degree (mild), second-degree (moderate), or third-degree (severe).

A consequence of a stretched or ruptured ligament can be instability of the joint. Not all injured ligaments require surgery, but if surgery is needed to stabilize the joint, the torn ligament can be repaired. Instability of a joint can, over time, lead to wear to the cartilage and eventually to osteoarthritis.

Joint inflammation from trauma or other medical reasons can stiffen the joint ligaments, resulting in restricted motion. In contrast, a group of rare inherited diseases called Ehlers-Danlos syndrome can lead to abnormal collagen, resulting in loss of joint stability because of laxity in the joint capsule.

Several immune diseases can affect the ligaments of the body's joints. Rheumatoid arthritis is a chronic disease that affects the synovial membrane of the joint, which produces the joint's lubricant synovium. This fluid becomes thickened and fleshy and erodes the joint structures, including the articular ligaments.

PERSPECTIVE AND PROSPECTS

The discovery of joint structures is credited to early anatomists such as Andreas Vesalius, who published *De fabrica humana* in 1543. Until this time, his contemporaries had claimed that ligaments and tendons were types of nerve units. Three centuries later, in 1858, Henry Gray's writings on dissection, *Gray's Anatomy,* described and illustrated the anatomy and function of the human body, including the role of ligaments.

Advances in orthopedic medicine and the development of sports medicine have introduced specific braces to protect major joint ligaments during athletic and nonathletic activities. In addition, the continuing development of surgical procedures for the repair of damaged ligaments can help the individual return to an optimal level of function after the ligament injury. Research is ongoing to provide information to treat and find a cure for the many pathologies that affect ligaments and associated connective tissues.

—*Jeffrey P. Larson, P.T., A.T.C.*

See also Arthritis; Bones and the skeleton; Cartilage; Connective tissue; Joints; Osteoarthritis; Sports medicine; Tendon disorders; Tendons.

FOR FURTHER INFORMATION:

Hoppenfeld, Stanley. *Physical Examination of the Spine and Extremities.* Norwalk, Conn.: Appleton-Century-Crofts, 1976.

Malone, T. R., T. McPoil, and A. J. Nitz. *Orthopedic and Sports Physical Therapy.* St. Louis: Mosby Year Books, 1997.

Norkin C. C. *Joint Structure and Function.* Philadelphia: F. A. Davis, 1992.

Scuderi, Giles R. *Sports Medicine: A Comprehensive Approach.* Philadelphia: Mosby/Elsevier, 2005.

Standring, Susan, et al., eds. *Gray's Anatomy.* 40th ed. New York: Churchill Livingstone/Elsevier, 2008.

LIGHT THERAPY

TREATMENT

ANATOMY OR SYSTEM AFFECTED: Brain, nervous system, psychic-emotional system, skin

SPECIALTIES AND RELATED FIELDS: Dermatology, gerontology, oncology, ophthalmology, psychiatry, psychology

DEFINITION: A noninvasive procedure using exposure to light as the mechanism for clinical treatment.

INDICATIONS AND PROCEDURES

Light therapy, or phototherapy, treats a variety of disorders. By exposing individuals to different kinds of light (for example, monochromatic, polychromatic, ultraviolet), symptoms can often be delayed, reduced, and eradicated. Immunological, neurotransmitter, and neuroendocrine systems play key roles in response to this type of treatment.

Best known in psychiatry, light therapy serves as a treatment for seasonal affective disorder (SAD), or winter depression; bulimia nervosa; sleep disorders; and "sundowner's syndrome," the late afternoon confusion and agitation sometimes accompanying Alzheimer's disease. Shift workers can also experience difficulties related to light exposure, and light therapies may provide some relief. Reduced environmental light is a factor in the etiology, onset, or maintenance of these problems. Thus, treatment involves exposing individuals to bright, full-spectrum light for specific time periods. Duration of exposure and light intensity vary by the disorder and individual treated.

In dermatology and oncology, light therapy treats psoriasis, skin ulcers, tumors, and esophageal cancers. The type of light and the intensities used, however, vary considerably from those applied for the treatment of psychiatric disorders.

USES AND COMPLICATIONS

The side effects of light therapy are best documented in psychiatry: Insomnia, mania, and (less frequently) morning hot flashes have been noted. Persons with other sensitivity to light, such as those prone to migraines, may also need to exercise caution with light therapy in order to avoid undesirable effects. Careful monitoring by medical providers of the patient's response to treatment is necessary. Additionally, professionals advise morning administrations of light therapy.

Users of light therapy must also be cautioned to adhere closely to recommended doses and intensity of exposure to light. Use of light outside prescribed parameters may be damaging to the eyes.

Light therapy is not effective universally; some patients may experience no improvement. For seasonal affective disorder, evidence suggests that younger individuals whose depression involves weight gain and increased sleep may be most likely to respond to treatment. For psoriasis, complementary treatments, such as psychotherapy, may facilitate a response to treatment.

PERSPECTIVE AND PROSPECTS

Light and dark cycles are a biological reality; thus, it is no surprise that light affects physical, emotional, and mental well-being. As the interest in noninvasive interventions increases, the attention given to environmental treatments such as light therapy is likely to increase as well. Recent developments in the use of light therapy for sleep and behavioral disorders are fueling clinical, research, consumer, and other business interests in this procedure. Experimentation with different frequencies or colors of light, doses, intensities, and sites on the body for application of light are ongoing and likely to increase the diversity of uses for this type of treatment. Additionally applications of light-based interventions in the workplace and elsewhere may prove useful in preventing disorders related to light deprivation and in helping to affect productivity, directly and indirectly.

—*Nancy A. Piotrowski, Ph.D.*

See also Alternative medicine; Alzheimer's disease; Bulimia; Chronobiology; Depression; Dermatology; Psoriasis; Psychiatry; Seasonal affective disorder; Skin disorders; Sleep; Sleep disorders.

FOR FURTHER INFORMATION:

Goldberg, Burton, John Anderson, and Larry Trivieri, eds. *Alternative Medicine: The Definitive Guide.* 2d ed. Berkeley, Calif.: Celestial Arts, 2002.

Hyman, Jane Wegscheider. *Light Book: How Natural and Artificial Light Affects Our Health, Mood, and Behavior.* Los Angeles: J. P. Tarcher, 1990.

Jacobs, Jennifer, ed. *The Encyclopedia of Alternative Medicine: A Complete Family Guide to Complemen-*

tary Therapies. Rev. ed. Boston: Journey Editions, 1997.

Kastner, Mark, and Hugh Burroughs. *Alternative Healing: The Complete A-Z Guide to over 160 Different Alternative Therapies.* New York: Henry Holt, 1996.

Marshall, Fiona, and Peter Cheevers. *Positive Options for Seasonal Affective Disorder.* New York: Hunter House, 2003.

Palmer, John D. *The Living Clock: The Orchestrator of Biological Rhythms.* New York: Oxford University Press, 2002.

LIPIDS

BIOLOGY

ANATOMY OR SYSTEM AFFECTED: Cells, gastrointestinal system

SPECIALTIES AND RELATED FIELDS: Biochemistry, cytology, nutrition, vascular medicine

DEFINITION: Organic compounds found in the tissues of plants and animals that serve as energy-storage molecules, function as solvents for water-insoluble vitamins, provide insulation against the loss of body heat, act as a protective cushion for vital organs, and are structural components of cell membranes.

KEY TERMS:

alcohol: an organic compound containing a hydroxyl (–OH) group attached to a carbon atom

carboxylic acid: an organic compound that contains the carboxyl (–CO$_2$H) group

ester: the relatively non-water-soluble compound formed when an alcohol reacts with a carboxylic acid

fatty acid: an organic compound that is composed of a long hydrocarbon chain with a carboxyl group at one end

glycerol: a three-carbon alcohol that has one hydroxyl compound on each carbon atom

hydrocarbon: an organic compound composed of only hydrogen and carbon atoms that does not dissolve in water (water-insoluble)

hydrophilic: "water-loving" or "water-attracting"; a term given to molecules or regions of molecules that interact favorably with water

hydrophobic: "water-hating" or "water-repelling"; a term given to molecules or regions of molecules that do not interact favorably with water

saponification: a reaction in which a strong basic solution splits a molecule into a carboxylic acid unit and an alcohol unit

STRUCTURE AND FUNCTIONS

Lipids are a class of bio-organic compounds that are typically insoluble in water and relatively soluble in organic solvents such as alcohols, ethers, and hydrocarbons. Unlike the other classes of organic molecules found in biological systems (carbohydrates, proteins, and nucleic acids), lipids possess a unifying physical property—solubility behavior—rather than a unifying structural feature. Fats, oils, some vitamins and hormones, and most of the nonprotein components of cell membranes are lipids.

There are two categories of lipids—those that undergo saponification and those that are nonsaponifiable. The saponifiable lipids can be divided into simple and complex lipids. Simple lipids, which are composed of carbon, hydrogen, and oxygen, yield fatty acids and an alcohol upon saponification. Complex lipids contain one or more additional elements, such as phosphorus, nitrogen, and sulfur, yielding fatty acids, alcohol, and other compounds on saponification.

The fatty acid building blocks of saponifiable lipids may be either saturated, which means that as many hydrogen atoms as possible are attached to the carbon chain, or unsaturated, which means that at least two hydrogen atoms are missing. Saturated fatty acids are white solids at room temperature, while unsaturated ones are liquids at room temperature, because of a geometrical difference in the long carbon chains. The carbon atoms of a saturated fatty acid are arranged in a zigzag or accordion configuration. These chains are stacked on top of one another in a very orderly and efficient fashion, making it difficult to separate the chains from one another. When carbons in the chain are missing hydrogen atoms, the regular zigzag of the chain is disrupted, leading to less efficient packing, which allows the chains to be separated more easily. Saturated fatty acids have a higher melting temperature because they require more energy to separate their chains than do unsaturated fatty acids. Unsaturated fatty acids can be converted into saturated ones by adding hydrogen atoms through a process called hydrogenation.

Simple lipids can be divided into triglycerides and waxes. Waxes such as beeswax, lanolin (from lamb's wool), and carnauba wax (from a palm tree) are esters formed from an alcohol with a long carbon chain and a fatty acid. These compounds, which are solids at room temperature, serve as protective coatings. Most plant leaves are coated with a wax film to prevent attack by microorganisms and loss of water through evaporation.

Animal fur and bird feathers have a wax coating. For example, the wax coating on their feathers is what allows ducks to stay afloat.

Edible fats and oils such as lard (pig fat), tallow (beef fat), corn oil, and butter are triglycerides. Triglyceride molecules are fatty acid esters in which three fatty acids (all saturated, all unsaturated, or mixed) combine with one molecule of the alcohol glycerol. Oils are triglycerides that are liquid at room temperature, while fats are solid at room temperature. The fluidity of a triglyceride is dependent on the nature of its fatty acid chains; the more unsaturated the triglyceride, the more fluid its structure. The triglycerides found in animals tend to have more saturated fatty acids than do those found in plants. Vegetable oils and fish oils are frequently polyunsaturated.

Complex lipids are classified as phospholipids or glycolipids. Structurally, phospholipids are composed of fatty acids and a phosphate group. Glycerol-based lipids called phosphoglycerides contain glycerol, two fatty acids, and a phosphate group. The phosphoglyceride structure contains a hydrophilic (polar) head, the phosphate unit, and two hydrophobic (nonpolar) fatty acid tails. The polar head can interact strongly with water, while the nonpolar tails interact strongly with organic solvents and avoid water. Egg yolks contain a large amount of the phosphoglyceride phosphatidylcholine (also called lecithin). This lipid is used to form the emulsion mayonnaise from oil and vinegar. Normally, oil and water do not mix. The hydrophobic oil forms a separate layer on top of the water. Since lecithin's structure contains both a hydrophobic and a hydrophilic region, it can attach to the water with its polar head and the oil with its nonpolar tail, preventing the two materials from separating. Lipids derived from the alcohol sphingosine are called sphingolipids. They contain one fatty acid, one long hydrocarbon chain and a phosphate group. Like the phosphoglycerides, sphingolipids have a head-and-two-tail structure. Sphingolipids are important components in the protective and insulating coating that surrounds nerves.

Glycolipids differ from phospholipids in that they possess a sugar group in place of the phosphate group. Their structure is again the polar head and dual tail arrangement in which the sugar is the hydrophilic unit. Cerebrosides, which are sphingosine-based glycolipids containing a simple sugar such as galactose or glucose, are found in large amounts in the white matter of the brain and in the myelin sheath. Gangliosides, which are found in the gray matter of the brain, in neu-

ral tissue, and in the receptor sites for neurotransmitters, contain a more complex sugar component.

Nonsaponifiable lipids do not contain esters of fatty acids as their basic structural feature. Steroids are an important class of nonsaponifiable lipids. All steroids possess an identical four-ring framework called the steroid nucleus, but they differ in the groups that are attached to their ring systems. Examples of steroids are sterols such as cholesterol, the bile acids secreted by the liver, the sex hormones, corticosteroids secreted by the adrenal cortex, and digitoxin from the digitalis plant, which is used to treat heart disease.

Lipids constitute about 50 percent of the mass of most animal cell membranes. Biological membranes control the chemical environment of the space they enclose. They are selective filters controlling what substances enter and exit the cell, since they constitute a relatively impermeable barrier against most water-soluble molecules. The three types of lipids involved are phospholipids (most abundant), glycolipids, and cholesterol. Phospholipids, when surrounded by an aqueous environment, tend to organize into a double layer of lipid molecules, a bilayer, allowing their hydrophobic tails to be buried internally and their hydrophilic heads to be exposed to the water. These phospholipids have one saturated and one unsaturated tail. Differences in tail length and saturation influence the packing efficiency of the molecules and affect the fluidity of the membrane. Short, unsaturated tails increase the fluidity of the membrane. Cholesterol is important in maintaining the mechanical stability of the lipid bilayer, thereby preventing a change from the fluid state to a rigid crystalline state. It also decreases the permeability of small water-soluble molecules.

The lipid bilayer provides the basic structure of the membrane and serves as a two-dimensional solvent for protein molecules. Protein molecules are responsible for most membrane functions; for example, they can provide receptor sites, catalyze reactions, or transport molecules across the membrane. These proteins may extend across the bilayer (transmembrane proteins) or be associated with only one face of the bilayer. Cell membranes also have carbohydrates attached to the outer face of the bilayer. These carbohydrates are bound to membrane proteins or part of a glycolipid. Typically, 2 to 10 percent of a membrane's total weight is carbohydrate. Evidence exists that cell-surface carbohydrates are used as recognition sites for chemical processes.

Lipids play an important role in health and well-being. The body acquires lipids directly from dietary lipids and indirectly by converting other nutrients into lipids. There are two fatty acids, linoleic and linolenic acids, which are called essential fatty acids. Since these fatty acids cannot be synthesized in the body in sufficient amounts, their supply must come directly from dietary sources. Fortunately, these acids are widely found in foodstuffs, so deficiency is rarely observed in adults.

About 95 percent of the lipids in foods are triglycerides, which provide 30 to 50 percent of the calories in an average diet. Triglycerides produce 4,000 calories of energy per pound, compared to the 1,800 calories per pound produced by carbohydrates or proteins. Since the triglyceride is such an efficient energy source, the body converts carbohydrates and proteins into adipose (reserve fatty) tissue for storage to be used when extra fuel is required.

While carbohydrates and proteins undergo major degradation in the stomach, triglycerides remain intact, forming large globules that float to the top of the mixture. Fats spend a longer time than other nutrients in the stomach, slowing molecular activity before continuing into the intestines. Thus, a fat-laden meal gives longer satiety than a low-fat one.

In the small intestine, bile salts split fat globules into smaller droplets, allowing enzymes called lipases to saponify the triglycerides. In some instances, the fatty acids at the two ends are removed, leaving one attached as a monoglyceride. About 97 percent of dietary triglycerides are absorbed into the bloodstream; the remainder are excreted. Although glycerol and fatty acids with short carbon chains are water-soluble enough to dissolve in the blood, the long-chain fatty acids and monoglycerides are not. These insoluble materials recombine to form new triglycerides. Since these hydrophobic triglycerides would form large globules if they were dumped directly into the blood, small triglyceride droplets are surrounded with a protective protein coat that can dissolve in water, taking the encapsulated triglyceride with it. This structure is an example of a lipoprotein.

Cholesterol is found in relatively small (milligram) quantities in foods, compared to triglycerides. Cholesterol supplies raw materials for the production of bile salts and to be used as a structural constituent of brain and nerve tissue. Since these functions are important to animals but serve no purpose in plants, cholesterol is found only in animals. Only about 50 percent of dietary cholesterol is absorbed into the blood; the rest is excreted. Much of the body's supply of cholesterol is produced in the liver. For most individuals, the amount of cholesterol synthesized in the body is larger than the amount absorbed directly from the diet.

Digested lipids released from the intestine and those synthesized in the liver compose the lipid content of the blood. The fatty acids required by the liver are obtained directly from the bloodstream or by synthesis from sources such as glucose, amino acids, and alcohol. Liver-synthesized triglycerides are incorporated into lipoprotein packages before entering the bloodstream. There are three types of lipoprotein packages that transport lipids to and from the liver. Very-low-density lipoproteins (VLDLs) transport triglycerides to tissues; low-density lipoproteins (LDLs) transport the cholesterol from the liver to other cells; and high-density lipoproteins (HDLs) transport cholesterol from other tissues to the liver for destruction.

Disorders and Diseases

Lipid consumption is an important dietary concern. Lipid deficiency is rarely observed in adults but can occur in infants who are fed nonfat formulas. Since fatty acids are essential for growth, lipid consumption should not be restricted in individuals under two years of age. Excess lipid consumption is associated with health problems such as obesity and cardiovascular disease. Although excess calories from any dietary source can lead to obesity, the body must expend less energy to store dietary fat than to store dietary carbohydrate as body fat. Thus, high-fat diets produce more body fat than do high-carbohydrate, low-fat diets.

Atherosclerosis, or "hardening of the arteries," is the leading cause of cardiovascular disease. A strong correlation exists between diets high in saturated fats and the incidence of atherosclerosis. In this condition, deposits called plaques, which have a high cholesterol content, form on artery walls. Over time, these deposits narrow the artery and decrease its elasticity, resulting in reduced blood flow. Blockages can occur, resulting in heart attack or stroke. High serum cholesterol levels (total blood cholesterol content) often result in increased plaque formation. Since dietary cholesterol is not efficiently absorbed into the bloodstream and the serum cholesterol level is largely determined by the amount of cholesterol synthesized in the liver, high serum cholesterol levels are frequently related to high saturated fat intake.

Since the measurement of the serum cholesterol level gives the total cholesterol concentration of the blood, it can be a somewhat misleading predictor of atherosclerosis risk; cholesterol is not free in blood, but is encapsulated in lipoproteins. Since the cholesterol packaged in the LDL, cholesterol that can be deposited in plaques ("bad" cholesterol), has a very different fate from that in the HDL, which is transporting cholesterol for destruction ("good" cholesterol), measuring the ratio of LDL cholesterol to HDL cholesterol has been found to be a better indicator of atherosclerosis risk. Decreasing dietary intake of cholesterol and saturated fats, increasing water-soluble fibers in the diet, removing excess body weight, and increasing the amount of aerobic exercise will all serve to improve the LDL-C/HDL-C ratio.

A number of hereditary diseases are known that result from abnormal accumulation of the complex lipids utilized in membranes. These diseases are called lipid (or lysosomal) storage diseases, or lipidoses. In normal individuals, the amount of each complex lipid present in the body is relatively constant; in other words, the rate of formation equals the rate of destruction. The lipids are broken down by enzymes that attack specific bonds in the lipid structure. Lipid storage diseases occur when a lipid-degrading enzyme is defective or absent. In these cases, the lipid synthesis proceeds normally, but the degradation is impaired, causing the lipid or a partial degradation product to accumulate, with consequences such as an enlarged liver and spleen, mental disability, blindness, and death.

Niemann-Pick, Gaucher's, and Tay-Sachs diseases are examples of lipidoses. Niemann-Pick disease is caused by a defect in an enzyme that breaks down sphingomyelin. The disease becomes apparent in infancy, causing mental retardation and death normally by age four. Gaucher's disease, a more common disease involving the accumulation of a glycolipid, produces two different syndromes. The acute cerebral form affects infants, causing severe nervous system abnormalities, retardation, and death before age one. The chronic form, which may become evident at any age, causes enlargement of the spleen, anemia, and erosion of the bones. In Tay-Sachs disease, a partially degraded lipid accumulates in the tissues of the central nervous system. Symptoms include progressive loss of vision, paralysis, and death at three or four years of age. Although Tay-Sachs disease is relatively rare (1 in 300,000 births), it has a high incidence in individuals of Eastern European Jewish descent (1 in 3,600 births). This defect is a recessive genetic trait that is found in one of every twenty-eight members of this population. For two parents who are both carriers of this trait, there is a one in four chance that their child will develop Tay-Sachs disease. Tests have been developed to detect the presence of the defective gene in the parent, and the amniotic fluid of a developing fetus can be sampled using a technique called amniocentesis to detect Tay-Sachs disease. Lipid storage diseases have no known cures; however, they can be prevented through genetic counseling.

PERSPECTIVE AND PROSPECTS

The ability of a cell to discriminate in its chemical exchanges with the environment is fundamental to life. How the cell membrane accomplishes this feat has been a subject of intense biochemical research since the beginning of the twentieth century.

In 1895, Ernst Overton observed that substances that are lipid-soluble enter cells more quickly than those that are lipid-insoluble. He reasoned that the membrane must be composed of lipids. About twenty years later, chemical analysis showed that membranes also contain proteins. Irwin Langmuir prepared the first artificial membrane in 1917 by mixing a phospholipid-containing hydrocarbon solution with water. Evaporation of the hydrocarbon left a phospholipid film on the surface of the water, which showed that only the hydrophilic heads contacted the water. When the Dutch biologists E. Gorter and F. Grendel deposited the lipids from red blood cell membranes on a water surface and decreased the occupied surface area with a movable barrier, a continuous film resulted that occupied an area approximately twice the surface area of the original red blood cells. In 1935, all these observations, along with the fact that the surfaces of artificial membranes containing only phospholipids are less water-absorbent than the surfaces of true biological membranes, were combined by Hugh Davson and James Danielli into a membrane model in which a phospholipid bilayer was sandwiched between two water-absorbent protein layers.

The technological advances of the 1950's in X-ray diffraction and electron microscopy allowed the structures of membranes to be probed directly. Such studies revealed that membranes are indeed composed of parallel orderly arrays of lipids, although many of the proteins are attached to one of the faces of the bilayer: The Davson-Danielli model was too simplistic. The freeze-fracture technique of preparing cells for electron microscopy has provided the most information about the nature of membrane proteins. In this technique, the two layers are separated so that the inner topography can be studied. Instead of the smooth surface predicted by the Davson-Danielli model, a cobblestone-like surface was observed that resulted from proteins penetrating into the interior of the membrane. All experimental evidence supports the fluid mosaic model for biological membranes, a model first proposed by Seymour Singer and Garth Nicholson in 1972. In this model, proteins are dispersed and embedded in a phospholipid bilayer that is in a fluid state. How membranes function was the next question to be considered.

Although most of the small molecules needed by cells cross the barrier via protein channels, some essential nutrients, such as cholesterol in its LDL package, are too large to pass through a small channel. In 1986, Michael Brown and Joseph Goldstein received the Nobel Prize for their discovery of specific protein receptors on the membranes of liver cells to which LDL molecules attach. These receptors move across the surface until they encounter a shallow indentation or pit. As the pit deepens, the membrane closes behind the LDL, forming a coating allowing transport across the hydrophobic membrane interior. The presence of insufficient numbers of these receptors causes abnormal LDL-cholesterol buildup in the blood.

Many questions remain unanswered concerning the roles of proteins and glycolipids in membranes. Membranes are involved in the movement, growth, and development of cells. How the membrane is involved in the uncontrolled multiplication and migration in cancer is one medically important question. Experiments that will answer questions about how membrane structure affects functioning should lead to the development of new medical treatments.

—*Arlene R. Courtney, Ph.D.*

See also Arteriosclerosis; Carbohydrates; Cholesterol; Digestion; Fluids and electrolytes; Food biochemistry; Gaucher's disease; Heart disease; Hypercholesterolemia; Hyperlipidemia; Metabolic disorders; Metabolic syndrome; Metabolism; Niemann-Pick disease; Nonalcoholic steatohepatitis (NASH); Obesity; Obesity, childhood; Plaque, arterial; Protein; Steroids; Tay-Sachs disease.

FOR FURTHER INFORMATION:

Bettelheim, Frederick A., et al. *Introduction to General, Organic, and Biochemistry.* 9th ed. Pacific Grove, Calif.: Brooks/Cole, 2010. A text designed for students with little previous chemistry background. Chapter 17 discusses the structure and function of lipids, chapter 21 discusses the conversion of biological molecules into energy, and chapter 22 gives details of the synthesis of lipids in the body.

Bloomfield, Molly M., and Lawrence J. Stephens. *Chemistry and the Living Organism.* 6th ed. New York: John Wiley & Sons, 1996. A text written for allied health students that has a well-written chapter on lipids. Other chapters provide good elementary coverage on organic compounds such as alcohols, carboxylic acids, and esters.

Brown, Michael S., and Joseph L. Goldstein. "How LDL Receptors Influence Cholesterol and Atherosclerosis." *Scientific American* 251 (November, 1984): 58-66. An article in which the Nobel laureates describe their work on LDL membrane receptors. This article is of an intermediate technical nature.

Christian, Janet L., and Janet L. Greger. *Nutrition for Living.* 4th ed. Redwood City, Calif.: Benjamin/Cummings, 1994. A human nutrition text written at a level requiring little or no technical knowledge. This book provides an elementary discussion of the nutritional aspects of fats and cholesterol.

Cornatzer, W. E. *Role of Nutrition in Health and Disease.* Springfield, Ill.: Charles C Thomas, 1989. Gives a comprehensive description of medical conditions in which lipids are involved.

Sikorski, Zdzisław E., and Anna Kołakowska, eds. *Chemical and Functional Properties of Food Lipids.* Boca Raton, Fla.: CRC Press, 2002. In seventeen chapters by international specialists, this book examines the nature, technological properties, reactivity, and health-related concerns and benefits of food lipids.

Vance, Dennis E., and Jean E. Vance, eds. *Biochemistry of Lipids, Lipoproteins, and Membranes.* 5th ed. Boston: Elsevier, 2008. First published in 1985, this edition details the startling advances made in lipid biochemistry and covers all aspects of lipids research.

LIPOSUCTION
PROCEDURE

ANATOMY OR SYSTEM AFFECTED: Abdomen, arms, hips, knees, legs

SPECIALTIES AND RELATED FIELDS: General surgery, plastic surgery

DEFINITION: The removal of fat deposits with a cannula and a suction pump in order to recontour body areas.

KEY TERMS:

abdomen: the area of the body between the diaphragm and the pelvis; it contains the visceral organs *adipose tissue:* the tissue that stores fat

cannula: a tube used to drain body fluids or to administer medications

general anesthesia: anesthesia that induces unconsciousness

local anesthesia: anesthesia that numbs the feeling in a body part; administered by injection or direct application to the skin

subcutaneous: under the skin

INDICATIONS AND PROCEDURES

The fat contained in adipose tissue makes up 15 to 20 percent of the body weights of most healthy individuals. Much adipose tissue is found inside the abdominal cavity, but significant amounts are located under the skin of the abdomen, arms, breasts, hips, knees, legs, and throat. The quantity of this subcutaneous fat at any such site is based on individual heredity, age, and eating habits. When excessive eating greatly elevates body fat, a patient becomes obese, a condition that can be life-threatening. Until recently, the sole means for decreasing fat content resulting from obesity was time-consuming dieting, which requires much patience and will power. In addition, the positive consequences of long diets can be easily obliterated if dieters begin to overeat again. Recurrent overeating is common and often followed by the rapid regaining of the fat.

Persons who have undesired, unattractive fat deposits as a result of age, heredity, or obesity may undergo cosmetic surgery, such as so-called tummy tucks, to remove them. Such major procedures, however, often remove muscle along with fat and cause considerable scarring. Liposuction is a relatively easy way to lose unattractive body fat; it also is seen as a fast way to reverse obesity and is touted as more permanent than dieting. A cannula connected to a suction pump is inserted under the skin in the desired area. Then a chosen amount of fat is sucked out, the cannula is withdrawn, and the incision is closed. The result is a recontouring of the body part. Hence, liposuction has become a very popular cosmetic surgery procedure for the abdomen, arms, breasts, hips, knees, legs, and throat; many pounds can be removed from large areas such as the abdomen.

Liposuction begins with the administration of antibiotics and the anesthesia of the area to be recontoured. Local anesthesia is safer, but general anesthesia is used when necessary. The process usually begins after a 1.3-centimeter (0.5-inch) incision is made in a fold of the treated body region, so that the scar will not be notice-able after healing. At this time, a sterile cannula is introduced under the skin of the treatment area. Next, the surgeon uses suction through the cannula to remove the fat deposits. Liposuction produces temporary tunnels in adipose tissue. Upon completion of the procedure, the incision is closed and the surgical area is wrapped with tight bandages or covered with support garments. This final stage of recontouring helps the tissue to collapse back into the desired shape during healing. In most patients, the skin around the area soon shrinks into the new contours. When this does not happen easily, because of old age or other factors, liposuction is accompanied by surgical skin removal.

USES AND COMPLICATIONS

Liposuction can be used for body recontouring only when undesired contours are attributable to fat deposits; those attributable to anatomical features such as bone structure cannot be treated in this manner.

A major principle on which liposuction is based is the supposition that the body contains a fixed number of fat cells and that, as people become fatter, the cells fill with droplets of fat and expand. The removal of fat cells by liposuction is deemed to decrease the future ability of the treated body part to become fat because fewer cells are available to be filled. Dieting and exercise are less successful than liposuction because they do not diminish the number of fat cells in adipose tissue, only decreasing fat cell size. Hence, when dieters return to eating excess food again or exercise stops, the fat cells expand again.

Another aspect of liposuction which is becoming popular is the ability to remove undesired fat from some body sites and insert it where the fat is wanted for recontouring. Most often, this transfer involves enlarging women's breasts or correcting cases in which the two breasts are of markedly different size. Liposuction also can be used to repair asymmetry in other body parts as a result of accidents.

Liposuction, as with any other surgery, has associated risks and complications. According to reputable practitioners, however, they are temporary and relatively minor, such as black-and-blue marks and the accumulation of blood and serum under the skin of treated areas. These complications are minimized by fluid removal during surgery and by the application of tight bandages or garments after the operation. Another related complication is that subcutaneous fat removal leads to fluid loss from the body. When large amounts of fat are removed, shock occurs if the fluid is not re-

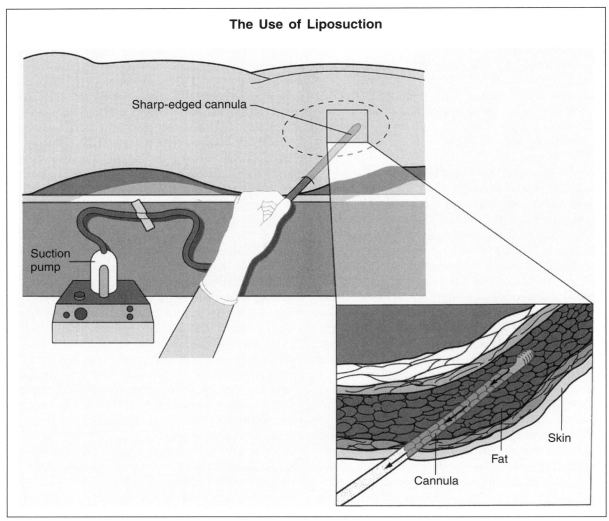

The Use of Liposuction

Sharp-edged cannula

Suction pump

Skin

Fat

Cannula

When unwanted areas of fat seem resistant to dieting and exercise, some patients turn to liposuction, the physical removal of fat deposits with a tube and a suction pump. The cosmetic results of this procedure may vary considerably.

placed quickly. Therefore, another component of successful liposuction is timely fluid replacement.

The more extensive and complex the liposuction procedure attempted, the more likely it is to cause complications. Particularly prone to problems are liposuction procedures in which major skin removal is required. Hence, surgeons who perform liposuction suggest that potential patients be realistic about the goals of the surgery. It is also recommended that patients choose reputable practitioners.

Perspective and Prospects

Liposuction, currently viewed as relatively safe cosmetic surgery, originated in Europe in the late 1960's.

In 1982, it reached the United States. Since that time, its use has burgeoned, and about a half million liposuction surgeries are carried out yearly. Although its first use was as a purely cosmetic procedure, liposuction is now done for noncosmetic reasons, including repairing injuries sustained in accidents. Women were once the sole liposuction patients. Now, men make up about one-quarter of treated individuals.

In the United States, liposuction is not presently accepted by insurance companies or considered tax deductible. This situation may change because several studies have found that obese people have a greater chance of developing cardiovascular disease and cancer. It must be noted, however, that liposuction offers only temporary relief from body fat. Although it does decrease fat deposition in a treated region, lack of proper calorie intake and exercise will deposit fat elsewhere in the body.

—*Sanford S. Singer, Ph.D.*

See also Bariatric surgery; Dermatology; Lipids; Nutrition; Obesity; Obesity, childhood; Plastic surgery; Skin; Weight loss and gain.

FOR FURTHER INFORMATION:

Schein, Jeffery R. "The Truth About Liposuction." *Consumers Digest* 30 (January/February, 1991): 71-74. Liposuction is the most popular type of cosmetic surgery, and that means that many people are assuming that liposuction can do more than it really can. Some facts about liposuction and physicians' certification are given.

Shelton, Ron M., and Terry Malloy. *Liposuction.* New York: Berkley, 2004. A consumer guide to liposuction that reviews the pros and cons and answers common questions.

Shiffman, Melvin A., and Alberto Di Giuseppe, eds. *Liposuction: Principles and Practice.* New York: Springer, 2006. A comprehensive book on the latest state-of-the-art methods.

Wilkinson, Tolbert S. *Atlas of Liposuction.* Philadelphia: Saunders/Elsevier, 2005. A helpful atlas covering liposuction. Includes bibliographical references and an index.

Zollinger, Robert M., Jr., and Robert M. Zollinger, Sr. *Zollinger's Atlas of Surgical Operations.* 8th ed. New York: McGraw-Hill, 2003. A comprehensive examination of surgery. Covers basic surgical anatomy and vascular, gynecologic, gastrointestinal, and miscellaneous abdominal procedures.

LISPING

DISEASE/DISORDER

ANATOMY OR SYSTEM AFFECTED: Mouth, teeth

SPECIALTIES AND RELATED FIELDS: Dentistry, speech pathology

DEFINITION: The defective pronunciation of the sibilants "s" and "z," usually substituted with a "th" sound.

CAUSES AND SYMPTOMS

A central or frontal lisp is caused by a child pushing the tongue past the teeth while speaking, which tends to occur in cases of an open bite. This produces the familiar lisp in which "s" and "z" sounds are pronounced like

---

INFORMATION ON LISPING

CAUSES: Physiological defects, dental problems, missing teeth

SYMPTOMS: Mispronunciation of sibilants *s* and *z*

DURATION: Typically short-term but may be chronic

TREATMENTS: Speech therapy

"th." Sometimes, the child tries to correct the protrusion of the tongue by pulling it in, but lisping still occurs because the correct position of the tongue has not been learned.

A lateral lisp involves the escape of air on both sides of the tongue, yielding an unpleasant "blubbering" sound. A possible cause is missing teeth, particularly the two upper front teeth.

A recessive lisp is caused by holding the tongue too far back in the mouth. The "s" and "z" sounds come out sounding more like "sh." This mild lisp is often associated in the popular media with the speech of an intoxicated person.

TREATMENT AND THERAPY

Speech therapists work with lisping children in two ways. In the phonetic placement method, the child is asked to pronounce the "t" sound and then prolong it. Once this is learned, the bite is closed and the child then practices moving the lips in a slightly protracted position; the tongue is moved back and forth until the "s" sound is achieved. This same process is used in learning to pronounce "z"; the "d" sound, however, is used in practice instead of a "t." In some cases, asking the child to pronounce "sh" first and then move the tongue forward along the roof of the mouth will produce an "s" sound.

In the auditory stimulation method, the speech therapist pronounces the correct sound repeatedly and compares it to the incorrect articulation. This method is very successful in young children with lisps.

After a sound has been practiced by itself, the child attaches it to nonsense syllables and practices pronouncing them. Gradually, the sound is introduced in familiar words, followed by sentences. The final test is the use of the newly acquired sound in spontaneous conversation.

—*Rose Secrest*

See also Developmental disorders; Developmental stages; Motor skill development; Speech disorders; Stuttering; Voice and vocal cord disorders.

FOR FURTHER INFORMATION:

Bleile, Ken M. *Manual of Articulation and Phonological Disorders: Infancy Through Adulthood.* 2d ed. Clifton Park, N.Y.: Thomson/Delmar Learning, 2004.

Gordon-Brannan, Mary E., and Curtis E. Weiss. *Clinical Management of Articulatory and Phonologic Disorders.* 3d ed. Philadelphia: Lippincott Williams & Wilkins, 2007.

Hamaguchi, Patricia McAleer. *Childhood Speech, Language, and Listening Problems: What Every Parent Should Know.* 2d ed. New York: Wiley, 2001.

Williams, A. Lynn. *Speech Disorders Resource Guide for Preschool Children.* Clifton Park, N.Y.: Thomson/Delmar Learning, 2003.

LISTERIA INFECTIONS

DISEASE/DISORDER

ALSO KNOWN AS: Listeriosis, *Listeria monocytogenes*

ANATOMY OR SYSTEM AFFECTED: Brain, nerves, nervous system

SPECIALTIES AND RELATED FIELDS: Bacteriology, obstetrics, pediatrics

DEFINITION: Infections caused by the bacterium *Listeria monocytogenes*.

CAUSES AND SYMPTOMS

Infection with *Listeria* bacteria is relatively rare and primarily affects pregnant women, newborn infants, and people with compromised immune systems. *Listeria* infection is a foodborne illness, meaning that infection occurs after eating a contaminated food product. Foods most commonly contaminated with *Listeria* are unpasteurized dairy products, uncooked meats, and raw, unwashed vegetables. For this reason, most pregnant women are advised by their doctors to make sure that all susceptible foods consumed during pregnancy are pasteurized and cooked thoroughly.

The symptoms of *Listeria* infection include fever, abdominal pain, diarrhea, and muscle aches, though some infections are completely asymptomatic. If infection progresses to reach the central nervous system, then symptoms can involve dizziness, headache, seizures, and death. Pregnant women who become infected can pass the bacteria to their unborn children. Shortly after birth, the newborn can become acutely ill and exhibit fever, irritability, and poor feeding. *Listeria* infection in the newborn is an emergency and can progress to death quickly. If the newborn survives the infection, then the child may suffer lifelong neurological damage.

> ### INFORMATION ON *LISTERIA* INFECTIONS
>
> **CAUSES:** Consumption of unpasteurized dairy products, uncooked meats, unwashed vegetables
> **SYMPTOMS:** Can be asymptomatic or include fever, abdominal pain, diarrhea, seizures, headache, death
> **DURATION:** Begins a day after ingestion of contaminated food, can last two to three days; more serious central nervous system infections can last much longer, with permanent damage
> **TREATMENTS:** Antibiotics

TREATMENT AND THERAPY

Diagnosis of *Listeria* infection is performed with a blood test or analysis of the spinal fluid through a spinal tap (lumbar puncture). Treatment for infection may require hospitalization and involves antibiotics. Ampicillin or penicillin G, often in conjunction with gentamicin, are the most commonly used antibiotics for these infections, but others such as trimethoprim-sulfamethoxazole and meropenem may be used in cases where the patient is allergic to penicillin or first-line treatments fail. Antibiotic treatment may last anywhere from ten days to eight weeks, depending on the patient's immune system and response to therapy.

Since the damage to newborn infants can be devastating, most infants presenting with fever, seizures, or other neurological symptoms receive a lumbar puncture to aid in diagnosis and are placed on prophylactic antibiotics that include ampicillin to treat *Listeria*. Ampicillin may be discontinued two to three days after treatment initiation if the spinal fluid is free of *Listeria* infection.

—*Jennifer Birkhauser, M.S., M.D.*

See also Bacterial infections; Botulism; *E. coli* infection; Enterocolitis; Food poisoning; Gastroenteritis; Gastroenterology; Gastroenterology, pediatric; Gastrointestinal disorders; Gastrointestinal system; Intestinal disorders; Intestines; Nausea and vomiting; Poisoning; Rotavirus; Salmonella infection; Shigellosis; Trichinosis; Tularemia.

FOR FURTHER INFORMATION:

Edelstein, Sari. "Foodborne Illness-Causing Pathogens." In *Food and Nutrition at Risk in America: Food Insecurity, Biotechnology, Food Safety, and Bioterrorism*, edited by Sari Edelstein. Sudbury, Mass.: Jones and Bartlett, 2008.

Stone, Joanne. "Pregnancy in Sickness and in Health." In *Pregnancy for Dummies*, edited by Mary Duenwald. Indianapolis: Wiley, 2008.

World Health Organization, ed. *Risk Assessment of Listeria Monocytogenes in Ready-to-Eat Foods: Interpretative Summary.* Rome: Food & Agricultural Organization of the United Nations, 2004.

LITHOTRIPSY

PROCEDURE

ANATOMY OR SYSTEM AFFECTED: Abdomen, bladder, kidneys, urinary system

SPECIALTIES AND RELATED FIELDS: Nephrology, urology

DEFINITION: A method of breaking up stones in the kidneys, ureters, and urinary bladder using shock waves or high-frequency sound waves.

INDICATIONS AND PROCEDURES

Stone fragmentation using shock waves or ultrasonic waves is less invasive, less painful, and less time consuming than conventional open surgery to remove stones or the organs that contain them. With lithotripsy, blood loss is minimal and recovery is quick, with a low morbidity (injury rate).

In extracorporeal shock-wave lithotripsy (ESWL), the patient is given either local or general anesthesia. A machine called a lithotripter is placed on the abdomen over the site of the stones. An emitter in the lithotripter sends out shock waves that break the stones into fine fragments that can pass through the urinary tract without harm to the patient, who is encouraged to drink copious amounts of fluid following the procedure.

In ultrasonic lithotripsy, an incision is made in the skin. The stone is approached and visualized with an endoscope, a hollow instrument with a telescope at one end for visualization. The other end of the instrument is introduced via the urethra into the bladder or ureter or via a small skin hole into the kidney. For kidney stones, a small needle is introduced into the kidney through the back under X-ray control, and a nephrostomy tract is established between the skin and the kidney. The ultrasonographic lithotripsy probe is intro-

duced through the endoscope and brought in contact with the stone.

A piezoceramic crystal is electrically stimulated, which generates ultrasonic waves that will fragment the stone. The design of the probe allows it to suction out the broken stone particles simultaneously. Larger stones can be fragmented into smaller pieces, which can then be grasped with forceps and pulled out. When a ureteral stone is treated by this method, a plastic tube (a double-J stent) is left in the ureter to prevent postoperative blockage and future scar formation. When a kidney stone is treated by this method, a large-caliber tube is left in the kidney (a nephrostomy tube) to drain the kidney and secure a tract for future X-ray studies

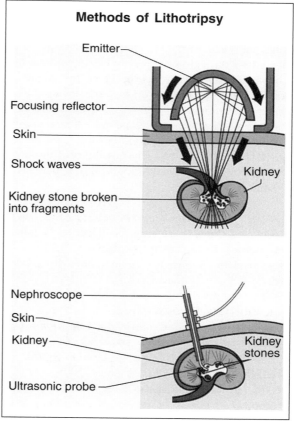

Kidney stones can be removed or broken into fragments using lithotripsy. In extracorporeal shock-wave lithotripsy (top), an emitter sends shock waves into tissues above the kidney stones, breaking the stones into very small fragments that can then be passed through the urine. In percutaneous lithotripsy (bottom), a nephroscope is inserted through the skin and into the kidney, where an ultrasonic probe breaks up and removes the stones.

and reinspection of the kidney for possible residual stone fragments.

USES AND COMPLICATIONS

The main morbidity associated with this procedure occurs during the establishment of the nephrostomy tract to gain access to the kidney, which can lead to bleeding, or during the introduction of the endoscope into the ureter, which can lead to perforation and future scarring. During stone fragmentation, it is imperative that the probe be in direct contact with the stone at all times, or it may cause ureteral perforation and bleeding. Overall, however, ultrasonographic lithotripsy is a safe and effective method of stone treatment, with few injuries and a quick recovery.

As with ultrasonic lithotripsy, few serious complications are associated with shock-wave lithotripsy. The presence of blood in the urine (hematuria) may be noted but is usually only temporary, as the stone fragments pass through the ureters, bladder, and urethra. Abdominal bruising may also occur, but this complication is minor in comparison to more invasive techniques. Severe pain that is unresponsive to medication may rarely signal perirenal hematoma. Other rare complications include pancreatitis and nerve palsy. Research is ongoing regarding the possibility of an association of ESWL with the development of hypertension in some patients.

—Saeed Akhter, M.D.;
updated by Victoria Price, Ph.D.

See also Cholecystectomy; Gallbladder; Gallbladder diseases; Kidney disorders; Kidneys; Nephrology; Stone removal; Stones; Ultrasonography; Urinary disorders; Urinary system; Urology.

FOR FURTHER INFORMATION:

Alexander, Ivy L., ed. *Urinary Tract and Kidney Diseases and Disorders Sourcebook: Basic Consumer Health Information About the Urinary System*. 2d ed. Detroit, Mich.: Omnigraphics, 2005.

Leikin, Jerrold B., and Martin S. Lipsky, eds. *American Medical Association Complete Medical Encyclopedia*. New York: Random House Reference, 2003.

Parker, James N., and Philip M. Parker, eds. *The 2002 Official Patient's Sourcebook on Kidney Stones*. San Diego, Calif.: Icon Health, 2002.

Tanagho, Emil A., and Jack W. McAninich, eds. *Smith's General Urology*. 17th ed. New York: McGraw-Hill, 2008.

Tierney, Lawrence M., Stephen J. McPhee, and Maxine A. Papadakis, eds. *Current Medical Diagnosis and Treatment 2006*. New York: McGraw-Hill Medical, 2006.

Walsh, Patrick C., et al., eds. *Campbell-Walsh Urology*. 4 vols. 9th ed. Philadelphia: Saunders/Elsevier, 2007.

LIVER

ANATOMY

ANATOMY OR SYSTEM AFFECTED: Abdomen, blood, circulatory system, endocrine system, gastrointestinal system, glands

SPECIALTIES AND RELATED FIELDS: Endocrinology, gastroenterology, hematology, internal medicine, toxicology

DEFINITION: A vital organ that contributes to control of blood sugar levels; metabolizes carbohydrates, lipids, and proteins; stores blood, iron, and some vitamins; degrades steroid hormones; and inactivates and/or excretes certain drugs and toxins.

KEY TERMS:

cirrhosis: a condition of the liver in which injured or dead cells are replaced with scar tissue

endoplasmic reticulum: a component of cells which in the liver is responsible for, among other things, the metabolism of xenobiotics

hepatitis: an infectious disease of the liver that is caused by a virus; at least three different types of hepatitis exist

hepatocyte: the functional cell of the liver; the liver contains only one type of functional cell

plasma proteins: any proteins found in the plasma of blood, which include those proteins necessary for blood clotting and some necessary for the transport of other molecules; most are produced by the liver

subclinical: referring to an infection in which the patient has no symptoms of disease; the infection is detected by other indicators, such as the presence of antibodies

virus: a subcellular particle that enters cells and causes cellular damage; it uses the cells' mechanisms to reproduce itself

xenobiotic: a nonbiological chemical that can enter a biological system; it could be a prescribed drug, a pollutant, or another substance

STRUCTURE AND FUNCTIONS

The liver, an accessory gland of the digestive system, is the largest organ in the human body. Located in the upper-right quadrant of the abdominal cavity, it abuts the diaphragm on the anterior surface. The liver is com-

The Anatomy of the Liver

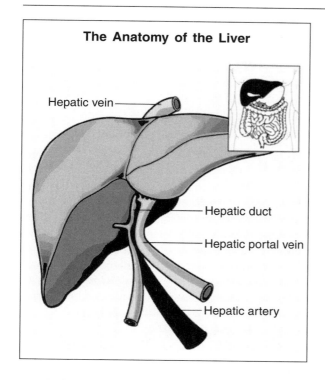

Hepatic vein

Hepatic duct

Hepatic portal vein

Hepatic artery

posed of two lobes of unequal size, with the large right lobe further divided into two smaller lobes. The organ is protected by the ribs, which cover nearly the entire surface. The liver contains only one type of functional cell, known as a hepatocyte. Closely associated with the organ is the gallbladder, a saclike structure that holds bile, a product of the hepatocytes. Bile is continually produced by the hepatocytes but is stored in the gallbladder until it is required for digestive products.

The liver is unique in that it receives blood from two different sources. The hepatic artery delivers blood to the liver from the systemic circulation. The liver also receives blood via the portal vein, which collects blood that has previously passed through the small intestine and has absorbed nutrients from the digestive system. As the blood enters the liver, it flows into dilated capillaries called sinusoids. Blood flow through sinusoids is much slower than through capillaries, and the exchange of materials between hepatocytes and the bloodstream is accomplished with little difficulty. This slower process also allows the liver to serve as a storage organ for blood, which gives the organ its characteristic dark red appearance.

The liver is essential to the normal functioning of the body. Its activities are many and varied: It regulates the metabolism of carbohydrates, lipids, and proteins; synthesizes proteins, particularly those of blood plasma

that control clotting; serves as a storage site for some vitamins and iron; degrades steroid hormones; and inactivates and/or excretes certain drugs and toxins.

The liver plays a major role in carbohydrate metabolism. As carbohydrates are absorbed from the small intestine, they are transported to the liver through the portal vein. The liver regulates blood sugar levels by removing excess quantities. If the diet includes too much glucose, this substance is stored in the liver or skeletal muscle as glycogen. If the blood sugar levels are low, the glycogen is broken down into glucose and released to the bloodstream. The liver is also capable of converting amino acids, lipids, or simple carbohydrates into glucose.

The principal functions of the liver in lipid metabolism are twofold. First, it is responsible for the breakdown of large fat molecules into small compounds that can be used for energy. Second, it synthesizes triglycerides, cholesterol, and phospholipids from other fats. All three of these compounds play important roles in cellular function.

The synthesis of proteins by the liver is of major importance for the body. The liver is capable of synthesizing not only a variety of proteins but also the nonessential amino acids that are the building blocks of proteins. Many of the proteins that the liver synthesizes are found in blood plasma, including those factors responsible for blood clotting. To protect the body against deficiencies in these substances, the liver stores vitamins A, D, and B_{12}. It is also capable of storing iron, the mineral necessary for the production of hemoglobin.

Located in the smooth endoplasmic reticulum of hepatocytes are nonspecific enzymes called the mixed-function oxidases. They are capable of metabolizing a wide variety of hormones, including some polypeptide hormones and the steroid hormones, such as cortisol, estrogen, and testosterone. These same enzymes are responsible for the degradation of many foreign substances that enter the body, such as prescription medications, illegal drugs, and toxins. Most of the materials metabolized are made more water-soluble, and therefore more easily excreted, by the kidney. Others are removed from the hepatocytes in the bile that the cells produce.

Production of bile by the hepatocytes is of utmost importance to the digestive system. Bile is composed of lecithin, cholesterol, bile pigments, proteins, and bile acids, along with an isotonic solution similar to blood plasma. Bile is produced continually and stored in the gallbladder. Several minutes after a meal begins, the gallbladder releases bile to the duodenum of the small intestine. The highest rate of bile release occurs during the duodenal digestion of food and is controlled by the hormone cholecystokinin. In the duodenum, bile acts as an emulsifier of fat in the diet. It breaks large lipid droplets into many small lipid droplets, which can more easily be digested by enzymes in the small intestine. About 95 percent of the bile is reabsorbed and returned to the liver, and the other 5 percent is excreted with the feces. This provides one mechanism for the body to use the digestive system for the removal of waste products. One important product that is excreted in this manner is bilirubin, a by-product of the normal destruction of old red blood cells.

DISORDERS AND DISEASES

The liver is unique among body organs because it has the ability to regenerate in cases of injury or disease. It is estimated that in a young, healthy individual a liver that has suffered a physical injury could regenerate as much as 80 percent of the total organ. Many important organs are paired, such as the lungs and kidneys. Though the liver is a single organ, its ability to regenerate ensures normal function even in cases of severe injury.

The presence of liver disease is detectable in many ways. With some diseases, the liver becomes enlarged and can be felt below the ribs. This swelling may be associated with localized discomfort or pain in the region. In more severe cases of liver disease, the organ may actually shrink and recede further under the ribs, a condition easily detected by a physician.

The pathophysiology of the liver is characterized by certain physiologic events that occur regardless of the underlying cause. Within the liver, disease may result in portal hypertension, blockage of bile ducts, and cellular injury or death. Cellular injury may be manifest by fatty infiltration and by interference with cellular functions, including the synthesis of proteins necessary for blood clotting, the metabolism of drugs or toxins, the regulation of glucose, and the production of bile. Any or all of these physiologic changes can lead to effects in other parts of the body.

Disease of the liver is often detectable by routine blood tests that include liver function tests. The patient may show decreased levels in the blood serum of proteins that are normally produced by the liver, an increased blood-clotting time, or increased serum levels of enzymes that are normally found only in the liver. A yellow skin tone known as jaundice has been associated with liver disease. This discoloration of skin and the sclera of the eye is a result of excessively high levels of bilirubin in the blood. Bilirubin is a by-product of the breakdown of red blood cells that are near the end of their 120-day life cycle.

The injury or death of liver cells may present a pathology unique to the liver, the disease cirrhosis. When hepatocytes are injured or diseased, they begin to accumulate lipids in vacuoles, giving the liver a whitish appearance. Associated with the development of a fatty liver, the cells may divide to produce more cells that will ensure normal function. Sometimes, however, this stimulation of cell division leads to an excess of hepatocytes, a condition that may result in abnormal patterns of blood flow through the liver. In addition, this phenomenon may include the production of large nodules of connective tissue to replace dead or dying cells, a condition comparable to scarring. The development of scars may cause increased blood pressure in the portal veins and may block bile ducts. Cirrhosis may be caused by a variety of conditions, including alcoholism, exposure to toxic substances, or infection. It is irreversible and ultimately causes the death of the patient.

Diseases of the liver can be classified according to the following scheme: congenital liver disorders, viral and nonviral infections, drug-induced and toxin-induced disease, vascular disorders, metabolic disorders, iron accumulation, alcoholic liver disease, and tumors.

The most common types of congenital diseases of the liver involve abnormalities of the bile ducts or of the portal vein, which may be associated with portal hypertension. More important, however, are those diseases that lead to the formation of cysts, such as polycystic liver disease or hepatic fibrosis. Jaundice of the newborn, a discoloration of the skin at birth, usually clears within a week or so with no long-term effects.

Viral infections of the liver may be associated with the hepatitis viruses or other viruses less specific for the liver. The four most common hepatitis viruses are hepatitis A, hepatitis B, hepatitis C, and hepatitis D. Hepatitis can also be associated with yellow fever, infectious mononucleosis, cytomegalovirus infection, and herpes simplex.

Hepatitis A is also known as infectious hepatitis. It is generally transmitted via fecal contamination of milk, water, or seafood. It is most common in the areas of the world where untreated sewage may come into contact with the water supply or food sources. It has a short incubation period and is usually not fatal; it does not lead to chronic hepatitis. Hepatitis B, also known as serum hepatitis, is transmitted from persons with an active form of the disease or from carriers via contaminated blood or blood products. It is particularly prevalent among drug users who share needles. The threat of contraction of hepatitis B from a transfusion has been greatly reduced by the screening of blood products. Hepatitis B has a long incubation period, up to six months. The severity of the disease varies greatly from subclinical hepatitis (showing no symptoms) to chronic hepatitis and in some cases may result in death. The course of hepatitis C disease resembles that of hepatitis B and may lead to chronic hepatitis. Hepatitis D is believed to be a defective virus that is found only in the presence of hepatitis B. It is transmitted via the same route and can result in chronic hepatitis. It occurs more commonly in Europe than in the United States.

Hepatitis from any cause may show subclinical or mild, influenza-like symptoms. Acute hepatitis may cause loss of appetite, vomiting, fever, jaundice, and enlargement of the liver. The viruses that cause hepatitis replicate within the liver cells, which could be the cause of the injury to these cells. Hepatocyte injury could also be a result of the immune system's attempt to fight the virus, which may injure the cells of the liver in the process. In either case, the damaged cells swell before they die. The liver can also be infected by bacterial cells, which usually reach the liver as a result of a systemic infection.

Many toxins or drugs can injure the liver, in a general pattern that is similar to the effects of infectious agents. The assault on the cell often leads to fatty infiltration, followed by swelling and finally by the death of the hepatocyte. Even in less severe cases of injury, those that do not lead to death of the hepatocyte, there is often impairment of the metabolic activities of the liver that can lead to diverse systemic effects. One of these effects is the ability to metabolize foreign compounds or naturally occurring steroids; the accumulation of these compounds throughout the body can have wide-ranging consequences.

The liver is adversely affected by the constant intake of excessive quantities of ethyl alcohol. In the early stages of alcoholism, the physiologic changes may be a result of improper nutrition or of vitamin deficiencies. During the more advanced stages of alcoholism, the patient is likely to suffer from a fatty liver and, ultimately, from cirrhosis. While those who stop drinking may slow down the advancement of cirrhosis, the disease appears to be irreversible.

There are more than five thousand metabolic enzymes in the liver, each of which is controlled geneti-

cally. Important in the treatment of metabolic disease is early diagnosis, which may prevent damage to other organs or to the liver. Dietary control may be used to minimize the effects of such conditions, leading to a near-normal life. Examples of treatable metabolic diseases are galactosemia, a condition which prevents the conversion of galactose to glucose; fructosemia, a condition that leads to the accumulation of fructose-1-phosphate; and Wilson's disease, an accumulation of copper in vital organs as a result of a defect in copper metabolism. In each case, the accumulation of a certain substance can lead to cellular damage, but dietary control of the substance can minimize the effects. Hemochromatosis is a similar disease that leads to accumulation of iron in the liver. As with Wilson's disease, the deposition of this element is not limited to the liver and can accumulate in other vital tissues of the body as well.

Cancer of the liver is usually caused by its spread from another site. Primary liver cancers are rare and usually do not occur until late in life. Risk factors may include exposure to hepatotoxins, chronic liver disease, or hepatitis B. There are two types of primary carcinomas of the liver: hepatocellular carcinoma, which develops in hepatocytes, and cholangiocellular carcinoma, which develops in bile ducts.

PERSPECTIVE AND PROSPECTS

The liver is a vital organ that plays a major role in the homeostasis of the body. Any condition that adversely influences the liver will have wide-ranging effects on other organs and the patient as a whole.

Because one of its functions is the metabolism of pollutants, drugs (including alcohol), and hormones, the liver is often exposed to substances that are toxic to its hepatocytes. When these compounds are encountered, the liver efficiently alters them for excretion. Sometimes, however, these substances may do damage to the cells before the liver can metabolize them.

When a liver cell is injured, the end result may be the death of the cell. Fortunately, liver cells are efficient at cell division and can replace those cells that have been injured or that have died. With continued damage to liver cells, however, the body can no longer replace them, and the resulting decrease in liver function leads to extensive complications throughout the body. A decrease in liver function will not only have an effect on the digestive system but will have wide-ranging effects on glucose and lipid metabolism (normal functions of the blood whose proteins are synthesized by the liver) and on the ability to remove certain foreign substances or toxins from the blood. For example, if the ability to metabolize medication is impaired by liver disease, the patient's body may accumulate high, even toxic, levels of drugs. These substances can have pronounced effects, particularly on the nervous system. With liver injury, the once-simple act of determining a medication dosage can become a critical problem.

Despite the liver's regenerative capacity, liver injury or disease can have permanent effects. However, some conditions previously thought incurable, such as chronic hepatitis B and C, can now be treated successfully in many cases with antiviral drugs and interferon. The medical community can treat the symptoms of hepatitis.

Cancer of the liver is also difficult to treat. Because it is not easily detected, the diagnosis is rarely early. Unless the cancer is restricted to one lobe that can be removed, surgery is rarely the answer. Treatment is further complicated by the fact that the liver cells are particularly sensitive to radiation and that the doses needed to treat the cancer would be deadly to hepatocytes. Chemotherapy has been the mainstay of treatment for both metastatic and primary liver cancer, but transplantation is increasingly recommended for patients with primary liver cancer.

With the discovery of immunosuppressive drugs, liver transplantation has become a positive procedure in the treatment of liver disease, and the results are promising. The availability of healthy livers for transplant, however, makes this an option limited to a small percentage of patients.

—Annette O'Connor, Ph.D.

See also Abdomen; Abdominal disorders; Alcoholism; Anatomy; Bile; Blood and blood disorders; Circulation; Cirrhosis; Gastroenterology; Gastroenterology, pediatric; Gastrointestinal disorders; Gastrointestinal system; Hematology; Hematology, pediatric; Hepatitis; Internal medicine; Jaundice; Liver cancer; Liver disorders; Liver transplantation; Metabolism; Nonalcoholic steatohepatitis (NASH); Systems and organs; Transplantation; Wilson's disease.

FOR FURTHER INFORMATION:

Chandrasoma, Parakrama, and Clive R. Taylor. *Concise Pathology.* 3d ed. Stamford, Conn.: Appleton & Lange, 1998. A pathology book written for health care personnel. It is well designed, and is appropriate for most laypersons.

Dollinger, Malin, et al. *Everyone's Guide to Cancer Therapy.* 5th ed. Kansas City, Mo.: Andrews McMeel, 2008. A well-organized book on therapy for various cancers, including a special section on liver cancers. Clearly describes the methods of treatment that are available and the treatment of choice. Written for the layperson.

Feldman, Mark, Lawrence S. Friedman, and Lawrence J. Brandt, eds. *Sleisenger and Fordtran's Gastrointestinal and Liver Disease: Pathophysiology, Diagnosis, Management.* New ed. 2 vols. Philadelphia: Saunders/Elsevier, 2010. A clinical text that covers basic liver anatomy; disorders of the gastrointestinal tract, biliary tree, pancreas, and liver; and related topics of nutrition and peritoneal diseases.

Guyton, Arthur C., and John E. Hall. *Guyton and Hall Textbook of Medical Physiology.* 12th ed. Philadelphia: Saunders/Elsevier, 2011. Although this is a text for medical students, the material is presented so well and with such a useful background that general readers will be able to understand the information that it contains. Offers good illustrations and tables that help to put everything in context.

McCance, Kathryn L., and Sue M. Huether. *Pathophysiology: The Biologic Basis for Disease in Adults and Children.* 6th ed. St. Louis, Mo.: Mosby/Elsevier, 2010. A very well written book on pathophysiology that not only presents the facts regarding certain diseases but also explains their physiological bases. Designed for student nurses, but its description of the physiology of the organ provides an extensive background for the less informed reader.

Scanlon, Valerie, and Tina Sanders. *Essentials of Anatomy and Physiology.* 5th ed. Philadelphia: F. A. Davis, 2007. A text designed around three themes: the relationship between physiology and anatomy, the interrelations among the organ systems, and the relationship of each organ system to homeostasis.

LIVER CANCER
DISEASE/DISORDER

ANATOMY OR SYSTEM AFFECTED: Liver

SPECIALTIES AND RELATED FIELDS: Gastroenterology, immunology, oncology, radiology

DEFINITION: Malignancies of the liver, which may be primary (arising in the organ itself) but are more likely to be secondary (metastasizing from another site).

CAUSES AND SYMPTOMS

The liver filters the blood supply, removing and breaking down (metabolizing) toxins and delivering them through the biliary tract to the intestines for elimination

INFORMATION ON LIVER CANCER

CAUSES: Metastasized tumors, genetic factors, radiation, occupational exposure to chemicals, dietary toxins, medical therapies, cirrhosis

SYMPTOMS: Ambiguous; typically includes jaundice and liver enlargement and tenderness

DURATION: One to twenty-nine months; often fatal

TREATMENTS: Chemotherapy, surgery

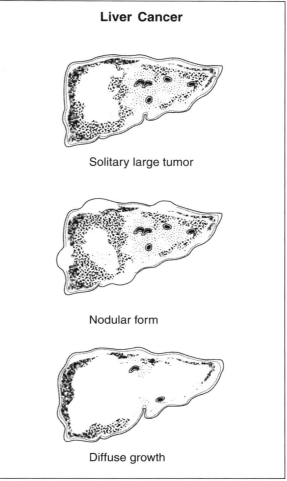

Liver Cancer

Solitary large tumor

Nodular form

Diffuse growth

The liver is a frequent site of cancer, most commonly from malignancies that have spread from their original site. The particular form the cancer takes depends on several factors, notably the primary source and its possible cause.

with other wastes. Because of the large volume of blood flowing through the liver (about a quarter of the body's supply), blood-borne toxins or cancer cells migrating from tumors elsewhere (the process called metastasis) pose a constant threat. In fact, in the United States most liver cancers are metastatic; only about 1 percent actually originate in the liver. In Southeast Asia and sub-Saharan Africa, primary liver cancer is the most common type, accounting for as much as 30 percent of all cancers.

Two major types of cancer affect the liver: those involving liver cells (hepatocellular carcinomas) and those involving the bile ducts (cholangiocarcinomas). The first is by far the more common, although tumors may contain a mixture of both, and their development is similar. Tumors may arise in one location, forming a large mass; arise in several locations, forming nodes; or spread throughout the liver in a diffuse form. Liver cancers occur in men about four to eight times more frequently than in women and in blacks slightly more than in whites, although the proportions vary widely among different regions of the world. In the United States, most cancers arise in people fifty years old or older; in other areas, people older than forty are at risk.

Primary liver cancer has so much regional and gender variation because causative agents are more or less common in different areas and men are more often exposed. A leading risk factor in the United States and Europe is cirrhosis, a scarring of liver tissue following destruction by viruses, toxins, or interrupted blood flow. In the United States, long-term alcohol consumption is the most common cause of cirrhosis, and men have long been more likely than women to become alcoholics. Likewise, hemochromatosis, a hereditary disease leading to the toxic buildup of iron, is a cancer precursor and more common in men than in women. In Africa and Southeast Asia, the hepatitis B and C viruses are leading precancer diseases because hepatitis has long been endemic in those areas, whereas in the United States it is not widespread (although the number of infected people began to rise in the 1980's).

Diet and medical therapies have also been implicated as liver carcinogens. Food toxins, especially aflatoxin from mold growing on peanuts (which are a staple in parts of Africa and Asia); oral contraceptives; anabolic steroids; and the high levels of sex hormones used in some treatments are thought to increase the likelihood of hepatobiliary tumors. Genetic factors, radiation, and occupational exposure to volatile chemicals may also play a minor role.

Although researchers generally agree about which agents are liver cancer precursors, the exact mechanism leading to tumor development is not thoroughly understood. Nevertheless, one factor may be universal. Viruses and toxins injure or destroy liver and bile duct cells; the body reacts to repair the damage with inflammation and an increased rate of new cell growth, a condition called regenerative hyperplasia. If the toxin damage continues, triggering ever more hyperplasia, as is the case with hepatitis and alcoholic cirrhosis, formation of a tumor becomes almost inevitable.

Like lymph nodes, the liver collects migrating cancer cells, so the cancers that physicians detect there often are metastases from cancers arising elsewhere in the body. In fact, liver involvement may be found before the primary cancer has been recognized. Colorectal cancer is especially given to metastasizing to the liver, since the digestive tract's blood supply is directly linked to the liver through the portal vein; similarly, lung and breast cancer may spread to the liver. Such metastases indicate advanced cancers that do not bode well for the patient's survival.

Symptoms may be ambiguous. Two common symptoms are jaundice and enlargement of the liver, with accompanying tenderness. Jaundice, a yellowing of the skin and eyes, is caused by an accumulation of bilirubin. Bilirubin builds up because a tumor has blocked the bile duct that normally empties it into the small intestine. (Both symptoms may also occur as a result of either gallstones or cirrhosis.) Patients with liver cancer may also have a fever and retain fluid in the abdominal cavities.

IN THE NEWS: PERCUTANEOUS HEPATIC PERFUSION (PHP)

In 2009, a much-anticipated clinical trial, sponsored by the National Cancer Institute, completed enrollment for testing percutaneous hepatic perfusion (PHP) as an improved method for treating liver cancer. PHP diverts the blood going into and out of the liver so that high doses of toxic drugs can be added without harming the rest of the body. This "regional chemotherapy" is used for cancers that are especially difficult to treat, which is frequently the case with liver cancer.

By the time that liver cancer has been diagnosed, it has typically spread to the whole organ, making it impossible to remove surgically (resection). Chemotherapy by that time is often futile as well, and any hope of success requires extreme measures. One such measure that has been around for nearly fifty years is to surgically reroute the blood vessels so that blood circulates through the liver via a pump that delivers the anticancer drug. After about thirty minutes, clean blood is reintroduced, and blood flow is rerouted back to normal. About ten years ago, investigators began experimenting with a nonsurgical procedure for rerouting the blood flow. The latest incarnation, and the subject of the clinical trial, is a system patented by Delcath Systems, Inc., that uses special catheters (ultra-fine tubing that can snake through veins and arteries) threaded up from the groin until they reach the liver. One catheter is then inflated to block normal blood flow into the liver while serving at the same as an artificial blood vessel for delivering the chemotherapy. The other catheter blocks the blood flow exiting the liver and provides a channel for sending the toxic blood through a filter that removes the drug. The filtered blood is returned to the patient through a third catheter in the neck. The big advantage of using catheters is that inserting them is relatively quick and easy. The absence of surgical trauma also permits repeated rounds of treatment so that oncologists can treat the cancer as aggressively as possible.

—Brad Rikke, Ph.D.

TREATMENT AND THERAPY

Doctors suspecting liver cancer conduct tests designed to distinguish this disease from other disorders. Palpation of the liver may reveal that the organ is enlarged or contains an unusual tissue mass, which is likely to be a tumor. A rubbing sound heard through the stethoscope may also come from a tumor. Hepatocellular carcinoma often elevates the alpha-fetoprotein level in blood. Abdominal ultrasound or computed tomography (CT) scans can provide good evidence of a tumor in the liver, and a biopsy will supply a tissue sample capable of proving the presence of cancer, especially if the biopsy is done with CT scan or ultrasound guidance. A tumor can also disrupt normal biochemical action in the body, which doctors may detect in blood tests. Liver function blood tests may be abnormal with both primary and secondary liver cancer.

Under even the most favorable circumstances, the outlook for patients with liver cancer is still not good. If a primary cancer is found while still fairly small, surgical removal is the surest and fastest treatment, although it is a difficult, risky procedure because of the liver's complex, delicate structure. Radiation and chemotherapy have not succeeded in shrinking tumors effectively. Because symptoms usually appear late in the development of primary liver cancer, it seldom is found early enough for surgical cure; patients usually live only one to two months after detection. Those found with small, removable cancers live an average of twenty-nine months. Most liver cancers are metastases, however, and removal of the liver tumor will not rid the patient of cancer. In general, hepatobiliary cancer patients have a 5 percent chance of living five years after diagnosis.

Liver cancer screening tests can locate tumors while they are still treatable, although routine physical examinations in Western nations seldom include such tests. Usually only patients with cirrhosis or chronic hepatitis are screened. The best ways to ward off liver cancer are to avoid viral infection and to abstain from alcohol. For those at risk for infection, such as health care workers, the most effective primary prevention is vaccination for hepatitis B.

—Roger Smith, Ph.D.

See also Alcoholism; Cancer; Carcinogens; Chemotherapy; Cirrhosis; Hepatitis; Jaundice; Liver; Liver disorders; Liver transplantation; Malignancy and metastasis; Oncology; Radiation therapy; Tumor removal; Tumors.

FOR FURTHER INFORMATION:

Curley, Steven A., ed. *Liver Cancer.* New York: Springer, 1998. Provides the general surgeon, surgical oncologist, radiation oncologist, and medical oncologist with current information regarding diagnosis and multimodality treatment approaches for patients with primary or metastatic hepatobiliary cancer.

Dollinger, Malin, et al. *Everyone's Guide to Cancer Therapy.* 5th ed. Kansas City, Mo.: Andrews Mc-Meel, 2008. A well-organized book on therapy for various cancers, including a special section on liver cancers. Clearly describes the methods of treatment that are available and the treatment of choice. Written for the layperson.

Eyre, Harmon J., Dianne Partie Lange, and Lois B. Morris. *Informed Decisions: The Complete Book of Cancer Diagnosis, Treatment, and Recovery.* 2d ed. Atlanta: American Cancer Society, 2002. The American Cancer Society endorses this excellent book, which provides a complete consumer reference for cancer diagnosis, treatment, and recovery.

Liver Cancer Network. http://www.livercancer.com. A group founded through and supported by Pittsburgh's Allegheny General Hospital. The group's mission is to provide liver cancer patients and their families with the basic knowledge needed to better communicate with their physicians and to give patients and families hope for the future. Gives excellent information about the liver's anatomy, and the disease's diagnosis and treatment.

Parker, James N., and Philip M. Parker, eds. *The Official Patient's Sourcebook on Adult Primary Liver Cancer.* San Diego, Calif.: Icon Health, 2002. Guides patients in using the Web to educate themselves about the disease and draws from public, academic, government, and peer-reviewed research to provide information on virtually all topics related to adult primary liver cancer, from the essentials to the most advanced areas of research.

Sachar, David B., Jerome D. Waye, and Blair S. Lewis. *Pocket Guide to Gastroenterology.* Rev. ed. Baltimore: Williams & Wilkins, 1991. Discusses such topics as gastroenterology, the digestive organs, and digestive system diseases. Includes bibliographical references and an index.

Shannon, Joyce Brennfleck. *Liver Disorders Sourcebook.* Detroit, Mich.: Omnigraphics, 2000. This book includes basic consumer health information about the liver and how it works; liver diseases, including cancer, cirrhosis, hepatitis, and toxic and drug-related diseases; tips for maintaining a healthy liver; laboratory tests; radiology tests and facts about liver transplantation; and a section on support groups, a glossary, and resources listing.

Steen, R. Grant. *A Conspiracy of Cells: The Basic Science of Cancer.* New York: Plenum Press, 1993. Thorough, lucid explanations of all physiological aspects of cancer make this book instructive for readers willing to slog through the subject's complexity and terminology.

LIVER DISORDERS

DISEASE/DISORDER

ANATOMY OR SYSTEM AFFECTED: Liver

SPECIALTIES AND RELATED FIELDS: Gastroenterology, internal medicine

DEFINITION: As one of the most complex organs in the body, the liver is the target of a wide variety of toxins, infectious agents, and cancers that lead to hepatitis, cirrhosis, abscesses, and liver failure.

KEY TERMS:

abscess: a localized collection of pus and infectious microorganisms

ascites: the presence of free fluid in the abdominal cavity

bilirubin: a major component of bile, derived from the breakdown products of red blood cells

cirrhosis: the fibrous scar tissue that replaces the normally soft liver after repeated damage by viruses, chemicals, and/or alcohol

hepatitis: inflammation of the liver, such as that caused by viruses or toxins

jaundice: a yellow discoloration of the skin, eyes, and membranes caused by excess bilirubin in the blood

portal hypertension: elevated pressures in the portal veins caused by resistance to blood flow through a diseased liver; produces many regional problems, including ascites

portal system: a system of veins, unique to the liver, that carry nutrient-rich blood from the digestive organs to the liver

CAUSES AND SYMPTOMS

The liver is the largest internal organ, lying in the upper-right abdominal cavity. Intricately attached to it by a system of ducts on its lower surface is the pear-shaped gallbladder. Unique to the liver is a blood supply that derives from two separate sources: the hepatic artery, carrying freshly oxygenated blood from the heart, and the portal vein, carrying blood rich in the products of digestion from the digestive organs. The liver cells, or hepatocytes, are arranged in thin sheets that are separated by large pores, blood vessels, and ducts. The result is a very soft, spongy organ filled with a large volume of blood.

The liver performs a wide variety of complex and diverse functions, more so than any other organ. Most commonly known is the production of bile, which is formed from the breakdown of red blood cells, cholesterol, and salts; stored in the gallbladder; and used in the small intestine to digest fats. The liver also serves the all-important purpose of detoxification by chemically altering harmful substances such as alcohol, drugs, and ammonia from protein digestion. Additionally, the liver is involved in the formation of such essential materials as blood proteins, blood-clotting factors, and sugar and fat storage compounds.

Because of the liver's many responsibilities and unique position as an intermediary between the digestive process and the blood (via the portal vein), it easily falls prey to many disease-causing agents. Chemicals, illegal drugs, alcohol, viruses, parasites, hormones, and even medical drugs can damage the liver and have widespread effects on the rest of the body. The liver is also the most frequent target of cancer cells that have spread beyond their primary site. In the United States and other industrialized countries, liver disease is usually related to alcoholism and cancer, while in the developing world it is often the result of infectious contamination by viruses and parasites.

There are two simplified methods of classifying liver disorders. The first is based on cause: infections (viruses and parasites), injury (alcohol and other toxins), inheritance (inability to perform certain functions), infiltration (iron and copper deposits), and tumors (both benign and malignant). The second method of classification is based on the result: hepatitis (inflammation), cirrhosis (permanent injury from alcohol or other toxins), and cancer, for example.

Each of these liver diseases produces a particular set of signs and symptoms depending on the length of time and the specific disruption of structure and function. Pain and swelling rarely occur alone and are usually associated with one or more of the following: nausea and vomiting, jaundice, ascites, blood-clotting defects, and encephalopathy. Indeed, in some cases liver failure ensues, leading to coma and death.

Jaundice, a yellow discoloration of the skin and whites (sclera) of the eyes, is caused by the secretion of bile precursors (bilirubin) from the damaged liver cells directly into the blood rather than into the ducts leading to the gallbladder. Consequently, bilirubin accumulates in the body's tissues, including the skin and eyes. Ascites, the collection of fluid beneath the liver in the abdomen, is an important sign of liver disease. This fluid comes primarily from the portal vein system, which lies between the liver and the digestive organs.

INFORMATION ON LIVER DISORDERS

CAUSES: Cirrhosis, infection, disease, abscess, liver failure, injury, genetic factors, tumors

SYMPTOMS: Vary; can include pain, swelling, nausea and vomiting, jaundice, easy bruising, excessive bleeding, blood clotting problems

DURATION: Acute to chronic

TREATMENTS: Drug therapy, surgery, transplant; most often symptomatic relief and supportive care

As the liver becomes congested and enlarged in response to injury or infection, blood flow becomes difficult and pressure begins to build, causing liquid to leak from the blood vessels into the abdominal cavity. Easy bruising, excessive bleeding, and other problems with blood clotting are important signs that reflect the failure of the liver to produce essential blood proteins. Neuropsychiatric symptoms such as a flapping hand tremor and encephalopathy (a state of mental confusion and disorientation that can quickly progress to coma) are not well understood, but it is likely that they result from an accumulation of toxic substances that would normally be cleared from the blood by the liver. Several other problems, such as the enlargement of male breasts, atrophy of the testicles, and other sexual changes, derive from the inability of the liver to clear the blood of hormones.

Hepatitis, an inflammation of the liver generally caused by viruses, is one of the most common diseases in the world. Hepatitis A, B, and C; Epstein-Barr virus (the causative agent of mononucleosis); and herpes are a few of the organisms that can infect the liver. Hepatitis A, transmitted through contaminated food, water, and shellfish, is usually a self-limited disease that resolves itself. Hepatitis B, transmitted through contact with infected blood and body secretions, is much more serious, with a carrier state, progressive organ damage, cancer, and death as possible sequelae. Hepatitis C is

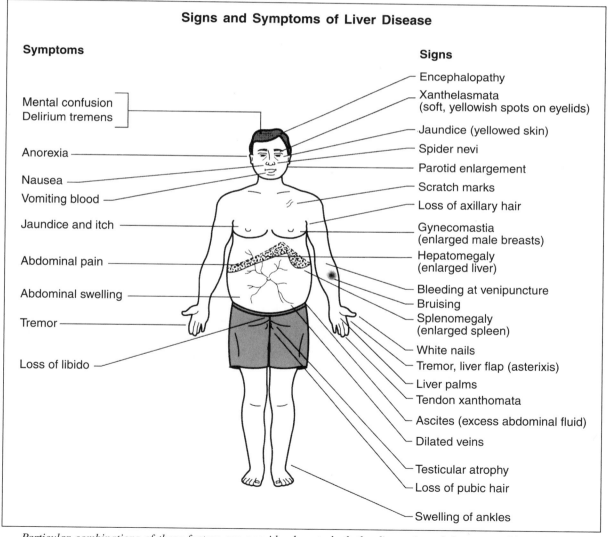

Signs and Symptoms of Liver Disease

Symptoms

- Mental confusion
- Delirium tremens
- Anorexia
- Nausea
- Vomiting blood
- Jaundice and itch
- Abdominal pain
- Abdominal swelling
- Tremor
- Loss of libido

Signs

- Encephalopathy
- Xanthelasmata (soft, yellowish spots on eyelids)
- Jaundice (yellowed skin)
- Spider nevi
- Parotid enlargement
- Scratch marks
- Loss of axillary hair
- Gynecomastia (enlarged male breasts)
- Hepatomegaly (enlarged liver)
- Bleeding at venipuncture
- Bruising
- Splenomegaly (enlarged spleen)
- White nails
- Tremor, liver flap (asterixis)
- Liver palms
- Tendon xanthomata
- Ascites (excess abdominal fluid)
- Dilated veins
- Testicular atrophy
- Loss of pubic hair
- Swelling of ankles

Particular combinations of these factors can provide clues to both the diagnosis and the extent of liver damage.

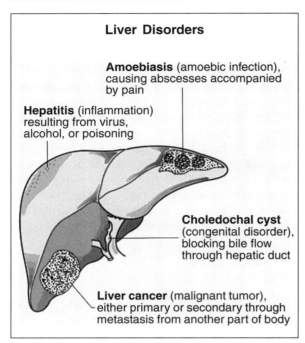

Liver Disorders

Amoebiasis (amoebic infection), causing abscesses accompanied by pain

Hepatitis (inflammation) resulting from virus, alcohol, or poisoning

Choledochal cyst (congenital disorder), blocking bile flow through hepatic duct

Liver cancer (malignant tumor), either primary or secondary through metastasis from another part of body

The liver's unique structure and functions leave it vulnerable to a wide range of diseases.

transmitted by intravenous drug use or blood transfusion. Infection most often causes no symptoms initially but leads to chronic infection in about 80 percent of individuals. Chronic infection progresses to cirrhosis in 20 to 30 percent of cases and may lead to liver cancer. Noninfectious causes of hepatitis in susceptible people include such frequently used substances as acetaminophen (Tylenol), halothane (general anesthesia), and oral contraceptives. Nonalcoholic steatohepatitis (NASH) is a disease that causes chronic inflammation and, upon biopsy, resembles alcoholic hepatitis. It is diagnosed in patients with persistent abnormal liver function tests, no evidence of hepatitis B or C, and consumption of less than 40 grams of ethanol per week. NASH is most often found in patients with obesity, type 2 diabetes, and hyperlipidemia.

Cirrhosis is the result of continuous toxic exposure that injures the liver beyond repair. Fibrous scar tissue replaces the normally soft, spongy organ, making it small and firm, with few hepatocytes capable of functioning normally. Chronic alcohol abuse is by far the most frequent factor in the development of cirrhosis. Severe ascites, bleeding disorders, encephalopathy, and sex organ changes often herald imminent liver failure and death from this disease.

Liver cancer is most often secondary to malignan-cies that have spread from other sites. In Asia and Africa, primary tumors of the liver itself are much more common, in part because of several factors: a high incidence of hepatitis B infection, food toxins, and parasite infestation. Chronic injury appears to play the critical role in liver cancer; hence the risk factors that have been established are cirrhosis, hepatitis B and C, and long-term exposure to a variety of chemicals, hormones, and drugs. Benign tumors may occur in young women who use oral contraceptives, but they are relatively infrequent.

Several other hepatic diseases warrant mention. Liver abscesses, encapsulated areas filled with infectious material, can be caused by bacteria, fungi, and parasites. These organisms enter the bloodstream through ingestion, skin puncture, or even intestinal rupture (as occurs in appendicitis and diverticulitis), and travel to the liver. Two unusual but notable disorders of iron and copper metabolism—hemochromatosis and Wilson's disease, respectively—have prominent liver involvement. While the disease mechanisms are not well understood, these essential metals are retained in excess and deposited in body tissues in toxic levels, causing damage. Finally, several genetic disorders of bile production run the gamut from mere nuisances to death in infancy. Disruption in bilirubin metabolism, the handling of red blood cell waste products by incorporation into bile, is affected to varying degrees. Severe jaundice reflects the accumulation of toxic levels of bilirubin in all body tissues, including the brain.

TREATMENT AND THERAPY

The diagnosis of a patient with suspected liver disease occurs in an orderly process that begins with a thorough history and physical examination, supported by a number of valuable blood tests and imaging techniques. Liver biopsy, the obtaining of a tissue sample for microscopic analysis, is often a final and definitive procedure if the disorder remains ambiguous. Both the cause and the chronology or state of the disease (whether of recent onset or advanced) determine treatment and outcome. While many signs and symptoms are nonspecific—nausea, vomiting, pain, hepatic enlargement, and jaundice—others such as ascites, encephalopathy, blood-clotting defects, and sex organ changes reflect significant organ damage and an advanced stage of disease. Careful questioning of the recent and past history of a patient can elicit facts that point to a diagnosis: exposure to known liver toxins such as alcohol, anesthetics, certain medications, and occupational chemicals;

travel to countries with known contaminated water supplies (hepatitis A); blood transfusions, kidney dialysis, sexual promiscuity, or intravenous drug abuse (hepatitis B and C); weight loss that is unexplained (cancer); or even a history of gallstones (blocked bile ducts between the liver and gallbladder). Armed with suspicions from the history, the physician uses the physical examination to note signs that confirm or reject the possibilities. A small and firm liver with ascites, tremor, enlarged male breasts, and small, shrunken testicles all point to an advanced stage of cirrhosis, for example. An enlarged painful liver, with vomiting, jaundice, fever, and recent raw shellfish ingestion, would likely suggest hepatitis A.

Blood tests play the second critical role in evaluating liver disease. An elevated bilirubin level would correlate with the severity of jaundice. Blood protein levels (albumin) and blood-clotting factors (prothrombin) may be dangerously low, revealing a near inability of the hepatocytes to synthesize these vital substances. Special chemicals that exist primarily in liver cells (hepatic enzymes and the aminotransferases) may be quite high, because the cells die and release their contents into the blood. Finally, elevated white blood cell counts and special tests for individual infections (viruses, bacteria, fungi, and parasites) can positively establish the diagnosis.

Depending on the suspected disease, confirmation may be needed from various imaging techniques, chosen specifically for a particular diagnosis. Plain X rays do little to visualize the liver, although they can reveal air in the abdomen, a consequence of a perforated intestine, appendix, or ulcer. A much more advanced method, the computed tomography (CT) scan, combines computer-generated views of multiple cross-sectional X rays, providing a highly detailed examination of the liver and thereby establishing a diagnosis in the majority of cases. Two other techniques that have more specific uses are ultrasound, which uses sound wave transmission, and magnetic resonance imaging (MRI), which uses magnetic fields to create an image. Ultrasound can readily distinguish solid masses from those that are fluid-filled (tumors versus abscesses) and can view the bile ducts. MRI is quite helpful in determining blood flow problems such as portal hypertension.

Finally, if a precise diagnosis remains ambiguous, a biopsy is performed. A sample of liver tissue is obtained using a large needle inserted through the skin, under the guidance of an ultrasound image. The sample is then viewed microscopically, and both the cause and the extent of liver damage are readily apparent. Treatment options for the majority of liver diseases are improving. If drug toxicity is suspected, especially from alcohol, immediate withdrawal of the agent can prevent further damage, as has been shown in cirrhosis. Obstructing gallstones can be surgically removed to relieve pressure in the bile ducts. Combinations of surgery, radiation, and chemotherapy are used in liver cancer, but the prognosis is poor. Little can be done for the inherited diseases of bilirubin metabolism, while some success has been achieved in treating the iron and copper storage diseases.

Infections of viral origin have specific treatment regimens. Prevention of hepatitis A and B is possible if pooled serum immunoglobulin is given immediately after exposure. This substance is a concentrated form of antibodies obtained from infected individuals whose diseases have completely resolved; essentially, it is a method of giving passive immunity. Chronic hepatitis B may be effectively treated with several antiviral medications or interferon. Chronic hepatitis C is treated with a combination of an antiviral medication (Ribavirin) plus interferon. Response rates to therapy depend upon the viral load, the genotype of the virus, and compliance with treatment and range between 50 and 80 percent. There are no specific therapies proven effective for treatment of NASH. Treatment is recommended for associated medical conditions, including weight loss, reduction of lipids (cholesterol and triglycerides), and control of diabetes. One area in which effective treatment does exist is in bacterial, fungal, and parasitic infections and abscesses. Appropriate antibiotics and surgical drainage yield dramatic improvement in most cases.

In many cases of liver disease, symptom relief and nutritional support, often carried out in the hospital, are the only options. Pain relief and the administration of intravenous fluid and nutrients to counteract vomiting and dehydration are the first steps. Ascites is relieved through bed rest, salt restriction, diuretics, and paracentesis, a procedure that uses ultrasound to guide a needle into the abdomen and withdraw fluid. Attempts to correct encephalopathy by removing toxins such as ammonia from the blood are generally ineffective, and mental changes, along with other intractable symptoms, often herald complete liver failure and imminent death.

Clearly, preventive measures are the most important factor in liver disease. One effective measure that is widely available is the hepatitis B vaccine, which is recommended during childhood in a three-injection series. Hepatitis A vaccine is available and recommended in children older than one year. Hepatitis A and B vaccines are recommended to any non-immune adult with chronic liver disease.

PERSPECTIVE AND PROSPECTS

Liver transplantation offers approximately four thousand patients per year replacement of the diseased organ with a normal, donated one. Begun experimentally in the early 1960's after decades of low success rates (less than 20 percent), it has finally been accepted as a lifesaving operation, with survival rates exceeding 70 percent at five years. Technical improvements, especially intraoperative blood circulation and cadaver organ preservation, have been combined with advances in immunosuppressive therapy that counteract rejection and refined patient selection and timing. The result is that liver transplantation has become the method of choice for patients whose liver disease is life-threatening, progressive, and unresponsive to other treatments.

Specific guidelines exist for both children and adults to be considered candidates for the procedure. It is imperative that the person is otherwise healthy and that the heart, lungs, kidneys, and brain are functioning well. Malignancy, human immunodeficiency virus (HIV) infection, incorrectable congenital defects, and continuing drug or alcohol abuse are obvious contraindications. However, infants with inherited, inevitably fatal liver disorders are good candidates, as are adults with end-stage liver failure from chronic hepatitis, for example. Controversial indications, requiring case-by-case evaluation, include advanced viral hepatitis (as recurrent infection in the donated organ often occurs) and alcohol-induced cirrhosis (because of the likelihood of damage to other organs and the high relapse rate after surgery). Relapse is also very common if the transplantation is done for a primary liver cancer.

Careful donor selection is equally important. The principal source of cadaver organs is victims of head trauma who are declared brain-dead. Organs are accepted from those sixty years of age or younger who had no viral, bacterial, or fungal infections and who were otherwise healthy up to the time of death. In the United States, recipient-donor matches are made through a nationwide organ transplantation registry, with highest priority going to those most critically ill. Only twelve to eighteen hours can elapse between organ retrieval and implantation—beyond that, liver tissue begins to degenerate.

The use of immunosuppressive therapy, drugs that keep the recipient's immune system in check, has contributed significantly to success and survival. Rejection of the transplanted organ remains one of the most feared postoperative complications, along with hemorrhaging. Because the body recognizes the organ as foreign tissue, the immune system's white blood cells attack and damage the implanted donor liver. The use of drugs to counteract this process allows the new liver to heal and the body to adapt to the presence of foreign tissue. Despite the use of these potent drugs, which themselves have serious side effects, rejection continues to be a problem. Nevertheless, one-year survival rates are 87 percent, and at five years, 73 percent of transplant patients are alive.

—Connie Rizzo, M.D., Ph.D.
updated by James P. McKenna, M.D.

See also Abdomen; Abdominal disorders; Alcoholism; Cirrhosis; Hepatitis; Jaundice; Liver; Liver cancer; Liver transplantation; Nonalcoholic steatohepatitis (NASH); Wilson's disease.

FOR FURTHER INFORMATION:

American Liver Foundation. http://www.liverfoundation .org. Provides physician referrals and information on support groups for persons with liver disease and their families.

Blumberg, Baruch S. *Hepatitis B: The Hunt for a Killer Virus*. Princeton, N.J.: Princeton University Press, 2003. A scientific memoir, the book traces the research and investigative twists and turns that led to the hepatitis B antigen, the elusive virus itself, and, finally, the vaccine.

Chopra, Sanjiv. *The Liver Book: A Comprehensive Guide to Diagnosis, Treatment, and Recovery*. New York: Simon & Schuster, 2002. Covers myriad information about liver disorders including how doctors diagnose liver ailments, what to expect from tests and screening, hepatitis B and hepatitis C, liver transplants, and the role of alternative treatments.

Feldman, Mark, Lawrence S. Friedman, and Lawrence J. Brandt, eds. *Sleisenger and Fordtran's Gastrointestinal and Liver Disease: Pathophysiology, Diagnosis, Management*. New ed. 2 vols. Philadelphia: Saunders/Elsevier, 2010. A clinical text that covers basic liver anatomy; disorders of the gastrointestinal tract, biliary tree, pancreas, and liver; and related topics of nutrition and peritoneal diseases.

Fishman, Mark, et al. *Medicine*. 5th ed. Philadelphia: Lippincott Williams & Wilkins, 2004. This excellent soft cover text is the perfect place to start. Used by medical students and other health professionals, it is clear and understandable, exploring normal biology and the process of disease.

Goldman, Lee, and Dennis Ausiello, eds. *Cecil Textbook of Medicine*. 23d ed. Philadelphia: Saunders/Elsevier, 2007. This bible of internal medicine has a superb section on liver diseases that is somewhat difficult but so well written and thorough that it is worth the effort. The text is well supplemented with diagrams and photographs.

Yamada, Todataka, et al., eds. *Textbook of Gastroenterology*. 5th ed. Hoboken, N.J.: Blackwell, 2009. The reference text used by specialists in the field, covering all aspects of the digestive system. A large section is devoted to the liver and gallbladder.

LIVER TRANSPLANTATION
PROCEDURE

ANATOMY OR SYSTEM AFFECTED: Abdomen, gallbladder, liver

SPECIALTIES AND RELATED FIELDS: Gastroenterology, general surgery

DEFINITION: Surgery performed to replace a diseased, nonfunctional liver with one that is healthy and capable of carrying out normal liver functions.

KEY TERMS:

bile: fluid produced by the liver and stored in the gallbladder to be secreted into the intestine; contains salts, bile pigments (bilirubin), cholesterol, and other waste products

cirrhosis: a severe degenerative condition in which healthy liver tissue is replaced with nonfunctional scar tissue; alcohol and drug abuse are the most common causes

hepatic: of or referring to the liver

hepatitis: inflammation of the liver

jaundice: a yellowish coloration of the skin and mucous membranes caused by high levels of bilirubin in the blood; the result of liver malfunction

INDICATIONS AND PROCEDURES

Liver transplantation is performed on individuals whose livers are severely diseased and unable to carry out normal liver functions. The most common cause of liver failure in adults is cirrhosis, which results from alcohol and/or drug abuse. In this condition, the liver becomes filled with tough, nonfunctional scar tissue. Symptoms of cirrhosis, as well as other liver diseases, include abnormal levels of liver enzymes in the blood,

jaundice, a lack of blood-clotting factors, the inability to dispose of bile, and the failure to detoxify metabolic by-products and other poisons, which can lead to coma and death. Other conditions that can lead to liver disease include hepatic cancer, long-term hepatitis B infection, and obstruction of the bile passages in the liver.

The donor liver may be obtained from a recently deceased individual, or a section of the liver can be obtained from a living donor. In either case, the donated organ must be a close immunological match to reduce the chance of transplant rejection. A preoperative injection is given to the recipient to dry up internal fluids and promote drowsiness, and general anesthesia is administered. A vertical incision is made from just below the breastbone to the navel. Muscles are moved aside, and a second incision is made through the outer membranous lining of the body cavity, revealing the internal organs. Bypass tubes are inserted into the hepatic veins and connected to veins in the arm to divert the flow of blood from the liver. When this is completed, the hepatic veins are cut, and the liver and gallbladder are removed from the body cavity. The veins of the donor liver are connected to the recipient veins, and the bypass tubes are removed. The new liver is then connected to the intestine, and the incisions are closed.

USES AND COMPLICATIONS

Liver transplantation is performed only when the individual has no other chance for survival. Typically, there is a long waiting list for available organs. Certain factors such as blood type and protein markers on cell surfaces must be matched as closely as possible in order to avoid rejection by the recipient's immune system. A liver from a recently deceased donor may be kept functioning only for five hours with specific cooling fluid, thus limiting its ability to be transported long distances. Because of the lack of available transplant organs and the necessity of compatibility, many people die before an appropriate organ becomes available. It is possible to transplant a segment of liver from a close relative; the liver can grow considerably and regenerate itself. This is a preferable situation and eliminates the pressure of transporting a donor liver between hospitals while attempting to keep it functioning.

After liver transplantation, the patient is kept in an intensive care unit for several days and in bed for at least a week. Pain from the incisions is alleviated with drugs. Rejection is the major danger, even with closely matched donor organs. Drugs such as cyclosporine are administered to suppress the immune system and, in most cases, must be taken for life. These immuno-suppressive drugs inhibit the normal functioning of the immune system, thus making the individual much more susceptible to frequent—and more severe—infections, including bacterial, fungal, and viral infections. Other possible complications of the long-term use of immunosuppressive drugs include cataracts, impaired wound healing, peptic ulcers, and steroid-induced diabetes mellitus. About 20 percent of patients suffer graft rejection, obstruction of the arteries, or infection. In the case of serious complications, another transplantation may be the patient's only hope for survival. In successful surgeries, patients are able to return to normal, active lives within a few weeks of the surgery.

Perspective and Prospects

The first successful liver transplantation procedure was performed in 1967. Nevertheless, this surgery was considered an experimental procedure until 1983, when a National Institutes of Health (NIH) conference on liver transplantation accepted it as a routine procedure. In 1984, more than 250 liver transplantations were performed in the United States. Within five years, that number increased dramatically, to 2,188 transplantation procedures performed in 1989, and by 2002, the number had climbed to more than 5,300 transplants. Long-term results are steadily improving; currently, more than half of recipients survive for five years or more. Improvements in survival rates are attributable to improved methods of preserving donor livers, the advent of living donor transplantation, better methods to prevent graft rejection, more suitable selection of recipients (for example, hepatic cancer patients typically have a high rate of recurrence of the disease in their transplanted liver), and improved surgical techniques.

Future prospects include further improvements in surgical techniques and advanced drug therapy to prevent graft rejection but not totally compromise the disease-fighting ability of the patient's immune system. Efforts at public education regarding the need for donor organs may cause more individuals to contact donor organ societies, family, and friends regarding their wishes to donate organs in the event of untimely death. In addition, improved treatments for the diseases that lead to liver failure may help to decrease the need for this surgical procedure.

—*Karen E. Kalumuck, Ph.D.*

See also Abdomen; Abdominal disorders; Alcoholism; Circulation; Cirrhosis; Gastroenterology; Gastro-enterology, pediatric; Gastrointestinal disorders; Gastrointestinal system; Hepatitis; Internal medicine; Jaundice; Liver; Liver disorders; Nonalcoholic steatohepatitis (NASH); Transplantation.

For Further Information:

Ahmed, Moustafa. *Surviving Liver Diseases: Life with a Liver Transplant*. London: MegaZette, 1999. Designed for the layperson, this resource offers guidance on the prevention of liver disease and offers personal narrative regarding liver transplantation.

Belzer, Folkert O., and Hans W. Sollinger. "Immunology and Transplantation." In *Basic Surgery*, edited by Hiram C. Polk, Jr., H. Harlan Stone, and Bernard Gardner. 5th ed. St. Louis, Mo.: Quality Medical, 1995. A chapter in a text discussing such topics as operative and diagnostical surgery.

Griffith, H. Winter. *Complete Guide to Symptoms, Illness, and Surgery*. Revised and updated by Stephen Moore and Kenneth Yoder. 5th ed. New York: Perigee, 2006. Covers more than five hundred diseases and disorders and includes information about causes and risk factors, preventive techniques, and diagnostic tests.

Mulholland, Michael W., et al., eds. *Greenfield's Surgery: Scientific Principles and Practice*. 4th ed. Philadelphia: Lippincott Williams & Wilkins, 2006. Covers the scope and practice of surgery and includes reviews of wound biology, immunology, the management of trauma and transplantation, surgical practice according to anatomic region and specialty, and musculoskeletal, neurologic, genitourinary, and reconstructive surgery.

United Network for Organ Sharing. http://www.unos .org. A site that provides detailed information for patients and family members about the procedure, living with a transplant, current transplant research, and how to donate organs.

Youngson, Robert M. *The Surgery Book: An Illustrated Guide to Seventy-three of the Most Common Operations*. New York: St. Martin's Press, 1997. In a clear, easy-to-follow format, this dependable, comprehensive sourcebook answers questions about and gives information on a wealth of operations, including mastectomy, vasectomy, prostatectomy, cesarean section, hernia repair, hip replacement, heart bypass, and dozens more.

Zollinger, Robert M., Jr., and Robert M. Zollinger, Sr. *Zollinger's Atlas of Surgical Operations*. 8th ed. New York: McGraw-Hill, 2003. A comprehensive examination of surgery. Covers basic surgical anatomy and vascular, gynecologic, gastrointestinal, and miscellaneous abdominal procedures.

LIVING WILL
HEALTH CARE SYSTEM

ALSO KNOWN AS: Health care directive, advance directive for health care, physician's directive

DEFINITION: A signed legal document that tells what medical treatment a person does or does not want, such as artificial nutrition and hydration, mechanical ventilation, or kidney dialysis. It is intended to be used only if a person is terminally ill or permanently unconscious and cannot speak.

KEY TERMS:

artificial nutrition and hydration: the medical intervention of giving a patient nutrients and/or fluids through a tube placed in the stomach, intestine, or a vein

dialysis machine: a machine that cleans the blood of toxins that can build up when the kidneys are not working well

mechanical ventilator: a machine that helps a person breath; a tube must be inserted down a person's throat or a procedure called a tracheotomy must be performed in which a hole is made in the throat for insertion of the tube

INTRODUCTION

A living will is a legal document, often part of a three-part advance directive that also includes a durable medical power of attorney and a do-not-resuscitate (DNR) order. A living will tells what medical treatment a person does or does not want, such as artificial nutrition and hydration, mechanical ventilation, or kidney dialysis. A durable medical power of attorney is a legal document that appoints a proxy to make medical-related decisions for a person if that person becomes unable to speak. A DNR is a document that directs medical staff not to use heroic measures, such as cardiopulmonary resuscitation (CPR), if a patient's heart stops or the patient stops breathing. Advance directives should be notarized, if possible, and a copy should be placed in a patient's medical record. A person must be eighteen years of age to sign a living will or advance directive. Most states will do not allow the withdrawal of life support from a pregnant patient.

The concept of a living will was first introduced in 1969 when it became apparent that medical technology had advanced to a level where a person could be kept alive in a permanently unconscious state for years using artificial life support machines. While artificial life support is an important medical tool that can save lives and help stabilize patients waiting to receive other medical treatments, many people do not want to receive artificial life support if it is intended only to prolong life rather than to treat or improve a medical condition.

FEATURES

A living will can be a simple form or a complex document describing specific treatment preferences for specific conditions. Living will forms are available at hospitals, nursing facilities, and many medical treatment centers. U.S. hospitals and nursing facilities are required by federal law to ask patients when they are admitted if they have a living will or would like to fill out a living will form. If a patient is unconscious or unable to communicate his or her wishes for medical treatment and does not have a living will, then the doctor is required to consult with family members to determine the patient's wishes regarding life-prolonging medical care. Living will forms are also available online at state health department Web sites. In addition, a lawyer can be hired to write a living will. State laws may vary for living wills, and a living will should be written to comply with the laws in the state in which medical care is provided.

The more specific a living will is, the easier it may be for the medical care team and the family to understand what a person wants. Discussing the living will with family and doctors can ensure that the intent of the living will is understood. Copies of the living will should be placed in the patient's medical record and shared with family members. Some living wills specify the need for two physicians to concur that the patient's medical condition is terminal with no chance of recovery before it is valid. A living will can be changed at any time, even when a patient is in the hospital receiving treatment. It is not intended to keep a person from receiving medical care for emergency treatment, even if terminally ill.

Most states offer a living will registry that allows state residents to store a copy of their living wills in a secure online database at no charge. Only authorized health care providers can view the database.

PERSPECTIVE AND PROSPECTS

The California Natural Death Act of 1976 was the first legislation to allow a patient to refuse medical treatment intended to prolong life. The same year, the New

Jersey Supreme Court established the right of a dying patient to refuse medical care in the case of Karen Ann Quinlan. Quinlan was twenty-one when she became unconscious, paramedics were unable to revive her, and she lapsed into a vegetative state. She was kept alive on a ventilator for several months. Her parents requested that she be removed from the ventilator, but the hospital refused. A court order was finally issued to remove her from the ventilator, but it allowed artificial nutrition and hydration. Quinlan lived in a nonresponsive coma until 1985, when she died of pneumonia.

Another well-publicized case involved Terri Schiavo, a twetny-six-year-old woman who experienced respiratory and cardiac arrest that left her in a vegetative state. When it became apparent that Schiavo would not recover, her husband requested that her artificial life support be discontinued. Schiavo's parents disagreed. A lengthy legal battle ensued. Without a living will, it was left to the courts to decide. In 2005, Schiavo was removed from life support and died a few weeks later.

An alternative to a living will supported by pro-life groups is a "will to live" form. The emphasis of the form is that the presumption should be for life, regardless of circumstances. Both living will and "will to live" documents can be used to provide details about the specific type of medical care desired by patients who are unable to communicate.

—*Sandra Ripley Distelhorst*

See also Cardiopulmonary resuscitation (CPR); Coma; Critical care; Death and dying; Ethics; Euthanasia; Hippocratic oath; Hospice; Law and medicine; Resuscitation; Terminally ill: Extended care.

FOR FURTHER INFORMATION:

Doukas, David John, and William Reichel. "How Advance Directives Work." In *Planning for Uncertainty: Living Wills and Other Advance Directives for You and Your Family*. 2d ed. Baltimore: Johns Hopkins University Press, 2007.

Mirarchi, Ferdinando. *Understanding Your Living Will: What You Need to Know Before a Medical Emergency*. Omaha, Nebr.: Addicus Books, 2006.

Whitman, Wynne A., and Shawn D. Glisson. "The Wants, Wishes, and Wills of Your Medical-Legal Affairs." In *Wants, Wishes, and Wills: A Medical and Legal Guide to Protecting Yourself and Your Family in Sickness and in Health*. Upper Saddle River, N.J.: FT Press, 2007.

LOCAL ANESTHESIA
PROCEDURE

ALSO KNOWN AS: Peripheral nerve block

ANATOMY OR SYSTEM AFFECTED: Nerves, nervous system

SPECIALTIES AND RELATED FIELDS: Anesthesiology, dentistry, dermatology, emergency medicine

DEFINITION: A method of numbing a small area of the body for pain relief or prevention during surgical procedures.

KEY TERMS:

anesthetic: a pharmacologic agent used to block nerve conduction and reduce sensations

injection: administration into the skin, muscle, or blood vessels via needle

local: for a drug effect, confined to a small area near the administration site

neurotoxicity: an excessive or unwanted effect of too much anesthetic drug on the nerves

topical: applied directly onto the skin to be absorbed into the area around the nerve tips

INDICATIONS AND PROCEDURES

Local anesthesia is an application of numbing agents to temporarily reduce or remove transmission of nerve sensations for short surgery or other localized procedures. A secondary use is continuous infusion administration for temporary relief of acute or chronic pain conditions. Local anesthesia in its truest form is limited to small body areas; conduction, or regional, anesthesia simply extends localized administration to a larger body area. The anesthetic agents can be applied to the skin topically or can be injected under the skin into tissue directly around a nerve ending. Both methods provide short-term blockage of sensations from peripheral nerve endings or bundles to the brain by interacting with sodium ion channels around the nerve conduction pathways; the local anesthetics alter ion gradients across cell walls at the site to prevent nerves from conducting the sensory information. However, local anesthetics in any form do not provide sedation or whole-body effects, because they affect the peripheral nervous system, in contrast with the sedative, central nervous system effects of general anesthesia. The duration of the nerve block may be proportional to the amount or rate of drug administered and the potency of the anesthetic selected; however, the intensity and duration of effect also may vary on the basis of type of drug, administration site and method (for example, topical administration is less intense than tissue injection), size of the nerve sheathes affected (for example, smaller sheaths or individual, rather than bundled, nerves may react more intensely to similar doses), and interactions with other drugs (for example, antihypertensive medications) or conditions.

The two main classes of local anesthetics are the esters and the amides, which have similar aromatic and amine groups in the chemical structures but differ in the intermediate group. Esters, which include procaine (Novocaine) and benzocaine, are hydrolyzed during breakdown, whereas amides, which include lidocaine and bupivicaine, are broken down by cytochrome enzymes in the liver. Both types come as sprays, patches, creams or lotions, and injections that generally have half-lives of less than two hours. Both can be given with vasoconstrictors, such as epinephrine, to slow blood vessel distribution of the anesthetic away from local tissue and to improve duration of numbing effect at the application site.

USES AND COMPLICATIONS

Local anesthesia use for surgical procedures most often encompasses dental, minor surgical, and emergency procedures. Emergency department techniques such as sutures may require topical agents or an injected form into the tissue for deeper or longer suturing. Many types of invasive dental procedures such as cavity fillings and root canals require anesthetic injection over a large area of nerve bundles in the oral cavity. Dermatologic procedures such as mole removal require topical or injected anesthetic nerve block at nerve endings. Topical skin numbing prior to drug injections is also common (such as topical lidocaine/prilocaine cream applied before vaccines given to children). Spinal anesthesia procedures block the peripheral nervous system conduction directly where the peripheral and central nervous systems meet to prevent sensation during cesarean section deliveries, cytoscopies, and other pelvic procedures for which general anesthesia is not required. After the anesthetic is administered by skin absorption or injection, nerve block typically occurs within approximately fifteen minutes and ranges from blockage of pain sensations only to full blockage of pain and temperature sensitivity. The extent of numbness is proportional to the potency and dose administered as well, with pain inhibition followed sequentially by touch, heat, and muscle control inhibition.

Use of local anesthesia for pain is less common. Continuous catheter infusion with low doses of local anesthetics provides relief of acute pain—for example,

during treatment of a patient who experienced trauma—and may have fewer side effects than analgesic treatments. Chronic pain may be successfully numbed by similar use of anesthesia, but as of the early twenty-first century there is no evidence of long-term effects beyond the time of administration.

Although topical or local injected applications are safer than generalized anesthesia, or sedation, risks are still present. Allergy to para-aminobenzoic acid (PABA) can cause a cross reaction to ester anesthetics, because hydrolysis of an ester anesthetic releases PABA as a breakdown product. Although rare, allergy to amide anesthetics is also possible; both allergies can manifest as rash, wheezing, or even anaphylactic shock. Common side effects of either anesthetic drug class are shallow breathing, altered heart rate, anxiety, tremors, dizziness, prolonged numbness, and tinnitus (ringing sensation in the ear). Although unlikely, central nervous system depression with associated bradycardia and cardiac depression are possible, especially with extremely high doses or rates of administration. Potentially irreversible nerve conduction block can occur within five minutes of toxic doses of anesthesia, and methemoglobinemia—evidenced by shortness of breath, fatigue, dizziness, and weakness—has occurred with benzocaine in particular. Such extreme side effects are more likely to occur if the patient has preexisting renal or liver problems that prevent adequate drug clearance, is pregnant, or is very young or very old. In addition, improper injection into the vascular system or directly into a nerve sheath can lead to these toxicities. Typically, however, nerve block from correct application of local anesthetics will reverse on its own within a few hours.

PERSPECTIVE AND PROSPECTS

Since the isolation of cocaine from coca plants in the late 1800's, interest in reducing sensory effects with chemical agents, and without sedation, has grown substantially. Procaine was derived from cocaine in 1904 by Alfred Einhorn to reduce toxicity associated with cocaine use; the more concentrated amide drug lidocaine, still one of the most widely used local anesthetic agents, followed in 1943, and others in the amide class have improved upon the potency of lidocaine. Local anesthetics have since played an expanding role in medicine, from large-area nerve blocks for cesarean deliveries to short-term relief as a treatment for chronic pain via catheter infusion. In the twenty-first century, efforts to standardize office-based anesthesia are developing because of the prevalence of local anesthesia administration for routine outpatient skin, dental, and minor surgical procedures.

Long-term local anesthesia is being developed, in particular with studies of a natural agent, saxitoxin, to provide numbing effects for as long as two to three days. Localized numbness in this manner would provide pain relief throughout a procedure and afterward during the period of most acute pain and recovery time. Saxitoxin is unrelated to cocaine and the other amide and ester agents; it is found in many varieties of fish and works by blocking transmission at extracellular, rather than intracellular, sodium channels.

—*Nicole M. Van Hoey, Pharm.D.*

See also Acupuncture; Anesthesia; Anesthesiology; Dermatology; Narcotics; Nervous system; Neurology; Neurology, pediatric; Pain; Pain management; Pharmacology; Surgery, general; Surgical procedures.

FOR FURTHER INFORMATION:

Anesthesia Patient Safety Foundation. *Spring 2000 Newsletter Special Issue: Office-Based Anesthesia Safety.* Indianapolis: Author, 2000.

Auletta, M., and R. Grekin. *Local Anesthesia for Dermatologic Surgery.* New York: Churchill Livingstone, 1991.

Dinehart, S. M. "Topical, Local, and Regional Anesthesia." In *Cutaneous Surgery*, edited by R. G. Wheeland. Philadelphia: W. B. Saunders, 1994.

Epstein-Barasha, H., et al. "Prolonged Duration Local Anesthesia with Minimal Toxicity." *Proceedings of the National Academy of Sciences* 106, no. 17 (2009): 7125-7130.

Huang, W., and A. Vidimos. "Topical Anesthetics in Dermatology." *Journal of the American Academy of Dermatology* 43, part 1 (2000): 286-298.

Larson, Merlin D. "History of Anesthetic Practice." In *Miller's Anesthesia*, edited by Ronald D. Miller. 7th ed. New York: Churchill Livingstone/Elsevier, 2010.

Marx, J. A., and R. S. Hockberger. "Management Principles." In *Rosen's Emergency Medicine.* 7th ed. Rockville, Md.: Mosby/Elsevier, 2009.

LOCKJAW. *See* TETANUS.

LOU GEHRIG'S DISEASE. *See* AMYOTROPHIC LATERAL SCLEROSIS.

LOWER EXTREMITIES

ANATOMY

ANATOMY OR SYSTEM AFFECTED: Bones, feet, hips, knees, legs, lymphatic system, musculoskeletal system, nerves, nervous system, skin

SPECIALTIES AND RELATED FIELDS: Neurology, orthopedics, physical therapy, podiatry

DEFINITION: The thighs, lower legs, and feet; the lower extremities are attached to the pelvis at the hip joint and consist of muscles, bones, blood vessels, lymph vessels, nerves, skin, and toenails.

KEY TERMS:

distal: farther away from the base or attached end

femur: the thigh bone

fibula: the smaller of the two bones in the lower leg, on the lateral side

knee: the joint between the thigh and the lower leg

lateral: on the outer side; toward the little toe when in reference to the leg

leg: the lower extremity, excluding the foot; the lower leg runs from the knee to the ankle

medial: on the side toward the midline; toward the big toe when in reference to the leg

proximal: closer to the base or attached end

tarsus: the ankle

thigh: the upper segment of the leg, from the hip joint to the knee

tibia: the larger of the two bones in the lower leg, on the medial side

STRUCTURE AND FUNCTIONS

The lower extremities consist of the thighs, lower legs, and feet. Each extremity attaches to the pelvis (innominate bone) at the hip joint. The lower extremity is made mostly of bones and muscles, but it also contains blood vessels, lymphatics, nerves, skin, toenails, and other structures. Important directional terms for the lower extremity include proximal (closer to the base or attached end), distal (further from the base or attached end), medial (on the same side as the tibia and big toe), and lateral (on the same side as the fibula and little toe). Along the foot, the lower surface is called plantar; the upper surface is called dorsal. The lower extremity is clothed in skin (or integument). The sole or plantar surface of the foot is unusual, along with the palm of the hand, in being completely hairless; it also contains the thickest outer skin layer (the stratum corneum) of any part of the body. Each toe has a hardened toenail on its dorsal surface.

The pelvic girdle that supports the lower extremity develops as three separate bones: the ilium, ischium, and pubis. All three help form the acetabulum, a socket into which the femur fits. Below the acetabulum, the ischium and pubis surround a large opening called the obturator foramen. The right and left pubis meet to form a pubic symphysis. The bones of the lower extremity include the femur, tibia, fibula, tarsals, metatarsals, and phalanges. The femur (thigh bone) is the largest bone in the body. Its rounded upper end, or head, fits into the acetabulum and is attached by a short neck. A rough-surfaced greater trochanter lies just beyond this neck and serves for the attachment of many muscles. The lesser trochanter, also for muscle attachments, lies just below the neck. The knee joint is covered and protected by the kneecap, or patella, the largest of the sesamoid bones formed within tendons at points of stress. The lower leg, from the knee to the ankle, contains two bones: the tibia on the medial side and the more slender fibula on the lateral side. The tarsus, or ankle, includes the talus, calcaneus, and five smaller bones. The talus (or astragalus) has a pulleylike facet for the tibia and other curved surfaces for articulation with the calcaneus and navicular. The calcaneus, or heel bone, is vertically enlarged in humans; the Achilles tendon attaches to its roughened lower tuberosity. Smaller tarsal bones include the navicular, the medial (or inner) cuneiform, the intermediate cuneiform, the lateral (or outer) cuneiform, and the cuboid. Beyond the tarsal bones, the foot is supported by five metatarsal bones. The big toe, or hallux, contains two phalanges; each of the remaining toes contains three phalanges.

The muscles of the lower extremity include extensors, which straighten joints, and flexors, which bend joints. Abductor muscles move the limbs sideways, away from the midline, while adductors pull the limbs back, toward the midline. The muscles of the iliac region attach the lower extremity to the body. The psoas major runs from the lumbar vertebrae to the lesser trochanter of the femur. The iliacus runs from the ilium and part of the sacrum to the femur, including the lesser trochanter. The anterior muscles of the thigh include the sartorius, the quadriceps femoris, and the articularis genus. The sartorius, the longest muscle in the body, flexes both hip and knee joints. It runs obliquely from the anterior border of the ilium across the front of the thigh to insert onto the medial side of the knee at the upper end of the tibia. The quadriceps femoris consists of the rectus femoris and the three vastus muscles; all four are strong extensors of the knee. The rectus femoris originates from the region surrounding the acetabulum. The vastus lateralis, vastus medialis, and vastus inter-

medius muscles all originate along the shaft of the femur. All four quadriceps muscles insert onto a common tendon which runs over the knee and inserts onto the top of the tibia. The patella is a sesamoid bone enclosed within this tendon where it runs over the front of the knee. The smaller articularis genus muscle originates on the anterior side of the shaft of the femur; it inserts onto the kneecap.

The extensor muscles of the hip and thigh help to maintain upright posture. The gluteus maximus, the largest of these muscles, originates from the posterior portion of the ilium and inserts high on the femur, especially onto the greater trochanter. The gluteus medius and gluteus minimis both originate from the outer surface of the ilium and insert onto the greater trochanter. The tensor fasciae latae originates along the iliac crest; it inserts onto a broad, sheetlike tendon (the fascia lata) which covers much of the lateral surface of the thigh. The piriformis runs from the sacrum to the greater trochanter of the femur. The obturator internus runs from the inner surface of the pelvis through the obturator foramen to the greater trochanter of the femur. The gemellus superior and the gemellus inferior originate from the rear margin of the ischium; they both insert onto the greater trochanter. The quadratus femoris originates from the lateral surface of the ischium; it inserts between the greater and lesser trochanters of the femur. The obturator externus originates along the outer surface of the pelvis below the obturator foramen and inserts near the greater trochanter.

The muscles on the medial (or inner) side of the thigh are all abductors of the thigh. The gracilis is a long, thin muscle that originates from the pubis, runs along the medial side of the thigh, and inserts high on the tibia. The pectineus originates anteriorly on the pubis and inserts onto the shaft of the femur below the lesser trochanter. The adductor longus originates from the pubis and inserts onto the posterior edge of the femur. The adductor brevis originates from the pubis and inserts onto the posterior edge of the femur. The adductor magnus is a large, triangular muscle that originates from the lower portion of the ischium and pubis; it expands to a long, thin insertion along the posterior edge of the femur.

The hamstring muscles run along the posterior side of the femur; they flex the knee and extend the hip joint. The biceps femoris originates from the posterior portion (the tuberosity) of the ischium and separately from the posterior edge of the femur. Both portions converge onto a common tendon that inserts primarily onto the top of the fibula. The semitendinosus originates from the posterior end of the ischium; it inserts by a long tendon onto the medial side of the tibia. The semimembranosus runs from the ischium to the posterior surface of the tibia.

The muscles on the front (anterior) side of the lower leg raise the foot by flexing it dorsally. At the ankle, their tendons are all held in place by two transverse bands, the extensor retinacula. The tibialis anterior originates along the anterior edge of the tibia; it inserts by a tendon onto the medial cuneiform and the base of the first metatarsal. The extensor hallucis longus originates from the anterior surface of the fibula; its tendon passes beneath the extensor retinacula to insert onto the distal phalanx of the big toe. The extensor digitorum longus originates near the top of the tibia and along the anterior side of the fibula. Its tendon passes beneath the extensor retinacula and splits into four tendons, inserted onto the second and third phalanges of the second through fifth digits. The peroneus tertius originates along the anterior edge of the fibula and runs alongside the extensor digitorum longus. It inserts onto the base of the fifth metatarsal bone.

The muscles on the posterior surface of the lower leg are mostly extensors of the foot; some also flex the knee. The gastrocnemius originates in two heads from opposite sides of the femur. It inserts onto the Achilles tendon, which attaches to the calcaneus. The soleus originates from the posterior surface of the fibula; it inserts onto the Achilles tendon. The plantaris originates from the posterior surface of the femur and inserts onto the posterior portion of the calcaneus. The popliteus runs from the lateral side of the femur across the back of the knee to insert onto the tibia. The flexor hallucis longus originates along the posterior surface of the fibula; its tendon runs around to the medial side of the ankle and inserts onto the base of the big toe. The flexor digitorum longus originates from the posterior surface of the tibia; its tendon crosses the sole of the foot obliquely and divides into four tendons that insert onto the distal phalanges of the second through fifth toes. The tibialis posterior originates from the posterior surfaces of the tibia, the fibula, and the interosseous membrane that joins them; its tendon passes around to insert onto the navicular bone. The peroneus longus originates along the lateral surface of the fibula; its tendon runs along a groove on the bottom of the cuboid to insert obliquely onto the base of the first metatarsal. The peroneus brevis originates along the lateral margin of the fibula; its tendon inserts onto the fifth metatarsal. The extensor digitorum brevis originates from the cal-caneus and runs obliquely across the dorsal side of the foot, dividing into four tendons. One tendon inserts onto the base of the big toe; the remaining tendons insert onto the tendons of the extensor digitorum longus.

Several flexor muscles of the foot are attached to the plantar aponeurosis, a flat ligament that runs from the calcaneus along the sole of the foot to the bases of the toes and to several flexor tendons. The abductor hallucis originates from the calcaneus and the plantar aponeurosis; it inserts onto the base of the big toe. The flexor digitorum brevis originates from the plantar aponeurosis and the calcaneus; it divides into four portions, each of which gives rise to a tendon. These tendons run into the second through fifth toes, each splitting in half to insert onto opposite sides of the second phalanx, separated by the tendons of the flexor digitorum longus, which emerge between them. The abductor digiti quinti originates from the calcaneus and the plantar aponeurosis; it inserts onto the base of the fifth toe. The quadratus plantae originates from the calcaneus and inserts onto the tendons of the flexor digitorum longus. The four small lumbricals run from the tendons of the flexor digitorum longus to the corresponding tendons of the extensor digitorum longus. The flexor hallucis brevis originates from the cuboid and lateral cuneiform bones; its two portions insert onto the big toe from opposite sides. The adductor hallucis originates from the second through fourth metatarsals and also from the bases of the third through fifth toes. Its tendon inserts onto the base of the big toe. The flexor digiti quinti originates from the base of the fifth metatarsal and inserts onto the base of the fifth toe. The four dorsal interossei originate from the bases of the metatarsal bones; they insert onto the bases of the second through fourth toes. The three plantar interossei originate from the third through fifth metatarsals and run beneath these bones to insert onto the bases of the corresponding toes.

Blood vessels of the lower extremity include both arteries and veins. The common iliac arteries arise from the dorsal aorta; each divides into an internal and an external iliac. The internal iliac artery supplies many muscles of the thigh region and pelvis. The external iliac artery branches into an inferior epigastric artery and a deep iliac circumflex artery; it then continues along the femur as the femoral artery. The femoral artery gives rise to a deep femoral artery running to the medial and posterior regions of the thigh; the base of this artery also gives rise to two circumflex arteries that send branches upward into many thigh muscles. Near the knee, the femoral artery branches into a descending geniculate artery to the knee, then continues as the popliteal artery, forming several branches to the thigh muscles and other small branches to the knee before splitting into anterior and posterior tibial arteries.

The anterior tibial artery descends along the front of the tibia, forming several small branches. It then continues into the foot as the dorsalis pedis artery, giving rise to a lateral tarsal artery and an arcuate artery, both of which form arches by joining with branches of the peroneal artery. The deep plantar artery and hallucis dorsalis artery also branch from the dorsalis pedis artery, while individual arteries to the second through fourth metatarsals arise from the arcuate artery. Arterial branches to all the toes arise from the individual metatarsal arteries, including the hallucis dorsalis, forming a system of collateral circulation in which multiple alternate routes permit blood flow even if one of the routes is temporarily blocked.

The posterior tibial artery gives rise to a peroneal artery; the two arteries then run down the posterior side of the lower leg, forming small branches to the muscles of the lower leg and nutrient arteries to the tibia and fibula. The posterior tibial artery branches to the calcaneus before it splits into a medial plantar artery, which runs along the medial margin of the foot into the big toe, and a much larger lateral plantar artery. The lateral plantar artery runs across the foot obliquely to the lateral side, then turns and runs obliquely in the other direction to the base of the big toe, where it runs into the deep plantar artery to form a loop. From this loop arise a series of plantar metatarsal arteries to all five toes. Blood can reach each toe from either side, and the arch that supplies this blood can receive its blood either by way of the posterior tibial and lateral plantar arteries or by way of the anterior tibial and deep plantar arteries, providing another example of collateral circulation.

There are several important veins draining the lower extremity. The deep veins originate from a series of plantar digital veins draining the individual toes into a deep plantar venous arch. This arch is drained to either direction by a lateral plantar vein and a medial plantar vein, which later unite to form a posterior tibial vein; this vein and the peroneal vein run parallel to the corresponding arteries along the posterior side of the lower leg. An anterior tibial vein drains the anterior side of the lower leg and the dorsal side of the foot. Near the knee, the peroneal vein and the anterior and posterior tibial veins unite to form the popliteal vein, which continues into the thigh as the femoral vein. The femoral vein receives the deep femoral vein as a tributary, then the

saphenous vein. The femoral vein then continues as the external iliac vein.

The lower extremity is also covered with a network of superficial veins that lie just beneath the skin. The vessels of this network are drained along the medial side of the lower leg and thigh by the great saphenous vein, which runs into the femoral vein just below the groin. The lateral side of the foot and the posterior surface of the lower leg are drained by the small saphenous vein, which drains into the popliteal vein.

The nerves to the lower extremity arise from two series of complex branchings, the lumbar plexus and sacral plexus. The largest nerve formed from the lumbar plexus is the femoral nerve, supplying muscles on the anterior side of the thigh and part of the lower leg. Other branches to the muscles include the obturator nerve to the adductor muscles and separate muscular branches to the psoas and iliacus muscles. Cutaneous sensory nerves to the skin include the lateral femoral cutaneous nerve to the lateral side of the thigh, the anterior cutaneous branches of the femoral nerve to the medial side of the thigh, and the saphenous nerve, a branch of the femoral nerve to the medial side of the lower leg.

The sacral plexus gives rise to the very large sciatic nerve and to several smaller nerves, including the superior gluteal and inferior gluteal nerves to the gluteal muscles, and separate muscular branches to the piriformis, quadratus femoris, obturator internus, and gemelli. Cutaneous branches such as the posterior femoral cutaneous nerve supply sensory fibers to the skin on the posterior surface of the thigh. The sciatic nerve, the largest nerve in the body, branches off to the hamstring muscles before splitting into tibial and peroneal nerves. The tibial nerve supplies the muscles on the posterior side of the lower leg and then runs onto the sole of the foot, where it splits into the medial and lateral plantar nerves, which together supply both cutaneous sensation and muscular innervation to the sole of the foot. The peroneal nerve divides into deep and superficial portions. The deep peroneal nerve supplies the muscles on the anterior side of the lower leg and the dorsal surface of the foot. The superficial peroneal nerve supplies cutaneous sensation to the lateral surface of the lower leg and the dorsal surface of the foot.

DISORDERS AND DISEASES

Many medical conditions and disorders affect the lower extremity; these include animal bites (including snakebites), injuries, fungus infections such as athlete's foot, contact dermatitis (including poison ivy), and an assortment of neuromuscular disorders, including nerve paralyses, muscular atrophies, and muscular dystrophies. Nerve paralyses of the lower extremities usually arise from traumatic injury.

Muscular atrophies are diseases in which muscle tissues become progressively weaker and smaller, usually beginning after the age of forty. Spastic movements sometimes occur. The small muscles of the hands and feet are usually affected sooner and more severely in comparison to the larger muscles of the legs and thighs. Amyotrophic lateral sclerosis (ALS), commonly known as Lou Gehrig's disease, is one such disease that usually begins with weakness and deterioration of the distal muscles. The disease proceeds to affect the rest of the extremities, then other parts of the body; it is usually fatal within three to five years after onset. A more rare type of atrophy, myelopathic muscular atrophy (or Aran-Duchenne atrophy), affects both upper and lower extremities and eventually spreads to the trunk. A degenerative lesion of the gray matter in the cervical region of the spinal cord is usually responsible.

Muscular dystrophy is a series of inherited diseases that begin in early childhood, affecting males more often than females. The most common type, Duchenne muscular dystrophy, is caused by a sex-linked recessive trait that impairs the body's ability to synthesize a large protein called dystrophin. Muscular dystrophy primarily affects the large muscles of the thigh and lower leg, impairing the ability to stand unassisted or to walk. The affected muscles become very weak but remain approximately normal in size and may even increase as muscle tissue is replaced by fatty and fibrous tissue. Progressive weakening makes walking and similar motor functions impossible, but, with proper care, patients can live for decades.

Sports injuries often occur in the lower extremities and are generally treated by orthopedic specialists. Fractured bones are generally set in casts and kept immobile until they heal. Injured or ruptured ligaments often require surgical treatment. Snakebites and other animal bites occur more often to the lower extremities than to other parts of the body. The bites of poisonous snakes must be treated quickly, before the venom reaches the heart. The patient must be kept calm and quiet, and experienced medical attention should be sought as soon as possible.

PERSPECTIVE AND PROSPECTS

The major muscles and bones of the lower extremities were studied in ancient societies by such individuals as Galen (or Caius Galenus), the physician to the Roman army in the second century. Ironically, the science of anatomy took many great strides because of the efforts of artists, who studied the human body in order to create realistic sculptures and paintings. During the Renaissance, Leonardo da Vinci (1452-1519) and Michelangelo (1475-1564) dissected human corpses illegally in their quest for this knowledge. Andreas Vesalius (1514-1564) produced the first well-illustrated anatomical texts, containing information that corrected many of the errors made by Galen.

Injuries to the leg are generally treated surgically. Whenever possible, broken bones are set in place, immobilized in a cast, and then allowed to heal. Muscles (or their tendons) must be sewn together. Nerve endings must be matched with their former locations if they are to grow back correctly. Gangrene, or tissue death from lack of circulation, occurs more often in the lower extremities than in the upper extremities. When the lower extremity is gangrenous or is injured beyond repair, an amputation is often performed. Artificial legs or partial legs are sometimes attached to the lower extremity.

—*Eli C. Minkoff, Ph.D.*

See also Amputation; Arthritis; Arthroplasty; Arthroscopy; Bone cancer; Bone disorders; Bone grafting; Bones and the skeleton; Bowlegs; Braces, orthopedic; Bunions; Bursitis; Casts and splints; Deep vein thrombosis; Feet; Flat feet; Foot disorders; Fracture and dislocation; Fracture repair; Frostbite; Grafts and grafting; Hammertoe correction; Hammertoes; Heel spur removal; Hemiplegia; Hip fracture repair; Hip replacement; Joints; Kneecap removal; Knock-knees; Ligaments; Liposuction; Motor skill development; Muscle sprains, spasms, and disorders; Muscles; Nail removal; Nails; Orthopedic surgery; Orthopedics; Orthopedics, pediatric; Osgood-Schlatter disease; Osteoarthritis; Osteochondritis juvenilis; Osteogenesis imperfecta; Osteopathic medicine; Paralysis; Paraplegia; Physical rehabilitation; Pigeon toes; Podiatry; Poliomyelitis; Prostheses; Quadriplegia; Restless legs syndrome; Rheumatoid arthritis; Rheumatology; Rickets; Tendon disorders; Tendon repair; Upper extremities; Varicose vein removal.

FOR FURTHER INFORMATION:

Agur, Anne M. R., and Arthur F. Dalley. *Grant's Atlas of Anatomy.* 12th ed. Philadelphia: Wolters Kluwer Health/Lippincott Williams & Wilkins, 2009. Excellent, detailed illustrations can be found in this standard reference work.

Crouch, James E. *Functional Human Anatomy*. 4th ed. Philadelphia: Lea & Febiger, 1985. A good beginning reference for an introduction to anatomy. This easy-to-read book provides clear explanations.

Currey, John D. *Bones: Structures and Mechanics*. 2d ed. Princeton, N.J.: Princeton University Press, 2006. Very accessible overview of a range of information related to whole bones, bone tissue, and dentin and enamel. Topics include stiffness, strength, viscoelasticity, fatigue, fracture mechanics properties, buckling, impact fracture, and properties of cancellous bone.

Marieb, Elaine N. *Essentials of Human Anatomy and Physiology*. 9th ed. San Francisco: Pearson/Benjamin Cummings, 2009. This text discusses the functional significance of various anatomical structures, including the foot. Readers will enjoy the excellent pictures and diagrams of the foot and associated body parts.

Rosse, Cornelius, and Penelope Gaddum-Rosse. *Hollinshead's Textbook of Anatomy*. 5th ed. Philadelphia: Lippincott-Raven, 1997. Helpful descriptions and illustrations mark this thorough, detailed reference source.

Standring, Susan, et al., eds. *Gray's Anatomy*. 40th ed. New York: Churchill Livingstone/Elsevier, 2008. This work stands as a classic in the field of anatomy. Thorough descriptions and excellent color illustrations are provided.

Van De Graaff, Kent M. *Human Anatomy*. 6th ed. New York: McGraw-Hill, 2002. Chapters 8 through 11 present a first-rate introduction to bones, the skeleton, and joints. The many clear illustrations, photographs, clinical commentaries, and X rays, as well as a pronunciation guide, a complete index, and a glossary, make this a very accessible book for the nonspecialist reader.

LUMBAR PUNCTURE

PROCEDURE

ALSO KNOWN AS: Spinal tap

ANATOMY OR SYSTEM AFFECTED: Brain, nerves, nervous system, spine

SPECIALTIES AND RELATED FIELDS: Anesthesiology, biochemistry, critical care, general surgery, neurology, oncology, pathology

DEFINITION: A process in which the physician places a hollow needle into the lower part of the spinal canal, either to harvest cerebrospinal fluid for diagnosis or to inject substances into the spinal canal.

KEY TERMS:

aneurysm: ballooning within an artery or vein that protrudes through a weak spot

angiogram: film on which images of blood vessels treated with a medium that is opaque to X rays become visible

cerebrospinal fluid (CSF): watery fluid that surrounds the brain and the spinal cord

meningeal irritation: inflammation of the meninges, or membranes surrounding the brain and spinal cord

meningitis: inflammation of the membranes of the brain or spinal cord

myelography: X-ray examination of the spinal cord, tissues, and nerves within the spinal canal

subarachnoid hemorrhage: a condition in which blood from a ruptured cranial blood vessel invades the surface of the brain

vertebrae: pieces of bone or cartilage of which the backbone or spine is composed

xanthochromic spinal fluid: yellowish CSF, indicating either an abnormally high protein level or a brain hemorrhage

INDICATIONS AND PROCEDURES

A lumbar puncture, often referred to as a spinal tap, is indicated for the diagnosis of meningitis because it is the best method for detecting meningeal irritation. A laboratory examination of the cerebrospinal fluid (CSF) harvested through a lumbar puncture can detect problems relating to the brain and spinal cord. Meningitis cannot be diagnosed through imaging methods such as computed tomography (CT) scanning.

Some subarachnoid (brain) hemorrhages involve the loss of so little blood that they are not detectable radiologically. When this is the case, the CSF may contain small amounts of blood that continues to be present in successive testing. If diagnosis is delayed, then the blood from a subarachnoid hemorrhage may have dissipated, making the CSF yellowish. This indicates that the blood in it is being metabolized. When this is the case, an immediate angiogram is indicated.

CSF withdrawn through a lumbar puncture should be examined immediately by a pathologist or hematologist to detect the presence of blood or, if it is xanthochromic or yellowish, to indicate either that the protein level is abnormally high or that a subarachnoid hemorrhage exists and blood is spreading over the surface of the brain. Such leakage may indicate an aneurysm and generally requires prompt surgery.

Although lumbar puncture is essentially a diagnostic

Lumbar Puncture

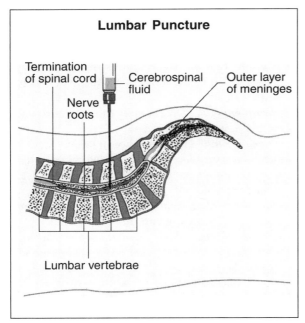

A lumbar puncture, commonly known as a spinal tap, is a diagnostic procedure in which cerebrospinal fluid is extracted from the meninges of the spine and analyzed for the presence of infection.

tool, it is sometimes indicated when CSF has built up to dangerous levels in the spinal canal and the patient is hydrocephalic. In such instances, excess CSF can be withdrawn from the spinal canal, but an immediate determination of the cause of the buildup is essential and treatment to eliminate the cause imperative.

Patients undergoing lumbar punctures lie sideways, chin down and knees drawn up to separate the vertebrae. Local anesthetic is used to numb the area surrounding the lower vertebrae. A hollow needle inserted between two lower vertebrae is pushed into the spinal canal. The entire procedure, involving minimal discomfort, takes about twenty minutes. The puncture wound left by the needle is covered with a sterile bandage. Patients may experience a headache following the procedure, but it usually disappears quickly. If it does not disappear within a few days, a small amount of the patient's blood can be injected into the site, creating a patch that should eliminate the headache.

USES AND COMPLICATIONS

Lumbar puncture is used to inject dyes into the spinal canal to serve as a contrast medium in diagnostic procedures involving X rays, particularly myelography. It is also used to introduce medications into the CSF for the treatment of certain types of cancer. This use, often appropriate in cases of leukemia and carcinomas of the nervous system, is frequently employed in pediatric care.

Some surgical procedures require that patients be awake during surgery. In such cases, local anesthetics are introduced into the spinal canal through lumbar puncture, rendering patients still conscious but insensate.

As with any invasive procedure, there is risk of infection, but it is minimal. The procedure is performed under sterile conditions. One danger, in the case of a subarachnoid hemorrhage, is blood loss. Bleeding, in rare cases, may become uncontrollable and result in death. One cautionary note is that lumbar puncture should never be performed in cases where a brain abscess is suspected unless reliable CT scans or other tests have failed to reveal a mass or reveal only a small mass.

Lumbar puncture in and of itself is not a high-risk procedure, although the conditions that require its use often involve high risks for the patient. It is advisable in most cases for the procedure to be performed where immediate surgery can be carried out if the patient's condition deteriorates suddenly.

PERSPECTIVE AND PROSPECTS

The earliest use of CSF in diagnosis was in the nineteenth century, when such primitive tools as sharpened bird quills were used to penetrate the lumbar region. The technique came into its own in the mid-twentieth century, when most problems of the central nervous system were diagnosed through an examination of the CSF.

Because of the importance of CSF in diagnosing meningitis, cerebral hemorrhages, and other dangerous conditions, considerable progress and sophistication have accompanied the development of lumbar puncture. The imaging tools currently available to surgeons, neurologists, hematologists, and pathologists are so advanced and accurate, however, that lumbar puncture is used as a diagnostic tool somewhat less than in the past.

—R. Baird Shuman, Ph.D.

See also Anesthesia; Anesthesiology; Bacterial infections; Bacteriology; Biopsy; Bleeding; Diagnosis; Fluids and electrolytes; Infection; Invasive tests; Meningitis; Nervous system; Neuroimaging; Neurology; Neurology, pediatric; Neurosurgery; Spine, vertebrae, and disks; Viral infections.

FOR FURTHER INFORMATION:

Bowden, Vicky R., and Cindy Smith Greenberg. *Pediatric Nursing Procedures*. Philadelphia: Lippincott Williams & Wilkins, 2003.

Colyar, Margaret R. *Well-Child Assessment for Primary Care Providers*. Philadelphia: F. A. Davis, 2003.

Doherty, Gerard M., and Lawrence W. Way, eds. *Current Surgical Diagnosis and Treatment*. 12th ed. New York: Lange Medical Books/McGraw-Hill, 2006.

Dougherty, Lisa, and Sara E. Lister, eds. *The Royal Marsden Hospital Manual of Clinical Nursing Procedures*. 7th ed. Malden, Mass.: Blackwell, 2008.

McAllister, Leslie D., et al. *Practical Neuro-oncology: A Guide to Patient Care*. Boston: Butterworth-Heinemann, 2002.

LUMPECTOMY. *See* MASTECTOMY AND LUMPECTOMY.

LUMPS, BREAST. *See* BREAST CANCER; BREAST DISORDERS; BREASTS, FEMALE.

LUNG CANCER

DISEASE/DISORDER

ANATOMY OR SYSTEM AFFECTED: Chest, lungs, lymphatic system, respiratory system

SPECIALTIES AND RELATED FIELDS: Environmental health, immunology, occupational health, oncology, pulmonary medicine, radiology

DEFINITION: The appearance of malignant tumors in the lungs, which is usually associated with cigarette smoking.

CAUSES AND SYMPTOMS

Most forms of lung cancer fall within one of four categories: squamous cell (or epidermoid) carcinomas and adenocarcinomas (each of which accounts for approximately 30 percent of all pulmonary cancers), small or oat cell carcinomas (accounting for about 25 percent of lung cancers), and large cell carcinomas (which represent about 15 percent of lung cancers). Each of these forms can be further categorized on the basis of cell differentiation within the tumor: either well differentiated (resembling the original cell type) or moderately or poorly differentiated. Upon biopsy, stage groupings are also determined on the basis of size, invasiveness, and possible extent of metastasis.

Oat or small cell carcinomas usually consist of small, tightly packed, spindle-shaped cells, with a high nucleus-to-cytoplasm ratio within the cell. Oat cell carcinomas tend to metastasize early and widely, often to the bone marrow or brain. As a result, by the time that symptoms become apparent, the disease is generally widely disseminated within the body. Coupled with a resistance to most common forms of radiation and chemotherapy, oat cell carcinomas present a particularly poor prognosis. In general, patients diagnosed with this form of cancer have a survival period measured, at most, in months.

Adenocarcinomas are tumors of glandlike structure, presenting as nodules within peripheral tissue such as the bronchioles. Often these forms of tumors may arise from previously damaged or scarred tissue, such as has occurred among smokers. The development of adenocarcinoma of the lung is not as dependent upon smoke inhalation, however, as are other forms of lung cancer.

Squamous cell, also called epidermoid, carcinomas tend to be slower-growing malignancies which form among the flat epithelial cells on the surface of a variety of tissues, including the bladder, cervix, or skin, in addition to the lung. The cells are often polygonal in shape, with keratin nodes on the surface of lesions. Squamous cell carcinomas tend to metastasize less frequently than other forms of lung cancer, allowing for a more optimistic prognosis.

Large cell carcinomas are actually a more general form of cancer in which the cells are relatively large in size, with the cell nucleus being particularly enlarged. Often these carcinomas have arisen as either squamous cell carcinomas or adenocarcinomas. Metastasis, when it occurs, is frequently within the gastrointestinal tract.

There is no question that the single leading cause or

INFORMATION ON LUNG CANCER

CAUSES: Smoking, exposure to other environmental toxins (asbestos, hydrocarbon products, nickel, vinyl chloride, uranium, pitchblende)

SYMPTOMS: Persistent cough (sometimes accompanied by blood), difficulty breathing, chest pain, repeated and long-lasting attacks of bronchitis or pneumonia

DURATION: Progressive and usually fatal

TREATMENTS: Depends on stage; may include alleviation of symptoms, surgery, chemotherapy, radiation therapy

factor resulting in lung cancer is smoking. Persons who do not smoke, and indeed even smokers who smoke fewer than five cigarettes per day, are at relatively low risk of developing any form of lung cancer. Those who smoke more than five cigarettes per day run an increased risk of developing lung cancer at rates approaching two hundred times that of the nonsmoker. This risk is greatest for oat cell carcinomas and least for adenocarcinomas (but still approximately a tenfold risk over that for nonsmokers). The relative risk is related to the number of cigarettes smoked: The more cigarettes, the greater the risk. In addition, though other environmental hazards can be related to the development of lung cancers, the risk associated with those hazards is without exception amplified by cigarette smoke.

Exposure to other specific environmental factors has also been associated with the formation of certain forms of pulmonary cancers. Individuals chronically exposed to materials such as asbestos, hydrocarbon products (coal tars or roofing materials), nickel, vinyl chloride, or radiochemicals (uranium and pitchblende) are at increased risk. Chronically damaged lungs, for whatever reason, are at significantly increased risk for development of cancer.

The symptoms of lung cancer may represent the damage caused by the primary tumor or may be the result of metastasis to other organs. The most common symptom is a persistent cough, sometimes accompanied by blood in the sputum or difficulty breathing. Chest pain may be present, especially upon inhalation. There may also be repeated attacks of bronchitis or pneumonia that tend to persist for abnormal periods of time.

TREATMENT AND THERAPY

Diagnosis of a tumor in the lung generally includes a chest X ray, along with use of a variety of diagnostic tests: bronchography (X-ray observation of the bronchioles following application of an opaque material), tomography (cross-sectional observation of tissue), and cytologic examination of sputum or bronchiole washings. Confirmation of the diagnosis, in addition to determination of the specific type of tumor and its clinical stage, generally requires a needle biopsy of material from the lung.

The treatment of the tumor is dependent on the form of the disease and on the extent of its spread. Surgery remains the preferred method of treatment, but because of the nature of the disease, less than half the cases are operable at the time of diagnosis. Of these, a large pro-

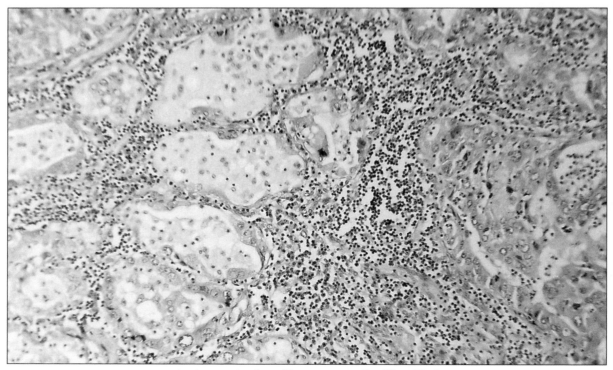

A microscopic view of lung cancer cells. (PhotoDisc)

In the News: Lack of Lung Cancer Symptoms in Some Women

In 2006, media stories reporting the death from lung cancer of Dana Reeve, widow of actor Christopher Reeve, focused on nonsmoking women who developed that disease. Reports concentrated on risk factors, including studies addressing the possible connection of estrogen with lung cancer, to educate women regarding screening. News accounts stressed that because lung cancer was often asymptomatic in women, female patients should not rely solely on symptoms to seek medical help, noting the work of researchers striving to develop effective methods to locate early-stage lung cancer. Articles noted the limitations of chest X rays, which do not detect most early-stage lung cancer tumors.

During 2005, the media had reported development of a potentially accurate lung cancer test in which dentists, physicians, or patients scraped samples of cheek cells inside the mouth to submit to medical laboratories for automated quantitative cytometry (AQC) evaluation. Researchers emphasized the low cost of this test, which did not need special equipment to take samples.

In the spring of 2006, the media reported on findings published in the journal *Chest* that indicated tests for chronic obstructive pulmonary disease (COPD) might not reveal women had lung cancer because their lungs seemed to function normally during those tests and no symptoms were apparent. Re-searchers emphasized women at risk of having lung cancer should undergo other types of tests and that physicians should consider patients' age, smoking history, and environment when screening for that disease.

The media discussed the October, 2006, issue of the *New England Journal of Medicine*, which printed information regarding a New York-Presbyterian Hospital/Weill Cornell Medical College study evaluating the benefits of computed tomography (CT) scanning to detect lung cancer in asymptomatic subjects who smoked or were exposed to risk factors. This method, using low radiation dosages, alerted researchers to cancerous lung tumors in 484 of the 31,567 subjects scanned, enabling surgical removal before the cancer spread. Reports noted that because physicians could focus on small tumors, healthy lung tissue could be preserved during surgery.

Critics expressed concerns that the study lacked a control group to evaluate whether CT scans helped extend patients' life spans. They criticized the approach for resulting in unnecessary biopsies and surgeries for scan-detected tumors which later were determined to be benign, stressing that additional studies examining the role of CT scanning for lung cancer should be considered. The Lung Cancer Alliance, however, endorsed CT scans.

—*Elizabeth D. Schafer, Ph.D.*

portion are beyond the point at which the surgical removal of the cancer and resection of remaining tissue are possible. A variety of chemotherapeutic measures are available and along with the use of radiation therapy can be used to produce a small number of cures or at least temporary alleviation of symptoms. Nevertheless, only a small proportion of lung cancers, perhaps 10 percent, respond with a permanent remission or cure.

Lung cancer represents the leading cause of cancer deaths among American men and women. In 2000, 164,000 new cases of lung cancer were reported, with 157,000 deaths reported. The prognosis for most forms of lung cancer remains poor.

—*Richard Adler, Ph.D.*

See also Addiction; Asbestos exposure; Bronchi; Bronchitis; Cancer; Carcinogens; Carcinoma; Chemotherapy; Lungs; Malignancy and metastasis; National Cancer Institute (NCI); Nicotine; Occupational health; Oncology; Pneumonia; Pulmonary diseases; Pulmonary medicine; Radiation therapy; Respiration; Smoking; Tumor removal; Tumors; Wheezing.

For Further Information:

Dollinger, Malin, et al. *Everyone's Guide to Cancer Therapy.* 5th ed. Kansas City, Mo.: Andrews McMeel, 2008. A well-organized book on therapy for various cancers. Clearly describes the methods of treatment that are available and the treatment of choice. Written for the layperson.

Eyre, Harmon J., Dianne Partie Lange, and Lois B. Morris. *Informed Decisions: The Complete Book of Cancer Diagnosis, Treatment, and Recovery.* 2d ed. Atlanta: American Cancer Society, 2002. This text from the American Cancer Society is intended for the layperson. It is exemplary in its discussion of cancer.

Henschke, Claudia I. *Lung Cancer: Myths, Facts, Choices—and Hope.* New York: W. W. Norton, 2003. An award-winning book that describes how the lungs work and how cancer develops. Reviews why early detection is so critical, provides questionnaires to pinpoint risk factors, and addresses practical concerns such as dealing with insurance issues.

Lung Cancer Online Foundation. http://www.lung canceronline.org. A Web site that strives to improve the quality of care and quality of life for people with lung cancer by funding lung cancer research and providing information to patients and families.

Parles, Karen, and Joan H. Schiller. *One Hundred Questions and Answers About Lung Cancer.* 2d ed. Sudbury, Mass.: Jones and Bartlett, 2010. A patient-oriented guide that covers a range of topics related to lung cancer, including risk factors and causes; methods of prevention, screening, and diagnosis; available treatments and how to choose among them; and ways of coping with common emotional and physical difficulties associated with the diagnosis and treatment.

Pass, Harvey I., et al., eds. *Lung Cancer: Principles and Practice.* 3d ed. Philadelphia: Lippincott Williams & Wilkins, 2005. This illustrated text addresses neoplasms of the lungs. Includes a bibliography and an index.

Steen, R. Grant. *A Conspiracy of Cells: The Basic Science of Cancer.* New York: Plenum Press, 1993. Provides a fine discussion of a variety of factors that cause cancers to develop.

LUNG DISEASES. *See* PULMONARY DISEASES.

LUNG SURGERY

PROCEDURE

ANATOMY OR SYSTEM AFFECTED: Lungs, respiratory system

SPECIALTIES AND RELATED FIELDS: Emergency medicine, general surgery, pulmonary medicine

DEFINITION: The correction and treatment of such lung problems as bronchiectasis, cancer, emphysema, and pneumothorax.

KEY TERMS:

catheter: a flexible tube inserted into a body cavity to distend it or maintain an opening

diaphragm: the muscular partition that separates the abdomen and the thorax

expiration: the act of breathing out, which partly collapses the lungs

inspiration: the act of breathing in, which expands the lungs

trachea: a cartilaginous, air-carrying tube that runs from the larynx to the bronchi of the lungs

INDICATIONS AND PROCEDURES

Located in the chest (or thoracic) cavity, the lungs rest on the diaphragm. Each lung is connected to the trachea, which brings air in on inspiration and carries it away on expiration. Prior to its entry into the lungs, the trachea forms two bronchi. Each enters a lung near its middle and subdivides into smaller and smaller passages called bronchioles. The smallest tubes open into tiny air sacs called alveoli. Each alveolus contains blood vessels called capillaries that take up oxygen and release carbon dioxide into the lungs to be expelled as waste. Alveoli are arranged into lobules, which are united into lung lobes. The left lung contains two such lobes, and there are three in the larger right lung. Appropriate alveolar function is essential to life. To optimize their action, the lungs are surrounded by a double membrane, the pleura, and supplied by nerves that control expansion on inspiration and contraction on expiration. This size change, accomplished by muscular action, normally occurs eighteen times per minute throughout life. It slows during sleep and accelerates during exercise.

Good health requires adequate lung operation, which can be compromised in many ways. The best-known lung disorders are abscesses, asthma, bronchiectasis, bronchitis, cancer, emphysema, pneumonia, pneumothorax, and tuberculosis. Of these, lung cancer, abscesses, bronchiectasis, and pneumothorax can be corrected surgically.

Lung cancer is a leading cause of cancer death among both men and women. The disease has been attributed primarily to smoking, although causative agents such as asbestos, radioactive substances, and other air pollutants also have been implicated. The development of lung cancer is slow until severe symptoms appear. An early warning is a persistent cough unassociated with asthma or emphysema, chest pain, shortness of breath, fatigue, and general listlessness. The detection of lung cancer in its beginning stages requires regular chest X rays. Early detection greatly enhances long-term survival.

Lung cancer is best treated by surgery. This requires the removal of a small wedge of lung tissue, a lobectomy (lobe removal), or a pneumonectomy (lung removal), depending on the stage of the cancer. During surgery, general anesthesia is followed by an incision around the rib cage on the affected side, along a lower rib. The rib is then detached to produce a gap, and the tumor and/or section of the lung is removed. Post-surgical patients are kept in an intensive care unit for several days, where they are fed and given therapeutic drugs intravenously. Chest drainage tubes are used to drain the incision site. Convalescence takes several months after leaving the hospital. Complications can include infection at the site of the incision and lung collapse.

Lung abscesses most often result from the inhalation of food or tooth fragments. The symptoms are chills, fever, chest pain, and a severe cough that brings up phlegm containing blood and pus. Abscesses are often located using X rays. In many cases, antibiotics are curative. Severe and/or large lung abscesses, however, require surgical drainage or—in extreme cases—the surgical removal of affected lung tissue. For lung abscesses to require surgery, the affected tissue must be thick-walled and antibiotic-resistant. The simplest such cases involve the placement of a catheter in the abscess to act as a drain. In very severe cases, the affected lung portion (usually a wedge) is removed surgically, as with lung cancer.

Bronchiectasis, the distortion of air tubes, is often the result of childhood lung infections and takes years to develop. In most cases, it causes the production of large amounts of foul-smelling phlegm and predisposes the patient to repeated severe lung infections following colds. Diagnosis is by X ray, and treatment is often the use of antibiotics at the first sign of any cold. In some cases, the problem is severe enough to require lung surgery. Bronchiectasis that is severe enough to cause recurrent pneumonia in the same lung segment is treated by surgery when the air tube involved can be removed as well. The potential dangers of this procedure are infection and lung collapse, but they are uncommon.

Pneumothorax occurs when air enters the space between the pleura layers around a lung, causing the afflicted lung parts to collapse. It may be attributable to chest injury (such as knife wounds) or to air from ruptured blisters on the surface of the lungs. The symptoms of pneumothorax are breathlessness, chest pain, and chest tightness. Minor pneumothorax often cures itself, but severe pneumothorax can be fatal if left untreated. Surgery to correct major pneumothorax, although rare, must be carried out quickly. Minor pneumothorax cases that require surgical intervention usually involve the insertion of a catheter to remove the intrapleural air. Patients are then monitored for several days to ensure proper healing. In cases in which the leakage of air persists or a pleural tear is responsible for the pneumothorax, surgical repair of the pleura is required.

USES AND COMPLICATIONS

Lung surgery is straightforward but potentially dangerous because it can lead to death as a result of respiratory failure. After major operations, it is important for patients to convalesce slowly and to comply with the physician's instructions. It is particularly important for the patient to ensure that infection does not occur, to report pain and other danger signs, and to convalesce carefully. The resumption of work and physical activity should be as directed by a physician.

Major advances in treating problems associated with lung surgery include better diagnosis of their extent via computed tomography (CT) scanning and magnetic resonance imaging (MRI). Furthermore, the use of cytotoxic drugs and radiotherapy to treat cancer, including lung cancer, seems to minimize the severity of the surgical treatment of these lesions.

—*Sanford S. Singer, Ph.D.*

See also Abscess drainage; Abscesses; Cancer; Chest; Edema; Embolism; Heart transplantation; Internal medicine; Lung cancer; Lungs; Pleurisy; Pneumothorax; Pulmonary diseases; Pulmonary medicine; Pulmonary medicine, pediatric; Respiration; Resuscitation; Thoracic surgery; Thrombosis and thrombus; Transplantation; Tumor removal; Tumors.

FOR FURTHER INFORMATION:

Beers, Mark H., et al., eds. *The Merck Manual of Diagnosis and Therapy.* 18th ed. Whitehouse Station, N.J.: Merck Research Laboratories, 2006. Contains a useful exposition of the characteristics, etiology, diagnosis, and treatment of lung disease. Designed for physicians, the material is also useful for less specialized readers.

Griffith, H. Winter. *Complete Guide to Symptoms, Illness, and Surgery.* Revised and updated by Stephen Moore and Kenneth Yoder. 5th ed. New York: Perigee, 2006. Covers more than five hundred diseases and disorders and includes information about causes and risk factors, preventive techniques, and diagnostic tests.

Matthews, Dawn D. *Lung Disorders Sourcebook*. Detroit, Mich.: Omnigraphics, 2002. A comprehensive overview of lung anatomy, physiology, and dysfunctions culled from government agencies, the American Academy of Family Physicians, the American Lung Association, and the Mayo Foundation. Discusses thirty-five lung disorders in depth.

Professional Guide to Diseases. 9th ed. Philadelphia: Lippincott Williams & Wilkins, 2008. A comprehensive yet concise medical reference covering more than six hundred disorders, this book includes information about the latest AIDS treatments, new parameters for defining diabetes, current information on cancers, updates on Alzheimer's disease, and more.

Tierney, Lawrence M., Stephen J. McPhee, and Maxine A. Papadakis, eds. *Current Medical Diagnosis and Treatment 2007*. New York: McGraw-Hill Medical, 2006. This text, updated yearly, is the point of reference for physicians and other health care practitioners. It incorporates each year's biomedical research discoveries that have immediate, relevant, and applicable use for the patient.

LUNGS

ANATOMY

ANATOMY OR SYSTEM AFFECTED: Chest, respiratory system

SPECIALTIES AND RELATED FIELDS: Environmental health, exercise physiology, oncology, pulmonary medicine, vascular medicine

DEFINITION: Vital organs that allow gas exchange between an organism and its environment.

KEY TERMS:

aerobic respiration: the chemical reactions that use oxygen to produce energy; some small organisms do not use oxygen and are called anaerobic

alveoli: small, thin-walled sacs at the end of the airways; most gas exchange with the blood occurs here

cellular respiration: the chemical reactions that produce energy in the cell; these reactions can be aerobic or anaerobic

cilia: hairlike structures on cells that sweep mucus containing bacteria and foreign particles out of the airways

diffusion: the constant motion of molecules that tends to spread them from places of high concentration to those of lower concentration; gases move across the alveoli by diffusion

gas exchange: the movement of oxygen and carbon dioxide across the membrane of the lungs; other gases, such as nitrogen, may also cross the membrane

mucus: a thick, clear, slimy fluid produced in many parts of the body; in the lungs, mucus catches foreign material and provides lubrication to allow smooth airflow

respiration: the exchange of gases in breathing or the cellular chemistry that involves the same gases in the cell and produces energy

STRUCTURE AND FUNCTIONS

Efficient gas exchange with the environment is critical for larger organisms because oxygen is required for the last step in a series of cellular chemical reactions which processes nutrients from food. These reactions, called aerobic respiration, provide most of the energy that maintains life. Furthermore, as these reactions proceed, parts of larger carbon molecules are removed. Carbon dioxide is produced as a by-product and must be removed from the body. Hence, oxygen and carbon dioxide must be exchanged.

Small aerobic organisms can simply absorb the oxygen from air or water across their moist membranes or skins. The oxygen travels from where it is more concentrated to where it is less concentrated, a process called diffusion. The carbon dioxide inside the cells also diffuses across the membrane in the opposite direction to the environment. Larger organisms, however, have relatively less outside surface area and require special structures for their gas exchange. Various types of gills, swim bladders, and lungs are all examples of ways to absorb more oxygen and release more carbon dioxide.

This article focuses on one of these specialized structures: the lung. The lung is found in air-breathing land creatures. It allows oxygen to enter the blood and carbon dioxide to be removed. Form reflects function: The lung provides large amounts of moist surface area, close to many small blood vessels for gas exchange. Humans have a joined pair of lungs suspended in the chest cavity. The two lungs are somewhat different in size: The left lung is divided into two lobes, while the right has three lobes. This difference reflects the fact that the left side of the chest cavity has less room because of the position and shape of the heart.

The pathway to the lungs begins with the nose. The air entering each nostril is temporarily divided among three pathways (nasal conchae) and then warmed and moisturized by contact with a mucous membrane containing many blood vessels. Bacteria and particles get caught on the sticky mucus on this membrane. If objects pass this point they can be trapped by mucus lower in the tract and be swept out by waving cilia, hairlike fibers extending from cells of the airway that move in unison to push particles backward. Large particles that irritate the mucous membranes can cause a sneeze, which may eject the offending particle at speeds up to 169 kilometers per hour.

The air then continues to the pharynx (throat), where the nasal passageways and the mouth meet, and moves into the larynx, the organ that produces the voice. Swallowing pulls the larynx upward, allowing the epiglottis to flip over the opening and prevent food from entering this part of the airway. This movement of the larynx during swallowing can be felt by light touch with the fingers.

The trachea, or windpipe, follows. It is 11 centimeters long and made rigid by rings of cartilage. The inside of the trachea has cilia and also produces mucus. As the trachea approaches the lungs, it branches into two bronchi, which enter sides of the lungs at a midpoint between top and bottom. The walls of the bronchi contain cartilage rings and smooth muscles. Irritation in the larynx, the trachea, or the bronchi may cause coughing. Coughing is a reflex, like sneezing, that attempts to cast out impurities.

The bronchi continue to branch until they contain only smooth muscle; at this point, they are called bronchioles. The smooth muscle can contract or relax to allow the diameter of the bronchioles to adjust. Hence, the airflow can be changed according to the needs of the body. The pathways inside the lungs resemble an upside-down tree. Millions of cilia line the bronchial "tree" and constantly beat to remove particles. Each bronchial tube branches into several alveolar ducts. Each duct ends with a grapelike cluster of sacs called alveoli. The irregular branching that has led to this point ranges from eight to twenty-five divisions, with an average of twenty-three. Each alveolus has walls that are only one cell thick. Because of the large number of these air sacs, the lungs are very light in weight.

Gas exchange occurs in the alveoli. These structures are closely associated with the body's smallest blood vessels, the capillaries. Oxygen dissolves into the moisture on the vast surface of the alveoli. It then crosses the thin tissue of the lungs and moves into the capillaries to enter the blood. Carbon dioxide moves in the other direction to the lungs. Direction is maintained by the principle of diffusion: Flow is always from a higher to a lower concentration. The surface tension of the watery film inside the alveoli can cause a problem in gas exchange. Water molecules have a strong attraction for one another and can cause the alveoli to collapse to a smaller volume, reducing the surface area available for gas exchange. Fortunately, among the regular cells of the lining of the alveoli is found a second type of cell, called the type II cell. Type II cells produce surfactant, a mixture of chemicals that lowers the overall surface tension in the alveoli by separating the water molecules. Therefore, the alveoli stay fully inflated.

Roaming white blood cells called macrophages are a final defense against foreign objects at the alveolar level. Macrophages protect the lungs by attacking and eating bacteria and particles. They can be found elsewhere in the body performing the same function.

The pleural membrane is a double covering, one layer lining the outside of the lungs and the other lining the inside of the chest cavity. These two layers, which are really the same membrane, move over each other as breathing occurs, reducing friction. If air enters the space between the double membrane, however, the lung will collapse, a condition known as pneumothorax.

Air enters the entire airway by expansion of the chest cavity, or thorax. The cavity can be thought of as a box in which the top cannot be moved upward but the bottom and the sides may move outward. The arched diaphragm muscle at the base of the cavity contracts to lower the bottom of the box. Muscles between the ribs, called intercostals, contract to elevate the chest. The ribs, which slant downward when relaxed, move outward. This expansion pushes the walls out, increases the volume of the chest cavity, and lowers its internal pressure, causing air to be pushed into the lungs. Exhalation results when the muscles relax and allow the natural recoil of the lungs to expel the air.

Young children breathe differently than do older children or adults. Babies and toddlers have ribs that are nearly horizontal. They depend mainly on the descent of the diaphragm muscle for breathing. By two years of age, the ribs have moved to the adult position and rib muscles increase in importance. In addition, a sexual difference in breathing has been observed. Females tend to rely mainly on rib movement, while males tend to use both rib and diaphragm movement, with an emphasis on the diaphragm.

The rate of breathing is controlled by the medulla of the brain, which checks the carbon dioxide content of the blood. Activity produces more carbon dioxide and affects the rate. The normal relaxed breathing rate is about twelve times a minute. A person resting in bed may inhale 8 liters of air per minute, while a runner may reach 50 liters per minute. If a person relaxes and falls into a very shallow rhythm, a yawn attempts to break the pattern. A yawn is a deeper breath that causes more gas exchange.

DISORDERS AND DISEASES

The lungs are the only major internal organs exposed to the outside environment, and they tend to show the effects of both age and type of use. A child's lungs are pink, but with age this color becomes darker and mottled because of particles that are trapped inside the macrophages of the lung. The lungs of city dwellers and coal miners show the greatest effects because of the poor quality of the air being inhaled. Understanding the pathologies of the lungs is linked to understanding the function of the lung itself.

For example, smoking and air pollution are known to cause chronic bronchitis. The repeated irritation of the bronchi by pollutants causes the linings of the air tubules to thicken, closing down the airways. Muscles contract, and the secretion of mucus increases. Poor drainage may lead to pneumonia. Smoking tobacco can also lead to cancer of the lung, mouth, pharynx, and esophagus. Tobacco smoke may contain as many as forty-three carcinogenic (cancer-causing) chemicals. Lung cancer usually begins with changes in the lining of the bronchi among the cells with cilia and those that produce mucus. The long-term irritation of smoking eventually destroys these cells faster than the bronchi can replace them. Abnormal cells, without cilia or the ability to produce mucus, begin to take their place. These cells offer less protection and, as irritation and replacement continues, may become cancerous. In the United States, lung cancer is the leading cause of cancer deaths in both men and women, and evidence has revealed the danger of inhaling smoke from someone else's cigarette. Smoking also leads to greater risk of various other lung diseases.

Pneumonia is a general term for any inflammation that produces a fluid buildup in the lungs. The excess fluid makes breathing difficult by blocking the alveoli. The cause of the inflammation can be bacterial, viral, fungal, or chemical. For example, Legionnaires' disease is a type of pneumonia caused by a bacterium that lives in air conditioners, humidifiers, and other water-storage devices. Because it causes a lack of oxygen in the body, pneumonia can be fatal if it is not controlled:

More than 70,000 deaths attributed to pneumonia occur in the United States each year. The very young and the very old are in the most danger, especially if they have already been weakened by other illnesses. Since the discovery of antibiotics, however, the majority of those infected recover.

Bronchitis is an inflammation of the mucous membrane of the bronchi that often follows a cold. A telltale symptom is a deep cough that eventually brings up gray or greenish phlegm. Bronchitis may be viral or bacterial; if the cause is bacterial, antibiotics can help in recovery. Chronic bronchitis can result from repeated attacks of bronchitis and is aggravated by smoking and air pollution.

Another lung disease is emphysema, which is usually caused by smoking. This condition is often seen in advanced cases of chronic bronchitis. In emphysema, the alveoli overinflate and break. Nearby alveoli are damaged and merge into larger units, leaving less surface area for gas exchange. Therefore, less of the air coming into the lungs comes into contact with the membrane. The increase in dead air space requires deeper breaths to obtain oxygen, and the lungs suffer further damage. Because the air sacs are permanently broken down, the damage is irreversible.

Tuberculosis is a highly contagious bacterial infection that damages the lungs and can spread to the kidneys and the bones. Immunization, screening for exposure, and antibiotics have controlled the number of cases found in countries with modern medical care systems. Worldwide, however, tuberculosis remains a major danger, and millions of lives are still lost to this disease every year.

According to the Mayo Clinic, cases of asthma appear to be increasing in the United States population. Asthma involves a hyperactive response of the airways. During an attack, the smooth muscles of the bronchi and bronchioles contract, and excess mucus is produced. In other cases, the airways may become inflamed and swollen. The cause may be allergies or other stimuli. Asthma is rarely fatal but interferes with normal functioning, as breathing becomes difficult. The blockage of breathing can be reversed with proper medications. Asthma does not lead to emphysema.

Respiratory distress syndrome occurs in about 50,000 premature infants every year. These infants have not yet developed the ability to produce sufficient surfactant in their alveoli to prevent collapse. The importance of surfactant can be illustrated by the difficulty of a baby's first breath. To inflate the alveoli requires up to twenty times the force of a normal breath. Without surfactant, the alveoli would collapse again and the next breath would be just as difficult. In 1990, a surfactant treatment derived from calf lungs became available. Treatment of premature babies with this surfactant before symptoms develop has resulted in an 88 percent survival rate.

Cystic fibrosis is a severe genetic problem in which the mucus produced in the airways (and the gastrointestinal tract) is abnormally thick. This thick mucus interferes with gas exchange, causing the heart to work harder and the valves to be damaged. As a result, the lung may collapse. Serious infections are more likely to occur. While about 50 percent of those with cystic fibrosis live only until their late teens and twenties, an increasing number of children and young adults with this disease are living into adult life. Progress on curing cystic fibrosis is being made: Researchers working in this area have located the gene that causes the condition.

If air is allowed to enter between the pleural membrane, the lungs will instantly collapse. The two lungs are independent enough so that one lung can be collapsed for healing while the other performs the gas exchange for the body. Furthermore, each lung subdivides into its lobes and then into ten bronchopulmonary segments. Each of these segments is a structural unit that can be removed surgically if diseased.

PERSPECTIVE AND PROSPECTS

The ancient Greeks established the first understandings of lung function. They rightly accepted that life depended on air but overgeneralized that air carried all disease. Empedocles of Agrigentum (c. 500-430 B.C.E.) demonstrated that air was a real substance by filling a wineskin with it. Empedocles erred, however, in explaining the mechanism of breathing. He compared the body to a pipe and thought that the movement of air in and out of the lungs caused vital air to move in and out of pores in the body's skin.

The writings of Galen of Pergamum (129-c. 199 C.E.) came to dominate Western medicine until the Renaissance. In his physiology, Galen attempted to connect the function of the lungs with the blood. He believed, however, that the liver produced a "vegetative" blood that traveled to the vena cava and then took different pathways. Some then flowed to other veins to nourish the whole body for growth. The rest entered the right side of the heart. Some of this substance entered the pulmonary artery into the lungs to allow impurities to be exhaled. The rest filtered to the left side of the heart through imagined pores in the septum.

In Galen's complicated scheme, the lungs were not only for exhaust: Vital air was inhaled there to be modified. The heart then pumped the modified air through the pulmonary vein to its left side. Here the air joined the blood to become "vital spirit," which traveled by arteries to warm the whole body. The brain converted this vital spirit into "animal spirit," distributing it by the nerves to cause movement and sensation. Galen did not know that blood traveled from one side of the heart to the other by moving through the lungs. He believed that the lungs acted as a reservoir of air for the heart. Galen also thought that breathing cooled the heart.

William Harvey (1578-1657) studied the position of valves in the veins and realized that Galen's vegetative blood traveled backward. Harvey then argued for a single blood that must go through the lungs to reach the other side of the heart. Blood travels in a circle, he bravely suggested. He was supported when the new microscopes discovered the necessary small vessels that connect arteries to veins.

Antoine-Laurent Lavoisier (1743-1794) noted that the lungs take in oxygen and that carbon dioxide is exhaled. He concluded that a slow combustion must occur in the lungs to warm the blood, while opponents noted that the lungs are not warmer than other parts of the body. By the 1790's, the idea was accepted that the lungs exchange Lavoisier's gases with the blood. Many believed that blood was the essence of life. In the 1850's, however, Georg Liebig and Hermann von Helmholtz showed that muscle tissue uses oxygen and releases carbon dioxide and heat. It was finally realized that the cells are the location of Lavoisier's slow fire of respiration and that the blood is the carrier of gases between the cells and the lungs.

—Paul R. Boehlke, Ph.D.

See also Abscess drainage; Abscesses; Allergies; Altitude sickness; Anatomy; Apnea; Asbestos exposure; Aspergillosis; Asphyxiation; Asthma; Avian influenza; Bacterial infections; Bronchi; Bronchiolitis; Bronchitis; Cancer; Chest; Childhood infectious diseases; Choking; Chronic obstructive pulmonary disease (COPD); Common cold; Coughing; Croup; Cyanosis; Cystic fibrosis; Diphtheria; Edema; Embolism; Emphysema; Environmental diseases; Environmental health; Exercise physiology; Heart transplantation; Hyperventilation; Influenza; Internal medicine; Interstitial pulmonary fibrosis (IPF); Kinesiology; Legionnaires' disease; Lung cancer; Lung surgery;

Measles; Multiple chemical sensitivity syndrome; Nicotine; Occupational health; Oxygen therapy; Physiology; Plague; Pleurisy; Pneumonia; Pneumothorax; Pulmonary diseases; Pulmonary edema; Pulmonary hypertension; Pulmonary medicine; Pulmonary medicine, pediatric; Respiration; Respiratory distress syndrome; Resuscitation; Smoking; Systems and organs; Thoracic surgery; Thrombolytic therapy and TPA; Thrombosis and thrombus; Toxoplasmosis; Transplantation; Tuberculosis; Tumor removal; Tumors; Wheezing; Whooping cough.

FOR FURTHER INFORMATION:

Corrin, Bryan, and Andrew G. Nicholson. *Pathology of the Lungs*. 2d ed. New York: Churchill Livingstone/Elsevier, 2006. This volume discusses such topics as lung development, infectious diseases, vascular disease, tumors, and transplantation.

Levitzky, Michael G. *Pulmonary Physiology*. 7th ed. New York: McGraw-Hill Medical, 2007. A clinical text that describes the structure and function of the respiratory system. Covers topics such as the physical process of respiration from the interrelationship of basic lung mechanics, the microscopic changes at the alveolar level of gas exchange, the "nonrespiratory" functions of the lungs, and how the lungs respond to stress.

Mason, Robert J., et al., eds. *Murray and Nadel's Textbook of Respiratory Medicine*. 5th ed. Philadelphia: Saunders/Elsevier, 2010. Details basic anatomy, physiology, pharmacology, pathology, and immunology of the lungs.

Sarosi, George A., and Scott F. Davies, eds. *Fungal Diseases of the Lung*. 3d ed. Philadelphia: Lippincott Williams & Wilkins, 2000. This resource covers a wide range of topics, including blastomycosis, coccidioidomycosis, cryptococcosis, and sporotrichosis.

Tapley, Donald F., et al., eds. *The Columbia University College of Physicians and Surgeons Complete Home Medical Guide*. Rev. 3d ed. New York: Crown, 1995. A comprehensive, practical health guide explaining all aspects of illness and treatment in common language. The section on respiratory diseases and lung health covers both the causes and the prevention of various diseases and problems.

West, John B. *Pulmonary Pathophysiology: The Essentials*. 7th ed. Philadelphia: Wolters Kluwer/Lippincott Williams & Wilkins, 2008. Examines lungs afflicted with obstructive, restrictive, vascular, and environmental diseases. Bronchoactive drugs,

the causes of hypoventilation, and the pathogenesis of asthma and pulmonary edema are new topics covered in this edition.

LUPUS. *See* SYSTEMIC LUPUS ERYTHEMATOSUS (SLE).

LYME DISEASE
DISEASE/DISORDER
ALSO KNOWN AS: Lyme borreliosis
ANATOMY OR SYSTEM AFFECTED: Eyes, heart, joints, knees, nerves, nervous system, skin
SPECIALTIES AND RELATED FIELDS: Bacteriology, cardiology, dermatology, epidemiology, neurology, ophthalmology, rheumatology
DEFINITION: Lyme disease is caused by bacteria transmitted by ticks. Initial symptoms include a spreading rash at the site of the tick bite; later, the central nervous system, heart, or joints may be affected.
KEY TERMS:
ectoparasite: an external parasite
seronegative Lyme disease: Lyme disease in which serum lacks a reaction with antibodies
spirochete: a long, helically coiled bacterial cell

CAUSES AND SYMPTOMS

Lyme disease is the most common tick-borne disease in the United States and Europe. It is caused by spirochete bacteria of the species complex *Borrelia burgdorferi sensu lato*. (This name refers to all bacteria causing Lyme disease.) *Borrelia burgdorferi sensu stricto* is the predominant cause of Lyme disease in the United States, while *Borrelia afzelii* and *Borrelia garinii* more often cause Lyme disease in Europe. The hard-bodied (Ixodes) tick transmits *Borrelia burgdorferi* to humans. Lyme disease is endemic in parts of New England, the upper Midwest, and Northern California. The tick species *Ixodes scapularis* (the black-legged tick or deer tick) transmits Lyme disease in the East and Midwest, while *Ixodes pacificus* (the Western black-legged tick) is the vector for Lyme disease in the West. In Europe, *Ixodes ricinus* (the sheep tick) is the vector.

Ticks are arachnid, obligate, blood-feeding ectoparasites with mouth parts that pierce the host skin. The tick saliva contains analgesics, anti-inflammatories, antihistamines, and anticoagulants that make it less likely that the tick bite will be detected. A tick takes three blood meals—as a larva, a nymph, and an adult—typically from different host species. The spirochete does not pass from the adult tick into the tick eggs.

INFORMATION ON LYME DISEASE

CAUSES: Bacterial infection from bite of infected ticks
SYMPTOMS: Fatigue, malaise, chills and fever, headache, muscle and joint pain, swollen lymph nodes, rash, arthritis, nervous system abnormalities
DURATION: Acute
TREATMENTS: Oral antibiotics

When a tick larva feeds on a host infected with *Borrelia burgdorferi*, that larva becomes infected, molts to the nymph stage, and passes on the spirochete when it takes its next blood meal. In the eastern United States, the hosts infected with *Borrelia burgdorferi* on which the tick feeds are white-footed mice (the reservoirs of infection) and deer. There is a receptor that binds an outer membrane protein of the bacterium to maintain the bacteria in the tick gut. When the tick begins feeding on another host, a bacterial protein is produced that aids in detaching the bacteria from the receptor, and bacteria begin multiplying. The bacteria then go to the salivary glands and via saliva go to the host skin. Initially, there is little or no transmission of bacteria to the host. It takes at least twelve hours and perhaps as long as three days before the efficient transfer of bacteria. Even though the adult tick is twice as likely as the nymph to be infected with the Lyme spirochete, most cases of Lyme disease are noted in the late spring and summer, when nymphs seek blood meals from hosts. This may be because the smaller nymph is more difficult to notice.

Within a month after *Borrelia burgdorferi* bacteria enter the skin, a bull's-eye-shaped, rapidly expanding rash may form at the bite site. Bacteria travel through the bloodstream to other organs. Viral infection-like symptoms may develop, such as fatigue, headache, and neck pain. Respiratory symptoms, such as coughing, and vomiting or diarrhea do not occur. Not all who have the viral infection-like symptoms develop the rash or note a tick bite. About 60 percent of those who had the skin rash and were not treated develop arthritis, usually of the knee. About 10 percent develop neurological problems, usually facial nerve palsy. About 5 percent develop a cardiac complication as a result of atrioventricular block. The eyes may also be affected.

Lyme disease experts disagree about other possible effects. In some individuals, months after initial infec-

tion and treatment, symptoms such as muscle pain and fatigue seem to develop. Bacteria in some parts of the body may be resistant to antibiotic treatment, causing a persistent infection. Such infections would benefit from additional antibiotic treatment. A Lyme infection may be more severe because of coinfection from the tick with other pathogens, such as the rickettsial infection human granulocytic anaplasmosis and the protozoan disease babesiosis.

TREATMENT AND THERAPY

To prevent Lyme disease, avoiding exposure to ticks is key. In a tick-infected area, one should wear protective clothing, use tick repellent such as DEET, check daily for ticks, and promptly remove any ticks. To reduce the population of ticks around a house, the lawn should be kept mowed and brush cleared.

The rash of Lyme disease is treated with antibiotics such as doxycycline, amoxicillin, or cefuroxime axetil. For those under eight years of age and pregnant women, however, doxycycline is not recommended.

In the late 1990's, a vaccine against Lyme disease was available. This vaccine induced the production of antibodies to a *Borrelia burgdorferi* outer cell membrane surface lipoprotein. In 2002, the manufacturers of the vaccine withdrew it from the market because of problems involving postvaccination fatigue.

PERSPECTIVE AND PROSPECTS

The clinical symptoms of Lyme disease have been documented in European medical literature as early as the 1880's, but each clinical sign was considered a separate illness. In the 1970's, an outbreak of apparent juvenile rheumatoid arthritis, in some cases preceded by a rash, occurred in Old Lyme and Lyme, Connecticut. In 1975, this range of different symptoms was recognized as a single illness. *Borrelia burgdorferi* was identified in 1982 by Willy Burgdorfer, a tick-borne disease expert from the Rocky Mountain Labs in Montana.

In 2006, the Infectious Diseases Society of America (IDSA) released updated diagnosis and treatment guidelines for Lyme disease. These guidelines recommend a bull's-eye, or erythema migrans (EM), rash or positive laboratory tests to diagnose Lyme disease. The IDSA guidelines do not recognize a chronic form of Lyme disease, nor do they recognize seronegative Lyme disease except in early infections. This stance has generated a great deal of controversy. Both the International Lyme and Associated Disease Society (ILADS), a professional medical society, and the Lyme

Disease Association, an all-volunteer association, have expressed concern about the stricter guidelines. They worry that patients with chronic Lyme disease will continue to suffer. There is much more to learn about the Lyme bacteria in order to aid patients.

—*Susan J. Karcher, Ph.D.*

See also Antibiotics; Arthritis; Bacterial infections; Bites and stings; Epidemiology; Lice, mites, and ticks.

FOR FURTHER INFORMATION:

American Lyme Disease Foundation. http://www.aldf .com.

Edlow, Jonathan A. *Bull's-Eye: Unraveling the Medical Mystery of Lyme Disease.* 2d ed. New Haven, Conn.: Yale University Press, 2004.

Edlow, Jonathan A., and Robert Moellering, Jr., eds. "Tick-borne Diseases, Part 1: Lyme Disease." *Infectious Disease Clinics of North America* 22, no. 2 (June, 2008).

International Lyme and Associated Disease Society. http://www.ilads.org.

Lyme Disease Association. http://www.lymedisease association.org.

Stricker, Raphael B., Andrew Lautin, and Joseph J. Burrascano. "Lyme Disease: The Quest for Magic Bullets." *Chemotherapy* 52 (2006): 53-59.

Wormser, Gary P., et al. "The Clinical Assessment, Treatment, and Prevention of Lyme Disease, Human Granulocytic Anaplasmosis, and Babesiosis: Clinical Practice Guidelines by the Infectious Diseases Society of America." *Clinical Infectious Diseases* 43, no. 9 (2006): 1089-1134.

Lymph

Biology

Anatomy or system affected: Blood, circulatory system, immune system, lymphatic system, spleen

Specialties and related fields: Hematology, immunology, internal medicine, oncology, serology

Definition: A milky fluid that carries cellular waste, nutrients, and pathogens for processing in the lymphatic system.

Structure and Functions

Blood flows from the heart through smaller and smaller arteries until it reaches capillaries. There the plasma (blood without red blood cells) oozes into the surrounding tissue, bathing the cells in oxygen, nutrients, and hormones. About 90 percent of this tissue fluid (also known as intercellular fluid or interstitial fluid) is absorbed back into the blood system via the veins. The remaining 10 percent enters the lymphatic system, and this is the milky fluid known as lymph. It carries with it cellular debris, minerals, proteins, and pathogens, such as viruses, bacteria, and cancer cells.

The lymphatic system is a network of vessels, similar to blood vessels, and lymph nodes. At some point, lymph passes through one of the hundred lymph nodes in the body, where it is cleansed of debris. White blood cells, primarily lymphocytes and macrophages, attack cancer cells and cells infected by microorganisms. Lymph therefore helps the immune system combat disease. The lymphatic system also plays a role in balancing the body's fluid load. Lymph exits the lymphatic system at the subclavian veins at the base of the neck, reentering the blood.

Disorders and Diseases

Problems associated with lymph arise when the lymphatic system fails to circulate it or when the fluid carries pathogens that cause an infection in the system. Lymphedema is the accumulation of lymph, which causes swelling. Congenital lymphedema is caused by an inadequate number of lymph vessels. It results in swelling in the legs, for the most part. The more common acquired lymphedema is usually the result of major surgery that involves removal of lymph nodes—as occurs, for instance, during surgery for breast cancer. Filariasis, a parasitical infection, can cause scarring and constriction in the lymphatic vessels and lymphedema. It may so distend the legs that they look like elephant legs, a rare condition known as elephantiasis.

Lymphadenitis is the inflammation of lymph nodes by a pathogen, typically bacteria or viruses spread from the skin or an orifice. Similarly, acute lymphangitis involves inflamed lymph vessels because of bacteria, usually streptococcus, in the skin.

—*Roger Smith, Ph.D.*

See also Blood and blood disorders; Circulation; Elephantiasis; Immune system; Immunology; Immunopathology; Lymphadenopathy and lymphoma; Lymphatic system; Vascular medicine; Vascular system.

FOR FURTHER INFORMATION:

Beers, Mark H., ed. *The Merck Manual of Medical Information: Second Home Edition.* Whitehouse Station, N.J.: Merck Research Laboratories, 2003.

Faiz, Omar, and David Moffat. *Anatomy at a Glance.* 2d ed. Malden, Mass.: Blackwell, 2006.

McDowell, Julie, and Michael Windelsprecht. *The Lymphatic System.* Santa Barbara, Calif.: Greenwood, 2004.

Parker, Steve. *The Human Body Book.* New York: DK Adult, 2001.

Thibodeau, Gary A., and Kevin T. Patton. *Structure and Function of the Human Body.* 13th ed. St. Louis: Mosby/Elsevier, 2008.

LYMPHADENOPATHY AND LYMPHOMA
DISEASE/DISORDER

ANATOMY OR SYSTEM AFFECTED: Lymphatic system

SPECIALTIES AND RELATED FIELDS: Hematology, internal medicine, oncology, vascular medicine

DEFINITION: Lymphadenopathy, or enlarged lymph nodes, refers to any disorder related to the lymphatic vessels of lymph nodes; lymphoma is a group of cancers consisting of unchecked multiplication of lymphatic tissue cells.

KEY TERMS:

B lymphocyte: a blood and lymphatic cell that plays a role in the secretion of antibodies

Hodgkin's disease: a malignant disorder of lymphoid tissue, generally first appearing in cervical lymph nodes, which is characterized by the presence of the Reed-Sternberg cell

lymphoma staging: a classification of lymphomas based upon the stage of the disease; used in the determination of treatment

non-Hodgkin's lymphoma: any malignant lymphoproliferative disorder other than Hodgkin's disease

Reed-Sternberg cell: a large atypical macrophage with multiple nuclei; found in patients with Hodgkin's disease

T lymphocyte: a blood and lymphatic cell that functions in cell-mediated immunity, which involves the direct attack of diseased tissues; subclasses of T cells aid B lymphocytes in the production of antibodies

CAUSES AND SYMPTOMS

The lymphatic system consists of a large complex of lymph vessels and groups of lymph nodes ("lymph glands"). The lymph vessels include a vast number of capillaries that collect fluid and dissolved proteins, carbohydrates, and fats from tissue fluids. The lacteals of the intestinal villi are lymph vessels that serve to absorb fats from the intestine and transport them to the bloodstream.

Lymph nodes are found throughout the body but are concentrated most heavily in regions of the head, neck, armpits, abdomen, and groin. Nodes function to filter out foreign materials, such as bacteria or viruses, which make their way into lymphatic vessels.

The sizes of lymph nodes vary: Some are as small as a pinhead, some as large as a bean. In general, they are shaped much like kidney beans, with an outer covering. Internally, they consist of a compartmentalized mass of tissue that contains large numbers of B and T lymphocytes as well as antigen-presenting cells (APC). The lymphatic circulation into the lymph nodes consists of a series of entering, or afferent, vessels, which empty into internal spaces, or sinuses. A network of connective tissue, the reticulum, regulates the lymph flow and serves as a site of attachment for lymphocytes and macrophages. The lymphatic circulation leaves the node through efferent, or exiting, vessels in the lower portion of the organ, the hilum.

Among the functions of lymph nodes are those of the immune response. B and T lymphocytes tend to congregate in specialized areas of the lymph nodes: B cells in the outer region, or cortex, and T cells in the underlying paracortex. When antigen is presented by an APC, T- and B-cell interaction triggers B-cell maturation and proliferation within the germinal centers of the cortex. The result may be a significant enlargement of the germinal centers and subsequently of the lymph node itself.

Lymphadenopathy, or enlarged lymph nodes, may signify a lymphoma, or cancer of the lymphatic system. More commonly, however, the enlarged node is secondary to other phenomena, usually local infections. For example, an ear infection may result in the entrance of bacteria into local lymphatic vessels. These vessels drain into regional nodes of the neck. The result is an enlargement of the nodes in this area, as an immune response is carried out.

Enlarged nodes caused by infections can, in general,

INFORMATION ON
LYMPHADENOPATHY AND LYMPHOMA

CAUSES: Disease, allergies, infection, viruses, genetic factors

SYMPTOMS: Enlarged lymph nodes, fatigue, mild fever, night sweats, weight loss

DURATION: Varies from acute to long-term

TREATMENTS: Vary; may include antibiotics, radiation therapy, chemotherapy, bone marrow transplantation

be easily differentiated from those caused by malignancies. Infectious nodes are generally smaller than 2 centimeters in diameter, soft, and tender. They usually occur in areas where common infections occur, such as the ears or the throat. Malignant lymph nodes are often large and occur in groups. They are generally firm and hard, and they often appear in unusual areas of the body (for example, along the diaphragm). To confirm a malignancy, a biopsy of material may be necessary.

Infectious nodes can also be caused by diseases such as infectious mononucleosis, tuberculosis, and acquired immunodeficiency syndrome (AIDS). Lymphadenopathy syndrome (LAS), a generalized enlargement of the lymph nodes, is a common feature of the prodromal AIDS-related complex (ARC).

Since lymphadenopathy can be caused by any immune proliferation in the germinal centers, allergy-related illnesses may also cause enlargement of the lymph nodes. Consequently, immune disorders such as rheumatoid arthritis, systemic lupus erythematosus, and even hay fever allergies may show enlarged nodes as part of their syndromes.

As is the case for any cell in the body, cells constituting the lymphatic system may undergo a malignant transformation. The broadest definition of these lymphoproliferative diseases, or lymphomas, can include both Hodgkin's disease and Hodgkin's lymphomas, in addition to acute and chronic lymphocytic leukemias (ALL and CLL). With the understanding of, and ability to detect, specific cell markers, it is possible to classify many of these lymphomas on the basis of their cellular origin. Such is the case for ALL, CLL, Burkitt's lymphoma, and many other forms of non-Hodgkin's lymphomas. The cell type that ultimately forms the basis for Hodgkin's disease remains uncertain.

Hodgkin's disease is a malignant lymphoma that first manifests itself as a painless enlargement of lymphoid tissue. Often, this is initially observed in the form of swollen lymph nodes in the neck or cervical region. Occasionally, the victim may exhibit a mild fever, night sweats, and weight loss. Untreated, the disease spreads from one lymphatic region to another, resulting in diffuse adenopathy. An enlarged spleen (splenomegaly) is a common result. As the disease spreads, other organs such as the liver, lungs, and bone marrow may be involved.

The disease is characterized by the presence of a characteristic cell type—the Reed-Sternberg cell. Reed-Sternberg cells appear to be of macrophage origin, with multilobed nuclei or multiple nuclei. They may also

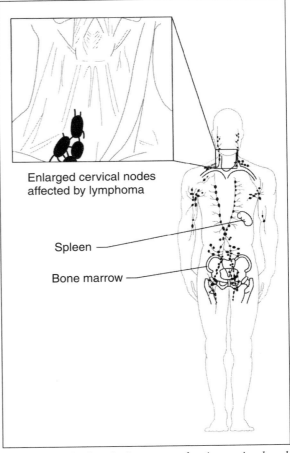

Enlarged cervical nodes affected by lymphoma

Spleen

Bone marrow

Anatomy of the lymphatic system, showing major lymph nodes; enlarged lymph nodes may occur for a wide variety of reasons, including but not limited to lymphoma (cancer).

be present in other lymphatic disorders, but their presence is considered to be indicative of all cases of Hodgkin's disease. The precise relationship of the cell to the lymphoma is unclear, but some researchers in the field believe that the Reed-Sternberg cell is the actual malignant cell of the disease. The other infiltrative cells present in the node, including many B and T lymphocytes, may simply represent the reaction to the neoplasm. This interpretation, however, has been disputed.

Lymphoma staging is a system of classifying lymphomas according to the stage of development of the disease. Staging is important in that the prognosis and basis for treatment are in part determined by the stage of disease. Characterizing the form of Hodgkin's disease, therefore, involves two forms of classification. The first is a four-part classification based on the histology or cell type (Rye Conference classification). This scheme is based upon the proportion of Reed-Sternberg cells, ranging from their being "hard to find" to their being the predominant type. The prognosis becomes less favorable as the proportion of these cells increases.

Clinical staging, like that based on histology, is a four-part classification scheme (it is actually six parts, since stage III can be divided into subclasses). In this system, classification is based upon the extent of spread or extralymphatic involvement. For example, stage I features the involvement of a single lymph node region or a single extralymphatic site. Stage IV involves multiple disseminated foci. Early-stage disease is more easily treated and has a better prognosis than late-stage disease.

Non-Hodgkin's lymphomas (NHLs) represent a multitude of malignant disorders. Unlike Hodgkin's disease, they frequently arise in lymphatic tissue that is not easily observed; for example, in the gastrointestinal tract, tonsils, bone, and central nervous system. They have a tendency to spread rapidly, with malignant cells being released into the bloodstream early in the disease. Consequently, by the time diagnosis of NHL is made, the disease has often spread and the prognosis may be poor.

Though the etiology of most forms of NHL remains unknown, certain characteristics are evident in some forms of these diseases. For example, a portion of chromosome 14 is elongated in about 60 percent of NHL patients. Nearly one-third of patients with NHLs of B-cell origin demonstrate a chromosomal translocation, often involving a piece of chromosome 14 being translocated to chromosome 18. Though the relationship of these changes to disease is unclear, one can surmise that chromosomal defects play at least some role in the development of some forms of these disorders.

At least two forms of NHL are either caused by viruses or related to their presence: Burkitt's lymphoma and adult T-cell lymphoma/leukemia. Burkitt's lymphoma, which was first described by Denis Burkitt in central Africa, is a B-cell tumor that occurs primarily in children. It is generally manifested as a large tumor of the jaw. This type of lymphoma is associated with early infection by the Epstein-Barr virus, or EBV (also the etiological agent of infectious mononucleosis). The relationship of the disorder to the virus remains unclear, and EBV may be either a specific cause or a necessary cofactor.

Specific chromosomal abnormalities are also associated with Burkitt's lymphoma. In 75 percent of cases, a translocation from chromosome 8 to chromosome 14 is evident, while in most other cases, a portion of chromosome 8 is translocated to either chromosome 2 or chromosome 22. Each of these translocations involves the transfer of the same gene from chromosome 8, the *c-myc* gene. The site to which the *c-myc* is translocated is in each instance a region that encodes protein chains for antibody production, proteins that are produced in large quantities. The *c-myc* gene product normally plays a role in committing a cell to divide. By being translocated into these specific regions, the *c-myc* gene product is overproduced, and the B cell undergoes continual replication.

Approximately 80 percent of NHL tumors are of B-cell origin; the remainder are primarily of T-cell origin. Those lymphomas that arise within the thymus, the organ of T-cell maturation, are called lymphoblastic lymphomas. Those that originate as more differentiated and mature T cells outside the thymus include a heterogeneous group of diseases (for example, peripheral T-cell lymphomas and Sézary syndrome). Often, by the time of diagnosis, these disorders have spread beyond the early stage of classification and have become difficult to treat.

Treatment and Therapy

Treatment and other means of dealing with lymphadenopathy depend on the specific cause. In the case of lymph node enlargement that is secondary to infections, treatment of the primary cause is sufficient to restore the normal appearance of the node. For example, in a situation in which nodes in the neck region are enlarged as the result of a throat infection, antibiotic treatment of the primary cause—that is, the bacterial infection—is sufficient. The nodes will resume their normal size after a short time.

Dealing with lymph node enlargement caused by lymphoma requires a much more aggressive form of treatment. There are many kinds of lymphomas, which differ in type of cell involvement and stage of differentiation of the involved cells. The manifestations of most lymphomas, however, are similar. In general, these disorders first present themselves as painless, enlarged nodes. Often, this occurs in the neck region, but in many forms of NHL, the lymphadenopathy may manifest itself elsewhere in the lymphatic system. As the disease progresses, splenomegaly (enlarged spleen) and hepatomegaly (enlarged liver) may manifest themselves. Frequently, the bone marrow becomes involved. If the enlarged node compresses a vital organ or vessel in the body, immediate surgery may be necessary. For example, if one of the veins of the heart is compressed, the patient may be in immediate, life-threatening danger. Treatment generally includes radiation therapy and/or chemotherapy.

As is true for lymphomas in general, Hodgkin's disease is found more commonly in males than in females. In the United States, it occurs at a rate of 2 per 100,000 population per year, resulting in more than 6,000 cases being diagnosed each year. Approximately 1,500 persons die of the disease each year. The cause of the disease is unknown, though attempts have been made to assign the Epstein-Barr virus to this role.

Hodgkin's disease has an unusual age incidence. The age-specific incidence exhibits a bimodal curve. The disease shows an initial peak among young adults between fifteen and thirty years of age. The incidence drops after age thirty, only to show an additional increase in frequency after age fifty. This is in contrast to NHL, which shows a sharp increase in incidence only after age forty-five. The reasons are unknown.

As noted earlier, the staging of Hodgkin's disease is important in determining methods of treatment; the earlier the stage, the better the prognosis. Patients in stage I (single node or site of involvement) or stage II (two or more nodes on the same side of the diaphragm involved, or limited extralymphatic involvement) have a much better prognosis than patients in stages III and IV (splenic or disseminated disease). Prior to the mid-1960's, a diagnosis of Hodgkin's disease was almost a death sentence. The development of radiation therapy and chemotherapy has dramatically increased the chances for survival; long-term remission can be achieved in nearly 70 percent of patients, and the "cure" rate may be higher than 90 percent with early detection. In part, this has been the result of understanding the progression of the disease (reflected in the process of staging) and utilizing a therapeutic approach to eradicate the disease both at its current site and at likely sites of spreading.

Radiation therapy is the treatment of choice for patients in stages I and II; spreading beyond local nodes is still unlikely in these stages. The body is divided into three regions to which radiation may be delivered: The mantle field covers the upper chest and armpits, the para-aortic field is the region of the diaphragm and spleen, and the third field is the pelvic area. For example, a patient manifesting lymphadenopathy in a single node in the neck region may undergo only "mantle" ir-

radiation. As noted above, with early detection, such treatment is effective 90 percent of the time (based on five-year disease-free survival).

Beyond stage II, a combination of radiation therapy and chemotherapy treatment is warranted. A variety of chemotherapy programs have been developed, the most common of which is known by the acronym MOPP (nitrogen mustard/Oncovin/procarbazine/prednisone). With combined radiation therapy and chemotherapy, even stage III disease may go into remission 60 to 70 percent of the time, while 40 to 50 percent of stage IV patients may enter remission. In general, therapy takes six to twelve months.

Non-Hodgkin's lymphomas represent a heterogeneous group of malignancies. Eighty percent are of B-lymphocyte origin. The wide variety of types has made classification difficult. The most useful method of classification for clinical purposes is based on the relative aggressiveness of the disease, low-grade being the slowest growing, followed by intermediate-grade and high-grade, which is the most aggressive.

NHLs often arise in lymphoid areas outside the mainstream. For example, the first sign of disease may be an abdominal mass or pain. Fever and night sweats are uncommon, at least in the early stages. Consequently, once the disease is manifested, it is often deep and widespread. Because the disorder is no longer localized by this stage, radiation therapy by itself is of limited use. For comparison, nearly half of Hodgkin's disease patients are in stage I at presentation; not quite 15 percent of NHL patients are in stages I and II. Consequently, treatment almost always involves extensive chemotherapy.

A variety of aggressive forms of chemotherapy may be applied. These may include either single drugs such as alkaloids (vincristine sulfate) and alkylating agents (chlorambucil) or combination programs such as that of MOPP. Low-grade types of NHL are frequently slow growing and respond well to less aggressive forms of therapy. Low-grade NHL patients often enter remission for years. Unfortunately, the disorder often recurs with time and may become resistant to treatment; remission may occur in 50 percent of the patients, but only about 10 percent survive disease-free after ten years. High-grade lymphomas are rapidly growing, and the prognosis for most patients in the short term is not good. Those patients who do achieve remission with aggressive therapy, however, often show no recurrence of disease. As many as 50 percent of these persons may be "cured." The difference in prognosis between low-grade and high-grade disease may relate to the characteristics of the malignant cell. A rapidly growing cancer cell may be more susceptible to aggressive therapy than a slow-growing cancer and more likely to die as a result. Thus, if a patient enters remission following therapy, there is greater likelihood that the cancer has been eradicated.

PERSPECTIVE AND PROSPECTS

What was likely Hodgkin's disease was first described in 1666 as an illness in which lymphoid tissues and the spleen had the appearance of a "cluster of grapes." The disorder was invariably fatal. In 1832, Thomas Hodgkin published a thorough description of the disease, including its progression from the cervical region of the body to other lymphatic regions and organs. The unusual histological appearance of the cellular mixture characteristic of Hodgkin's disease was noted during the nineteenth century. It was early in the twentieth century, however, that Dorothy Reed and Karl Sternberg described the cell that is characteristic of the disorder: the Reed-Sternberg cell. As noted earlier, the number and proportion of such cells are the bases for the classification of the disease.

Two forms of non-Hodgkin's lymphoma are known to be associated with specific viruses: Burkitt's lymphoma (BL) and adult T-cell leukemia (ATL). BL was described by Denis Burkitt, who studied the pattern of certain forms of lymphomas among Ugandan children during the late 1950's. He noted that nearly all cases were found in children between the ages of two and fourteen, and noted that most cases in Africa were found in the malarial belt. Burkitt suspected that a mosquito might be involved in the transmissions of BL. Though no link has been found with arthropod transmission, the idea that BL might be associated with a viral agent bore fruit. In 1964, Michael Epstein and Yvonne Barr reported the presence of a particle in BL tissue that resembled the herpes virus. The Epstein-Barr virus was eventually linked to BL, though the specific role played by the virus remains elusive.

Adult T-cell leukemia was first noted in Japan during the 1970's. Japanese scientists observed that the majority of NHLs there were of T-cell origin and exhibited a similar clinical spectrum. The disease was later observed in the Caribbean basin, the southeastern United States, South America, and central Africa. In 1980, Robert Gallo isolated the etiological agent, the human T-cell lymphotrophic type I virus (HTLV-I).

The treatment of Hodgkin's disease represents one of the few success stories in dealing with cancers. In addition, some forms of NHL—notably, Burkitt's lymphoma—respond well to treatment. The prognosis for most patients with NHL, however, is less than optimal. In addition, the specific causes of most NHL syndromes are not known. Those with which a virus is linked may, in theory, be prevented by means of vaccination. The etiological agents or factors associated with the development of other forms of lymphomas remain elusive.

—Richard Adler, Ph.D.

See also Burkitt's lymphoma; Cancer; Carcinogens; Chemotherapy; Epstein-Barr virus; Hodgkin's disease; Infection; Lymph; Lymphatic system; Malignancy and metastasis; Oncology; Radiation therapy.

FOR FURTHER INFORMATION:

Cerroni, Lorenzo, Kevin Gatter, and Helmut Kerl. *Skin Lymphoma: The Illustrated Guide.* 3d ed. Hoboken, N.J.: Wiley-Blackwell, 2009. This book is an extremely practical guide to diagnosis that will help any pathologist spot skin lymphoma. It combines stunning pictures of histopathology (tissue specimens) with the clinical features, making it attractive and useful to pathologists and clinicians.

Delves, Peter J., et al. *Roitt's Essential Immunology.* 11th ed. Malden, Mass.: Blackwell, 2006. An outstanding textbook on immunology. The early chapters on the lymphatic system, lymph nodes, and the immune response provide an excellent background for the subject.

Greer, John, et al., eds. *Wintrobe's Clinical Hematology.* 12th ed. Philadelphia: Wolters Kluwer/Lippincott Williams & Wilkins Health, 2009. A textbook of hematologic disorders, with an excellent review of lymphatic diseases, including Hodgkin's disease. Written for clinicians and students of medicine.

Holman, Peter, and Jodi Garrett. *One Hundred Questions and Answers About Lymphoma.* 2d ed. Sudbury, Mass.: Jones and Bartlett, 2011. A patient-oriented guide that covers a range of topics related to lymphatic diseases, including risk factors and causes; methods of prevention, screening, and diagnosis; available treatments and how to choose among them; and ways of coping with common emotional and physical difficulties associated with the diagnosis and treatment.

Jandl, James H. *Blood: Textbook of Hematology.* 2d ed. Boston: Little, Brown, 1996. A textbook on hematology. The book is quite detailed but is recommended for anyone who is seriously interested in the subject. Though the lymphatic system is not specifically covered, blood and lymphatic cells are extensively covered.

Knowles, Margaret A., and Peter J. Selby. *Introduction to the Cellular and Molecular Biology of Cancer.* 4th ed. New York: Oxford University Press, 2006. A general description of cancer and areas of research. The text discusses features of cancer and its possible origins. The possible role of oncogenes in the disease is also included. Though not intended for the layperson, the book does present a good overview of the subject.

Leukemia and Lymphoma Society. http://www.leukemia.org. A group dedicated to funding blood cancer research, education, and patient services for patients with leukemia and other lymphatic diseases.

Lymphoma Information Network. http://www.lymphomainfo.net. Offers information on the diagnosis and treatment options for adult and childhood Hodgkin's disease and resources for further research.

National Cancer Institute. *What You Need to Know About Non-Hodgkin's Lymphoma.* Rev. ed. Bethesda, Md.: Department of Health and Human Services, Public Health Service, National Institutes of Health, 1999. Aimed at the patient who has been diagnosed with non-Hodgkin's lymphoma, this publication offers the latest advice.

LYMPHATIC DISORDERS. *See* LYMPHADENOPATHY AND LYMPHOMA.

LYMPHATIC SYSTEM
ANATOMY
ANATOMY OR SYSTEM AFFECTED: Circulatory system, immune system, spleen

SPECIALTIES AND RELATED FIELDS: Hematology, immunology, vascular medicine

DEFINITION: A network of vessels, paralleling those of the circulatory system, and nodules that collects extravascular materials and fluids from tissue in order to return them to the bloodstream.

KEY TERMS:

antigen-presenting cell (APC): a type of macrophage or interstitial cell that initiates the immune response by "presenting" processed antigen to B and T lymphocytes

edema: an abnormal accumulation of fluids around tissues

lacteals: lymphatic capillaries in the villi of the small intestine that absorb fat, producing a milky substance called chyle

lymph: the straw-colored fluid of the lymphatic system; as much as 1 to 2 liters is collected from tissue each day and returned to the bloodstream

lymph node: a small, oval structure that filters tissue fluids; lymph nodes are found in areas such as the armpits, groin, mouth, and neck, and serve as sites of immune response

lymphocytes: cells of the lymphatic system; B lymphocytes function in antibody production, while T lymphocytes function in cellular immunity

Peyer's patches: lymphatic nodules in the ileum of the intestine; Peyer's patches are one kind of mucosal associated lymphoid tissue (MALT), which, unlike lymph nodes, are not enclosed by tissue capsules

spleen: a lymphatic organ found between the stomach and the diaphragm; destroys old blood cells and filters foreign material from the blood

thoracic duct: the largest lymphatic vessel, which collects lymphatic fluid and returns it to the bloodstream at the left subclavian vein in the region of the neck

thymus: the lymphatic gland in which T lymphocytes mature; located in humans just below the thyroid

STRUCTURE AND FUNCTIONS

The lymphatic system is a complex of capillaries, ducts, nodes, and organs that filters and maintains interstitial fluid—that is, fluid from body tissues. Fluid is collected from body tissues and returned to the bloodstream. In addition, the system functions as a site of the immune response, primarily in the spleen and the lymph nodes, and transports fat and protein to the bloodstream.

The organs of the lymphatic system are divided into primary lymphoid organs and secondary organs. The primary organs include the thymus and the bone marrow, which are sites where lymphocytes are produced and mature. Secondary lymphoid organs are those in which the immune response is carried out. These include both encapsulated organs such as the spleen and lymph nodes and unencapsulated organs such as the mucosal associated lymphoid tissue, which includes Peyer's patches in the intestine and Waldemeyer's ring in the throat (the tonsils and adenoids), which encircles the pharynx. Lymph nodes are found throughout the body, but they occur in large numbers in the head, neck, armpits (the axillary nodes), and abdomen and groin (the inguinal nodes).

The lymphatic vessels essentially parallel those of the bloodstream. The system originates in peripheral tissue as small openings, or sinuses, within the tissue. Fluid that drains from the tissue collects in these sinuses and forms lymph. In addition, a significant amount of liquid (1 to 2 liters) that is lost from blood capillaries each day also collects in the interstitial fluid. The lymph is physiologically similar to blood plasma in that it is a balanced solution of electrolytes containing some carbohydrates, lipids, and proteins. In general, the protein level is about half that found in blood, since most blood proteins are too large to pass through the endothelial walls of blood capillaries. Arguably, the major function of the lymphatic system is the return of this fluid, and its constituent materials, to the blood. The buildup of abnormal amounts of fluid in tissue results in swelling, or edema. Approximately 60 percent of lost fluid is returned to the blood through the lymphatics, and the remainder is collected directly into small blood capillaries.

Generally speaking, the peripheral portion of the lymphatic system is completely separate from that of the blood. Once the interstitial fluid is collected, it begins to move toward the thoracic duct. Since the duct is found in the neck region, this movement is primarily in an upward direction. The fluid moves through regional lymph nodes, such as those found in the groin or armpits, and gradually collects in the larger ducts of the major lymphatics. Though an extensive system of valves is found in the lymphatic system to prevent the movement of lymph in the wrong direction, no internal pumping mechanism analogous to the heart exists. The movement of the lymph is mediated by the musculature of the body: respiratory pressure, muscular movement, and the pulsing or motion of nearby organs. Lymphatic fluids from all portions of the body, except for the upper-right quadrant, eventually collect in the thoracic duct. Lymph from the upper-right quadrant of the body collects in the right lymphatic duct. The endothelia of these major lymphatic ducts are contiguous with those of the veins in the neck, and it is here that the fluid is returned to the bloodstream. Valves present in the lymphatic ducts serve to prevent the backup of blood from the bloodstream into the lymphatic system.

In addition to the electrolytes and proteins that collect in lymph, foreign materials such as infectious agents may also penetrate the skin or internal surfaces of the body. These materials pass into tissue fluids and also collect in the lymphatic system. From here, they travel to regional lymph nodes, where they are filtered out by phagocytic cells such as macrophages. In addition, antigen-collecting cells in the skin, including dendritic cells, may transport foreign materials such as bacteria to these regional nodes. These cells may intercalate, or interdigitate, among the lymphocytes of the lymph nodes and, along with the macrophages, "present" antigen to B and T cells. In this manner, the immune response is initiated.

An analogous situation exists in the blood sys-

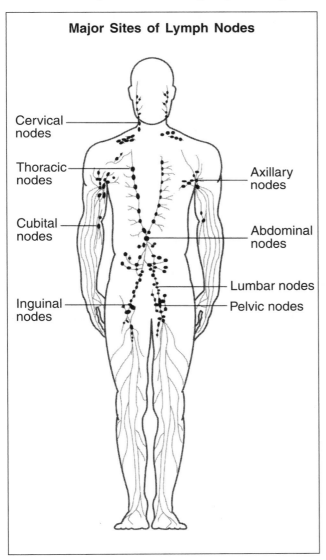

Major Sites of Lymph Nodes

Cervical nodes

Thoracic nodes

Cubital nodes

Inguinal nodes

Axillary nodes

Abdominal nodes

Lumbar nodes

Pelvic nodes

tem. In this case, however, it is the macrophages of the spleen that serve to filter foreign material, such as infectious agents, from the blood. Damaged or old red blood cells are removed in a similar manner. The macrophages then degrade the foreign material and "present" it to B and T lymphocytes in the spleen.

Most of the immune response occurs in the lymph nodes and the spleen. Once the interaction has occurred between the APCs and the lymphocytes, differentiation of the B and T cells begins. The B cells develop into plasma cells, which are essentially antibody-producing factories, while T cells may undergo proliferation. Within the nodes, B and T cells are generally confined to specific areas: the outer cortex for B cells and the underlying paracortex for T cells. Embedded within the cortex are collections of primary nodules, which consist primarily of B cells. Once antigenic stimulation occurs, the cells within the nodules enlarge and proliferate, forming secondary follicles that surround germinal centers. These germinal centers enlarge as B lymphocytes mature and proliferate, and they account for the enlargement of regional lymph nodes in the event of infection. In addition, blood vessels within the node may become enlarged, increasing blood flow. Though some of the activated lymphocytes eventually find their way to the bloodstream, most remain within the lymphatic system. Antibodies produced in response to an infection, however, are transported to the blood.

Since lymph nodes serve as regions of drainage for local tissue, they also represent a route through the body for cancer cells that break away from a tumor. For example, cells from a breast cancer may lodge in regional lymph nodes of the neck or armpit and travel from there to other areas of the body. Although specialized types of lymphocytes capable of killing tumor cells are found in the nodes, some cancer cells may survive. It is for this reason that, during the removal of tumors, localized nodes are examined for evidence of metastasis. If no cancer cells are observed in the nodes, the chances are high that the cancer has not spread.

Mucosal associated lymphatic tissue (MALT) is found along mucosal membranes in regions of the intestines (Peyer's patches and the appendix) and the throat (tonsils). The tonsils actually consist of a network of three groups of tissues that are located at the base of the tongue, at the back of the throat, and at the roof of the nasopharynx (adenoids). Like the spleen and the lymph nodes, MALT tissues may be sites of germinal centers. Unlike the spleen and lymph nodes, however, these tissues are not enclosed by defined capsules of connective tissue. They may be loosely organized, like the mucosa of the intestinal villi, or they may form organized regions like those of the tonsils and adenoids.

MALT appears to function to protect the body against respiratory or gastrointestinal agents. For example, agents such as bacteria or viruses that enter through the oral or respiratory route may stimulate an immune response by the tonsils. The swelling of the tonsils, tonsillitis, is the result of a localized immune response much like that found in the spleen or the lymph nodes. Germinal centers within the tissue represent areas of B cell maturation and proliferation. In the same way, the Peyer's patches consist of approximately thirty to forty nodules along the wall of the intestines. Gastrointestinal antigens that penetrate the intestinal wall stimulate germinal centers in these regions.

Digestion products of carbohydrates and proteins are actively transported into the villi of the small intestine and enter the bloodstream directly. Fats, however, enter the blood in a more roundabout way through the lymphatic system. Fats are digested in the small intestine and diffuse into underlying cells. There they are assembled into triglycerides and, along with cholesterol, are enclosed in protein envelopes; the resulting bodies are called chylomicrons. Once these bodies pass into the lacteals of the lymphatic system, the whitish fluid, chyle, is transported to a region at the beginning of the thoracic duct called the cisterna chyli. It is here that the fat enters the bloodstream.

DISORDERS AND DISEASES

If the interstitial fluid—that is, the fluid in the tissues—increases beyond the capacity of the lymphatic system to handle the situation, an abnormal accumulation of fluid will build up in the tissue. This creates a situation known as edema. A variety of etiological factors can cause edema. For example, burns, inflammation, and certain allergic reactions may increase the level of capillary permeability. This is particularly true if a large amount of protein is lost as the result of a serious burn.

An increase in capillary hydrostatic pressure may also increase the rate of fluid buildup in the tissues. This may be a by-product of several conditions: congestive heart failure, renal failure, or the use of a variety of drugs (estrogen, phenylbutazone). For example, an increase in the sodium concentration of the blood caused by retention resulting from renal failure or simply an excess of salt in the diet may cause water retention and increased blood volume. The sequelae include increased fluid leakage and edema. It is for this reason that a reduction in sodium intake is often recommended for those who suffer from this problem. Diuretics may be prescribed to promote the excretion of sodium and water. Similarly, venous obstruction as serious as phlebitis or as minor as the pressure from a tight bandage or clothing may increase hydrostatic pressure and lead to edema.

A buildup of fluid in the lungs, or pulmonary edema, may occur as a result of congestive heart failure. Hydrostatic pressure in the capillaries of the lungs is relatively low when compared with that of the circulation elsewhere. As a result, the "wetness" of lung tissue is minimal. In patients with serious congestive heart disease, capillary fluid is backed up into the lung (and, indeed, in tissues of the extremities). The result is fluid leakage into the alveoli and bronchioles. Though the lymphatics are capable of removing small amounts of excess fluids, at some point the leakage of plasma and dissolved proteins exceeds the capacity of the lymphatic system to handle the problem. The result is a vicious circle. Since less oxygen is taken up through the lungs, capillary permeability increases. More fluid and protein are then lost. Unless intervention is carried out, the patient may eventually drown in his or her own fluids.

Intervention for pulmonary edema generally involves elevating the head and knees of the patient (Fowler's position) and the administration of diuretics. A low-sodium diet, allowing for decreased fluid retention, may also relieve some of the stress on the lymphatic system. With time, the number of lymphatic vessels in the lungs may increase, allowing for a greater capacity to remove fluids.

A variety of disorders may directly involve the lymphatic system itself. Lymphedema, or the accumulation of lymph in tissue with subsequent swelling, may result from the absence of lymphatic vessels or from obstructions within the vessels. The symptoms of lymphedema, particularly in the lower extremities, include mild swelling that becomes increasingly severe with time. The problem may be exacerbated by menstruation or pregnancy. In some instances, lymphatic vessels may be absent, either congenitally or because of surgical removal. Diagnosis of the problem often requires the use of lymphangiography (lymphography). In this procedure, a contrast medium is injected, and the lymphatic vessels are examined by means of X rays.

The etiologic factors associated with lymphatic obstruction may either be congenital or have external causes. Milroy's disease is a hereditary lymphedema characterized by chronic obstructions. The obstruction of lymphatic vessels may also be caused by the presence of tumor cells or the infiltration of parasites. For example, elephantiasis is caused by an infestation of a parasitic worm that obstructs the flow of fluid. The affected limb or region of the body may swell to an astounding degree.

The treatment of most of these disorders is essentially symptomatic. An obstruction may be treated or removed. Often, lymphedema may be treated by having the patient sleep with the feet elevated. A low-salt diet or diuretics may be indicated, and a light massage in the direction of lymph flow may also be helpful.

As is true for all tissues in the body, the cells and organs of the lymphatic system may also undergo malignant transformation. Any neoplasm of lymphoid tissue is referred to as a lymphoma. In general, these are malignant. Though lymphomas may be of different forms and involve different types of cells, they are characterized by enlarged lymph nodes (generally in the neck), fever, and weight loss. Among the more common forms of lymphomas are Hodgkin's disease and non-Hodgkin's lymphomas, a mixed collection of malignant solid tumors originating among the secondary lymphoid tissues of the lymph nodes. Hodgkin's disease generally appears first among the cervical or axillary lymph nodes. Its manner of presentation usually allows for early diagnosis and treatment. As a result, the prognosis with early intervention has significantly improved since the 1960's.

Non-Hodgkin's lymphomas often develop in less obvious areas of the lymphatic system, such as the gastrointestinal tract, the central nervous system, and the oral and nasal pharynx. The result is that diagnosis is often delayed until the disease has spread, and therefore the prognosis is less optimistic. More than 80 percent of non-Hodgkin's lymphomas are of B-lymphocyte origin, and they often arise within the follicles of the lymph node. There is some evidence that neoplastic transformation may be related to antigen exposure. In some instances, molecular defects of the cell DNA may result in the neoplastic event. Non-Hodgkin's lymphomas may also be of T-lymphocyte or, less commonly, macrophage origin. Most treatments of lymphomas include both radiation therapy and chemotherapy.

PERSPECTIVE AND PROSPECTS

The first description of the lymphatic system was made by the Italian anatomist Gasparo Aselli in 1622. Aselli observed the lacteals in the intestinal walls of dogs that he had dissected, and he included diagrams of the lacteals in his text *De Lactibus* (1627), the first anatomical medical text with color plates.

The role of the lymphatic system in maintaining the fluid dynamics of the body was understood by the beginning of the twentieth century. Much of this knowledge resulted from the early work of the British physiologist Ernest Henry Starling.

Beginning about 1900, Starling's research centered on the secretion and circulation of lymph. It was known that the lymphatic system as a parallel to blood circulation was found only among the higher vertebrates. This indicated that it had developed relatively late during the course of evolution. There occurred, along with the increasing development of the body's circulatory system as organisms evolved, an increase in the hydrostatic pressure within the system—that is, as the circulatory system became more complex, blood vessels branched into smaller and thinner capillaries. The pressure within those capillaries became higher. Starling pointed out the significance of the hydrostatic pressures within the capillaries: Fluids and dissolved materials leak out of the capillaries into the tissues.

Starling did not believe, however, that protein was able to leak through the capillary walls. In the 1930's, Cecil Drinker demonstrated that protein is a major constituent of dissolved material in lymph and suggested that an important role of the lymphatic system is the return of this protein to the bloodstream. Drinker was unable to prove definitively that the protein in lymph originated with the blood, and it remained for H. S. Mayerson to confirm this point in the 1940's.

Lymphocytes had been observed in the blood as early as the nineteenth century. Their role in the immune process was not readily apparent, however, and various functions were assigned to them. In 1948, Astrid Fagraeus demonstrated that lymphocytes mature into antibody-producing plasma cells. It remained unclear whether this was the sole purpose of these cells.

In 1956, Bruce Glick and Timothy Chang, working with chickens, discovered that an organ called the bursa, found near the cloaca in the region of the tail, was the site of the production of antibody-producing cells. Their discovery, along with those of Robert Good and Jacques Miller some years later, showed that lymphocytes are not all identical; at least two distinct populations exist. It remained for Henry Claman and his coworkers, in 1966, to demonstrate that these two pop-

ulations of lymphocytes act cooperatively in the production of antibodies.

In 1969, Ivan Roitt called those lymphocytes that mature in the thymus gland T cells. The lymphocytes that mature in the bursa, an organ found only in birds, were called B cells. Since mammals lack the bursa, B cells in these organisms mature within the bone marrow (considered a bursa equivalent). Once the cells are released from the marrow, they migrate into both the lymphatic system and the bloodstream.

—Richard Adler, Ph.D.

See also Angiography; Bacterial infections; Bladder cancer; Blood and blood disorders; Breast cancer; Breast disorders; Burkitt's lymphoma; Cancer; Cervical, ovarian, and uterine cancers; Chemotherapy; Circulation; Colon cancer; DiGeorge syndrome; Edema; Elephantiasis; Epstein-Barr virus; Gallbladder cancer; Histology; Hodgkin's disease; Immune system; Immunology; Immunopathology; Kawasaki disease; Kidney cancer; Liver cancer; Lower extremities; Lung cancer; Lymph; Lymphadenopathy and lymphoma; Malignancy and metastasis; Mononucleosis; Mouth and throat cancer; Oncology; Prostate cancer; Pulmonary edema; Skin cancer; Sleeping sickness; Splenectomy; Stomach, intestinal, and pancreatic cancers; Systems and organs; Testicular cancer; Tonsillectomy and adenoid removal; Tonsillitis; Tumors; Upper extremities; Vascular medicine; Vascular system.

FOR FURTHER INFORMATION:

Delves, Peter J., et al. *Roitt's Essential Immunology.* 11th ed. Malden, Mass.: Blackwell, 2006. A standard immunology text. Though the lymphatic system is not singled out in any particular section of the book, its role in the immune response is an underlying theme throughout the text.

Dwyer, John M. *The Body at War: The Story of Our Immune System.* 2d ed. London: J. M. Dent, 1993. Provides a good general description of the immune system. The immune function of the lymphatic system, the roles of lymph nodes in the immune response, and the functions of lymphatic cells are described in a basic manner for the nonscientist.

Eales, Lesley-Jane. *Immunology for Life Scientists.* Hoboken, N.J.: John Wiley & Sons, 2003. A highly readable text for the nonspecialist that covers such topics as antigens, hypersensitivity, autoimmunity, reproductive immunity, and immunodeficiency.

Janeway, Charles A., Jr., et al. *Immunobiology: The Immune System in Health and Disease.* 6th ed. New

York: Garland Science, 2005. An excellent text that provides a lucid and comprehensive examination of the immune system, covering such topics as immunobiology and innate immunity, the recognition of antigen, the development of mature lymphocyte receptor repertoires, the adaptive immune response, and the evolution of the immune system.

Kindt, Thomas J., Richard A. Goldsby, and Barbara A. Osborne. *Kuby Immunology.* 6th ed. New York: W. H. Freeman, 2007. An excellent textbook on the subject of immunology. The section on the cells and organs of the immune system is well organized and includes the latest information on lymphatic circulation. The immune function of the lymphatic system is the major emphasis.

LYMPHOMA. *See* **LYMPHADENOPATHY AND LYMPHOMA.**

MACRONUTRIENTS

BIOLOGY

ANATOMY OR SYSTEM AFFECTED: All

SPECIALTIES AND RELATED FIELDS: Biochemistry, nutrition, public health, sports medicine

DEFINITION: The dietary ingredients required in large quantities for health and activity.

KEY TERMS:

carbohydrates: organic substances with the general formula of $(CH_2O)n$; the primary dietary carbohydrates are starches and sugars

fiber: organic substances resistant to digestion by human enzymes; a common dietary fiber is cellulose

gluconeogenesis: the synthesis within the body of glucose from noncarbohydrate precursors

kwashiorkor: a condition caused by inadequate dietary protein intake

lipids: organic substances insoluble in water but soluble in alcohol, ether, chloroform and other fat solvents; the primary dietary lipids are triglycerides

marasmus: a condition caused by inadequate dietary macronutrient intake, both protein and energy

proteins: organic substances consisting of linked amino acids, nitrogen-containing molecules

triglycerides (triacylglycerides): three fatty acids covalently attached to a glycerol moiety

STRUCTURE AND FUNCTIONS

Macronutrients are generally considered to include carbohydrates, lipids, and proteins; these are dietary constituents consumed in the largest quantities. While water and oxygen are also needed in large amounts, they are not usually considered to be food. Although fiber ingested in substantial quantity is desirable for optimum health, it is, by definition, a non-nutritive dietary constituent. In addition, calcium, sodium and chloride (salt), magnesium, potassium, phosphorus, and sulfur are sometimes added to the list of macronutrients because they are needed in large amounts compared to vitamins and other minerals; however, they are best referred to as macrominerals.

Carbohydrates, lipids, and proteins provide the energy (calories) needed for maintenance, growth, thermoregulation, and physical activity, as well as pregnancy and lactation. All three also provide for other needs: Carbohydrates are components of structural polysaccharides inside cells and on their surfaces; lipids are important in cellular membrane structure and function and as precursors of some hormones; and proteins are a source of amino acids needed for the synthesis of body proteins, nucleic acids, and other hormones. Lipids also facilitate the uptake of the fat-soluble vitamins A, D, E, and K. As sources of energy, all three macronutrients are virtually interchangeable, although the nitrogen of the amino acid constituents of proteins must be concomitantly disposed of, mostly in the form of urinary urea. The carbon in these substances is combusted with oxygen, producing carbon dioxide, and during the process the metabolic energy and heat are generated that support living processes. Total dietary intake of macronutrients (and hence energy) should be kept in balance with energy expenditure. Excess intake over expenditure will lead to overweight and eventually obesity, which is detrimental to health, as it is associated with some cancers, coronary heart disease, diabetes, and other chronic diseases. Acceptable macronutrient distribution ranges in human diets have been set for carbohydrates, lipids, and proteins to prevent frank deficiencies and minimize incidences of chronic diseases from overconsumption.

Dietary carbohydrates, primarily starches and sugars, are digested to monosaccharides (primarily glucose and fructose), and transported into the blood. Carbohydrate uptake in excess of that needed for immediate use is stored as glycogen, principally in liver and skeletal muscle, or is converted to fatty acids and stored as triglycerides in adipose depots. Subsequently, glycogen can be broken down to glucose for use as a ready fuel source for the body. Humans do not have a dietary requirement for carbohydrates. However, a diet devoid of carbohydrates would have to compensate with much larger quantities of protein. Some amino acids can be converted to the glucose needed in the body by a process termed gluconeogenesis, whereas little of the fat content can be so converted. However, a high-protein diet would be ketotic, disrupting mineral balance. Because the brain and nervous tissue have a requirement for glucose, an acceptable macronutrient distribution range for carbohydrates has been set at 45 to 65 percent of the energy content of the diet. Furthermore, no more than 25 percent of the energy needs should be met with added sugar, which is metabolized rapidly and can thereby disrupt whole body metabolism. Added sugar is also associated with a lower intake of essential vitamins and minerals, as well as with a high risk of dental caries (cavities).

Dietary lipids, primarily triglycerides, are essentially digested to their constituent fatty acids for absorption and then are reconstituted to triglycerides in intestinal tissue. Because triglycerides are insoluble in water, they are transported in the body via a complex system of lipoproteins—chylomicra, low-density lipoproteins (LDLs), and high-density lipoproteins (HDLs). Their constituent fatty acids are used as fuel by various tissues, and any excess triglycerides are stored in adipose tissue. Two fatty acids, linoleic and α-linolenic, termed essential fatty acids because they cannot be synthesized by the human body, are required in small quantities. Human diets should contain a minimum of 10 percent diversified lipids (linoleic is found in a variety of plant oils and α-linolenic in fish oil) to ensure that the requirement for these essential fatty acids is met. The acceptable macronutrient distribution range for lipids has been set at 20 to 35 percent of the energy content of the diet for adults. Lipid intake should be slightly higher for infants and children because of the demands of growth.

Dietary proteins generally serve as energy sources once the need for their constituent amino acids as precursors of body protein has been met. Dietary proteins are digested to their constituent amino acids and absorbed across the intestinal tract into the blood, where they are taken up by various tissues for synthesis of body proteins, which are continually being broken down and resynthesized. Amino acids absorbed in excess of that need are used as fuel, either directly or after conversion to glucose by gluconeogenesis. Adult humans have a requirement for 0.8 grams (g) of well-balanced protein per kilogram (kg) of body weight each day; this corresponds to 56 g of protein per day for the average man and 46 g per day for the average woman. The acceptable macronutrient distribution range for proteins has been set at 10 to 35 percent of the energy content of the diet. Protein intake should be slightly lower for infants and children to compensate for the higher proportion of lipid intake and to minimize the need to dispose of excess nitrogen.

Disorders and Diseases

The main disorders associated with macronutrients result from their inadequate or excess consumption, namely starvation and obesity. The former is particularly problematic for infants and children because of their higher demands for growth and brain development; some early deficits lead to permanent impairment. Two general types of starvation are recognized; marasmus is due to a general deficiency of macronutrients, also referred to as protein-calorie malnutrition, whereas kwashiorkor is primarily attributed to a deficiency of dietary protein.

Anorexia nervosa (restricted intake) and bulimia nervosa (binge eating followed by purging, vomiting, or misuse of laxatives or diuretics) are two eating disorders with complex and variable etiologies that can lead to reduced macronutrient intake, starvation, and even death.

Ironically, calorie-restricted diets that reduce macronutrient intakes by 20 to 40 percent primarily from carbohydrate and lipids, while maintaining adequate intakes of protein and other nutrients, appear to be associated with increased longevity and decreased incidence of some cancers and other diseases of aging. However, few people are willing to restrict their intake voluntarily to such an extent and to live with a continuous feeling of hunger.

Obesity is a modern epidemic largely because of the ready availability and consumption of inexpensive food coupled with a more sedentary lifestyle. While particularly a problem in Western societies, it is making inroads in the rest of the world. Obesity is associated with increased risk of coronary heart disease, some cancers, and type 2 diabetes. Excessive weight also puts added stress on knee and ankle joints. Obesity is, by definition, an energy imbalance, where energy intake (from macronutrients) exceeds energy expenditure, as from physical exercise. Obesity is a multifactorial disease, however, influenced by both genetic and environmental factors. Some people appear to be more susceptible to weight gain, as genetic factors have an impact on appetite, endocrinology, metabolism, and activity. The environmental factors include access to palatable food and lack of exercise. While not a major contributor to the current epidemic, binge eating disorder can lead to obesity.

Perspective and Prospects

The ancient Greeks noted that a wide variety of foods were converted into the organs and tissues of people consuming them. They concluded that the differences between food and human protoplasm must be superficial and that they must be made from the same substance. They also assumed that the need for food after growth had ceased was caused by the wearing out of organs and tissues and the continuous need to replace them. In the late 1700's, Antoine Lavoisier demonstrated that carbon dioxide expiration increased with exercise and that the oxidation of fats and carbohydrates accounted for most of the energy needed for animal heat production. In the nineteenth century, the need for nitrogen in the diet was demonstrated for dogs and by analogy for humans; proteins were first described as the main nitrogen-containing substances in food. Sophisticated calorimetry equipment large enough for humans to live in for several days made it possible to quantitate energy balance and, by 1900, permitted the conclusion that the metabolism of lipids and carbohydrates could be used for mechanical work with similar efficiency. In that same period, dietary proteins were shown to be broken down to amino acids in the digestive tract, absorbed, and used to rebuild body protein.

Relative to macronutrient consumption, the dilemma of undernutrition and overnutrition in the world, often within a country and even within the same household, makes it difficult for nutritionists and public health professionals to tailor recommendations and to inform political decisions. The concept of an optimum intake of macronutrients, while easy to grasp, is difficult to enact. A further complication is the individual variation in metabolism and taste, even within the same culture. Cases have been confirmed where individuals with distinct genotypes respond differently, even oppositely, to the same macronutrient intervention. In the future, one can foresee personalized genomic-based nutrition advice.

—*James L. Robinson, Ph.D.*

See also Anorexia nervosa; Antioxidants; Beriberi; Carbohydrates; Cholesterol; Digestion; Eating disorders; Enzymes; Food biochemistry; Gastroenterology; Gastroenterology, pediatric; Gastrointestinal system; Kwashiorkor; Lactose intolerance; Lipids; Malabsorption; Malnutrition; Metabolism; Obesity; Obesity, childhood; Phytonutrients; Protein; Supplements; Vitamins and minerals; Weight loss and gain.

FOR FURTHER INFORMATION:

Gibney, Michael J., et al. *Clinical Nutrition.* Malden, Mass.: Blackwell Science, 2005. Published by the Nutrition Society, this authoritative text deals with the clinical aspects of macronutrients and other nutrients.

Mahan, L. Kathleen, and Sylvia Escott-Stump. *Krause's Food, Nutrition, and Diet Therapy.* 11th ed. Philadelphia: W. B. Saunders, 2004. Edited by two registered dieticians, it contains a separate chapter on the macronutrients.

Otten, Jennifer J., Jennifer Pitzi Hellwig, and Linda D. Meyers. *Dietary Reference Intakes: The Essential Guide to Nutrient Requirements.* Washington, D.C.: National Academies Press, 2006. Published by the Institute of Medicine, it is intended as a practical reference for health professionals and includes a section on macronutrients.

Shils, Maurice E., et al. *Modern Nutrition in Health and Disease.* 10th ed. Baltimore: Lippincott Williams & Wilkins, 2006. A comprehensive text with separate chapters on each of the three macronutrients.

MACULAR DEGENERATION
DISEASE/DISORDER
ANATOMY OR SYSTEM AFFECTED: Eyes
SPECIALTIES AND RELATED FIELDS: Ophthalmology
DEFINITION: A degenerative disease of the central portion of the retina that results primarily in loss of central vision.

CAUSES AND SYMPTOMS

The macula is located in the center of the retina, the light-sensitive tissue at the back of the eye. The retina instantly converts light, or an image, into electrical impulses. The retina then sends these impulses, or nerve signals, to the brain. One of the earliest signs of age-related macular degeneration (ARMD) seen by physicians during a dilated eye examination is deposits of tiny, bright yellow material called drusen, which is harder as a result of aging or softer and larger if associated with ARMD and vision loss. As parts of the eye in the retina and choroid become thinner or lose tissue, central vision and/or peripheral vision is affected, depending on the area of damage. Central vision is needed to see clearly and to perform everyday activities such as reading, writing, driving, and recognizing people and things. Peripheral vision, needed for walking, is much less commonly affected.

There are two forms of ARMD: early and advanced. About 90 percent of cases are early ARMD, although the advanced type affects 7 percent of those seventy-five years or older. Advanced ARMD is further categorized into two distinct types based on their clinical features: dry and wet. The dry form involves thinning of the macular tissues and disturbances in its pigmentation. About 70 percent of patients have the dry form. The remaining 30 percent have the wet form, which can involve bleeding within and beneath the retina, opaque deposits, and eventually scar tissue. The wet form accounts for 90 percent of all cases of legal blindness in macular degeneration patients.

Neither dry nor wet macular degeneration causes pain. The most common early sign of dry macular degeneration is blurring vision that prevents people from

INFORMATION ON MACULAR DEGENERATION

CAUSES: Unclear; possibly aging, genetic factors, nutrition, smoking, sunlight exposure

SYMPTOMS: Dependent on form; can include blurred or distorted central vision, bleeding within and beneath retina, development of scar tissue, eventual blindness

DURATION: Typically long-term

TREATMENTS: Vision aids (e.g., magnifying glasses, special lenses, electronic systems); laser photocoagulation; surgery; low-level radiation; injection of photosensitive chemicals into bloodstream

seeing details clearly that are in front of them, such as faces or words in a book. In the early stages of wet macular degeneration, straight lines appear wavy or crooked. This is the result of fluid leaking from blood vessels and lifting the macula, distorting vision.

A number of risk factors can affect the initial development of ARMD: age, smoking, genetic predisposition, and ethnicity. Two risk factors have also been studied and suggested in causing a progression of ARMD: nutrition and high blood pressure. Age is the most important risk factor for macular degeneration: The older the patient, the higher the risk. Studies have shown that having a family with a history of macular degeneration raises the risk factor. Because macular degeneration affects most patients later in life, however, it has proven difficult to study cases in successive generations of a family. Heavy smoking, at least a pack of cigarettes a day, can double a person's risk of developing ARMD. The more a person smokes, the higher the risk of macular degeneration. Moreover, the adverse effects of smoking persist, even fifteen to twenty years after quitting. Those with a family history of ARMD are more likely to develop the disease due to a genetic mutation of part of a gene called the complement factor H gene. With a family history of the disease, the risk is greater for developing the wet type than the dry type of ARMD. Studies have shown that non-Hispanic Caucasians have a greater risk of developing ARMD than do African Americans or Hispanics.

Poor dietary habits contribute to ARMD as well. A diet high in saturated fats may clog the vessels leading to the eyes, thus reducing the flow of nutrient-rich blood. Excess fat may deposit itself directly in the membrane behind the retina. In this case, nutrients might not be able to reach the cells that nourish the retina. High blood pressure has also been shown to increase the risk of developing ARMD in the second eye in those having ARMD in one eye.

An effective test to determine if a person has wet macular degeneration is fluorescent angiography. A special dye is injected into a vein in the patient's arm and then flows to the blood vessels in the eye. Photographs are taken of the retina. The dye highlights any problems in the blood vessels and allows the doctor to determine if they can be treated. Annual eye examinations that include dilation of the pupils are also useful in early detection. Early detection is important because a person destined to develop macular degeneration can sometimes be treated before symptoms appear, which may delay or reduce the severity of the disease. Anyone who notices a change in vision should contact an ophthalmologist immediately.

TREATMENT AND THERAPY

New and exciting treatments are in development for ARMD as extensive research is being done. Currently, there is no cure, and no treatment recommendations exist for those with dry type ARMD, the type that is much less threatening to vision. Some treatments, however, can slow the progression of wet type ARMD. Research has shown that stopping smoking is the most effective preventive measure in regard to developing ARMD and slowing its progression.

Antioxidants have proved promising in recent studies which show that they can lower the risk of progression to more advanced ARMD in those who have moderate or advanced disease. In a major clinical trial called the Age-Related Disease Study (AREDS), it was shown that patients with moderate or severe ARMD taking antioxidants vitamin C, vitamin E, and beta carotene plus zinc and copper had a lower risk of progression among both nonsmokers and smokers. Since the group of smokers who took zinc alone had the same lowered risk of progression as those smokers taking antioxidants plus zinc and copper, it was recommended that smokers with ARMD take zinc alone, as some antioxidants have shown to increase the risk of lung cancer and coronary heart disease when used at high doses.

Although no treatments can reverse the actual pathologic process of the disease of wet type ARMD, some treatments used by ophthalmologists are aimed at containing the damaged vessels that cause the loss of vision. They include laser photocoagulation, photodynamic therapy, intravitreous injections, and, as a last resort, macular translocation surgery.

Laser photocoagulation involves using a high-intensity thermal laser to burn off the blood supply to abnormal choroidal membranes. The benefits of this treatment are that it is done in the outpatient setting using only topical anesthetic drops and that it prevents the formation of new abnormal vessels associated with ARMD for two or three years. It is limited, however, to only those patients with well-defined abnormal areas (only about 15 percent of patients with ARMD). It cannot restore lost vision and may actually destroy normal retinal tissue along with the neovascular formation that is targeted.

Photodynamic therapy involves the injection of a dye called verteporfin which, when activated by a photo laser, forms substances that destroy the abnormal newly formed vessels associated with wet type ARMD. Thus, by the use of this dye and laser combination, the normal vessels are protected and the abnormal vessels are destroyed. It has also been shown that this treatment can be repeated safely.

The vascular endothelial growth factor (VEGF) inhibitors are a class of agents that block a factor involved in the disease process of ARMD. VEGF is essential for the formation of the new abnormal vessels that cause the loss of vision and the anatomic destruction associated with ARMD. The VEGF inhibitors block this factor, thereby limiting those destructive effects. Studies involving these agents have shown that a majority of patients showed improvement in their vision and marked anatomic improvement of their retinas.

Macular translocation surgery involves surgically removing the macula from a diseased area and attaching it to a healthier area of the retina. Although currently an experimental therapy and not well studied, it can be used for those patients in which no other treatment options are left. If performed successfully, macular translocation surgery can improve central vision and allow a majority of patients to read. Great risks are associated with this type of treatment, however, including detachment of the retina and the development of double vision. In addition, use of a steroid injection into the vitreous and/or the posterior sub-Tenon's space has shown short-term improvement in vision.

Many visual aids have been developed for patients with ARMD to make the most of their remaining vision, including magnifying glasses, powerful special lenses, and large-print books and reading materials. Voice synthesizers in electronic devices such as calculators, clocks, and phones are also very helpful. Maximizing room lighting by the use of stronger lights, opening windows, and painting walls brighter colors can help patients see better at home.

PERSPECTIVE AND PROSPECTS

Blindness or low vision affects 3.3 million Americans aged forty and over, or one in twenty-eight, according to the Eye Disease Prevalence Research Group study, sponsored by the National Eye Institute. This figure is projected to reach 5.5 million by the year 2020. The study reports that low vision and blindness increase significantly with age, particularly in people over age sixty-five. People eighty years of age and older currently make up 8 percent of the population but account for 69 percent of blindness. ARMD affects about 15 percent of the U.S. population by age fifty-five and more than 30 percent by age seventy-five. It is the most common cause of legal blindness in people over the age of sixty-five.

Although there is no cure for ARMD, many treatments are available to curtail progression of the disease. As extensive research continues in this area, advances in the diagnosis and treatment of this debilitating condition are anticipated by many in the field of ophthalmology. Currently, the National Eye Institute is studying the possibility of transplanting healthy cells into a diseased retina, evaluating families with a history of ARMD to understand genetic and hereditary factors that may cause the disease, and looking at certain anti-inflammatory treatments for the wet form of ARMD.

—*Kenneth Dill, M.D.*

See also Aging; Blindness; Blurred vision; Cataracts; Eye infections and disorders; Eye surgery; Eyes; Laser use in surgery; Myopia; Ophthalmology; Smoking; Vision; Vision disorders.

FOR FURTHER INFORMATION:

American Macular Degeneration Foundation. http://www.macular.org. Provides information to clinicians and patients regarding the latest in research regarding ARMD. Offers an award-winning video for helping patients with ARMD cope with this debilitating illness.

D'Amato, Robert, and Joan Snyder. *Macular Degeneration: The Latest Scientific Discoveries and Treatments for Preserving Your Sight*. New York: Walker, 2000. Ophthalmologist and noted researcher D'Amato teams up with macular degeneration patient Snyder to write a reassuring, hopeful, and informative book providing the facts that sufferers need in order to understand the disorder, handle treatment options, and live successfully with low vision.

Kansai, Jack. *Diseases of the Macula.* New York: Elsevier, 2002. A clinical text that covers diseases that primarily affect the macula, such as age-related macular degeneration, together with secondary diseases that might have an indirect effect on macular function, such as vascular and inflammatory disorders.

Macular Degeneration Foundation. http://www.eye sight.org. Describes this charitable educational and research foundation dedicated to discovering the cause of and developing cures for macular degeneration.

MayoClinic.com. "Macular Degeneration." http://www.mayoclinic.com/health/macular-degeneration/DS00284. Provides a comprehensive overview of the risk factors, symptoms, and treatment of ARMD.

Sardegna, Jill, et al. *The Encyclopedia of Blindness and Vision Impairment.* 2d ed. New York: Facts On File, 2002. All aspects of vision impairment are covered in five hundred entries, including health and social issues, surgery and medications, adaptive aids, education, and helpful organizations. Twelve appendixes provide myriad resources for research, support, and services.

Sutton, Amy L., ed. *Eye Care Sourcebook: Basic Consumer Health Information About Eye Care and Eye Disorders.* 3d ed. Detroit, Mich.: Omnigraphics, 2008. A complete guide to eye care that includes such topics as eye anatomy, preventive vision care, refractive disorders and eye diseases, current research and clinical trials, and a list of organizations.

MAGNETIC FIELD THERAPY
TREATMENT

ANATOMY OR SYSTEM AFFECTED: Cells, immune system

SPECIALTIES AND RELATED FIELDS: Alternative medicine

DEFINITION: A practical and inexpensive modality that uses magnets to relieve chronic and acute pain incurred through overuse or trauma.

INDICATIONS AND PROCEDURES

In this treatment method, which is based on physics principles called the Hall effect and Faraday's law, magnetic pads are placed on or near the site of injury or soreness in order to stimulate local circulation by attracting positive and negatively charged ions in the blood and lymph. This biomagnetic attraction of electrolytes utilizes an alternating pattern of polarities that penetrate 5 to 20 centimeters into the body's tissues, depending on field strength (which is normally between 300 and 950 gauss). A common magnet will not produce this effect because only the ions and fluid in vessels that are precisely in line with the north-south poles will be attracted. Many advocates claim that magnetic therapy works faster than diathermies such as ultrasound. A warm tingling sensation is often felt minutes after application because of the increase of microcirculation, which brings more oxygen, nutrients, white blood cells, and antibodies to the damaged tissues and which removes metabolic waste products.

USES AND COMPLICATIONS

Several forms of magnetic field therapy (including pulsed electromagnetic therapy) have been used for years in Japan, Germany, and other countries, and double-blind studies are being conducted in the United States to determine the validity of numerous testimonials. Disorders that are regularly treated with magnetic therapy in other countries include carpal tunnel syndrome, osteoarthritis, tendinitis, bursitis, migraine headaches, and energy problems such as chronic fatigue syndrome and malaise. Magnetic deficiency syndrome is now documented in Japanese medical literature, and many American physicians agree that proper magnetic balance in the tissues is an overlooked ingredient of health.

Magnetic pads come in several sizes and shapes to allow for comfortable attachment to any area of the body, including silver-dollar-sized pads that are one-eighth of an inch thick, for concentrated force, and 5-by-7-inch pads for larger areas such as the back. Magnetic massage balls, mattress pads, pillows, seat cushions, and orthotic insoles are also sold. The magnets are permanently charged and have no harmful side effects, although they are not recommended for pregnant women or patients wearing pacemakers. In 2005 and 2006, some respected medical journals reported positive treatment outcomes for the healing of surgical wounds. Because this result defies conventional medical wisdom, however, the use of magnetic field therapy in mainstream medicine remains controversial.

—*Daniel G. Graetzer, Ph.D.;*
updated by LeAnna DeAngelo, Ph.D.

See also Alternative medicine; Bursitis; Carpal tunnel syndrome; Chronic fatigue syndrome; Circulation; Fatigue; Migraine headaches; Osteoarthritis; Pain management; Tendon disorders.

For Further Information:

Burroughs, Hugh, and Mark Kastner. *Alternative Healing: The Complete A-Z Guide to Over 160 Different Alternative Therapies.* La Mesa, Calif.: Halcyon, 1996.

Jacobs, Jennifer, ed. *The Encyclopedia of Alternative Medicine: A Complete Family Guide to Complementary Therapies.* Rev. ed. Boston: Journey Editions, 1997.

Null, Gary. *Healing with Magnets.* New York: Carroll & Graf, 2006.

Pelletier, Kenneth. *The Best Alternative Medicine.* New York: Fireside, 2002.

Trivieri, Larry, Jr., and John W. Anderson, eds. *Alternative Medicine: The Definitive Guide.* 2d ed. Berkeley, Calif.: Ten Speed Press, 2002.

Vegari, G. *Magnetic Therapy.* Christchurch, New Zealand: Caxton, 2004.

White, R., K. Cutting, and P. Beldon. "Magnet Therapy: Opening the Debate." *Journal of Wound Care* 15, no. 5 (May, 2006): 208-209.

Magnetic resonance imaging (MRI)
Procedure

Anatomy or system affected: All

Specialties and related fields: Biotechnology, nuclear medicine, radiology

Definition: A noninvasive, nonradiological method of obtaining detailed information concerning normal and diseased tissue.

Key terms:

electromagnetic waves: a convenient way of understanding energy as a wave; visible light, X rays, and radiowaves, which have the longest wavelength and lowest energy, are the most familiar examples

Fourier transform: a mathematical method which allows MRI to utilize one radio frequency pulse and thereby examine all wavelengths, as opposed to examining each wavelength individually with a continuous wave

nucleus: the dense, positively charged, central core of an atom, containing its massive protons and neutrons

zeugmatography: a name applied to MRI characterizing the close relationship of nuclear magnetic forces and electromagnetic waves (from the Greek *zeugma*, meaning "to yoke together")

Indications and Procedures

In 1901, Wilhelm Conrad Röntgen won the first Nobel Prize in Physics for his discovery of X rays. Twentieth

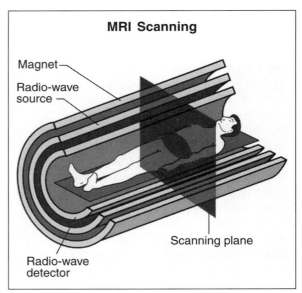

MRI Scanning

Magnet—
Radio-wave source—
Scanning plane
Radio-wave detector

This diagnostic imaging technique employs a powerful magnet to generate a magnetic field that is capable of aligning the protons in the body's hydrogen atoms, which are then knocked out of alignment by radio-wave pulses; as the protons realign, they emit radio signals that can be detected and used to create a cross-sectional image of the body.

century applications of this radiation have produced medical miracles. Magnetic resonance imaging (MRI), often called nuclear magnetic resonance (NMR or nmr) imaging, differs in fundamental ways from X rays and other imaging methods. It is capable of producing a far richer array of three-dimensional images without the dangers attendant on ionizing radiation or the introduction of radioactive chemicals. MRI allows both safe diagnosis and study in healthy subjects. Furthermore, the method can be used to examine flowing matter, such as in the circulatory system.

The nuclei of hydrogen atoms behave like tiny magnets when they are placed in a magnetic field. When radio waves are superimposed on the magnetic waves, hydrogen atoms can be made to change their alignment with the magnetic field. The time required for the atoms to return to their original orientation, after the radio waves cease, varies with the nature of the tissue in which the hydrogen atoms reside. This combination of natural circumstances together with the marvels of modern electronics have made it possible to obtain detailed images of brain tumors, spinal fluid, and blood vessels.

The discovery, in the mid-1940's, by Edward M. Purcell and Felix Bloch of the basic techniques of nuclear magnetic resonance won for them the 1952 Nobel

Prize in Physics. Their innovation changed dramatically the practice of chemistry, biochemistry, and biology. Following new theoretical and practical contributions, diagnostic medicine is participating fully in this revolution.

Both permanent magnets and electromagnets are used, and each has advantages, but the superconducting magnet is rapidly becoming the standard. The essential factors in producing detailed images are constant field strength and a highly uniform field. A transmitter, connected to a radio frequency transmitter-receiver, is used to broadcast the signal and to receive the signal returned from the patient. A short but intense pulse of radio frequency power is required, and its duration is critical to control electronic noise, which obscures the signal required to form the final image. These signals must be processed by complex computer methods to allow the final image to be displayed.

During the 1970's, several innovations were introduced allowing broad application of the MRI technique. Paul Lauterbur demonstrated the generation of spatial maps by rotating the object to obtain a series of projections from which an image can be reconstructed. His method, called nmr zeugmatography, introduced a radically new approach to MRI. By superimposing a magnetic field gradient on the main magnetic field, it is possible to make the resonance frequency a function of the spatial origin of the signal. Later, Richard R. Ernst

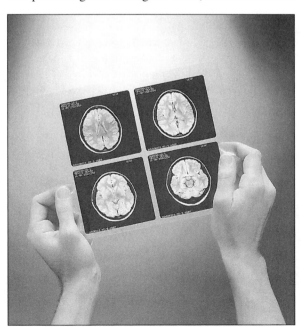

MRI scans of the head. (Digital Stock)

built on his earlier introduction of Fourier-transform NMR to develop methods of "two-dimensional nmr." Such techniques provide detailed information concerning the local structure of large molecules of biological importance. He was awarded the 1991 Nobel Prize in Chemistry because this same method laid the groundwork for the clinical use of MRI. Methods are now available for the creation of three- and four-dimensional MRI, which are important in protein studies and which will pave the way for future applications in nonchemical research.

Uses and Complications

MRI has been used in the evaluation of a wide variety of medical situations. The earliest uses involved the brain and the spinal cord, where it is absolutely necessary to avoid high-energy radiation or radioactivity. Since MRI is capable of providing excellent soft-tissue images and of penetrating bony and air-filled structures, it is also well suited to examination of the chest and abdomen. In these applications, it was first necessary to overcome problems associated with motion. A further important modification, the flow imaging technique, allows the use of MRI in studies of the vascular system and has led to magnetic resonance angiography. This latter approach has clear advantages over the invasive X-ray procedure. Additional modifications allow the direct study of tissues of various living organisms under physiological conditions.

Functional MRI is a developing technique that allows neuroradiologists and neurosurgeons to evaluate the activity of the brain and cerebral blood vessels in real time, observing brain activity while the patient is asked questions or asked to perform various functions. This technique is especially helpful in coma patients or in patients in a persistent vegetative state. There are even rare instances of functional MRI demonstrating active brain function in paralyzed patients who were thought to be brain dead or comatose.

Despite the broad applicability of MRI, there are limitations. Patients on life-support systems or with unstable physiological conditions must be evaluated with other imaging techniques. The presence of a magnetic metal apparatus in the body is another limitation. There have also been discussions concerning effects that might be related to the electrical currents induced by magnetic gradient fields.

—K. Thomas Finley, Ph.D.

See also Computed tomography (CT) scanning; Imaging and radiology; Neuroimaging; Noninvasive tests; Nuclear medicine; Positron emission tomography (PET) scanning; Radiopharmaceuticals; Single photon emission computed tomography (SPECT); Ultrasonography.

FOR FURTHER INFORMATION:

Bongard, Frederick, and Darryl Y. Sue, eds. *Current Critical Care Diagnosis and Treatment*. 3d ed. New York: McGraw-Hill Medical, 2008. A medical text that combines medical and surgical perspectives with diagnostic and treatment knowledge. Covers forty topics in critical care basics, medical critical care, and essentials of surgical intensive care and includes information on imaging procedures.

Bushong, Stewart C. *Magnetic Resonance Imaging: Physical and Biological Principles*. 3d ed. St. Louis, Mo.: Mosby, 2003. An introductory text that describes the fundamentals of electricity and magnetism, explains how the MRI system works, and reviews the latest imaging techniques.

Buxton, Richard B. *An Introduction to Functional Magnetic Resonance Imaging: Principles and Techniques*. 2d ed. New York: Cambridge University Press, 2009. Designed for the medical professional, this guide covers all aspects of magnetic resonance imaging.

Cahill, Donald R., Matthew J. Orland, and Gary M. Miller. *Atlas of Human Cross-Sectional Anatomy: With CT and MR Images*. 3d ed. New York: Wiley-Liss, 1995. Discusses such topics as X-ray computed tomography and magnetic resonance imaging. Includes bibliographical references and an index.

Griffith, H. Winter. *Complete Guide to Symptoms, Illness, and Surgery*. Revised and updated by Stephen Moore and Kenneth Yoder. 5th ed. New York: Perigee, 2006. Covers more than five hundred diseases and disorders and includes information about causes and risk factors, preventive techniques, and diagnostic tests such as the MRI.

Pagana, Kathleen Deska, and Timothy J. Pagana. *Mosby's Diagnostic and Laboratory Test Reference*. 9th ed. St. Louis, Mo.: Mosby/Elsevier, 2009. A clinical handbook that gives alphabetically organized laboratory and diagnostic tests for easy reference. Each listing includes such things as alternate or abbreviated test names, type of test, normal findings, possible critical values, test explanation and related physiology, and potential complications.

Smith, Michael B., K. Kirk Shung, and Timothy J. Mosher. "Magnetic Resonance Imaging." In *Principles of Medical Imaging*, edited by Shung, Smith, and Benjamin M. W. Tsui. San Diego, Calif.: Academic Press, 1992. A chapter in a text devoted to biophysics and diagnostic imaging. Includes bibliographical references and an index.

MALABSORPTION
DISEASE/DISORDER

ANATOMY OR SYSTEM AFFECTED: Gallbladder, gastrointestinal system, intestines, liver, pancreas, stomach

SPECIALTIES AND RELATED FIELDS: Biochemistry, biotechnology, family medicine, gastroenterology, genetics, neonatology, nutrition, pediatrics

DEFINITION: The impaired absorption of nutrients from food into the bloodstream.

CAUSES AND SYMPTOMS

The nutritive components of food—carbohydrates, protein, fats, vitamins, and minerals—must be digested in the gastrointestinal tract and absorbed into the circulatory system to be of use to the body. Malabsorption of these nutrients is caused by specific defects in any one of the many separate processes involved in the digestion and absorption of food. It is also the result of general impairment of the structure or function of the gastrointestinal tract.

Malabsorption leads to poor growth when it affects the uptake of any essential nutrient, which is one that must be obtained from the diet. It may cause diarrhea if one of the more abundant constituents of food is not absorbed; carbohydrate malabsorption will usually lead to a watery diarrhea, while protein and fat malabsorption will cause a foul-smelling diarrhea that is dark or whitish, respectively. Diarrhea itself may reduce the absorption of nutrients.

Cystic fibrosis is one of the most common causes of malabsorption in children. The mucus accompanying this disease is secreted into the gastrointestinal tract; it is largely indigestible and can obstruct the passage of nutrients.

TREATMENT AND THERAPY

Treatment for malabsorption depends entirely on its cause. In the case of bacterial infections that affect intestinal function, treatment with appropriate antibiotics will return this function to normal. In celiac sprue, an intolerance to the gluten found in wheat and other grains that alters the absorptive surface of the intestines, the removal of gluten from the diet restores

---

INFORMATION ON MALABSORPTION

CAUSES: Cystic fibrosis, infection, physiological defects
SYMPTOMS: Diarrhea, poor growth
DURATION: Ranges from acute to chronic
TREATMENTS: Depends on form; may include antibiotics, dietary changes

---

normal activity. Some specific defects can be cured by the elimination or replacement of the dietary constituent that is not well digested or absorbed. In other cases, no curative treatment is known, as with cystic fibrosis.

PERSPECTIVE AND PROSPECTS

In 1825, William Beaumont, a U.S. Army surgeon, was the first to study human digestion in the stomach. Since then, the processes of digestion and absorption have become well understood, as have many of the causes of acquired and inherited malabsorption. Effective treatment has been developed in all but the most intractable cases. It is hoped that progress in understanding the genetic basis for inherited malabsorption will lead to earlier and definitive identification of affected individuals and eventually to suitable therapies.

—*James L. Robinson, Ph.D.*

See also Allergies; Bariatric surgery; Carbohydrates; Celiac sprue; Cystic fibrosis; Diarrhea and dysentery; Digestion; Gastroenterology; Gastroenterology, pediatric; Gastrointestinal system; Gluten intolerance; Malnutrition; Nutrition; Protein; Vitamins and minerals.

FOR FURTHER INFORMATION:

Bonci, Leslie. *American Dietetic Association Guide to Better Digestion.* New York: Wiley, 2003.

Christian, Janet L., and Janet L. Greger. *Nutrition for Living.* 4th ed. Redwood City, Calif.: Benjamin/Cummings, 1994.

Jackson, Gordon, and Philip Whitfield. *Digestion: Fueling the System.* New York: Torstar Books, 1984.

Janowitz, Henry D. *Indigestion: Living Better with Upper Intestinal Problems, from Heartburn to Ulcers and Gallstones.* New York: Oxford University Press, 1994.

Mayo Clinic. *Mayo Clinic on Digestive Health: Enjoy Better Digestion with Answers to More than Twelve Common Conditions.* 2d ed. Rochester, Minn.: Author, 2004.

Peikin, Steven R. *Gastrointestinal Health.* Rev. ed. New York: Quill, 2001.

Sharon, Michael. *Complete Nutrition: How to Live in Total Health.* London: Prion, 2001.

MALARIA

DISEASE/DISORDER

ALSO KNOWN AS: Paludism

ANATOMY OR SYSTEM AFFECTED: Blood, immune system, liver, spleen

SPECIALTIES AND RELATED FIELDS: Biochemistry, immunology, internal medicine, pathology, public health

DEFINITION: One of the world's most serious and potentially fatal diseases, malaria is the result of a parasite transmitted into the bloodstream by mosquito bites. It is most common in subtropical zones, especially in Africa, Asia, and Latin America.

KEY TERMS:

Anopheles: the genus of mosquitoes that, by depositing infected saliva into the blood of humans, serves as a vector for transmission of the parasite that causes malaria

merozoites: products of a multistage reproductive process in the malarial parasite's life span; released into the bloodstream, where they destroy red blood cells

Plasmodium falciparum: one of several parasites that cause malarial symptoms; the species that is most dangerous, and lethal, for humans

CAUSES AND SYMPTOMS

Malaria in humans is caused by transfer into the bloodstream, through the saliva of the *Anopheles* mosquito, of the protozoan (single-cell) *Plasmodium* parasite. There are several different strains of the malaria parasite, all belonging to the phylum Sporozoa, a classification connected with the importance of spores in the organism's reproductive cycle. Serious and potentially lethal malarial infections in humans are primarily associated with *P. falciparum*. Other *Plasmodium* parasites that can produce infection are *P. vivax* (formerly present in temperate climate zones but now found only in the subtropics), *P. malariae* (also only subtropical), and *P. ovale* (quite rare, and mainly limited to West Africa). Other *Plasmodium* parasites infect only nonhuman primates (*P. knowlesi* and *P. cynomolgi*, for example), only rodents (four different species), or only birds (*P. cathemerium* and *P. gallinaceum*). The latter two species have been used widely in experimental testing of antimalarial vaccines.

It is important to note that only one mosquito genus, *Anopheles*, and only the female *Anopheles* mosquito, serves the vector function in transmitting malaria. The explanation of the female's role is surprisingly simple: Only the female *Anopheles* nourishes itself (usually in the night hours) by piercing the skin of its victim and sucking small quantities of blood. The male of the species feeds mainly on fruit juices.

In the most common scenario, the mosquito ingests the *Plasmodium* parasite when it sucks the blood of an already infected human. This phase is followed by several others—all connected with the reproductive processes of the same organism (both sexual and asexual)—until subsequent generations of the parasite are passed on by the mosquito to another human host, who then becomes infected. The protozoan's first, sexual stage of reproduction occurs when male gametes emit flagella that seek out and join their female counterpart, producing a fertilized zygote. Once lodged in the gut tissue of the mosquito in the form of an oocyst, a further, asexual stage of reproduction occurs through what is called sporogony: the release from the oocyst of myriad spores. They spread rapidly throughout the body of the mosquito. Many enter the insect host's salivary glands, from which they are transferred into the blood of the next human bitten by the mosquito. It is the further development of the spores in the human organism that produces the disease symptoms associated with malaria.

Once transmitted into the human host through the mosquito saliva, the parasite spores flow quickly through the blood, entering the liver. Their next transformation occurs once they lodge themselves in the cells of the liver, becoming what are called hepatic trophozoites. As they feed off of the liver cells, the trophozoites grow and burst open. This process of asexual multiplication in the liver is referred to as hepatic schozogony. At that stage, the parasite has multiplied many hundreds of times, producing the actual agent of malarial disease, merozoites. If the parasite is *P. vivax*, then this phase may not occur immediately, as a result of a state of dormancy in the parasitic trophozoites. In this case, months or even years can pass before the merozoites are released. Even then, the delayed release is still not final. This explains why some malaria-infected individuals experience a cyclical disappearance of symptoms, followed some time later by a resurgence of the latent disease.

When released from the trophozoites, the merozoites quickly invade the red blood cells of the host. The

---

INFORMATION ON MALARIA

CAUSES: Transmission of parasitic infection via mosquitoes
SYMPTOMS: Recurrent bouts of severe fever, chills, sweating, vomiting; damage to kidneys, blood, brain, and liver
DURATION: Acute to long-term
TREATMENTS: Drug therapy (chloroquine, mefloquine)

---

damage that they inflict leads to anemic reactions as the number of healthy blood cells in the organism decreases. It is not only the liver that is affected; the disease can also spread to the spleen.

Once the effects of malaria begin to take hold in the blood and various organs of the body, certain symptoms will appear. There is an onset of fever, probably caused by the release of a pyrogen (a fever-inducing agent) by the white blood cells reacting to the diseased situation of red blood cells that have been attacked by the malaria parasite. Since this release of pyrogens may follow an irregular pattern, fever can come and go, seemingly sporadically. Meanwhile, as the number of parasitized red blood cells increases, infected red blood cells begin to attach themselves to the inside tissue of capillaries of the internal organs. The effect is blockage of the necessary free flow of blood. If pressure builds because of this blockage, then blood vessels themselves may burst. Such internal hemorrhages allow the directionless dispersion of infected blood within the body, increasing the anemic symptoms that are characteristic of malaria. Perhaps the most dramatic sign of blocked blood vessels occurs if and when the parasitized cells affect the blood flow to the brain. In such cases, convulsions occur, eventually leading to coma.

TREATMENT AND THERAPY

Long before researchers were able to explain the causes of malaria, treatment of its symptoms, primarily manifested in spells of fever, involved giving the patient doses of quinine. As knowledge of the disease increased, different forms of treatment evolved. Such developments occurred not only as new discoveries emerged; they also became necessary as the malaria parasite itself evolved genetically, in effect developing its own immunity to quinine-based treatment.

Several compounds were developed in the later decades of the twentieth century to complement or, more recently, to replace complete dependence on quinine.

Depending on the *Plasmodium* species coming into contact with it, the alkaloid quinine could kill the parasitical organism at key stages in its reproductive activity. Sometimes, however, toxic side effects accompanied the use of quinine in malaria cases. These negative effects eventually sparked research aimed at producing synthetic drugs that could be as effective as quinine in preventing malaria, even though they might not be as effective in treating the disease once contracted. The earliest synthetic antimalarials, introduced between 1926 and the early 1950's, included pamaquine, the first synthetic; mepacrine; and chloroquine and primaquine, two well-known drugs from the mid-1940's through the 1950's. These synthetic agents intervened to stop reproduction of the malaria parasite at different points in its life span. Depending on which preventive drug was taken, treatment might have to begin well before expected exposure, during the period of exposure, or for a certain period after being present in a malaria-infected area. Several generations of antimalarial drugs are on the market, but such progress in pharmaceutical options has not effectively resolved the problem of endemic malaria in regions of the world where those most in need lack either public health information programs or the financial means to obtain necessary drugs.

Research involving vaccination to protect against malarial infection has tended to follow one of two main approaches: vaccines to combat the diffusion of spores directly, and vaccines to block one or several stages of in the parasite's life cycle. Some vaccines have been developed by extracting spores from the blood of infected patients and using methods such as radiation to reduce their potency. Injection of these weakened agents into the blood can induce formation of antibodies that are able to fight invasive spores coming from an outside source (mosquito saliva) into a potential host organism.

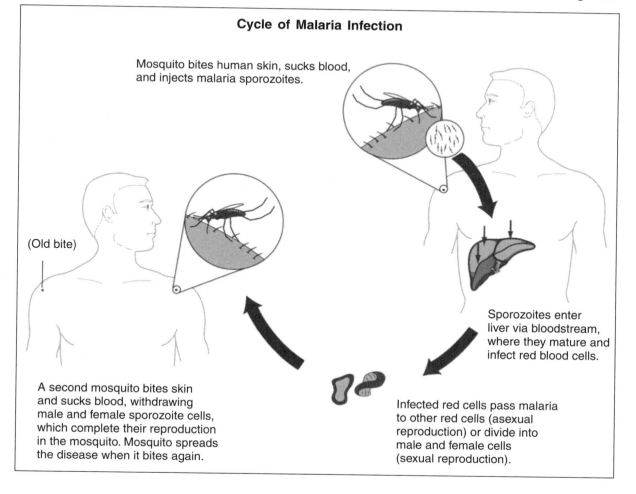

Cycle of Malaria Infection

Mosquito bites human skin, sucks blood, and injects malaria sporozoites.

Sporozoites enter liver via bloodstream, where they mature and infect red blood cells.

Infected red cells pass malaria to other red cells (asexual reproduction) or divide into male and female cells (sexual reproduction).

A second mosquito bites skin and sucks blood, withdrawing male and female sporozoite cells, which complete their reproduction in the mosquito. Mosquito spreads the disease when it bites again.

(Old bite)

Commercial production of such vaccines, however, would require finding an economically viable way of obtaining and treating large quantities of *Plasmodium* spores, not only from *P. falciparum* but also from other malaria parasites that are less deadly but an important threat to large numbers of people around the world. For this reason, researchers have tended to concentrate more on isolating antigens that the body produces naturally to fight invasive spores and merozoites, analyzing them, and attempting to use biotechnology to produce effective synthetic antigens.

Observation over a long period of time has provided statistical evidence that, in a number of subtropical areas where malaria is endemic, fatalities from the disease are more frequent among children than among adults. The reason for this is linked to the adult population's prior exposure to one or more nonlethal malarial infections. In essence, the adult body's production of natural antigens seems to neutralize the effects of blood cells that have become carriers. If they remain in the bloodstream, these antigens reduce the susceptibility to what, in children, takes the form of a sudden invasion of infected and (for the body's immune system) unrecognizable blood cells transmitted through *Anopheles* mosquito bites.

There is, therefore, an entire field of malaria research dealing with the body's own immune responses. Where malaria is concerned, researchers pay particular attention not only to the challenge of understanding how immunity can build in populations living in endemic zones but also to the possibility of increasing the efficiency of certain body organs that naturally affect the bloodstream in ways that can impede the spread of the parasite's damage. Attention has focused, for example, on the internal functions of the spleen. The spleen can prevent the progress of intravascular pathogens in general by reducing the flow of infected red blood cells to other organs and isolating them in a chemical state that renders them less directly dangerous to the body. This capacity is called splenic filtration. Although research has not yet identified an effective way to use externally applied medications to enhance this facet of the spleen's natural defense system, it is agreed that here there is a serious prospect for another area of treatment to complement, if not replace, preventive drugs and synthetic antigens.

Once it was clear that malaria was transmitted by mosquitoes, the most logical tactic to prevent spread of the disease involved campaigns to eradicate, or at least diminish the life chances of, *Anopheles*. Thus, drainage of swamp areas (a costly but effective measure where possible), public health measures to guard against insalubrious concentrations of stagnant water, and insecticide spraying have been practiced throughout the world to combat *Anopheles*. During World War II and until the late 1950's, DDT was the insecticide of choice. When the harmful side effects of DDT for humans and the environment became apparent, legislation in most but not all countries banned the chemical. Research has since aimed at, but not fully succeeded in, developing safer insecticides that can approach DDT's levels of efficiency.

PERSPECTIVE AND PROSPECTS

Research in the field of malarial disease and its biological origins advanced rather slowly, with most major advances occurring fairly late in the nineteenth century. It was in 1897 that a surgeon in the British Indian army, Sir Ronald Ross, following British tropical disease expert Sir Patrick Manson's suggestions, announced his discovery that malaria was transmitted to humans by mosquitoes. There had been earlier theories concerning the role of mosquitoes, some going back as far as the early eighteenth century in Italy (where the term "malaria," meaning "bad air," had originated). It took the work of a French military doctor in Algeria, Alphonse Laveran, to show, under a microscope, the ongoing activity of parasites in the blood of malaria patients. Laveran also did postmortem studies of malaria victims' blood and organs and found a dark pigment composed mainly of iron which came from the parasites' apparent digestion and waste disposal of vital hemoglobin in the red blood cells. He became the first to posit that malaria was a disease of red blood cells and that it was caused by an invasion of parasites.

From there, it was a question of finding how the parasites entered the human bloodstream. This was the result of Ross's observation in India of a particular variety of mosquito larvae (later identified as the small brown *Anopheles*, distinct from *Culex* varieties commonly observed in the daytime) collected from stagnant waters in the region. When Ross followed Manson's suggestion that mosquitoes hatched from these larvae should be induced to feed from a known malaria patient, he found that only a few insects survived the next few days. When these were dissected, he found oocysts embedded on the wall of the mosquitoes' gut. Microscopic analysis showed that they contained the same dark pigment that Laveran had found in the blood of malaria victims in Algeria.

Both Ross (in 1902) and Laveran (in 1907) received Nobel Prizes in recognition of their work, Ross in medicine and Laveran in physiology or medicine. Other contributors, notably the Italian Giovanni Batista Grassi, carried on significant work in the same first decade of the twentieth century that paralleled (or, according to Grassi, may have been accomplished before) Ross's studies. The most important suggestion by Grassi—which was correct but which took much more work to prove in the laboratory—was that there must be significant transformations, in fact multiple stages of reproduction, between the sporozoite phase of dissemination of the parasite via mosquito saliva and the merozoite phase, when the actual attacking parasite can destroy red blood cells in the human host. Later researchers finally provided, in 1934, convincing evidence that there was a sequence of sexual and asexual phases of reproduction (the later labeled "schizogony") in the life cycle of the *Plasmodium* parasite.

Over the years, other researchers helped broaden the understanding of malaria, its causes, and treatment. Despite the obvious costs paid during the first half of the twentieth century involving debilitation and loss of human lives in areas where malaria was endemic, truly major breakthroughs occurred only during the extraordinary conditions created by World War II. The fact that large numbers of troops were sent to areas in East, South, and Southeast Asia as well as Africa meant that the danger of widespread malarial infection could hamper strategic operations. Distribution of all forms of preventive equipment, including both mosquito nets and insect repellents, was destined to become standard procedure in tropical zones. Doses of quinine were also part of each soldier's medical supply packet.

—*Byron D. Cannon, Ph.D.*

See also Bites and stings; Centers for Disease Control and Prevention (CDC); Epidemics and pandemics; Epidemiology; Fever; Insect-borne diseases; Parasitic diseases; Protozoan diseases; Tropical medicine; Zoonoses.

FOR FURTHER INFORMATION:

Farmer, Paul. *Infections and Inequalities: The Modern Plagues*. Berkeley: University of California Press, 2001. This book surveys the past history of, and future prospects for, attempts to address the imbalance between malarial (and other disease) risk factors characteristic of developed and less developed tropical regions of the world.

Honigsbaum, Mark. *The Fever Trail: In Search of the Cure for Malaria*. New York: Farrar, Straus and Giroux, 2002. A popular science book that chronicles the history of malaria and its effect on the world.

Malaria Foundation International. http://www.malaria.org. A group that funds global outreach projects designed to fight malaria and raises public awareness and provides education about the disease.

Rocco, Fiammetta. "Corrections and Clarification: The Global Spread of Malaria in a Future, Warmer World." *Science* 289 (September, 2000): 2283-2284. This graphically illustrated article attempts to predict which areas of the globe now vulnerable to malarial infections may not be vulnerable by 2050, and, conversely, which areas now free of the disease may become malaria zones.

_____. *The Miraculous Fever-Tree: Malaria and the Quest for a Cure That Changed the World*. New York: HarperCollins, 2003. A historical view of scientific advances in the treatment of malaria since the centuries-old use of bark from the cinchona tree.

MALIGNANCY AND METASTASIS
DISEASE/DISORDER

ANATOMY OR SYSTEM AFFECTED: All

SPECIALTIES AND RELATED FIELDS: Internal medicine, oncology, pathology, plastic surgery

DEFINITION: "Malignancy" is the uncontrolled growth of tumor cells that invade and compress surrounding tissues and break through the skin or barriers within the body; "metastasis" describes the tendency of malignant cells to break loose from their tumor of origin to travel to other locations within the body.

KEY TERMS:

benign tumors: tumors that grow relatively slowly, do not interfere with normal body functions, and do not metastasize

carcinogen: a natural or artificial substance inducing the transformation of cells toward the malignant state

chemotherapy: the use of chemicals to kill or inhibit the growth of cancer cells

multistep progression: the typical pathway of induction of cancer, beginning with an initial alteration to a gene and progressing to the fully malignant state

oncogene: a gene directly or indirectly inducing the transformation of cells from the normal to the malignant state; most oncogenes have normal counterparts in body cells

retrovirus: a virus infecting mammalian and other cells that sometimes carries and introduces oncogenes into host cells

transfection: a technique used to introduce genes into cells by exposing the cells to fragmented deoxyribonucleic acid (DNA) under conditions that promote the uptake and incorporation of DNA

tumor suppressor gene: a gene that, in its normal form, inhibits cell division

CAUSES AND SYMPTOMS

Cancer cells are characterized by two primary features. One of these is uncontrolled cell division: Cells enter an unregulated, rapid growth phase by losing the controls that normally limit division rates to the amount required for normal growth and maintenance of body tissues. The second feature is metastasis, in which tumor cells lose the connections that normally hold them in place in body tissues, break loose, and spread from their original sites to lodge and grow in other body locations. Tumor cells with these characteristics are described as malignant.

The detrimental effects of solid malignant tumors result from the interference of rapidly growing masses of cancer cells with the activities of normal tissues and organs, or from the loss of vital functions because of the conversion of cells with essential functions to nonfunctional forms. Some malignant tumors of glandular tissue upset bodily functions by producing and secreting excessive quantities of hormones.

Solid malignant tumors, as they grow, compress surrounding normal tissues; they destroy normal structures by cutting off blood supplies and interrupting nerve function. They may also break through barriers that separate major body regions, such as internal membranes and epithelia or the gut wall. They may also break through the skin. Such breakthroughs cause internal or external bleeding and infection, and they destroy the organization and separation of body regions necessary for normal function. Both compression and breakthroughs can cause pain that, in advanced cases, may become extreme.

Malignant tumors of blood tissues involve cell lines that normally divide to supply the body's requirements for red and white blood cells. Cancer in these cell lines crowds the bloodstream with immature, nonfunctional cells that are unable to accomplish required activities, such as the delivery of oxygen to tissues or the activation of the immune response.

When the total mass of actively growing and dividing malignant cells becomes large, their demands for nutrients may deprive normal cells, tissues, and organs of their needed supplies, leading to generally impaired functions, fatigue, weakness, and weight loss.

Not all unregulated tissue growths are malignant. Some tumors, such as common skin warts, are benign—they do not usually interfere with normal body functions. They grow relatively slowly and do not metastasize. Often, benign tumors are surrounded by a closed capsule of connective tissue that prevents or retards expansion and breakup. Some initially benign tumors, however, including even common skin warts, may change to malignant forms.

Individual cells of a malignant tumor exhibit differences from normal cells in activity, biochemistry, physiology, and structure. First and foremost is the characteristic of uncontrolled division. Cancer cells typically move through the division cycle much more rapidly than normal cells. The rapid division is accompanied by biochemical changes characteristic of dividing cells such as high metabolic rates; increases in the rate of transport of substances across the plasma membrane; increases in protein phosphorylation; raised cytoplasmic concentrations of sodium, potassium, and calcium ions; and an elevated pH. Often chromosomal abnormalities are present, including extra or missing chromosomes, exchanges of segments between chromosomes, and breakage.

Cancer cells also typically fail to develop all the characteristics and structures of fully mature cells of their type. They may also lose mature characteristics if these were attained before conversion to the malignant state. Frequently, loss of mature characteristics involves disorganization or disappearance of the cytoskeleton. Alterations are also noted in the structure and

INFORMATION ON MALIGNANCY AND METASTASIS

CAUSES: Genetic factors, carcinogens, retroviruses

SYMPTOMS: Vary; can include loss or impairment of normal bodily functions, interrupted nerve function, internal or external bleeding and infection, pain, swelling, fatigue, weakness, weight loss

DURATION: Often chronic with recurrent episodes

TREATMENTS: Surgery, radiation, chemotherapy

density of surface carbohydrate groups. Cancer cells lose tight attachments to their neighbors or to supportive extracellular materials such as collagen; some cancer cells secrete enzymes that break cell connections and destroy elements of the extracellular material, aiding their movement into and through surrounding tissues. If removed from the body and placed in test-tube cultures, most cancer cells have the capacity to divide indefinitely. In contrast, most normal body cells placed in a culture medium eventually stop dividing.

The conversion of normal cells to malignant types usually involves multiple causes inducing a series of changes that occur in stages over a considerable length of time. This characteristic is known as the multistep progression of cancer. In most cases, the complete sequence of steps leading from an initiating alteration to full malignancy is unknown.

The initial event in a multistep progression usually involves the alteration of a gene from a normal to an aberrant form known as an oncogene. The gene involved is typically one that regulates cell growth and division or that takes part in biochemical sequences with this effect. The alteration may involve substitutions or the loss of DNA sequences, the movement of the gene to a new location in the chromosomes, or the movement of another gene or its controlling elements to the vicinity of the gene. In some cases, the alteration involves a gene that in normal form suppresses cell division in cells in which it is active. Loss or alteration of function of such genes, known as tumor suppressor genes, can directly or indirectly increase growth and division rates.

An initiating genetic alteration may be induced by a long list of factors, including exposure to radiation or certain chemicals, the insertion of viral DNA into the chromosomes, or the generation of random mutations during the duplication of genetic material. In a few cancers, the initiating event involves the insertion of an oncogene into the DNA by an infecting virus that carries the oncogene as a part of its genetic makeup.

In some cases, about 5 percent in humans, an initiating oncogene or faulty tumor suppressor gene is inherited, producing a strong predisposition to the development of malignancy. Among these strongly predisposed cancers are familial retinoblastoma, familial adenomatous polyps of the colon, and multiple endocrine neoplasia, in which tumors develop in the thyroid, adrenal medulla, and parathyroid glands. In addition to the strongly predisposed cancers, some, including breast, ovarian, and colon cancers other than familial adenomatous polyps, show some degree of disposition

in family lines—members of these families show a greater tendency to develop the cancer than individuals in other families.

Subsequent steps from the initiating change to the fully malignant state usually include the conversion of additional genes to oncogenic form or the loss of function of tumor suppressor genes. Also important during intermediate stages are further alterations to the initial and succeeding oncogenes that increase their activation. The initial conversion of a normal gene to oncogenic form by its movement to a new location in the chromosomes may be compounded at successive steps, for example, by sequence changes or the multiplication of the oncogene into extra copies. The subsequent steps in progression to the malignant state are driven by many of the sources of change responsible for the initiating step. Because genetic alterations often occur during the duplication and division of the genetic material, an increase in the cell division rate by the initiating change may increase the chance that further alterations leading to full malignancy will occur.

A change advancing the progression toward full malignancy may take place soon after a previous change or only after a long delay. Moreover, further changes may not occur, leaving the progression at an intermediate stage, without the development of full malignancy, for the lifetime of the individual. The avoidance of environmental factors inducing genetic alterations—such as overexposure to radiation sources such as sunlight, X rays, and radon gas and chemicals such as those in cigarette smoke—increases the chance that progressions toward malignancy will remain incomplete.

The last stage in progression to full malignancy is often metastasis. After the loss of normal adhesions to neighboring cells or to elements of the extracellular matrix, the separation and movement of cancer cells from a primary tumor to secondary locations may occur through the development of active motility or from breakage into elements of the circulatory system.

Relatively few of the cells breaking loose from a tumor survive the rigors of passage through the body. Most are destroyed by various factors, including deformation by passage through narrow capillaries and destruction by blood turbulence around the heart valves and vessel junctions. Furthermore, tumor cells often develop changes in their surface groups that permit detection and elimination by the immune system as they move through the body. Unfortunately, the rigors of travel through the body may act as a sort of natural selection for the cells that are most malignant—that is, those most able to resist destruction—and that can grow uncontrollably and spread by metastasis.

Many natural and artificial agents trigger the initial step in the progression to the malignant state or push cells through intermediate stages. Most of these agents, collectively called carcinogens, are chemicals or forms of radiation capable of inducing chemical changes in DNA. Some, however, may initiate or further this progression by modifying ribonucleic acids (RNAs) or proteins, or they may act by increasing the rate of DNA replication and cell division.

Treatment and Therapy

Cancer is treated most frequently by one or a combination of three primary techniques: surgical removal of tumors, radiation therapy, and chemotherapy. Surgical removal is most effective if the growth has remained localized so that the entire tumor can be detected and removed. Often, surgery is combined with radiation or chemotherapy in an attempt to eliminate malignant cells that have broken loose from a primary tumor and lodged in other parts of the body. Surgical removal followed by chemotherapy is presently the most effective treatment for most forms of cancer, especially if the tumor is detected and removed before extensive metastasis has taken place. Most responsive to surgical treatments have been skin cancers, many of which are easily detected and remain localized and accessible.

Radiation therapy may be directed toward the destruction of a tumor in a specific body location. Alternatively, it may be used in whole-body exposure to kill cancer cells that have metastasized and lodged in many body regions. In either case, the method takes advantage of the destructive effects of radiation on DNA, particularly during periods when the DNA is under duplication. Because cancer cells undergo replication at higher rates than most other body cells, the technique is more selective for tumors than for normal tissues. The selection is only partial, however, so that body cells that divide rapidly, such as those of the blood, hair follicles, and intestinal lining, are also affected. As a consequence, radiation therapy often has side effects ranging from unpleasant to serious, including hair loss, nausea and vomiting, anemia, and suppression of the immune system. Because radiation is mutagenic, radiation therapy carries the additional disadvantage of being carcinogenic—the treatment, while effective in the destruction or inhibition of a malignant growth, may also initiate new cancers or push cells through intermediate stages in progression toward malignancy.

When possible, radiation is directed only toward the body regions containing a tumor in order to minimize the destruction of normal tissues. This may be accomplished by focusing a radiation source on the tumor or by shielding body regions outside the tumor with a radiation barrier such as a lead sheet.

Chemotherapy involves the use of chemicals that retard cell division or kill tumor cells more readily than normal body cells. Most of the chemicals used in chemotherapy have been discovered by routine screening of substances for their effects on cancer cells in cultures and test animals. Several hundred thousand chemicals were tested in the screening effort that produced the thirty or so chemotherapeutic agents available for cancer treatment.

Many of the chemicals most effective in cancer chemotherapy alter the chemical structure of DNA, produce breaks in DNA molecules, slow or stop DNA duplication, or interfere with the natural systems repairing chemical lesions in DNA. The effects inhibit cell division or interfere with cell functions sufficiently to kill the cancer cells. Because DNA is most susceptible to chemical alteration during duplication and cancer cells duplicate their DNA and divide more rapidly than most normal tissue cells, the effects of these chemicals are most pronounced in malignant types. Normal cells, however, are also affected to some extent, particularly those in tissues that divide more rapidly. As a result, chemotherapeutic chemicals can produce essentially the same detrimental side effects as radiation therapy. The side effects of chemotherapy are serious enough to be fatal in 2 to 5 percent of persons treated. Because they alter DNA, many chemotherapeutic agents are carcinogens and carry the additional risk, as with radiation, of inducing the formation of new cancers.

Not all chemicals used in chemotherapy alter DNA. Some act by interfering with cell division or other cell processes rather than directly modifying DNA. Two chemotherapeutic agents often used in cancer treatment, vinblastine and taxol, for example, slow or stop cell division through their ability to interfere with the spindle structure that divides chromosomes. The drugs can slow or stop tumor growth as well as the division of normal cells.

Tumors frequently develop resistance to some of the chemicals used in chemotherapy, so that the treatment gradually becomes less effective. Development of resistance is often associated with random duplication of DNA segments, commonly noted in tumor cells. In some, the random duplication happens to include genes that provide resistance to the chemicals employed in chemotherapy. The genes providing resistance usually encode enzymes that break down the applied chemical or its metabolic derivatives, or transport proteins of the plasma membrane capable of rapidly excreting the chemical from the cell. One gene in particular, the multidrug resistance gene (MDR), is frequently found to be duplicated or highly activated in resistant cells. This gene, which is normally active in cells of the liver, kidney, adrenal glands, and parts of the digestive system, encodes a transport pump that can expel a large number of substances from cells, including many of those used in chemotherapy. Overactivity of the MDR pump can effectively keep chemotherapy drugs below toxic levels in cancer cells. Cells developing resistance are more likely to survive chemotherapy and give rise to malignant cell lines with resistance. The chemotherapeutic agents involved may thus have the unfortunate effect of selecting cells with resistance, thereby ensuring that they will become the dominant types in the tumor.

Success rates with chemotherapy vary from negligible to about 80 percent, depending on the cancer type. For most, success rates do not range above 50 to 60 percent. Some cancer types, including lung, breast, ovarian, and colorectal tumors, respond poorly or not at all to chemotherapy. The overall cure rate for surgery, radiation, and chemotherapy combined, as judged by no recurrence of the cancer for a period of five years, is about 50 percent.

It is hoped that full success in the treatment of cancer will come from the continued study of the genes controlling cell division and the regulatory mechanisms that modify the activity of these genes in the cell cycle. An understanding of the molecular activities of these genes and their modifying controls may bring with it a molecular means to reach specifically into cancer cells and halt their growth and metastasis.

PERSPECTIVE AND PROSPECTS

Indications that malignancy and metastasis might have a basis in altered gene activity began to appear in the nineteenth century. In 1820, a British physician, Sir William Norris, noted that melanoma, a cancer involving pigmented skin cells, was especially prevalent in one family under study. More than forty kinds of cancer, including common types such as cancer of the breast and colon, have since been noticed to occur more frequently in some families than in others. Another indication that cancer has a basis in altered gene activity

was the fact that the chromosomes of many tumor cells show abnormalities, such as extra chromosomes, broken chromosomes, or rearrangements of one kind or another. These abnormalities suggested that cancer might be induced by altered genes with activities related to cell division.

These indications were put on a firm basis by research with tumors caused by viruses infecting animal cells, most notably those caused by a group of viruses infecting mammals and other animals, the retroviruses. Many retroviral infections cause little or no damage to their hosts. Some, however, are associated with induction of cancer. (Another type of pathogenic retrovirus is responsible for acquired immunodeficiency syndrome, or AIDS.) The cancer-inducing types among the retroviruses were found to carry genes capable of transforming normal cells to the malignant state. The transforming genes were at first thought to be purely viral in origin, but DNA sequencing and other molecular approaches revealed that the viral oncogenes had normal counterparts among the genes directly or indirectly regulating cell division in cells of the infected host. Among the most productive of the investigators using this approach were J. Michael Bishop and Harold E. Varmus, who received the 1989 Nobel Prize in Physiology or Medicine for their research establishing the relationship between retroviral oncogenes and their normal cellular counterparts.

The discovery of altered host genes in cancer-inducing retroviruses prompted a search for similar genes in nonviral cancers. Much of this work was accomplished by transfection experiments, in which the DNA of cancer cells is extracted and introduced into cultured mouse cells. Frequently, the mouse cells are transformed into types that grow much more rapidly than normal cells. The human oncogene responsible for the transformation is then identified in the altered cells. Many of the oncogenes identified by transfection turned out to be among those already carried by retroviruses, confirming by a different route that these genes are capable of contributing to the transformation of cells to a cancerous state. The transfection experiments also identified some additional oncogenes not previously found in retroviruses.

In spite of impressive advances in treatment, cancer remains among the most dreaded of human diseases. Recognized as a major threat to health since the earliest days of recorded history, cancer still counts as one of the most frequent causes of human fatality. In technically advanced countries, it accounts for about 15 to 20 percent of deaths each year. In a typical year, more persons die from cancer in the United States than the total number of Americans killed in World War II and the Vietnam War combined. Smoking, the most frequent single cause of cancer, is estimated to be responsible for about one-third of these deaths.

—*Stephen L. Wolfe, Ph.D.*

See also Biopsy; Cancer; Carcinogens; Carcinoma; Cytology; Cytopathology; Imaging and radiology; Laboratory tests; Lymphadenopathy and lymphoma; Mammography; Oncology; Pathology; Radiation therapy; Tumor removal; Tumors.

FOR FURTHER INFORMATION:

Alberts, Bruce, et al. *Molecular Biology of the Cell*. 5th ed. New York: Garland, 2008. Describes the development and characteristics of malignance and metastasis. The text is clearly written at the college level and is illustrated by numerous diagrams and photographs.

Dollinger, Malin, et al. *Everyone's Guide to Cancer Therapy*. 5th ed. Kansas City, Mo.: Andrews McMeel, 2008. An excellent source of medical information about cancer, written for the general public. Describes various cancer sites in the body. Includes a helpful glossary of medical terminology.

Eyre, Harmon J., Dianne Partie Lange, and Lois B. Morris. *Informed Decisions: The Complete Book of Cancer Diagnosis, Treatment, and Recovery*. 2d ed. Atlanta: American Cancer Society, 2002. This text from the American Cancer Society is intended for the layperson. It is exemplary in its discussion of cancer.

Lackie, J. M., and J. A. T. Dow, eds. *The Dictionary of Cell and Molecular Biology*. 4th ed. Boston: Academic Press, 2007. Encompasses cytology and molecular biology. Includes bibliographical references.

Lodish, Harvey, et al. *Molecular Cell Biology*. 6th ed. New York: W. H. Freeman, 2008. An excellent textbook written at the college level. Includes an unusually complete discussion of the characteristics and causes of malignancy and metastasis. Many highly illustrative diagrams and photographs are included.

Weinberg, Robert. "Finding the Anti-Oncogene." *Scientific American* 259 (September, 1988): 44-51. A lucidly written description of tumor suppressor genes and their possible use as a means to inhibit tumor growth. Many innovative and informative illustrations are included with the article.

Wolfe, Stephen L. *Molecular and Cellular Biology*. Belmont, Calif.: Wadsworth, 1993. Chapter 22,
"The Cell Cycle, Cell Cycle Regulation, and Cancer," describes the cellular factors and processes regulating the growth and division of both normal and malignant cells. Written at the college level, the book is readable and illustrated with many useful and informative diagrams and photographs.

MALNUTRITION

DISEASE/DISORDER

ANATOMY OR SYSTEM AFFECTED: Gastrointestinal system, intestines, nails, stomach, all bodily systems

SPECIALTIES AND RELATED FIELDS: Gastroenterology, nutrition, pediatrics, public health

DEFINITION: Impaired health caused by an imbalance, either through deficiency or excess, in nutrients.

KEY TERMS:

anemia: a condition in which there is a lower-than-normal concentration of the iron-containing protein in red blood cells, which carry oxygen

famine: a lack of access to food in a population, the cause of which can be a natural disaster, such as a drought, or a situation created by humans, such as a civil war

kwashiorkor: the condition that results from consuming a diet that is sufficient in energy (kilocalories) but inadequate in protein content

marasmus: the condition that results from consuming a diet that is deficient in both energy and protein

osteoporosis: a bone disorder in which the bone's mineral content is decreased over time, resulting in a weakening of the skeleton and susceptibility to bone fractures

protein energy malnutrition (PEM): a deficient intake of energy (kilocalories) and/or protein, the most common type of undernutrition in developing countries; the two major types of PEM are kwashiorkor and marasmus

undernutrition: continued ill health caused by a long-standing dietary deficiency of the energy (kilocalories) and the nutrients that are required to maintain health and provide protection from disease

CAUSES AND SYMPTOMS

Malnutrition literally means "bad nutrition." It can be used broadly to mean an excess or deficiency of the nutrients that are necessary for good health. In industrialized societies, malnutrition typically represents the excess consumption characterized by a diet containing too much energy (kilocalories), fat, and sodium. Malnutrition is most commonly thought, however, to be undernutrition or deficient intake, the consumption of inadequate amounts of nutrients to promote health or to support growth in children. The most severe form of undernutrition is called protein energy malnutrition, or PEM. It commonly affects children, who require nutrients not only to help maintain the body but also to grow. Two types of PEM occur: kwashiorkor and marasmus.

Kwashiorkor is a condition in which a person consumes adequate energy but not enough protein. It usually is seen in children between one and four who are weaned so that the next baby can be breast-fed. The weaning diet consists of gruels made from starchy foods that do not contain an adequate supply of amino acids, the building blocks of protein. These diets do, however, provide enough energy.

Diets in many developing countries are high in bulk, making it nearly impossible for a child to consume a sufficient volume of foods such as rice and grain to obtain an adequate amount of protein for growth. The outward signs of kwashiorkor are a potbelly, dry unpigmented skin, coarse reddish hair, and edema in the legs. Edema results from a lack of certain proteins in the blood that help to maintain a normal fluid balance in the body. The potbelly and swollen limbs often are misinterpreted as signs of being "fat" among the developing world cultures. Other signs requiring further medical testing include fat deposits in the liver and decreased production of digestive enzymes. The mental and physical growth of the child are impaired. Children with kwashiorkor are apathetic, listless, and withdrawn. Ironically, these children lose their appetites.

INFORMATION ON MALNUTRITION

CAUSES: Limited diet, possibly related to poverty, famine, or war; chronic diarrhea; vitamin and mineral deficiency; iron-deficiency anemia; certain diseases

SYMPTOMS: Vary; may include dry and unpigmented skin, coarse reddish hair, swollen limbs, impaired mental and physical development, apathy, listlessness, increased susceptibility to upper respiratory infection and diarrhea, gaunt appearance, muscle wasting

DURATION: Can be short-term or chronic

TREATMENTS: Refeeding with diet adequate in protein, calories, and other essential nutrients; fluid restoration; vitamin and mineral supplements

---

They become very susceptible to upper respiratory infection and diarrhea. Children with kwashiorkor also are deficient in vitamins and minerals that are found in protein-rich foods. There are symptoms caused by these specific nutrient deficiencies as well.

Marasmus literally means "to waste away." It is caused by a deficiency of both Calories (kilocalories) and protein in the diet. This is the most severe form of childhood malnutrition. Body fat stores are used up to provide energy, and eventually muscle tissue is broken down for body fuel. Victims appear as skin and bones, gazing with large eyes from a bald head with an aged, gaunt appearance. Once severe muscle wasting occurs, death is imminent. Body temperature is below normal. The immune system does not operate normally, making these children extremely susceptible to respiratory and gastrointestinal infections.

A vicious cycle develops once the child succumbs to infection. Infection increases the body's need for protein, yet the PEM child is so protein deficient that recovery from even minor respiratory infections is prolonged. Pneumonia and measles become fatal diseases for PEM victims. Severe diarrhea compounds the problem. The child is often dehydrated, and any nourishment that might be consumed will not be adequately absorbed.

The long-term prognosis for these PEM children is poor. If the child survives infections and is fed, PEM returns once the child goes home to the same environment that caused it. Children with repeated episodes of kwashiorkor have high mortality rates.

Children with PEM are most likely victims of famine. Typically, these children either were not breast-fed or were breast-fed for only a few months. If a weaning formula is used, it has not been prepared properly; in many cases, it is mixed with unsanitary water or watered down because the parents cannot afford to buy enough to use it at full strength.

It is difficult to distinguish between the cause of kwashiorkor and that of marasmus. One child ingesting the same diet as another may develop kwashiorkor, while the other may develop marasmus. Some scientists think this may be a result of the different ways in which individuals adapt to nutritional deprivation. Others propose that kwashiorkor is caused by eating moldy grains, since it appears only in rainy, tropical areas.

Another type of malnutrition involves a deficiency of vitamins or minerals. Vitamin A is necessary for the maintenance of healthy skin, and even a mild deficiency causes susceptibility to diarrhea and upper respiratory infection. Diarrhea reinforces the vicious cycle of malnutrition, since it prevents nutrients from being absorbed. With a more severe vitamin A deficiency, changes in the eyes and, eventually, blindness result. Night blindness is usually the first detectable symptom of vitamin A deficiency. The blood that bathes the eye cannot regenerate the visual pigments needed to see in the dark. Vitamin A deficiency, the primary cause of childhood blindness, can result from the lack of either vitamin A or the protein that transports it in the blood. If the deficiency of vitamin A occurs during pregnancy or at birth, the skull does not develop normally and the brain is crowded. An older child deficient in vitamin A will suffer growth impairment.

Diseases resulting from B-vitamin deficiencies are rare. Strict vegetarians, called vegans, who consume no animal products are at risk for vitamin B_{12} deficiency resulting in an anemia in which the red blood cells are large and immature. Too little folate (folic acid) in the diet can cause a similar anemia. Beriberi is the deficiency disease of thiamine (vitamin B_1) in which the heart and nervous systems are damaged and muscle wasting occurs. Ariboflavinosis (lack of riboflavin) describes a collection of symptoms such as cracks and redness of the eyes and lips; inflamed, sensitive eyelids; and a purple-red tongue. Pellagra is the deficiency disease of niacin (vitamin B_3). It is characterized by "the Four Ds of pellagra": dermatitis, diarrhea, dementia, and death. Isolated deficiency of a B vitamin is rare, since many B vitamins work in concert. Therefore, a lack of one hinders the function of the rest.

Scurvy is the deficiency disease of vitamin C. Early signs of scurvy are bleeding gums and pinpoint hemorrhages under the skin. As the deficiency becomes more severe, the skin becomes rough, brown, and scaly, eventually resulting in impaired wound healing, soft bones, painful joints, and loose teeth. Finally, hardening of the arteries or massive bleeding results in death.

Rickets is the childhood deficiency disease of vitamin D. Bone formation is impaired, which is reflected in a bowlegged or knock-kneed appearance. In adults, a brittle bone condition called osteomalacia results from vitamin D deficiency.

Malnutrition of minerals is more prevalent in the world, since deficiencies are observed in both industrialized and developing countries. Calcium malnutrition in young children results in stunted growth. Osteoporosis occurs when calcium reserves are drawn upon to supply the other body parts with calcium. This occurs in later adulthood, leaving bones weak and fragile.

General loss of stature and fractures of the hip, pelvis, and wrist are common, and a humpback appears. Caucasian and Asian women of small stature are at greatest risk for osteoporosis.

Iron-deficiency anemia is the most common form of malnutrition in developing societies. Lack of consumption of iron-rich foods is common among the poor, and this problem is compounded by iron loss in women who menstruate and who thus lose iron monthly. This deficiency, which is characterized by small, pale red blood cells, causes weakness, fatigue, and sensitivity to cold temperatures. Anemia in children can cause reduced ability to learn and impaired ability to think and to concentrate.

Deficiencies of other minerals are less common. Although these deficiencies are usually seen among people in developing nations, they may occur among the poor, pregnant women, children, and the elderly in industrialized societies. Severe growth retardation and arrested sexual maturation are characteristics of zinc deficiency. With iodine deficiency, the cells in the thyroid gland enlarge to try to trap as much iodine as possible. This enlargement of the thyroid gland is called simple or endemic goiter. A more severe iodine deficiency results from a lack of iodine that leads to a deficiency of thyroid hormone during pregnancy. The child of a mother with such a deficiency is born with severe mental and/or physical retardation, a condition known as congenital hypothyroidism or cretinism.

The causes of malnutrition, therefore, can be difficult to isolate, because nutrients work together in the body. In addition, the underlying causes of malnutrition (poverty, famine, and war) often are untreatable.

TREATMENT AND THERAPY

Treatment for PEM involves refeeding with a diet adequate in protein, Calories, and other essential nutrients. Response to treatment is influenced by many factors, such as the person's age, the stage of development in which the deprivation began, the severity of the deficiency, the duration of the deficiency, and the presence of other illnesses, particularly infections. Total recovery is possible only if the underlying cause that led to PEM can be eliminated.

PEM can result from illnesses such as cancer and acquired immunodeficiency syndrome (AIDS). Victims of these diseases cannot consume diets with enough energy and protein to meet their body needs, which are higher than normal because of the illness. Infections also increase the need for many nutrients. The first step

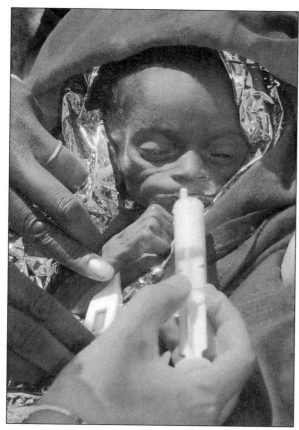

A seven-month-old child suffering from severe malnutrition is helped by a medic in Angola in 2002. (AP/Wide World Photos)

in treatment must be to cure the underlying infection. People from cultures in which PEM is prevalent believe that food should not be given to an ill person.

Prevention of PEM is the preferred therapy. In areas with unsafe water supplies and high rates of poverty, women should be encouraged to breast-feed. Education about proper weaning foods provides further defense against PEM. Other preventive efforts involve combining plant proteins into a mixture of high-quality protein, adding nutrients to cereal products, and using genetic engineering to produce grains with a better protein mix. The prevention of underlying causes such as famine and drought may not be feasible.

Prekwashiorkor can be identified by regular plotting of the child's growth. If treatment begins at this stage, patient response is rapid and the prognosis is good. Treatment must begin by correcting the body's fluid imbalance. Low potassium levels must be corrected. Restoration of fluid is followed by adequate provision of Calories, with gradual additions of protein that the

patient can use to repair damaged immune and digestive systems. Treatment must happen rapidly yet allow the digestive system to recover—thus the term "hurry slowly." Once edema is corrected and blood potassium levels are restored, a diluted milk with added sugar can be given. Gradually, vegetable oil is added to increase the intake of Calories. Vitamin and mineral supplements are given. Final diet therapy includes a diet of skim milk and other animal protein sources, coupled with the addition of vegetables and fat.

The residual effects of PEM may be great if malnutrition has come at a critical period in development or has been of long duration. In prolonged cases, damage to growth and the digestive system may be irreversible. Mortality is very high in such cases. Normally, the digestive tract undergoes rapid cell replacement; therefore, this system is one of the first to suffer in PEM. Absorptive surfaces shrink, and digestive enzymes and protein carriers that transport nutrients are lacking.

Another critical factor in the treatment of PEM is the stage of development in which the deprivation occurs. Most PEM victims are children. If nutritional deprivation occurs during pregnancy, the consequence is increased risk of infant death. If the child is carried to term, it is of low birth weight, placing it at high risk for death. Malnutrition during lactation decreases the quantity, but not always the nutritional quality, of milk. Thus, fewer Calories are consumed by the baby. Growth of the child is slowed. These babies are short for their age and continue to be shorter later in life, even if their diet improves.

During the first two years of life, the brain continues to grow. Nutritional deprivation can impair mental development and cognitive function. For only minimal damage to occur, malnutrition must be treated in early stages. Adults experiencing malnutrition are more adaptive to it, since their protein energy needs are not as great. Weight loss, muscle wasting, and impaired immune function occur, and malnourished women stop menstruating.

Successful treatment of a specific nutrient deficiency depends on the duration of the deficiency and the stage in a person's development at which it occurs. Vitamin A is a fat-soluble vitamin that is stored in the body. Thus, oral supplements or injections of vitamin A can provide long-term protection from this deficiency. If vitamin A is given early enough, the deficiency can be rapidly reversed. By the time the patient is blind, sight cannot be restored, and frequently the patient dies because of other illnesses. Treatment also is dependent upon adequate protein to provide carriers in the blood to transport these vitamins. Treatment of the B-vitamin deficiencies involves oral and intramuscular injections. The crucial step in treatment is to initiate therapy before irreversible damage has occurred. Scurvy (vitamin C deficiency) can be eliminated in five days by administering the amount of vitamin C found in approximately three cups of orange juice. Treatment of vitamin D deficiency in children and adults involves an oral dose of two to twelve times the recommended daily allowance of the vitamin. Halibut and cod liver oils are frequently given as vitamin D supplements.

Successful treatment of a mineral deficiency depends on the timing and duration of the deficiency. Once the bones are fully grown, restoring calcium to optimal levels will not correct short stature. To prevent osteoporosis, bones must have been filled to the maximum with calcium during early adulthood. Estrogen replacement therapy and weight-bearing exercise retard calcium loss in later years and do more than calcium supplements can.

Iron supplementation is necessary to correct iron-deficiency anemia. Iron supplements are routinely prescribed for pregnant women to prevent anemia during pregnancy. Treatment also includes a diet with adequate meat, fish, and poultry to provide not only iron but also a factor that enhances absorption. Iron absorption is also enhanced by vitamin C. Anemias caused by lack of folate and vitamin B_{12} will not respond to iron therapy. These anemias must be treated by adding the appropriate vitamin to the diet.

Zinc supplementation can correct arrested sexual maturation and impaired growth if it is begun in time. In areas where the soil does not contain iodine, iodine is added to salt or injections of iodized oil are given to prevent goiter. Cretinism cannot be cured—only prevented.

In general, malnutrition is caused by a diet of limited variety and quantity. The underlying causes of malnutrition—poverty, famine, and war—are often untreatable. Overall treatment lies in prevention by providing all people with a diet that is adequate in all nutrients, including vitamins, minerals, and Calories. Sharing the world's wealth and ending political strife and greed are essential elements of the struggle to end malnutrition.

PERSPECTIVE AND PROSPECTS

Over the years, the study of malnutrition has shifted to include the excessive intake of nutrients. In developing countries, the primary causes of death are infectious diseases, and undernutrition is a risk factor. In industrialized societies, however, the primary causes of death are chronic diseases, and overnutrition is a risk factor. The excessive consumption of sugar is linked to tooth decay. Also, overnutrition in terms of too much fat and Calories in the diet leads to obesity, high blood pressure, stroke, heart disease, some cancers, liver disease, and one type of diabetes.

Historically, the focus of malnutrition studies was deficiencies in the diet. In the 1930's, classic kwashiorkor was described by Cicely Williams. Not until after World War II was it known that kwashiorkor was caused by a lack of protein in the diet. In 1959, Derrick B. Jelliffe introduced the term "protein-calorie malnutrition" to describe the nutritional disorders of marasmus, marasmic kwashiorkor, and kwashiorkor.

PEM remains the most important public health problem in developing countries. Few cases are seen in Western societies. Historically, the root causes have been urbanization, periods of famine, and the failure to breast-feed or early cessation of breast-feeding. Marasmus is prevalent in urban areas among infants under one year old, while kwashiorkor is prevalent in rural areas during the second year of life.

Deficiencies of specific nutrients have been documented throughout history. Vitamin A deficiency and its cure were documented by Egyptians and Chinese around 1500 B.C.E. In occupied Denmark during World War I, vitamin A deficiency, caused by dairy product deprivation, was common in Danish children. Beriberi, first documented in Asia, was caused by diets of polished rice that were deficient in thiamine. Pellagra was seen in epidemic proportions in the southern United States, where corn was the staple grain, during World War I.

Zinc deficiency was first reported in the 1960's. The growth and maturation of boys in the Middle East were studied. Their diets were low in zinc and high in substances that prevented zinc absorption. Consequently, the World Health Organization recommended increased zinc intake for populations whose staple is unleavened whole grain bread. Goiter was documented during Julius Caesar's reign. Simply adding iodine to salt has virtually eliminated goiter in the United States.

If classic malnutrition is observed in industrialized societies, it usually is secondary to other diseases, such as AIDS and cancer. Hunger and poverty are problems that contribute to malnutrition; however, the malnutrition that results is less severe than that found in developing countries.

Specific nutrients may be lacking in the diets of the poor. Iron-deficiency anemia is prevalent among the poor, and this anemia may impair learning ability. Other deficiencies may be subclinical, which means that no detectable signs are observed, yet normal nutrient pools in the body are depleted. Homelessness, poverty, and drug or alcohol abuse are the major contributing factors to these conditions. In addition, malnutrition as a result of poverty is exacerbated by lack of nutritional knowledge and/or poor food choices.

—Wendy L. Stuhldreher, Ph.D., R.D.

See also Anemia; Anorexia nervosa; Appetite loss; Bariatric surgery; Beriberi; Breast-feeding; Bulimia; Carbohydrates; Celiac sprue; Cholesterol; Congenital hypothyroidism; Eating disorders; Failure to thrive; Food biochemistry; Fructosemia; Galactosemia; Gluten intolerance; Goiter; Growth; Hirschsprung's disease; Hypercholesterolemia; Hyperlipidemia; Kwashiorkor; Lactose intolerance; Lead poisoning; Macronutrients; Malabsorption; Metabolism; Nutrition; Osteoporosis; Protein; Scurvy; Supplements; Thyroid disorders; Vitamins and minerals; Weaning; Weight loss and gain; Weight loss medications.

FOR FURTHER INFORMATION:

Barasi, Mary E. *Human Nutrition: A Health Perspective.* 2d ed. New York: Oxford University Press, 2003. A text that emphasizes basic nutrition information and the application of this information to health maintenance and disease prevention.

Christian, Janet L., and Janet L. Greger. *Nutrition for Living.* 4th ed. Redwood City, Calif.: Benjamin/ Cummings, 1994. This introductory textbook of nutrition is easy to understand. It provides brief explanations of various vitamin and mineral deficiencies, as well as of PEM. Photographs showing symptoms are included.

Garrow, J. S., W. P. T. James, and A. Ralph, eds. *Human Nutrition and Dietetics.* 10th ed. New York: Churchill Livingstone, 2000. Several chapters in this book provide information on malnutrition, from PEM to specific nutrient deficiencies. History, causes, symptoms, and treatments of the disorders are covered. Includes an excellent list of references.

Kreutler, Patricia A., and Dorice M. Czajka-Narins. *Nutrition in Perspective.* 2d ed. Englewood Cliffs, N.J.: Prentice Hall, 1987. This textbook provides a chapter on the food supply, including issues for meeting the problem of undernutrition. It also de-

scribes the deficiency diseases for vitamins and minerals and PEM in various chapters.

Wardlaw, Gordon M., and Anne M. Smith. *Contemporary Nutrition.* 7th ed. New York: McGraw-Hill, 2008. One chapter of this text covers undernutrition and emphasizes the types of undernutrition and hunger found in the United States.

Whitney, Ellie, and Sharon Rady Rolfes. *Understanding Nutrition.* 12th ed. Belmont, Calif.: Wadsworth, 2009. This is an introductory nutrition textbook. Various chapters have information about the different nutrient deficiencies and malnutrition.

MALPRACTICE
ETHICS

DEFINITION: The failure to care for patients in accordance with professional standards, for which injured patients are allowed to sue for compensation.

KEY TERMS:

damages: compensation awarded to a plaintiff for an injury incurred because of a defendant's action or lack of action

defendant: a person or corporation alleged in a lawsuit to have committed a wrong

liability: responsibility for a wrongdoing

plaintiff: a person or corporation that brings legal action against another person or corporation

tort: an action or the result of an action that is defined by law to be a wrong or injury

CONTROVERSIES SURROUNDING MALPRACTICE LITIGATION

In the United States, few medical topics arouse more anger in physicians, more debate in state legislatures, or more confusion in the public than malpractice. In part, the media encourages this attention when it reports multimillion-dollar jury awards for damages, sensational stories that often make all the parties involved—lawyers, the defendant doctor, the plaintiff patient, and juries—look somehow reprehensible. In part, the rise in malpractice insurance, which has contributed to the increasing cost of medical care, has upset both doctors and the public. Yet inflation and the rare spectacular settlement obscure the value of a system that since the late eighteenth century has given patients legal redress for injury, has helped maintain professional standards of medical care, and has allowed state governments some control over the local health care industry.

As the word's elements imply, "malpractice" simply

means the poor execution of duties. The definition bears close examination, however, on one key feature: what "poor" entails. The first recourse of a patient who feels inadequately cared for is to discuss the complaint with the doctor (or dentist, chiropractor, or other health care provider). This measure clears up many complaints, since most are based on simple misunderstandings. A patient receiving no satisfaction from the doctor may file a complaint with the state board of medical examiners, which is each state's official government body, staffed by doctors, that issues medical licenses and disciplines physicians and surgeons. In both cases, the doctor or a panel of peers will decide if the patient's complaint meets the professional standards of "poor." A patient who is not pleased with this decision may bring suit in civil court. No patient, however, can press a lawsuit for malpractice simply because he or she feels wronged. For legal action to have any chance of succeeding, the doctor must have injured the patient because of negligent care. Even then, lawyers for the patient must rely on expert testimony from other doctors to establish that the physician gave the patient poor care. All official avenues of redress therefore depend on the medical profession's own standards.

Four basic standards guide doctors in ethically performing their professional duties, and failure in any one of them may constitute malpractice. First, doctors must inform their patients about treatments for an ailment and receive their explicit consent. The patient must understand the doctor's plan of treatment and any procedure's potential risks and benefits; if a patient cannot understand because of age or mental condition, a guardian must consent, except in some emergency situations. The consent may be verbal unless an invasive technique, such as surgery, is involved, in which case the law requires a signed consent form. Without the patient's consent, a physician performing a medical procedure not only may be subject to a malpractice lawsuit but also can be charged with assault under criminal law. Second, a doctor must treat a patient with reasonable skill, as defined by accepted medical practice. This point is crucial. Doctors do not have to render the best aid possible, or even the best aid of which they are capable; they must only meet professional guidelines for any specific diagnostic, palliative, or corrective measure. Both the key terms in this standard—"reasonable" and "accepted medical practice"—have been notoriously hard to define in court because they vary from region to region and from school of medicine to school of medicine. Rural physicians, for example, cannot be

expected to give the level of care available in cities, since cities have more specialists available and support technology; nor are general practitioners expected to have the skill of a specialist, such as a cardiologist. Third, physicians are responsible for what other health care workers under their charge do to patients. If other doctors (such as medical residents), nurses, physical therapists, or medical technicians act on a doctor's orders, that doctor is ultimately responsible for supervising their performance. Fourth, a doctor accepting responsibility for a patient enters a contractual obligation and may not abandon that obligation without either finding another physician to take his or her place or notifying the patient well in advance so the patient can engage another doctor. At the same time, however, the patient's obligation is to follow the doctor's medical advice.

Doctors are not the only health care workers who can be charged with malpractice. If other medical personnel act as a team with a doctor or surgeon, they may also be held liable. For example, during surgery a surgeon is assisted by an anesthesiologist and various nurses, any of whom may separately fail in his or her duties and be sued as a result. Thus, whenever a patient suffers at the hands of a medical team, the trend has been to sue each member. Furthermore, if the facilities or personnel employed by a hospital prove substandard, the hospital itself may be liable.

Tort liability and contractual responsibility govern the legal treatment of malpractice, both of which fall under civil law. (This classification assumes that doctors inadvertently cause harm; if they intentionally injure a patient, they are subject to charges under criminal law.) A patient may sue for breach of contract if his or her doctor has broken that contract—usually by abandoning the patient without proper notice. This sort of lawsuit is by far the least common. Tort liability means that the doctor is responsible for any injury (tort) caused to the patient through negligence. The patient may seek compensation for a tort by suing the doctor for damages. The presumption is that money, which is almost always the form of compensation sought, can make up for the harm done. Damages can be awarded for two types of injury. Concrete physical injury is the most typical, and damages may include money to cover medical bills, lost wages, convalescent care, and other expenses relating directly to the disability. A jury may also grant damages for pain and suffering, a difficult type of injury on which to place a price; such damages account for some of the largest monetary awards.

Because damages may amount to millions of dollars, most doctors who lose a malpractice suit cannot hope to pay them without help. Insurance provides that help, which usually takes one of three forms. First, for monthly payments (premiums), traditional insurance companies offer policies to doctors that will guarantee money up to a certain amount to pay damages. Also, if its client is sued, the insurance company assigns attorneys who handle the legal negotiations and the defense in court. Second, hospitals or other large organizations may pay for malpractice damages from a pool of money reserved for that purpose alone. Third, doctors and other health care providers may set up an insurance company of their own for mutual coverage, often called "bedpan mutuals."

Malpractice litigation in the United States is a ponderous, expensive business. In the mid-1970's, malpractice insurance prices began to rise sharply; between 1983 and 1985 alone, the cost increased 100 percent. Malpractice premiums remained relatively flat during the 1990's. By the end of the decade, however, physicians began to be hit with unexpectedly large increases. In 2001, eight states saw two or more liability insurers raise rates by at least 30 percent, according to the American Medical Association, and doctors in more than a dozen states saw one or more insurers charge at least 25 percent more for medical malpractice insurance. The George W. Bush presidential administration released a report in 2002 that found the price of malpractice insurance for certain high-risk specialists increased about 10 percent in 2001 alone and was expected to rise another 20 percent between 2002 and 2003. From 1996 to 1999, jury awards for medical malpractice claims jumped 76 percent, according to Jury Verdict Research. Doctors pass on some or all of these costs to patients by charging higher fees. If a patient sues, however, the insurance cannot cover every type of loss. The amount of time that a doctor must spend with lawyers, the time in court, and the overall distraction from practicing mean reduced earnings. Yet the cost is not only to the doctor. The plaintiff pays attorneys by contingency fee, which means that the attorney receives a percentage (usually 20 to 30 percent) of money from any settlement. A patient losing a suit does not pay the attorney but still must pay court costs and expenses, which can quickly amount to thousands of dollars. Finally, when suits reach court, public funds contribute to the court's expenses, and those expenses climb if a decision is appealed or retried, as is sometimes the case.

Patients and doctors alike complain that soaring malpractice litigation in the United States since 1960 has been destructive, introducing suspicion into the doctor-patient relationship. In addition to its emotional impact, the suspicion concretely affects medical practice, most medical economists claim. Because physicians fear lawsuits, they perform more diagnostic tests than are called for by medical protocols. Often the chances are remote that these tests will reveal any useful information, yet doctors order them to show that they have done everything possible for the patient if they are sued. The extra tests cost money, which either the patient or the insurance company must pay. In either case, the expenditures inflate the cost of medicine. The practice of such "defensive medicine" has also led some doctors to refuse to perform high-risk procedures except in hospitals that have extensive facilities. Obstetricians provide a signal case in point. Fearing lawsuits for any complications that may arise, many obstetricians will not deliver babies at home or in small hospitals, forcing rural patients to rush long distances to the nearest big-city hospital for delivery.

One scholar of the malpractice system has remarked that it seems designed to protect the interests of everyone except the person who most needs help: the injured patient. While this is surely a rhetorical exaggeration, all studies have found that only a fraction of injuries are ever compensated. Moreover, the system, based on adversarial disputation, seems hostile and dauntingly complex to both patient and physician. Yet, although no one thinks it perfect, the system evolved in accordance with two widely held American attitudes toward regulation in general: It limits abuses, and it preserves professional autonomy.

TRIAL PROCEDURES IN MALPRACTICE CASES

Few malpractice claims actually end in jury awards for damages. Only about 10 percent of patients injured by doctors file lawsuits, of which about 20 percent end in payment to the plaintiff. Overwhelmingly the payments come from out-of-court settlements that win the plaintiff only a part of the money sought in the suit. Taking a suit all the way to a jury settlement is risky for plaintiffs; they win only about two in ten cases.

From the outset, then, the chances are against the injured patient, and for this reason malpractice litigation is not popular among lawyers. To have a reasonable chance to win a case in court, or at least to force the doctor's insurance company to offer a settlement out of court, the lawyer must first be sure that a causal connection can be made between the patient's injury and physician negligence. In other words, patients cannot sue simply on the hope of winning damages; courts try to reject such "frivolous" suits before they come to trial.

A lawyer believing that a reasonable causal link can be established will write up a summons and complaint on the client's behalf and send them to the doctor. The summons warns the doctor that the patient is filing a lawsuit. The complaint explains the patient's allegation of harm and the amount of damages that the patient demands in compensation. The doctor must answer in a specific time—about a month in most states—and the answer, issued through the doctor's lawyers or those of his or her insurance company, almost always denies responsibility for any injury. The legal battle is then joined.

During a pretrial period known as discovery, each side investigates the other, hoping to find facts that will support arguments in court. Lawyers rely on three investigative methods. The first is documentary disclosure. The plaintiff's lawyer will demand records, especially the patient's medical record, and the doctor must furnish them in a reasonable time. In the second method, written interrogatories, the plaintiff's lawyer sends the doctor a list of questions that must be answered in writing. Third is the deposition, a formal legal proceeding. Lawyers from both sides meet and together question, in separate sessions, the defendant, plaintiff, and key witnesses, all of whom answer the questions under oath, so that they are guilty of perjury if they lie. Many suits are dropped during discovery, with or without monetary settlement. If the suit continues but one side has little evidence on which to base arguments, the other side will probably file a motion for summary judgment, which essentially asks a judge to end the litigation by disqualifying the weak case. Discovery and pretrial motions may take years to complete.

Trials follow a pattern, with some variations, designed to allow each side to present claims and counterclaims systematically. A trial starts with opening statements in which the lawyers describe the general plan for their cases; no actual arguments are made. Next, to clarify matters for the jury, the judge may summarize the applicable legal principles for the case. Then witnesses are called and questioned, first by the plaintiff's lawyer. After he or she finishes with each witness, the defendant's lawyer may also ask questions, a procedure called cross-examination. When the plaintiff's side is done calling witnesses, then the defense lawyer calls and questions more, which the lawyer for the plaintiff may also cross-examine.

During the questioning, two types of evidence are admitted: testimony, the oral or written statements of what people have seen or heard, and "real" or "demonstrative" evidence, physical objects such as an X ray or a needle that have a bearing on the case. The testimony is crucial for the plaintiff, because at this point an expert witness must swear that the defendant was negligent to a "medical certainty" by failing to adhere to one or more medical standards of practice. Since only a doctor is qualified to make this judgment, expert witnesses are always physicians. Finally, the lawyers make closing statements, each insisting that the evidence supports the position of his or her client, and the jury retires to decide on a verdict. If the jurors decide in favor of the plaintiff, they can also lower or raise the amount of requested damages. If they decide for the defendant, the doctor, then the case ends without a monetary settlement. A victorious plaintiff cannot expect immediate payment. Appeals to higher courts may last years, and the appellate courts, after examining the trial records, can reverse a verdict, change the amount of damages, or order a new trial.

Even if a trial does get under way, however, it may not end in a verdict. At any point in the proceedings, one side or the other may give up. Insurance companies regularly send observers to malpractice trials who assess the progress of arguments objectively. An observer detecting a weakness in the defense or noticing that the jury favors the plaintiff for any reason will offer a settlement to the plaintiff's lawyer, because such a settlement will save court costs and probably involve less money than a jury award for damages. Likewise, the plaintiff's lawyer, recognizing that the chances of winning are slim, may try to make a deal with the insurance company. Such dickering may even continue after a verdict is announced, if it is appealed. Also, at any point in the trial the judge may end the case if he or she thinks that one side cannot possibly win; similarly, the judge may reverse a verdict or change the amount of damages if the jury's decision shocks his or her professional conscience.

PERSPECTIVE AND PROSPECTS

By the mid-1970's, the entire American health care system, in the view of most health care observers, was in a state of crisis. Costs had risen, and facilities, especially in urban areas, were strained, while rural areas were often underserved. Critics have blamed the problems on increasingly costly technology and drugs, government regulation, professional salaries, and inadequate preventive medicine. Few doubt that malpractice litigation has contributed significantly as well.

Estimates in 1993 claimed that defensive medicine alone had increased the annual cost of American health care from $10 billion to $36 billion. Combined with increasing fees for medical services and other costs, defensive medicine has helped drive up the cost of medical insurance. Because of these financing problems, legislatures around the country have tried to control the increasing numbers of malpractice suits with tort reform, arbitration or review panels, and legal fee limits. In 2002, lawmakers in Ohio and other states began attempting to drive down premiums by passing laws that limit the jury awards injured patients can be given for pain and suffering. The Bush administration also supported a nationwide limit of $250,000 on these damages, although questions remain about how well the caps work.

Tort reforms include a number of measures that modify the procedures or awards of malpractice litigation. Two reforms are designed to shorten the process. One method is to reduce the statute of limitations for malpractice claims—the period after injury when a lawsuit can be started. The second involves limiting the rules governing the discovery phase of pretrial action. Two further reforms restrict the amount of damages. The most popular of these is to impose maximum amounts for types of injury, especially pain and suffering. In the second reform, jury damages must be reduced by the amount of money from other sources, such as health insurance, that a patient receives for the injury.

Several states have instituted review panels or required arbitration before a suit can proceed to court. Laypeople and judges, as well as doctors, make up the review panels, which try to identify and disallow frivolous suits. Arbitration panels actually decide on the amount of damages, if any, to be made, and their decisions cannot be appealed.

These reforms have only slowed the rate of lawsuits and the rise in the amount of money spent on paying damages and fees. Whatever its defects, the tort system has succeeded in making doctors wary of negligence. Critics insist, however, that the system for addressing malpractice has punished all physicians, not simply the incompetent, and has contributed to the increasingly litigious tenor of American society.

—Roger Smith, Ph.D.;
updated by Martha Oehmke Loustaunau, Ph.D.

See also American Medical Association (AMA); Autopsy; Critical care; Critical care, pediatric; Emergency medicine; Ethics; Euthanasia; Forensic pathology; Health care reform; Health maintenance organizations (HMOs); Hippocratic oath; Hospitals; Iatrogenic disorders; Law and medicine; Living will; Managed care; Obstetrics; Pathology; Resuscitation.

FOR FURTHER INFORMATION:

Furrow, Barry R., et al. *Health Law: Cases, Materials and Problems*. 6th ed. St. Paul, Minn.: Thomson/West, 2008. Covers a range of issues related to health and the law, including cost control, prospective payment, health care antitrust, and federal and state regulation of health care delivery; legal and ethical issues created by reproductive technology and by the dilemmas of death and dying; and the core topics of professional liability and the physician-patient relationship.

Groopman, Jerome E. *Second Opinions: Stories of Intuition and Choice in the Changing World of Medicine*. New York: Viking, 2000. Among other examples, Groopman describes the case of a woman with leukemia wrongly diagnosed as having asthma, a patient with melanoma who became the object of professional infighting about the availability and advisability of interferon treatment, and a young physicist told that he had fewer than six months to live and the ensuing tussle between specialists about the usefulness of bone marrow transplant.

Jonsen, Albert R., Mark Siegler, and William J. Winslade. *Clinical Ethics: A Practical Approach to Ethical Decisions in Clinical Medicine*. 6th ed. New York: McGraw-Hill, 2006. Discusses the whole range of medical ethics, including legal issues, confidentiality, care of the dying patient, and euthanasia and assisted suicide.

Merry, Alan, and Alexander McCall Smith. *Errors, Medicine, and the Law*. New York: Cambridge University Press, 2003. Argues that many medical accidents are linked to the complexity of modern health care and calls for a more informed alternative to the "blaming culture" in medicine.

Pence, Gregory. *Classic Cases in Medical Ethics: Accounts of Cases That Have Shaped Medical Ethics, with Philosophical, Legal, and Historical Backgrounds*. 4th ed. New York: McGraw-Hill, 2004. Surveys important cases that have defined and shaped the field of medical ethics. Each case is accompanied by careful discussion of pertinent philosophical theories and legal and ethical issues.

Sage, William M., and Rogan Kersh, eds. *Medical Malpractice and the U.S. Health Care System*. New York: Cambridge University Press, 2006. Examines medical liability with regard to American health policy. Offers ideas for reform in the areas of patient safety, liability insurance, and tort litigation.

Sharpe, Virginia F., and Alan I. Faden. *Medical Harm: Historical, Conceptual, and Ethical Dimensions of Iatrogenic Illness*. New York: Cambridge University Press, 1998. Of the many seekers after a healthier life or of relief from suffering who rightfully expect benefit from the health care system, some are more harmed than helped. This book deals mostly with harmful medical events which happen in hospitals.

Zobel, Hiller B., and Stephen N. Rous. *Doctors and the Law: Defendants and Expert Witnesses*. New York: W. W. Norton, 1993. Zobel, a judge, and Rous, a physician, give advice to physicians on how best to endure a malpractice suit. The step-by-step account of the legal proceedings, evidential requirements, and possible psychological effects on the physician make insightful reading for nonphysicians as well.

MAMMOGRAPHY

PROCEDURE

ANATOMY OR SYSTEM AFFECTED: Breasts

SPECIALTIES AND RELATED FIELDS: Gynecology, oncology, preventive medicine, radiology

DEFINITION: The use of X rays of the female breast, primarily in the detection and diagnosis of malignant breast tumors.

INDICATIONS AND PROCEDURES

X-ray mammography is a complicated procedure. The quality of the mammographic image is proportionately dependent upon the imaging equipment in use and the way in which it is utilized.

Critical factors include compression of the breast, positioning of the breast, the use of the right image receptor, and exposure of the X-ray tube. Improper use of equipment and procedures contributes to an image that is suboptimal. With proper care and thorough knowledge in the use of instruments designed for mammography, however, excellent image quality can be obtained.

In mammography, four physical constraints must be considered when evaluating the performance of the systems. First, contrast is of utmost importance because minute differences in soft tissue density are essential. Second, resolution is important because of the need to identify microcalcifications as small as 100 micrometers, which are often associated with abnormalities. Third, an adequate X-ray dose is vital to obtain an image with the proper signal-to-noise ratio. Too much radiation, however, means added risk for the patient. Fourth, a decrease in noise (background) is important to achieve an image with an adequate signal-to-noise ratio for proper diagnosis.

The examination can be conducted with the patient standing or sitting. To achieve the desired radiographic projection, the X-ray tube is set at an optimal angle. The mammography unit has a support plate onto which the breast is positioned. A plastic paddle assists in compressing the breast onto this plate. The pressure applied to achieve proper compression can be applied manually, but most mammography technicians prefer power-assisted compression, as this permits the radiographer to use both hands to position the breast properly. The shape, rigidity, and composition of the compression or support plate are crucial factors. The support plate is composed of a carbon-fiber composite capable of a high X-ray transmission. The support is in front of the tunnel, and the tunnel receives the image receptor. The standard image receptor uses a high-resolution mammographic screen-film combination. With receptor technology advancing rapidly, however, digital receptors are fast becoming available. The big advantage of digital receptors is that they offer either a limited field of view for stereotactical localization or a full field of view for standard mammographic imaging.

Since all mammography units are intended to show the soft tissue of the breast while displaying differences in contrast and since proper compression is vital, the natural mobility of the breast should be considered. The breast is easiest to compress from the inferior and lateral aspects. The preliminary automatic compression between the paddle and the support plate should never go beyond 45 pounds of pressure, and the patient should not be in pain. Nevertheless, the breast must be taut to the touch.

Improper compression can lead to erroneous results. The outcome of proper compression is a reduction of X-ray radiation to the breast by reducing tissue thickness; the bringing of lesions closer to the film, thus facilitating an accurate reading; a reduction in movement blurriness because the breast is held immobile; increased contrast as a result of flattened breasts, thereby decreasing thickness; elimination of confusion caused by superimposition shadows; and easier visualization of the borders of circumscribed lesions.

It is helpful if magnification of the image is possible, particularly if small areas are being examined. Magnification is of greater importance in areas of suspicious microcalcifications or at surgical sites. Unfortunately, the greater the magnification, the higher the patient's radiation dose because the breast is placed much closer to the source of radiation.

In addition to compression, image quality depends on a number of factors: positioning, radiation exposure, contrast, sharpness, noise, artifacts, and labeling. The craniocaudal position (compression of the breast from top to bottom) and the mediolateral oblique position (compression of the breast from side to side) are the two standard positions employed in mammography. Each position provides specific views, and proper positioning reveals as much of the tissue as possible for diagnosis. Any area that is omitted will create false results that may endanger the patient's life. Adequate exposure to radiation is essential. If this is not acheived, then it is difficult to identify the skin and subcutaneous tissue. Usually, contrast is highest for thinner breasts and lowest for thicker breasts; this is primarily the result of more scattered radiation and greater tissue absorption of low radiation in thicker breasts. Without contrast, particularly in thicker breast tissue, different tissue densities will have very similar appearances.

Sharpness, or the visualization of fine details in the image, is one of the central factors in achieving a correct diagnosis. If the desired sharpness is not obtained, then the image is referred to as unsharp. Unsharpness may be the result of motion blur, poor screen-film contrast, or other technical factors. Noise and sharpness are closely linked. Noise is defined as increased background and a decreased ability to see tiny structures, such as calcifications. The major contributors of noise are scatter and quantum mottle, which is fluctuation in the number of X-ray photons needed to form the image. Examples of artifacts are scratches, fingerprints, dirt, lint, and dust. Standardized labeling in mammography to identify the left side from the right side, so that the films cannot be subject to misinterpretation, is vital, especially because mammograms can be legal documents.

A slightly different approach is used to screen women with breast implants. Two craniocaudal views are obtained, one with the implant in the field of view and one with the implant as much out of the field as pos-

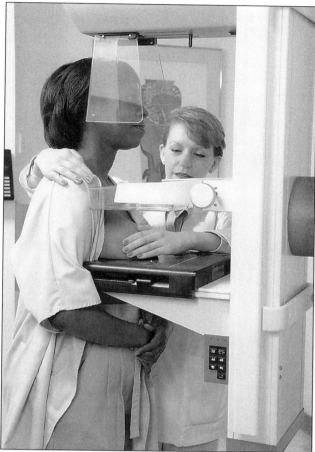

A woman receives a mammogram. It is recommended that regular screenings take place beginning in middle age. (PhotoDisc)

sible. In a similar way, two mediolateral oblique views are imaged.

Digital mammography differs from regular mammography in that in the former, electronic detectors capture and facilitate the display of the X-ray signals on a computer or laser-printed film. In all other aspects, it is still the same procedure—proper positioning and compression of the breast are still critical for obtaining quality digital images. The goal of digital mammography also remains the same, to detect and localize breast abnormalities.

As exposure to radiation is a major concern with traditional mammography, the primary force to developing digital X-ray mammography is the idea that it has the potential to enhance image quality, and therefore lesion detection (especially for dense breasts), with a lower dose of radiation. The greatest advantage in digital mammography is its ability to separate image acquisition from image display, thus providing the ability to manipulate contrast, brightness, and magnification with one exposure.

Dynamic or real-time imaging, especially with biopsies, is possible with digital mammography, providing a better understanding of breast tumors with regard to localization and boundaries. This procedure can also facilitate the direct use of computers for detection and diagnosis. In addition, with this technology it is possible to form three-dimensional images by combining images from all angles. The ease of digital image archiving, retrieval, and transmission is another advantage.

Uses and Complications

There are two basic types of mammographic examinations: screening mammography and diagnostic mammography. Screening mammography refers to examinations of women with no obvious symptoms to detect breast cancers. A standard screening examination includes two views of each breast, sometimes referred to as the standard views.

General agreement has been reached that screening mammography reduces mortality from breast cancer in women fifty years of age or older, but an ongoing debate exists over the effectiveness of screening mammography in women aged forty to forty-nine. Randomized clinical trials have confirmed the validity of screening mammography. Deaths attributable to breast cancer have been reduced. The American Cancer Society and most other well-known professional societies have continued to recommend mammography screening for women in the younger age group because of the results of several studies that advocate the benefits of screening in this age group. For example, a fourteen-year follow-up to the Edinburgh trial has shown a mortality reduction of 21 percent for women aged forty-five to forty-nine who were screened with mammography. A sixteen-year follow-up to the UK Trial of Early Detection of Breast Cancer revealed a 27 percent decrease in mortality in women who were screened with mammography, and no evidence was found that women aged forty-five to forty-six at the start of screening received less benefit than did older women. Breast self-examination alone does not bring down the rate of mortality.

A negative result produced by screening mammography would not include straight lines, unless there is a history of surgery or trauma, and would not show bulging contours from tissue into fatty areas. Charac-

teristics in a screening view that suggest the need for follow-up diagnostic screening are masses, microcalcifications, architectural distortion, and parenchymal asymmetry. Palpable abnormalities described by the patient, focal tenderness, and spontaneous nipple discharge also warrant diagnostic screening.

As with all preventive measures, screening mammography cannot eliminate all deaths from breast cancer, for several reasons. It does not detect all types of cancers, including some that are actually detected by physical examination. Also some tumors may appear and develop too quickly to be detected and identified at an early, more curable stage. Mammograms are particularly difficult to interpret for women with dense breast tissue, which is especially common in young women. The dense tissue prevents the identification of abnormalities associated with tumors, thereby leading to a higher rate of false-positive and false-negative test results.

Diagnostic mammography, also referred to as consultative or problem-solving mammography, is the type of study preferred when there are clinical findings, such as a palpable lump or an abnormal screening mammogram requiring additional analysis. Additionally, each diagnostic mammography examination is performed to suit the individual patient who has symptoms or abnormal findings. Diagnostic mammography may warrant additional views of the breast, such as spot compression and magnification, a correlative clinical examination, and ultrasonography. In almost all instances, barring a few exceptions, a radiologist is present during the performance of a diagnostic mammography study.

Diagnostic mammography should be carried out when a biopsy is being considered for a palpable lump in a woman over thirty years of age. The reason for doing a mammogram preceding a biopsy is to define the nature of the clinical abnormality better and to find other unexpected lesions.

Mammographic characteristics of possible benign lesions are a cluster of small round or oval calcifications; nonpalpable, noncalcified, and solid round or oval, and predominantly well-circumscribed, masses; nonpalpable focal symmetry with concave margins and interspersed fat; asymptomatic single dilated duct (no nipple discharge); and multiple (three or more) similar findings, distributed randomly and often bilaterally. Mammographic characteristics of malignant lesions are a mass with no history of previous surgery, trauma, or mastitis that is ill-defined and microtubulated; malignant-type microcalcifications; skin thickening and retraction; nipple retraction; and architectural distortion with no history of previous surgery or trauma.

The ruling concern in mammography is the amount of radiation to which the patient is exposed. Therefore, an automatic radiation exposure control device is necessary to avoid overexposure. The radiation detector is placed behind the image receptor so that its image does not appear on the mammogram. Exposure is terminated when the signal recorded by the monitor reaches a predefined level. Unfortunately, the X-ray photons reaching the detector fluctuate considerably depending on the size and composition of the breast. As a result, the signal recorded by the detector is only an approximate indication of the energy absorbed. Therefore, it is unlikely that an accurate reading will be available.

In any therapeutic model that is considered a source of risk to the patient, it is essential to bear in mind the number of deaths caused by the technique as opposed to the number of deaths that it actually prevents. Fortunately, the benefits of mammography supersede the risk of radiation exposure. Furthermore, risk estimates have decreased following the adoption of a relative risk model and allowance for the variation of risk with age at exposure.

PERSPECTIVE AND PROSPECTS

Though much progress has been made in the field of cancer medicine, early detection is the best approach in the war against breast cancer. Ample clinical data have shown that women diagnosed with breast cancers in the early stages are more likely to survive than those diagnosed with more advanced stages of the same disease. A systematic physical breast examination by a clinician once a year and breast self-examination once a month can help in identifying tumors that are fairly small and that can go unnoticed in the absence of such examinations.

Nearly all medical experts agree that in women over fifty, routine X-ray mammography, with or without clinical examination, has been valuable in detecting tumors and at earlier stages. This has been very effectively shown in randomized clinical trials to reduce disease-specific mortality. In the United States, women undergo screening mammography as part of their routine health maintenance, and mammography is considered to be a necessary procedure in the annual physicals of women over fifty. Subsequently, routine, annual mammographic screening has been actively promoted in many countries and nongovernmental agencies.

Breast imaging technologies that are being developed are progressing with three distinct goals in mind: to identify the most minute tumor lesions; to localize abnormalities to aid further examination, analysis, or treatment; and to characterize the abnormalities and assist in the decision-making process following identification. Radiologists and patients alike dream of an ideal imaging modality that would achieve all three goals in a single use. In reality, most current technologies fail to do so; hence, many developers are intent on perfecting one goal at a time. In addition to these technical goals, developers hope to generate methods that are more practical, inexpensive, harmless, and appealing to the patient.

—Giri Sulur, Ph.D.

See also Breast biopsy; Breast cancer; Breast disorders; Breast surgery; Breasts, female; Cancer; Cyst removal; Cysts; Glands; Gynecology; Imaging and radiology; Mastectomy and lumpectomy; Mastitis; Noninvasive tests; Oncology; Pathology; Screening; Tumor removal; Tumors; Women's health.

FOR FURTHER INFORMATION:

Bassett, Lawrence W., et al. *Film-Screen Mammography: An Atlas of Instructional Cases.* New York: Raven Press, 1991. This teaching atlas is an anthology of high-quality mammograms with a wide variety of pathologically proved cases.

Gamagami, Parvis. *Atlas of Mammography: New Early Signs in Breast Cancer.* Cambridge, Mass.: Blackwell Science, 1996. Provides many examples of images that will help laypeople understand a mammogram.

Kopans, Daniel B. *Breast Imaging.* 3d ed. Baltimore: Lippincott Williams & Wilkins, 2007. Well written and comprehensive. An important reference in the field.

Love, Susan, and Karen Lindsey. *Dr. Susan Love's Breast Book.* Rev. 4th ed. Cambridge, Mass.: Da Capo Press, 2005. One of the most influential books in women's health written for a general audience. Details breast development, changes with age, and breast cancer detection and treatment.

Mitchell, George W., Jr., and Lawrence W. Bassett, eds. *The Female Breast and Its Disorders.* Baltimore: Williams & Wilkins, 1990. A comprehensive text offers the expertise of representatives from obstetrics and gynecology, diagnostic radiology, pathology, surgery, medicine, therapeutic radiology, and psychiatry.

Sutton, Amy L., ed. *Cancer Sourcebook for Women: Basic Consumer Health Information About Leading Causes of Cancer in Women.* 3d ed. Detroit, Mich.: Omnigraphics, 2006. An excellent overview of female cancers, including screening.

MANAGED CARE

HEALTH CARE SYSTEM

SPECIALTIES AND RELATED FIELDS: Organizations and programs, public health

DEFINITION: A health insurance system that oversees or manages the access, quality, and cost of medical care of its participants.

STRUCTURE AND SUBTYPES

Managed care organizations are health insurance plans that aim to provide efficient, quality health care by management of services. The main goals of managed care organizations include providing quality of health care services and providing the services at the best cost to the insurance company. These goals are met by direct oversight over an individual's care, such as determining medical necessity of health services and evaluating the appropriateness of specialists' referrals.

There are three general types of managed care organizations: the health maintenance organization (HMO), the preferred provider organization (PPO), and the point-of-service organization (POS). Each of these different types of insurance plans has its own distinct characteristics and carries its own advantages and disadvantages to its participants. HMOs focus on preventive medicine and place strong emphasis on the role of the primary care physician. HMOs are structured into networks of providers, or physicians and hospitals that participate in their program. Patients pay a set monthly fee and in order to be covered by the insurance company, must see only physicians within the approved network. HMOs are unique in that they serve as the insurance company (the payer) and the provider at the same time, in that the physicians, hospitals, and insurers that participate in the HMO are also employed by the organization. The primary care physician serves as a gatekeeper to other physicians in the system. Therefore, the primary care physician must approve and coordinate all contact with any medical care for his or her patients. This includes access to specialists (such as cardiologists, dermatologists, or psychiatrists) and any medical procedures. The only exception to this rule is during an emergency or crisis situation. In this way, HMOs are considered the strictest and most restricting type of managed care organization available.

One advantage of HMOs is low out-of-pocket costs for the patient. The fixed monthly fee that is charged to the patient does not depend on the amount of care given and cannot increase with increased visits. Similarly, HMOs do not have maximum lifetime payouts, unlike some other health insurance structures. Therefore, any amount of care that is deemed necessary will be provided to the patient with no maximum cap. Another advantage of an HMO plan is the focus on preventive medicine and wellness, encouraging visiting a physician regularly and healthy lifestyle choices. However, there are some disadvantages to HMO plans. These can include a limited access to specialty care in a timely manner and no coverage for physicians outside the network.

Health maintenance organizations operate in a variety of subtypes. These subtypes may overlap in style and operation. In the staff model, physicians are salaried and are direct employees of the HMO. Their offices are typically in buildings that belong exclusively to the HMO company and are operated by other physicians in the system. In this type of system, the physicians only see patients under the specific managed care of the HMO. In the group model of the HMO, the company does not employ the physicians directly; they are contracted together. Physicians practice under a group practice format, and the group practice is employed itself by the HMO. Traditionally, the group practice model physicians also only see patients who are part of the HMO program. The last subtype of HMO structure is an independent practice association (IPA), in which the association serves as an intermediate between the physician and the HMO. In this model, the physician may see his or her own patients as well as patients with the HMO plan.

The PPO, also called an "open access HMO," is managed differently than a health maintenance organization. In a PPO, the physicians and hospitals are contracted to provide services only to a specific group of individuals who participate in the PPO. The system is similar to the HMO in that the group of physicians and hospitals form a network for care, but there is no primary care physician who serves as a gatekeeper in the PPO. A patient may see a specialist without approval or management from another physician. Also, in a PPO, patients are permitted to visit a physician outside the network for an increased cost. Therefore, seeing a physician who is in the network usually has a lower out-of-pocket cost for the patient than seeing a physician out of the network. Unlike the HMO, in a PPO the patient does not pay monthly regardless of the services provided but pays out of pocket in deductibles and copays based on how many visits they incur.

One advantage of the PPO system is more freedom in choosing the provider of choice, as well as the ability to see a specialist without prior approval of a primary care physician. Also, out-of-pocket expenses, such as deductibles, are capped each year, limiting the amount a patient or family has to pay for health care services. However, a disadvantage of a PPO system is that there is limited coverage for providers who are outside the network. Also, a lot of paperwork and time may be involved in reimbursement for services out of the network.

A POS plan is a type of managed health care that integrates features of both the HMO and the PPO. These systems involve both in network (contracted) physicians and hospitals, with freedom to visit physicians outside of the network. In this type of insurance plan, similar to an HMO, there is no deductible paid by the patient and usually only a minimal copayment when a health care provider in network is used. Also, a primary care physician is chosen who makes referrals to specialists. If one chooses to go outside the network for health care, POS coverage functions more like a PPO. By using an out-of-network provider, the patient may have an annual deductible and be responsible for copays to the out-of-network physician. The advantages of the POS system include the maximum amount of freedom in choosing which physician to see and allowing the patient to control out-of-pocket costs. Out-of-network costs can be significant, however, and serve as a disadvantage to POS systems.

OPERATION AND COST CONTAINMENT

Health maintenance organizations manage their costs by restricting covered medical care to their in network providers. The participating providers, as employees of the HMO, have agreed to practice medicine in accordance with the HMO's guidelines and restrictions. These guidelines and restrictions may be incorporated into primary care physicians' decisions regarding approval for specialty care visits.

Another way that HMOs manage costs is through utilization review, a process by which the HMO monitors the physicians' practice. By comparing the physician's practices with other physicians, such as number of referrals and cost of services, the HMO can measure the most efficient practice techniques.

Another technique for cost containment in HMO systems is case management. In case management, the goal is preventive medicine before a catastrophic event can occur. The theory behind case management is that it is cheaper to prevent a disease than to treat it. Case management may also include disease management, such as management of chronic conditions to prevent them from progressing into worsening conditions.

While many professionals argue that one main goal of health maintenance organizations is to save money, many HMOs themselves argue that they do not have a significant increase in profit over their PPO or POS plans. The research supporting this theory suggests that although the out-of-pocket expense is smaller for the patient, the patient may take advantage of the unlimited use of in-network providers and visit more often than those patients who participate in other programs. Therefore, with increased utilization from some patients, the cost to the HMO rises to that of other plans.

PERSPECTIVE AND PROSPECTS

In 1929, the first health maintenance organization in the United States was organized by Michael Shadid. Shadid was a medical and business pioneer who provided medical care for rural farmers in Elk City, Oklahoma. The members who enrolled in his plan paid a predetermined fee and received medical care from Dr. Shadid. In the same year, the Ross-Loos Medical Group was established in Los Angeles to provide prepaid medical services to county employees and employees of the city's department of water and power. In 1982, the Ross-Loos Medical Group was purchased by CIGNA, and it is still in business today. The enactment of Medicare and Medicaid legislation in 1965 served as a landmark in the history of managed health care by extending coverage to millions of additional Americans who could otherwise not afford medical coverage.

The first mandated health care act by government was the Health Maintenance Organization Act of 1973, which required employers with twenty-five or more employees to offer federally certified HMO options. Dr. Gordon K. Macleod served as the first director of this program and also performed many research studies in other countries regarding health maintenance organization and structure. Today, there are more than six hundred managed care programs with more than 25 percent of the United States's population covered under their care.

—Leah M. Betman, M.S., C.G.C.

See also Allied health; Ethics; Health care reform; Health maintenance organizations (HMOs); Law and medicine; Malpractice; Medicare.

For Further Information:

Dorsey, J. L. "The Health Maintenance Organization Act of 1973 and Prepaid Group Practice Plan." *Medical Care* 13 (January, 1975): 1-9. This article gives an outline of the first mandated health care act by government in the United States. It outlines the need for such an act and the standards that employers must maintain for the health care of their employees.

Kongstvedt, P. R. *The Managed Health Care Book.* 4th ed. Aspen, Colo.: Aspen, 2001. This text gives a complete overview of managed health care. The author discusses different subtypes of managed care, cost saving techniques, oversight, legal responsibilities, and operations. This book also discusses the history of managed health care in the United States.

Longest, B. B. "Health and Health Policy." In *Health Policymaking in the United States.* 4th ed. Chicago: Health Administration Press, 2006. This chapter provides a framework for discussing health policy in its relation to different types of insurance plans in the United States, including health maintenance organizations. It discusses the history of insurance companies in the United States, as well as structure and function of health maintenance organizations and other forms of managed care.

MANIC-DEPRESSIVE DISORDER. *See* BIPOLAR DISORDERS.

MAPLE SYRUP URINE DISEASE (MSUD)
DISEASE/DISORDER

ALSO KNOWN AS: Branched-chain ketoaciduria
ANATOMY OR SYSTEM AFFECTED: Nervous system
SPECIALTIES AND RELATED FIELDS: Family medicine, genetics, neonatology, pediatrics
DEFINITION: A recessive autosomal genetic disease resulting in the absence, partial activity, or inactivity of a multisubunit enzyme responsible for metabolizing the branched-chain amino acids leucine, isoleucine, and valine.

CAUSES AND SYMPTOMS

As a result of deficient branched-chain alpha-ketoacid dehydrogenase (BCKD), the essential branched chain amino acids leucine, isoleucine, and valine are not metabolized in patients with maple syrup urine disease

---

> ### INFORMATION ON MAPLE SYRUP URINE DISEASE (MSUD)
>
> **CAUSES:** Genetic defect resulting in accumulation of amino acids leucine, isoleucine, and valine
> **SYMPTOMS:** Within three to seven days after birth, poor weight gain, high-pitched cry, irritability, lethargy, characteristic maple syrup smell of urine; if untreated, mental retardation, seizures, and death
> **DURATION:** Lifelong
> **TREATMENTS:** Diet with controlled amounts of isoleucine, leucine, and valine

(MSUD). The branched-chain amino acids and their ketoacid products accumulate in the blood and interfere with brain function. High levels of leucine are especially toxic. The classic form of the disease results in little (less than 2 percent) or no BCKD activity. Symptoms develop within three to seven days after birth and include poor weight gain, a high-pitched cry, irritability, lethargy, and a characteristic maple syrup smell to the urine. If the disease is untreated, then mental retardation, various neurological symptoms such as seizures, and even death can result.

Variant forms of the disease in which there is some (3 to 12 percent) BCKD activity result in milder symptoms. A rare variant form of the disease called thiamine-responsive MSUD responds to high doses of thiamine.

TREATMENT AND THERAPY

The treatment of severe MSUD, which should begin immediately after diagnosis, involves a special diet with controlled amounts of isoleucine, leucine, and valine to ensure metabolic control. Enfamil, a special dietary formula, provides leucine but may have to be supplemented with isoleucine and valine to provide adequate intake of all three amino acids and permit normal growth and development.

Treatment of the milder forms of MSUD also involves management through diet therapy. Diet therapy should be continued throughout life, and the levels of the branched-chain amino acids should be monitored often.

PERSPECTIVE AND PROSPECTS

MSUD was first described in 1954. The name derives from the sweet, maple syrup smell of the patient's urine. Because MSUD is caused by a recessive gene, there is a

1 in 4 chance that two heterozygous carriers will have an affected child. MSUD affects about 1 in 180,000 newborns in the United States, but in some populations, such as Mennonites, it may be as high as 1 in 176.

Some states test for the disease in their newborn screening programs. Testing should be done within the first twenty-four hours after birth, since early diagnosis is essential. Some of the milder variant forms are missed in the screening programs. The detection of alloisoleucine is diagnostic for MSUD but may not appear until the sixth day of life. Carrier testing is available for the Mennonite variant of the disease.

—*Charles L. Vigue, Ph.D.*

See also Enzyme therapy; Enzymes; Food biochemistry; Genetic counseling; Genetic diseases; Metabolic disorders; Metabolism; Neonatology; Nutrition; Screening.

FOR FURTHER INFORMATION:

Clarke, Joe T. R. *A Clinical Guide to Inherited Metabolic Diseases.* 3d ed. New York: Cambridge University Press, 2006.

Icon Health. *Maple Syrup Urine Disease: A Medical Dictionary, Bibliography, and Annotated Research Guide to Internet References.* San Diego, Calif.: Author, 2004.

Jorde, Lynn B., et al. *Medical Genetics.* 3d ed. St. Louis, Mo.: Mosby/Elsevier, 2006.

Pritchard, Dorian J., and Bruce R. Korf. *Medical Genetics at a Glance.* 2d ed. Malden, Mass.: Blackwell Science, 2008.

MARBURG VIRUS

DISEASE/DISORDER

ALSO KNOWN AS: Green monkey fever

ANATOMY OR SYSTEM AFFECTED: Immune system

SPECIALTIES AND RELATED FIELDS: Epidemiology, virology

DEFINITION: Marburg hemorrhagic fever is a rare, highly lethal disease caused by Marburg filovirus.

CAUSES AND SYMPTOMS

Marburg hemorrhagic fever is caused by a filovirus. Filoviruses are separated into two distinct types, Marburg and Ebola. All filoviruses are classified as biohazard level 4 agents based on their high mortality rate, potential transmissibility, and absence of effective vaccines or treatments. The systemic nature of filovirus infections suggest they may have immunosuppressive effects.

Human-infecting viruses usually appear as small, round, or oval organisms. Filoviruses are unique among human viruses, appearing as long, cylindrical organisms with twists and loops. The natural reservoir for filoviruses is unknown but is presumed to be wild animals (zoonotic). Research suggests that filoviruses may possibly be linked to bats, from which the viruses are occasionally introduced into primate populations. The primary transmission of Marburg filovirus from its natural reservoir appears to occur only in sub-Saharan Africa within five degrees of the equator.

Human transmission of Marburg hemorrhagic fever is by direct contact with infected blood, semen, urine, mucus, and organs. Some evidence suggests that aerosol transmission may also occur. The virus enters the body through lesions and initially infects the lymph nodes, spleen, and liver. Marburg filovirus can survive several weeks in corpses and blood samples.

The incubation period of Marburg hemorrhagic fever is three to ten days after infection, and symptoms include high fever, severe headache, painful sore throat, rashes, muscle pain (myalgia), inflamed lymph nodes, dementia, and bloody vomiting and diarrhea from internal hemorrhaging. Symptoms usually progress to bleeding from the gums and nose, puncture openings in the skin, small hemorrhages in the whites of the eyes, and eventual red blood cell immobilization. Hair, skin, and nail loss, as well as searing body pain from inflamed nerves, occur in later stages of infection. The infection may last as long as three weeks and is often described as agonizing. In fatal cases, the patient's blood pressure undergoes a final severe drop resulting in surgical shock prior to death.

TREATMENT AND THERAPY

There is no vaccine or specific therapy available for filoviral infections. Specific symptoms are treated during the course of infection; the patient either responds

---

INFORMATION ON MARBURG VIRUS

CAUSES: Infection with a filovirus

SYMPTOMS: High fever, headache, sore throat, rashes, muscle pain, inflamed lymph nodes, dementia, bloody vomiting and diarrhea, bleeding from gums and nose, small hemorrhages in eyes

DURATION: Up to three weeks, often fatal

TREATMENTS: None; alleviation of symptoms

or does not. Secondary prevention requires total isolation of infected patients. Primary infected patients show a higher mortality rate than do secondary infected patients. The mortality rate for humans infected with Marburg hemorrhagic fever ranges from 23 to 90 percent, with some outbreaks being more deadly than others.

PERSPECTIVE AND PROSPECTS

Marburg hemorrhagic fever was first described in 1967 during outbreaks at research laboratories in Marburg and Frankfurt, Germany, and Belgrade, Yugoslavia, and linked to African Green monkeys imported from Uganda. Since the initial outbreaks, sporadic cases of Marburg hemorrhagic fever have been identified in eastern and southern Africa, with the largest outbreak occurring in the Democratic Republic of the Congo in 1998. One of the most frightening aspects of Marburg hemorrhagic fever is its ongoing inclusion in some nations' biological weapons programs.

—*Randall L. Milstein, Ph.D.*

See also Bleeding; Centers for Disease Control and Prevention (CDC); Ebola virus; Epidemiology; Hemorrhage; Tropical medicine; Viral hemorrhagic fevers; Viral infections; Zoonoses.

FOR FURTHER INFORMATION:

Garrett, Laurie. *The Coming Plague: Newly Emerging Diseases in a World out of Balance.* New York: Penguin, 1995.

Klenk, Hans-Dieter, ed. *Marburg and Ebola Viruses.* New York: Springer, 1999.

Levy, Elinor, and Mark Fischetti. *The New Killer Diseases: How the Alarming Evolution of Mutant Germs Threatens Us All.* New York: Crown, 2003.

McCormick, Joseph B., Susan Fisher-Hoch, and Leslie Alan Horvitz. *Level 4: Virus Hunters of the CDC.* Rev. ed. New York: Barnes & Noble, 1999.

MARFAN SYNDROME
DISEASE/DISORDER

ANATOMY OR SYSTEM AFFECTED: Bones, eyes, heart, musculoskeletal system, spine

SPECIALTIES AND RELATED FIELDS: Cardiology, genetics, ophthalmology, orthopedics

DEFINITION: A condition in which the connective tissue does not form correctly and tends to be too flexible. The abnormal chemical composition, especially of the skeleton and heart, leads to major medical characteristics that are sometimes in evidence only at puberty.

CAUSES AND SYMPTOMS

Recent studies have located the gene that causes the inherited form of Marfan syndrome. About 25 percent of Marfan syndrome cases result from spontaneous mutation. While this knowledge promises better future recognition of the condition, the range and severity of the condition is so variable that diagnosis remains difficult.

Usually, Marfan syndrome is discovered through a detailed family history. The observation that a person is tall and slender and has unusually long fingers or arms is often an early clue. The presence of loose joints with great suppleness is characteristic of the disease. Manifestations of this condition may occur in any part of the body, but the heart, eyes, and spinal column are the most common.

TREATMENT AND THERAPY

Because a variety of organs may be involved in Marfan syndrome, it is essential that several specialists form a team to evaluate and monitor the patient during his or her lifetime. The most serious, and most common, problem area is the heart. Mitral valve problems may lead to leakage or regurgitation of blood. The aortic valve can develop a backflow into the heart.

In the eyes, a characteristic sign is the dislocation of the lens. This symptom is difficult to detect and, like many others, can vary widely in intensity. Cataracts are also associated with this condition.

Other characteristics are found in the skeleton. Spinal curvature, or scoliosis, and a breastbone that either protrudes or indents are observed. Crowded teeth and an arched palate are not uncommon.

Any of these symptoms can lead to serious consequences and should be discovered as early as possible. Regular examinations by specialists in cardiology, ophthalmology, and orthopedics are essential. Most of

---

INFORMATION ON MARFAN SYNDROME

CAUSES: Genetic mutation

SYMPTOMS: Tall and slender appearance, long fingers or arms, loose joints, heart problems, dislocation of eye lens, scoliosis, crowded teeth

DURATION: Lifelong

TREATMENTS: Dependent on severity and structures affected; may include surgery and medications

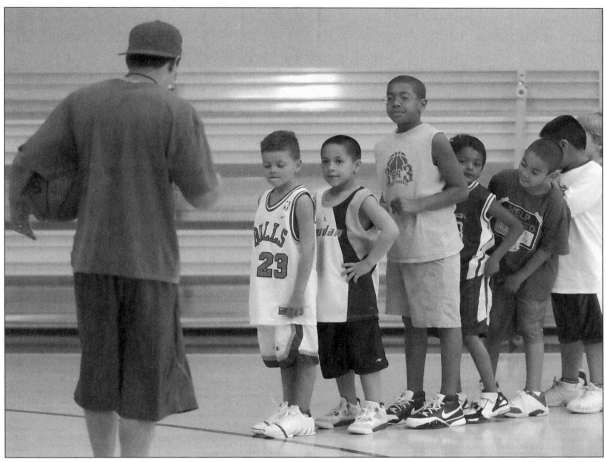

A seven-year-old (third child from left) who was born with Marfan syndrome, an inherited connective tissue disease that causes defects in the skeleton, eyes, and heart. (AP/Wide World Photos)

the possible progressive aspects of the condition can be treated effectively.

—*K. Thomas Finley, Ph.D.*

See also Bones and the skeleton; Cardiology; Cardiology, pediatric; Eye infections and disorders; Eyes; Genetic diseases; Growth; Heart; Joints; Mitral valve prolapse; Optometry; Optometry, pediatric; Orthopedics; Orthopedics, pediatric; Scoliosis; Vision disorders.

FOR FURTHER INFORMATION:

Hetzer, R., P. Gehle, and J. Ennker, eds. *Cardiovascular Aspects of Marfan Syndrome*. New York: Springer, 1995.

National Marfan Foundation. http://www.marfan.org.

Parker, James N., and Philip M. Parker, eds. *The Official Patient's Sourcebook on Marfan Syndrome*. San Diego, Calif.: Icon Health, 2002.

Pyeritz, Reed E., and Julia Conant. *Marfan Syndrome*. 5th ed. Port Washington, N.Y.: National Marfan Foundation, 2001.

Robinson, Peter N., and Maurice Godfrey, eds. *Marfan Syndrome: A Primer for Clinicians and Scientists*. New York: Kluwer Academic/Plenum, 2004.

MARIJUANA

DISEASE/DISORDER, TREATMENT

ALSO KNOWN AS: *Cannabis sativa*, hemp, various popular names (pot, ganja, weed)

ANATOMY OR SYSTEM AFFECTED: Brain, circulatory system, eyes, gastrointestinal system, heart, lungs, musculoskeletal system, nerves, nervous system, psychic-emotional system, respiratory system

SPECIALTIES AND RELATED FIELDS: Alternative medicine, ethics, neurology, pharmacology, psychiatry, psychology, public health

Definition: A plant containing a psychoactive substance with the potential for both recreational abuse and medical use.

Introduction

The term "marijuana" refers to both the illegal drug and the plant itself. The hemp plant, *Cannabis sativa*, is a fast-growing (to fifteen feet), bushy annual with finely branched leaves further divided into lance-shaped, sawtooth-edged leaflets. The species was first classified in 1735 by the Swedish botanist Carolus Linnaeus. Both male and female plants produce tetrahydrocannabinol (THC), the psychoactive ingredient in the drug. THC collects in tiny droplets of sticky resin produced by glands located at the base of fine hairs covering most of the plant's surface, with the most highly concentrated THC found in the female flower heads. When pollinated, however, the female flower heads produce highly nutritious seeds containing no THC.

Recreational and Medicinal Uses

Marijuana ranks as the third most commonly used recreational drug in the Western world, behind alcohol and tobacco. It is usually smoked, but it can be eaten or brewed as tea. Responses vary according to dosage and experience using the drug, but most people experience a mild euphoria, or "high." Mood, short-term memory, motor coordination, thought, sensation, and time sense can all be affected. Hunger, known as "the munchies," frequently occurs soon after exposure. The heart rate increases, the blood pressure increases while supine but drops when standing, and the eyes can become bloodshot. The most rapid onset with most temporary effect occurs with smoked marijuana. Unlike alcohol or tobacco, no deaths have been directly attributed to marijuana use alone.

Marijuana has been cultivated and used as a medicine for thousands of years. The Food and Drug Administration (FDA) has approved a synthetic formulation of THC, Marinol (brand name of the generic drug dronabinol), that doctors can prescribe legally for the treatment of nausea and vomiting associated with cancer chemotherapy and the loss of appetite and weight loss characteristic of patients with acquired immunodeficiency syndrome (AIDS). In addition, both Marinol and marijuana are used to alleviate pain, muscle spasms, neurological disorders, and glaucoma. Many users of medicinal THC prefer to smoke marijuana despite its illegality rather than take the legal pill because orally delivered THC is not well absorbed by the body. Research is being conducted into a patch or some other method of delivering the legal drug more effectively. Previously classified among drugs such as cocaine and morphine with a high potential for abuse, Marinol was moved to a less restricted category that includes anabolic steroids in July, 1999.

Perspective and Prospects

Despite the FDA's tacit acknowledgment of the medicinal value of marijuana by the approval of Marinol, marijuana itself is classified as a substance with high potential for abuse and no accepted medical use under federal drug laws, stifling research into other potential medical benefits. Scientific evidence, including the 1990 report of the National Academy of Sciences *Marijuana and Medicine: Assessing the Science Base*, strongly supports further research.

—*Sue Tarjan*

See also Addiction; Alcoholism; Alternative medicine; Chemotherapy; Club drugs; Eye infections and disorders; Glaucoma; Herbal medicine; Intoxication; Narcotics; Nausea and vomiting; Pain management; Pharmacology; Self-medication; Smoking; Substance abuse; Tobacco.

For Further Information:

Earleywine, Mitch. *Understanding Marijuana: A New Look at the Scientific Evidence.* New York: Oxford University Press, 2002.

ElSohly, Mahmoud A., ed. *Marijuana and the Cannabinoids.* Totowa, N.J.: Humana Press, 2007.

Iversen, Leslie L. *The Science of Marijuana.* New York: Oxford University Press, 2000.

Mack, Alison, and Janet Joy. *Marijuana as Medicine? The Science Beyond the Controversy.* Washington, D.C.: National Academy Press, 2001.

Onaivi, Emmanuel S., ed. *Marijuana and Cannabinoid Research: Methods and Protocols.* Totowa, N.J.: Humana Press, 2006.

Shohov, Tatiana, ed. *Medical Use of Marijuana: Policy, Regulatory, and Legal Issues.* New York: Nova Science, 2003.

MASSAGE

TREATMENT

ANATOMY OR SYSTEM AFFECTED: All

SPECIALTIES AND RELATED FIELDS: Alternative medicine, exercise physiology, geriatrics and gerontology, oncology, pediatrics, physical therapy, preventive medicine, sports medicine

DEFINITION: The intentional and systematic manipulation of the soft tissues of the body to promote health and healing.

INDICATIONS AND PROCEDURES

Massage is used in both wellness and treatment models of health care. Wellness implies the achievement of an optimal state of well-being. The health enhancing effects of massage such as relaxation, stress reduction, and increased body conditioning or awareness contribute to general wellness. In the treatment model, massage is considered a modality indicated to alleviate the symptoms and/or pain of a specific condition. A particular massage technique can be more or less effective for each illness or injury. The treatment model includes the subspecialty of sports massage, a beneficial intervention for athletes and people engaged in strenuous physical activity.

Two men were instrumental in the development of classic Western massage: Pehr Henrik Ling (1776-1839) and Johann Mezger (1838-1909). Ling developed an approach for treating medical conditions called the Swedish movement cure in the nineteenth century. Mezger defined four categories of massage using French terminology: *effleurage*, *petrissage*, *tapotement*, and *frictions*. The work of these men was further developed by their students and was incorporated into both regular and alternative medicine.

The physical effects of massage include healthy skin, relaxation, increased blood circulation and immune system functioning, metabolic balance in the muscles, connective tissue pliability, increased joint mobility and flexibility, and pain reduction. The mental and emotional benefits include increased mental clarity, reduced anxiety, and emotional release.

USES AND COMPLICATIONS

Massage has proven benefits for mind and body health. Research in the twentieth century showed a positive relationship between the reduction of pain and stress after massage. Other studies revealed that massage promoted weight gain in premature infants and reduced anxiety in adolescents hospitalized for psychi-atric conditions. It can help slow the aging process among older adults and bring comfort to the terminally ill.

A basic tenet of massage practice is "Do no harm." Massage practitioners are trained to identify "endangerment sites." These are areas of the body which are less protected and more vulnerable to damage. "Contraindications" are conditions under which receiving massages are not advisable, such as when it could worsen a condition or spread infection. Health history information is essential for a safe massage session.

As of the year 2000, twenty-five states and the District of Columbia had licensing requirements for massage therapists. The American Massage Therapy Association (AMTA) had thirty thousand members who had to have a minimum of five hundred hours of training from a recognized school. Every practitioner must adhere to a code of ethics and standards of practice.

PERSPECTIVE AND PROSPECTS

Massage has been used for centuries in native and folk cultures all over the world. It has periodically lost and regained popularity in the Western world. After a decline in the 1950's, it experienced a revival of credibility and value during the human potential movement of the late 1960's. Since then, it has been increasingly incorporated into medical treatment and prevention programs. The Office of Alternative Medicine was established by the National Institutes of Health to explore alternative medical practices. Massage therapy was included in the comprehensive 1994 report.

—*Susan L. Sandel, Ph.D.*

See also Acupressure; Alternative medicine; Headaches; Muscle sprains, spasms, and disorders; Muscles; Pain; Pain management; Physical rehabilitation; Stress; Stress reduction.

FOR FURTHER INFORMATION:

American Massage Therapy Association. http://www .amtamassage.org.

Beck, Mark F. *Theory and Practice of Therapeutic Massage*. Clifton Park, N.Y.: Thomson/Delmar Learning, 2006.

Fritz, Sandy. *Mosby's Fundamentals of Therapeutic Massage*. 3d ed. St. Louis, Mo.: Mosby Year Book, 2004.

Salvo, Susan G., and Maureen Pfeiffer, eds. *Massage Therapy: Principles and Practice*. 3d ed. Philadelphia: Saunders/Elsevier, 2007.

Trivieri, Larry, Jr., and John W. Anderson, eds. *Alternative Medicine: The Definitive Guide*. 2d ed. Berkeley, Calif.: Ten Speed Press, 2002.

Werner, Ruth. *A Massage Therapist's Guide to Pathology*. 4th ed. Philadelphia: Wolters Kluwer/Lippincott Williams & Wilkins, 2009.

MASTECTOMY AND LUMPECTOMY

PROCEDURES

ANATOMY OR SYSTEM AFFECTED: Breasts

SPECIALTIES AND RELATED FIELDS: General surgery, oncology, pathology, plastic surgery, radiology

DEFINITION: Mastectomy involves the surgical removal of one or both breasts, whereas lumpectomy involves the removal of one or more tumors and surrounding tissue from the breast.

KEY TERMS:

BRCA1: an abbreviation for breast cancer 1; the mutant chromosomal factor, when found in chromosome 17, which indicates that a woman is vulnerable to developing breast cancer

estrogen: any of several hormones produced by the ovaries that regulate some female reproductive processes and maintain secondary sex characteristics in the female

fibrocystic breasts: the lumpy breasts that some women routinely develop, particularly in the seven or eight days before menstruation

mammography: an X-ray examination of the breasts, the purpose of which is to reveal tumors and other abnormalities

metastasis: the spreading of cancer cells from the original site to other parts of the body

palpation: a digital examination of affected parts of the body

quadrantectomy: a form of lumpectomy that removes more tissue than the usual lumpectomy, leaving little visible scarring but slightly diminishing the size of the affected breast

sonogram: an image of body organs produced through focusing sound waves on the part to be examined

ultrasound: a method of diagnostic imaging that focuses sound waves inaudible to humans on a given organ to produce detailed images of that organ

INDICATIONS AND PROCEDURES

The early indications of breast cancer are often quite subtle, although in this stage it may be revealed by routine mammograms. In some cases, no overt symptoms exist until the cancer is well advanced. Women between forty and fifty years of age without risk factors are advised to have a mammogram every two years. Women over fifty or in the high-risk category because of a family history of breast cancer should have a mammogram once every year. If palpation of the breast reveals a lump, then immediate mammography is indicated.

It is necessary to be constantly vigilant for any sign that an abnormality exists in the breast. Clear indications of possible breast cancer include lumps or thickening of the tissue in the breast or in the area under the arms. Symptoms such as discoloration of the breasts or dimpling, thickening, scaling, or puckering of one or both breasts may also arouse suspicion of breast cancer. A significant change in the shape of the breast or a swelling of it are also symptomatic. A bloody discharge from the nipple, scaly skin on the nipple or surrounding area, inversion of the nipple, or discoloration of the area surrounding the nipple may presage the presence of breast cancer.

Monthly palpation of the breasts, preferably seven or eight days after menstruation, may reveal lumps that could be harmless growths but that might be cancerous. This procedure is referred to as breast self-examination (BSE). Because the female breast contains many glands, it is not uncommon in some women for lumps to appear regularly—often profusely—particularly in the week prior to menstruation. Women with notably lumpy breasts are said to have fibrocystic breasts. Often, the lumps diminish in size in the week following menstruation. If they do not recede, however, then these lumps should be regarded with suspicion and the patient should be examined by a physician, preferably a surgeon, gynecologist, or oncologist.

Once a problem is detected, a number of procedures must be considered for dealing with it. The initial procedure in treating suspected breast cancer usually involves a mammogram to reveal irregularities in the breast. If the results of the mammogram are negative and the patient is still convinced that there is a lump in the breast, an ultrasound or sonographic examination may be indicated. In such tests, harmless sound waves are focused on the breast. These sound waves are reflected so that they create an image of formations within the breast. Although ultrasound cannot definitively indicate whether a lump is cancerous, it can at least verify whether a lump exists. It can also show whether the lump is hollow and filled with fluid, in which case it is usually a benign cyst rather than a cancerous growth.

If a growth is detected, the next, least-invasive means of determining whether it is cancerous is through a needle biopsy. In this procedure, the patient, under local anesthetic, has a hollow needle inserted into the growth. Fluids and cells are then harvested from it. If the growth is a cyst, a clear or light yellow fluid will be withdrawn, causing the cyst to collapse. This may be all the treatment required. In all cases, however, the substances withdrawn from the growth are examined by a pathologist for the presence of cancer cells.

Not all growths are so positioned that needle biopsies are possible. In such cases, a surgical biopsy is probably necessary. If the lump is small, then a lumpectomy, or the removal of the entire lump, may occur. Larger lumps often cannot be removed at this stage, so portions are excised for pathological examination. A pathologist carefully studies the tissue removed to determine whether it contains cancer cells.

In the past, biopsies often occurred while patients were anesthetized and, if the pathological report was positive for cancer, then a radical mastectomy was performed immediately while the patient was still under anesthetic. Since the late twentieth century, however, a two-step procedure has usually replaced this one-step method. If cancer is detected, then surgery is delayed, giving physicians the opportunity to consult with their patients about the treatments available to them.

The major decision in such cases usually is whether a total mastectomy or a partial mastectomy, commonly referred to as a lumpectomy, should be performed. Total mastectomy involves the total removal of the breast and the surrounding lymph nodes.

A radical mastectomy, done under general anesthetic, involves making a large, elliptical incision on the breast, including the nipple and often the entire breast. The incision normally extends into the armpit. All the breast tissue is excised, including the skin and the fat down to the chest muscles. The incision extends into the armpit to remove as much of the breast tissue as possible, including the lymph nodes, which may be cancerous. Once the bleeding has been controlled, a drainage tube is inserted and the incision is closed with sutures, clips, or adhesive substances.

This drastic form of treatment can be traumatic both physically and psychologically to patients. Many women fear the disfigurement that follows it. Some women, especially those with a family history of breast cancer, may decide that the total removal of the breast is their safest option. In some cases, to prevent future threats of breast cancer, they demand the removal of both breasts.

A lumpectomy, usually performed under local anesthetic, involves the removal only of cancerous tissue. The incision is made under the breast, and the lump, with surrounding tissue, is removed. The appearance of the breast remains much the same as it was before the surgery. In some cases, physicians recommend a quadrantectomy, which involves the removal of the cancerous tissue as well as significant amounts of the surrounding tissue. Quite often, the lymph nodes are removed as well. When this treatment is used, the breast will appear slightly smaller than it previously was, but it can be enhanced through plastic surgery.

Subcutaneous mastectomy is frequently indicated in situations where the tumor is small. In this procedure, the surgeon makes an incision under the breast. Most of the skin and the nipple remain intact, although the milk ducts that lead into the nipple are cut. Following the surgery, sometimes immediately, a breast implant can be inserted, restoring the breast to its normal appearance. Mastectomy and lumpectomy are routinely followed by a course of radiation and/or chemotherapy designed to kill any fugitive cancer cells that the surgery has missed.

While the goal of mastectomy is to create as little scarring as possible, considerable scarring may occur, particularly with radical mastectomy, and the absence of one or both breasts usually requires significant psychological adjustments on the part of women who have undergone the procedure. The breast reconstruction performed by a plastic surgeon following a mastectomy is often accompanied by treatment from a psychologist or psychiatrist.

Some women with family histories of breast cancer, particularly if the disease has occurred in first-level relatives (mother or sisters), may opt for a mastectomy rather than a lumpectomy to relieve themselves of the fear of contracting the disease, although most oncologists make such women fully aware of other, less drastic procedures available to them.

Certainly a consideration in reaching a decision about whether to have a lumpectomy or the more drastic mastectomy must include many factors. High on the list of such factors is heredity. In many patients who suffer from this disease, *BRCA1*, a mutated gene found on chromosome 17, is an early indication that breast cancer may eventually occur. *BRCA1* is a gene frequently present in the female members of families with histories of breast cancer and ovarian cancer. About 85 percent of women with the *BRCA1* gene will develop breast cancer if they live a normal life span. Women who have the *BRCA1* gene may decide to have a prophylactic mastectomy before symptoms occur, although many women in this situation prefer treatment with tamoxifen, which appears to hold breast cancer at bay.

Advances in treating cancers of all kinds progressed rapidly during the last half of the twentieth century, and even greater impetus characterizes current advances. The four major treatments—often used in combination with each other—are surgery, radiation therapy, chemotherapy, and hormonal therapy. In the treatment of breast cancer, radiation may be used initially to shrink existing tumors that, once reduced in size, will be removed surgically. Although, when surgeons remove cancerous tumors, they also remove large numbers of surrounding cells that might be affected, such a procedure is usually followed by additional radiation aimed at killing any lingering cancer cells the surgery has missed.

Uses and Complications

The salient use of surgery in cases of breast cancer is to remove its source, not only clearing away any tumors that may be found but also removing additional cancerous tissue as well as lymph nodes that might be affected.

Cancer cells can exist either in the breast's lobules, which contain the cells that produce milk, or in the ducts that carry the milk to the nipples. Cancer cells in either of these locations can be of two types, invasive or noninvasive (also called in situ). The major complication with invasive cancer is that it can and usually does metastasize, spreading often to the lymph nodes, into the lungs and to other parts of the body. In such cases, a radical mastectomy is indicated. It must be performed as quickly as possible and followed by a strenuous course that typically includes radiation or chemotherapy. Noninvasive cancer is less likely to metastasize, although it sometimes does. Lumpectomy or quadrantectomy is often used to treat such cancers, but these procedures must be followed by close monitoring over the rest of the patient's life and by radiation or chemotherapy following surgery.

Chemotherapy is used less often than radiation in the postsurgical treatment of breast cancer but is occasionally used along with it. Some physicians use anticancer drugs to reduce the possibility of recurrence. This treatment, as well as hormone treatment, is designed to kill any fugitive cancer cells that have strayed from the immediate site of the cancer that has been removed. Whereas surgery and radiation are local, affecting only the part of the body being focused upon, chemotherapy is systemic: The drugs used in chemotherapy travel through the bloodstream to all parts of the body. The disadvantage of chemotherapy is that it nearly always has significant side effects. In rare cases, complications are so extreme that they result in death. Usually, chemotherapy is indicated only for women who have not yet undergone the menopause and whose tumors are an inch or larger in size. It may also be employed in cases in which the patient's tumor shows signs of growing rapidly and aggressively invading and attacking other parts of the body.

Related to chemotherapy is hormonal therapy. Hormones are chemicals produced by the body for various purposes. For example, when one is under sudden, undue stress, the body produces adrenaline, which provides a rush of energy and causes the heartbeat to accelerate. In women, the body produces estrogen every month during the menstrual cycle. Estrogen causes the cells in the milk ducts and lobules to grow in preparation for pregnancy. This chemical stimulates the growth of normal cells but can also stimulate the growth of cancer cells. Hormonal therapy is systemic. It involves introducing into the bloodstream a synthetic chemical, usually tamoxifen, which makes it impossible for the body's natural estrogen to find its way to cancer cells that would be nourished by it. A complete biopsy report can determine whether hormonal therapy is appropriate in individual cases.

Perspective and Prospects

Until the middle of the twentieth century, a diagnosis of cancer, particularly of breast cancer, was viewed as a death sentence. Diagnosis generally occurred after the cancer had metastasized. In the first half of the century, general practitioners were much more prevalent than the specialists who, working as a team, are now generally mustered to provide cancer treatment once a diagnosis is made.

With the proliferation of sophisticated medical equipment, including the highly sensitive X-ray machines used in mammography and the various forms of ultrasound and sonograph equipment that are part of nearly every hospital's arsenal of diagnostic equipment, an increasing number of cancers are discovered before they become symptomatic, so that they can be treated with considerable success.

Historically, mastectomies have been performed for centuries. President John Adams's daughter underwent this excruciating surgery early in the nineteenth century, enduring this procedure without the benefit of anesthesia. As was usually true in such cases, the surgery extended her life for only a little while because her cancer was discovered in an advanced stage and had metastasized.

By the late nineteenth and early twentieth centuries, accepted treatment for breast cancer was a radical mastectomy that involved the removal of the affected breast and of as many surrounding cancer cells and lymph nodes as possible. William Halsted, a pioneer in the field of breast cancer surgery and a professor of surgery at the highly respected Johns Hopkins University Medical School, championed the cause of the radical mastectomy, which he viewed as a procedure that could extend substantially the survival of his patients. Little was said about curing breast cancer patients of their cancers. The radical surgery that physicians across the country performed following Halsted's lead was viewed simply as a means of adding months or years to the life of the cancer patient. Until 1970, about 70 percent of women in the United States who had breast cancer were subjected to radical mastectomy.

Several factors brought about a major change in the treatment of breast cancer during the 1960's and 1970's, when social activism was very much in the forefront of American life. Feminists pointed out that most of the surgeons treating breast cancer were men. As an increasing number of women entered medical schools and eventually established medical practices, greater attention was paid to treating breast cancer in less disfiguring ways than had been common earlier.

Along with this change came advances in medical technology that made early diagnosis and more focused treatment a reality. As the chemical treatment of all cancers came to be better understood and more widely employed, the focus was more on preventing and curing cancer than on merely prolonging the lives of those who suffered from it.

Laboratory tests for detecting a woman's predisposition for breast cancer became increasingly sophisticated and accurate. Where the *BRCA1* gene was present, the possibility of developing breast cancer was greatly increased, so that women shown to possess this gene were made more vigilant than ever before in monitoring their conditions and in seeking immediate medical intervention if even the slightest symptom appeared.

Shortly after the end of World War II, some oncologists rejected Halsted's emphasis on radical mastectomy. Surgeon Jerome Urban garnered numerous followers in his call for superradical surgeries in cancer cases. His procedures involved the removal of ribs, various internal organs, and even limbs in order to find and destroy every cancer cell. Surgeon Bernard Fisher stood in opposition to Urban, championing the effectiveness of smaller surgeries, such as the simple mastectomy, which involved the removal of one breast but not of all the lymph nodes and, in some cases, the lumpectomy, involving the removal only of the tumor and its surrounding cells.

The lumpectomy has gained acceptance through the intervening years. It is less disfiguring than either the radical or the simple mastectomy, leaving only a small scar on the underside of the breast. In cases where lumpectomy is viewed as a viable option, survival rates and cure rates are comparable to those of patients who have undergone more radical surgery.

Advances in medical science are accelerating substantially. Stem cell research offers great promise in the treatment and cure of diseases such as breast cancer. Researchers appear to be on the threshold of developing cells designed to destroy specific errant cells, such as those that cause cancer, while leaving healthy cells intact.

—*R. Baird Shuman, Ph.D.*

See also Breast biopsy; Breast cancer; Breast disorders; Breast surgery; Breasts, female; Cancer; Chemotherapy; Gender reassignment surgery; Gynecology; Malignancy and metastasis; Mammography; Oncology; Plastic surgery; Radiation therapy; Tumor removal; Tumors; Women's health.

FOR FURTHER INFORMATION:

Fowble, Barbara, et al. *Breast Cancer Treatment: A Comprehensive Guide to Management.* St. Louis: Mosby Year Book, 1991. Although the presentations in this book are somewhat outdated, they do offer excellent general information, particularly in regard to specific means of performing breast surgery in minimally disfiguring ways.

Friedewald, Vincent, and Aman U. Buzdar, with Michael Bokulich. *Ask the Doctor: Breast Cancer.* Kansas City, Mo.: Andrews McMeel, 1997. Written at a level that laypersons can easily understand, this comprehensive presentation of causes, treatment, and overall outlook for people suffering from breast cancer is strongly recommended.

Hirshaut, Yashar, and Peter I. Pressman. *Breast Cancer: The Complete Guide*. 5th ed. New York: Bantam Books, 2008. This user-friendly book is thorough and accurate in its presentations of the diagnosis and pathology of breast cancer and in its extensive discussion of various means used to treat it. The chapter entitled "Prognosis" is especially cogent.

Judd, Sandra J., ed. *Breast Cancer Sourcebook: Basic Consumer Health Information About Breast Cancer*. 2d ed. Detroit: Omnigraphics, 2004. One of the most extensive treatments of the topic of breast cancer. Its glossary of terms relating to breast cancer is helpful.

Lange, Vladimir. *Be a Survivor: Your Guide to Breast Cancer Treatment*. Los Angeles: Lange Productions, 1999. Directed toward those who are dealing with breast cancer, this upbeat book focuses on managing the disease with an eye toward survival. It deals with the psychology of breast cancer victims and suggests coping mechanisms. A valuable and encouraging book for those who are in the early stages of dealing with their diagnoses. Its guide to cancer centers around the United States is helpful.

Lerner, Barron H. *The Breast Cancer Wars: Hope, Fear, and the Pursuit of a Cure in Twentieth-century America*. New York: Oxford University Press, 2001. The author provides a medical and cultural history of how breast cancer was dealt with during the twentieth century. Lerner uses his extensive knowledge of the field to show the progress made over a hundred-year period.

Mayer, Musa. *Examining Myself*. London: Faber & Faber, 1994. This first-person account of a woman who has suffered from breast cancer is well written. It presents valuable medical information at a level that the average reader will easily comprehend.

Morris, Peter J., and William C. Wood, eds. *Oxford Textbook of Surgery*. 2d ed. New York: Oxford University Press, 2000. Perhaps the most extensive and complete book available on surgery. It deals fully with every surgical aspect of breast cancer.

Phippen, Mark L., and Maryann Papanier Wells, eds. *Patient Care During Operative and Invasive Procedures*. Philadelphia: W. B. Saunders, 2000. Aimed primarily at nurses and other support staff, this book is thorough and offers excellent information about the instruments that must be available to surgeons for various procedures, including radical mastectomy and lumpectomy.

Sproul, Amy, ed. *A Breast Cancer Journey: Your Personal Guidebook*. 2d ed. Atlanta: American Cancer Society, 2004. This authoritative book is particularly valuable for its presentation of the options that breast cancer patients have available to them. The presentation is up to date and timely. Impeccably accurate.

MASTITIS

DISEASE/DISORDER

ANATOMY OR SYSTEM AFFECTED: Breasts, glands
SPECIALTIES AND RELATED FIELDS: Bacteriology, family medicine, gynecology, nutrition, obstetrics
DEFINITION: A bacterial infection of the mammary gland.

CAUSES AND SYMPTOMS

Mastitis is usually caused by a staphylococcal infection of the breast. The bacteria may enter the breast through a sore or crack in the nipple, although some patients do not report having sore or cracked nipples. Generally, mastitis occurs in women who are breast-feeding babies, but women who are not breast-feeding may also experience the disease. Onset of the infection is often associated with stress, reduced immunity, or missed or increased intervals between breast-feedings of a baby.

Common symptoms of mastitis are swelling, redness, hotness, tenderness, an area of hardness, and pain in part or all of the infected breast. In some cases, there is a localized area of soreness in the breast, while in other cases, the entire breast may be inflamed. The victim typically has flulike symptoms, such as tiredness, aches, chills, fever, and fatigue. These feelings often occur prior to breast soreness. If the cause is simple

---

INFORMATION ON MASTITIS

CAUSES: Bacterial infection (usually staphylococcal) typically through cracks in nipples during breast-feeding; also, engorgement with breast milk or plugged duct

SYMPTOMS: Breast swelling, redness, hotness, tenderness, hard area, pain; typically begins with flulike symptoms (tiredness, aches, chills, fever, fatigue)

DURATION: Two to five days for bacterial infection; one to two days for blocked duct

TREATMENTS: Alternate hot and cold packs, gentle massage, acetaminophen or ibuprofen for fever; continued breast-feeding; antibiotics if necessary (cephalexin, cloxacillin, erythromycin, flucloxacillin)

engorgement with breast milk or a plugged duct, then the patient will start feeling better instead of worse. Blocked ducts usually resolve themselves naturally within twenty-four to forty-eight hours, although a blocked duct may sometimes lead to mastitis.

TREATMENT AND THERAPY

Alternate hot and cold packs applied to the sore area of the infected breast help reduce the inflammation and pain and provide comfort. Gently massaging the tender area increases circulation and helps loosen any plugged ducts. Fever can be treated with acetaminophen or ibuprofen without any harm to a breast-feeding baby. Patients should also drink plenty of fluids. For nursing mothers, unless the pain is too intense, breast-feeding should be continued during the treatment of mastitis. If breast-feeding is discontinued, then the breast should be drained regularly with a breast pump.

Once a diagnosis of mastitis is made, proper antibiotics should be administered, if necessary. Cephalexin, cloxacillin, erythromycin, and flucloxacillin are effective drugs against the *Staphylococcus* bacteria. Once they are administered, the soreness usually starts to disappear within two to five days. Redness may continue for up to a week or more. Bed rest helps relieve stress and builds up the immune system. If not treated properly and in a timely manner, mastitis can lead to a breast abscess that requires surgical draining.

PERSPECTIVE AND PROSPECTS

Mastitis is most common among nursing mothers during the first three months postpartum. The most important preventive measure against mastitis for these women is regular breast-feeding. Recurrent mastitis is associated with irregular breast-feeding patterns, fatigue, and stress. Frequent breast-feeding and lifestyle changes that promote good health and a strengthened immune system are key ingredients for reducing the occurrence of mastitis.

If antibiotics are prescribed for treatment, it is important that the full course be taken even though the patient improves quickly; otherwise, the risk of mastitis returning increases. Two newer drugs, clindamycin and ciprofloxacin, have proven effective in treating mastitis if the patient is allergic to penicillin-derived medication.

—*Alvin K. Benson, Ph.D.*

See also Abscess drainage; Abscesses; Antibiotics; Bacterial infections; Breast biopsy; Breast disorders; Breast-feeding; Breasts, female; Hormones; Mammography; Women's health.

FOR FURTHER INFORMATION:

Colson, Jenni Lynn, ed. *Breastfeeding Sourcebook.* Detroit, Mich.: Omnigraphics, 2002.

Icon Health. *Mastitis: A Medical Dictionary, Bibliography, and Annotated Research Guide to Internet References.* San Diego, Calif.: Author, 2004.

Marz, Russell B. *Medical Nutrition from Marz.* 2d ed. Portland, Oreg.: Quiet Lion Press, 1999.

Reddy, Pavani. "Postpartum Mastitis and Community-Acquired Methicillin-Resistant *Staphylococcus aureus.*" *Emerging Infectious Diseases* 13, no. 2 (February 1, 2007): 298.

Swenson, Deborah E. *Telephone Triage for the Obstetric Patient: A Nursing Guide.* Philadelphia: W. B. Saunders, 2001.

MASTURBATION

DEVELOPMENT

ANATOMY OR SYSTEM AFFECTED: Genitals

SPECIALTIES AND RELATED FIELDS: Psychiatry

DEFINITION: A manual stimulation of one's own or another person's genital organs usually resulting in orgasm without engaging in sexual intercourse.

PHYSICAL AND PSYCHOLOGICAL FACTORS

Masturbation is the first sexual experience among a great majority of people. Some young people inadvertently stumble on sexual arousal and orgasm in the course of engaging in some other physical activity. Others purposefully stimulate themselves, aroused by curiosity after reading erotic literature, watching sexually explicit films, or listening to imaginary or real sexual adventures of their peers.

Most men and women practice masturbation to relieve sexual tension, achieve sexual pleasure, enjoy sexual stimulation in the absence of an available partner, and experience relaxation. When masturbating, men tend to focus on the stimulation of the penis. Stimulation of the clitoral shaft and clitoral area with a hand or an object is the method that women most commonly employ. Some women masturbate by using a vibrator. Mutual masturbation provides a satisfying and pleasurable form of sexual intimacy and release for many couples. It is also one of the most common techniques that gay and lesbian couples use during sexual intimacy.

DISORDERS AND EFFECTS

Under certain circumstances, masturbation may result in some undesirable consequences. If a child masturbates constantly, it may be an indication of excessive anxiety and tension. Compulsive and frenzied masturbation may reflect abuse or maltreatment in a child's home life. Frequent masturbation may be a child's way of relieving tension or unconsciously re-enacting past or present traumatic sexual episodes. Among adults, excessive masturbation may point toward a person's lack of self-esteem and the resultant fear and inability to develop healthy interpersonal relationships with persons of the opposite sex. Psychiatry, psychotherapy, and sex therapy have proven helpful in successfully alleviating these problems.

PERSPECTIVE AND PROSPECTS

Throughout history, attitudes toward the practice of masturbation have been riddled with misconceptions, guilt, and fear. Fear of masturbation and its supposed harmful effects, such as loss of memory and intelligence, was widespread in the nineteenth century. Semen was considered a vital fluid important for bodily functioning, and wasting it through masturbation was considered as contributing to weakening of the body and production of illness. Medical authorities today do not find any evidence of physical damage from masturbation. In fact, many modern sex therapists encourage self-stimulation as part of healthy sexuality. In modern sex therapy, masturbation has become part of the therapeutics used in treating certain sexual dysfunctions. Patients with difficulties or inability to have orgasm are encouraged by their therapists to engage in masturbation. It is widely believed that orgasm once achieved through masturbation will eventually generalize and transfer to satisfactory sexual intercourse.

—*Tulsi B. Saral, Ph.D.*

See also Aphrodisiacs; Domestic violence; Men's health; Puberty and adolescence; Rape and sexual assault; Reproductive system; Sexual dysfunction; Sexuality; Women's health.

FOR FURTHER INFORMATION:

Bockting, Walter, and Eli Coleman, eds. *Masturbation as a Means of Achieving Sexual Health*. New York: Haworth Press, 2003.

Dodson, Betty. *Sex for One: The Joy of Selfloving*. New York: Harmony Books, 1996.

Laqueur, Thomas Walter. *Solitary Sex: A Cultural History of Masturbation*. New York: Zone Books, 2003.

Marcus, Irwin M., and John J. Francis, eds. *Masturbation: From Infancy to Senescence*. New York: International Universities Press, 1975.

Rowan, Edward L. *The Joy of Self-Pleasuring: Why Feel Guilty About Feeling Good?* Amherst, Mass.: Prometheus Books, 2000.

Sarnoff, Suzanne, and Irving Sarnoff. *Masturbation and Adult Sexuality*. Bridgewater, N.J.: Replica Books, 2001.

MEASLES

DISEASE/DISORDER

ALSO KNOWN AS: Morbilli, rubeola

ANATOMY OR SYSTEM AFFECTED: Ears, lungs, mouth, nervous system, respiratory system, skin

SPECIALTIES AND RELATED FIELDS: Family medicine, internal medicine, pediatrics, public health, virology

DEFINITION: A highly contagious disease contracted through a virus transmitted in respiratory secretions and characterized by a spreading skin rash.

KEY TERMS:

desquamation: the sloughing off of the outer layers of skin

Koplik's spots: small red spots with white centers generally found in the mouth during early stages of measles

maculopapular rash: reddish skin eruptions characterized by small, flat discolorations that may progress into small pimples

otitis media: infection or inflammation of the middle ear, an occasional complication of measles infection

paramyxoviruses: a group of ribonucleic acid (RNA) viruses that includes the etiological agents for measles, mumps, and a variety of respiratory infections

pharyngitis: infection or inflammation of the pharynx, or throat

photophobia: abnormal sensitivity of the eyes to light, a condition common to a variety of illnesses, including measles

prodromal stage: the early stage of a disease during which symptoms first appear

viremia: a condition characterized by the presence of a virus in the bloodstream

CAUSES AND SYMPTOMS

Measles is a highly contagious viral disease characterized by a maculopapular (pimply) rash that develops on the skin and spreads rapidly over much of the cutaneous surface of the body. Measles virus is classified with the paramyxoviruses, a class of viruses in which ribonucleic acid (RNA) serves as the genetic material. Closely related viruses in the same group include rinderpest and distemper virus, agents associated with dis-

INFORMATION ON MEASLES

CAUSES: Viral infection
SYMPTOMS: Spreading rash, malaise, fever, respiratory difficulty
DURATION: One to two weeks
TREATMENTS: Alleviation of symptoms

ease in ruminants such as cows and in dogs or cats, respectively. It is likely that measles originated when one of these other animal viruses became adapted to humans several thousand years ago.

In modern times but before the advent of measles vaccination, measles was a common disease of childhood, usually appearing between the ages of five and ten. The illness is among the most contagious of infections, and the virus was generally spread among children in schools. Widespread immunization of children, begun in the 1960's, tended to push the age of exposure into the teenage years. Most outbreaks since the 1980's have occurred among college students. Since recovery from the disease confers lifelong immunity, infection among older adults is infrequent. In developing nations, places where vaccination may be haphazard, measles is still a disease of early childhood; malnutrition and related problems of poverty have resulted in a significant level of mortality among infected children.

Exposure generally follows an oral-oral means of transmission, as the person inhales contaminated droplets from an infected individual. The incubation period for active measles ranges from seven to fourteen days. During this early stage, the infected individual becomes increasingly contagious. The lack of any obvious symptoms during these early stages lends itself to the spread of the disease.

Contact by the virus with the surface cells of the respiratory passages, or sometimes the conjunctiva (the outer surface of the eye), allows the infectious agent to enter the body. The virus spreads through the local lymph nodes into the blood, producing a primary viremia. During this period, the virus replicates both in the lymph nodes and in the respiratory sites through which the virus entered the body. The virus returns to the bloodstream, resulting in a secondary viremia and widespread passage of the virus throughout the body by the fifth to seventh day after the initial exposure. Viral levels in the blood reach their peak toward the end of the incubation period, some fourteen days after infection. Once symptoms begin, the virus is widely disseminated throughout the body, including sites in small blood vessels, lymph nodes, and even the central nervous system.

The initial incubation period is followed by a prodromal stage, in which active symptoms appear. This stage is characterized by a fever that may reach as high as 103 degrees Fahrenheit, coughing, sensitivity of the eyes to light (photophobia), and malaise. Koplik's spots appear on the buccal mucosa in the mouth one to two days prior to development of the characteristic measles rash.

The maculopapular rash first appears on the head and behind the ears and gradually spreads over the rest of the body during the course of twenty-four to forty-eight hours. Clear signs of respiratory infection appear, including a cough, pharyngitis, and occasional involvement of the bronchioles or even pneumonia. While malaise and anorexia (appetite loss) are common during the fever period, diarrhea and vomiting generally do not occur. Over time, the rash becomes increasingly dense, exhibiting a blotchy character. Desquamation is common in many affected areas of the skin. Gradually, over a period of three to five days, the rash begins to fade, usually following the sequence by which it first appeared. The rash fades first on the forehead, then on the extremities.

Complications, while they do occur, are unusual in otherwise healthy individuals. Most result from secondary bacterial infections. Occasionally, these complications may manifest themselves as infections of the ear. Pulmonary infections are common among cases of measles and account for most of the rare deaths that follow development of the disease. Photophobia is also common, accounting for the former belief that measles patients had to be kept in a dark room; as long as the patient is comfortable, this step is unnecessary.

The obvious manifestations of measles infection make the isolation of the virus unnecessary for diagnosis. Ironically, the near disappearance of measles in the United States has made most physicians unfamiliar with the disease; it is not unusual for an attending physician to mistake the rash for another illness. For this reason, laboratory diagnosis is often useful. Laboratory confirmation is generally based on a serological assay for measles antibodies in the blood of infected persons.

A rare sequela to measles infection is the development of subacute sclerosing panencephalitis, a disease characterized by progressive neurological deterioration. The specific mechanism by which measles infection may develop into this disease remains unclear, but

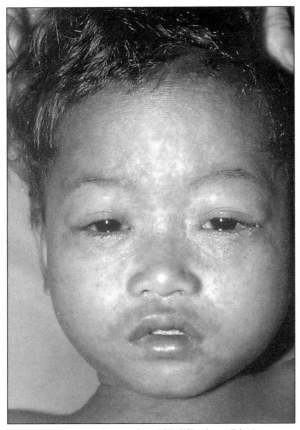

A child with measles. (CDC/Barbara Rice)

it may be the result of a rare combination of events in the victim. Since spread of the virus into the central nervous system is common during measles infection whereas the development of subacute sclerosing panencephalitis is rare (approximately one case per 100,000 measles infections), it is likely that some form of immune impairment is at the root of this disease. Diagnosis of subacute sclerosing panencephalitis is difficult and is based on developing dementia accompanied by unusual levels of measles antibodies in cerebrospinal fluid.

TREATMENT AND THERAPY

No specific treatment for measles is available; therapy consists of symptomatic intervention. Bed rest is recommended, and the patient should not come into contact with persons not previously exposed to the virus through either natural infection or immunization.

Itching of the rash is common and may be treated with cool water or the standard regimen of cornstarch or baking soda applications. The most common com-

plications result from secondary bacterial infections, which generally take the form of otitis media (middle-ear infection), pharyngitis, or pneumonia. Appropriate use of antibiotics is usually sufficient to prevent or treat such complications.

Immunization with the measles virus may be either passive or active. Children less than one year of age and patients who are immunocompromised or chronically ill may be protected if human immunoglobulin is administered within a week after exposure. While effective immunity is short term, it is capable of protecting these individuals during this period. Since no active disease or infection develops, however, immunity to future infection remains minimal in these cases.

During the early 1960's, an effective vaccine was developed to immunize children against measles. The vaccine consists of an attenuated form of the virus. Although early forms of the vaccine were inconsistent in producing a lifelong immunity, they were effective in decreasing the prevalence of the disease. Later generations of the attenuated vaccine proved more effective in developing long-term immunity among the recipients.

Since maternal antibodies are present in newborns, it is recommended that measles immunization begin between twelve and fifteen months of age. Often, this program is part of a combination MMR vaccine, for measles, mumps, and rubella (German measles). A second booster is given following elementary school. The American Academy of Pediatrics does not consider a third vaccination to be necessary if the approved routine has been followed. It is recommended that children who were first immunized prior to their first birthday should receive boosters at fifteen months of age and again at age twelve. Indications are that immunity from vaccination is long term, if not lifelong. Recovery from natural infection results in a lifelong immunity to measles.

Inconsistency of the first generation of vaccine resulted in ineffective immunity among some individuals vaccinated during the 1960's. A number of small outbreaks during the 1980's were the result. Most cases of measles, however, have occurred in individuals who failed to be immunized.

PERSPECTIVE AND PROSPECTS

The origin and early history of measles is uncertain, as the first authentic description of measles as a specific entity was that by the Arab physician al-Razi (Rhazes) in a 910 C.E. treatise on smallpox and measles. Rhazes quoted earlier work by the Hebrew physician El Yehudi, so it is likely that familiarity with these respective illnesses had existed for some time.

Measles is entirely a human disease, with no known animal reservoir. Consequently, the paucity of human populations of sufficient size to maintain transmission means that the spread of such an epidemic disease would have been unlikely before 2500 B.C.E. It is probable that the disease entered the human species through adaptation of the similar animal viruses of rinderpest or distemper. The absence of any description of a disease like measles in the writings of Hippocrates (c. fourth century B.C.E.) likewise renders it unlikely that the disease was widespread before that date.

Epidemic disease with a rash characteristic of measles is known to have spread through the Roman Empire during the early centuries of the common era. The difficulty in differentiating measles from smallpox by the physicians of the time contributes to the difficulty in understanding the history of the illness. It is certain that by the time of Rhazes, measles had become common in the population.

The terminology of measles lent further confusion during the Middle Ages. Measles was often referred to as *morbilli*, a Latin term meaning "little disease," to distinguish it from *il morbo*, or plague. The word "measles" first appeared in the fourteenth century treatise *Rosa Anglica*, by John of Gaddesden. The term may have been applied initially to the sores on the legs of lepers (*mesles*), and it was only later that illnesses characterized by similar rashes (measles, smallpox, and rubella) were clearly differentiated by European physicians. The significance of a rash with a white center in the mouth was probably recognized by John Quier in Jamaica and Richard Hazeltine in New England during the latter portion of the eighteenth century, but it was in 1896 that the American pediatrician Henry Koplik firmly reported its role in early stages of the disease.

Measles followed the path of European explorers to the Americas during the sixteenth century. Repeated outbreaks of measles devastated the native populations, which had minimal immunity to the newly introduced disease. The most thorough epidemiological investigation of measles newly introduced into a population was that by Peter Panum in his study *Observations Made During the Epidemic of Measles on the Faroe Islands in the Year 1846* (1940). In the population of 7,864 persons, 6,100 became ill, with 102 deaths. Mortality rates as high as 25 percent were not unusual in previously unexposed populations. In Hawaii in 1848, 40,000 deaths occurred among the population of 150,000

persons following the introduction of measles. Even higher mortality rates probably occurred among the populations of Peru and Mexico in 1530-1531, following their exposure to infected Spanish explorers.

The earliest attempt at immunization was probably that of Francis Home of Edinburgh in 1758. Home soaked cotton in the blood of measles patients and placed it on the small cuts on the skin of children. The viral nature of measles was first demonstrated by John Anderson and Joseph Goldberger of the United States Public Health Service, who in 1911 induced the disease in monkeys using filtered extracts from human tissue. In 1954, the virus itself was isolated by John Enders, who grew the agent in human and monkey tissue in a laboratory.

The first effective vaccine was developed by Enders in 1958 using an attenuated (live) form of the virus. The vaccine was tested and then licensed in 1963. Several variations of the vaccine that proved superior in producing long-term immunity were developed in the decades that followed. In 1974, the World Health Organization introduced a widespread vaccination program within developing countries.

The absence of any natural reservoir for measles other than humans has made the eradication of the disease possible. Active immunization of children in the United States reduced the annual incidence of the disease from 482,000 reported cases in 1962 to fewer than 1,000 in the late 1990's. Widespread vaccination and worldwide surveillance has made global eradication of the disease a realistic possibility.

—*Richard Adler, Ph.D.*

See also Childhood infectious diseases; Epidemics and pandemics; Fever; Immunization and vaccination; Mumps; Rashes; Rubella; Viral infections.

FOR FURTHER INFORMATION:

American Medical Association. *American Medical Association Family Medical Guide.* 4th rev. ed. Hoboken, N.J.: John Wiley & Sons, 2004. An excellent general source for information about illnesses and questions about medical problems.

Bernstein, David, and Gilbert Schiff. "Viral Exanthems and Localized Skin Infections." In *Infectious Diseases*, edited by Sherwood L. Gorbach, John G. Bartlett, and Neil R. Blacklow. Philadelphia: W. B. Saunders, 2004. This book contains extensive discussions of bacterial and viral illnesses. The section addressing measles contains much information about the symptoms and progression of the disease.

Biddle, Wayne. *A Field Guide to Germs*. 2d ed. New York: Anchor Books, 2002. This comprehensive book is easily accessible to the nonspecialist and includes a discussion of nearly every virus, bacterium, and fungus known to cause human and nonhuman animal disease. The history of the microbe and the treatment of diseases are included.

Kiple, Kenneth F., ed. *The Cambridge World History of Human Disease*. New York: Cambridge University Press, 1999. In addition to being an encyclopedia describing human diseases, this book provides an epidemiological history of disease and discusses possible origins and treatments. The authors target a general population.

Madigan, Michael T., and John M. Martinko. *Brock Biology of Microorganisms*. 12th ed. San Francisco: Pearson/Benjamin Cummings, 2009. A college textbook on the subject of microbiology. An extensive section on microbial diseases provides a concise description of measles and its prevention.

Wagner, Edward K., and Martinez J. Hewlett. *Basic Virology*. 3d ed. Malden, Mass.: Blackwell Science, 2008. A very readable undergraduate text covering issues of virology and viral disease, properties of viruses and virus-cell interaction, working with viruses, and replication patterns of specific viruses.

Woolf, Alan D., et al., eds. *The Children's Hospital Guide to Your Child's Health and Development*. Cambridge, Mass.: Perseus, 2002. An authoritative and comprehensive guide to children's health, providing a guide to every common illness or condition that affects children and a carefully designed emergency section.

MEDICAL COLLEGE ADMISSION TEST (MCAT)

HEALTH CARE SYSTEM

DEFINITION: A computer-based standardized exam used by medical and other health professions' schools for assessment of student readiness in a medical curriculum.

KEY TERMS:

assessment: the process of measuring the knowledge, skills, and attitudes of an individual or group

biological sciences: the branch of natural science that deals with structure and behavior of living organisms; includes disciplines such as zoology, genetics, cell biology, biochemistry and molecular biology, and anatomy and physiology

physical sciences: the branch of natural science that analyzes the nature and properties of energy and nonliving matter; includes disciplines such as physics, chemistry, astronomy, and geology

PURPOSE AND USE

The MCAT is administered by the Association of American Medical Colleges (AAMC), the body that represents the 131 allopathic medical schools (those granting doctor of medicine, or M.D. degrees) in the United States and 17 schools in Canada. The purpose of the MCAT is to assess prospective medical school applicants on the knowledge that they have attained during their undergraduate education. The test has been devised by looking at what is required for success in medical school and in the practice of medicine, as determined by medical educators and practicing physicians. In addition to AAMC schools, the MCAT is used by the American Association of Colleges of Osteopathic Medicine (AACOM), comprised of 26 schools granting osteopathic medical (D.O.) degrees, and the American Association of Colleges of Podiatric Medicine (AACPM), comprised of 8 schools granting podiatric medical (D.P.M.) degrees. The MCAT is also used by many veterinary medical schools and other allied health programs in lieu of other standardized assessments.

CONTENT, COVERAGE, AND SCORING

The MCAT consists of three multiple-choice sections (physical sciences, verbal reasoning, and biological sciences) and a writing sample. Each of the three multiple-choice sections is scored on a basis of 1 to 15. The writing assessment is scored using a letter system, ranging from J through T. Scores are reported to students and medical schools as a combination of the four parts; thus, a typical composite score might be reported as 31P, with subset scores also reported.

The physical sciences section assesses problem-solving ability in the areas of general chemistry and general physics. There are fifty-two questions with seventy minutes to answer them. This includes seven passage-based sets of questions (four to seven questions each) and thirteen independent questions. The biological sciences section of the exam is constructed in a similar fashion, with fifty-two questions with seventy minutes. This portion assesses problem-solving ability in the biological sciences (including general biology, genetics, and biochemistry/molecular biology) as well as in organic chemistry. The biological sciences section of the exam has been shown to correlate best with scores on the USMLE Step 1 Exam, the exam taken by medical students after their basic courses in medical school.

The verbal reasoning section of the exam includes forty multiple-choice questions in a period of sixty minutes designed to assess one's ability to understand, evaluate, and apply information and arguments presented in prose style. This section consists of seven passages taken from the humanities, social sciences, and natural sciences and is included partly to encourage undergraduates with broad educational backgrounds to consider careers in the health professions. Each passage is followed by five to seven questions assessing the ability to extrapolate and use information. No specific content knowledge is required to do well on this section.

The multiple-choice sections of the MCAT are not adaptive (unlike the Graduate Record Exam, or GRE); therefore, students who finish early may go back through any of the questions in that particular section, since they are set and do not change according to how well the test taker has done.

For the writing sample, examinees are given sixty minutes to compose an expository response to two different prompts. Each prompt is designed to assess one's ability to develop an idea, present that idea cohesively and logically, and write clearly and properly.

Perspective and Prospects

The MCAT has been part of the medical school admissions process for more than sixty years. Today all medical schools in the United States and most in Canada require applicants to submit recent MCAT scores. Many other health professions and graduate programs also accept MCAT scores in lieu of other standardized tests. Because of its widespread acceptance, more than seventy thousand students take the exam each year.

The forerunner of the MCAT was developed by F. A. Moss in 1928. Responding to unacceptably high dropout rates of up to 50 percent in U.S. medical schools, he and his colleagues prepared the Scholastic Aptitude Test for Medical Students. This test assessed visual memory, content knowledge, scientific vocabulary and definitions, logical reasoning, and knowledge of required premedical courses. Following introduction of this test, the national dropout rate decreased by more than two-thirds.

Following advancements in test-measurement technology and testing psychology, the Medical College Admission Test was rolled out in 1948. Four subtests were used, measuring verbal ability, quantitative ability, scientific understanding, and knowledge of modern society (broad liberal arts skills and knowledge). Most medical schools at the time deemed the scientific and quantitative knowledge to be much more important than verbal ability or societal knowledge and often used only those two scores to determine admissions. In 1977, the societal knowledge section (renamed general knowledge in the 1960's) was eliminated, and subscores began being reported for biology, chemistry, and physics. In 1991, the MCAT was changed to its present form, and the current scoring scale was adopted. In 2007, the MCAT became a computer-based assessment.

Although the MCAT has remained relatively stable in its content and format (multiple-choice questions) over a long period of time, periodic changes in the content and style of questions have kept the exam fresh and taken advantage of research on how students learn and demonstrate that learning. In 2007, the AAMC convened a task force to revamp the content of the exam one more time, taking into consideration new skills and knowledge needed for twenty-first century medicine. That exam, expected to be released in 2013, will likely have increased emphasis on molecular areas of biology and decreased emphasis on some areas of the physical sciences.

—*Kerry L. Cheesman, Ph.D.*

See also American Medical Association (AMA); Education, medical; Hippocratic oath.

For Further Information:

Association of American Medical Colleges (AAMC). *MCAT Essentials.* Washington, D.C.: AAMC, 2010. Also available at http://www.aamc.org/students/mcat/mcatessentials.pdf.

McGaghie, William. "Assessing Readiness for Medical Education: Evolution of the MCAT." *Journal of the American Medical Association* 288, no. 9 (September 4, 2002).

Miller, Robert, and Dan Bissell. *Med School Confidential: A Complete Guide to the Medical School Experience—By Students, for Students.* New York: St. Martin's Press, 2008.

MEDICARE

PROGRAM

DEFINITION: A federal health insurance program for persons over sixty-five, persons with end-stage renal disease, and some disabled individuals. Medicare is part of the Social Security system, and participation is closely tied to Social Security eligibility.

KEY TERMS:

beneficiary: the person who receives the benefits of an insurance policy; for health insurance, the beneficiary is the patient receiving health care

coinsurance: an arrangement in which a percentage of the total bill for health services is paid by the insurer and the rest is paid by the beneficiary

deductible: the amount that the patient must pay before the insurance pays any amount

managed care organization: a health care organization that combines the functions of insurer and provider; it reduces redundancy of services and uses primary care providers as gatekeepers to reduce cost

medically necessary: services and supplies that are appropriate and needed for the diagnosis or treatment of the person's medical condition

Medicare Trust Fund: accumulated contributions from Social Security payroll taxes that are used to pay for the Medicare program

premiums: periodic payments for insurance coverage

primary care provider: a doctor or nurse practitioner who is trained to provide basic medical care

skilled nursing care: a level of care that requires the skills of a registered nurse

INTRODUCTION

Medicare is a federal health insurance program for individuals who are sixty-five or older, persons who have end-stage renal disease (irreversible kidney failure), and some individuals who have disabilities. In addition to age and special conditions, eligible individuals or their spouses must have been employed for at least ten years in a job where they paid Social Security payroll taxes and must be citizens or permanent residents of the United States. Medicare was passed into law as Title XVIII of the Social Security Act of 1965. The intent of the Medicare law was to provide financial protection to elderly individuals against the high cost of illness and hospitalization.

In 2002, more than forty million Americans were covered by Medicare services, making it the largest health insurance program in the United States. Medicare is administered through the Centers for Medicare and Medicaid Services (CMS), formerly the Health Care Financing Administration (HCFA). CMS is an agency of the Social Security Administration within the Department of Health and Human Services (DHHS).

Medicare is financed through a combination of Social Security payroll tax, premiums, and general revenue funds. Services for the Original Medicare Plan are available nationwide, and the insured person can go to any provider that accepts Medicare. The original program operates in the same way as other fee-for-service medical insurance plans, which means the insured person is charged a fee each time that person receives health care services. The person providing the service files a claim for payment. These fees, or claims, are paid fully or partially by Medicare. The Social Security Administration does not pay the claims directly; it has contractual arrangements with private insurance organizations that handle all payments. Fiscal intermediaries process claims from hospitals and other inpatient facilities, and carriers process claims from physicians and suppliers.

CMS has the responsibility to interpret and clarify the provisions of the laws and regulations governing Medicare. Its responsibility includes making determinations as to whether a particular service will be approved for payment by Medicare. However, the majority of decisions about whether a specific type of service will be covered are made at the local level by the fiscal intermediaries or carriers who process claims.

The structure of the Medicare program has remained basically unchanged since its inception. There are two parts to the Original Medicare Plan: Part A and Part B. Part A, called Hospital Insurance (HI), pays for inpatient services. Most people do not pay for Medicare Part A; it is financed through the Social Security payroll taxes that are earmarked for the Medicare Trust Fund. At age sixty-five, individuals receive Part A automatically if they are already receiving Social Security retirement benefits or retirement benefits through the Railroad Retirement Board, or if they are eligible to receive either of these benefits but have not yet filed for them. Individuals who had Medicare-covered government employment also receive Part A without paying premiums, as do their spouses. Individuals under sixty-five can receive Part A benefits without paying if they have had Social Security or Railroad Retirement Board disability benefits for twenty-four months. Other individuals entitled to Part A benefits without paying are those with end-stage renal disease (ESRD) who are receiving kidney dialysis or who have had a kidney transplant.

Part A benefits include a semiprivate room, in a hospital or skilled nursing facility, with related services and supplies including laboratory and diagnostic procedures, nursing care, surgical care, and rehabilitative services. Skilled nursing home services are paid for after the person has been hospitalized for three days for a related health condition. Medicare pays for medications given to the patient while in the hospital or skilled nursing facility. In situations of medical necessity, a private room is allowed. Part A pays for part-time skilled nursing care in the home, as well as for physical, occupational, and speech-language therapy. Hospice care for people with a terminal illness is paid for through Part A. Hospice care includes medical and support services such as drugs for the control of pain or other symptoms and skilled nursing care.

Part B, called Supplemental Medical Insurance (SMI), pays for outpatient services, including services from primary care providers, specialist physicians, clinical psychologists, and social workers. Part B also pays for outpatient mental health services, surgical services and supplies, diagnostic tests, procedures, outpatient therapies, and durable medical equipment such as canes, wheelchairs, walkers, and oxygen-delivery equipment. These services and supplies are covered when they are medically necessary. Medicare helps pay for ambulance services when other sources of transportation would endanger the person's health, artificial limbs and prosthetic devices, braces, chiropractic services, emergency care, immunosuppressive drugs for patients who have undergone organ transplantation, kidney dialysis, nutritional therapy services for diabetics or patients with ESRD, and telemedicine in rural areas. Medicare pays for approved medications that are administered as part of physicians' services.

Preventive services are also covered under Part B. These preventive services are bone density tests, colorectal cancer screening, diabetes services and supplies, glaucoma screening, mammography, clinical breast examinations, Pap tests and pelvic examinations, prostate cancer screening, and vaccinations. Rules apply as to who qualifies and the frequency of these services.

Under the Original Medicare Plan, neither Part A nor Part B will pay for any of the following: services that Medicare does not consider medically necessary, private-duty nursing, routine physical examinations, dental care or dentures, custodial care (basic maintenance care such as bathing and feeding), hearing aids and hearing examinations, outpatient medications (with some limited exceptions), cosmetic surgery,

glasses (except following cataract surgery), orthopedic shoes, or alternative medicine such as acupuncture. Medicare does not pay for medical services outside the United States (with some very limited exceptions).

A provider or supplier must inform the beneficiary if a specific service will likely not be paid for by Medicare. If the person still chooses to receive the service, the person will be asked to sign an advance beneficiary notice (ABN). By signing the ABN, the person is agreeing to pay out-of-pocket if Medicare does not pay.

Part B is optional, and individuals have a choice of whether to enroll in Part B at the same time that they enroll in Part A. Most people do have to pay for coverage under Part B. In 2000, approximately 75 percent of eligible seniors had Part B. Approximately one-fourth of the total cost for these services is financed through premiums, and the remainder is financed through general federal revenue funds. The charge for the premium is adjusted yearly; in 2007, the monthly premium for Part B was $93.50, which is deducted from the person's Social Security, railroad retirement, or civil service retirement check. If individuals do not receive a retirement check, then Medicare bills them for the Part B premiums on a quarterly basis. Eligible persons can postpone enrolling in Part B if they or their spouses are working and have group health insurance through their employment. However, if they do not have group health insurance and delay enrolling in Part B, then their monthly payments will be increased by 10 percent for every year that they did not enroll but could have done so.

For services under both Part A and Part B, the insured person is responsible for paying the deductible, coinsurance, and copayment. The deductible for Part B is $131 per year. As an example, a patient has surgery on January 2 costing $531. Since he has not paid his deductible for the year, he must first pay that amount ($131); then Medicare pays its share, which is usually 80 percent, of the remaining amount ($320). The patient pays the remainder ($80). One exception to the usual 20 percent paid by beneficiaries is in the case of outpatient mental health services, in which beneficiaries pay 50 percent of the fees.

Private insurance can be purchased separately to help pay coinsurance amounts, deductibles, and other out-of-pocket expenses for individuals who have the Original Medicare Plan. They are called Medigap policies, since they are used to fill the gaps in the Original Medicare Plan. Medigap policies are regulated by federal and state laws. There are ten standard plans referred to as Plans A through J, each of which has a different set of benefits. Some Medigap policies pay a portion of prescription medication fees.

In 2007, Medicare Part A had a $992 deductible for a hospital stay for each benefit period. A benefit period begins the day the person becomes an inpatient in either a hospital or a skilled nursing facility and ends when the person has not received inpatient care for sixty consecutive days. If the person is hospitalized after one benefit period has ended, then a new benefit period begins. In 2007, for each benefit period the costs were an initial deductible of $992 for days one through sixty and $248 per day for days sixty-one through ninety. After ninety days, the person can use lifetime reserve days, which means that Medicare will pay all covered costs, except for a coinsurance payment of $496 a day, for up to sixty days. These reserve days can be used only once during the person's lifetime. For care in a skilled nursing facility, for each benefit period the beneficiary pays nothing for the first twenty days, up to $124 per day for days twenty-one through one hundred, and all costs after one hundred days.

Medicare beneficiaries sometimes have additional health care coverage that pays bills first, then Medicare pays the remainder; this is called Medicare Secondary Payer. Examples of primary payers are veterans' benefits, workers' compensation, union health coverage, or employer-sponsored insurance. To conserve Medicare funds, the Coordination of Benefits program monitors and manages the payment process when beneficiaries have more than one policy.

Physician services and supplies will cost more if the physician or supplier does not accept assignment. Assignment is an agreement from a physician, other health care provider, or supplier of medical equipment whereby they accept the Medicare-approved fee as full payment for rendered services. The approved fee is the cost that has been established by Medicare as reasonable for the particular service. Even if the physician or other providers do not accept assignment, a maximum is placed on what they can charge, called the limiting charge. The maximum, or limit, is 15 percent over Medicare's approved amount.

To reflect the changes occurring in health care delivery, Medicare law was amended in 1997 to allow beneficiaries to choose among several different health insurance plans based on their needs. The Original Medicare Plan remained as it was originally implemented. Another option, Medicare+Choice, enables beneficiaries to enroll in a managed care plan or private fee-for-service plan. In managed care plans, a specified group of providers render services to all members enrolled in the plan. All Medicare+Choice plans must include services covered by Parts A and B of the Original Medicare Plan. These plans can also provide additional services such as prescription medication, dental care, preventive care, and glasses. The cost for additional services depends on the specific plan. With Medicare private fee-for-service plans, no restriction is placed on which providers the beneficiary can use for services, as long as the provider is willing to accept the plan's payment. Under these plans, the beneficiary may be required to pay a premium, in addition to what is paid for Part B, and a copayment when services are rendered.

To enroll in a Medicare+Choice program, the individual must have Part A and B of the Original Medicare Plan, live in an area where a particular plan is available, and not have ESRD. Medicare pays a determined amount of money monthly to these private plans for beneficiaries' coverage. In 2002, 11 percent of Medicare beneficiaries were enrolled in a Medicare+Choice plan.

All Medicare beneficiaries, regardless of the type of plan, have the right to appeal a decision related to the amount of payment for a service, whether a particular service or item should be covered, or the length of time that a service should be provided. After filing an appeal, the beneficiary must receive a response within seventy-two hours if a delay would cause medical harm.

In addition to the right to appeal decisions, beneficiaries have a right to information, to know their treatment choices and be involved in treatment decisions, to file complaints, and to nondiscriminatory treatment that reflects sensitivity to cultural differences. Medicare is required by law to protect the privacy of medical information as set forth in the Health Insurance Portability and Accountability Act (HIPAA) of 1996.

If a person qualifies for Medicare but cannot afford to pay for Medicare deductibles and coinsurance, that person may be eligible for the Medicare Savings Programs available through the State Medical Assistance Office. If the person's income and resources are severely limited, then the individual may qualify for Medicaid in addition to Medicare.

In 2000, Medicare expenditures were $131.1 billion for Part A and $90.7 billion for Part B. Since 1965, benefits have expanded, and there has been an increase in both expenditures per person and the number of beneficiaries in the program. These factors have caused continuing concern in Congress regarding the cost and financing of Medicare. Cost-containment measures over the years have included instituting a prospective payment system for hospitals, nursing home care, and home care; providing more options through managed care organizations; and shifting services previously covered by Part A to Part B.

PERSPECTIVE AND PROSPECTS

In June, 2003, both houses of Congress passed bills to amend Medicare to include coverage for prescription medications and give individuals more choice in the selection of health insurance plans. These bills reflected Congress's attempt to monitor and improve the quality of health care services for Medicare recipients while maintaining the integrity of the Medicare Trust Fund. The resulting Part D drug benefit received mixed reviews.

—*Roberta Tierney, M.S.N., J.D., A.P.N.*
See also Aging: Extended care; American Medical Association (AMA); Department of Health and Human Services; Geriatrics and gerontology; Health care reform; Hospice; Hospitals; Terminally ill: Extended care.

FOR FURTHER INFORMATION:

Blevins, Sue A. *Medicare's Midlife Crisis*. Washington, D.C.: Cato Institute, 2001. The author provides a history of government-sponsored health insurance, the background leading to the passage of Medicare, the cost trends of Medicare, and the ongoing effort to maintain a sound and responsive program.

Medicare: The Official U.S. Government Site for People with Medicare. http://www.medicare.gov. Includes information on the quality of care provided by health care facilities approved by Medicare.

Rettenmaier, Andrew J., and Thomas R. Saving. *The Economics of Medicare Reform*. Kalamazoo, Mich.: W. E. Upjohn Institute for Employment Research, 2000. An in-depth discussion of health insurance financing; examines present costs and alternative methods of financing as applied to the Medicare program.

U.S. Department of Health and Human Services. Centers for Medicare and Medicaid Services. *Medicare and You 2010*. Washington, D.C.: Author, 2010. Updated yearly, this easy-to-understand booklet provides information about enrollment, coverage, options, and contact persons. Essential reading for those who are, or will be, eligible for Medicare benefits. Also available at http://www.medicare.gov/publications/pubs/pdf/10050.pdf.

MEDITATION

TREATMENT

ANATOMY OR SYSTEM AFFECTED: All
SPECIALTIES AND RELATED FIELDS: Alternative medicine, preventive medicine
DEFINITION: Techniques involving controlled breathing, visualization, and repeated words or phrases that are used to achieve relaxation and reduce muscle tension, which may have health benefits.

INDICATIONS AND PROCEDURES

One of the most popular techniques used in meditation is concentration, in which one focuses attention on a single object such as the function of breathing, a candle flame, or a visualized image. When attention wanders, the practitioner brings it gently back to the original focus. Sometimes a mantra, a chosen word or phrase given by a teacher or chosen by the practitioner, is repeated silently or aloud. Mantras are central to the practice of meditation. A typical mantra is the om mantra of Tibetan Buddhism.

Guided imagery utilizes listening to a voice, taped or live, that guides the practitioner to visualize a beautiful and peaceful place, where one feels calm and secure. Walking or dancing meditation focuses on movement and ritual, and the practice of yoga incorporates breathing and movement or physical postures to help relax body and mind. Soothing music may also be used with any of the techniques. Teachers recommend starting slowly with five-minute sessions, working up to twenty minutes once or twice a day.

USES AND COMPLICATIONS

Meditation techniques, which are thousands of years old, are being promoted as a benefit to health and well-being, primarily in stress-related conditions. Meditation traditionally has been and is used in a religious sense to deepen one's understanding and involvement with the spiritual, mystical, and sacred aspects of life. It is also used as an exercise in self-discovery and revelation, helping the practitioner turn inward, temporarily shutting out worldly cares and strife to find inner peace and calm. Being religious, however, is not essential to meditation; in fact, anyone can learn the techniques and reap the health benefits of this age-old practice.

Numerous studies confirm that prolonged or interpersonal stress can produce such conditions as constriction of blood vessels, pain and swelling in joints, suppression of the immune system, decreases in white blood cells and changes in their function, and high cholesterol levels. Chemicals such as adrenaline, produced when the body is under stress, can raise blood pressure, increase heart rate, and cause other harmful physiological responses when stress is persistent or sustained. Stress is also linked to many diseases and conditions, including heart attacks, diabetes, cancer, allergies, and skin disorders.

Meditation, in helping the patient to relax, reduces muscle tension and decreases the release of these harmful chemicals. A number of stress-related conditions have been shown to benefit from meditation, including chronic pain, arthritis, infertility, psoriasis, respiratory conditions such as asthma and emphysema, premenstrual syndrome (PMS), tension headaches, irritable bowel syndrome (IBS), ulcers, insomnia, and fibromyalgia.

—*Martha Oehmke Loustaunau, Ph.D.*
See also Alternative medicine; Anxiety; Biofeedback; Hypnosis; Stress; Stress reduction; Yoga.

FOR FURTHER INFORMATION:

Benson, Herbert, and Miriam Z. Klipper. *The Relaxation Response.* Updated and expanded ed. New York: Avon Books, 2000.

Harmon, Robert, and Mary Ann Myers. "Prayer and Meditation as Medical Therapies." *Physical Medicine and Rehabilitation Clinics of North America* 10, no. 3 (August, 1999): 651-662.

Kabat-Zinn, Jon. *Wherever You Go, There You Are: Mindfulness Meditation in Everyday Life.* 10th anniversary ed. New York: Hyperion, 2005.

Trivieri, Larry, Jr., and John W. Anderson, eds. *Alternative Medicine: The Definitive Guide.* 2d ed. Berkeley, Calif.: Ten Speed Press, 2002.

MELANOMA

DISEASE/DISORDER

ANATOMY OR SYSTEM AFFECTED: Skin

SPECIALTIES AND RELATED FIELDS: Dermatology, internal medicine, pathology

DEFINITION: A malignant disease which originates with the melanocytes in the skin. While there may be a variety of causes, the primary risk factor is extent of exposure to sunlight.

KEY TERMS:

dysplasia: the aberrant growth or development of cells

melanocytes: cells in the upper layer of skin which produce the pigment melanin

metastasis: the spread of cells from a primary site of cancer to areas throughout the body

---

> ### INFORMATION ON MELANOMA
>
> **CAUSES:** Exposure to ultraviolet light and resulting mutations
> **SYMPTOMS:** Nevus (usually a mole) that changes in shape, size, or pigmentation; may spread to lymphatic system and other regions
> **DURATION:** Chronic, sometimes fatal
> **TREATMENTS:** Surgery, chemotherapy, radiation, biological therapy using protein extracts from the melanoma

nevus: a pigmented site on the skin which is composed of melanocytes

CAUSES AND SYMPTOMS

Melanocytes are cells in the skin which produce the melanin, most commonly recognized as the basis of skin color. Following exposure to ultraviolet (UV) light, particularly that found in sunlight, melanocytes begin the synthesis of increased levels of pigment, some of which is transferred to the surrounding cells. The process is a response to the potential damage induced by UV light and helps disperse the damaging effects of the rays.

Ultraviolet light is relatively high in energy, and significant exposure, especially exposure sufficient to cause sunburn, is damaging to deoxyribonucleic acid (DNA), the genetic material in the cell. The genetic changes that result have the potential to produce mutations which develop into cancer. Much of current research into the biology of melanomas has involved an understanding of these molecular changes.

The first alteration in physical appearance of the site is the formation of a nevus, a benign lesion consisting of replicating melanocytes. Generally speaking, nevi do not often evolve beyond the benign stage, and they rarely progress to cancer. Depending upon the extent of mutation or the accumulation of genetic changes over time with continued exposure to sunlight, however, melanocytes within the lesion may grow increasingly dysplastic. Growth regulation is disrupted, and, on a microscopic level, they no longer appear normal. It is during this period that the first symptoms of an abnormal condition may appear.

Most melanomas start at the site of a mole. Often the initial indication a mole has progressed to a malignant form is a change in its shape, size, or pigmentation. The phrase "ABCD" is often recommended as a means to remember the symptoms: *a*symmetry, in which one side of the mole differs from the other; *b*order, in which the edge is no longer sharp and pigmentation begins to spread; *c*olor, in which the pigmentation may develop hues of different shades; and *d*iameter, in which the size of the mole increases.

Analysis of what have become malignant cells, and therefore the decision as to the course of treatment, is indicated by a staging designation ranging from stage 0 to stage IV. Stage 0 designates a melanoma that is limited to the outer layer of skin, the epidermis. Stage IV indicates that a cancer has undergone metastasis, spreading into the lymphatic system and other regions of the body.

TREATMENT AND THERAPY

Initial treatment remains the surgical removal of the melanoma itself. Since this is an aggressive form of cancer, early diagnosis, prior to the stage at which metastasis has begun, is critical. The National Cancer Institute has recommended four methods of treatment, the choice dependent upon the stage of the disease. If surgery is insufficient, usually because of metastasis, then chemotherapy remains the second choice. Chemotherapeutic drugs are either taken orally or injected directly into the bloodstream. If the tumor is localized, then the drug may be perfused directly into the local tissue. The relatively nonspecific nature of the chemotherapy often produces severe side effects.

An alternative treatment may involve radiation. Radiation therapy may be directed into the cancer either externally or from an implanted radiation source within the cancerous region itself. This form of directed treatment may help avoid the side effects of chemotherapy, but it is most effective only if the cancer is in a limited area.

In recent years, some success has been achieved using new forms of biological treatment. A cancer "vaccine" is prepared using protein extracts from the melanoma itself, the idea being that by allowing the immune system to react against the vaccine, the cancer itself may also be targeted.

PERSPECTIVE AND PROSPECTS

Melanoma is a particularly deadly form of skin cancer. While only approximately 4 percent of skin cancers are actually melanomas, this form of cancer accounts for some 80 percent of skin cancer deaths.

While research into the molecular nature of melanoma has provided significant insight into the cause and progress of the disease, at least at the molecular level, prevention remains of primary importance. Most cases result from exposure to the UV light found in sunlight. Since sensitivity to sunlight is in part a function of the level of pigmentation of the skin, individuals, especially those with light skin, must be more cognizant of the danger of overexposure to the sun. If sun exposure cannot be avoided or is desired, then people must be careful to use proper sunscreens to at least limit the level of exposure to UV rays. Whether it is the myth of the "healthy tan" or simply the psychological desire to show a tanned body, however, people will continue to expose themselves to the sun. Until such behaviors change, it remains likely that the incidence of melanoma will remain at current levels.

Since the earlier the stage of development, the better the prognosis, recognition of the ABCD warning signs is critical for those who have had extensive exposure to the sun. Current treatments for advanced or recurrent melanoma are primarily palliative, an attempt to prolong and improve the quality of life. Improved prognosis depends upon the effectiveness of new and combined forms of therapy, most notably combinations of immune therapy and chemotherapy.

—*Richard Adler, Ph.D.*

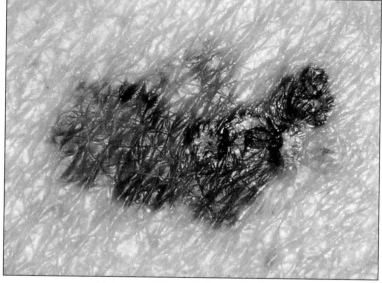

Melanoma. (National Cancer Institute)

See also Cancer; Carcinogens; Chemotherapy; Dermatology; Dermatopathology; Lesions; Malignancy and metastasis; Moles; Oncology; Radiation therapy; Skin; Skin cancer; Skin disorders; Skin lesion removal.

FOR FURTHER INFORMATION:

Gilchrest, B., et al. "The Pathogenesis of Melanoma Induced by Ultraviolet Radiation." *New England Journal of Medicine* 340, no. 17 (April 29, 1999): 1341-1348.

Gore, Martin, and Julie Newton-Bishop. *Melanoma: Critical Debates*. Malden, Mass.: Blackwell, 2002.

Melanoma Research Foundation. http://www.melanoma.org.

Miller, Arlo, and Martin C. Mihm, Jr. "Melanoma." *New England Journal of Medicine* 355, no. 1 (July 6, 2006): 51-65.

Poole, Catherine. *Melanoma: Prevention, Detection, and Treatment*. 2d ed. New Haven, Conn.: Yale University Press, 2005.

MELATONIN

BIOLOGY

ANATOMY OR SYSTEM AFFECTED: Brain, endocrine system, glands

SPECIALTIES AND RELATED FIELDS: Alternative medicine, endocrinology, neurology, pharmacology, preventive medicine

DEFINITION: A substance produced by the pineal gland that has been used as a controversial therapeutic agent.

KEY TERMS:

endocrine system: the glands that produce hormones

hormone: a substance produced in one part of the body that has effects in other parts of the body

melatonin: the hormone produced by the pineal gland

pineal gland: a small organ inside the brain that produces melatonin

STRUCTURE AND FUNCTIONS

Melatonin, also known as N-acetyl-5-methoxytryptamine, is a hormone found in a wide variety of living organisms. In vertebrates (animals with backbones), including humans, it is produced by the pineal gland. The pineal gland is located deep within the center of the brain. Although it is inside the brain, it is considered part of the endocrine system rather than the nervous system. In humans, the pineal gland is a gray or white organ less than 1 centimeter long and shaped like a pinecone.

The pineal gland produces varying amounts of melatonin in response to changes in light. Light inhibits the production of melatonin, and darkness stimulates it. In some small animals, light reaches the pineal gland directly through the skull. In larger animals, including humans, information about lightness and darkness is transmitted by the nervous system from the eyes to the suprachiasmatic nucleus, a cluster of nerve cells in a region of the brain known as the hypothalamus. The suprachiasmatic nucleus regulates the secretion of melatonin by the pineal gland.

Melatonin is believed to be involved in regulating the sleep cycle in response to changes in light. Because the amount of melatonin produced by the pineal gland declines sharply at puberty, it is believed to be involved in the development of the reproductive system. Because melatonin production continues to decline with age, some researchers believe that it is associated with the process of aging.

DISORDERS AND DISEASES

Disorders of melatonin production other than its normal decline with age are rare. Tumors of the pineal gland may reduce melatonin production. Some evidence suggests that this may lead to premature aging. Children with tumors of the pineal gland may reach puberty at a very early age.

Some researchers suggest that the normal decline in melatonin production with age is associated with diseases of the elderly. Animal studies suggest that loss of melatonin is associated with increased cell damage. Melatonin is believed to act as an antioxidant, a substance that protects cells from free radicals, which are produced when cells use oxygen. Cell damage has been linked to a large number of diseases of the elderly, including various forms of cancer, heart disease, and Alzheimer's disease.

Based on this evidence, melatonin has been used to treat and prevent a wide variety of illnesses. In the 1990's, melatonin became widely used in the United States. Because it was classified as a dietary supplement rather than as a drug, it was available without a prescription and with little government regulation. While some researchers suggested caution until more was known about melatonin, others suggested taking small daily doses of the hormone to slow down the aging process. Popular books such as *The Melatonin Miracle* (1995), by Walter Pierpaoli, William Regelson, and Carol Colman, claim that melatonin can stimulate the immune system, prevent cancer and heart disease, improve sexual relations, reduce the effects of stress, act as a contraceptive, and add years to the human life span. Critics argue that these claims are greatly exaggerated.

The least controversial suggested use for melatonin is as a sleeping aid. Human studies have indicated that melatonin is safe and effective for this use. Unlike many other sleeping pills, melatonin seems to have no effect on normal sleep patterns and few side effects. Melatonin has also been shown to be effective in treating jet lag, the difficulty that travelers have adjusting to a new time zone.

Critics of routine melatonin use point out that little is known about its long-term effects. They also point to evidence that some people may experience short-term side effects such as nightmares, headaches, daytime sleepiness, and mild depression. A major concern is the lack of regulation of melatonin products, leading to the possibility that other, unknown substances may be present.

Even the most optimistic proponents of melatonin suggest certain precautions. Many products contain more melatonin than researchers believe is necessary, leading to the possibility of a greater risk of side effects with no increase in benefit. Melatonin should only be taken at bedtime to avoid unwanted sleepiness. It should not be used by children, who already produce high levels of melatonin. It should not be used by pregnant women because its effect on the fetus is unknown. Because it is believed to stimulate the immune system, melatonin should be avoided in people with severe allergies, autoimmune disorders, or cancer of the immune system.

PERSPECTIVE AND PROSPECTS

The pineal gland was known to exist in ancient times. It was first described scientifically by the Greek physician Galen in the second century. The French philosopher René Descartes (1596-1650) suggested that it was the location of the human soul. The true function of the pineal gland remained unknown until the middle of the twentieth century.

Melatonin was discovered in 1958 and first described as a hormone in 1963. Research into its effects began in the 1970's and 1980's. Interest in this hormone increased dramatically in 1995, with the publication of several books and articles publicizing its possible benefits. Research on melatonin is expected to continue for many years, particularly in regard to its long-term effects.

—*Rose Secrest*

See also Aging; Antioxidants; Brain; Chronobiology; Endocrine disorders; Endocrine glands; Endocrinology; Endocrinology, pediatric; Glands; Hormone therapy; Hormones; Light therapy; Pharmacology; Sleep disorders.

FOR FURTHER INFORMATION:

Brzezinski, Amnon. "Melatonin in Humans." *New England Journal of Medicine* 336, no. 3 (January 16, 1997): 186-195. Discusses the evidence that melatonin has a role in the biologic regulation of circadian rhythms, sleep, and mood, and perhaps in reproduction, tumor growth, and aging.

Goodman, H. Maurice. *Basic Medical Endocrinology*. 4th ed. Boston: Academic Press/Elsevier, 2009. Focuses on research advances in the understanding of hormones involved in regulating most aspects of bodily functions. Includes coverage of the pineal gland and its regulatory principles.

Holt, Richard I. G., and Neil A. Hanley. *Essential Endocrinology and Diabetes*. 5th ed. Malden, Mass.: Blackwell, 2007. This text addresses the field of endocrinology, describing the physiology of the endocrine glands and the hormones that they produce. Includes an index.

"Melatonin: Questions, Facts, Mysteries." *University of California, Berkeley, Wellness Letter* 16, no. 8 (May, 2000): 1-2. Argues that too little is known about the dosage and health effects of melatonin.

Olcese, James, ed. *Melatonin After Four Decades: An Assessment of Its Potential*. New York: Kluwer Academic/Plenum, 1999. Nearly sixty contributions review the research advances made in the understanding of melatonin's role in health and disease and discuss the future uses of melatonin.

Pandi-Perumal, S. R., and Daniel P. Cardinali, eds. *Melatonin: Biological Basis of Its Function in Health and Disease*. Georgetown, Tex.: Landes Bioscience, 2006. Wide-ranging chapters explore the latest research on melatonin.

MEMORY LOSS
DISEASE/DISORDER

ANATOMY OR SYSTEM AFFECTED: Brain, nervous system, psychic-emotional system

SPECIALTIES AND RELATED FIELDS: Geriatrics and gerontology, neurology, psychiatry, psychology

DEFINITION: Total or limited impairment of memory that may be sudden or gradual.

CAUSES AND SYMPTOMS

Memory impairment is a common problem, and often a concern among older individuals. Memory problems are not, however, restricted to older adults. They may occur at any age and may be attributable to numerous conditions and behaviors, including the use of alcohol and other drugs. Memory loss occurs in various degrees and may be associated with other evidence of brain dysfunction and other physical and emotional problems. Memory loss may be partial, limited to events immediately before or after a traumatic event. Memory loss may also be complete. Amnesia is the term used to describe complete memory loss. Memory loss may also be permanent or temporary, or may vacillate, with a person slipping in and out of being able to remember appropriately.

Benign senescent forgetfulness. In this condition, the memory deficit affects mostly recent events, and although a source of frustration, it seldom interferes with the individual's professional activities or social life. An important feature of benign forgetfulness is that it is selective and affects only trivial, unimportant facts. For example, one may misplace the car keys or forget to return a phone call, respond to a letter, or pay a bill. Cashing a check or telephoning someone with whom one is particularly keen to talk, however, will not be forgotten. The person is aware of the memory deficit, and written notes often are used as reminders. Patients with benign forgetfulness have no other evidence of brain dysfunction and maintain their ability to make valid judgments.

Dementia. In dementia, the memory impairment is global, does not discriminate between important and trivial facts, and interferes with the person's ability to pursue professional or social activities. Patients with dementia find it difficult to adapt to changes in the workplace, such as the introduction of computers. They also find it difficult to continue with their hobbies and interests.

The hallmark of dementia is no awareness of the memory deficit, except in the very early stages of the disease. This is an important difference between dementia and benign forgetfulness. Although patients with early dementia may write themselves notes, they usually forget to check these reminders or may misinterpret them. For example, a man with dementia who is invited for dinner at a friend's house may write a note to that effect and leave it in a prominent place. He may then go to his host's home several evenings in succession because he has forgotten that he already has fulfilled this social en-

gagement. As the disease progresses, patients are no longer aware of their memory deficit.

In dementia, the memory deficit does not occur in isolation but is accompanied by other evidence of brain dysfunction, which in very early stages can be detected only by specialized neuropsychological tests. As the condition progresses, these deficits become readily apparent. The patient is often disoriented regarding time and may telephone relatives or friends very late at night or not realize the time of day. As the disease progresses, the disorientation affects the patient's environment: A woman with dementia may wander outside her house and be unable to find her way back, or she may repeatedly ask to be taken back home when she is already there. In later stages, patients may not be able to recognize people whom they should know: A man may think that his son is his father or that his wife is his mother. In fact, it is possible for the patient to not even recognize his or her own reflection in a mirror. This stage is particularly distressing to the caregivers. Patients with dementia may often exhibit impaired judgment. They may go outside the house inappropriately dressed or at inappropriate times, or they may purchase the same item repeatedly or make donations that are disproportional to their funds. Alzheimer's disease is one of the most common causes of dementia in older people.

Multiple infarct dementia. Multiple infarct dementia is caused by the destruction of brain cells by repeated strokes. Sometimes these strokes are so small that neither the patient nor the relatives are aware of their occurrence. When many strokes occur and significant brain tissue is destroyed, the patient may exhibit symptoms of dementia. Usually, however, most of these strokes are quite obvious because they are associated with weakness or paralysis in a part of the body. One of the characteristic features of multiple infarct dementia is that its onset is sudden and its progression is by steps. Every time a stroke occurs, the patient's condition dete-

---

INFORMATION ON MEMORY LOSS

CAUSES: Aging, head trauma, certain diseases, repeated strokes, depression

SYMPTOMS: Vary; can include benign forgetfulness, disorientation and impaired judgment, weakness or paralysis in body part

DURATION: Acute to chronic

TREATMENTS: Varies; can include medication, surgery

riorates. This is followed by a period during which little or no deterioration develops until another stroke occurs, at which time the patient's condition deteriorates further. Very rarely, the stroke affects only the memory center, in which case the patient's sole problem is amnesia. Multiple infarct dementia and dementia resulting from Alzheimer's disease should be differentiated from other treatable conditions which also may cause memory impairment, disorientation, and poor judgment. It is important to recognize, however, that both conditions may exist in the same person.

Depression. Depression may cause memory impairment as a result of problems related to concentration and attention. This condition is quite common and at times is so difficult to differentiate from dementia that the term "pseudo-dementia" is used to describe it. One of the main differences between depression that presents the symptoms of dementia and dementia itself is insight into the memory deficit. Whereas patients with dementia are usually oblivious of their deficit and not distressed (except those in the early stages), those with depression are nearly always aware of their deficit and are quite distressed. Patients with depression tend to be withdrawn and apathetic and to show a marked disturbance of affect. In contrast, those with dementia demonstrate emotional blandness and some degree of emotional lability, or a lack of stableness in expressed emotion. One of the problems characteristic of depressed patients is their difficulty in concentrating. This is typified by poor cooperation and effort in carrying out tasks with a variable degree of achievement, coupled with considerable anxiety. Further, anxiety may disrupt memory, compounding any other problems.

Head trauma. Amnesia is sometimes seen in patients who have sustained a head injury. The extent of the amnesia is usually proportional to the severity of the injury. In most cases, the complete recovery of the patient's memory occurs, except for the events just preceding and following the injury. With traumatic brain injury, however, amnesia may not be the only symptom. Other memory deficits can be observed and experienced. As such, following any head injury, evaluation is advisable, even if the injury is a closed head injury.

PERSPECTIVE AND PROSPECTS

Memory impairment is a serious condition that can interfere with one's ability to function independently, and sometimes at all. Any time that memory loss develops, identification of underlying causes should occur because a treatable cause may be found, preventing further memory loss or perhaps reducing the amount of memory loss. In some cases, proper treatment may even reverse memory loss, such as in some conditions related to alcohol-related memory loss. Research examining memory continues to differentiate among conditions involving memory loss. Efforts to better assess conditions and make distinctions earlier in the process of such conditions remain important. The earlier that problems such as dementia can be identified, for instance, the earlier treatment may be able to occur, potentially increasing quality of life.

Research has also identified ways to slow the progression of some diseases related to memory loss. As the root causes of memory impairment and brain changes are understood, future research may be able to arrest the progress of amnesia and memory loss and even to treat dementias now considered irreversible, such as Alzheimer's disease and multiple infarct dementia. Exciting research in the area of inflammation and immunological functioning may prove to be productive.

*—Ronald C. Hamdy, M.D.,
and Louis A. Cancellaro, M.D.;
updated by Nancy A. Piotrowski, Ph.D.*

See also Addiction; Aging; Alcoholism; Alzheimer's disease; Amnesia; Anxiety; Brain; Brain damage; Brain disorders; Club drugs; Concussion; Dementias; Depression; Geriatrics and gerontology; Head and neck disorders; Intoxication; Marijuana; Pick's disease; Psychiatry; Psychiatry, geriatric; Shock therapy; Strokes; Substance abuse.

FOR FURTHER INFORMATION:

Hamdy, Ronald C., J. M. Turnbull, and M. M. Lancaster, eds. *Alzheimer's Disease: A Handbook for Caregivers.* 3d ed. St. Louis, Mo.: Mosby Year Book, 1998. This handbook offers nursing tips for people caring for Alzheimer's patients. Includes bibliographical references and an index.

Masoro, Edward J., and Steven N. Austad, eds. *Handbook of the Biology of Aging.* 6th ed. Boston: Academic Press/Elsevier, 2007. This is part of a handbook on aging series. This edition significantly revises earlier versions of this work. Varied theories of aging are discussed, along with additions exploring whether diseases associated with aging are necessarily part of the aging process.

Mendez, Mario F., and Jeffrey L. Cummings. *Dementia: A Clinical Approach.* 3d ed. Philadelphia:

Butterworth-Heinemann, 2003. This is a standard textbook, comprehensively presenting the clinical, diagnostic, therapeutic, and basic science aspects of the dementias. This edition has been revised and updated with nearly one thousand new references and revised descriptions of all major dementia syndromes.

O'Brien, John, et al., eds. *Dementia*. 3d ed. New York: Oxford University Press, 2006. Text that covers advances in the research of degenerative disorders, current diagnostic criteria, rating scales, investigations, neurobiological mechanisms, therapeutic options and services, and all aspects of management, including psychosocial and psychological approaches, among other topics.

West, Robin L., and Jan D. Sinnott, eds. *Everyday Memory and Aging*. New York: Springer, 1992. This work discusses the methodology of research into the human memory. Focuses on the changes in memory that occur naturally with age, as well as those that are brought about by various forms of dementia in the older individual.

MÉNIÈRE'S DISEASE
DISEASE/DISORDER
ALSO KNOWN AS: Endolymphatic hydrops
ANATOMY OR SYSTEM AFFECTED: Ears
SPECIALTIES AND RELATED FIELDS: Audiology, otorhinolaryngology
DEFINITION: A disease of the inner ear caused by excessive pressure in the cochlear fluid. Its symptoms are hearing loss, tinnitus (ringing in the ear), nausea, and episodes of vertigo.

CAUSES AND SYMPTOMS
Ménière's disease results from excess pressure caused by surplus fluids in the cochlea (inner ear) or the semicircular canals concerned with the sense of balance. Typically this condition results when the structure that reabsorbs excess fluid from the inner ear ceases to function properly. The cause may be an infection, allergies, a spasm of one of the tiny blood vessels in the semicircular canal, or a small hemorrhage in the cochlear duct. Ménière's syndrome affects both the vestibular nerve (causing attacks of vertigo) and the auditory nerve (causing hearing impairment).

The classic symptoms of Ménière's disease are tinnitus, a sensation of fullness in the ears, dizziness, hearing impairment (including fluctuating distortions of sound), and a rapidly progressing loss of hearing.

> ## INFORMATION ON MÉNIÈRE'S DISEASE
>
> **CAUSES:** Excess fluid in inner ear as result of infection, allergies, blood vessel spasm, or small hemorrhage in cochlear duct
>
> **SYMPTOMS:** Ringing and fullness in ears, dizziness, hearing impairment, rapidly progressing hearing loss, vertigo, loss of equilibrium, nausea and vomiting, rhythmic jerking motion of eyes, sometimes deafness
>
> **DURATION:** Often chronic with recurrent attacks lasting thirty minutes to several hours
>
> **TREATMENTS:** Diuretics, blood vessel dilators, low-salt diet, motion sickness medications, antihistamines, bed rest; in severe cases, destruction of cochlea through surgery or ultrasound

The attacks are typically abrupt and momentary, but recur frequently. Dizziness may range from a mild whirling sensation and unsteady balance to severe attacks of vertigo and complete loss of equilibrium accompanied by nausea and vomiting. The eyes often show a rhythmic jerking motion.

TREATMENT AND THERAPY
The treatment selected for Ménière's disease depends on the theoretical diagnosed cause, as no single remedy is universally successful. Infections and allergies can often be treated by diuretic drugs, sedative and blood vessel dilators, or low-salt diets, all intended to reduce cochlear fluid pressure. Motion sickness and antihistamine drugs may be used to treat the symptoms. Since attacks of violent dizziness can occur suddenly, the affected person must immediately lie down to avoid falling. During a severe attack, the patient should be confined to bed since any movement of the head produces the disturbing sensation that the room is rotating. A bout may last several weeks, during which time bed rest and medication are recommended. Attacks, which recur at irregular intervals of weeks, or months, may last a half hour to several hours. Mild attacks usually disappear within a year, but more severe cases require a medical regimen. In some cases surgery may be necessary to decompress the cochlea and/or semicircular canals. If all other medical measures fail, the disability is severe, and deafness is well advanced, destruction of the cochlea by surgery or ultrasound may be a last resort.

PERSPECTIVE AND PROSPECTS

Ménière's disease was first described and recorded in detail in 1861 by French physician Prosper Ménière. Formerly only the most severe and disabling cases were treated surgically because the operation required destruction of the hearing nerve. Since the advent of microsurgical instruments it has become possible to separate the hearing and balance filaments in the main nerve and clip only the balance filaments when the problem is in the semicircular canals. It is also now possible to utilize ultrasonic beams to selectively destroy balance filaments without damaging the sensitive auditory nerves.

—*George R. Plitnik, Ph.D.*

See also Audiology; Balance disorders; Dizziness and fainting; Ear infections and disorders; Ears; Hearing; Hearing loss; Nausea and vomiting; Otorhinolaryngology; Tinnitus.

FOR FURTHER INFORMATION:

Griffith, H. Winter. *Complete Guide to Symptoms, Illness, and Surgery.* Revised and updated by Stephen Moore and Kenneth Yoder. 5th ed. New York: Perigee, 2006.

Harris, Jeffrey P., ed. *Ménière's Disease.* The Hague, the Netherlands: Kugler, 1999.

Paparella, Michael M., ed. *Pathogenesis of Ménière's Disease: Treatment Considerations.* Philadelphia: W. B. Saunders, 2002.

Weber, Peter C., ed. *Ménière's Disease.* Philadelphia: W. B. Saunders, 1997.

MENINGITIS

DISEASE/DISORDER

ANATOMY OR SYSTEM AFFECTED: Brain, head, nervous system, spine

SPECIALTIES AND RELATED FIELDS: Emergency medicine, neurology, public health

DEFINITION: An inflammation of the meninges of the brain and spinal cord.

CAUSES AND SYMPTOMS

The meninges is the three-layered covering of the spinal cord and brain. The layers are the outer dura mater, inner pia mater, and middle arachnoid. Meningitis is the inflammation or infection of the arachnoid and pia mater. It is characterized by severe headaches, vomiting, and pain and stiffness in the neck. These symptoms may be preceded by an upper respiratory infection. The age of the patient may affect which signs and symptoms are displayed. Newborns may exhibit either fever or hypothermia, along with lethargy or irritability, disinterest in feeding, and abdominal distension. In infants, examination may find bulging of the fontanelles (the soft areas between the bones of the skull found in newborns). The elderly may show lethargy, confusion, or disorientation. As pressure in the skull increases, nausea and vomiting may occur. With meningococcal meningitis, a rash of pinpoint-sized or larger dots appears.

Most cases of meningitis are the result of bacterial infection. These cases are sometimes referred to as septic meningitis. The bacteria invade the subarachnoid space and may have traveled from another site of infection, having caused pneumonia, cellulitis, or an ear infection. It is unclear if the bacteria make their way from the original area of infection to the meninges by the bloodstream or the lymphatic system. Once they have entered the subarachnoid space, they divide without inhibition since there is no impediment posed by defensive cells. In other words, the cerebrospinal fluid (CSF) contains very few white blood cells to inactivate the bacteria. More rarely, some bacteria may be introduced into the area by neurological damage or surgical invasion.

The most common cause of bacterial meningitis in adults and older children is meningococcus (*Neisseria meningitidis*). It is a diplococcus that typically does its damage inside the cell. The incidence of meningococcal meningitis is 2 to 3 cases per 100,000 people per year, and it most often affects schoolchildren and military recruits. *Haemophilus influenzae* is the most common culprit infecting babies between two months and one year of age. Complications or residual effects often follow bacterial meningitis. These may include deafness, delayed-onset epilepsy, hydrocephalus, cerebritis, and brain abscess. In addition, for several weeks after resolution of the disease the patient may experience headaches, dizziness, and lethargy.

INFORMATION ON MENINGITIS

CAUSES: Bacterial or viral infection

SYMPTOMS: Severe headaches, vomiting, pain and stiffness in the neck, upper-respiratory infection, lethargy, confusion, disorientation

DURATION: Acute

TREATMENTS: Antibiotics, surgery, supportive therapy (blood transfusions, subdural taps)

Aseptic meningitis is meningitis attributable to causes other than bacteria. These causes include neurotropic viruses, such as those that cause poliomyelitis or encephalitis; other viruses such as those that cause mumps, herpes, mononucleosis, hepatitis, chickenpox, and measles; spirochetes; bacterial products from brain abscesses or previous cases of bacterial meningitis; and foreign bodies, such as those found in the air or chemicals, in the CSF. Most cases of aseptic meningitis are viral in origin. The signs and symptoms are similar to those of bacterial meningitis. Onset is usually gradual, with symptoms starting mildly. The slight headache becomes worse over the course of several days, the neck becomes characteristically stiff, and photophobia (dislike of bright light) occurs.

Tuberculous meningitis is different from most other forms of meningitis because it lasts longer, has a higher mortality rate, and affects the CSF less. It mostly strikes children and is usually the result of a bacillus infection from the respiratory tract or the lymphatic system that has relocated to the meninges. When the bacilli are translocated to the central nervous system, they form tubercles that release an exudate. If tuberculous meningitis is left untreated, death may occur within three weeks. Even with treatment, it may result in neurologic abnormalities.

Treatment and Therapy

If meningitis is suspected, the first testing procedure is an examination of the CSF. To obtain CSF, a lumbar puncture, sometimes called a spinal tap, is made. Opening pressure, protein and glucose concentrations, total cell count, and cultures of microbes are determined. In cases of meningitis, the CSF is almost always cloudy and generally comes out under higher-than-normal pressure. An elevated white blood cell count in the CSF would be one indication that the patient has bacterial meningitis; another would be lowered serum glucose but slightly raised protein concentration, especially albumin. About 90 percent of bacterial meningitis cases show gram-positive staining. The examination of this slightly atypical fluid, along with presenting symptoms and signs, gives the diagnostician some confidence in diagnosing meningitis accurately. Further cultures and a repeat puncture are necessary to pinpoint the kind of meningitis and to check the effect of the treatment.

Bacterial meningitis should be treated promptly with antibiotics specific for the causative bacteria. The suc-

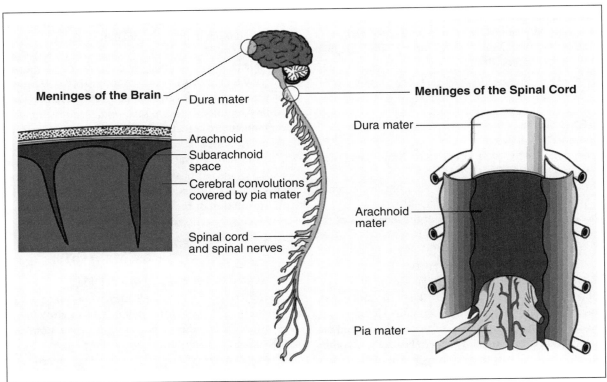

Meninges of the Brain
- Dura mater
- Arachnoid
- Subarachnoid space
- Cerebral convolutions covered by pia mater
- Spinal cord and spinal nerves

Meninges of the Spinal Cord
- Dura mater
- Arachnoid mater
- Pia mater

Meningitis attacks the meninges of the brain or the spinal cord or both.

cess of treatment is contingent on the magnitude of the bacterial count and the quickness with which the bacteria can be controlled. Virtually all bacterial cases are treated with ampicillin or penicillin. Cases aggressively treated with very large doses of antibiotics are the most successful. If antibiotics do not destroy the areas of infection, surgery should be considered. Surgery is especially effective if meningitis is recurrent or persistent. Viral meningitis may be treated with adenine arabinoside if the cause is herpes simplex. No medication will kill other viruses causing the infection. The condition usually resolves itself in a few days, even without treatment. When necessary, supportive therapy should be employed, including blood transfusions. Young children with open fontanelles often undergo subdural taps to relieve pressure caused by CSF buildup.

Mortality rates in meningitis vary with age and the pathogen responsible. Those suffering from meningococcal meningitis (without overwhelming bacterial numbers) have a fatality rate of only 3 percent. Newborns suffering from gram-negative meningitis, however, have a 70 percent mortality rate. In addition, the younger the patient, the more likely the incidence of lasting neurological damage.

There are two basic ways to prevent meningitis: chemoprophylaxis for likely candidates of the disease and active immunization. Those exposed to a known case are usually treated with rifampin for four days; rifampin is especially useful in inactivating *H. influenzae*. Active immunization is suggested for toddlers eighteen to twenty-four months of age, especially for those in situations where there is a high risk of exposure (such as day care centers).

—*Iona C. Baldridge*

See also Abscesses; Antibiotics; Bacterial infections; Brain; Brain damage; Brain disorders; Chickenpox; Encephalitis; Hepatitis; Herpes; Immunization and vaccination; Lumbar puncture; Measles; Mononucleosis; Mumps; Nervous system; Neuroimaging; Neurology; Neurology, pediatric; Poliomyelitis; Spinal cord disorders; Spine, vertebrae, and disks; Viral infections; West Nile virus.

FOR FURTHER INFORMATION:

American Medical Association. *American Medical Association Family Medical Guide.* 4th rev. ed. Hoboken, N.J.: John Wiley & Sons, 2004.

Bloom, Floyd E., M. Flint Beal, and David J. Kupfer, eds. *The Dana Guide to Brain Health.* New York: Dana Press, 2006.

Ferreiros, C. *Emerging Strategies in the Fight Against Meningitis.* New York: Garland Science, 2002.

Meningitis Research Foundation. http://www.meningitis.org.

Shmaefsky, Brian. *Meningitis.* Rev. ed. Philadelphia: Chelsea House, 2010.

Tunkel, Allan R. *Bacterial Meningitis.* Philadelphia: Lippincott Williams & Wilkins, 2001.

Wilson, Michael, Brian Henderson, and Rod McNab. *Bacterial Disease Mechanisms: An Introduction to Cellular Microbiology.* New York: Cambridge University Press, 2002.

MENOPAUSE

BIOLOGY

ANATOMY OR SYSTEM AFFECTED: Psychic-emotional system, reproductive system, uterus

SPECIALTIES AND RELATED FIELDS: Endocrinology, gynecology

DEFINITION: The time during a woman's life when her ability to conceive ends; menopause is marked by irregular, and eventually complete cessation of, menstruation, accompanied by hormonal changes such as the dramatic reduction in the body's production of estrogen.

KEY TERMS:

climacteric: that phase in the aging process of women marking the transition from the reproductive stage of life to the nonreproductive stage

estrogen: the female hormones estradiol and estrone, produced by the ovaries and responsible for the development of secondary sex characteristics

exogenous: originating outside an organ or part

osteoporosis: a condition characterized by a loss of bone density and an increased susceptibility to fractures

progesterone: a hormone, released by the corpus luteum and placenta, responsible for changes in the uterine endometrium

PROCESS AND EFFECTS

The word "menopause" comes from two Greek words meaning "month" and "cessation." It is used medically to mean a cessation of, not a "pause" in, menstrual periods. Technically, the menopause begins the moment a woman has had her final menstrual period; until then, her menstrual periods may have shown a wide variety of irregularities, including missed periods.

Medical experts refer to the time when the body is noticeably preparing for the menopause as the perimenopause, which can begin anywhere from five to ten years before the menopause. While estrogen levels begin to decrease gradually, periods are normal but memory may be less sharp and mood swings may occur. During that time, a woman still experiences menstrual periods, but they are erratic. Some women stop menstruating suddenly, without irregularities; however, they are in the minority. For some women, signs of the menopause, such as hot flashes, may begin during the perimenopause. For even more women, such signs begin, or at least increase in intensity, at the menopause.

The term "climacteric" covers a longer span and includes all the years of diminishing estrogen production, both before and after a woman's last menstrual period. Some experts believe that women may undergo declines in their levels of estrogen even when they are in their late twenties; almost all experts believe that estrogen levels drop at least by a woman's mid-thirties, and the process accelerates in the late forties.

The average age at which the menopause occurs in women from the United States is 51.4 years, with the usual range between ages forty-five and fifty-five. For some it occurs much earlier, for others much later. Only 8 percent of women reach the menopause before age forty, and only 5 percent continue to menstruate after age fifty-three. A very few have menstrual periods until they are sixty.

Even after the menopause, the climacteric continues. Declining hormonal levels bring more changes, until the situation stabilizes. A decade or more of noticeable changes can take place before the climacteric is completed. Unlike the climacteric, the menopause itself is usually considered completed after one full year without a period. After two years, a woman can be reasonably certain that her periods have ceased permanently. The signs and symptoms of the menopause, however, can linger for years longer.

Starting in her mid-forties, a woman's ovaries gradually lose their ability to respond to the follicle-stimulating hormone (FSH), which is released by the pituitary into the blood, triggering the release of estrogen from the ovaries. A few eggs do remain even after menstrual flows have ceased, and the production of estrogen does not stop completely after the menopause; in much smaller amounts, it continues to be released by the adrenal glands, in fatty tissue, and in the brain. At the menopause, however, the blood levels of estrogen are drastically reduced—by about 75 percent.

About two to four years before the menopause, many women stop ovulating or ovulate irregularly or only oc-

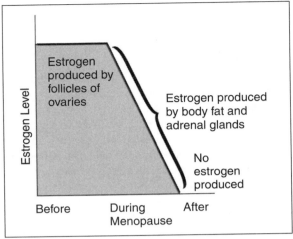

During the menopause, which may last for several years, estrogen production diminishes; after the menopause, estrogen is no longer produced by the body.

casionally. Although almost all the follicles enclosing the eggs are depleted by this time, the ovaries continue to produce estrogen. Estrogen continues to build up the endometrium (the lining of the uterus), but without ovulation no progesterone is produced to shed the extra lining. Therefore, instead of regular periods, a woman may bleed at unexpected times as the extra lining is shed sporadically.

During the perimenopause, menstrual periods may be late or early, longer than usual or shorter, and lighter than before or heavier. They may disappear for several months, then reappear for several more. It has been noted that in 15 to 20 percent of women the typical menopausal symptoms, sometimes accompanied by noticeable mood swings similar to premenstrual tension, begin during the perimenopausal period.

According to the National Institutes of Health (NIH), about 80 percent of women experience mild or no signs of the menopause. The rest have symptoms troublesome enough to seek medical attention. The two most important factors in determining how a woman will fare are probably the rate of decline of her female hormones and the final degree of hormone depletion. A woman's genes, general health, lifetime quality of diet, level of activity, and psychological acceptance of aging are also major influences. The most severe symptoms occur in women who lose their ovaries through surgery or radiation when they are perimenopausal.

When only the uterus is removed (hysterectomy) and the ovaries remain intact, menstrual periods stop but all other aspects of the menopause occur in the same way and at the same age. When only one ovary is removed, the menopause occurs normally. If both ovaries are removed, a complete menopause takes place abruptly, sometimes with intense effects. Women who have had a tubal ligation to prevent pregnancy will experience a normal menopause because tubal ligation does not affect ovaries, the uterus, or hormonal secretions.

Although experts disagree about the causes of a variety of symptoms that may appear at the menopause, there is no disagreement about the fact that the majority of women experience hot flashes, or flushes. For two out of three women, hot flashes can start well before the last menstruation. Generally, however, hot flashes increase dramatically at menopause and continue to occur, with intermittent breaks (sometimes lasting several months), for five years or so.

While hot flashes are not dangerous, they are uncomfortable. Many women have only three or four episodes a day—or even a week—and hardly notice them. Others have as many as fifty severe flashes a day. The intense waves of heat generally last several minutes, but some unusual flashes have been reported to last as long as an hour. Usually there is some perspiration; with a severe flash, there is heavy perspiration. Because the blood vessels dilate (expand) and then contract, the hot flash is often followed by chills, even intense shivering. Since the flashes are usually worse at night, they can cause insomnia.

Other vasomotor symptoms can also appear with the menopause. Experts believe that they are the result of disruptions of the same mechanisms—vasomotor instability—that are manifested as hot flashes. Palpitations, which are distinct and rapid heartbeats, may also occur. A woman may experience dizziness or may feel faint or nauseated at times. She may have peculiar sensations in her arms and hands, especially her fingers. Some feel these sensations as tingling, or pins and needles, while others say that their fingers occasionally feel numb. One of the oddest, most frightening sensations associated with the menopause is formication, a feeling of insects crawling over the skin.

Headaches, depression, mood swings, insomnia, and weight gain often affect women at the menopause and may be related to the body's hormonal readjustments. Insomnia is second only to hot flashes as the symptom that causes women to seek out their doctors' help at the menopause. The hypothalamus controls sleep as well as temperature and hormone production; insomnia is caused by changes in sleep patterns and brain waves from the same hypothalamic disturbances that result in

the hot flashes and an overstimulated central nervous system.

COMPLICATIONS AND DISORDERS

During the menopause, the walls of the vagina become smooth and dry and produce less lubrication, producing a condition called atrophic vaginitis. It has been assumed that this condition is attributable to a lack of estrogen. Despite doubts concerning the relationship between circulating estrogen and objective measures of vaginal atrophy, estrogen (often topical) is frequently prescribed and effectively used in the alleviation or elimination of symptoms.

One of the problems that women encounter with the menopause is calcium deficiency. Many experts believe that before the menopause a woman requires a minimum of 1,000 milligrams of calcium a day in food or supplements. At the menopause, however, a woman who is not taking estrogen needs 1,500 milligrams of calcium a day. Since it is very difficult to obtain these daily allotments from food without consuming considerable amounts of milk or milk products, calcium supplements are often recommended for menopausal and postmenopausal women.

If the calcium deficiency is allowed to persist, osteoporosis, a loss of bone density that can lead to dangerous fractures, can result. Osteoporosis is known to have less of a damaging effect on women who are somewhat overweight because estrogen continues to be produced in fatty tissues after the menopause. Cigarettes, alcohol, and caffeine increase bone loss because they interfere with the body's ability to absorb calcium. A well-balanced diet, calcium supplements, and regular exercise—especially weight-bearing exercise—are effective ways of controlling osteoporosis. Hormone therapy is another means of coping with osteoporosis brought on by the menopause. Since nearly half of all women do not develop osteoporosis, however, many physicians do not believe that administering estrogen therapy to combat this disease is worth the risks, except in women at high risk for osteoporosis.

Although estrogen was isolated as a substance in the 1920's, the modern study of hormones—how they work, where they are produced, what their benefits are—began in the 1940's. Originally, estrogen was administered cautiously to women who had lost their ovaries through surgery and to those with severe distress after the menopause. It was not until the 1960's that estrogen replacement therapy became widespread, however, when books such as Robert A. Wilson's *Feminine*

Forever (1966) promoted its use as the newfound "fountain of youth" for women. The replacement of estrogen was suddenly fashionable, with the hormone being viewed as a miracle drug that could keep women looking and feeling youthful well into their later years. Physicians began prescribing it for women well before the menopause, and it was recommended for use throughout life. Often, large doses were prescribed.

By the mid-1970's, twenty million women in the United States were taking estrogen. A decade later, however, the number had fallen to four or five million. Beginning in 1975, research studies began documenting dramatic increases—sometimes as high as 500 percent—in cases of cancer of the lining of the endometrium among women taking estrogen, compared with those not taking it. Other studies at that time found higher rates of breast cancer as well as other problems, such as gallbladder conditions, among women taking estrogen.

Some studies found the overall risk of contracting uterine cancer increased 350 percent for women who took estrogen for a year or more. Some women who were on the therapy for long periods were judged to be as much as 100 percent more likely to contract uterine cancer. Furthermore, contrary to expectations, some studies claimed that the risk persisted even ten years after the estrogen use was discontinued. Other studies also found that the risk of cancer persisted, though for a shorter period.

These studies were based on replacement therapy using estrogen only. Estrogen stimulates the growth of cells in the endometrium, which is one of the aspects of the development of cancer. Consequently, a treatment was developed in which estrogen was combined with a form of progesterone in an effort to reduce the risk of uterine cancer and other diseases. Today, the most widely used regimen calls for estrogen in the lowest effective dose three weeks each month. During the last week to thirteen days of this therapy, a form of progesterone called progestin is added, and then both hormones are stopped. Uterine bleeding, similar to that of a menstrual period, may occur, allowing the progesterone to break down any excess buildup of cells in the endometrium.

In the past, a number of women were given hormone therapy to alleviate menopausal symptoms, and they may have received longer-term therapy with the intention of preventing cardiac disease and osteoporosis. Some clinicians prescribed estrogen therapy for women with severe symptoms after a surgical menopause.

In the early twenty-first century, however, the use of hormone therapy—either long-term or short-term—was questioned. A study called the Women's Health Initiative, funded by the NIH, compared thousands of women who took combination hormone therapy to women who were given placebos. Those on the combination treatment had an increased risk for heart disease, stroke, and blood clots in the lungs. As a result, organizations such as the American Heart Association, the American College of Obstetricians and Gynecologists, and the North American Menopause Society recommended that combination therapy not be used for the prevention of cardiac disease, osteoporosis, or dementia. Today, combination hormone therapy is offered only to women with vasomotor symptoms (hot flashes and associated discomforts) that are severe enough to negatively impact life, and dosages are intended to be the lowest possible dose for the shortest period of time. Other drugs can be used to prevent or treat osteoporosis, drugs such as bisphosphonates and selective estrogen receptor modulators (SERMs), which do not carry the same risks as hormone therapy.

Anecdotal evidence and some research studies suggest that stress reduction and exercise can relieve some of the symptoms of the menopause, including hot flashes and mood swings. In addition, a host of herbal remedies on the market claim to improve menopausal symptoms, although caution should be used in choosing these products. A double-blind pilot study of women using soy as a natural estrogen replacement therapy turned out positive; hot flashes decreased significantly in women taking soy powder for six weeks. The isoflavones in soy are chemically similar to estrogens. Vitamin E, which is structurally similar to estrogen at the molecular level, decreases hot flashes in some women, but the evidence so far is anecdotal and no large studies have been conducted. Black cohosh is the best documented of all the herbal remedies. Studies suggest that it can relieve menopause-related headaches, depression, anxiety, hot flashes, night sweats, heart palpitations, and vaginal dryness and thinning. Black cohosh suppresses the secretion of luteinizing hormone, a hormone that is believed to be at the root of many menopausal symptoms. One European study of eighty women found that black cohosh relieved menopausal symptoms more effectively than estrogen replacement therapy.

PERSPECTIVE AND PROSPECTS

The menopause, in various guises, was referred to in many early cultures and texts. Initially, an association was made between age and the loss of fertility. By the sixth century, written records on the cessation of menstruation were well documented. At that time, it was believed that menstruation did not cease before the age of thirty-five, nor did it usually continue after the age of fifty. It was thought that obese women ceased menstruation very early and that the periods remained normal or abnormal and increased in flow or became diminished depending on age, the season of the year, the habits and peculiar traits of women, the types of food eaten, and complicating diseases. Similar descriptions of menstrual cessation and its age of onset continued for another thousand years. It was not until the late eighteenth and early nineteenth centuries, however, that much advancement in the knowledge of the topic took place.

John Leake, influenced by William Harvey's historic description of the circulatory system, made one of the first reasonable attempts to explain the etiology of the menopause in his 1777 book *Medical Instructions Towards the Prevention and Cure of Chronic or Slow Diseases Peculiar to Women*. He believed that as long as the "prime of life" continued, along with the circulating force of the blood being more than equal to the resistance of the uterine vessels, the menses would continue to flow. When these vessels became firm from the effect of age, however, the diminished current of blood would be insufficient to force the uterine vessels open, and then periodic discharge would cease.

A later development in the history of menstruation studies was to link menstruation with all sorts of other problems, both emotional and organic. Leake commented that at the time of cessation of menses, women were often afflicted by various chronic diseases. He added that some women were prone to pain and lightheadedness, others were plagued by an intolerable itching at the neck of the bladder, and some were affected by low spirits and melancholy. Leake thought, because it seemed extraordinary that so many disorders should result from such a natural occurrence in a woman's life, that these symptoms could be explained away by indulgence in excesses, luxury, and an "irregularity" in the passions. Laying the blame for complications with the menopause on societal (in particular, female) excesses continued for some time.

Specific disease associations were also made; in 1814, John Burns announced that the cessation of menses seemed to cause cancer of the breast in some women. Edward John Tilt, a British physician, wrote one of the first full-length books on *The Change of Life in Health and Disease* (1857). Some of his views were that women should adhere to a strict code of hygiene during menstruation because they are often afflicted with cancer, gout, rheumatism, and nervous disorders.

These beliefs reflect a tendency from the mid-nineteenth century onward for medical literature to associate the menopause with many negative sociological features. For example, Colombat de l'Isère, in his book *Traité des maladies des femmes et de l'hygiène spéciale de leur sexe* (1838; *A Treatise on the Diseases and Special Hygiene of Females*, 1845), expressed his belief that during the menopause women ceased to live for the species and lived only for themselves. He thought that it was prudent for men to avoid having erotic thoughts about women in whom these feelings ought to have become extinct; he believed that after the menopause sexual enjoyment for women was ended forever.

Not all physicians, however, took such a negative attitude. Some believed that examining this phase in a woman's life presented a challenge. They believed that the boundaries between the physiological and the pathological in this field of study were ill-defined and that it was in the interest of the male gender that more research into this stage of a woman's life be done. The narrow boundary between normal physiology and pathology had not been fully defined nearly a hundred years later, nor did the many negative and unsubstantiated theories cease. Well into the 1960's, the menopause was still considered "abnormal" and a "negative" state by some physicians.

Three major milestones exist in the history of menopause research in the twentieth century. The first event was the achievement of Adolf Butenandt, a Nobel Prize winner in chemistry. He succeeded in 1929 in isolating and obtaining, in pure form, a hormone from the urine of pregnant women which was eventually called estrone. The second development was the publication of *Feminine Forever* in 1966, which became an instant best seller. As a result of the book's publication, physicians were prompted to take sides in a heated and continuing debate. The third landmark was the publication of an editorial and two original articles in *The New England Journal of Medicine* of December 4, 1975, claiming an association between exogenous estrogens and endometrial cancer. This claim brought about legal action by initiating, at least in the United States, a series of health administration inquiries.

—Genevieve Slomski, Ph.D.;
updated by Karen E. Kalumuck, Ph.D.

See also Aging; Arteriosclerosis; Breast cancer; Cervical, ovarian, and uterine cancers; Endocrinology; Endometrial cancer; Gynecology; Heart disease; Herbal medicine; Hormone therapy; Hormones; Hot flashes; Hysterectomy; Infertility, female; Menstruation; Midlife crisis; Obesity; Osteoporosis; Ovarian cysts; Ovaries; Sterilization; Women's health.

FOR FURTHER INFORMATION:

Corio, Laura E., and Linda G. Kahn. *The Change Before the Change: Everything You Need to Know to Stay Healthy in the Decade Before Menopause.* 2d ed. London: Piatkus Books, 2005. An engaging and well-researched book that discusses what to expect during perimenopause, from the first sign of menstrual irregularity to the onslaught of physiological and emotional changes. Appendixes on herbs, phytoestrogens, and hormone therapy are particular strengths.

Doress-Worters, Paula B., and Diana Laskin Siegal. *The New Ourselves, Growing Older: Women Aging with Knowledge and Power.* New York: Simon & Schuster, 1994. In this updated version of a classic work developed in collaboration with the Boston Women's Health Book Collective, a host of issues related to maturing in women are addressed, including the menopause, osteoporosis, and estrogen replacement therapy. The positive aspects of changes are emphasized, and the book is filled with practical advice and resource lists.

Greenwood, Sadja. *Menopause, Naturally: Preparing for the Second Half of Life.* Updated ed. Volcano, Calif.: Volcano Press, 1996. This classic book gives a clear description of the natural changes in the menopause and holistic approaches to its management.

Love, Susan, and Karen Lindsey. *Dr. Susan Love's Menopause and Hormone Book: Making Informed Choices.* Rev. ed. New York: Three Rivers Press, 2003. Renowned physician Love reviews recent research on hormone therapy and offers advice about when such therapy is recommended. Also covers diet, exercise, stress management, alternative therapies, and medications other than hormones.

Maas, Paula, Susan E. Brown, and Nancy Bruning. *The Mend Clinic Guide to Natural Medicine for Menopause and Beyond.* New York: Dell, 1997. After giving a concise and lucid description of the physiological changes that occur during the menopause, this concisely written text addresses a host of symptoms and dispenses the current wisdom from a host of alternative medical traditions, including ancient Chinese medicine, acupressure, herbal therapy, and homeopathy.

North American Menopause Society. http://www .menopause.org. Web site run by a scientific research organization. Includes an excellent "consumers" section covering the range of menopause symptoms and treatments and providing referral lists and resource links, among other features.

Sheehy, Gail. *The Silent Passage: Menopause.* Rev. ed. New York: Pocket Books, 1998. Expanding on her article published in the October, 1991, issue of *Vanity Fair*, Sheehy draws from more than one hundred interviews conducted with women experiencing various stages of menopause, as well as interviews with dozens of experts in many disciplines.

Stoppard, Miriam. *Menopause.* 2d ed. London: DK, 2002. A thorough exploration of the physiology, symptoms, medical complaints, and medical management of menopause, which also discusses maintaining sexuality, monitoring health, and preparing for the years beyond menopause.

MENORRHAGIA
DISEASE/DISORDER
ANATOMY OR SYSTEM AFFECTED: Blood, reproductive system, uterus

SPECIALTIES AND RELATED FIELDS: Gynecology

DEFINITION: Excessively heavy or prolonged menstrual flow.

CAUSES AND SYMPTOMS

Menorrhagia can be caused by many disorders: anatomic abnormalities of the uterus, hormonal imbalances, certain medical conditions, medications, and malignancy. Common anatomic causes are uterine fibroids and adenomyosis. Irregular menstrual cycles resulting from hormonal imbalances can be associated with menorrhagia. Medical conditions such as blood clotting disorders and liver or thyroid disease contribute to menorrhagia. Medications that prevent blood clotting, such as coumadin or heparin, can lead to increased menstrual flow. Uterine and other reproductive tract cancers can result in unusually heavy menstrual flow.

Symptoms of menorrhagia are uterine bleeding that is excessive (more than 80 milliliters) and/or bleeding that lasts for more than seven days. Unlike metrorrhagia, bleeding occurs at regular intervals. The patient can become anemic and exhibit symptoms of either acute or chronic blood loss. Symptoms and signs which

INFORMATION ON MENORRHAGIA

CAUSES: Uterine abnormalities (fibroids, adenomyosis); hormonal imbalances; blood clotting disorders; liver or thyroid disease; blood thinners (coumadin, heparin); uterine and other reproductive tract cancers

SYMPTOMS: Excessive uterine bleeding, sometimes anemia

DURATION: Chronic

TREATMENTS: Depends on cause and severity; may include iron supplements, oral contraceptives or medroxyprogesterone, hormone injections to induce menopause, high-dose estrogens, dilation and curettage (D & C), thermal ablation, endometrial polyp or fibroid resection, placement of progesterone-impregnated IUD, myomectomy, hysterectomy

suggest the cause of menorrhagia may be present, such as large palpable fibroids, or evidence of hypothyroidism or liver disease.

TREATMENT AND THERAPY

Menorrhagia can be treated via a medical or a surgical approach. The selection of treatment often depends on the cause and severity of the menorrhagia. If menorrhagia is the result of conditions amenable to medical treatment (such as a thyroid disorder), then control of these conditions may decrease the bleeding. If the patient has irregular cycles (for example, because of lack of ovulation), then hormones such as oral contraceptive pills or medroxyprogesterone may be used to regulate the cycles and decrease menstrual flow. A patient who is nearing the menopause can receive hormone injections that place her into an earlier artificial menopause, and hence eliminate menstrual bleeding altogether. If the patient encounters acute and profuse bleeding, then high-dose estrogens may be given.

If menorrhagia is resistent to medical management, then surgical treatment may be necessary. Examples of procedural treatments for menorrhagia are dilation and curettage (D & C), for acute, profuse bleeding; thermal ablation of the endometrial lining; hysteroscopic resection of endometrial polyps or fibroids; and placement of a progesterone-impregnated intrauterine device (IUD). Hysterectomy is the definitive surgery for menorrhagia, no matter what the cause, since menstrual bleeding cannot occur without the uterus. Patients with

large fibroids or adenomyosis often are not responsive to medical management. These patients would be candidates for hysterectomy. In patients with large fibroids and menorrhagia who wish to retain childbearing potential, a myomectomy may be performed instead of hysterectomy. If a patient is suspected or known to have a malignancy of the reproductive tract that is causing menorrhagia, then surgical management is the appropriate treatment.

Finally, patients can become severely anemic from menorrhagia, and blood transfusion may be necessary. Mild anemia can be treated with iron supplementation.

—*Anne Lynn S. Chang, M.D.*

See also Anemia; Bleeding; Cervical, ovarian, and uterine cancers; Dysmenorrhea; Endometriosis; Genital disorders, female; Hysterectomy; Menstruation; Myomectomy; Polyps; Reproductive system; Uterus; Women's health.

FOR FURTHER INFORMATION:

Golub, Sharon. *Periods: From Menarche to Menopause.* Newbury Park, Calif.: Sage, 1992.

Icon Health. *Menorrhagia: A Medical Dictionary, Bibliography, and Annotated Research Guide to Internet References.* San Diego, Calif.: Author, 2004.

Kasper, Dennis L., et al., eds. *Harrison's Principles of Internal Medicine.* 16th ed. New York: McGraw-Hill, 2005.

O'Donovan, Peter, Paul McGurgan, and Walter Prendiville, eds. *Conservative Surgery for Menorrhagia.* San Francisco: Greenwich Medical Media, 2003.

Stenchever, Morton A., et al. *Comprehensive Gynecology.* 4th ed. St. Louis, Mo.: Mosby/Elsevier, 2006.

Tierney, Lawrence M., Stephen J. McPhee, and Maxine A. Papadakis, eds. *Current Medical Diagnosis and Treatment 2006.* New York: McGraw-Hill Medical, 2006.

MEN'S HEALTH

OVERVIEW

ANATOMY OR SYSTEM AFFECTED: All

SPECIALTIES AND RELATED FIELDS: All

DEFINITION: Issues related to the health and well-being of men.

KEY TERMS:

colonoscopy: examination of the colon using an endoscope inserted into the rectum

digital rectal exam: examination in which a gloved finger is placed in the rectum to feel the prostate gland for lumps, enlargement, or irregularities

endoscope: a flexible tube with a camera device that is inserted into the body

epididymis: the coiled tube behind the testicles that stores and transports sperm

high-risk behaviors: behaviors that increase the chance of injury, disease, or harm

Klinefelter syndrome: a disease in which an extra X chromosome in males causes abnormal development of the testicles

prostate diseases: diseases that affect the prostate gland

prostate-specific antigen (PSA): a glycoprotein produced by the prostate gland; its levels in the blood can indicate the presence of cancer

screening: tests to detect health problems and diseases

sexually transmitted diseases (STDs): contagious diseases that can be spread through sexual contact

sigmoidoscopy: examination of the lower portion of the colon (sigmoid) using an endoscope inserted in the rectum

MAJOR HEALTH CONCERNS

Men in the United States have a lower life expectancy than do women. Generally, men smoke, drink, and participate in more activities that may result in physical trauma. According to the Centers for Disease Control and Prevention (CDC), the ten leading causes of death among men are accidents, cancer, diabetes, heart disease, lung disease, liver disease, suicide, and homicide.

Accidents or unintentional injuries are the fifth leading cause of death in the United States. The risk of death as a result of a motor vehicle accident is twice as high among men and is highest within the age range of fifteen to twenty-four.

Cancer can occur in anyone at any age, but 76 percent of all cancers are diagnosed in those age fifteen and older. Nonmelanoma skin cancer is the most common cancer. Lung cancer is the leading cause of death among both men and women. Other cancers that affect men include prostate cancer, colon cancer, and testicular cancer.

Skin cancer may be identified as melanoma or nonmelanoma skin cancer. Skin cancers are more common in people with fair skin, hair, and eyes. The most important cause and risk factor for developing skin cancer is excessive sun exposure. Symptoms of skin cancer include skin areas that are crusty, scaly and rough, firm and red, shiny, or waxy, as well as nonhealing sores. The borders of cancerous areas are asymmetrical (un-

even). The color is uneven, and the abnormal area is usually larger than six millimeters.

Lung cancer develops from abnormal cell growth in the lining of the lungs. Survival rates of lung cancer are poor. The earlier lung cancer is found, the better the chance for survival. Approximately one in ten survive five years after being diagnosed. Smoking is the number-one cause of lung cancer. Other risk factors include environmental pollution; exposure to radon, asbestos, and gases in closed areas, as in mining; and a family history of lung cancer. At first, one may have no symptoms, but as cancer grows, wheezing, shortness of breath, a persistent cough that worsens over time, coughing blood, chest pain, hoarseness, fatigue, decreased appetite, and neck and face swelling occur.

Colon cancer (colorectal cancer) develops from abnormal cell growth in the lining of the colon. It is the fourth most common cancer in men. About 90 percent of all colorectal cancers are diagnosed after age fifty. Risk factors and causes of colon cancer include a high-fat and low-fiber diet, alcohol abuse, smoking, lack of exercise, diabetes, colitis, irritable bowel, family history of colon cancer, and rectal polyps (growths on the lining of the colon). Polyps are common among those aged fifty and older. In the early stages, there may be no symptoms, but as the cancer grows, symptoms may include a change in bowel movements (diarrhea, constipation, bloody stools that are bright red or very dark, a feeling that the bowel does not empty completely, thin stools), abdominal discomfort (gas pains, cramping, bloating, sense of fullness), vomiting, weight loss, and fatigue.

Prostate cancer is caused by the growth of cancer cells in the prostate gland. Prostate cancer is the third most common cause of death from cancer in men, and it is the most common cause of death from cancer in men over age seventy-five. A definitive cause of prostate cancer is still under investigation. It has been linked to a high-fat diet and elevated testosterone levels. African American men older than age sixty, farmers, tire plant workers, painters, and those exposed to cadmium are at high risk for prostate cancer. Symptoms result from the blocking of urine flow because of prostate enlargement and include frequent urge to urinate (micturia), dribbling urine, painful or burning urination (dysuria), difficulty or inability to urinate, bloody urine or semen, painful ejaculation, and pain or stiffness in the thighs, hips, or lower back.

Testicular cancer is caused by the growth of cancer cells in one or both testicles. It is the most common cancer in men between ages fifteen and thirty-four and is most common in Caucasians. Approximately eight thousand men are diagnosed with testicular cancer annually in the United States. The causes of testicular cancer are still under investigation, but risks include cryptorchidism (undescended testicles) and a family history of testicular cancer. Symptoms of testicular cancer include a dull ache in the groin or low abdomen, pulling or heaviness in the scrotum, testicular or scrotal pain, and testicular enlargement.

Diabetes mellitus is a metabolic disorder in which the pancreas does not produce enough insulin to process and maintain proper blood sugar levels. Over time, poorly controlled diabetes can cause eye, heart, kidney, and nerve damage. About two-thirds of those with diabetes die of heart disease. There are two main types of diabetes. In type 1 diabetes, the body produces no insulin. It affects 10 percent of those with diabetes and is most often seen in males under age thirty. Type 1 diabetes is more prevalent among North Europeans, African Americans, and Hispanics, respectively. The causes of type 1 diabetes are not completely understood, but it is thought to be linked to an inherited, genetic predisposition that is activated by an environmental trigger from exposure to environmental chemicals or viruses that attack the immune system.

In type 2 diabetes, the body either does not produce enough insulin or does not use insulin efficiently. Approximately 90 percent of those with diabetes have type 2 diabetes. The risk of developing this type increases with age and most often affects those over age forty. One-third of men with type 2 diabetes are unaware of it until problems such as erectile dysfunction (impotence), vision loss, or kidney disease develop. Causes and risk factors for developing type 2 diabetes include a family history of diabetes, lack of exercise, a high-fat diet, elevated cholesterol levels, obesity, advancing age, high blood pressure, and being of African American, Hispanic, American Indian, Asian American, or Pacific Islander descent. Symptoms of both types of diabetes include blurred vision, headache, excessive thirst and hunger, unexplained weight loss, dry and itchy skin, slow-healing cuts and bruises, frequent urination, recurring infections, tingling in the hands and feet, mood swings, irritability, depression, and fatigue.

Cardiovascular disease refers to problems that affect the heart (heart disease) and circulation (vascular disease). Heart disease is the number-one killer of men. Being male increases the risk of developing heart dis-

ease. The mortality rate for African American men with heart disease is twice as high as for Caucasian men. Causes and risk factors include advancing age, family history, diabetes, elevated cholesterol, high blood pressure, a high-fat diet, lack of regular exercise, obesity, and smoking. Common cardiovascular diseases include coronary artery disease, cardiomyopathy, heart valve disease, heart failure, hyperlipidemia, high blood pressure, and stroke.

Coronary artery disease is the leading cause of heart attacks. In this condition, blood flow through the arteries of the heart is blocked. The most common cause is the buildup of fatty deposits (plaque) in the lining of an artery, called arteriosclerosis. Symptoms include shortness of breath, chest pain (angina), and/or a heart attack (myocardial infarction). Risk factors include smoking, elevated cholesterol, diabetes, high blood pressure, obesity, physical inactivity, and stress.

Cardiomyopathy involves conditions that enlarge the heart and weaken the heart muscle so that it does not pump efficiently. Causes and risk factors for developing cardiomyopathy are aging, alcoholism, high blood pressure, obesity, and smoking. Symptoms include chest pain, shortness of breath, irregular heartbeat, abdominal distention, swelling in the lower legs, fatigue, dizziness, and fainting.

Heart valve disease refers to conditions that damage the heart valves that may result in inadequate closure (prolapse), leaking (regurgitation), or narrowing (stenosis) of the valves so that blood does not circulate adequately. Causes and risk factors for the development of heart valve disease include rheumatic fever, heart attack (myocardial infarction), infections of connective tissue such as systemic lupus erthyematosus (SLE), poliomyelitis, rheumatoid arthritis, aging, congenital birth defects, medications, or radiation treatment. Symptoms of heart valve disease include shortness of breath, chest pain, irregular heart beat, high or low blood pressure, fatigue, and dizziness or faintness upon physical activity.

Heart failure is a condition in which the heart is unable to pump blood to organs and tissues efficiently. Heart failure may develop suddenly or gradually. Congestive heart failure is a condition in which the inability of the heart to pump blood to organs and tissues efficiently leads to a buildup of fluid in the body. Causes and risk factors for heart failure include coronary artery disease, heart valve disease, or cardiomyopathy. Symptoms of heart failure include shortness of breath, chest pain, heart palpitations, fluid retention that causes swelling in the lower legs and abdomen, weight gain (from fluid retention), weakness, dizziness, and fatigue.

Hyperlipidemia refers to elevated fats (lipids) in the blood that eventually form fatty deposits (plaque) on the walls of arteries that lead to coronary artery disease. The most common lipids include high-density lipoprotein (HDL) cholesterol, low-density lipoprotein (LDL) cholesterol, and triglycerides. Hypercholesterolemia refers to elevated blood cholesterol levels (higher than 200 milligrams) and is the leading risk factor for heart disease. High levels of HDL (higher than 60 milligrams) protect against heart disease. High levels of LDL (higher than 100 milligrams) can lead to heart disease. Hypertriglyceridemia refers to elevated triglyceride blood levels (higher than 150 milligrams). Hyperlipidemia increases the risk for heart attack, stroke, and diabetes. Causes and risk factors for hyperlipidemia include diabetes, high blood pressure, hypothyroidism, kidney or liver disease, aging, sex (men have a higher risk for elevated lipids), smoking, a high-fat diet, alcohol abuse, obesity, lack of exercise, heredity, stress, and medications such as corticosteroids, diuretics, and some blood pressure pills.

High blood pressure (hypertension) occurs when the pressure of the blood in the arteries is too high. High blood pressure is referred to as the silent killer because it often creates no symptoms. It is a major risk factor for heart disease. Untreated hypertension can lead to heart failure, heart attack, stroke, and kidney failure. A normal blood pressure is 120/80 or below. Blood pressure above 140/90 is considered high blood pressure. Prehypertension refers to blood pressures between 120/80 and 140/90. In those with diabetes and kidney disease, a blood pressure of 130/80 or higher is too high, and if it is not decreased, then high blood pressure is likely to develop. Causes and risk factors for high blood pressure include aging; race; sex (higher incidence in men); heredity; alcohol or drug abuse; obesity; stress; socioeconomic status; kidney, thyroid, or adrenal gland diseases; diabetes; sensitivity to salt; lack of exercise; and some medications, such as cold, allergy, and migraine medications.

Stroke (also called a brain attack or cerebral vascular accident) can be either ischemic or hemorrhagic. Both prevent oxygen and nutrients from reaching the brain. Ischemic strokes are caused by blockage or narrowing of blood vessels leading to the brain, while hemorrhagic strokes are broken blood vessels that bleed into the brain. Causes and risk factors for a stroke include aging, arteriosclerosis, family history, race (higher incidence in African Americans), sex (higher incidence in men), diabetes, heart disease, high blood pressure, elevated blood lipids, a high-fat diet, lack of regular exercise, obesity, and smoking. Symptoms of a stroke include weakness or numbness of the face, arm, or leg on one side of the body; loss of vision; loss of speech; inability to understand what is being said; headache; dizziness; and walking problems or falling.

Pulmonary or lung diseases affect the health of the lungs. Common lung diseases are chronic obstructive pulmonary disease (COPD), bronchitis, emphysema, asthma, influenza, pneumonia, and lung cancer. Men are vulnerable to these diseases because they are more likely to smoke and to have jobs that involve exposure to hazardous materials.

COPD is the fourth leading cause of death in the United States. There is a strong link between COPD and lung cancer. Causes and risk factors for COPD include smoking; a history of childhood respiratory infections; asbestos, radon, and other air pollutants; and heredity. Symptoms of COPD include coughing, shortness of breath, chest tightness, and wheezing.

Chronic bronchitis occurs when the lining of the lungs become inflamed and swollen so that the airways become small and clogged with excess mucus and oxygen cannot be absorbed. Smoking and exposure to secondhand smoke are the main causes of bronchitis. Allergies, air pollution, infections, and pollutants from mining, farming, and working with textiles are also factors. Symptoms of chronic bronchitis include shortness of breath, coughing, and increased mucus that occurs most days for three months in a year over two consecutive years.

Emphysema occurs when the air sacs (alveoli) that exchange oxygen and carbon dioxide become damaged. Fifty-five percent of those with emphysema are men. Emphysema develops slowly over time, so symptoms do not become evident until it is well established. Smoking and exposure to secondhand smoke are the main causes of emphysema. Allergies, aging, heredity, air pollution, and pollutants from mining, farming, and working with textiles are also factors. Symptoms include a chronic cough with or without mucus production, fatigue, and loss of appetite.

Asthma results in inflammation and swelling in the airways that causes narrowing, preventing air from passing through them. Causes and risk factors for developing asthma include smoking, gastric reflux disease, lung infections, exercise, heredity, allergies, pollution, cold air, and environmental triggers. Symptoms of asthma include wheezing, chest tightness, coughing, and shortness of breath.

Influenza is a contagious viral infection caused by the influenza virus that can be deadly. The elderly, young children, and those with weakened immune systems are at highest risk for serious complications. Symptoms include headache, fever, sore throat, dry cough, nausea, vomiting, diarrhea, fatigue, and muscle weakness and aching. Pneumonia is a deadly infection and/or inflammation of the lungs in which the airways become blocked by pus or fluid so that oxygen cannot be passed to and from the lungs. Individuals affected by heart disease, diabetes, age, or weakened immune systems are at a higher risk of dying from pneumonia. Risk factors and causes of pneumonia include chemicals, bacteria, viruses, and other microbes. Symptoms of pneumonia include fever, chills, sweating, shaking, cough, chest pain, and shortness of breath.

Chronic liver disease is the gradual failure of the liver to function effectively. Cirrhosis of the liver results from scar tissue that replaces healthy liver tissue and hinders the blood flow through the liver so that nutrients, hormones, and drugs are not processed normally. It is the eighth leading cause of death in the United States. Fibrosis of the liver is the overgrowth of scar tissue in the liver (usually from cirrhosis) that results from an infection, inflammation, or injury that prevents the liver from storing vitamins and minerals, regulating blood clotting, producing proteins and enzymes, maintaining hormone balance, and metabolizing or detoxifying substances. Risk factors for chronic liver disease include alcoholism, obesity, a low-fiber and high-fat diet, high blood pressure, elevated blood lipids, family history, and some medications. Symptoms include weakness, fatigue, confusion, loss of appetite, abdominal pain, excessive bruising, swelling in abdomen and legs, gastric bleeding, and yellow skin coloring (jaundice).

Suicide is the eighth leading cause of death among men in the United States. Men are four times more likely to commit suicide than are women. Suicide risk is related to depression, chronic illness, living alone, history of physical or sexual abuse, unemployment, age (highest among men in their twenties, sixties, and seventies), and marital status (higher among the never married, divorced, or recently widowed). Many men do not readily identify their depression and so do not seek treatment. It is estimated that each year more than six million men are affected with depression. Risk factors

and causes of depression include loss of a loved one, stress, financial problems, relationship problems, positive or negative life changes, and heredity. Symptoms of depression include feelings of hopelessness, guilt, worthlessness, or helplessness; persistent sadness or anxiety; loss of interest in daily life activities and hobbies; difficulty concentrating; memory loss; indecisiveness; irritability; increased or decreased sleep; loss of energy; fatigue; weight loss or gain; physical ailments; and thoughts of death or suicide.

Men face unique diseases and disorders of the reproductive system. Testicular trauma is most often related to injuries acquired from contact sports or accidents. Symptoms of testicular trauma include pain, swelling, and bruising of one or both testes. Testicular rupture is rare, but it can cause blood to leak into the scrotum and requires surgical repair. Testicular torsion occurs when the spermatic cord twists and cuts the blood supply to the testicle. Adolescent males are often affected as a result of injuries sustained from strenuous activities. Symptoms of testicular torsion are sudden and severe testicular pain, tenderness, and testicular swelling.

Epididymitis is an inflammation of the epididymis. Males ages nineteen to forty are most often affected. Epididymitis is usually caused by an infection and can be the result of a sexually transmitted disease. Symptoms include scrotal pain and swelling, abscess (collection of pus), dysuria, frequent urination, urgency to urinate, abdominal pain, fever, and chills.

Hypogonadism occurs when the testicles do not produce enough testosterone. There are two types. Primary hypogonadism results from an abnormality in the testicles. Secondary hypogonadism results from a problem with the pituitary gland. Causes and risk factors of hypogonadism include undescended testicles, testicular trauma, hemochromatosis (excess iron in the blood), pituitary disorders from a head injury or pituitary tumor, mumps infection, Klinefelter syndrome, aging, chemotherapy or radiation therapy, and medications. Symptoms of hypogonadism include impaired growth of the penis and testicles, decreased muscle mass and body hair, enlarged breasts, infertility, erectile dysfunction, decreased sex drive, fatigue, difficulty concentrating, hot flashes, and depression.

Prostatitis is an inflammation in the prostate gland that is usually caused by a bacterial infection. Risk factors include urinary tract infections, medical procedures requiring insertion of objects into the penis, anal intercourse, benign prostatic hyperplasia (BPH), or prostate enlargement. Symptoms of prostatitis include a tender and swollen prostate, fever; chills; low back, joint, and muscle pain; urinary frequency; dysuria; bloody urine (hematuria); difficulty starting the stream of urine (hesitancy); frequent urination at night (nocturia); and painful ejaculation.

BPH is an enlargement of the prostate gland. It naturally occurs with age and affects 50 percent of men after age sixty and 70 percent of men in their seventies and eighties. When an enlarged prostate presses against the urethra, it blocks the flow of urine. Symptoms of BPH include hesitant urination, frequent urination, urgency to pass urine, weak stream of urine, dribbling urine, dysuria, nocturia, straining to urinate, inability to pass urine (retention), and/or feeling that the bladder is not completely emptied.

Sexually transmitted diseases (STDs) are infections that are transferred through sexual acts such as intercourse, oral sex, sharing sexual objects such as vibrators, and intimate skin-to-skin contact. The United States has the highest number of STDs in the world, with more than 15 million cases reported each year. Almost two-thirds of all STDS occur in adults younger than age twenty-five. STDs include hepatitis B, genital herpes, human papilloma virus (HPV), chlamydia, gonorrhea, and syphilis. STDs can cause infertility and damage to the heart, kidneys, and brain, as well as an increased chance of contracting acquired immunodeficiency syndrome (AIDS). AIDS, the most serious STD, has no cure and can be fatal. STD symptoms may include discharge from the penis; painful sex; dysuria; sore throat from oral sex; pain in the anus from anal intercourse; chancres (painless red sores) on the genitals, tongue, throat, and anus; blisters or warts around the genitals; dark urine; light-colored bowel movements; and yellow skin (jaundice).

PREVENTION AND TREATMENT OPTIONS

The best way for men to manage these health concerns is prevention through education, healthy living, and screenings to identify diseases in their early stages, when they are most treatable.

Skin cancer can be prevented by minimizing sun exposure, wearing protective clothing that covers exposed skin, avoiding the sun during midday, and using sunscreen with SPF 15 or stronger year-round. Men should apply sunscreen at least one-half hour before going into the sun and then reapply it frequently. The American Academy of Dermatology recommends annual screening for skin cancer by a dermatologist. Treatment for skin cancer includes surgery to remove cancerous cells, radiation to shrink and kill cancerous cells, chemotherapy, and photodynamic therapy, in which a light-activated drug that targets cancerous cells is injected and then activated by lasers to destroy cancer cells.

Lung cancer is treated through the surgical removal of tumors, radiation therapy to shrink tumors, chemotherapy, photodynamic therapy, electrosurgery (which concentrates high-energy electromagnetic radiation to destroy tissue), and cryotherapy (which destroys cancerous tissue using extreme cold).

Colon cancer screening includes a rectal examination and stool test for blood every year, sigmoidoscopy every five years, barium enema every five years, and colonoscopy every ten years. Colon cancer screening should begin at age fifty, or sooner if there is a personal or family history of colon cancer or bowel disease. Treatment for colon cancer includes surgical removal of cancerous tissue, chemotherapy, and radiation therapy.

Prostate cancer screening recommendations are annual screenings after age fifty. For high-risk men, annual screenings should begin at age forty. Screenings include a digital rectal exam (DRE) and a prostate-specific antigen (PSA) test. The level of PSA is elevated when there are problems in the prostate. A biopsy may also show abnormal cells in the prostate. Treatment for prostate cancer includes prostatectomy (surgical removal of the prostate), radiation therapy, monthly hormone injections to shrink the prostate cancer cells, or "watchful waiting" until the tumor becomes larger.

Testicular self-examination (TSE) can help identify testicular cancer early. The American Cancer Society recommends that men over the age of fifteen perform monthly TSEs. These examinations are best done after a warm shower. Using both hands, the testicles should be rolled between thumbs and fingers to feel for any lumps. Abnormalities should be reported to a doctor. Treatment for testicular cancer includes orchiectomy (surgical removal of the testes), radiation therapy, and chemotherapy.

Diabetes is screened by a fasting blood glucose test, which measures blood glucose (sugar) after not eating for at least eight hours; a glucose tolerance test, which measures blood glucose two hours after drinking a concentrated sugar beverage; or a random blood glucose test, which checks the level of blood sugar without fasting. It is recommended that men over age forty-five be tested for diabetes every three years and those at high risk for diabetes be tested at age thirty. Treatment of diabetes may require taking hypoglycemic (low blood sugar) medications or insulin injections in addition to following a diabetic diet, monitoring blood glucose, and getting regular exercise.

Coronary artery disease is treated with lifestyle changes such as smoking cessation, exercise, medications, weight control, and a low-fat, high-fiber diet. Angioplasty (the opening of coronary arteries) or coronary artery bypass surgery may be needed. Cardiomyopathy and heart failure are treated with a low-salt, low-fat diet and medications to regulate and strengthen the heartbeat and decrease fluid retention. A cardiac pacemaker can improve the heart rhythm, while an implantable cardiac device (ICD) monitors heart rhythms and gives an electrical shock when a deadly heart rhythm occurs. Heart transplantation is a last resort when heart failure cannot be controlled. Heart valve disease can be treated with medication to regulate heart rhythm and strengthen the heartbeat, relax blood vessels (vasodilators), control blood pressure (antihypertensives), and reduce fluid retention (diuretics). A balloon valvuloplasty introduces an uninflated balloon into the heart valve that is inflated to open the valve and then removed. If symptoms cannot be controlled, surgery may be necessary to repair or replace the affected valve.

Hyperlipidemia treatment includes lifestyle changes to reduce dietary fats and increase fiber in the diet, weight control, and regular exercise. Lipid-reducing medications may be used if lifestyle changes are not effective. If blood lipids are normal, then screening should be done at least every five years starting at age thirty-five. Screening should be done annually for elevated levels. Men who smoke, who have diabetes, or who have heart disease in their family should have their lipids checked starting at age twenty.

Blood pressure screenings should be done at each health care visit for men aged eighteen and older. Treatment for high blood pressure begins with lifestyle changes such as weight control, smoking cessation, limited alcohol consumption, regular exercise, and a low-fat, high-fiber diet. Antihypertensive medications are generally used if lifestyle changes are not effective.

Stroke can be treated with medications, surgical intervention and rehabilitation to restore optimum function. A carotid endarterectomy removes fatty deposits (plaque) in the artery that leads to the brain. Cerebral angioplasty opens the carotid artery by inflating a balloon into it to compress plaque, remove plaque with a rotating blade, or implant coils (stents) to keep the vessel open. Tissue plasminogen activator (TPA or tPA) is effective in treating strokes caused by blood clots by dissolving the clot and restoring circulation to the brain, but there is only a three-hour window of time in which it will be effective.

Bronchitis treatment is focused on reducing its symptoms, including avoiding smokers and air pollution, increasing fluids to keep mucus thin, humidifying the air to keep the airways open, deep breathing at least every hour to clear airways, and taking medications to open the airways, encourage coughing, and reduce inflammation, swelling, and mucus. If bronchitis worsens, then oxygen may be required to relieve shortness of breath and maintain adequate oxygen levels.

Emphysema treatment includes stopping smoking, avoiding smokers and air pollution, exercising to strengthen the lungs and diaphragm, maintaining a constant comfortable temperature in the home, increasing fluids to keep mucus thin, taking medications to open the airways and thin mucus, and pursed lip breathing (lips partially closed while slowly breathing out to keep airways open). As emphysema worsens, supplemental oxygen may be required.

Asthma treatment begins with controlling the environment. Wearing a mask while cleaning; avoiding fur, feathers, and materials known to cause an attack; humidifying the air; and using an air conditioner in hot weather are some methods of avoiding an asthma attack. Medications for treating asthma include those that open the airways for quick relief; daily medications to control symptoms of inflammation, open airways, and block release of chemicals that cause inflammation; and those that decrease the reaction to irritants. Desensitization is helpful in allergy-induced asthma, in which small amounts of substances that cause an allergic reaction are injected weekly over several months to develop immunity to them. Finally, anti-IgE monoclonal antibody medications help block antibodies that cause asthma attacks.

Men can lower the chances of developing influenza by getting a flu shot every year. Treatment for the flu is based on treating the symptoms and includes drinking adequate fluids, bed rest, and taking medications for fever, aches, cough, congestion, and nausea. Over-the-counter medications can minimize the discomfort of flu symptoms but do not treat the virus. Antiviral medications are helpful in preventing and treating the flu, but they must be given as soon as symptoms begin in order to be effective. Pneumonia can be prevented by having a pneumonia vaccination. It is 90 percent effective, and one dose prevents infection for five to ten years. Treatment for pneumonia includes drinking adequate fluids, bed rest, taking antibiotics for bacterial pneumonia, and taking medications to relieve fever, aches, cough, and congestion.

Liver disease treatment depends on the problem. Alcohol abuse is the primary cause of liver disease in men. Those at risk for exposure to hepatitis can be vaccinated against hepatitis B and hepatitis A. Treatment may include high blood pressure medication (antihypertensives), chemotherapy, radiation therapy, bile duct drainage, placing coils (stents) in the bile duct or blood vessels in the liver to keep them open, and liver transplantation.

Depression is most often treated by psychological counseling, cognitive behavioral therapy, interpersonal therapies, and antidepressant medications, with generally good results. Other treatments may include exercise, meditation, and light therapy. Treating depression in men can help to prevent suicide.

Testicular trauma can be evaluated by ultrasound or Doppler to identify the extent of injury. Treatment includes ice packs, scrotal support, anti-inflammatory medications, and bed rest for twenty-four hours. Surgical exploration may be warranted if the injury is severe. Testicular torsion is an emergency situation and should be evaluated by a urologist as soon after the injury as possible to prevent irreversible damage to the testicles. Treatment includes pain relief and manual rotation of the testicle to untwist the cord. This procedure is successful 70 percent of the time. If manual rotation does not work, then surgical intervention is necessary.

Treatment for epididymitis includes ice for swelling, a scrotal supporter, antibiotics, bed rest, and anti-inflammatory medicines (ibuprofen, naprosyn). Untreated epididymitis can cause scarring resulting in infertility. If the cause is related to a sexually transmitted disease, then any partners should be checked and provided treatment as well. Using condoms during sex can help to prevent infections.

Treatment for hypogonadism depends on its cause. Testosterone replacement helps in sexual function, increases muscle strength, and prevents bone loss. Pituitary hormones may help increase testosterone levels and sperm production. Surgical removal of a pituitary tumor may help restore testosterone levels as well.

Benign prostatic hypertrophy is treated with medications to lower the tension in the valve under the bladder to allow urine to pass, or to decrease the amount of testosterone so that the prostate shrinks. Surgical removal of the prostate and radiation therapy to shrink the prostate are also optional treatments. There are no screening guidelines for BPH, and digital rectal examination is the only tool.

Prostatitis is not an easy diagnosis to make because symptoms are usually vague. Bacterial cultures of the urine and prostate secretions may or may not show an infection, but antibiotics are usually prescribed, along with medications to relax the prostate and relieve discomfort. Men are encouraged to increase their fluid intake for adequate hydration.

The only way to prevent STDs is through abstinence. Alternative means include education about STDs and their effects and using latex condoms during vaginal, anal, and oral sex. Polyurethane condoms are not as effective as latex, but they are the only alternative for those with latex allergies. Being with one partner (monogamy) who has tested negative for STDs is another way to prevent STDs. Regular screening for STDs are essential for those with multiple sexual partners. When diagnosed early, most STDs can be treated effectively.

PERSPECTIVE AND PROSPECTS

Men's health as a discrete subject within medicine began in the twenty-first century, modeled on the women's health movement. The *Journal of Men's Health and Gender* was founded in 2004. Its goals are to provide information and education about treatment and preventive care specifically for men. The Men's Health Act of 2005 established the Office of Men's Health in the Department of Health and Human Services.

Current men's health issues are in part attributable to the fact that men still tend to participate in risky activities, smoke, drink more alcohol, and be less likely to seek medical attention or participate in health screenings than are women. African American men are twice as likely to develop heart disease than the general population, one-third of men with Type II diabetes are not aware of it, suicide rates among men are four times higher than for women, and almost 69 percent of American men are overweight or obese.

In 2006, the National Center for Health Statistics reported that male life expectancy was seventy-five, about five years less than for women. Lifestyle changes play a large role in improving the life expectancy of men. Eating healthy, staying physically active, having regular medical checkups, and avoiding behaviors that are more prone to end in injury, illness, and death can increase men's life expectancy beyond the present average. Education and program development to engage more men in developing healthy lifestyles are essential for preventing disease and improving quality of life.

—*Sharon W. Stark, R.N., A.P.R.N., D.N.Sc.*

See also Accidents; Alcoholism; Asbestos exposure; Cancer; Cholesterol; Chronic obstructive pulmonary disease (COPD); Circumcision, male; Cirrhosis; Colon cancer; Color blindness; Concussion; Depression; Diabetes mellitus; Erectile dysfunction; Exercise physiology; Gender reassignment surgery; Genital disorders, male; Gulf War syndrome; Gynecomastia; Hair loss and baldness; Hair transplantation; Heart attack; Heart disease; Heart valve replacement; Hemophilia; Hermaphroditism and pseudohermaphroditism; Hormones; Hydroceles; Hypercholesterolemia; Hyperlipidemia; Hypertension; Hypertrophy; Hypospadias repair and urethroplasty; Incontinence; Infertility, male; Klinefelter syndrome; Lung cancer; Mumps; Occupational health; Orchitis; Penile implant surgery; Posttraumatic stress disorder; Proctology; Prostate cancer; Prostate enlargement; Prostate gland; Prostate gland removal; Puberty and adolescence; Pulmonary diseases; Screening; Semen; Sexuality; Sexually transmitted diseases (STDs); Skin cancer; Smoking; Sperm banks; Sports medicine; Steroid abuse; Suicide; Testicles, undescended; Testicular cancer; Testicular surgery; Testicular torsion; Vas deferens; Vasectomy; Women's health.

FOR FURTHER INFORMATION:

Donatelle, Rebecca J. *Health: The Basics.* 7th ed. San Francisco: Benjamin Cummings, 2006. Provides information for lifestyle changes based in current health promotion and disease prevention trends for specific health issues.

Kasper, Dennis L., et al., eds. *Harrison's Principles of Internal Medicine.* 16th ed. New York: McGraw-Hill, 2005. Offers a comprehensive and detailed discussion of most diseases, symptoms, causes, diagnosis, treatment, and expected outcomes.

Litin, Scott C., ed. *Mayo Clinic Family Health Book.* 4th ed. New York: HarperResource, 2009. This handbook provides information regarding healthy living, diseases, and medical care from birth to old age.

Lunenfeld, Bruno, and Louis Gooren, eds. *Textbook of Men's Health.* Boca Raton, Fla.: Parthenon, 2007. Discusses the effects of hormone decline on aging and disease in men.

MedlinePlus. "Men's Health Issues." http://www.nlm .nih.gov/medlineplus/menshealthissues.html#over views. This Web site provides links to news, overviews, and research into conditions affecting men.

National Institutes of Health. "Men's Health." http:// health.nih.gov/category/menshealth. This site provides links to other Web sites with information and resources on a variety of issues related to men's health.

Simon, Harvey B. *The Harvard Medical School Guide to Men's Health.* New York: Free Press, 2004. Offers a comprehensive guide based on research for men to improve their health through healthy living and lifestyle changes.

U.S. Department of Health and Human Services. *Healthy People 2010: Understanding and Improving Health.* Rev. ed. Boston: Jones and Bartlett, 2001. A guide for reaching national goals to improve health in the United States. Specific areas of concern are identified, with discussions of physical, social, and psychological factors in disease and the means to address them.

MENSTRUATION

BIOLOGY

ANATOMY OR SYSTEM AFFECTED: Reproductive system, uterus

SPECIALTIES AND RELATED FIELDS: Endocrinology, gynecology, pediatrics

DEFINITION: The monthly discharge of blood and tissue (menses) by women of childbearing age, caused by changes in hormonal levels.

KEY TERMS:

endometrium: the layer of cells lining the inner cavity of the uterus; the source of menstrual discharge

feedback: a system in which two parts of the body communicate and control each other, often through hormones; can be either negative (inhibitory) or positive (stimulatory)

follicle: a spherical structure within the ovary that contains a developing ovum and that produces hormones; each ovary contains thousands of follicles

hormone: a chemical signal produced in some part of the body that is carried in the blood to another body part, where it has some observable effect

menstrual cycle: the cycle of hormone production, ovulation, menstruation, and other changes that occurs on an approximately monthly schedule in women

ovary: the organ that produces ova and hormones; the two ovaries lie on either side of the uterus, within the abdominal cavity

ovulation: the process by which an ovum is released from its follicle in the ovary; occurs in the middle of each menstrual cycle

ovum (pl. ova): the egg or reproductive cell produced by the female, which when fertilized by a sperm from the male will develop into an embryo

prostaglandins: chemical signals that have local effects on the organ that produces them

uterus: the organ that nourishes and supports the developing embryo; also called the womb

Process and Effects

Menstruation is the monthly discharge of bloody fluid from the uterus. It occurs in humans and in other primates (apes and monkeys), but not in all mammals; for example, horses, cats, and dogs do not menstruate. The menstrual fluid consists of blood, cells and debris from the endometrial lining of the uterus, and mucus and other fluids. The color of the discharge varies from dark brown to bright red during the period of flow. The menstrual discharge does not normally clot after leaving the uterus, but it may contain endometrial debris that resembles blood clots. The flow lasts from four to five days in most women, with spotting (the discharge of scant fluid) possibly continuing another day or two. The volume of fluid lost ranges from 10 to 80 milliliters, with a median of about 40 milliliters. The blood in the menstrual discharge amounts to only a small fraction of the body's total blood volume of about 5,000 milliliters, so normal physiological functioning is not usually impaired by the blood loss that occurs during menstruation.

The first menstruation (menarche) begins when a girl goes through puberty at the age of twelve or thirteen; the last episodes of menstruation occur some forty years later at the time of menopause. Menstruation does not occur during the months of pregnancy or for the first few months after a woman has given birth.

Menstruation is the most visible event of the woman's monthly menstrual cycle. The average length of the menstrual cycle in the population is about 29.1 days, but it may vary from 16 to 35 days, with variation occurring between different individuals and in one individual from month to month. Girls who have just gone through puberty and women who are approaching the menopause tend to have more variation in their cycles than do women in the middle of their reproductive years. There is also an age-related change in cycle length: Cycles tend to be relatively long in teenagers, then decrease in length until a woman is about forty years old, after which cycles tend to lengthen and become irregular.

Hormones cause menstruation to be coordinated with other events in the menstrual cycle. Uterine function is regulated by two hormones, estrogen and progesterone, that are produced in the ovaries. In turn, the production of estrogen and progesterone is controlled by follicle-stimulating hormone (FSH) and luteinizing hormone (LH), both of which are produced in the pituitary gland. The hormones from the ovaries and from the pituitary have mutual control over each other: They participate in a feedback relationship. The fact that females produce ova only once a month, in a cycle, rather than continuously, is the result of a change in the feedback relationships between the ovarian and pituitary hormones as the menstrual cycle proceeds.

In the first half of the cycle, the follicular phase, a predominant negative feedback effect keeps pituitary hormone levels low while allowing estrogen to increase. Day 1 of the menstrual cycle is defined as the day of the onset of the menstrual flow. During the days of menstrual bleeding, levels of estrogen and progesterone are low, but FSH levels are high enough to cause the growth of follicles in the ovary. As the follicles start to grow, they secrete estrogen, and increasing amounts are secreted as the follicles continue to enlarge over the next five to ten days. The estrogen exerts negative feedback control over the pituitary: FSH and LH production is inhibited by estrogen, so levels of these hormones remain low during the follicular phase. Besides producing estrogen, the growing follicles contain ova that are maturing and preparing for ovulation. Meanwhile, estrogen acts on the uterus to cause the growth of the endometrial lining. The lining becomes thicker and its blood supply increases; glands located in the lining also grow and mature. These uterine changes are known as endometrial proliferation.

As the woman nears the middle of her cycle, a dramatic change in hormonal feedback occurs. The increasing secretion of estrogen shifts the hormonal system into a positive feedback mode, whereby an increase in estrogen stimulates the release of LH and FSH from the pituitary instead of inhibiting it. Thus, at the middle of the cycle (around day 14), simultaneous peaks in levels of estrogen, LH, and FSH occur. The peak in LH triggers ovulation by causing changes in the wall of the follicle, allowing it to break open to release its ovum. Although a group of follicles had matured up to this point, usually only the largest one ovulates, and the remainder in the group die and cease hormone production.

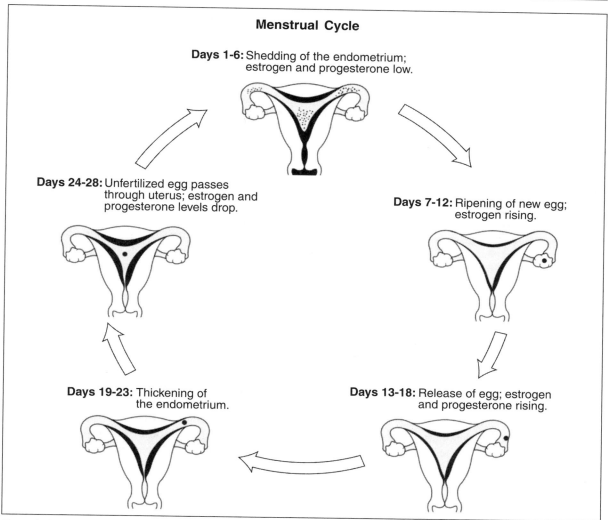

Menstrual Cycle

Days 1-6: Shedding of the endometrium; estrogen and progesterone low.

Days 24-28: Unfertilized egg passes through uterus; estrogen and progesterone levels drop.

Days 7-12: Ripening of new egg; estrogen rising.

Days 19-23: Thickening of the endometrium.

Days 13-18: Release of egg; estrogen and progesterone rising.

Exact timing varies from woman to woman; day 1 is defined as the day of onset of menstrual flow; ovulation occurs in mid-cycle (around day 14). Hormonal levels are rising and falling throughout the cycle.

Following ovulation, negative feedback is reestablished. The follicle that just ovulated remains as a functional part of the ovary; it becomes transformed into the corpus luteum, a structure which produces estrogen and progesterone throughout most of the second half of the cycle, the luteal phase. During this phase, the combined presence of estrogen and progesterone reestablishes negative feedback over the pituitary, and LH and FSH levels decline. A second ovulation is prevented because an LH peak is not possible at this time. The combined action of estrogen and progesterone causes the uterus to enter its secretory phase during the second half of the cycle: The glands in the thickened endometrium secrete nutrients that will support an embryo if

the woman becomes pregnant, and the ample blood supply to the endometrium can supply the embryo with other nutrients and oxygen. If the woman does in fact become pregnant, the embryo will secrete a hormone that will ensure the continued production of estrogen and progesterone, and because of these hormones, the uterus will remain in the secretory condition throughout pregnancy. Menstruation does not occur during pregnancy because of the high levels of estrogen and progesterone, which continually support the uterus.

If the woman does not become pregnant, the corpus luteum automatically degenerates, starting at about the twenty-fourth day of the menstrual cycle. As the corpus luteum dies, it fails to produce estrogen and progesterone, so levels of these hormones decrease. As the amounts of estrogen and progesterone drop, the uterus begins to produce prostaglandins, chemicals that act as local signals within the uterus. The prostaglandins cause a number of changes in uterine function: Blood flow to the endometrium is temporarily cut off, causing the endometrial tissue to die, and the uterine muscle begins to contract, causing further changes in blood flow. The decreased blood flow and the muscle contractions contribute to the cramping pain that many women feel just before and at the time of menstrual bleeding. Menstrual bleeding starts when the blood flow to the endometrium is reestablished and the dead tissue is sloughed off and washed out of the uterus. This event signals the start of a new menstrual cycle.

COMPLICATIONS AND DISORDERS

Many disorders involving menstruation exist. Toxic shock syndrome is a disease that, while not caused directly by menstruation, sometimes occurs during menstruation in women who use tampons to absorb the menstrual flow. The symptoms of toxic shock syndrome—fever, rash, a drop in blood pressure, diarrhea, vomiting, and fainting—are caused by toxins produced by the bacterium *Staphylococcus aureus*. This bacterium is normally present in limited numbers within the vagina, but the use of high-absorbency tampons is associated with a higher-than-normal bacterial growth and toxin production. Toxic shock syndrome requires immediate medical attention, since it may be fatal if left untreated. Women can reduce the risk of toxic shock syndrome by changing tampons often, using lower-absorbency types, and alternating the use of tampons and sanitary napkins.

Amenorrhea is defined as the absence of menstruation. It is usually, but not always, coincident with lack of ovulation. Amenorrhea may be primary (the woman has never menstruated) or secondary (menstrual cycles that were once normal have stopped). The condition is usually associated with abnormal patterns of hormone secretion, but the problem in hormone secretion may itself be merely the symptom of some other underlying disorder. One of the most common situations leading to both primary and secondary amenorrhea is low body weight, caused by malnutrition, eating disorders, or sustained exercise. Body fat has two roles in reproduction: It provides energy needed for tissue growth and cell functions, and it contributes to circulating estrogen levels. Loss of body fat may create a situation in which the reproductive system ceases to function because of

low estrogen levels and because of lack of needed energy. The result is seen as amenorrhea. Emotional or physical stress may also cause amenorrhea, because stress results in the release of hormones that interfere with the reproductive hormones. Ideally, amenorrhea is treated by removing its cause; for example, a special diet or a change in an exercise program can bring about an increase in body fat stores, or stress level can be reduced through changes in lifestyle or with counseling. Ironically, sometimes birth control pills are prescribed for women with amenorrhea. The pills do not cure the amenorrhea, but they counteract some of the long-term problems associated with it, such as changes in the endometrial lining and loss of bone density.

Dysmenorrhea refers to abnormally intense uterine pain associated with menstruation. It is estimated that 5 to 10 percent of women experience pain intense enough to interfere with their school or work schedules. Dysmenorrhea may be primary (occurring in women with no known disease) or secondary (caused by a disease condition such as a tumor or infection). Studies have shown uterine prostaglandin levels to be correlated with the degree of pain perceived in primary dysmenorrhea, and drugs that interfere with prostaglandins offer an effective treatment for this condition. These drugs include aspirin, acetaminophen, ibuprofen, and naproxen; some formulas are available without a doctor's prescription, but the stronger drugs require one. Secondary dysmenorrhea is best managed by removing the underlying cause; if this is not possible, the antiprostaglandin drugs may be useful in controlling the pain.

Menorrhagia is excessive menstrual blood loss, usually defined as more than 80 milliliters of fluid lost per cycle. This condition can have serious health consequences because of the loss of red blood cells, which are essential for carrying oxygen to tissues. Women who have given birth to several children are more likely to suffer from menorrhagia, possibly because of enlargement of the uterine cavity and interference with the mechanisms that limit menstrual blood flow. Women who have diseases that interfere with blood clotting may also have menorrhagia. Although the menstrual discharge itself does not usually form clots after it leaves the uterus, clots do form within the uterine endometrium; these clots normally prevent excessive blood loss. Treatment for menorrhagia may begin with iron and vitamin supplements to induce increased red blood cell production, or transfusions may be used to replace the lost red blood cells. If this is unsuccessful, treatment with birth control pills, destruction of the endometrium by laser surgery, or a hysterectomy (surgical removal of the uterus) may be necessary.

Endometriosis is a condition in which endometrial cells from the uterus become misplaced within the abdominal cavity, adhering to and growing on the surface of internal organs. The outside of the uterus, the oviducts (Fallopian tubes), the surface of the ovaries, and the outer surface of the intestines can all support the growth of endometrial tissue. Endometriosis is thought to arise during menstruation, when endometrial tissue enters the oviducts instead of being carried outward through the cervix and vagina. Through the oviducts, the endometrial tissue has access to the abdominal cavity. Since the misplaced endometrial tissue responds to hormones in the same way that the normal endometrium does, it undergoes cyclic changes in thickness and attempts to shed at the time of menstruation. Endometriosis results in intense pain during menstruation and can cause infertility because of interference with ovulation, ovum or sperm transport, or uterine function. Endometriosis is treated with birth control pills or with drugs that suppress menstrual cycles, or the endometrial tissue may be removed surgically.

Premenstrual syndrome (PMS) is a set of symptoms that occurs in some women in the week before the start of menstruation, with the symptoms disappearing once menstruation begins. Researchers and physicians who study PMS have struggled to devise a standard definition for the disorder, but the list of possible symptoms is lengthy and varies from woman to woman and even within one woman from month to month. The possible symptoms include both psychological and physical changes: irritability, nervous tension, anxiety, moodiness, depression, lethargy, insomnia, confusion, crying, food cravings, fatigue, weight gain, swelling and bloating, breast tenderness, backache, headache, dizziness, muscle stiffness, and abdominal cramps. A diagnosis of PMS requires that the symptoms show a clear relation to the timing of menstruation and that they recur during most menstrual cycles. Researchers estimate that 3 to 5 percent of women have PMS symptoms that are so severe that they are incapacitating, but that milder symptoms occur in about 50 percent of all women.

Because of the variability in symptoms between women, some researchers believe that there are several subtypes of PMS, each with its own cluster of symptoms. It is possible that each subtype has a unique cause. Suggested causes of PMS include an imbalance in the ratio of estrogen to progesterone following ovulation, changes in the hormones that control salt and water balance (the renin-angiotensin-aldosterone system), increased levels of prolactin (a hormone that acts on the breast), changes in amounts of brain chemicals, altered functioning of the biological clock that determines daily rhythms, poor diet or sensitivity to certain foods, and psychological factors such as attitude toward menstruation, stresses of family or professional life, and underlying personality disorders. Studies evaluating these theories have yielded contradictory results, so that no one cause of PMS has yet been found. Current treatments for PMS include dietary therapy, hormone administration, and psychological counseling, but no treatment has been found effective in all PMS patients.

An interesting phenomenon associated with menstruation is menstrual synchrony, also known as the "dormitory effect." Among women who live together, menstrual cycles gradually become synchronized, so that the women begin to menstruate within a few days of one another. Researchers have found that this phenomenon probably occurs because of pheromones, chemical signals that are produced by an individual and that have an effect on another individual. Pheromones act on the brain through the sense of smell, even though there may not be an odor that is consciously perceived.

PERSPECTIVE AND PROSPECTS

Early beliefs about menstruation were based on folk magic and superstition rather than on scientific evidence. Even today, some cultures persist in believing that menstruating women possess deleterious powers: that the presence of a menstruating woman can cause crops to fail, farm animals to die, or beer, bread, jam, and other foods to be spoiled. Some people believe that these incidents will occur even if the menstruating woman has no evil intention. Because of the possibility of these events, some cultures prohibit menstruating women from interacting with others. In the most rigorous example of such a taboo, some societies require that menstruating women live in special huts for the duration of the bleeding period.

Folk beliefs about menstruating women have been bolstered by religious views of menstruating women as "unclean" and in need of purification. In Orthodox Judaism, there are detailed proscriptions to be observed by a menstruating woman, including the avoidance of sexual intercourse. Seven days after her menstrual flow has stopped, the Orthodox Jewish woman undergoes a ritual purification, after which she may resume sexual relations with her husband. Early Christians absorbed the Jewish belief in the uncleanliness of a menstruating woman and prohibited her from entering church or receiving the sacraments. These injunctions were lifted by the seventh century, but the view of women as spiritually and bodily impure persists in some Christian groups to this day.

In the United States, most couples abstain from intercourse during the woman's menstrual period. There is no medical justification for this behavior; in fact, research has demonstrated that intercourse can alleviate menstrual cramping, at least temporarily. Still, surveys have shown that a majority of both men and women think that it is wrong for a woman to have intercourse while menstruating.

There are also persistent beliefs that women's physical and mental abilities suffer during menstruation. In fact, this was the predominant medical opinion up through the nineteenth and early twentieth centuries. Medical writings from this time are filled with injunctions for women to rest and refrain from exercise and intellectual strain while menstruating. It was a common belief that education could actually cause physical harm to women. Some men used this advice as justification for excluding women from equal opportunities in education and employment. Starting in the late nineteenth century, however, scientific studies clearly demonstrated that education has no harmful effects and that there is no diminution of intellectual or physical performance during menstruation. Nevertheless, the latter finding has been one that the general population finds difficult to accept.

The latest view of menstruation is that, far from being harmful, menstrual bleeding is directly beneficial to a woman's health. Margie Profet, an evolutionary biologist at the University of California, theorizes that menstruation evolved as a means of periodically removing disease-causing bacteria and viruses from the woman's uterus. These organisms might enter the uterus along with sperm after sexual activity. In Profet's view, the energetic cost of replacing the blood and tissue lost through menstruation is more than outweighed by the protective benefits of menstruation. Her theory implies that treatments which suppress menstruation, as birth control drugs sometimes do, are not always advantageous.

Suppression of menstruation through extended or continuous cycling with combined hormonal contraception has recently been reexamined for various benefits, including increased contraceptive efficacy. Some clinicians and consumers have embraced this concept, which can be done with any continuous (no placebo or no-pill interval) use of a monophasic combined oral contraceptive pill, the Ortho Evra patch, or NuvaRing. New formulations of combined oral contraceptives include Seasonale and Seasonique, both of which result in menstrual bleeding every three months, and Lybrel, which eliminates cycles for one year. Other formulations have shortened the one week pill-free interval, resulting in shorter and lighter menses.

—*Marcia Watson-Whitmyre, Ph.D.*

See also Amenorrhea; Cervical, ovarian, and uterine cancers; Childbirth; Conception; Contraception; Dysmenorrhea; Endocrinology; Endometriosis; Genital disorders, female; Gynecology; Hormones; Hot flashes; Infertility, female; Menopause; Menorrhagia; Ovarian cysts; Ovaries; Pregnancy and gestation; Premenstrual syndrome (PMS); Puberty and adolescence; Reproductive system; Toxic shock syndrome; Uterus; Women's health.

FOR FURTHER INFORMATION:

Ammer, Christine. *The New A to Z of Women's Health: A Concise Encyclopedia.* 6th ed. New York: Checkmark Books, 2009. A respected classic that covers the full spectrum of women's health issues, including reproduction, the aging process, methods of contraception, and childbearing. Helpful charts and illustrations.

Berek, Jonathan S., ed. *Berek and Novak's Gynecology.* 14th ed. Philadelphia: Lippincott Williams & Wilkins, 2007. A standard text covering all aspects of gynecology including biology and physiology, family planning, sexuality, and benign gynecologic conditions.

Covington, Timothy R., and J. Frank McClendon. *Sex Care: The Complete Guide to Safe and Healthy Sex.* New York: Pocket Books, 1987. Parts 1 and 2 deal with contraception and sexually transmitted diseases, but part 3 covers some topics directly related to menstruation: premenstrual syndrome, toxic shock syndrome, feminine hygiene, and various myths.

Golub, Sharon. *Periods: From Menarche to Menopause.* Newbury Park, Calif.: Sage, 1992. An exceptionally complete book that presents information on all aspects of the menstrual cycle. The chapters dealing with scientific studies are accurate and easy to read. The author includes her thoughts on how society could make menstruation easier for women and on further research that needs to be done.

Loulan, JoAnne, and Bonnie Worthen. *Period: A Girl's Guide to Menstruation.* Rev. ed. Minnetonka, Minn.: Book Peddlers, 2001. A guide for young women that thoroughly covers questions about puberty and menstruation and includes diagrams to familiarize readers with the inner workings of their bodies.

Quilligan, Edward J., and Frederick P. Zuspan, eds. *Current Therapy in Obstetrics and Gynecology.* 5th ed. Philadelphia: W. B. Saunders, 2000. A standard medical reference on treatment for women's disorders, arranged in an encyclopedia format, with short articles on each topic. There is a particularly good description of premenstrual syndrome, written by Guy E. Abraham and Richard J. Taylor.

Rako, Susan. *No More Periods? The Risks of Menstrual Suppression and Other Cutting-Edge Issues in Women's Reproductive Health.* New York: Harmony Books, 2003. Argues that menstrual suppression and the manipulation of women's hormones for the purposes of birth control is "bad science" and can lead to bone loss, sexual dysfunction, sterility, and depression.

Weschler, Toni. *Taking Charge of Your Fertility.* Rev. ed. New York: Collins, 2001. An excellent book that encourages women to become responsible for their own reproductive health. Includes discussions of menstrual cycles and the hormones involved.

MENTAL RETARDATION
DISEASE/DISORDER

ANATOMY OR SYSTEM AFFECTED: Brain, nervous system, psychic-emotional system

SPECIALTIES AND RELATED FIELDS: Genetics, psychiatry, psychology

DEFINITION: Significant subaverage intellectual development and deficient adaptive behavior often accompanied by physical abnormalities.

KEY TERMS:

educable mentally retarded (EMR): individuals with mild-to-moderate retardation; they can be educated with some modifications of the regular education program and can achieve a minimal level of success

inborn metabolic disorder: an abnormality caused by a gene mutation that interferes with normal metabolism and often results in mental retardation

mental handicap: the condition of an individual classified as "educable mentally retarded"

mental impairment: the condition of an individual classified as "trainable mentally retarded" and typically distinguished from mentally ill

neural tube defects: birth defects resulting from the failure of the embryonic neural tube to close; usually results in some degree of mental retardation

trainable mentally retarded (TMR): individuals with moderate-to-severe retardation; only low levels of achievement may be reached by such persons

CAUSES AND SYMPTOMS

Mental retardation is a condition in which a person demonstrates significant subaverage development of intellectual function, along with poor adaptive behavior. Diagnosis can be made at birth if physical abnormalities also accompany mental retardation. An infant with mild mental retardation, however, may not be diagnosed until problems arise in school. Estimates of the prevalence of mental retardation vary from 1 to 3 percent of the world's total population.

Diagnosis of mental retardation takes into consideration three factors: subaverage intellectual function, deficiency in adaptive behavior, and early-age onset (before the age of eighteen). Intellectual function is a measure of one's intelligence quotient (IQ). Four levels of retardation based on IQ are described by the American Psychiatric Association. An individual with an IQ between 50 and 70 is considered mildly retarded, one with an IQ between 35 and 49 is moderately retarded, one with an IQ between 21 and 34 is severely retarded, and an individual with an IQ of less than 20 is termed profoundly retarded.

A person's level of adaptive behavior is not as easily determined as an IQ, but it is generally defined as the ability to meet social expectations in the individual's own environment. Assessment is based on development of certain skills: sensorimotor, speech and language, self-help, and socialization skills. Tests have been developed to aid in these measurements.

To identify possible mental retardation in infants, the use of language milestones is a helpful tool. For example, parents and pediatricians will observe whether children begin to smile, coo, babble, and use words during the appropriate age ranges. Once children reach school age, poor school achievement may identify those who are mentally impaired. Psychometric tests appropriate to the age of the children will help with diagnosis.

Classification of the degree of mental retardation is never absolutely clear, and dividing lines are often somewhat arbitrary. There has been debate about the value of classifying or labeling persons in categories of mental deficiency. On one hand, it is important for professionals to understand the amount of deficiency and to determine what kind of education and treatment would be appropriate and helpful to each individual. On the other hand, such classification can lead to low self-esteem, rejection by peers, and low expectations from teachers and parents.

There has been a marked change in the terminology used in classifying mental retardation from the early days of its study. In the early twentieth century, the terms used for moderate, severe, and profound retardation were "moron," "imbecile," and "idiot." In Great Britain, the term "feeble-minded" was used to indicate moderate retardation. These terms are no longer used by professionals working with the mentally retarded. "Idiot" was the classification given to the most profoundly retarded until the middle of the twentieth century. Historically, the word has changed in meaning, from William Shakespeare's day when the court jester was called an idiot, to an indication of psychosis, and later to define the lowest grade of mental deficiency. The term "idiocy" has been replaced with the expression "profound mental retardation."

Determining the cause of mental retardation is much more difficult than might be expected. More than a thousand different disorders that can cause mental retardation have been reported. Some cases seem to be entirely hereditary, others to be caused by environmental stress, and others the result of a combination of the two. In a large number of cases, however, the cause cannot be established. The mildly retarded make up the largest proportion of the mentally retarded population, and their condition seems to be a recessive genetic trait with no accompanying physical abnormalities. From a medical standpoint, mental retardation is considered to be a result of disease or biological defect and is classified according to its cause. Some of these causes are infections, poisons, environmental trauma, metabolic and nutritional abnormalities, and brain malformation.

Infections are especially harmful to brain development if they occur in the first trimester of pregnancy. Rubella is a viral infection that often results in mental retardation. Syphilis is a sexually transmitted disease that affects adults and infants born to them, resulting in progressive mental degeneration.

Poisons such as mercury, lead, and alcohol have a very damaging effect on the developing brain. More recent concerns about mercury in the diets of those who frequently consume fish and other seafood have encouraged some individuals, such as pregnant women, to change their dietary behavior in an effort to avoid potential harm to fetal development. Lead-based paints linger in older houses and are even on toys, causing poisoning in children or otherwise affecting the mental functioning of all persons in the home. Children may mouth or suck on these lead-painted toys, or they may eat chipped house paint and plaster or put them in their mouths; all of these actions possibly cause mental retardation, cerebral palsy, and convulsive and behavioral disorders as a result of lead exposure.

Traumatic environmental effects that can cause mental retardation include prenatal exposure to X rays, lack of oxygen to the brain, or a mother's fall during pregnancy. During birth itself, the use of forceps can cause brain damage, and labor that is too brief or too long can cause mental impairment. After the birth process, head trauma or high temperature can affect brain function.

Poor nutrition and inborn metabolic disorders may cause defective mental development because vital body processes are hindered. One of these conditions, for which every newborn is tested, is phenylketonuria (PKU), in which the body cannot process the amino acid phenylalanine. If PKU is detected in infancy, subsequent mental retardation can be avoided by placing the child on a carefully controlled diet, thus preventing buildup of toxic compounds that would be harmful to the brain.

The failure of the neural tube to close in the early development of an embryo may result in anencephaly (an incomplete brain or none at all), hydrocephalus (an excessive amount of cerebrospinal fluid), or spina bifida (an incomplete vertebra, which leaves the spinal cord exposed). Anencephalic infants will live only a few

---

INFORMATION ON MENTAL RETARDATION

CAUSES: Often unknown; may include genetic factors, disease, infections, poisons, environmental trauma, metabolic and nutritional abnormalities, brain malformation

SYMPTOMS: Physical abnormalities, subaverage intellectual function, deficiency in adaptive behavior

DURATION: Lifelong

TREATMENTS: None; supportive therapy may include special education, physical therapy, family counseling

hours. About half of those with other neural tube disorders will survive, usually with some degree of mental retardation. Research has shown that if a mother's diet has sufficient quantities of folic acid, neural tube closure disorders will be rare or nonexistent.

Microcephaly is another physical defect associated with mental retardation. In this condition, the head is abnormally small because of inadequate brain growth. Microcephaly may be inherited or caused by maternal infection, drugs, irradiation, or lack of oxygen at birth.

Abnormal chromosome numbers are not uncommon in developing embryos and will cause spontaneous abortions in most cases. Those babies that survive usually demonstrate varying degrees of mental retardation, and incidence increases with maternal age. A well-known example of a chromosome disorder is Down syndrome (formerly called mongolism), in which there is an extra copy of the twenty-first chromosome. Gene products caused by the extra chromosome cause mental retardation and other physical problems. Other well-studied chromosomal abnormalities involve the sex chromosomes. Both males and females may be born with too many or too few sex chromosomes, which often results in mental retardation.

Mild retardation with no other noticeable problems has been found to run in certain families. It occurs more often in the lower economic strata of society and probably reflects only the lower end of the normal distribution of intelligence in a population. The condition is probably a result of genetic factors interacting with environmental ones. It has been found that culturally deprived children have a lower level of intellectual function because of decreased stimuli as the infant brain develops.

Treatment and Therapy

Diagnosis of the level of mental retardation is important in meeting the needs of the intellectually handicapped. It can open the way for effective measures to be taken to help these persons achieve the highest quality of life possible for them.

Individuals with an IQ of 50 to 70 have mild-to-moderate retardation and are classified as "educable mentally retarded" (EMR). They can profit from the regular education program when it is somewhat modified. The general purposes of all education are to allow for the development of knowledge, to provide a basis for vocational competence, and to allow opportunity for self-realization. The EMR can achieve some success in academic subjects, make satisfactory social ad-

justment, and achieve minimal occupational adequacy if given proper training. In Great Britain, these individuals are referred to as "educationally subnormal" (ESN).

Persons with moderate-to-severe retardation generally have IQs between 21 and 49 and are classified as "trainable mentally retarded" (TMR). These individuals are not educable in the traditional sense, but many can be trained in self-help skills, socialization into the family, and some degree of economic independence with supervision. They need a developmental curriculum which promotes personal development, independence, and social skills.

The profoundly retarded are classified as "totally dependent" and have IQs of 20 or less. They cannot be trained to care for themselves, to socialize, or to be independent to any degree. They will need almost complete care and supervision throughout life. They may learn to understand a few simple commands, but they will be able to speak only a few words. Meaningful speech is not characteristic of this group.

EMR individuals need a modified curriculum, along with appropriately qualified and experienced teachers. Activities should include some within their special class and some in which they interact with students of other classes. The amount of time spent in regular classes and in special classes should be determined by individual needs in order to achieve the goals and objectives planned for each. Individual development must be the primary concern.

For TMR individuals, the differences will be in the areas of emphasis, level of attainment projected, and methods used. The programs should consist of small classes that may be held within the public schools or outside with the help of parents and other concerned groups. Persons trained in special education are needed to guide the physical, social, and emotional development experiences effectively.

A systematic approach in special education has proven to be the best teaching method to make clear to students what behaviors will result in the successful completion of goals. This approach has been designed so that children work with only one concept at a time. There are appropriate remedies planned for misconceptions along the way. Progress is charted for academic skills, home-living skills, and prevocational training. Decisions on the type of academic training appropriate for a TMR individual are not based on classification or labels, but on demonstrated ability.

One of the most important features of successful special education is the involvement of parents. Parents faced with rearing a retarded child may find the task overwhelming and have a great need of caring support and information about their child and the implications for their future. Parental involvement gives the parents the opportunity to learn by observing how the professionals facilitate effective learning experiences for their children at school.

Counselors help parents identify problems and implement plans of action. They can also help them determine whether goals are being reached. Counselors must know about the community resources that are available to families. They can help parents find emotional reconciliation with the problems presented by their special children. It is important for parents to be able to accept the child's limitations. They should not lavish special or different treatment on the retarded child, but rather treat this child like the other children.

Placing a child outside the home is indicated only when educational, behavioral, or medical controls are needed that cannot be provided in the home. Physicians and social workers should be able to do some counseling to supplement that of the trained counselors. Those who offer counseling should have basic counseling skills and relevant knowledge about the mentally retarded individual and the family.

EMR individuals will usually marry, may have children, and often become self-supporting. The TMR will live in an institution or at home or in foster homes for their entire lives. They will probably never become self-sufficient. The presence of a TMR child has a great impact on families and may weaken family closeness. It creates additional expenses and limits family activities. Counseling for these families is very important.

Sheltered employment provides highly controlled working conditions, helping the mentally retarded to become contributing members of society. This arrangement benefits the individual, the family, and society as the individual experiences the satisfaction and dignity of work. The mildly retarded may need only a short period of time in the sheltered workshop. The greater the degree of mental retardation, the more likely shelter will be required on a permanent basis. For the workshop to be successful, those in charge of it must consider both the personal development of the disabled worker and the business production and profit of the workshop. Failure to consider the business success of these ventures has led to failures of the programs.

There has been a trend toward deinstitutionalizing the mentally retarded, to relocate as many residents as possible into appropriate community homes. Success will depend on a suitable match between the individual and the type of home provided. This approach is most effective for the mentally retarded if the staff of a facility is well trained and there is a fair amount of satisfactory interaction between staff and residents. It is important that residents not be ignored, and they must be monitored for proper evaluation at each step along the way. Top priority must be given to preparation of the staff to work closely with the mentally impaired and handicapped.

In the past, there was no way to know before a child's birth if there would be abnormalities. With advances in technology, however, a variety of prenatal tests can be done, and many fetal abnormalities can be detected. Genetic counseling is important for persons who have these tests conducted. Some may have previously had a retarded child, or have retarded family members. Others may have something in their backgrounds that would indicate a higher-than-average risk for physical and/or mental abnormalities. Some come for testing before a child is conceived; others do not come until afterward. Tests can be done on the fetal blood and tissues that will reveal chromosomal abnormalities or inborn metabolic errors.

Many parents do not seek testing or genetic counseling because of the stress and anxiety that may result. Though most prenatal tests result in normal findings, if problems are indicated the parents are faced with what may be a difficult decision: whether to continue the pregnancy. It is often impossible to predict the extent of an abnormality, and weighing the sanctity of life in relation to the quality of life may present an ethical and religious dilemma. Others prefer to know what problems lie ahead and what their options are.

Finally, it is important to realize that problems such as mental retardation may not occur in isolation from other problems. Concurrent physical and mental illnesses may add complexity to managing treatment and services for individuals with more than one condition. Assessment to rule out other conditions remains an important step in ongoing and evolving care for individuals with mental retardation and similar conditions.

PERSPECTIVE AND PROSPECTS

Throughout history, the mentally retarded were first ignored, and then subjected to ridicule. The first attempts to educate the mentally retarded were initiated in France in the mid-nineteenth century. Shortly afterward, institutions for them began to spring up in Europe and the United States. These were often in remote rural areas, separated from the communities nearby, and were usually ill-equipped and understaffed. The institutions were quite regimented, and harsh discipline was kept. Meaningful interactions usually did not occur between the patients and the staff.

The medical approach of the institutions was to treat the outward condition of the mentally retarded and ignore them as people. No concern for their social and emotional needs was shown. There were no provisions for children to play, nor was there concern for the needs of the family of those with mental handicaps.

Not until the end of the nineteenth century were the first classes set up in some U.S. public schools for education of the mentally retarded. The first half of the twentieth century brought about the expansion of the public school programs for individuals with both mild and moderate mental retardation. After World War II, perhaps in response to the slaughter of mentally handicapped persons in Nazi Germany, strong efforts were made to provide educational, medical, and recreational services for the mentally retarded.

Groundbreaking research in the 1950's led to the normalization of society's attitude about the mentally retarded in the United States. Plans to help these individuals live as normal a life as possible were made. The National Association for Retarded Citizens was founded in 1950 and had a very strong influence on public opinion. In 1961, U.S. president John F. Kennedy appointed the Panel on Mental Retardation and instructed it to prepare a plan for the United States to help meet the complex problems of the mentally retarded. The panel presented ninety recommendations in the areas of research, prevention, medical services, education, law, and local and national organization. Further presidential commissions on the topic were appointed and have had far-reaching effects for the well-being of the mentally retarded.

A "Declaration of the Rights of Mentally Retarded Persons" was adopted by the General Assembly of the United Nations in 1971, and the Education for All Handicapped Children Act was passed in the United States in 1975, providing for the development of educational programs appropriate for all handicapped and disabled children and youth. These pieces of legislation were milestones in the struggle to improve learning opportunities for the mentally retarded.

Changes continue to take place in attitudes toward greater integration of the retarded into schools and the community, leading to significant improvements. The role of the family has increased in emphasis, for it has often been the families themselves that have worked to change old, outdated policies. The cooperation of the family is very important in improving the social and intellectual development of the mentally retarded child. Because so many new and innovative techniques have been used, it is very important that programs be evaluated and compared to one another to determine which methods provide the best training and education for the mentally retarded.

—Katherine H. Houp, Ph.D.;
updated by Nancy A. Piotrowski, Ph.D.

See also Batten's disease; Birth defects; Brain; Brain damage; Congenital hypothyroidism; Cornelia de Lange syndrome; Developmental disorders; Down syndrome; Endocrine disorders; Fetal alcohol syndrome; Fragile X syndrome; Genetic diseases; Genetics and inheritance; Learning disabilities; Phenylketonuria (PKU); Prader-Willi syndrome; Pregnancy and gestation; Psychiatry; Psychiatry, child and adolescent; Rubinstein-Taybi syndrome.

FOR FURTHER INFORMATION:

American Association of Intellectual and Developmental Disabilities. http://www.aaidd.org. Formerly the American Association of Mental Retardation, this group for professionals in the mental health field promotes progressive policies, research, effective practices, and universal human rights for the mentally retarded, or for people with intellectual and developmental disabilities, a term preferred by this organization.

Beirne-Smith, Mary, James R. Patton, and Shannon H. Kim, eds. *Mental Retardation.* 7th ed. Upper Saddle River, N.J.: Prentice Hall, 2006. Covers the causes and characteristics of individuals with mental retardation across the life span, explores the benefits of assistive technology, and surveys related legislation and policy issues.

Best Buddies International. http://www.bestbuddies.org. Facilitates support among people with mental retardation and involving them in their communities.

Drew, Clifford J., ed. *Mental Retardation: A Lifespan Approach to People with Intellectual Disabilities.* 8th ed. Boston: Allyn & Bacon, 2004. An introductory and interdisciplinary text that examines all aspects of diagnosis and intervention and discusses multicultural issues related to assessment bias, language differences, and mental retardation in all stages of life.

Dudley, James R. *Confronting the Stigma in Their Lives: Helping People with a Mental Retardation Label.* Springfield, Ill.: Charles C Thomas, 1997. This book is written for those concerned with combating the negative effects of being labeled as having a mental disorder.

Glidden, Laraine Masters. *International Review of Research in Mental Retardation.* New York: Elsevier, 2006. An interdisciplinary text, updated regularly, that surveys recent research into the causes, effects, classification systems, and syndromes of mental retardation. Contributions from nutrition, genetics, psychology, education, and other health and behavioral sciences are included.

Matson, Johnny L., and Rowland P. Barrett, eds. *Psychopathology in the Mentally Retarded.* 2d ed. Boston: Allyn & Bacon, 1993. This book addresses an often-neglected topic: the psychological problems that may be found in those with mental retardation. Discusses special emotional problems based on the causation of deficiencies.

Schalock, Robert, et al. *Intellectual Disability: Definition, Classification, and Systems of Supports.* 11th ed. Washington, D.C.: American Association on Intellectual and Developmental Disabilities, 2010. Written by a committee of experts, this work provides updated, authoritative information on mental retardation, "including best practice guidelines on diagnosing and classifying intellectual disability [mental retardation] and developing a system of supports for people living with an intellectual disability."

MENTAL ILLNESS. *See* **PSYCHIATRIC DISORDERS;** *specific diseases.*

MERCURY POISONING

DISEASE/DISORDER

ANATOMY OR SYSTEM AFFECTED: Nervous system

SPECIALTIES AND RELATED FIELDS: Environmental health, epidemiology, neurology, occupational health, pediatrics

DEFINITION: Mercury is a naturally occurring element that can cause neurological damage in humans exposed to it.

KEY TERMS:

methylmercury: a neurotoxin that is the form of mercury that accumulates most easily in biological tissues

neuropathy: any disease of the nervous system

INFORMATION ON MERCURY POISONING

CAUSES: Exposure to mercury through inhalation or ingestion

SYMPTOMS: Neurological damage; may include tremors, slurred speech, cognitive problems

DURATION: Chronic

TREATMENTS: None; avoidance or limiting of exposure

CAUSES AND SYMPTOMS

Mercury is a metallic element once used in a wide variety of applications, ranging from industrial use in processing ore to serving as the indicator fluid in thermometers. In its pure form, mercury is a soft silver-colored metal with a melting point of a frigid −40 degrees Celsius. Consequently, mercury is liquid at room temperature. Mercury and mercury compounds such as methylmercury are known neurotoxins. Prolonged exposure to mercury, either through inhaling mercury vapors or through ingesting it as a contaminant in foodstuffs, will lead to permanent neurological damage. Ingested mercury can also irritate the gastrointestinal tract and has been known to damage kidneys.

Occupational neuropathy has long been anecdotally associated with mercury exposure. The phrase "mad as a hatter," for example, became common in the nineteenth century when workers in the hat industry developed tremors, slurred speech, and problems thinking clearly following exposure to fumes produced by the felting process. A mercury nitrate compound was used to remove animal hair from hides in hat factories. In some cases of long-term exposure, neuropathy progressed to the point where the sufferers experienced hallucinations.

Despite the widespread prevalence of occupational illness among hatters, the nineteenth century medical community did not recognize the dangers of mercury exposure. Mercury was, in fact, used for a variety of medical applications, ranging from treating syphilis to being applied as a topical antiseptic in the form of mercurochrome. Mercurochrome continued to be used as late as the 1990's, although the Food and Drug Administration (FDA) ruled in 1998 that it would be treated as a "new drug," meaning that any company wishing to manufacture it for nationwide distribution had to submit it for FDA review first.

The mining industry also used mercury extensively.

Mercury amalgamates readily with gold dust, making it heavier and causing it to sink in to the bottom of rocker boxes as ore is washed as part of placer mining. During the California gold rush, at least 7,600 tons of mercury were deposited into Sierra Nevada streams. Similar amounts were used elsewhere globally, leading to large quantities of mercury being deposited on streambeds and ocean floors. That mercury is now making its way back into the environment in the form of methylmercury, the organic form of mercury that causes most concern among health care professionals today.

Methylmercury is formed when mercury forms a mercury-carbon compound through bacterial action. Manufactured methylmercury and dimethylmercury were common fungicides until the 1970's, when they were banned due to their toxicity.

TREATMENT AND THERAPY

With mercury poisoning, prevention is the best form of treatment. Occupational exposure to mercury rarely takes place, and the biggest risk of mercury poisoning today comes from its ingestion within the food chain. Methylmercury bioaccumulates readily and has been found in large concentrations in seafood such as tuna, swordfish, and shark. Numerous studies have shown that when pregnant women consume fish containing high levels of methylmercury the resulting mercury poisoning can cause permanent neurological damage to the developing fetus. Young children are also at risk of developing neuropathy if they eat fish with high mercury levels. This problem was first recognized in the 1970's, but did not become widely publicized until the early twenty-first century. Pregnant women, nursing mothers, and young children are all now advised to avoid some varieties of fish completely, while limiting their consumption of others.

PERSPECTIVE AND PROSPECTS

Although the use of mercury for many applications was discontinued as evidence mounted regarding the dangers of mercury exposure, thimerosal, a mercury compound, continued to be used as a preservative in vaccines used in human medicine into the twenty-first century. In the 1990's, many parents became convinced that thimerosal, which metabolizes readily to ethylmercury, was responsible for the rising rate of autism in American children. Some health activists argued that the increase in autism in the late twentieth century correlated with the increase in the number of vaccines that young children received in the first few years of life. The use of thimerosal as a preservative was discontinued by manufacturers for most vaccines, with the exception of influenza, but research showed that vaccines were not the cause of autism.

One use of mercury that does continue despite several decades of debate over its safety is the application of mercury amalgam tooth fillings in dentistry. The typical "silver" tooth filling is actually 50 percent mercury. Health activists argue that the practice should be stopped, as mercury leaching from the filling into the body could lead to mercury poisoning. In 2002, the FDA concluded that research to date had shown no evidence of ill effects other than rare cases of allergic reactions.

Given the widespread dispersion of mercury into the environment through pollution from numerous industries, mercury exposure will continue to be a health issue for many generations to come. Marine estuaries and ocean floors, as well as inland lakes and rivers, remain contaminated, and methylmercury will continue to work its way up the food chain.

—*Nancy Farm Mannikko, Ph.D.*

See also Autism; Cavities; Dentistry; Dentistry, pediatric; Environmental diseases; Environmental health; Food poisoning; Immunization and vaccination; Lead poisoning; Nervous system; Neurology; Neurology, pediatric; Occupational health; Poisoning; Toxicology.

FOR FURTHER INFORMATION:

Booth, Shawn. "Mercury, Food Webs, and Marine Animals: Implications of Diet and Climate Change for Human Health." *Environmental Health Perspectives* 113, no. 5 (May, 2005): 521-526. Discusses the effect of changes in diet on a specific population in the Faroe Islands, and shows how the amount of methylmercury exposure in utero affected cognitive development in children.

Davidson, Philip W., Gary J. Myers, and Bernard Weiss, eds. *Neurotoxicity and Developmental Disabilities*. New York: Elsevier, 2006. An anthology that includes articles on mercury exposure as well as other environmental toxins.

Friberg, Lars. *Inorganic Mercury*. Geneva: World Health Organization, 1991. Looks at mercury and environmental pollution.

WHO Task Group on Environmental Health Criteria for Mercury. *Mercury: Environmental Aspects*. Geneva: World Health Organization, 1989. Discusses mercury toxicity and toxicology.

Mesothelioma

Disease/Disorder

Anatomy or system affected: Abdomen, lungs, respiratory system

Specialties and related fields: General surgery, occupational health, oncology, pathology, pharmacology, preventive medicine, pulmonary medicine, radiology

Definition: A malignancy originating from the mesothelial surfaces (the lining cells) of the pleural and peritoneal cavities, the pericardium, or the tunica vaginalis. The distribution of mesothelioma may be unifocal or multifocal or may involve the lining cells in a continuous manner. Approximately 80 to 90 percent of all cases have a pleural origin (malignant pleural mesothelioma).

Key terms:

asbestos: a term for a group of naturally occurring silicate minerals with long, thin fibers

ascites: accumulation of fluid in the peritoneal cavity

chemotherapy: treatment of disease by chemicals; usually, systemic therapy of some types of cancer

dyspnea: difficulty or shortness of breathing

pericardium: a fluid-filled conical sac of fibrous tissue that surrounds the heart and the roots of the great blood vessels

peritoneum: a serous membrane that forms the lining of the abdominal cavity

pleura: a serous membrane that covers and protects the lungs

Causes and Symptoms

Mesothelioma is directly attributable to occupational asbestos exposure, with a history of exposure in more than 90 percent of cases. Para-occupational exposure (for example, women whose husbands work in an asbestos environment) has also been suggested. Idiopathic or spontaneous mesothelioma has been reported to occur in the absence of any exposure to asbestos. Other types of mineral fibers, such as erionite or tremolite, have also been shown to induce mesothelioma. The causative role of radiation, genetic factors, and Simian virus 40 is under investigation.

Mesothelioma usually occurs in the fifth to seventh decades of life, and 70 to 80 percent of cases occur in men. Rarely, it can be diagnosed between the ages of twenty and forty; these individuals usually have a history of childhood exposure to asbestos. In industrial countries, the incidence of mesothelioma is 2 in 1 million per year among women and 10 to 30 in 1 million per year among men.

The primary sites of mesothelioma include the pleura (about 90 percent), the peritoneum (about 5 percent), and the pericardium (0.4 percent). Pleural mesothelioma spreads via the fissures of the pleura to encase the lung surfaces. Peritoneal mesothelioma rapidly spreads within the confines of the abdominal cavity to involve most accessible peritoneal and omental surfaces.

Chest pain and/or dyspnea are the typical presenting features of pleural mesothelioma. Pleuritic-type pain can occur in the presence of pleural effusions. Involvement of the mediastinal structures, hoarseness of the voice, and superior vena caval obstruction is possible. Dysphagia (difficulty swallowing) is usually a late finding. Hemoptysis (coughing up blood), lymphadenopathy, and metastatic symptoms are rare. Additional features include chest wall mass, fatigue, fever, sweats, and weight loss. Very rarely, patients may be asymptomatic.

Peritoneal involvement may be found in up to one-third of mesothelioma cases at autopsy. Peritoneal mesothelioma presents with nonspecific symptoms such as loss of appetite, nausea and vomiting, diarrhea or constipation, and, occasionally, ascites. Small bowel obstruction is a late feature.

Physical examination is usually unremarkable except for signs of pleural effusion and pleural thickening as a result of tumor infiltration. Infiltration of the pericardium can result in signs of cardiac tamponade, compression of the heart because of fluid buildup. Blood tests can reveal an elevated erythrocyte sedimentation rate. Immunohistochemical markers calretinin, WT-1, and cytokeratin are established diagnostic mark-

---

Information on Mesothelioma

Causes: Primarily occupational asbestos exposure; role played by radiation, genetic factors, possibly simian virus 40

Symptoms: Chest pain, dyspnea, fatigue, fever, sweats, dysphagia and weight loss (pleural mesothelioma); loss of appetite, nausea, vomiting, diarrhea or constipation, ascites (peritoneal mesothelioma)

Duration: Fatal in four to eight months if untreated; survival of sixteen to nineteenth months with treatment

Treatments: Surgery, radiotherapy, chemotherapy

ers. Osteopontin and mesothelin have recently been introduced as new markers for mesothelioma.

Diagnosis is based on the combination of accurate history, examination, radiology, and laboratory testing. Radiological imaging is essential for the diagnosis, staging, and management of mesothelioma. X rays, computed tomography (CT), magnetic resonance imaging (MRI), and positron emission tomography (PET) can be used to evaluate the disease. In most cases, mesothelioma is readily identified or strongly suspected on routine hematoxylin-eosin histology. The three major histological patterns are sarcomatous, epithelial, and mixed (biphasic).

Treatment and Therapy

Management under a multidisciplinary team consisting of respiratory physicians, oncologists, radiologists, palliative care physicians, and lung cancer specialist nurses should be offered to all patients with mesothelioma. It generally includes multimodality treatment options that combine surgery, chemotherapy, and radiation.

Surgical resection and radiotherapy represent the standard treatment in a patient with resectable malignant pleural mesothelioma. The three most common surgical procedures used are pleurodesis, debulking surgery (cytoreductive surgery or pleurectomy/decortication) and extrapleural pneumonectomy. Radiation therapy can be used to control local tumor growth or as a prophylaxis to reduce the incidence of recurrence and pain at sites of diagnostic or therapeutic instrument insertion, or as part of multimodal definitive treatment. In some cases, it may lead to regression of the disease. Chemotherapy is used to reduce the incidence of distant metastases, to lengthen survival, to improve quality of life, and to provide symptomatic relief. Drugs with single-agent activity include pemetrexed, raltitrexed, vinorelbine, and vinflunine. The addition of pemetrexed or raltitrexed to cisplatin has been shown to prolong survival. For patients with unresectable mesothelioma, the combination of cisplatin and pemetrexed or ralitrexed is the standard treatment.

Most patients need palliation of symptoms early on in the course of the disease and recognition of this by the patient, family, and primary care physician, together with end-of-life care, are essential in the management of patients with mesothelioma.

Life expectancy is poor, with median survival between eight and fourteen months after diagnosis. Identified and verified indicators of poor prognosis include nonepithelioid histology, poor performance status, chest pain, age older than seventy-five, male gender, white blood cell count of 8.3 × 109/liters or greater, platelets greater than 400,000 microliterss (L), and a lactate dehydrogenase (LDH) test of 500 international units per liter (IU/L). With surgery, radiotherapy, and chemotherapy,) the survival may be sixteen to nineteen months. In general, the prognosis of peritoneal mesothelioma is worse than that for pleural mesothelioma, with a mean survival time of about seven months.

Perspective and Prospects

Asbestos is considered the main cause of mesothelioma in the Western world. The link between asbestos exposure and mesothelioma was not recognized until 1960, when the disease was first described in South African asbestos miners. The insulating properties of asbestos, however, have been known long before. The pathogenetic role of asbestos has been linked to its ability to cause the release of tumor necrosis factor alpha and other cytokines and growth factors, and to generate mutagenic oxygen radicals from exposed mesothelial cells and nearby macrophages. As of 2009, approximately two thousand to three thousand cases of mesothelioma occur in the United States annually. The incidence of mesothelioma is expected to peak between 2010 and 2020 due to the long latency period (thirty-five to forty-five years after asbestos exposure). Cases of mesothelioma are also expected in those exposed to dust created by the collapse of the Twin Towers in New York following the terrorist attacks of September 11, 2001, particularly among first responders.

Over the past decade, significant advances have been made toward an improved ability to diagnose and stage the disease, define the prognosis, and treat mesothelioma. Novel treatment modalities such as intrapleural chemotherapy, photodynamic therapy, and hyperthermic perfusion have already been used with some success. Immunomodulating, cytokine-targeted treatments (antigrowth factor drugs), and gene therapy are currently under investigation worldwide. These experimental treatments may in the future be combined with standard therapy in multimodality protocols.

—*Katia Marazova, M.D., Ph.D.*

See also Asbestos exposure; Cancer; Chronic obstructive pulmonary disease (COPD); Environmental diseases; Environmental health; Interstitial pulmonary fibrosis (IPF); Lung cancer; Lungs; Occupational health; Pulmonary diseases; Pulmonary medicine; Pulmonary medicine, pediatric.

FOR FURTHER INFORMATION:

Belli, C., et al. "Malignant Pleural Mesothelioma: Current Treatments and Emerging Drugs." *Expert Opinion on Emerging Drugs* 14, no. 3 (September, 2009): 423-437.

Hesdorffer, M. E., et al. "Peritoneal Mesothelioma." *Current Treatment Options in Oncology* 9, nos. 2/3 (June, 2008): 180-190.

Ray, M., and H. L. Kindler. "Malignant Pleural Mesothelioma: An Update on Biomarkers and Treatment." *Chest* 136, no. 3 (September, 2009): 888-896.

Tsao, A. S., et al. "Malignant Pleural Mesothelioma." *Journal of Clinical Oncology* 27, no. 12 (April, 2009): 2081-2090.

Yang, H., J. R. Testa, and M. Carbone. "Mesothelioma Epidemiology, Carcinogenesis, and Pathogenesis." *Current Treatment Options in Oncology* 9, nos. 2-3 (June, 2008): 147-157.

Zervos, M. D., C. Bizekis, and H. I. Pass. "Malignant Mesothelioma 2008." *Current Opinion in Pulmonary Medicine* 14, no. 4 (July, 2008): 303-309.

METABOLIC DISORDERS

DISEASE/DISORDER

ANATOMY OR SYSTEM AFFECTED: All

SPECIALTIES AND RELATED FIELDS: Biochemistry, endocrinology, genetics, nutrition, pediatrics, perinatology

DEFINITION: Disorders resulting from alterations in the pathways by which the body derives energy and synthesizes other molecules from carbohydrates, lipids, and proteins in food; usually caused by genetic defects that result in a missing or faulty enzyme.

KEY TERMS:

anabolic: the metabolic processes by which small molecules are combined to produce larger molecules; used for energy storage or growth of the organism

catabolic: the metabolic processes by which food and stored products are broken down to release energy for use by the cell

enzyme: a protein whose job is to enable chemical reactions to occur in the cell in a timely manner; a biological catalyst

essential: referring to an amino acid, lipid, or vitamin that is necessary for proper cell functioning, but which the human body is ordinarily unable to produce on its own; must be supplied through the diet

metabolism: the process of extracting energy that can be used to power the cells of the body; includes both anabolic and catabolic processes

prenatal/neonatal screening: a tool whereby small volume fluid samples (prenatal) or blood samples (neonatal) are drawn and studied to determine the genetic traits carried by the child; neonatal screening is often mandated by law and used to find metabolic diseases as early in life as possible

CAUSES AND SYMPTOMS

Metabolic disorders of all types are usually inherited from one or both parents who carry a defective gene; the gene is one that codes for an enzyme responsible for a part of the metabolic pathway (either anabolic or catabolic). Much like an assembly line that takes raw material and produces a final product through multiple steps, the metabolism of proteins, lipids, and carbohydrates in the human body requires multiple steps, each with its own enzyme. In some cases, there are multiple pathways to metabolize a particular starting product. In this case, lack of one enzyme may not have a dramatic effect. Other pathways are exclusive, however, and any disruption of an enzyme will lead to disease. In addition to loss of a particular product, some enzyme defects lead to the accumulation of precursor molecules that may be toxic or may interfere with normal function of the cell.

When the deoxyribonucleic acid (DNA) coding for a particular gene is altered, one of three outcomes may be seen: no change (silent mutation), partial loss of ability of the enzyme to do its job (mild disease), or complete loss of enzyme function (mild to severe disease). Diseases in the human are not known for all enzymes that could potentially be lost; this is most likely because disruption of an enzyme that is absolutely necessary in early development of the fetus will lead to early (and undetected) loss of the fetus.

Disorders of metabolism may be classified according to the pathways that are disrupted. Disorders associated with protein/amino acid metabolism may be seen when amino acids cannot be effectively broken down or when they cannot be transported into the cells of the body for use in building new proteins. Most of these disorders are seen early in life, since many proteins are essential for growth and development of the body. Examples of amino acid metabolism disorders are phenylketonuria (PKU) and maple syrup urine disease (MSUD). Other amino acid/protein disorders are homocystinuria, citrullinemia, alkaptonuria, and tyrosinemia.

Phenylalanine is an essential amino acid involved in the production of tyrosine, which in turn is converted to dopamine and serotonin. In PKU, the absence of this conversion means that phenylalanine accumulates in the body, causing toxic reactions within the brain and other organs. Mental retardation is the most obvious effect of this toxicity; other symptoms may include seizures, skin rashes, nausea and vomiting, and aggressive behavior. Phenylacetate (a by-product of excess phenylalanine) is secreted in sweat and urine, giving a distinctive odor to the child.

Leucine, isoleucine, and valine are amino acids that have a branched side chain. As a result of the presence of this special shape, an enzyme that can convert these enzymes is needed in order to metabolize food containing them. In MSUD, that enzyme is absent or deficient and these amino acids accumulate in the urine, giving a distinctive smell for which the disorder is named. If left untreated, this can lead to vomiting, staggering, confusion, coma, and eventual death from degeneration of the developing nerves early in life. A total of six different genes are responsible for production of the branched-chain alpha-ketoacid dehydrogenase enzyme complex, thus leading to some variation in the severity of the disease. While this disease is rare in the general population, the Mennonite community of Pennsylvania has a high rate of carriers for these mutations and thus is particularly affected.

Lipids (fats) are used in numerous ways in the human body, including for energy, temperature regulation, cell membrane structure, and nerve function. A variety of enzymes are responsible for breaking down and processing both stored and dietary lipids. In the absence of efficient processing of lipids, accumulations occur that can be extremely harmful to the organs of the body. Examples of lipid metabolism disorders are fatty acid oxidation disorders and Tay-Sachs disease. Other lipid metabolism disorders include Gaucher's disease, Refsum's disease, Niemann-Pick disease, Tangier dis-

---

INFORMATION ON METABOLIC DISORDERS

CAUSES: Missing or faulty enzymes
SYMPTOMS: Depends on enzyme affected; may include mental retardation, seizures, rashes, nausea, vomiting, coma, delayed development, organ damage, paralysis, dementia, blindness
DURATION: Chronic and often fatal
TREATMENTS: Ranges from none to dietary restrictions to enzyme therapy

---

ease, carnitine uptake defect, and trifunctional protein deficiency.

Several enzymes are involved in pathways that help stored lipids to be broken down and turned into energy. In the most common fatty acid oxidation disorder the enzyme deficient in this pathway is medium-chain acyl-coenzyme A dehydrogenase (MCAD). This is one of the most common errors of metabolism among people of northern European descent. A buildup of acyl-coenzyme A leads to delayed development, heart muscle weakness, and enlarged liver; death may occur. Symptoms develop shortly after birth and are most severe if the child goes without food for a prolonged period of time, or following exercise and the need for more energy to the cells (thus triggering the lipid breakdown pathways).

Perhaps the best known of the lipid metabolism disorders, Tay-Sachs disease results from errors in the enzyme β-hexosaminidase, which is responsible for breaking down the lipid GM2 ganglioside. The gene for this enzyme is known to reside on chromosome 15, and the absence of this enzyme allows large amounts of the ganglioside to accumulate in neurons. This accumulation leads to neurodegeneration that often results in floppy muscle tone, then paralysis, dementia, blindness, and death by age three or four. Less severe forms lead to long-term problems in the nervous system that progress throughout life. Tay-Sachs disease is most commonly seen in the Ashkenazi Jewish community but is also seen in the French Canadian population of Quebec and the Cajun population of Louisiana.

Carbohydrates (especially glucose) are the principal fuels for the body on a daily basis. Carbohydrate metabolism requires a variety of intracellular enzymes, as well as those responsible for transport and entry into the cell. Diseases or disorders of carbohydrate metabolism can be quite severe. Examples of carbohydrate metabolism disorders are type 1 diabetes mellitus and glycogen storage diseases.

The ability to get glucose (the primary carbohydrate) into the cells of the body requires the hormone insulin. A lack in the production of insulin in the pancreas (type 1 diabetes) leads to hyperglycemia (high blood levels of glucose) and a lack of glucose for energy within the cells. In addition to lack of cellular energy, this can lead to increased risk of blindness, heart disease, kidney failure, neurological diseases, and problems with circulation in the extremities. Type 1 diabetes may result from any one of several known mutations in DNA, the most common of which has been tracked

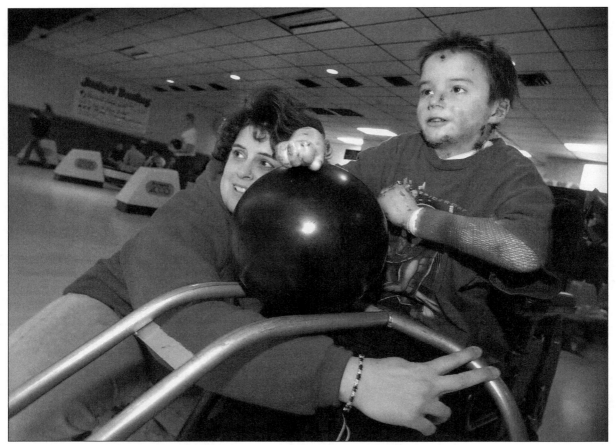

This child suffers from an incurable inborn metabolic error known as epidermolysis bullosa, which makes his skin blister at the touch. (AP/Wide World Photos)

to chromosome 6. In some forms of type 1 diabetes, the body attacks either the insulin or the pancreatic cells that produce it, making this an autoimmune disease.

Glycogen is the branched-chain storage form of glucose in the liver and muscles of the body. Glycogen storage diseases are actually a group of eleven similar diseases that result in the inability of the body to produce sufficient glucose for the bloodstream to be used by cells of the body to produce energy. In addition to low blood sugar levels, children with these diseases often have enlarged livers, swollen abdomens, and weak muscles. Elevated levels of lipids in the blood (taking the place of glucose as an energy source), may lead to acidosis and stress on the heart and kidneys.

In addition to the transport, storage, and breakdown of proteins, lipids, and carbohydrates, metabolism involves alterations in the use of elements such as iron and copper and the synthesis, storage, and use of the components of DNA and ribonucleic acid (RNA). Diseases and disorders in each of these areas are known as well. Examples include Wilson's disease, Menkes disease, hereditary hemochromatosis, and Lesch-Nyhan syndrome.

Copper is necessary in cells for energy metabolism, bone production, and nerve maturation. Wilson's disease and Menkes disease are disorders of copper transport and absorption that lead to a buildup of copper to toxic levels in the liver and the brain. Both liver disease and neurological damage can be present if they are not diagnosed early on; eventually, toxicity can be seen in many other organs as well. Menkes disease is usually fatal during infancy. Both diseases have been mapped to chromosome 13 and appear to be the result of proteins that are part of a transmembrane pump system. Menkes disease is transmitted as an X-linked recessive trait, while Wilson's disease is autosomal recessive.

Hereditary hemochromatosis is a disorder of iron metabolism seen predominantly in those of Northern European, Caucasian descent and traceable to a mutation on chromosome 6. Because iron is not adequately metabolized, the levels stored in the body grow over time, leading to symptoms that include cirrhosis of the liver, cardiomyopathy (heart muscle disease), alterations in skin pigmentation, joint damage, and decreased functioning of the gonads. Because men generally retain iron better than women do, symptoms often occur earlier in men. Symptoms also occur early in alcoholics, as alcohol consumption affects uptake of dietary iron.

Both DNA and RNA are constructed in part from nitrogen-containing bases; these bases are chemically grouped as purines and pyrimidines. The body can both make and recycle these bases. One of the genes involved in the recycling of purines (HPRT1) is located on the X chromosome. In Lesch-Nyhan syndrome, several known mutations result in low levels of the enzyme, and thus a lack of purine recycling. The resulting disease is seen almost exclusively in males and causes accumulation of uric acid (the starting point in purine synthesis). Uric acid leads to gout (painful deposits in the skin and joints) and kidney stones. For unknown reasons, this enzyme deficiency also leads to self-mutilation (biting of the fingers and tongue). Severe muscle weakness and mental retardation generally occur.

TREATMENT AND THERAPY

The most important diagnostic tool available for metabolic disorders is routine neonatal genetic screening. In 2005, a report by the American College of Medical Genetics recommended a core panel of twenty-eight metabolic disorders that should be screened for in all newborn children. This list includes disorders of protein metabolism, carbohydrate metabolism, and lipid metabolism, as well as a few multisystem disorders. Such screening does not prevent disorders but does allow early detection and therefore early intervention with diet, drugs, and other regimens that allow extended life spans for those afflicted.

Once detected, treatment of metabolic disorders is quite varied and is related to the underlying cause of the disorder. For protein/amino acid disorders, dietary restrictions are a key element in treatment. For instance, in PKU, phenylalanine intake must be restricted starting in the first few weeks of life. This means elimination of most forms of natural protein and substitution with phenylalanine-free foods. Patients with homocysteinuria often improve with vitamin B_6 (pyridoxine) or vitamin B_{12} (cobalamin). In maple syrup urine disease, restricting the dietary intake of the three branched-chain amino acids to the minimal amount required for growth and development allows for the best improvement. Vitamin B_1 (thiamine) is helpful in those with mild disease; dialysis is used in those with severe disease. Gene therapy is a possibility in the future.

In lipid disorders, control of diet is also essential. With fatty acid oxidation disorders it is important that patients eat often, never skip meals, and consume a diet high in carbohydrates and low in lipids. Treatment with intravenous glucose is helpful during attacks. The long-term outcome is very good in those who follow a strict dietary regimen. Likewise, in Refsum disease, a diet with little or no phytanic acid (carefully controlled plant products that contain no chlorophyll) is the key; plasmapheresis may be also be helpful. Other lipid disorders, including Gaucher's and Tay-Sachs, require drug intervention. Gaucher's type I patients (especially those without nervous system damage) can be treated with enzyme replacement therapy; the modified enzyme is given intravenously every two weeks. Enzyme therapy has been shown to stop, and even reverse, many of the symptoms of this disease. The late-onset (less severe) form of Tay-Sachs has seen some promise from treatment with a ganglioside synthesis inhibitor. Treatment of the infantile form has shown little promise, since much of the neurological damage occurs prior to birth and reversing neurological damage that has already occurred has proven to be extremely difficult.

Type 1 diabetes can usually be controlled well with daily insulin (artificial) and control of diet (to match the amount of energy needed for daily activities). Although islet cell transplantation or immunosuppression has been on the drawing board for several years, no real success has yet been obtained.

Other metabolic disorders run the gamut from easy to impossible to treat. Hereditary hemochromatosis, for instance, is easy to control, with therapeutic phlebotomy (blood-letting) to remove excess iron that has built up. Early diagnosis and treatment leads to a normal life span. By contrast, there is no cure for Niemann-Pick disease, and these children generally die of infection or degeneration of the central nervous system. For Menkes disease, administration of copper histidinate has shown promise, but it increases the patient's life span only by a few years (less than ten). In Lesch-Nyhan syndrome, medications are used to decrease the levels of uric acid; restraint against self-mutilation is commonly needed. Advances in gene therapy look promising for several of these conditions as well.

Perspective and Prospects

Metabolic disorders have existed since the earliest humans roamed the earth, but it was not until the early twentieth century that the mechanism for these disorders was recognized. The term "inborn error of metabolism" was coined by Archibold Garrod, a British physician who published a classic text on the subject in 1923, following a study of children with alkaptonuria. This was the first such treatise to explain how symptoms often seen in sickly children could be explained on the basis of enzyme defects. Many of these diseases, such as diabetes, had been well established and named years before but not yet understood in terms of their biochemistry. The genetic basis for these disorders was not determined until much later—the 1970's and beyond.

Another early pioneer in this field was the German pediatrician Albert Niemann, who in 1914 described in detail a child with nervous system impairment. This condition later became known as Niemann-Pick disease, when Luddwick Pick took tissue samples from several such children after their deaths and provided chemical evidence of a distinct lipid storage problem.

The discovery of insulin in the 1920's provided the first opportunity to treat a metabolic disease in a standardized way, as insulin could be extracted and purified in a controlled laboratory setting. The availability of insulin has saved millions of lives since its discovery.

The hope for the future is gene therapy. The first gene therapy successes were recorded in children with enzyme deficiencies, and there are many trials throughout the world aimed at improving the chances of survival and healthy lives of those with similar metabolic disorders through correction of the genetic defect. In the future, such therapy might even be available in utero.

—*Kerry L. Cheesman, Ph.D.*

See also Arthritis; Diabetes mellitus; Digestion; Endocrinology; Endocrinology, pediatric; Enzyme therapy; Enzymes; Fatty acid oxidation disorders; Food biochemistry; Fructosemia; Gastroenterology; Gastroenterology, pediatric; Gastrointestinal system; Gaucher's disease; Genetic diseases; Glands; Glycogen storage diseases; Glycolysis; Gout; Hemochromatosis; Hormones; Kidney disorders; Lipids; Maple syrup urine disease (MSUD); Mental retardation; Metabolic syn-

drome; Metabolism; Mucopolysaccharidosis (MPS); Niemann-Pick disease; Nonalcoholic steatohepatitis (NASH); Obesity; Obesity, childhood; Phenylketonuria (PKU); Tay-Sachs disease; Wilson's disease.

For Further Information:

Gilbert, Hiram F. *Basic Concepts in Biochemistry.* 2d ed. New York: McGraw-Hill, 2000. Although written as a review for medical students, its simple, nononsense approach to metabolism makes it a useful tool for anyone seeking an introduction to human metabolic systems.

Machalek, Alisa Zapp. *The Structures of Life.* Bethesda, Md.: Department of Health and Human Services, Public Health Service, National Institutes of Health, National Institute of General Medical Sciences, 2000. General introduction to proteins and how errors in manufacturing them can create problems in the body. Also discusses development of new drugs and other research. Also available at http://publications.nigms.nih.gov/structlife.

Nussbaum, Robert L., Roderick R. McInnes, and Willard F. Huntington. *Thompson and Thompson Genetics in Medicine.* 7th ed. Philadelphia: Saunders/Elsevier, 2006. An excellent text meant primarily for medical students but readable by anyone with a background in basic biology, it describes many of the important metabolic diseases of the human and their basis in genetic defects.

Scriver, Charles R., et al., eds. *The Metabolic and Molecular Bases of Inherited Disease.* 8th ed. New York: McGraw-Hill, 2001. Probably the most important text in its field, this is an exhaustive look at metabolic diseases, their causes, and their treatment.

Metabolic syndrome
Disease/disorder

Also known as: Insulin resistance syndrome, Syndrome X, Deadly Quartet

Anatomy or system affected: All

Specialties and related fields: Cardiology, endocrinology, internal medicine, nutrition

Definition: A constellation of metabolic changes that affect most major organ systems and may impinge on practically all systems of the body, often beginning with excess weight or obesity.

Key terms:

atherosclerosis: fat deposition and pathologic changes in the arterial surface and walls of major blood vessels of the body

diabetes mellitus type 2: peripheral resistance to insulin and increases in serum glucose and insulin concentrations, with damage to arteries in various organs

dyslipidemia: abnormal blood lipid levels, especially characterized by high serum triglycerides and very low-density lipoproteins (VLDLs) and depressed serum high-density lipoprotein (HDL) cholesterol

hyperinsulinemia: an abnormally high serum insulin concentration

obese: having a body mass index (BMI), calculated as weight in kilograms divided by height in meters squared, that is greater than 30

overweight: having a BMI that is between 25 and 29.9

steatohepatitis: an increased fat content in the liver independent of alcohol consumption

CAUSES AND SYMPTOMS

Metabolic syndrome is a complex medical disorder. According to guidelines issued by the National Cholesterol Education Program/Adult Treatment Panel III (NCEP/ATP III), diagnosis of metabolic syndrome is made when an individual displays at least three of the following risk factors: abdominal obesity, elevated triglycerides, low levels of the high-density lipoprotein (HDL) type of cholesterol, high blood pressure, and the presence of more than 100 milligrams per deciliter (mg/dL) of glucose in the blood after fasting.

The National Heart, Lung, and Blood Institute (NHLBI) estimates that as many as forty-seven million adults in the United States suffer from metabolic syndrome, which is around 25 percent of the total adult population. Age plays a large role in metabolic syndrome, with the likelihood of being diagnosed increasing as an individual gets older. Total body weight is also an indicator of the likelihood of the metabolic syndrome criteria being met. Males who are overweight are six times as likely as normal-weight males to be diagnosed with metabolic syndrome, and those who are obese are thirty-two times as likely.

In females, being overweight leads to a fivefold increase in the chances of being diagnosed with metabolic syndrome and obesity a seventeen-fold increase, compared to women of normal weight. Disturbingly, metabolic syndrome is now being recognized in children and adolescents; this is probably related to the increase in obesity and type 2 diabetes mellitus seen in this age group over recent years. There is also evidence to demonstrate a genetic component to metabolic syndrome; further research will clarify this.

INFORMATION ON METABOLIC SYNDROME

CAUSES: Unknown; possibly poor utilization of glucose and abnormal cellular metabolism

SYMPTOMS: Lipid abnormalities, insulin resistance, abdominal obesity, high blood pressure; may result in diabetes, heart disease, stroke, colon cancer, nonalcoholic steatohepatitis (NASH), polycystic ovary disease, chronic renal failure

DURATION: Chronic

TREATMENTS: Weight loss, diet modification, drug therapy

Key aspects of the metabolic syndrome are an energy imbalance and resultant altered metabolic pathways. The abnormal metabolic reactions seen in metabolic syndrome confer an increased risk for type 2 diabetes mellitus and cardiovascular disease (CVD). Several other diseases—colon cancer, nonalcoholic steatohepatitis (NASH), polycystic ovary disease, and chronic renal failure—can also be a consequence of this syndrome.

The National Health and Nutrition Examination Survey determined that the most prevalent risk factor displayed by individuals with metabolic syndrome is abdominal obesity. This is when fat is stored in the abdominal region of the body as opposed to in the buttocks and thighs. People with abdominally stored fat are often said to have "apple" type bodies; those with fat stored lower, in the buttocks and thighs, are said to be "pear" shaped. Men are typically apples and women are pears. Cortisol is a stress response hormone that promotes fat deposition in the abdominal area in individuals with chronic stress. Nearly all cases of overweight and obesity, including abdominal obesity, are due to excess calorific intake (overeating) combined with a sedentary lifestyle. In the United States, around one-third of the adult population is obese. Obesity greatly increases the risk for type 2 diabetes and cardiovascular disease.

Abnormal levels of fats in the blood is called dyslipidemia. In people who are overweight or obese, the levels of lipids in the body are so high that the pathways involved in fat synthesis and breakdown cannot keep up, and chronically high blood lipids are seen.

In addition, due to impaired insulin action and incorrect handling of glucose by their cells, individuals with type 2 diabetes tend to have high levels of blood triglyceride and low HDL cholesterol levels. This puts type 2 diabetics and obese individuals at high risk for CVD.

The second most prevalent factor seen in patients diagnosed with metabolic syndrome is hypertension, or high blood pressure. One in four Americans suffers from hypertension. If untreated, it can lead to CVD and kidney failure. The atherosclerotic process is accelerated in the metabolic syndrome and in type 2 diabetes because of the presence of multiple metabolic abnormalities. In insulin resistance, plaque formation may be enhanced because of the increased expression of adhesion molecules on endothelial cells and an increased rate of monocyte adhesion to endothelial cells. Circulating plasminogen is also more likely activated, which typically leads to increased clotting. In addition, hypertension may contribute to an increased risk of stroke in those with the metabolic syndrome.

The third most prevalent factor is hyperglycemia, or impaired fasting glucose. To satisfy the criterion for metabolic syndrome the glucose level in the blood after fasting must be over 100 mg/dl. A person with 100 to 125 mg/dl would be considered prediabetic, and diabetes is diagnosed when the fasting level of glucose is 126 mg/dl or above. Increases in blood glucose are indicative of a phenomenon called insulin resistance. Here, the cells of the body do not respond properly to insulin, and as a result glucose cannot enter the cells for use or storage so it remains in the circulating blood. Chronically elevated blood glucose concentration permits glucose molecules to combine with diverse proteins in the body, including hemoglobin within red blood cells, by a process known as glycation or glycosylation. Glycation also leads to blood vessels becoming rigid, a factor that contributes to CVD.

Any one of the risk factors listed on the NCEP/ATP III guidelines can cause chronic health problems, specifically type 2 diabetes mellitus and CVD. Diagnosis of metabolic syndrome requires that at least three out of the five criteria are met. This translates into a vastly increased risk for these chronic health problems; the reason why the life span of individuals diagnosed with metabolic syndrome is an average of fourteen years shorter than those without the disease.

Treatment and Therapy

Treatment strategies for the metabolic syndrome focus on weight loss through a comprehensive program utilizing behavioral changes, including improved nutrition and an increase in physical activities. The long-term goal of therapy is a better balance between the intake of food energy sources and energy expenditure, so that a healthier body weight can be achieved. Dietary treatment typically requires the involvement of nutritionists and registered dieticians to provide educational information and institute changes in food selection.

Physicians provide overall care, and concomitant with lifestyle changes use the prescription of medications for one or more of the components of metabolic syndrome. Metformin is a drug used to treat type 2 diabetes mellitus; it works by improving insulin action, and has also been shown to stop the development of impaired fasting glucose to type 2 diabetes in patients with metabolic syndrome. Angiotensin-converting enzyme (ACE) inhibitors are used in the treatment of hypertension. They are successful in treating hypertension and, in addition, have a beneficial effect on insulin resistance in metabolic syndrome. Another class of drugs is the statins, which are used to improve cholesterol levels in people with metabolic syndrome. Statins also appear to cause a reduction in inflammation seen in metabolic syndrome, leading to a reduction in CVD.

Since the emerging epidemic of the metabolic syndrome is expected to continue, both preventive and treatment strategies are needed. Prevention aimed toward reducing the development of this syndrome in children and adolescents should involve schools and community agencies.

Perspective and Prospects

Recognition of the metabolic syndrome essentially paralleled the increases in overweight and obesity in the United States in the early 1990's. Physicians were diagnosing many overweight and obese patients with the major components of the metabolic syndrome without linking them to a major health trend. Other countries of affluence were also reporting cases.

The metabolic syndrome was first defined in 1998 by the World Health Organization (WHO). The WHO criteria included a BMI of more than thirty; a blood triglyceride level greater than or equal to 150 mg/dl; HDL cholesterol level under 35 mg/dl in men and 39 mg/dl in women; blood pressure over 140/90 mm Hg; impaired glucose tolerance, insulin tolerance or type 2 diabetes; insulin resistance; and microalbuminuria (protein in the urine). In 2001 the NCEP/ATP III released their guidelines for the diagnosis of metabolic syndrome, which quickly became the most widely accepted. These differed from the WHO guidelines in several ways. Firstly, BMI measurement was replaced with waist circumference measurement when it became clear that it was not necessarily the total body fat content, but the way in which it is deposited in the body that is important to pathogenesis. A waist circumference of over forty inches for men and over thirty-five inches for women is considered a risk factor for metabolic syndrome. Secondly, the HDL values were changed to less than 40 mg/dl for men and 50 mg/dl for women, and blood pressure limit was lowered to 130/85 mm Hg. A fasting glucose level of over 110 mg/dl was defined as a risk for metabolic syndrome. Finally, insulin resistance and microalbumiuria were removed from the criteria. In 2005 the guidelines were updated by American Heart Association (AHA) and NHLBI; the fasting blood glucose level was lowered to 100 mg/dl. These are the currently used criteria for the diagnosis of metabolic syndrome.

The metabolic syndrome has deadly consequences because of the nature of the chronic diseases that it spawns. This problem will worsen in the future in the United States because excessive calorific intake, eating the wrong kinds of food (for example highly processed food containing high fructose corn syrup, trans fats, or too much salt), and too little physical activity continue to dominate society. The epidemic nature of this syndrome requires that new public health measures be initiated and implemented as soon as possible. Preventive strategies need to be instituted to reduce the enormous impact of this syndrome anticipated in the United States in the coming decades. The overall cost of treatment will be enormous.

—*Claire L. Standen, Ph.D.; additional material by John J. B. Anderson, Ph.D.*

See also Arteriosclerosis; Diabetes mellitus; Endocrine disorders; Endocrinology; Endocrinology, pediatric; Hormones; Hyperlipidemia; Hypertension; Metabolic disorders; Obesity; Obesity, childhood; Weight loss and gain.

FOR FURTHER INFORMATION:

Byrne, Christopher D., and Sarah H. Wild, eds. *The Metabolic Syndrome.* Hoboken, N.J.: John Wiley & Sons, 2005.

Chrousos, George P., and Constantine Tsigos, eds. *Stress, Obesity, and Metabolic Syndrome.* Boston: Blackwell/New York Academy of Sciences, 2006.

Codario, Ronald A. *Type 2 Diabetes, Pre-diabetes, and the Metabolic Syndrome: The Primary Care Guide to Diagnosis and Management.* Totowa, N.J.: Humana Press, 2005.

Hansen, Barbara C., and George A. Bray, eds. *The Metabolic Syndrome: Epidemiology, Clinical Treatment, and Underlying Mechanisms.* Totowa, N.J.: Humana Press, 2008.

Houston, Mark C. *The Handbook of Hypertension.* Hoboken, N.J.: Wiley-Blackwell, 2009.

Levine, T. Barry, and Arlene Bradley Levine. *Metabolic Syndrome and Cardiovascular Disease.* Philadelphia: Saunders/Elsevier, 2006.

METABOLISM

BIOLOGY

ANATOMY OR SYSTEM AFFECTED: Gastrointestinal system, intestines, kidneys, liver, pancreas, spleen, stomach

SPECIALTIES AND RELATED FIELDS: Biochemistry, cytology, exercise physiology, gastroenterology, nutrition, pharmacology

DEFINITION: The processes by which the substance of plants and animals incidental to life is built up and broken down.

KEY TERMS:

adipose tissue: tissue that stores fat; occurs in humans beneath the skin, usually in the abdomen or in the buttocks

anabolism: the metabolic activity through which complex substances are synthesized from simpler substances

basal metabolic rate (BMR): the standardized measure of metabolism in warm-blooded organisms

calorie: a measurement of heat, particularly in measuring the value of foods for producing energy and heat in an organism

catabolism: the complete breaking down of molecules by an organism for the purpose of obtaining chemical building blocks

essential nutrients: molecules that an organism needs for survival but cannot manufacture itself

standard metabolic rate (SMR): the standardized measure of metabolism in cold-blooded organisms

storage compounds: areas in the body that store nutrients not immediately required by an organism

STRUCTURE AND FUNCTIONS

Metabolism is an ongoing process in living organisms. It is fundamentally concerned with the chemistry of life. An organism's metabolic rate is the rate at which it consumes the energy it derives from the nutrients that sustain it. Organisms consume energy by converting chemical energy to heat and external work; most of the latter is converted to heat also, as external work, such as walking or moving in any way, overcomes friction. A workable measure of metabolic rate, therefore, is the rate at which an organism produces heat. The food that organisms ingest is measured in Calories, each Calorie being the measure of what is required to raise the temperature of one kilogram of water by one degree Celsius.

Metabolism consists of two essential underlying processes, anabolism and catabolism. In vertebrates, the food ingested is immediately mixed with digestive enzymes in the mouth. These enzymes are produced by the salivary glands. As a ball of food, a bolus, passes through the digestive system, additional enzymes found in the stomach, the pancreas, and the small intestine work upon it, accelerating the digestive process.

Some nonenzymes are also vital to the digestive process. Most notable are hydrochloric acid, which, in the stomach, is a necessary ingredient for the efficient use of the stomach's pepsin, and bile salts in the small intestine, nonenzymes essential to the digestive process. The action of the digestive apparatus results in catabolism, or the breaking down of the components of food, notably lipids, carbohydrates, and proteins, into small molecules used to build and repair cells. Such molecules, through absorption, traverse the wall of the small intestine to enter the blood or the lymph so that they can be distributed throughout the body to meet its immediate requirements.

Amino acids break down protein, permitting it to enter the bloodstream, whereas glucose and other enzymes act to break down the large carbohydrates into small molecules that are absorbed into the bloodstream. After they are catabolized into smaller molecules, the lipids or fats, unlike proteins and carbohydrates, enter the lymphatic system rather than the bloodstream, which they can enter only after they have passed through the lymphatic system.

Organisms typically cannot digest all the types of nutrients they ingest. Most vertebrates, for example, are incapable of digesting cellulose, the major carbohydrate component of most plants. This material, therefore, simply passes through the digestive system and is excreted. Fiber, which passes through the digestive tract essentially undigested, performs a valuable function in keeping the colon clear and, over the long term, in preventing colon cancer.

A remarkably complex biochemical process occurs when the circulatory system delivers its absorbed sugars, lipids, and amino acids to the parts of the body where they are needed to build new cells and repair existing cells. Sometimes, this process requires the conversion of sugar molecules to fat molecules or animo acids. For a cell to construct a protein, it must connect in a specific, complex order the many animo acid molecules that the process requires. While some of the requisite amino acids result directly from ingesting nutrients, others are not available in this way and must be obtained through the synthesis of sugar molecules.

Molecules that an organism needs for survival but that it cannot manufacture itself are obtained through ingestion. Such molecules are called essential nutrients. It takes twenty different kinds of amino acids, for example, to manufacture protein, but the body is capable of producing only half of these. Because green plants can synthesize all twenty forms of amino acids, they are a major and ready source of the essential nutrients required to sustain life.

Also, as part of a nutritional chain, one can note that although neither humans nor chickens can synthesize valine, a vital amino acid, chickens obtain valine by eating grain that is rich in it. Humans, in turn, eat chickens, through which they obtain valine. This amino acid is also available to humans through the green vegetables they eat.

The food that organisms ingest is used both to provide the necessary building blocks for the synthesis of membranes, enzymes, and other parts of cells and to provide energy. If the nutrients ingested are greater than the body's requirements for such synthesis and for the production of energy, then food molecules may be husbanded for future use in storage compounds within the organism. The excess stored in this way is usually in the form of lipids. In humans, such excesses are stored essentially around the abdomen and buttocks, where they can accumulate in considerable quantity.

If a human's food supply is severely reduced or completely cut off, the body draws on these reserves, using the stored fat cells until they have been completely depleted. Afterward, nutrients, mostly proteins, will be drawn from muscle mass, the sudden reduction of which can quickly eventuate in death.

The survival of organisms is usually dependent upon the work that they perform. Energy to carry out this work is derived through the splitting of the chemical bonds of adenosine triphosphate (ATP) and the splitting of the bonds of food molecules. Highly sophisticated and refined series of biochemical reactions called

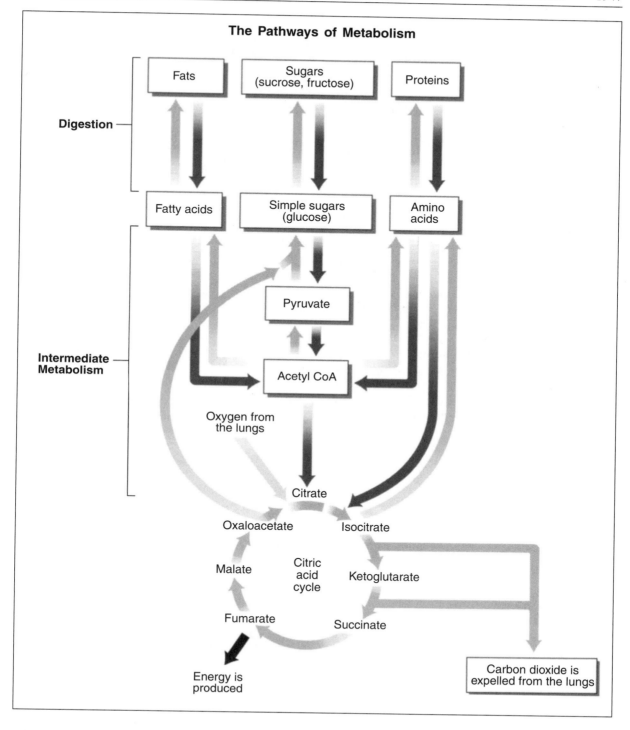

The Pathways of Metabolism

cellular respiration and aerobic catabolism permit most animals to transfer energy from the chemical bonds of nutrient molecules to the bonds of ATP.

Every cell in the body has the enzymes and cellular equipment to carry out aerobic catabolism and to manufacture its own ATP. Oxygen, carried through the blood, is the essential ingredient in aerobic catabolism, which results in the oxidization of nutrient molecules and their being broken up into small molecules composed largely of carbon dioxide and water. In this process, energy is released, some of it lost as heat and some of it conserved in the bonds of ATP.

As amino acids, lipids, and carbohydrates are catabolized in humans, the lipids and carbohydrates are used by the muscles, whereas the brain gains its energy almost exclusively through the glucose that catabolized carbohydrates produce. Excess amino acids are converted by the liver and, to a smaller extent, by the kidneys to carbohydrates or lipids.

In a process called anaerobic glycolysis, which involves the creation of ATP without the presence of oxygen, energy is produced by converting glucose or glycogen into lactic acid. The body cannot excrete lactic acid, thereby making impossible its accumulation in its original form in the body. Lactic acid is released into the bloodstream after exercise and, now subjected to oxygen, is metabolized by the liver and either converted to glucose or oxidized aerobically in order to release additional energy.

As vertebrates age, their metabolic rate often decreases. In humans, a decreased metabolic rate, reduced activity in old age, and a failure to reduce caloric intake can result in substantial weight gain. Therefore, as humans age, their physicians usually encourage them to engage in physical activity and to reduce the overall number of calories that they consume. Physical activity generally helps to sustain the basal metabolism at levels higher than those found among the sedentary.

DISORDERS AND DISEASES

All metabolic disorders stem either from genetic or environmental origins, or from a combination of the two. For example, a person with a predisposition for diabetes, an inherited genetic disorder, may exacerbate this predisposition by indulging in a diet high in fats and carbohydrates, by overindulging in alcoholic beverages, and by engaging in little physical activity.

Environmental factors such as diet and exercise can hasten the onset of a disease that lurks in one's genes. People with this predisposition who control diet and alcohol consumption and who make strenuous exercise regular parts of their daily activity, however, may forestall the onset of the disease, possibly keeping it at bay for their entire lifetimes.

Significant advances were first made in the 1960's in tracing the genetic origins of diseases. The discovery that deoxyribonucleic acid (DNA), the molecular basis of heredity, exists in the nucleus of every cell of living organisms was a major biochemical discovery. It has led to vastly increased insights into heredity and into metabolic disorders of genetic origin, certainly the overwhelming majority of all such disorders. Among the many metabolic disorders attributable to inheritance are diabetes, arthritis, gout, phenylketonuria (PKU), Tay-Sachs disease, Niemann-Pick disease, and hemochromatosis.

Microbiologists can detect a number of abnormalities in fetuses by analyzing the amniotic fluid that surrounds them in the womb. This process, known as amniocentesis, can identify more than twenty inherited metabolic disorders before an infant is born. Genetic manipulation in utero can alter some metabolic disorders, thereby bypassing or modifying faulty or abnormal genes. The genes of a person carrying a predisposition for a metabolic defect usually do not carry the information required for the synthesizing of a particular protein, usually an enzyme. This deficiency inhibits catalytic activity and blocks a metabolic pathway, resulting in a genetic abnormality.

In a minority of cases, the protein serves a role in transport or acts as a cell-surface receptor. Whatever role the protein in question serves, a delicate balance exists within the cells. When this balance is disturbed, metabolic problems ensue. For example, a gene may be responsible for producing an enzyme that converts one substance to another substance. If this gene is defective, the enzyme derived from it may be deficient and may fail to carry out the conversion or carry it out so slowly as to result in an inefficient conversion. While the first substance, a protein, accumulates in the cell, causing a surplus, it will be in short supply in the cell involved in the conversion, resulting in a deficiency. The surplus or the shortage may eventuate in a metabolic disorder, the genetic disbalance often revealing itself in overt symptoms.

Evidence of metabolic disorders can occur at any time in a person's life. They sometimes are detectable prenatally, but they may occur in early childhood, adolescence, adult life, or old age. In some cases, the onset of a serious metabolic disorder will be followed quickly by death. Many people suffering from such disorders, however, live long, active, full lives, many of them exceeding the average life span. Some metabolic disorders, such as diabetes, are manageable over long periods through diet and medication.

Some types of metabolic disorders can be treated successfully with massive doses of vitamins. At least twenty fairly common disorders respond favorably to such treatment. For example, Wilson's disease, which results in excessive amounts of copper being accumulated in the tissues, is generally treated successfully with D-penicillamine, a compound that removes copper from the tissues and deposits it into the urinary system for excretion as urine.

Certain nutrients trigger metabolic disorders in some organisms. The avoidance of these nutrients can prevent the triggering of the disorder on a permanent basis. Also, where the disorder results from a deficiency of an end product in a reaction, the disorder may be forestalled by replacing the end product.

PERSPECTIVE AND PROSPECTS
The metabolism was scarcely understood until the 1770's, when Joseph Priestley discovered oxygen and set other researchers on the path to understanding its role in the biochemical aspects of all life. In the next decade, Antoine-Laurent Lavoisier and Adair Crawford were the first researchers to measure the heat produced by animals and to suggest convincingly that animal catabolism is a form of combustion.

These early, tentative steps toward understanding how organisms derive energy and how they expend it led to further research that, in 1828, resulted in Friedrich Wohler's synthesis of an organic compound, urea, from inorganic substances, demonstrating that the compounds that living organisms produce can be converted from inorganic to organic through metabolism.

It was not until 1842 that Justus von Liebig categorized foods as falling into three essential types, carbohydrates, lipids, and proteins. He measured the caloric values of nutrients and advanced considerably what was known about nutrition and its role in metabolism. At about the same time, Julius Robert von Mayer and James Joule discovered that motion, heat, and electricity are all forms of the same thing, energy. It was not until the 1890's, however, that Max Rubner and Wilbur Atwater demonstrated conclusively through empirical data that animals release energy according to thermodynamic and biochemical principles established through studies of inanimate systems.

Landmark discoveries about metabolism proceeded into the twentieth century. In 1907, Walter Fletcher and Frederick Gowland Hopkins discovered that lactic acid results when glucose is subjected to the anaerobic contraction of muscles. Five years later, Hopkins discovered substances that are now recognized as vitamins, a term invented in 1912 by Casimir Funk. Ten years later,

Frederick Banting and others pinpointed insulin as a substance that could be synthesized and used to reduce levels of blood sugar in humans, thereby making diabetes a manageable rather than a clearly fatal disorder.

A turning point in the understanding of metabolism and especially of metabolic disorders came in 1926 when James B. Sumner purified the first enzyme, showing it to be a protein, clearly leading to the realization that metabolic disorders result from a faulty protein in the genes. In 1941, Fritz Lipmann established the central role of ATP as a carrier of energy in living organisms, and the following year, Rudolf Schoenheimer demonstrated that the adult body's chemical constituents are in constant flux, suggesting that normal, healthy organisms are constantly renewing themselves.

As one surveys the future in terms of the rapidly increasing knowledge of metabolism and genetics, it is clear that genetic engineering offers daunting biological challenges. Birth defects can be detected well before birth, and many of them, through genetic manipulation, can be prevented. It is now within the capability of genetic engineering to predetermine the sex of a fetus and to control matters of gender. Amniocentesis can reveal abnormalities by the second trimester of pregnancy, revealing such conditions as metabolic disorders.

The capabilities that currently lie within reach pose substantial ethical problems and challenges. For example, if a fetus clearly shows evidence of being afflicted with a metabolic disorder, what use should be made of this information? Some parents would elect to terminate the pregnancy, given the challenges of raising such a child.

—R. Baird Shuman, Ph.D.

See also Acid-base chemistry; Arthritis; Caffeine; Carbohydrates; Cholesterol; Diabetes mellitus; Digestion; Endocrinology; Endocrinology, pediatric; Enzyme therapy; Enzymes; Exercise physiology; Fatty acid oxidation disorders; Food biochemistry; Fructosemia; Gastroenterology; Gastroenterology, pediatric; Gastrointestinal system; Gaucher's disease; Genetic diseases; Glands; Glycogen storage diseases; Glycolysis; Gout; Hemochromatosis; Hormones; Kidney disorders; Lipids; Macronutrients; Maple syrup urine disease (MSUD); Metabolic disorders; Metabolic syndrome; Mucopolysaccharidosis (MPS); Niemann-Pick disease; Nonalcoholic steatohepatitis (NASH); Obesity; Obesity, childhood; Phenylketonuria (PKU); Protein; Tay-Sachs disease; Wilson's disease.

FOR FURTHER INFORMATION:

Barasi, Mary E. *Human Nutrition: A Health Perspective.* 2d ed. New York: Oxford University Press, 2003. A text that emphasizes basic nutrition information, its role in metabolism, and the application of this information to health maintenance and disease prevention.

Becker, Kenneth L., et al., eds. *Principles and Practice of Endocrinology and Metabolism.* 3d ed. Philadelphia: Lippincott Williams and Wilkins, 2001. The treatment of metabolic disorders is extensive and accurate. The contributors are well informed and current in their information.

Devlin, Thomas M., ed. *Textbook of Biochemistry: With Clinical Correlations.* 6th ed. Hoboken, N.J.: Wiley-Liss, 2006. This college textbook presents considerable information on genetic engineering, hormones, and related topics. Includes chemical structures, diagrams, and references useful to the reader. All descriptions are simple but scholarly.

Edwards, Christopher R., and Dennis W. Lincoln, eds. *Recent Advances in Endocrinology and Metabolism.* 4th ed. New York: Churchill Livingstone, 1992. Particularly thorough in its treatment of such common metabolic disorders as diabetes, arthritis, and thyroid problems. The contributors also treat the less common metabolic disorders directly and clearly.

Feek, Colin, and Christopher Edwards. *Endocrine and Metabolic Disease.* New York: Springer, 1988. This comprehensive volume presents information about every conceivable sort of metabolic disorder. The language is sometimes technical, but readers not specifically schooled in the field will be able to comprehend the salient points the authors make.

Hoffmann, Georg F., et al. *Inherited Metabolic Diseases.* Philadelphia: Lippincott Williams & Wilkins, 2002. A clinical text that details medical history, symptoms, the process of diagnosis and therapy, and organ-specific treatment of metabolic disorders.

Isaacs, Scott, and Neil Shulman. *The Hormonal Balance: Understanding Hormones, Weight, and Your Metabolism.* Boulder, Colo.: Bull, 2007. Details how metabolic and hormonal imbalances can affect weight and perpetuate obesity. Examines diet and lifestyle changes to address menstrual irregularities and diseases such as diabetes.

King, Richard A., Jerome I. Rotter, and Arno G. Motulsky, eds. *The Genetic Basis of Common Diseases.* 2d ed. New York: Oxford University Press, 2002. Covers advances in the understanding of molecular processes involved in genetic susceptibility and disease mechanisms. Examines a range of diseases in detail and includes a chapter on genetic counseling.

Kronenberg, Henry M., et al., eds. *Williams Textbook of Endocrinology.* 11th ed. Philadelphia: Saunders/Elsevier, 2008. Text that covers the spectrum of information related to the endocrine system, including thyroid disorders, diabetes, endocrinology and aging, female reproduction and fertility control, sexual function and dysfunction, kidney stones, and endocrine hypertension.

Whitehead, Roger G. *New Techniques in Nutritional Research.* San Diego, Calif.: Academic Press, 1991. This book provides the most thorough treatment of the nutritional aspects of metabolic disorders. It is especially strong in its presentation of disorders stemming from the accumulation of trace minerals, suggesting ways of treating such situations with vitamins or by other means.

METASTASIS. *See* CANCER; MALIGNANCY AND METASTASIS.

METHICILLIN-RESISTANT *STAPHYLOCOCCUS AUREUS* (MRSA) INFECTIONS

DISEASE/DISORDER

ALSO KNOWN AS: Methicillin-resistant staph infections

ANATOMY OR SYSTEM AFFECTED: Blood, blood vessels, bones, circulatory system, feet, hands, heart, joints, kidneys, legs, liver, muscles, musculoskeletal system, nose, respiratory system, skin, spine, spleen

SPECIALTIES AND RELATED FIELDS: Bacteriology, cardiology, critical care, dermatology, epidemiology, family medicine, general surgery, internal medicine, microbiology, nursing, orthopedics, pediatrics, pharmacology, podiatry, public health, pulmonary medicine, radiology, rheumatology, sports medicine

DEFINITION: An infection caused by a virulent and destructive bacteria that is resistant to common antibiotics and difficult to treat. It may be localized to one area of the body or may become systemic (spread throughout the body).

KEY TERMS:

abscess: a collection of pus

bacteremia: bacterial infection of the blood

bacterial endocarditis: bacterial infection of the heart valves

cellulitis: infection of the skin and underlying tissue
culture: growth of bacteria in laboratory conditions
osteomyelitis: infection of bone
septic arthritis: infection of a joint
surgical debridement: removal of diseased tissue
surgical drainage: removal of pus

CAUSES AND SYMPTOMS

Staphylococcus aureus is an organism commonly found on skin, especially in the nose, axilla (underarm), groin, and rectal areas. Methicillin resistance is the genetically acquired ability of some strains to withstand exposure to a class of antibiotics designed to treat staphylococci. Methicillin-resistant *Staphylococcus aureus* (MRSA) infections occur when a visible or microscopic break in the skin allows these bacterial organisms to enter the body. Such points of entry may be the result of injury, such as an abrasion sustained wrestling or playing football, or surgical, as in a cesarean section or a joint replacement. Needles used to inject medication or illicit drugs can also introduce these bacteria. Sometimes the source is as innocuous as a hair follicle, and occasionally the source of a bloodstream infection is never identified.

Many strains of MRSA are virulent and destructive. Infections are characterized by fever and by pain, redness, and swelling at the site. Pus may drain from the area or may build up as an abscess within infected tissue. MRSA may be invasive, meaning that it spreads deep into tissues and into the bloodstream, traveling through the body and infecting other sites. The most common site of infection is the skin, where MRSA may cause cellulitis (infection of the skin layers), folliculitis (infection of hair follicles), or a boil (an abscess complicating folliculitis). It is a common cause of foot and leg infections in patients with diabetes. Osteomyelitis (bone infection) can occur by direct invasion from an overlying skin infection or through trauma (fracture or foreign body such as shrapnel). When bacteria enter the bloodstream, they may find a focus in any organ or tissue and infect that area, sometimes even forming abscesses in these secondary sites. The spine, spleen, and kidneys are common secondary sites. Bacterial endocarditis, or infection of the heart valves and linings, is a particularly dangerous form of MRSA infection and is very difficult to treat. MRSA infections can complicate surgical procedures, causing infection of the incision and sometimes invading deeper tissues or spreading systemically. MRSA infection of surgically placed foreign bodies (artificial joints, bone plates and pins, heart valves) sometimes occurs. MRSA pneumonia can occur in hospitalized patients who require respirators and is a rare but sometimes fatal complication of influenza.

TREATMENT AND THERAPY

Treatment of MRSA infections is challenging both because of the organism's resistance to antibiotics and because of its aggressive and persistent nature. When possible, laboratory testing of the infecting organism can help guide the selection of antibiotics most likely to be effective. Specimens from the infected site (pus, infected tissue, blood) can be cultured for bacterial growth and the bacteria subjected to testing for susceptibility to a variety of antibiotics. Those shown in the laboratory to kill or inhibit growth of the cultured bacteria are those most likely to be effective in treating infection.

The antibiotics most commonly used for treating MRSA infections are vancomycin, linezolid, daptomycin, quinupristin/dalfopristin, clindamycin, and various forms of sulfa drugs and tetracyclines. Intravenous (IV) treatment is necessary for severe infections. Some infections, such as bacterial endocarditis and osteomyelitis, require antibiotics for six weeks or more, and relapse is not unusual. Surgical debridement to remove diseased tissue or surgical drainage of an abscess may be necessary in addition to antibiotics. MRSA infection involving a foreign body (for example, a prosthetic joint) is particularly difficult to eradicate; removal of the foreign body is often recommended in addition to antibiotics.

PERSPECTIVE AND PROSPECTS

Since the discovery of microorganisms as a cause of disease, *Staphylococcus aureus*, a common inhabitant of normal skin, has been shown capable of causing se-

---

INFORMATION ON MRSA INFECTIONS

CAUSES: Bacteria entering through break in skin from trauma, surgery, injection; point of entry may be unidentifiable

SYMPTOMS: Fever, pain, redness, swelling, pus if localized

DURATION: days to weeks; can be fatal if systemic

TREATMENTS: Antibiotics, surgery

vere, life-threatening infection under some conditions. The introduction of antibiotics proved it able to adapt rapidly through mutation, as some strains became resistant first to penicillin and later to the semi-synthetic penicillins (such as methicillin) designed to treat penicillin-resistant staphylococci. Initially, these antibiotic-resistant strains were found almost entirely in hospitals and nursing homes, where exposure to antibiotics and evolutionary pressure favored their existence. Since the 1990's, MRSA has become widespread outside these settings. Some of these "community-acquired" strains, or CA-MRSA, have caused severe infections and even death in young, healthy people who became infected through minor sports injuries or following influenza. Public health authorities have instituted more stringent guidelines for cleaning athletic equipment, immediate showering after practices and competitions, excluding infected athletes from participation, covering open wounds with bandages, and so on. Education and public awareness of appropriate hygiene and infection control measures will be important in reducing spread of infection through communities. Efforts to reduce unnecessary (treatment of a common cold) or inappropriate (premature discontinuation) antibiotic use may help to prevent further antibiotic resistance. Research and development of more effective antibiotics are essential for improving cure rates for severe MRSA infections.

—*Margaret Trexler Hessen, M.D.*

See also Antibiotics; Bacterial infections; Bacteriology; Drug resistance; Epidemiology; Hospitals; Iatrogenic disorders; Infection; Staphylococcal infections.

FOR FURTHER INFORMATION:

Bowman, M. C., D. A. Wohl, and A. H. Kaplan. "Staphylococcal Infections." In *Netter's Internal Medicine*, edited by M. S. Runge and M. A. Greganti. 2d ed. Philadelphia: Saunders/Elsevier, 2009.

Brooks, G. F., et al., eds. *Jawetz, Melnick, and Adelberg's Medical Microbiology*. 24th ed. New York: McGraw-Hill, 2007.

Yok, Q. al-, and P. Moreillon. "*Staphylococcus aureus* (Including Staphylococcal Toxic Shock)." In *Mandell, Douglas, and Bennett's Principles and Practice of Infectious Diseases*, edited by G. L. Mandell, J. E. Bennett, and R. Dolin. Philadelphia: Churchill Livingstone/Elsevier, 2009.

MICROBIOLOGY

SPECIALTY

ANATOMY OR SYSTEM AFFECTED: Cells, immune system

SPECIALTIES AND RELATED FIELDS: Bacteriology, environmental health, epidemiology, immunology, pathology, public health, virology

DEFINITION: The study of organisms too small to be seen by the unaided human eye, especially the identification, transmission, and control of microorganisms that cause disease.

KEY TERMS:

deoxyribonucleic acid (DNA): the genetic material of a cell that directs the synthesis of proteins; ribonucleic acid (RNA) is the intermediary needed to complete protein synthesis

flora: the microorganisms that are commonly found on or in the human body; also called microflora

infectious disease: an illness caused by a microorganism or its products, in contrast to diseases caused by factors such as heredity or poor nutrition

microorganism: an organism that is too small to be seen without a magnifying lens; also known as a microbe

pathogen: an organism that causes an infectious disease

SCIENCE AND PROFESSION

Microbiology is the field of science that focuses on microorganisms, living things that can be studied only by using microscopes and other special equipment. Microorganisms have an important place in the ecology of the planet. They form a basis for food chains and, as decomposers, recycle many materials in the environment. Because microbes are everywhere, humans come in contact with a wide variety every day; many live on or in the human body. Most of these organisms either are harmless or are prevented from multiplying by the immune system and other defenses. Others are able to penetrate these defenses and cause an illness. Medical microbiologists study microorganisms that cause these diseases. These pathogens come primarily from four groups: bacteria, fungi, protozoans, and viruses.

Bacteria, along with blue-green algae, belong to the Monera kingdom and are the simplest organisms that exist in cellular form. The bacterial chromosome consists of a loop of deoxyribonucleic acid (DNA) containing several hundred genes. Because it is unprotected by a nuclear membrane, bacterial DNA can be manipulated more easily than can DNA in plants and animals. Several traits are used to identify bacterial species.

There are three basic shapes: coccus (round), bacillus (rod), and spirillum (spiral). Gram's stain procedure divides bacteria into two main groups based on their cell wall content. Other staining procedures can identify the presence of such structures as flagella, capsules, and endospores, which may have implications for control measures. For example, endospores are resistant to many common disinfectants, and boiling them for up to four hours may not destroy them. In addition to staining, chemical and metabolic tests are used to differentiate bacterial species.

Although the fungi kingdom includes larger organisms such as mushrooms, the ones of interest to medical microbiology are the yeasts, molds, and related microorganisms. Like plants, they have cell walls. They cannot manufacture their own food by photosynthesis, however, and must either be saprophytes, living on dead organic material, or parasites, obtaining nutrients from another living organism. Fungi reproduce by means of spores that are released and carried by the air to a suitable medium. They thrive in a warm, moist environment with a carbohydrate source of food.

Protozoa, members of the Protista kingdom, are often referred to as one-celled animals. They have no cell walls and must ingest or absorb their food. Their ability to move enables them to spread more quickly than can nonmotile microbes. Four main categories exist. The amoebas move by means of projections called pseudopodia. The flagellates move by means of long hairlike structures (flagella) that whip back and forth. Ciliates are covered with short hairlike structures (cilia) that beat in a synchronized way to cause movement. Sporozoans must move by means of the circulation of blood and tissue fluids within a host. Of all the microorganisms, protozoa are the ones that most resemble human cells. Treatment for a protozoal disease must be monitored closely; most chemicals that are effective against protozoa are also toxic to humans.

Viruses are on the borderline between living and nonliving things. They are not cellular in form, unlike all other forms of life. Each virus particle, called a virion, is made up of a protein coat and a nucleic acid core of either DNA or RNA. Viruses are classified by size, shape, type of nucleic acid in their core, and type of cell they invade or disease they cause.

To reproduce, a virion attaches itself to a living cell and injects its core into the cell. The nucleic acid then takes over the cell's protein-manufacturing apparatus to make new virus particles. The host cell ruptures as these viruses are released to infect other cells. Some viral DNA can incorporate itself into the host DNA and remain dormant until some factor triggers a new reproductive cycle. Viruses usually can attack only one type of cell or species; however, mutations can occur that allow them to infect other species. For example, human immunodeficiency virus (HIV), the cause of acquired immunodeficiency syndrome (AIDS), is believed to have mutated from simian immunodeficiency virus (SIV) in monkeys.

DIAGNOSTIC AND TREATMENT TECHNIQUES

When the type of microorganism causing an infectious disease is unknown, a medical microbiologist follows a series of procedures known as Koch's postulates. Named for Robert Koch, who proposed them, these procedures identify and confirm that a particular microorganism is the cause of the disease. First, the microorganism must be present in the tissues of all individuals who have the disease. This means that all the microorganisms in a sample of diseased tissue must be identified and classified so that a possible pathogen may be differentiated from the normal flora. Second, the suspected pathogen must be isolated and grown in a pure culture. Many microorganisms can be grown on a simple medium called nutrient agar. Some microorganisms may need specific nutrients added to the medium or may be obligate parasites—that is, they can grow only on or in living cells. Anaerobic organisms cannot grow at all if oxygen is present. Since these special needs are not known in advance, the detection of some pathogens may be difficult.

The third step the researcher takes is to inoculate an animal with the organism in an effort to duplicate the disease. In the case of human diseases, mammals—such as rabbits, guinea pigs, and mice—are used. Finding the right animal subject may also pose a problem, since not all animals are susceptible to human diseases. For example, armadillos must be used to study leprosy, because the more common laboratory animals are not susceptible to it. In the last of Koch's procedures, the organism must be reisolated from the diseased animal. This step verifies the identity of the pathogen and confirms that it is the same as the original form. If the organism has been identified correctly as the cause of the disease, researchers can then proceed to learn more about the microorganism and its role in the disease process.

The identification of a pathogen as the cause of a specific disease and knowledge of its biological characteristics aid medical researchers in finding prevention and treatment strategies. To cause illness, a microorganism must meet several criteria. First, it must survive transfer to the new host. Some pathogens can form protective structures, such as endospores, that will keep them alive outside a host for a long period of time. A pathogen that cannot survive outside a host must be passed directly in some way from an infected person to a healthy one. Second, a pathogen must overcome the host's defenses. Some may enter through a wound, bypassing the skin barrier that protects the human body from many infections. Some produce chemicals that damage cells and weaken the body. Still others may be able to cause illness only if the person's defenses are weakened by some factor such as age, malnutrition, or another existing illness. Finally, the organism must cause some damage to the host, resulting in the symptoms and signs associated with that illness. The disease process can best be understood by examining several examples of pathogens, the diseases they cause, and the strategies used against them.

The members of the genus *Clostridium* are all anaerobic, form endospores, and produce toxins. Among the bacteria in this group are the pathogens that cause gangrene, tetanus, and botulism. Gangrene usually occurs when a wound has cut off the blood supply to an area of the body. *Clostridium perfringens* enters the body and is able to survive because the lack of blood has created an anaerobic condition. It produces a toxin that destroys surrounding tissue, allowing it to spread. Antibiotics may be effective in preventing the bacteria from spreading to healthy tissue but, because drugs are transported in the blood, may not be able to reach the infected site. Placing the patient in a chamber containing oxygen under high pressure is one strategy used to destroy anaerobic bacteria. *Clostridium tetani* also enters the body through a wound—sometimes a very small one. Since this organism is common and a small wound may go unnoticed, regular immunizations with tetanus vaccine are recommended. Once *C. tetani* bacteria enter the body, they produce a neurotoxin. This nerve poison causes the muscles to stiffen, resulting in a condition called tetanus, or lockjaw. In addition to antibiotics, an antitoxin must be given to neutralize the poison. *Clostridium botulinum* causes botulism, a type of food poisoning. If proper canning techniques are not used, the endospores will germinate. The food then provides a medium on which they can grow, and the sealed can provides the perfect anaerobic conditions. *C. botulinum* produces a neurotoxin that, if it is not destroyed by adequate cooking, will produce neurological symp-

toms such as double vision and dizziness. This disease must be treated by an appropriate antitoxin or death from respiratory failure can occur in a matter of days.

The human intestine contains large numbers of microorganisms. Some of them provide benefits to their host by producing vitamins and inhibiting the growth of other, potentially harmful, microorganisms. Disease can result if the balance is changed. *Escherichia coli*, part of the normal intestinal flora, can cause infections when it is transferred to another part of the body, such as the urinary bladder. In developing countries, *E. coli* bacteria contaminate drinking water in such large numbers that they result in infantile diarrhea, a common cause of death in those countries. A 1993 epidemic in the United States involved a particularly virulent strain of *E. coli* that had been ingested in improperly cooked ground beef. The characteristics of the strain, combined with the large number of bacteria in the meat, disrupted the intestinal balance of those who ingested it, caused hundreds of people to become ill, and resulted in the deaths of three young children.

The use of antibiotics can disrupt the natural balance by destroying beneficial bacteria as well as pathogens. *Candida albicans*, a yeastlike fungus, is part of the normal human flora. Its growth in the intestine is controlled by certain kinds of bacteria. When antibiotics are used, these beneficial bacteria are destroyed, and the *Candida* begins to multiply. This may not only result in intestinal yeast infections but also contribute to yeast infections in the vagina and other areas where *Candida* can be found. Strategies used to restore the balance may involve eating yogurt or capsules containing *Acidophilus*, one of the beneficial bacteria. Sugars, an important source of food for yeast, should be eliminated from the diet. If these measures do not work, antifungal medication may have to be used.

Fungi that cause skin infections such as athlete's foot are called dermatophytes. When an infected person takes a shower, dermatophyte spores are left in the shower stall. The warm, moist environment then allows the spores to survive until a potential new host comes. Since feet are usually enclosed in shoes and socks, the dermatophytes are again provided with an ideal warm, moist environment. Prevention strategies involve using fungicidal disinfectants to kill the spores and wearing sandals in the shower to avoid coming in contact with the spores. Treatment includes antifungal medication and making the environment less suitable for fungi by keeping the feet dry.

Protozoa are also vulnerable to dry conditions. *Entamoeba histolytica*, the cause of amebic dysentery, is usually ingested in contaminated water. It can, however, form cysts, which allows it to resist drying and freezing. An individual can become ill after eating food rinsed in contaminated water or drinking a "safe" beverage that contained ice made from contaminated water.

Plasmodium species are responsible for malaria, which kills two million people in the world each year. Because this protozoan cannot live outside a host, it is dependent on the female *Anopheles* mosquito to transmit it from one person to another. When a mosquito "bites," it actually pierces the skin with a hypodermic-like mouth and injects a local anesthetic to prevent the host from feeling its presence. At the same time, if it is infected with *Plasmodium*, it will inject malarial parasites into the bloodstream. These parasites spend most of their life cycle inside red blood cells, where they are protected from normal immune defenses. When they have multiplied, they rupture the cells as they leave. Treatment involves maintaining sufficiently high levels of medicine, such as quinine, in the plasma that the parasites die. The most important public health strategy is to control the mosquito population and prevent transmission.

Other than bacteria, viruses are the most common pathogens. The mode of transmission of viruses from one host to another depends on the type of virus. Some can survive for a long period of time outside a host, others must be transferred quickly through the air or by contact, and others can survive only when passed directly into the host by body fluids or insect bites. The damage done to the host depends on the type of tissue that is infected by the virus. For example, the Epstein-Barr virus invades the lymphatic system. It causes the enlarged lymph nodes and abnormal lymphocytes that are characteristic of mononucleosis. It is also associated with Burkitt's lymphoma and Hodgkin's disease, both of which are cancers of the lymphatic system. The human immunodeficiency virus (HIV) invades the T lymphocytes, the white blood cells that are crucial to the functioning of the immune system. Damage to the immune system not only makes the individual vulnerable to disease organisms coming from outside the body but also disrupts the balance between the host and normal human flora. This allows other viruses, bacteria, protozoa, and fungi such as *Candida* to multiply and cause potentially fatal secondary infections.

PERSPECTIVE AND PROSPECTS

Infectious diseases have had devastating effects on human populations and societies. For example, during the eighty-year period starting in 1347, recurrent plague epidemics resulted in the deaths of 75 percent of the European population. For many centuries, some physicians and others hypothesized that invisible creatures were the cause of disease. In 1546, Girolamo Fracastoro suggested the presence of germs (seeds) of disease that could be passed from person to person. Because these creatures could not be seen, this "germ" theory was not widely accepted. Then, in 1673, Antoni van Leeuwenhoek began sending descriptions and pictures of what he called "animalcules" to the Royal Society of London. An amateur scientist, Leeuwenhoek made simple microscopes and systematically studied the objects and materials around him. His discoveries of what are now known to be protozoa and bacteria were verified, and they opened the field of microbiology as a science. Using their new knowledge of the microbial world, nineteenth century researchers began to reexamine the germ theory of disease. In 1857, Louis Pasteur, a chemist, discovered that certain bacteria caused wine to spoil. A few years later, he isolated a protozoan as a cause of a silkworm disease and predicted that microbes could cause human illness. In 1875, Robert Koch, a German physician, devised a procedure by which he demonstrated that anthrax was caused by a specific type of bacterium: *Bacillus anthracis*. His experiments led to widespread acceptance of the germ theory of disease, and his procedures provided a systematic method by which researchers could identify those germs. The twenty-five years that followed are referred to as the golden age of microbiology; one by one, nearly all the major bacterial pathogens were identified.

During this intense period of discovery, researchers soon found that, although fine porcelain filters were used to trap microorganisms, in some cases the liquid filtrate was capable of causing disease. The term "virus," meaning poison, was used because it was thought at first that the liquid contained a toxic substance. Pasteur hypothesized that there might be an organism too small to be seen using the light microscope. Later, this was verified, when researchers were able to remove the water from the filtrate, leaving crystals. After the invention of the electron microscope in 1933, individual virions could be seen.

The discovery of pathogens quickly led to research aimed at finding ways to prevent and treat infectious diseases. The contagious nature of disease was known in ancient times. This is illustrated by the practices of Greek physicians and Jewish hygiene laws. Prior to Koch's work, Ignaz Phillipp Semmelweis in the 1840's and Joseph Lister in the 1860's showed that antiseptic techniques could control transmission of diseases. In 1849, John Snow traced the source of a cholera epidemic to a water pump in London. The knowledge that a specific pathogen was involved made it possible for more specific means of prevention to be applied. Within ten years of Koch's report, Louis Pasteur developed vaccines for anthrax and rabies. Immunizations for many infectious diseases were developed, public sanitation measures were taken to reduce the contamination of food and water, and surgeons adopted techniques to control surgical and wound infection.

Although progress in disease prevention was being made, once a person became ill, treatment was still primarily a matter of keeping the patient alive until the disease ran its course. In the early twentieth century, a German physician named Paul Ehrlich began to search for what he called a "magic bullet"—a chemical that would specifically treat a disease by killing the pathogens that caused it. After several years of work, compound 606, an arsenic derivative, was made available to treat syphilis. Sulfa drugs were developed in the 1920's. In 1929, Alexander Fleming discovered penicillin, a substance produced by the mold *Penicillium* that could destroy bacteria in cultures. In 1939, Ernst Chain and Howard Florey used penicillin successfully to treat bacterial infections. In 1944, Selman Waksman discovered streptomycin and used the term "antibiotic" to refer to a substance manufactured by a living organism that kills or inhibits the growth of a pathogen.

By the 1970's, it seemed that the end of infectious disease as a major medical problem was in sight. Several developments brought an end to this complacency. Strains of *Staphylococcus* appeared that were resistant to common antibiotics and caused an increase in postsurgical infections. Antibiotic-resistant strains of gonorrhea and syphilis also became widespread. Childhood diseases, once thought to be under control, reappeared as a result of neglected vaccination programs. Increased world travel also facilitated the spread of disease from country to country. Then, in 1981, AIDS was first described; within a few years, it became a worldwide health problem. As people with AIDS began to succumb to previously uncommon secondary diseases, these diseases had to be studied. A new antibiotic-resistant strain of tuberculosis also appeared as a direct result of the AIDS epidemic. These developments have reemphasized the study of microbiology and demonstrated its importance to human health.

—*Edith K. Wallace, Ph.D.*

See also Antibiotics; Bacterial infections; Bacteriology; Bionics and biotechnology; Cells; Cytology; Cytopathology; Diagnosis; DNA and RNA; Drug resistance; Epidemiology; Fungal infections; Gastroenterology; Gastroenterology, pediatric; Gastrointestinal disorders; Gastrointestinal system; Genetic engineering; Gram staining; Immune system; Immunization and vaccination; Immunology; Laboratory tests; Microscopy; Mutation; Pathology; Pharmacology; Pharmacy; Prion diseases; Protozoan diseases; Serology; Toxicology; Tropical medicine; Urinalysis; Urinary system; Urology; Urology, pediatric; Viral infections.

FOR FURTHER INFORMATION:

Alcamo, I. Edward. *Microbes and Society: An Introduction to Microbiology*. 2d ed. Sudbury, Mass.: Jones and Bartlett, 2008. A nonscientific text for the liberal arts student that explores the importance of microbes to human life and their role in food production and agriculture, in biotechnology and industry, in ecology and the environment, and in disease and bioterrorism.

Biddle, Wayne. *A Field Guide to Germs*. 2d ed. New York: Anchor Books, 2002. This comprehensive book is easily accessible to the nonspecialist and includes a discussion of nearly every virus, bacterium, and fungus known to cause human and nonhuman animal disease. The history of the microbe and the treatment of diseases are included.

Gallo, Robert. *Virus Hunting*. New York: Basic Books, 1991. Written for the general reader by one of the discoverers of the AIDS virus. It examines the field of virology and the methods used to study viruses, especially cancer-causing viruses. The search for the AIDS virus is detailed. Name and subject indexes are included.

Gladwin, Mark, and Bill Trattler. *Clinical Microbiology Made Ridiculously Simple*. 4th ed. Miami: MedMaster, 2009. The authors explain the principles behind microbiology in easy-to-understand terms. Includes a bibliography and an index.

Jensen, Marcus M., and Donald N. Wright. *Introduction to Microbiology for the Health Sciences*. 4th ed. Englewood Cliffs, N.J.: Prentice Hall, 1997. An introductory college textbook that focuses on the field of medical microbiology. It reviews the general characteristics of microorganisms, but the emphasis is on pathogenic species and the prevention and treatment of disease. Each chapter contains case histories illustrating the direct application of principles.

Madigan, Michael T., and John M. Martinko. *Brock Biology of Microorganisms.* 12th ed. San Francisco: Pearson/Benjamin Cummings, 2009. An outstanding microbiology text. The authors provide a thorough description of bacteria and the means by which they are studied. Relevant to this topic are chapters on methods of isolation and characterization.

Murray, Patrick R., Ken S. Rosenthal, and Michael A. Pfaller. *Medical Microbiology.* 6th ed. Philadelphia: Mosby/Elsevier, 2009. Focuses on microbes that cause disease in humans. Each chapter consistently presents the etiology, epidemiology, host defenses, identification, diagnosis, prevention, and control of each disease.

MICROSCOPY

PROCEDURE

ANATOMY OR SYSTEM AFFECTED: Cells

SPECIALTIES AND RELATED FIELDS: Bacteriology, cytology, histology, microbiology, pathology, virology

DEFINITION: The use of a microscope to make extremely small objects appear larger in order to make them visible.

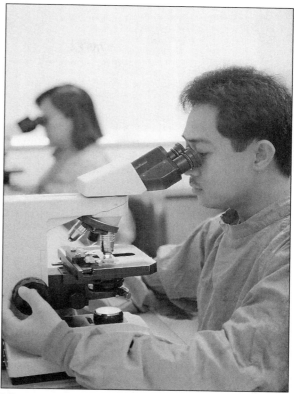

Microscopes are essential in the analysis of laboratory specimens. (PhotoDisc)

INDICATIONS AND PROCEDURES

Conventional microscopy uses a beam of light to illuminate a thin slice of material to be viewed. The material may be stained to provide contrast among its components. The visible light is aimed through the material and collected in a lens. Additional lenses magnify the image until it is visible to the eye of the viewer.

Electron microscopy is a procedure in which a beam of electrons, rather than visible light, is projected toward an object to be viewed. The object is prepared by coating it with a fine layer of metal, frequently gold, that is one or two atoms thick. The electrons reflect off the coated object and hit a screen. The image on the screen is magnified and becomes visible to the human eye. An alternative procedure involves a very thin section of material that is dried and put into a vacuum chamber. A beam of electrons is directed through the prepared specimen. A coated screen receives the electron beam and transforms the image into one visible to the human eye.

Fluorescence microscopy is a procedure that is based on the fact that fluorescent materials emit visible light when they are irradiated with ultraviolet light, which is outside the spectrum visible to the human eye. Some materials manifest this property naturally; others may have to be treated with fluorescent solutions in a process similar to staining. When the absorption of the specimen is in the relatively long ultraviolet range, two filters are also used. The first is placed over the light source to eliminate all but the desired long ultraviolet rays. The second is placed over the eyepiece. The result is a field that becomes dark and allows any red or yellow fluorescence to be visible.

USES AND COMPLICATIONS

Microscopy has extended the range of understanding for physical objects. Intracellular organelles are routinely made visible. Microscopy has made possible the science of microbiology. Fluorescence allows immunoglobulins to be routinely assayed. Viruses are too small to be seen with a light microscope, but electron microscopy has enabled virologists to view and classify viruses.

The drawbacks of current microscopy techniques

are primarily that only small samples of material can be viewed at a time. Usually, the material must be destroyed while it is being prepared. Living tissue may be viewed, but only at levels of magnification below those possible at the limits of normal microscopy and far below those possible with electron microscopy.

Electron microscopy allows the greatest amount of magnification for objects. Because the wavelength of electrons is thousands of times shorter than that of visible light, the resulting magnification is several thousand times greater than that possible with visible light. The use of subatomic particles theoretically increases the potential of magnification, but a continuous source of subatomic particles is difficult and quite expensive to supply.

—L. Fleming Fallon, Jr., M.D., Ph.D., M.P.H.
See also Antibiotics; Bacteriology; Cells; Cytology; Cytopathology; Diagnosis; Gram staining; Laboratory tests; Microbiology; Microscopy, slitlamp; Pathology.

FOR FURTHER INFORMATION:
Hawkes, Peter W., and John C. H. Spence, eds. *Science of Microscopy.* New York: Springer, 2007.
Madigan, Michael T., and John M. Martinko. *Brock Biology of Microorganisms.* 12th ed. San Francisco: Pearson/Benjamin Cummings, 2009.
Murray, Patrick R., Ken S. Rosenthal, and Michael A. Pfaller. *Medical Microbiology.* 6th ed. Philadelphia: Mosby/Elsevier, 2009.
Singleton, Paul, and Diana Sainsbury. *Dictionary of Microbiology and Molecular Biology.* Rev. 3d ed. Hoboken, N.J.: John Wiley & Sons, 2007.
Spector, David L., and Robert D. Goldman, eds. *Basic Methods in Microscopy: Protocols and Concepts from Cells—A Laboratory Manual.* Cold Spring Harbor, N.Y.: Cold Spring Harbor Laboratory Press, 2006.

MICROSCOPY, SLITLAMP
PROCEDURE
ALSO KNOWN AS: Biomicroscope
ANATOMY OR SYSTEM AFFECTED: Eyes
SPECIALTIES AND RELATED FIELDS: Ophthalmology
DEFINITION: The use of a special instrument to examine the tissues of the eye.

INDICATIONS AND PROCEDURES
The slitlamp microscope, or biomicroscope, is used to examine and evaluate tissues of the eye with both stereopsis and multiple values of optical magnification.

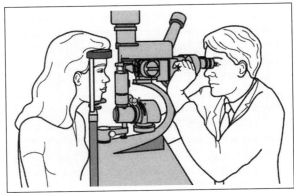

The slitlamp microscope, or biomicroscope, is used by ophthalmologists to examine the health of the eye.

The anterior segment of the eye is observed with several types of illumination: diffuse, direct (both broad and narrow beam, the latter allowing an almost slidelike examination of the clear corneal layers), indirect (side illumination), retroillumination (in which abnormalities are back-illuminated with light reflected from more internal structures), specular (in which light is reflected off various layers to show the detail of each surface), and sclerotic scatter (internal illumination). Various dyes (such as fluorescein or rose bengal) may be employed to help differentiate normal from abnormal tissues.

The instrument has two coaxial rotating arms controlled by a joystick level; one arm carries the adjustable slitlamp illumination system, with attendant filters and optical stops, and the other arm carries the observation optics (a binocular microscope). An adjustable chin and forehead rest positions the subject's head.

Auxiliary devices allow the measurement of intraocular pressure (tonometer) and corneal thickness (pacometer) and the evaluation of the angle between the cornea and iris (gonioscope lens). Cameras, both still and video, may be attached at various sites. High-powered auxiliary optical lenses have also been developed, which allow the clinician to use the slitlamp microscope to observe the posterior pole of the eye (through the pharmacologically dilated pupil), including the optic nerve and most of the retina. Ophthalmic lasers can also be attached to this system in order to treat the various structures of the eye as they are observed directly through the same optics, using the principle of the reversibility of the path of light.

Allvar Gullstrand received a Nobel Prize in 1911 for his contributions to optics, and the same year he introduced his refinement of the slitlamp microscope. Modern instruments and techniques are largely based on his work.

—*Barry A. Weissman, O.D., Ph.D.*

See also Eye infections and disorders; Eye surgery; Eyes; Laser use in surgery; Microscopy; Ophthalmology; Optometry; Vision; Vision disorders.

FOR FURTHER INFORMATION:

Kaufman, Paul L., and Albert Alm. *Adler's Physiology of the Eye: Clinical Application.* 10th ed. St. Louis, Mo.: Mosby, 2003.

Ledford, Janice K., and Valerie N. Sanders. *The Slit Lamp Primer.* 2d ed. Thorofare, N.J.: SLACK, 2006.

Newell, Frank W. *Ophthalmology: Principles and Concepts.* 8th ed. St. Louis, Mo.: Mosby, 1996.

Riordan-Eva, Paul, and John P. Whitcher. *Vaughan and Asbury's General Ophthalmology.* 17th ed. New York: Lange Medical Books/McGraw-Hill, 2007.

Sutton, Amy L., ed. *Eye Care Sourcebook: Basic Consumer Health Information About Eye Care and Eye Disorders.* 3d ed. Detroit, Mich.: Omnigraphics, 2008.

Wenzel, Martin. *Specular Microscopy of Intraocular Lenses: Atlas and Textbook for Slit-Lamp and the Specular Microscopic Examinations.* New York: Thieme Medical, 1993.

MIDLIFE CRISIS

DISEASE/DISORDER

ANATOMY OR SYSTEM AFFECTED: Psychic-emotional system

SPECIALTIES AND RELATED FIELDS: Psychiatry, psychology

DEFINITION: The emotional, psychological, physical, spiritual, and relationship crises that arise during the transition from early to later adulthood.

KEY TERMS:

development: a generally predictable process of physical, emotional, cognitive, and/or spiritual growth or differentiation

developmental stressors: the events or other characteristics associated with the developmental process, which may be experienced as causing subjective or objectively measurable discomfort

midlife crisis: a crisis resulting from stressors related to the transition from early adulthood to later adulthood

situational stressors: the events or characteristics that may be experienced unpredictably during life and that may cause subjective or objectively measurable discomfort

CAUSES AND SYMPTOMS

Before the nature of the midlife crisis can be explored, it is first helpful to identify what is meant by "midlife." As the average life expectancy has changed throughout history, so has the period termed midlife. For example, current human life expectancy in the United States had risen to 77.5 years of age; this breaks down to 74.8 years for men and 80.1 for women of all races. These figures are more than twice as long as the average life expectancy during the time of the Massachusetts Bay Colony, and more than three and a half times as long as someone in ancient Greece could have expected to live.

Life expectancy changes as it is influenced by any number of factors, including nutrition, health care and prevention, stress and lifestyle issues, historical period, culture, race, individual variability, gender, and social context. Consequently, there is no precise age at which midlife commences. It is also difficult to state unequivocally when the possibility for a midlife crisis ends. Nevertheless, some developmental theorists, such as D. J. Levinson, suggest the period from forty to forty-five is the time of the midlife transition or "crisis." Others have indicated that this time period may last until the age of fifty-three. Yet the results of these studies, collected primarily from Caucasian males in the United States, may not be applicable to the general population.

Other researchers, Carol Gilligan among them, have engaged in a critique of the assumptions underlying previous comments on midlife crises and theories of how human beings develop, pointing out how this research may be based on outdated and/or incomplete studies of human development and experience. Gilligan's line of research demonstrates, for example, how it may be that women have an experience of the aging process that is different from the one commonly experienced by men. As a result, the process of normal adult development and the nature of this crisis remain less than crystal clear.

Midlife crisis experiences seem to arise in response to a variety of precipitating factors, including both normal developmental changes and severe or numerous stressors. This variability raises another interesting challenge to the notion of a midlife crisis. Is experience of a midlife crisis a predictable event or an aberration? Some experts claim that the belief in a "midlife crisis" is one of the many myths about the aging process.

Some argue that that many adults do not experience

an unusually severe crisis at midlife, or instead that midlife may be a tremendous period of growth. Others suggest that those who do experience a significant midlife crisis tend to have suffered similar crises throughout their adulthood. The stress involved in the transitions in midlife may be similar to, and not necessarily occurring more frequently than, those experienced by the same individual in any stage of life. If so, the adjective "midlife," as indicative of a qualitatively or quantitatively different kind of crisis, may be misleading.

On the other hand, some clinical studies reveal the male population in midlife to have a significant increase in mental health problems, including depression, alcoholism, and suicide. In fact, most studies of adulthood display something atypical among middle-aged men, whether dramatic or subtle. In addition, discussions around midlife changes for women are becoming more popular. With these discussions, however, the age range examined is advancing.

Caution is necessary when making general statements about a phenomenon such as midlife crisis, but for the sake of this discussion, a more general perspective is taken. It is assumed that midlife crises, however varied in form, intensity, or duration, do commonly occur. In addition, they are best understood from a holistic and contextual perspective on the individual's life.

A developmental framework that describes the cycle that an individual experiences in life further clarifies an understanding of midlife crises. The life changes of an individual may be seen as summative and consecutive. During this life cycle, one stage, with its tasks and crises, is lived and resolved before another is reached. Erik Erikson developed one framework for understanding the individual life cycle and its tasks, crises, and stages. Life crises are attributable in large part to the stress of transitioning from one part of life to another. The stage relevant to a discussion of midlife crises is termed generativity versus stagnation; in other words, midlife is the period of time during which individuals strive to come to terms with whether they are and may continue to be productive, or whether they will stagnate.

Development is also a physical experience. Therefore, an individual's psychological and emotional responses are influenced by changing physiology and health. One common midlife example in women is the menopause and its attendant hormonal changes. At few other times in a woman's life is there such a complex interaction between physical and psychological fac-

---

INFORMATION ON MIDLIFE CRISIS

CAUSES: Interrelated biological, emotional, psychological, and social components
SYMPTOMS: Anxious or depressed mood; loss of interest in normal activities; intensified reevaluation of life; sudden changes in relationships; difficulty with organic processes (sleeping, eating, concentration); spiritual reevaluation
DURATION: Ranges from short-term to long-term
TREATMENTS: Highly individualized; may include medication and/or psychotherapy

---

tors. Along with the physical stresses brought about by hormonal changes, the psychological and emotional reactions of each woman to this normal transition vary depending on her lifestyle, attitudes, self-image, and network of supportive relationships. This type of experience may contribute to crises in midlife.

In addition to the impact of changing physiology, the experience of midlife is emotional, cognitive, and spiritual. Midlife crises may be precipitated by an individual's reflection on or reevaluation of the meaning of life. Similarly, midlife may be a time during which people begin or intensify the process of spiritual evaluation and reckoning. It is a time during which people take stock of their lives and come to grips with their mortality.

A decline or change in physical functioning may trigger thoughts about mortality and death. A frequent phenomenon is evident in the change of one's perspective on time, from a focus on "time since birth" to one on "time left to live." Self-assessment may lead to greater emphasis on long-neglected aspects of the self or relationships with others.

All these issues are known as developmental issues or stressors, which are more or less predictable in life according to the person's stage of development. Situational stressors also contribute to the development of life crises. Situational stressors include such things as unexpected illness or injury, unemployment, and war—all things which are not necessarily related to the person's chronological age or development through time. Consequently, it is reasonable to conclude that these factors may be potent in midlife as well.

Typically, individuals live not in isolation from one another but within the context of relationships. The most common network of relationships is the family. A discussion of issues that have biological, emotional, psychological, and social components, therefore, must include an examination of what is happening with other family members and the family as a group. These factors, including what is termed the family life cycle, may influence the development or severity of the subjective experience of midlife crisis. In fact, the crises of midlife often arise from the interaction between individual and family factors.

Those experiencing midlife crisis are usually members of what has become known as the "sandwich generation"—a generation sandwiched between, and with the responsibility for taking care of, those in two others. For example, a middle-aged woman may have responsibilities with aging parents on one hand and with an adolescent son on the other. The coincidence of adolescence, with her son's focus on the development of an identity and his constant evaluation of his own and his parents' values, beliefs, and behaviors, may only exacerbate her similar search for meaning. She also may be reevaluating her accomplishments and striving to do more of what she believes has been meaningful so far in life. In contrast, the elder generation may be struggling to find some sense of integrity about a life ending. Each individual in the family becomes a point of contact, contrast, or conflict with the other.

The various manifestations of a midlife crisis are much like the symptoms exhibited by people in response to stress. The symptoms include an anxious or depressed mood, loss of interest in normal activities, an intensified reevaluation of life (both past and future), sudden changes in relationships, difficulty with organic processes (such as sleeping, eating, and concentration), and a subjective feeling of the need for a change. Extreme reactions may be a function of the psychology and emotional makeup of a particular individual in the context of his or her life. In addition, people who have less social support or who are living a lifestyle which they have long been aware was unfulfilling are more likely to experience a more significant crisis.

Not only do people and family groups vary in their reactions to midlife stress, but different ethnic and cultural groups do as well. The meaning associated with life events is generated within the context of these various social groups. Each social group develops its own culture with its own rules and regulations regarding how to respond or behave. In other words, individuals understand and respond to stressors as they do because of their experience within larger social groups. For example, within the Caucasian culture in the United States, a certain mythology has developed around the

midlife crisis. Midlife is sometimes seen as a time when a man will buy a sports car and leave his middle-aged wife for a younger woman, or when a woman will leave her husband for a younger man or to start a business. Someone else might give up her booming career and begin working with the underprivileged. As a result, within the context of this particular culture, dramatic lifestyle changes are predicted, explained, and possibly even supported. It must be understood, however, that not all the changes that occur are pathological; in fact, some may be signs of new and important growth.

In summary, midlife crises are those crises that may arise during the developmental stage associated with midlife. Like crises or other stress reactions, midlife crises vary in timing, intensity, duration, and character from one person, family, and social group to another. Crises in midlife seem to be no more frequent than crises at other stages of development.

TREATMENT AND THERAPY

Medical science has contributed to the understanding of the concept of midlife crisis through research, theory building, and the development and testing of treatment strategies, including the use of medication and psychotherapeutic techniques. Yet there are no specific treatments for a midlife or any other kind of crisis because the needs of the individual and the family group vary considerably. The range of possible treatments or clinical applications of medical science to this area are largely in the form of supporting the preexisting resources and coping skills of the individual and his or her family and other social support systems.

As with other life skills, an individual's ability to cope with and manage crises depends on the nature of one's character and personality, past experiences in managing crises, and degree of social support. The more well developed the person's character and coping mechanisms, the more numerous his or her experiences in successfully resolving past crises, and the greater amount of perceived support from family and friends, the more likely he or she will be able to resolve conflicts and crises in the present and future successfully.

Since midlife crises can differ from those in other stages, because of the particular tasks to be negotiated at this stage, resolution may involve the need to address certain tasks constructively. An individual may be called on to reevaluate or reassess his or her life, putting into perspective what is hoped for relative to what has transpired. An individual struggling with crises associated with midlife should be encouraged to explore the contributing situational and developmental issues openly. This process may involve cognitive reevaluation, working through feelings, or spiritual and existential reassessment.

Professionals often suggest that several tasks must be addressed in order to facilitate the successful resolution of a midlife crisis. The individual must reckon with his or her own mortality, go through a process of self-assessment, examine sex role obligations and expectations, and gain perspective on his or her generativity. Self-assessment involves taking stock and putting life into perspective. Life's polarities and contradictions must be examined and resolved in some manner.

One central polarity involves sex roles. The traditional differences between men and women often break down during the period of midlife. This process is facilitated by the life review accompanying a midlife crisis. For example, a woman may decide that she has devoted much of her life to the care and nurture of others while putting her own needs second. As a result, she may attempt to remedy the situation by developing the more stereotypical male characteristics of being assertive and goal-directed. Similarly, a male may turn away from his career as the primary source of self-esteem and gratification to developing richer interpersonal relationships.

Clinical and research evidence demonstrates a solid link between life crisis and disease onset. Consequently, medical health professionals may be called on to assist individuals struggling with the effects of a midlife crisis. These professionals, as well as other concerned individuals, may intervene in a variety of ways.

In a preventive fashion, helpers may offer what is termed anticipatory guidance to the individual approaching midlife transitions. In other words, conversations can include predictive or educative content orienting the person toward what to expect as he or she approaches or anticipates these changes. Individuals in the midst of midlife review and crisis may also need assistance, support, and/or direction in resolving generativity issues. The individual needs to resolve how he or she will make a significant contribution to others, rather than stagnate and become increasingly self-absorbed. Accomplishment of these tasks may involve repercussions in work, family, and social relationships.

Sometimes physicians are called on to treat individuals exhibiting physical and/or psychological symptoms related to midlife crises. Antidepressant and antianxiety medications are very effective with some conditions, including those in which the symptoms are impairing the person's ability to function over an extended period.

Various forms of assistance also may be offered through informal conversation, in an office visit for brief counseling, or within the process of psychotherapy for a longer-term approach. Regardless of the context, however, being able to anticipate or come to grips with the issues involved helps individuals to feel less out of control and to believe that the problems are being handled constructively.

Family and social support are very helpful in times of crisis. The degree to which these relationship contexts are flexible and supportive can either exacerbate problems or ameliorate struggles. A balance between permission and validation, with encouragement for the individual to continue managing daily functioning and obligations, is important. In the absence of an individual's ability to negotiate and resolve successfully the conflicts associated with the crisis, and perhaps without the presence of a supportive network of family and friends, individual and/or family therapy or a support group may be of help. These modes of therapy and support provide helpful perspective, normalization of the experience, and training or advice regarding constructive problem-solving and conflict resolution techniques.

PERSPECTIVE AND PROSPECTS

In many areas of medical science pertaining to human behavior and emotional experience, important ideas from different theories are often integrated to yield a more comprehensive understanding. Congruently, several theoretical frameworks shape approaches to and perspectives on the understanding of midlife crises. Evolutionary theory, human growth and development, sociocultural theories, theories about the life cycle, behavior theory, family systems theory, learning theory, and theories of stress and coping all contribute to this understanding.

The theory of evolution proposed by Charles Darwin provides the understanding of human beings as living interdependently, as well as adapting to their changing environment. The development of effective coping strategies ensures survival and promotes human community. Midlife crises present the individual and his or her social context with an opportunity for testing the effectiveness of these strategies.

The work of psychologist Abraham Maslow emphasized the tendency of human beings to strive toward the maintenance of life and the promotion of growth. An individual negotiating transitions in life taps into this growth motivation in order to maximize and enrich personal experience. In the midst of crisis, basic necessities of life are the first priority. Once the fundamental needs for food, shelter, and physical survival are satisfied, an individual will strive toward fulfilling what Maslow termed higher-level goals, such as emotional security and spiritual enlightenment.

According to Rupolf H. Moos, crisis theory deals with the impact of disruptions on established patterns of personal and social identity. This framework suggests that, in addition to seeking to maximize human growth and potential, each individual first struggles to maintain a state of social and psychological equilibrium. In crisis, the midlife adult will seek homeostasis or balance prior to exploring opportunities for productive change. Thus, the similarity between crisis theory and theories of human growth and development may be apparent. The crises involved in midlife are more often related to the higher-level goals defined within each of these frameworks.

The stage or developmental theories described previously provide a framework within which to understand some of these transitions and the emotional, psychological, and physical changes that are involved. In addition, the perspective of the individual as developing, growing, evolving, and coping within the context of a family system enriches the view of midlife crisis. Further sociocultural theories help one to see how individuals within specific cultures may or may not view change at midlife as a crisis. Change is relative with regard to cultural mores. For instance, to the extent that individuals within a culture have a history of having one job or one spouse or one home throughout a lifetime, changes brought on by any number of factors that might change this could be viewed as a crisis. In other cultures, where such change is more the norm, such events may be seen not as crisis-related but more in accord with what is viewed as normal. In this way, the experience of midlife crises may be saying as much about a culture as it does about individuals within that culture.

The resulting context for an understanding of midlife crisis, then, is one of an integration of ideas and theories. This integration supports an understanding of midlife crisis as a product of the normative development and transitions in life. An individual's reaction to the required transitions depends on his or her personal characteristics, coping skills, family and social relationships, aspects of the transition or crisis itself, and other features of the physical and social environments.

—*Layne A. Prest, Ph.D.;*
updated by Nancy A. Piotrowski, Ph.D.

See also Aging; Antianxiety drugs; Antidepressants; Anxiety; Death and dying; Depression; Factitious disorders; Hypochondriasis; Menopause; Neurosis; Panic attacks; Psychiatric disorders; Psychiatry; Psychoanalysis; Psychosomatic disorders; Sexual dysfunction; Sexuality; Stress; Stress reduction.

FOR FURTHER INFORMATION:

Bee, Helen L., and Barbara L. Bjorklund. *The Journey of Adulthood*. 6th ed. Upper Saddle River, N.J.: Prentice Hall, 2009. A comprehensive text that explores the major theories of adult development and covers health and medicine, behavior genetics, cognitive development, social psychology, and social development in the context of adult development. Topics related to midlife crisis include dealing with stress, conceptualizing the transitions of adulthood, and adult anxiety and depression.

Berk, Laura E. *Development Through the Life Span*. 4th ed. Boston: Allyn & Bacon, 2002. This book examines basic theories, research findings, current applications of theory, and social policies as they relate to development across the life span.

Gaudette, Pat, and Gay Courter. *How to Survive Your Husband's Midlife Crisis*. New York: Berkley, 2003. Uses personal stories and an engaging sense of humor to explore the reasons for midlife crises and to offer resources for support.

Gilligan, Carol. "New Maps of Development: New Visions of Maturity." *American Journal of Orthopsychiatry* 52 (April, 1982): 199-212. In this article, Gilligan begins to map out her alternatives to previously accepted theories of adult development. These alternatives are based on comparative research that contrasts male and female experiences. The author suggests that a woman's development cannot be measured according to the same yardstick as a man's.

Holmes, Thomas H., and E. M. David, eds. *Life Change, Life Events, and Illness*. New York: Praeger, 1989. The editors of this book have compiled an important collection of research and clinical applications of stress and coping theories to practical and everyday experience. The authors of the various papers clarify the connection between life stressors and both psychological and physical illness.

Moos, Rudolf H., ed. *Coping with Life Crises*. Cambridge, Mass.: Springer, 1986. Moos is a pioneer in the field of stress, families, and development. The book and its authors provide a view of midlife crises within the larger context of life development and transitions, as well as of crises in general. The authors emphasize the perspective that many crises are normal or normative.

Schulz, Richard, and Robert B. Ewen. *Adult Development and Aging*. 3d ed. New York: Macmillan, 1999. This textbook can be easily understood by the general reader and includes a comprehensive view of the development and aging processes.

Migraine headaches

Disease/disorder

Anatomy or system affected: Blood vessels, brain, eyes, head, nerves, nervous system

Specialties and related fields: Family medicine, internal medicine, neurology, occupational health, pharmacology, vascular medicine

Definition: Chronic, severe, and throbbing vascular headaches.

Key terms:

armamentarium: the arsenal of drugs aimed at preventing or lessening the impact of a disease or disorder

aura: sensory symptoms that proceed and indicate the onset of a migraine

ergot: a fungal parasite on rye that contains ergoline alkaloid; ergot poisoning in the Middle Ages gave rise to dry gangrene, insanity, and St. Anthony's Fire, but derivatives of ergot may be medically prescribed to treat migraines

tyramine and tyrosine: amino acids that may trigger the onset of migraines in some patients

Causes and Symptoms

Migraine is the name given to a particularly severe, chronic, and painful headache that occurs often on one side but sometimes on both sides of the head, usually just behind or above one or both eyes. Until the early twenty-first century, migraines were medically described as vascular headaches resulting from the dilation of blood vessels that supply nervous tissue in the brain. Recent research indicates that the primary source of migraines may be neurological rather than vascular. It appears that neuron messages that control the size of blood vessels in the brain are interrupted as a result of chemical changes in the brain. The dilated vessels become swollen and press on adjacent nerves, neurons, and other brain tissue, which in turn become irritated

and inflamed. The result is a throbbing headache that is often debilitating.

Between 18 and 28 percent of Americans suffer from migraines, although the number may be much higher as many cases remain undiagnosed or are mistaken for sinus headaches or bouts of colds or influenza. Migraines are three times more common in women than in men. More than half of the women experiencing migraines have more headaches near or during their menstrual cycle; these are referred to as menstrual migraines. The peak incidence of migraines occurs between the ages of thirty to forty and wanes after the age of fifty, but they also occur in some children and elderly people. The incidence of migraine headaches is increasing in all age groups, and it is estimated that at least one out of every four individuals suffers from migraines at some point in life. Some recent medical research has linked certain genes to migraines, indicating that the source might be genetic. This correlates with the fact that 70 to 80 percent of migraine sufferers have family members who also experience migraines.

At least fourteen distinct types of migraine headaches are recognized by the International Headache Society. They can be grouped broadly into three categories: classical migraines, which are preceded by a warning aura; common migraines, which are not preceded by an aura; and atypical migraines.

Migraine symptoms often vary greatly from patient to patient and sometimes from one migraine episode to another. Warning aura symptoms of classic migraines occur within an hour of migraine onset and may include sensitivity to bright lights and sound, especially flashing lights, strobe lights, and laser lights. Some people are disturbed by loud or unexpected noise. Other aura symptoms may include hallucinations, hot flashes, a tingling of limbs that may extend in the hands and feet, numbness or weakness on one side of the body, and cravings for certain kinds of foods. Women experience classic migraines less often than do men.

Aura symptoms are followed by the onset of migraine headache. In most types of migraines, the pain is concentrated on one side of the head and then may radiate into the face, eyes, and sinuses. As the migraine becomes increasingly severe, nausea, vomiting, and dizziness are manifested, along with increased urination and sometimes diarrhea. Some patients report vision problems including blind spots, sensitivity to bright and flickering lights, double vision, or tunnel vision.

Three types of migraines occur mostly in children: hemiplegic, basilar, and retinal migraines. Sufferers of hemiplegic migraines sometimes experience temporary paralysis on the same side of the head as the migraine pain. Basilar migraine may last several days, and the pain is centered in the eye and the nerves that control vision. The patient may experience double vision, hearing loss, vertigo, and a bulging, enlarged eye. In both basilar migraine and retinal migraine, temporary blindness or vision blurring may occur.

Two other atypical types of migraines are complicated migraines, in which both symptoms and aura persist for a week or more, and abdominal migraines, in which migraine pain is transferred to the abdominal area. Abdominal migraine is a recurrent disorder that occurs mainly in children. Moderate to severe abdominal pain and nausea may last for up to three days. The source of this type of migraine is unknown. Most children who experience abdominal migraines suffer migraine headaches later in life.

The causes of migraines are varied. Heredity, lifestyle, environmental factors, and changes in hormone levels have all been implicated, and probably all contribute to some degree to the onset and severity of migraines. Some specific migraine triggers include lights, weather changes, certain foods, food additives, certain beverages, odors, lack of sleep, loud noises, and stress. In many patients, a single factor may trigger a migraine, while in other patients several factors may work

in tandem, each contributing to the onset of the migraine. It is recommended that migraine victims keep a headache log or diary. This will help to identify individual triggers and narrow down the causes. As much as possible, these triggers should be avoided or limited. A few patients report no obvious triggers that initiate their migraine headaches.

Bright or strong lights, especially when glaring or flickering, are incipient migraine triggers in some patients. In others, the flickering of a television or computer screen or strobe lighting may start a migraine. Changes in weather also initiate migraines, at least in some patients, especially the rapid temperature and humidity changes during the fall/winter and spring/summer transition periods.

Foods that trigger migraines in some patients include dairy products, eggs, red wines and other alcoholic drinks, and caffeinated and carbonated drinks. Preserved foods that contain high levels of nitrates, such as hot dogs or pepperoni, and pickled foods have also been implicated as migraine triggers. Some migraine sufferers also react to foods that contain a high content of specific amino acids such as tyramine and tyrosine.

Probably the most compelling correlation can be made between the amount of stress in a person's life and the onset and frequency of migraines. Emotional factors that have been implicated as migraine triggers include frustration, anger, and depression. In addition, emotional stress may exacerbate response to other migraine triggers as well.

Unlike tension headaches, migraines are so frequent and so painful that most patients seek medical attention. Migraines are clinically diagnosed by health care specialists who employ radiological and laboratory tests to ensure that other factors such as tumors or epilepsy are not the cause of headaches.

TREATMENT AND THERAPY

The treatment of migraines fall roughly into two categories: prescription drugs or changes in lifestyle to prevent migraines, and various strategies to alleviate the pain and duration of migraines. For many migraine sufferers, taking over-the-counter nonsteroidal anti-inflammatory drugs (NSAIDs) as needed (such as Advil, Motrin, Aleve, or Excedrin Migraine), drinking plenty of water, and eating regularly spaced meals helps to prevent or minimize the occurrence of migraines.

To prevent the onset of migraines, powerful antidepressants may be prescribed, particularly drugs that shut down terminal nerve receptors, thereby stopping further pain transmission sequences. Most effective are tricyclic antidepressants, such as amitriptyline, nortriptyline (Pamelor), and protriptyline (Vivactil). They appear to reduce the effect of migraines by changing the level of serotonin and other brain chemicals. These medications are considered to be first-line treatment agents. In some cases, these medical treatments have met with mixed success and have limited effectiveness.

Therapeutic strategies for sufferers of severe migraines employ some of the armamentarium of medically prescribed drugs now available, including beta-blockers, barbiturates, ergotamines, triptans, botulinum toxin type A (Botox) injections, antidepressants, serotonin inhibitors, and anticonvulsants. Of these drugs, some of the most powerful are ergotamines, which are derivatives of ergot alkaloids. They are injected into the muscle or vein or placed under the tongue. Ergot-derived drugs are potentially dangerous, however, and should be taken with caution. They should never be taken if the patient is pregnant or has a blood disease. Any medication that constricts blood vessels can be very dangerous if the victim already suffers from narrowing of the blood vessels, such as high blood pressure or coronary artery disease.

The triptans, including sumatriptan (Imitrix), rizatriptan (Maxalt), zolmitriptan (Zomig), almotriptan (Axert), naratriptan (Amerge), frovatriptan (Frova), and eletriptan (Relpax), can help to lessen the effects of migraines quickly. The first of the triptans to be used, Imitrix, acts to balance chemicals in the brain by binding to serotonin receptors and causing blood vessels to constrict. The others act similarly. Imitrix can be administered orally, by nasal spray, or by injection. Since triptans are not addictive narcotics or barbiturates, migraine pain can be relieved while the victim is still alert and in control. Side effects of triptans can include nausea, dizziness, and muscle weakness. On rare occasion, they can lead to stroke or heart attack. The triptan drugs should not be used with ergotamines or with antidepressants, particularly monoamine oxidase inhibitors (MAOIs) or selective serotonin reuptake inhibitors (SSRIs) such as Prozac. When used with antidepressants, triptans can produce serotonin syndrome, an excessive release of serotonin, which can result in weakness, tremors, and lack of coordination. A physician should be consulted before mixing any migraine drugs.

Self-care remedies aimed at preventing migraines include stress management, aerobic exercise, yoga, meditation, acupuncture, anger management, fasting, psychotherapy aimed at developing a positive attitude, emotional repair and stabilization, biofeedback, and the use of herbal and flower extracts. Magnesium supplements help some migraine victims.

A few migraine sufferers resort to folk remedies such as vinegar compresses, warm salt packs, herbal or ice footbaths, or headache tonics. One popular headache tonic consists of fresh ginger root, coriander seeds, diced garlic, and honey. Folk remedies should never be substituted for medical attention.

During and immediately following a migraine, most patients attempt to lessen or alleviate pain by ice packs and aspirin, acetaminophen (Tylenol), or other nonprescription drugs.

PERSPECTIVE AND PROSPECTS

Although the pain is sometimes debilitating for short periods following attacks, migraines are not life-threatening. Furthermore, there are typically no serious afteraffects of migraine headaches, although the individual is often wan, fatigued, and sometimes confused following a migraine episode. Some recent medical studies have shown that some migraine sufferers are at increased risk of stroke.

The incidence and intensity of migraine headaches wanes with age; most patients report that migraines either disappeared or become infrequent after the age of fifty. Many female patients also report that migraines stopped following the menopause.

—Dwight G. Smith, Ph.D.;
updated by Alvin K. Benson, Ph.D.

See also Auras; Brain; Brain disorders; Cluster headaches; Fatigue; Headaches; Multiple chemical sensitivity syndrome; Nausea and vomiting; Pain; Pain management; Stress; Stress reduction.

FOR FURTHER INFORMATION:

American Council for Headache Education. *Migraine: The Complete Guide.* New York: Dell, 1994. A thorough account aimed at educating the general public.

Davidoff, Robert A. *Migraine: Manifestations, Pathogenesis, and Management.* 2d ed. New York: Oxford University Press, 2002. This comprehensive and scientific treatment is written by a clinician. Emphasizes the many different types and severity of migraines and their causes, pathophysiology, and treatment.

Evans, Randolph W., and Ninan T. Mathew. *Handbook of Headache.* 2d ed. Philadelphia: Lippincott Williams & Wilkins, 2005. Written by two medical doctors, this book contains a comprehensive discussion about migraines, including causes, symptoms, and treatments.

Henry, Katherine A., and Anthony P. Bossis. *One Hundred Questions and Answers About Migraine.* 2d ed. Sudbury, Mass.: Jones and Bartlett, 2009. A patient-oriented guide that covers causes, symptoms, diagnosis, treatments, and coping skills.

Milne, Robert D., and Blake More, with Burton Goldberg. *Definitive Guide to Headaches: An Alternative Medicine.* Tiburon, Calif.: Future Medicine, 1997. The authors emphasize the alternative therapy approach to eliminating migraines and other types of headaches.

Paulino, Joel, and Ceabert J. Griffith. *The Headache Sourcebook.* Chicago: McGraw-Hill/Contemporary Books, 2001. This paperback is billed as the complete guide to managing migraines and other sources of headache.

MISCARRIAGE

DISEASE/DISORDER

ALSO KNOWN AS: Spontaneous abortion

ANATOMY OR SYSTEM AFFECTED: Psychic-emotional system, reproductive system, uterus

SPECIALTIES AND RELATED FIELDS: Embryology, gynecology, obstetrics, perinatology, psychology

DEFINITION: A pregnancy that self-terminates within the first twenty weeks of gestation; the same condition occurring after twenty weeks is termed a stillbirth.

KEY TERMS:

abortion: the medical term for intended and unintended pregnancy loss

blighted ovum: a condition in which the gestational sac and placenta grow without a developing child inside

ectopic pregnancy: a pregnancy in which the implantation of the fertilized egg occurs anywhere outside the uterus, usually in the Fallopian tube

human chorionic gonadotropin (hCG): the hormone, produced only in pregnancy, that makes the uterine lining receptive for the developing embryo or fetus; pregnancy tests determine its presence

molar pregnancy: abnormal, cystlike placental tissue that grows either in place of the developing child (complete mole) or in addition to the developing child (partial mole)

recurrent miscarriage: a condition in which a woman experiences three consecutive miscarriages

threatened abortion: when the symptoms of a miscarriage first occur

CAUSES AND SYMPTOMS

Approximately 15 to 20 percent of all known pregnancies will end in miscarriage. Furthermore, it is estimated that 50 to 75 percent of all fertilized eggs fail to implant in the uterus—a situation generally unknown to the woman. The likelihood of a miscarriage drops during the pregnancy's duration: approximately 10 percent in the first four weeks after implantation, 5 percent for the next six weeks, and 3 percent for the following eight weeks. (The stillbirth rate is approximately 1 percent.)

The symptoms of a threatened abortion may include spotting of blood, which may turn into heavier bleeding; cramping, possibly accompanied by lower back pain and vaginal discharge of tissue, clots, or pinkish fluid. A completed miscarriage may also demonstrate changes in pregnancy signs, such as nausea and breast sensitivity. A hormonal sign of a threatened abortion is the failure of human chorionic gonadotropin (hCG) levels to double every two days.

There are three conditions where a woman experiences a miscarriage and the developing child is missing in the sac. About 30 percent of miscarriages before the eighth gestational week are blighted ova, as an embryo has failed to develop. Complete molar pregnancies arise when a sperm (or two) fertilize an egg that has lost its genes. The resulting development of pregnancy tissues—absent the developing child—usually leads to the symptoms of a miscarriage in the first several gestational weeks, but expulsion of the placenta may not occur. Because of the higher likelihood of residual disease (including cancer) in the abnormal tissue if any is left behind, surgical removal of the molar tissue is often warranted. Women who have aborted a molar pregnancy are advised to not get pregnant again for a year, and then they must be closely monitored for subsequent pregnancies, as they are at increased risk for further abnormalities that can become malignant. Finally, a woman may have a recognized pregnancy yet not realize that she was actually pregnant with twins and that one died. This "vanishing twin syndrome" occurs in an estimated 3.5 percent of all twin pregnancies.

Analyses reveal the probability of the most common causes of miscarriages: 50 to 60 percent, genetic abnormalities; 10 to 15 percent, defects in the uterus (such as double or septal uterus) or the cervix (such as incomplete closure); and 10 to 15 percent, hormonal (such as low progesterone or thyroxin) and/or immune disorders (such as lupus or antiphosphid antibody syndrome). A woman's poor health, history of disease (such as endometriosis), history of miscarriages, and advanced age (a 75 percent miscarriage rate for women forty-five and older) also increase the probability of a miscarriage. Recent studies have indicated that the presence of bacterial vaginosis is associated with late-onset miscarriages and preterm deliveries. The presence of the bacteria known as beta strep in the mother's birth canal is tied to preterm labor when it goes untreated. Lifestyle choices that can compromise a successful pregnancy may involve the abuse of substances such as caffeine, cocaine, or nicotine; the contraction of sexually transmitted diseases (STDs), such as chlamydia, human immunodeficiency virus (HIV), or human papillomavirus (HPV); or exposure to harmful agents, such as radiation.

TREATMENT AND THERAPY

Little can be done to stop a miscarriage in the first two months of pregnancy, though some effective interventions are possible in later gestational periods. Magnesium sulfate is effective in combating preeclampsia (high blood pressure during pregnancy) and premature labor contractions. A cervical stitch (cerclage) can rectify an incompetent cervix (premature dilation). Most medical efforts, however, are directed toward the prevention of future miscarriages—the treatment of disease, lifestyle changes, RhO shots for Rh problems—and recovery from the present miscarriage.

There are two aspects of recovery from a miscarriage. The physical part involves the natural or artificial removal of pregnancy tissue—either chemically, as with pitocin, or surgically, as with dilation and curettage (D & C)—and the establishment of a new menstrual cycle. A typical physical recovery ranges from a few days to a few weeks for the miscarriage itself and one to two months after the miscarriage for the next period. Women are usually advised to wait one to two normal periods before trying to conceive again. Approximately 60 percent of women trying to conceive will be successful within six months of the miscarriage.

The psychological recovery may take longer than the physical recovery. Social support, good mental health prior to the miscarriage, deeper religious faith, and successful grieving (mourning, not denying, the loss and then moving forward in life) are some of the factors correlated with a better psychological recovery. Support groups exist for individuals who have suffered miscarriage, stillbirth, or infant death. Similar groups exist to provide support to individuals who are pregnant after the loss of an earlier pregnancy. Such support is essential in decreasing anxiety.

PERSPECTIVE AND PROSPECTS

Until the latter half of the twentieth century, miscarrying women received little satisfaction from the medical community. In fact, many of the drugs introduced in the mid-twentieth century, such as diethylstilbestrol (DES) and its numerous estrogenic cousins, caused more harm than good. However, by the latter part of the twentieth century significant progress was made in diagnosing and preventing miscarriages.

In the early twenty-first century, three avenues of research appear to be promising. Studies are revealing certain genetic predispositions for miscarriages, such as the low production of nitric oxide, resulting in less blood to the uterus. Miscarriages are also being linked to autoimmune disorders and hormonal deficiencies. Use of hormone injections to women who are found to have a hormonal imbalance can help to prevent miscarriage. Finally, assisted reproductive technologies offer intriguing possibilities, such as the ethically controversial opportunity to screen preimplantation embryos for chromosomal abnormalities. In these and other areas of research, new hopes are being raised for old griefs.

—*Paul J. Chara, Jr., Ph.D.,*
and Kathleen A. Chara, M.S.;
updated by Robin Kamienny Montvilo, R.N., Ph.D.

See also Abortion; Addiction; Assisted reproductive technologies; Ectopic pregnancy; Fetal alcohol syndrome; Genetic diseases; Genetics and inheritance; Obstetrics; Placenta; Pregnancy and gestation; Pre-

---

INFORMATION ON MISCARRIAGE

CAUSES: Genetic abnormalities, uterine or cervical defects, hormonal or immune disorders; risks increase with poor health, history of reproductive tract disease or miscarriage, age over forty-five, certain substances (caffeine, cocaine, nicotine), radiation exposure, STDs

SYMPTOMS: Spotting that turns into heavier bleeding; cramping and lower back pain; vaginal discharge (tissue, clots, pinkish fluid); nausea; loss of pregnancy signs

DURATION: Acute

TREATMENTS: None in first two months of pregnancy; later, magnesium sulfate for preeclampsia or premature contractions, cervical stitch for incompetent cervix

mature birth; Stillbirth; Teratogens; Uterus; Women's health.

FOR FURTHER INFORMATION:

Eisenberg, Arlene, Heidi E. Murkoff, and Sandee E. Hathaway. *What to Expect When You're Expecting.* 4th ed. New York: Workman, 2009.

Friedman, Lynn, and Irene Daria. *A Woman Doctor's Guide: Miscarriage—The Support and Facts You Need to Get Through Pregnancy Loss.* New York: Kensington, 2001.

Jutel, A. "What's in a Name? Death Before Birth." *Perspectives in Biology and Medicine* 49, no. 3 (2006): 425-434.

Lanham, Carol Cirruli. *Pregnancy After a Loss: A Guide to Pregnancy After a Miscarriage, Stillbirth, or Infant Death.* New York: Berkley, 1999.

Ugwumadu, A. H., and P. Hay. "Bacterial Vaginosis: Sequelae and Management." *Current Opinions in Infectious Disease* 12, no. 1 (1999): 53-59.

MITES. *See* BITES AND STINGS; LICE, MITES, AND TICKS; PARASITIC DISEASES.

MITRAL VALVE PROLAPSE
DISEASE/DISORDER

ANATOMY OR SYSTEM AFFECTED: Circulatory system, heart

SPECIALTIES AND RELATED FIELDS: Cardiology, family medicine, internal medicine, vascular medicine

DEFINITION: The inability of the mitral valve in the heart to close properly.

CAUSES AND SYMPTOMS

The mitral valve connects the heart's left ventricle and left atrium. The oxygenated blood, having already passed through the right heart chambers and the lungs, arrives in the left atrium through the pulmonary veins and then passes through the mitral valve into the left ventricle. Compression of the left ventricle pumps the blood into the aorta and on to the rest of the body. A properly functioning mitral valve closes and prevents regurgitation or backflow into the left atrium. Mitral valve prolapse occurs when the two leaves of the mitral valve close imperfectly, allowing leakage. This condition, known also as mitral valve insufficiency prolapse, is the most common cardiac syndrome. Found in all segments of society, it is most common in young adult women.

> ## INFORMATION ON MITRAL VALVE PROLAPSE
>
> **CAUSES:** Rheumatic fever, inflammation of heart lining (endocarditis), cardiac tumors, genetic error
>
> **SYMPTOMS:** Undue fatigue after exercise, shortness of breath, chest pain
>
> **DURATION:** Chronic
>
> **TREATMENTS:** Regular exercise; good eating habits; occasionally, surgery

Mitral valve prolapse has several possible causes including rheumatic fever, inflammation of the heart lining (endocarditis), cardiac tumors, or most often, genetic error. Its symptoms are undue fatigue after exercise, shortness of breath, and chest pain. Other common complaints are anxiety, depression, and panic, all related to stress. The number of diagnosed cases in Western countries is rising markedly and may be the result of more sophisticated diagnostic techniques or the increasing stress in modern society.

PERSPECTIVE AND PROSPECTS

Until the 1960's, the detection of mitral valve prolapse was through a characteristic "click" heard by the physician when the mitral leaves attempted to close. Now the

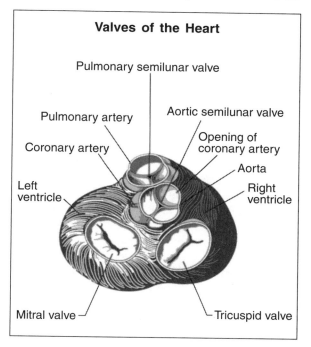

Valves of the Heart

Pulmonary semilunar valve

Pulmonary artery

Aortic semilunar valve

Coronary artery

Opening of coronary artery

Aorta

Left ventricle

Right ventricle

Mitral valve

Tricuspid valve

use of echocardiograms, allowing ultrasound images of the beating heart and blood flow, is standard practice.

People with mitral valve prolapse lead a normal life, and many are unaware that they have the condition. Repeated irregularity in breathing or an inexplicable shortness of breath is a sign to see one's physician. Regular exercise and good eating habits are recommended for this mild condition. Only in severe cases is mitral valve prolapse treated surgically or considered life-threatening.

—*K. Thomas Finley, Ph.D.*

See also Anxiety; Cardiac surgery; Cardiology; Cardiology, pediatric; Circulation; Congenital heart disease; Echocardiography; Endocarditis; Fatigue; Heart; Heart disease; Rheumatic fever; Stress.

FOR FURTHER INFORMATION:

Alpert, Joseph S., James E. Dalen, and Shahbudin H. Rahimtoola, eds. *Valvular Heart Disease*. 3d ed. Philadelphia: Lippincott Williams & Wilkins, 2000. Discusses diseases of the heart valve and their treatments. Includes bibliographical references and an index.

Boudoulas, Harisios, and Charles F. Wooley, eds. *Mitral Valve: Floppy Mitral Valve, Mitral Valve Prolapse, Mitral Valvular Regurgitation*. 2d ed. Armonk, N.Y.: Futura, 2000. A thorough study of mitral valve insufficiency. Includes bibliographical references and an index.

Crawford, Michael, ed. *Current Diagnosis and Treatment—Cardiology*. 3d ed. New York: McGraw-Hill Medical, 2009. Discusses advances in cardiac diagnostics, treatments, and prognostic indicators and includes extensive information on prevention techniques.

Eagle, Kim A., and Ragavendra R. Baliga, eds. *Practical Cardiology: Evaluation and Treatment of Common Cardiovascular Disorders*. 2d ed. Philadelphia: Lippincott Williams & Wilkins, 2008. Details advances in cardiac medicine.

Frederickson, Lyn. *Confronting Mitral Valve Prolapse Syndrome*. New York: Warner Books, 1992. Designed for the lay reader, this guide offers concise coverage of mitral valve prolapse. Includes bibliographical references and an index.

Gersh, Bernard J., ed. *The Mayo Clinic Heart Book*. 2d ed. New York: William Morrow, 2000. One of the most respected texts for laypeople on heart disease. Covers all aspects of anatomy, physiology, diagnosis, treatment, and prevention.

MOLD AND MILDEW
BIOLOGY, DISEASE/DISORDER

ANATOMY OR SYSTEM AFFECTED: Immune system, lungs, nose, respiratory system, skin

SPECIALTIES AND RELATED FIELDS: Environmental health, microbiology, pediatrics, pulmonary medicine, toxicology

DEFINITION: Mold is a generalized term describing nonfruiting fungi, often microscopic and living in moist areas both outdoors and inside buildings, which consume nutrients and produce spores. Mold, which thrives in humid and closed spaces, has contributed to the development of effective pharmaceuticals but has also been blamed for various health problems and diseases.

KEY TERMS:

conidiophore: a spore-creating area on hyphae in fungi
conidium: spores
hyphae: thin tubes in fungi that secure food and grow, expanding mold size
mycelium: mold colonies consisting of numerous meshed hyphae
mycologists: scientists who study the biological field specializing in fungi and similar spore producers that do not undergo photosynthesis
mycotoxins: poisons released by fungi

STRUCTURE AND FUNCTIONS

Mold grows in wet environments where abundant food, primarily organic materials such as cellulose, provides nourishment. Although mycologists consider mildew to be an outdoor fungal plant disease, that term is popularly used to designate mold found indoors on cloth and wooden objects. Thousands of mold species and millions of strains exists. Scientists have found molds both on Earth and in space. Mold spores are always present in air, moving with currents and surrounding humans. They cannot totally be eliminated inside buildings.

Fungi release enzymes to digest food in hyphae to create cells and energy. Mold eats dust, paper, and leather products, living in basements and cooling and heating systems. It can be found in walls, in insulation, and on ceilings. Flooding intensifies mold growth. Mold perishes if food sources are completely devoured or if mites that eat mold spores are present.

Mold hyphae have conidiophores that make conidium. Shaped as spirals, ovals, or spheres, mold spores can be barbed or smooth. If spores have access to nutrients, moisture, air, and sufficiently warm temperatures, then germination starts within twelve to forty-eight hours of being discharged from the conidiophore, and an initial hyphae emerges from the spore. As the hyphae consumes food, a mycelium forms in a period ranging from several days to almost two weeks later for *Stachybotrys chartarum*, also called black mold.

Although some molds such as penicillin are helpful, many molds are toxic. In their spores usually, but sometimes in hyphae, molds create mycotoxins, which protect them from bacteria and can cause sickness in other organisms. The access of molds to food and water affects their production of mycotoxins, which are not created by every mold. Molds do not discharge mycotoxins every place that they grow, nor do they always create toxic quantities of mycotoxins. Molds are mostly benign when outdoors because mycotoxins frequently scatter in the air. Inside, however, mycotoxins can accumulate in dangerous amounts.

DISORDERS AND DISEASES

Scientists have proven that outdoor molds can cause many human, plant, and animal illnesses. Some researchers have considered inside molds to be detrimental to human health, associating them with weakened immune systems and various ailments because people have suspected that exposure to indoor molds intensified their allergies and asthma. Some have blamed contact with molds in their homes and other buildings for triggering headaches, skin rashes, nosebleeds, and fevers.

Based on animal testing and cases of humans exposed to moldy agricultural products, medical researchers recognize known mold dangers. For example, black mold produces satratoxin, which can attack and destroy brain cells, particularly neurons, impeding the ability to smell and detect odors. *Trichothecenes* mycotoxins created by *Stachybotrys* and *Fusarium* molds can cause sore throats, blistered skin, and exces-

sive bleeding. *Aspergillus flavus* produces aflatoxins, which can be carcinogenic. Aspergillosis, a disease affecting the lungs, is triggered by mycotoxins created by *Aspergillus* molds. *Claviceps purpurea*, referred to as ergot, produces mycotoxins that can be hallucinogenic. Some forms of that mycotoxin are useful, however, in soothing migraines or inducing childbirth.

Although individual mold mycotoxins might be harmless, mixtures of mycotoxins can be potentially damaging as their adverse effects combine. The degree to which molds might cause health problems depends on the concentration of mycotoxins and how they invade body systems, specifically whether humans breathe or ingest spores and where the spores settle within their bodies. The size of spores influences their impact on people's health. Researchers hypothesize that some mycotoxins might reach vulnerable lung tissues because they are too tiny to be stopped by nasal defenses that block other harmful microorganisms.

PERSPECTIVE AND PROSPECTS

In 1837, scientists initially became aware that black mold existed when it was found in wallpaper in a Prague, Czechoslovakia, residence. By 1986, William Croft, B. B. Jarvis, and C. S. Yatawara presented the first scientific paper, published in *Atmospheric Environment*, discussing the toxicity of indoor mold. They suggested that black mold spores located in a Chicago house, which later proved lethal to laboratory animals, might be linked to health issues that the residents experienced.

During 1993 and 1994, physicians treated infants whose lungs bled at a Cleveland, Ohio, children's hospital. An investigation by hospital physicians and Centers for Disease Control and Prevention (CDC) personnel revealed that the infants lived in homes containing black mold spores. The media printed stories blaming black mold for the infants' sickness, while hospital officials emphasized the complexity of the situation and the need for a thorough investigation to verify if mold had caused the medical conditions.

The possible dangers of indoor molds again became news in 1999, when *USA Weekend* magazine warned of health hazards allegedly attributed to black mold. Lawsuits resulting in several million dollars in damages increased public awareness of the mold health issue as the media sensationalized the topic. Litigation and mold-related services escalated; con artists took advantage of people's fears of toxic mold. Some legislation relevant to mold and health concerns required house sellers to reveal whether mold had ever existed in structures for sale.

In 2004, the Institute of Medicine of the National Academies in the United States published a consensus report on damp indoor spaces and health. The report concluded that an association exists between damp indoor environments and problems such as upper respiratory-tract symptoms, coughing, wheezing, and asthma symptoms in some human populations. Research in this area continues to lead to healthier work and home environments. Reductions in dampness in indoor spaces improve health and also address known problems such as mold, bacteria, and dust.

—Elizabeth D. Schafer, Ph.D.

See also Allergies; Aspergillosis; Asthma; Blisters; Coughing; Environmental diseases; Environmental health; Fungal infections; Headaches; Immune system; Immunology; Lungs; Microbiology; Multiple chemical sensitivity syndrome; Nasopharyngeal disorders; Pulmonary diseases; Pulmonary medicine; Rashes; Respiration; Sinusitis; Skin; Skin disorders; Sore throat; Wheezing.

FOR FURTHER INFORMATION:

Lankarge, Vicki. *What Every Home Owner Needs to Know About Mold (And What to Do About It)*. New York: McGraw-Hill, 2003.

May, Jeffrey C., and Connie L. May. *Mold Survival Guide for Your Home and for Your Health*. Baltimore: Johns Hopkins University Press, 2004.

Money, Nicholas P. *Carpet Monsters and Killer Spores: A Natural History of Toxic Mold*. New York: Oxford University Press, 2004.

Shoemaker, Ritchie C. *Mold Warriors: Fighting America's Hidden Health Threat*. Baltimore: Gateway Press, 2007.

MOLES

DISEASE/DISORDER

ALSO KNOWN AS: Nevi pigmentosa

ANATOMY OR SYSTEM AFFECTED: Skin

SPECIALTIES AND RELATED FIELDS: Dermatology, family medicine, plastic surgery

DEFINITION: Nonmalignant marks, pigmented spots, or growths on the skin.

CAUSES AND SYMPTOMS

The common mole, also known as a nevus pigmentosus, is a mark, spot, or growth found on the skin that is generally benign and may be either congenital (present

---

> ## INFORMATION ON MOLES
>
> **CAUSES:** Congenital and environmental factors, aging
> **SYMPTOMS:** Flat or raised mark, spot, or growth on skin
> **DURATION:** Short-term to chronic
> **TREATMENTS:** Removal through cauterization, laser treatment

at birth) or developmental. Moles may be various colors, shapes, and sizes, and they can be flat or raised. Caucasian adults usually have about twenty pigmented nevi, the majority of which are less than 0.5 inch in diameter, with fewer pigmented ones evident at birth.

A mole is primarily the result of an accumulation of melanocytes, cells that form the skin pigment melanin. The greater the number of melanocytes, the darker the brown color of the mole. When the melanocytes are located deep below the skin surface, the mole appears dark bluish in color. Melanocytes also form the relatively larger vascular nevi (birthmarks) that derive from abnormal vascular construction in the skin. Types of birthmarks include the strawberry hemangioma and the port-wine stain, which arise from poorly developed blood vessels, and the nevus anemicus, which is attributed to a reduced blood flow.

TREATMENT AND THERAPY

In most cases, moles are benign, but occasionally they develop into malignant melanoma, especially after puberty. This transformation may be indicated by the development of a flat, pigmented zone around the base of a mole or the progressive enlargement of an existing mole. Other evidence of skin cancer involves increased darkening and loss of the hair surrounding a mole, as well as ulceration and bleeding.

A newly formed mole is usually flat. If it arises between the dermis and the epidermis, then the mole is called a junction nevus; this type may become malignant. A dermatologist's care in a timely manner is usually recommended. The main treatment involves removal of the mole by cauterization or laser treatment.

Moles occasionally disappear with age. Generally, however, more nevi form with aging, such as freckles, and they are usually permanent. The growth of new moles and darkening or other changes in existing ones should be monitored. New moles are usually dome-shaped and elevated slightly above the surrounding skin. Plucking the hair associated with moles is not recommended, as this may damage the skin and lead to ulceration and bleeding.

—*Soraya Ghayourmanesh, Ph.D.*

See also Birthmarks; Dermatology; Dermatology, pediatric; Melanoma; Skin; Skin cancer; Skin disorders; Warts.

FOR FURTHER INFORMATION:

Burns, Tony, et al., eds. *Rook's Textbook of Dermatology*. 7th ed. Malden, Mass.: Blackwell Science, 2004.

McClay, Edward F., and Jodie Smith. *One Hundred Questions and Answers About Melanoma and Other Skin Cancers*. Boston: Jones and Bartlett, 2004.

Mackie, Rona M. *Clinical Dermatology*. 5th ed. New York: Oxford University Press, 2003.

Marks, James G., Jr., and Jeffrey J. Miller. *Lookingbill and Marks' Principles of Dermatology*. 4th ed. Philadelphia: Saunders/Elsevier, 2006.

Schofield, Jill R., and William A. Robinson. *What You Really Need to Know about Moles and Melanoma*. Baltimore: Johns Hopkins University Press, 2000.

Turkington, Carol, and Jeffrey S. Dover. *The Encyclopedia of Skin and Skin Disorders*. 3d ed. New York: Facts On File, 2007.

Weedon, David. *Skin Pathology*. 3d ed. New York: Churchill Livingstone/Elsevier, 2010.

MONKEYPOX

DISEASE/DISORDER

ANATOMY OR SYSTEM AFFECTED: Immune system, respiratory system, skin

SPECIALTIES AND RELATED FIELDS: Dermatology, emergency medicine, internal medicine, public health, virology

DEFINITION: A rare disease, originating in the rain forests of Central and West Africa, that affects animals and humans and is caused by a virus.

CAUSES AND SYMPTOMS

Monkeypox is a poxvirus in the *Orthopoxvirus* genus, which contains three other species affecting humans: variola (smallpox), vaccinia (the current smallpox vaccine), and cowpox (the original smallpox vaccine). The virion is large and brick-shaped, containing double-stranded deoxyribonucleic acid (DNA) that has been decoded and comprises 196,858 base pairs. Since smallpox was declared eradicated in 1979, monkeypox is regarded as the most serious naturally occurring poxvirus infection.

Bites or direct contact with an infected animal may result in transmission. Person-to-person spread also occurs through respiratory droplets, requiring close contact with an infected host. Direct contact with body fluids or skin lesions may also transmit the virus. Less commonly, virus-contaminated objects from infected humans, pets, or laboratory animals may spread the disease indirectly.

The disease can affect persons of any age, but children are more common. The incubation period is about twelve days, and the illness commences with a fever that may be accompanied by headache and enlarged lymph nodes. One to three days later, a maculopapular rash develops. The rash primarily involves the periphery (head and extremities) and resembles smallpox more than chickenpox, which is more centrally (trunk) located. However, lymphadenopathy is not usually seen in smallpox. The rash of monkeypox may involve the palms and soles. The skin lesions progress through a vesiculopustular stage before finally crusting. Secondary infection and scarring may occur. Lesions may also be seen in the mouth and upper respiratory tract, producing a cough and occasionally respiratory distress. Spread of the infection to the brain, causing encephalitis, is a rare but serious complication. The illness typically lasts two to four weeks, and while mortality rates as high as 10 percent have been reported from Africa, fatal cases are rare with modern health care.

TREATMENT AND THERAPY

Smallpox vaccine is about 85 percent protective against monkeypox infection, and individuals at risk should receive the vaccine. Exposed individuals should receive vaccine within four days of exposure but may

---

INFORMATION ON MONKEYPOX

CAUSES: Viral infection transmitted by bite or direct contact with infected animal (primarily African rodents); also transmitted person-to-person through respiratory droplets, direct contact with body fluids or skin lesions

SYMPTOMS: Rash, fever, headache, lymph node enlargement, coughing; may spread to brain, causing encephalitis

DURATION: Two to four weeks

TREATMENTS: Protection with smallpox vaccine before or after exposure; antiviral drug cidofovir only in severe cases

benefit up to two weeks after exposure. Vaccinia immunoglobulin may be considered for treatment or prophylaxis, although its effectiveness is unproven. The antiviral agent cidofovir is active against monkeypox in vitro and in animals. Unfortunately, the efficacy of cidofovir for human cases is unknown. Because cidofovir is a toxic drug, it should be considered for treatment only in severe cases and should not be used for prophylaxis.

PERSPECTIVE AND PROSPECTS

In 1958, monkeypox was first described in captive *Cynomolgous* monkeys in Copenhagen, Denmark. The first human case was identified in 1970 in the Democratic Republic of Congo. African squirrels are the main reservoir of monkeypox, but the virus has been found in a number of other African rodents.

A shipment of eight hundred African rodents from Ghana to an animal distributor in Texas during April, 2003, resulted in the infection of coinhabiting captive prairie dogs. Many of these animals were sold as pets, and the result was eighty-one human cases of monkeypox in six states. All patients survived, but 25 percent required hospitalization and two children had severe disease.

Low herd immunity, along with repeated introduction of monkeypox from the African wild reservoir, will likely produce more human illness, both in Africa and at distant sites. The use of smallpox vaccine in high-risk and exposed persons, along with antiviral agents such as cidofovir for severe cases, should limit disease and improve outcomes.

—*H. Bradford Hawley, M.D.*

See also Immunization and vaccination; Rashes; Smallpox; Viral infections; Zoonoses.

FOR FURTHER INFORMATION:

Bernard, Susan M. "Qualitative Assessment of Risk for Monkeypox Associated with Domestic Trade in Certain Animal Species, United States." *Emerging Infectious Diseases* 12, no. 12 (December 1, 2006): 1827.

Centers for Disease Control and Prevention. "Multistate Outbreak of Monkeypox—Illinois, Indiana, and Wisconsin, 2003." *Morbidity and Mortality Weekly Report* 52 (June 13, 2003): 537-540.

_____. "Update: Multistate Outbreak of Monkeypox—Illinois, Indiana, Kansas, Missouri, Ohio, and Wisconsin, 2003." *Morbidity and Mortality Weekly Report* 52 (July 2, 2003): 1-3.

Hutlin, Yvan J. F., et al. "Outbreak of Human Monkeypox, Democratic Republic of Congo, 1996-1997." *Emerging Infectious Diseases* 7 (May/June, 2001): 434-438.

Ježek, Zdeněk, and Frank Fenner, eds. *Human Monkeypox*. New York: S. Karger, 1988.

MONONUCLEOSIS

DISEASE/DISORDER

ALSO KNOWN AS: Infectious mononucleosis, the kissing disease

ANATOMY OR SYSTEM AFFECTED: Heart, lymphatic system, spleen, throat

SPECIALTIES AND RELATED FIELDS: Family medicine, pediatrics, virology

DEFINITION: An acute viral infectious disease that produces lymph node enlargement (hyperplasia).

KEY TERMS:

anorexia: loss of appetite

dysphagia: difficulty in swallowing

lymph nodes: glandlike masses or knots of lymphatic tissue that are distributed along the lymphatic vessels to filter bacteria or foreign bodies from the body

periorbital: referring to the region around the eyes

spleen: a large lymphatic organ in the abdominal cavity that forms lymphocytes and other blood cells and stores blood

splenomegaly: enlargement of the spleen

CAUSES AND SYMPTOMS

Mononucleosis is caused by the Epstein-Barr virus, which is transmitted through infected saliva or by blood transfusions. It has an incubation period of four to six weeks. The saliva may remain infective for as long as eighteen months, and after the primary infection, the virus may be present in the nasal secretions and shed periodically for the rest of the host's life. Many cases occur in adolescents—hence the popular name "the kissing disease." The virus can be cultured from the throat of 10 to 20 percent of most healthy adults. The incidence of mononucleosis varies seasonally among high school and college students but does not vary among the general population. The disease is fairly common in the United States, Canada, and Europe and occurs in both sexes.

Mononucleosis is characterized by fever, fatigue, anorexia, a sore throat, chills, a skin rash, bleeding gums, red spots on the tonsils, malaise, and periorbital edema. Lymph nodes in the neck enlarge, and splenomegaly develops in about half of patients. In a small number of patients, liver involvement with mild jaundice occurs.

The diagnosis is made by several different tests, such as the differential white blood count. In mononucleosis, lymphocytes and monocytes make up greater than 50 percent of the blood cells, with a figure of more than 10 percent being atypical. The leukocyte count is normal early in the disease but rises during the second week. Serology studies show an increase in the heterophile antibody titer, although the monospot test is more rapid and can detect the infection earlier and is widely used. Children under four years of age often test negative for heterophil antibodies, but the test will identify 90 percent of cases in older children, adolescents, and adults.

TREATMENT AND THERAPY

The treatment of mononucleosis is mainly supportive, since the disease is self-limiting. The patient is usually placed on bed rest during the acute stage of the disease, and activity is limited to prevent rupture of the enlarged spleen, usually for at least two months. Acetaminophen (Tylenol) is given for the fever, and saline gargles or lozenges may be used for the sore throat. Patients need to increase their fluid intake. Many doctors use corticosteriods such as prednisone during the course of the disease to lessen the severity of the symptoms. If rupture of the spleen occurs, emergency surgery is necessary to remove the organ.

Complications are uncommon but may include rupture of the spleen, secondary pneumonia, heart involvement, neurologic manifestations such as Guillain-Barré syndrome, meningitis, encephalitis, hemolytic anemia, and orchitis (inflammation of the testes).

PERSPECTIVE AND PROSPECTS

Viruses, such as the one responsible for mononucleosis, were first studied in the 1930's, and they remain a challenge to laboratory investigators. Most information about viruses has come from studying their effects, rather than the viruses themselves. The majority of methods for destroying or controlling viruses are ineffective. There is no prevention for many of the diseases caused by viruses, such as infectious mononucleosis. It may be reassuring to know that the disease seldom causes severe complications if the symptoms are treated and medical care is given to those infected with the Epstein-Barr virus.

—*Mitzie L. Bryant, B.S.N., M.Ed.*

See also Childhood infectious diseases; Chronic fatigue syndrome; Epstein-Barr virus; Fatigue; Fever; Hodgkin's disease; Immune system; Jaundice; Lymphadenopathy and lymphoma; Lymphatic system; Otorhinolaryngology; Sore throat; Viral infections.

FOR FURTHER INFORMATION:

Beers, Mark H., et al., eds. *The Merck Manual of Diagnosis and Therapy*. 18th ed. Whitehouse Station, N.J.: Merck Research Laboratories, 2006. Contains a useful exposition of the characteristics, etiology, diagnosis, and treatment of mononucleosis. Designed for physicians, the material is also useful for less specialized readers.

Dreher, Nancy. "What You Need to Know About Mono." *Current Health 2* 23, no. 7 (March, 1997): 28-29. Infectious mononucleosis is an illness that is most common among young people ages fifteen to twenty-five. The infection is caused by the Epstein-Barr virus. Facts about mono are presented.

Harkness, Gail, ed. *Medical-Surgical Nursing: Total Patient Care*. 10th ed. St. Louis, Mo.: Mosby, 1999. This textbook briefly covers the cause, symptoms, diagnosis, and treatment of infectious mononucleosis. The clinical pathology and possible complications of the disease are discussed as well.

Kimball, Chad T. *Colds, Flu, and Other Common Ailments Sourcebook*. Detroit, Mich.: Omnigraphics, 2001. A comprehensive guide for general readers covering treatment issues and controversies surrounding common ailments and injuries. Includes discussions on mononucleosis.

Litin, Scott C., ed. *Mayo Clinic Family Health Book*. 4th ed. New York: HarperResource, 2009. Perhaps the best general medical text for the layperson, this book covers the entire medical field. While the information is derived from a wide variety of highly technical sources, the articles are written to be easily understood by a general audience.

Shrader, Laurel, and John Zonderman. *Mononucleosis and Other Infectious Diseases*. Rev. ed. New York:

Chelsea House, 2000. Part of the Twenty-first Century Health and Wellness series for young adults. Covers symptoms, diagnosis, treatment, historical perspective, and conditions that lead to the spread of mononucleosis and other infectious diseases.

Sompayrac, Lauren. *How Pathogenic Viruses Work*. Boston: Jones and Bartlett, 2002. Engaging exploration of the basics of virology. The author uses twelve of the most common viral infections to demonstrate how viruses "devise" various solutions to stay alive.

Woolf, Alan D., et al., eds. *The Children's Hospital Guide to Your Child's Health and Development*. Cambridge, Mass.: Perseus, 2002. An authoritative and comprehensive guide to children's health, providing a guide to every common illness or condition that affects children and a carefully designed emergency section.

Morgellons disease

Disease/disorder

Anatomy or system affected: Psychic-emotional system, skin

Specialties and related fields: Dermatology, neurology, psychiatry

Definition: A skin disorder characterized by a pattern of dermatologic symptoms described as insectlike sensations, with skin lesions varying from very minor to disfiguring, and associated with disabling fatigue, joint pain, and various neuropsychiatric symptoms. In the first decade of the twenty-first century, the cause, transmission, and treatment remained under investigation.

Key terms:

obsession: a recurrent and persistent thought or impulse associated with continuous and involuntary preoccupation that cannot be expunged by logic or reasoning

psychosomatic illness: a disorder in which physical symptoms are caused or aggravated by psychological factors

skin biopsy: a removal of a piece of skin for the purpose of further microscopic examination

skin lesion: superficial growth or patch of the skin that differs from the surrounding area surrounding

Causes and Symptoms

Morgellons disease is a pattern of dermatologic symptoms first described several centuries ago. Patients typically complain of insectlike sensations, such as persisting itching, stinging, biting, pricking, burning, and crawling. They often have skin lesions that can vary from very minor to disfiguring. Some patients, however, have no visible changes in the skin. In some cases, fiberlike material can be obtained from the skin lesions; patients describe this material as "fibers," "fiber balls," and "fuzz balls." In other cases, "granules" can be removed from the skin, described by the patients as "seeds," "eggs," and "sands." The majority of patients report disabling fatigue, reduced capacity to exercise, joint pain, and sleep disturbances. Additional symptoms may include hair loss, neurological symptoms, weight gain, recurrent fever, orthostatic intolerance, tachycardia, decline in vision, memory loss, and endocrine abnormalities (such as diabetes type 2, Hashimoto's thyroiditis, hyperparathyroidism, or adrenal hypofunction).

The disease may occur at any age and has a large geographic distribution. It occurs in both males and females. Cases of elderly women living alone seem more frequently reported. Physical stress was reported to be a common precursor. Rural residence and exposure to unhygienic conditions (contact with soil or waste products) are often described. Results from routine laboratory tests are often variable and inconsistent.

The vast majority of these patients have been diagnosed with psychosomatic illness. Prior psychiatric diagnosis (such as bipolar disorder, paranoia, schizophrenia, depression, and drug abuse) has been recorded in more than 50 percent of patients in a recent case study. Patients are obsessively focused on the skin symptoms in terms of complaints and measures to eradicate the disease and to prevent contagion. They usually seek help from between ten and forty physicians and complain of being not understood or taken seriously. Usually, patients are intensely anxious and not open to the idea that they may have a psychological

---

Information on Morgellons Disease

Causes: Unknown; under investigation

Symptoms: Insectlike skin sensations of stinging, persisting itching, biting, pricking, burning, and crawling; minor to disfiguring skin lesions; disabling fatigue; joint pain; psychosomatic and neurological symptoms

Duration: Chronic

Treatments: Symptomatic and supportive skin care, antipsychotic medications

or neurological pathology. They often experience extreme frustration.

Morgellons disease has also been reported in association with conditions that are characterized by itching, such as renal disease, malignant lymphoma, or hepatic disease.

The etiology of Morgellons disease remains under investigation. So far, no examinations, biopsies, and tests have been able to provide evidence supporting any possible cause. Skin biopsies from patients with Morgellons disease typically reveal nonspecific pathology or inflammatory process/reaction with no observable pathogen.

TREATMENT AND THERAPY

The management of patients with Morgellons disease is symptomatic and supportive. It can include skin care with baths, topical ointments, and emollients. It is important for the treating physician (in most cases, a dermatologist) to refer the patient to a psychiatrist or to prescribe appropriate psychoactive medication. Long-term treatment with pimozid (0.5 to 2 milligrams once daily) has been suggested. Risperidone and aripiprazone have also been reported to be efficient. Patients should be convinced that the medication may be needed for months or years.

PERSPECTIVE AND PROSPECTS

Morgellons disease was initially described in France, in 1674, by Sir Thomas Browne. "The Morgellons" was the term used to describe dermal complaints such as hairlike extrusions and sensations of movement beneath the skin reported by children. By the early seventeenth century, this condition was thought to be caused by the parasite *Dranculus* (later called *Dracontia*), and the suggested treatment consisted of filament removal from the skin. Michel Ettmuller produced the only known drawing dating from 1682 of "The Morgellons," the objects associated with what was then believed to be a parasitic infestation in children.

The name "Morgellons disease" was created in 2002 to describe patients presenting with this clinical set of symptoms and to provide an alternative to "delusion of parasitosis." Although the condition was first described many centuries ago, much attention has recently been given to the disease because of the Internet, mass media, and the online support group Morgellons Research Foundation at www.morgellons.com. There is still a discussion whether Morgellons disease is very similar, if not identical, to "delusion of parasitosis." Thus,

whether Morgellons disease is a delusional disorder or even a disease has been a mystery for more than three hundred years. So far, research about Morgellons is sparse and limited. General practitioners, mental health professionals, and the general public need to be aware of the signs and symptoms of this mysterious condition. Recently, some authors suggest the term "syndrome" instead of "disease."

—*Katia Marazova, M.D., Ph.D.*

See also Antidepressants; Anxiety; Bipolar disorders; Body dysmorphic disorder; Delusions; Dermatology; Factitious disorders; Hallucinations; Hypochondriasis; Itching; Neurology; Neurology, pediatric; Neurosis; Psychiatric disorders; Psychiatry; Psychosis; Psychosomatic disorders; Skin; Skin disorders; Stress.

FOR FURTHER INFORMATION:

Harvey, William T., et al. "Morgellons Disease: Illuminating an Undefined Illness—A Case Series." *Journal of Medical Case Reports* no. 3 (2009): 8243.

Koblenezer, Caroline S. "The Challenge of Morgellons Disease." *Journal of the American Academy of Dermatology* 55 (2006): 920-922.

Savely, Virginia R., Mary M. Leitao, and Raphael B. Stricker. "The Mystery of Morgellons Disease: Infection or Delusion?" *American Journal of Clinical Dermatology* 7, no. 1 (2006): 1-5.

MOSQUITO BITES. *See* BITES AND STINGS; INSECT-BORNE DISEASES.

MOTION SICKNESS

DISEASE/DISORDER

ALSO KNOWN AS: Carsickness, airsickness, seasickness

ANATOMY OR SYSTEM AFFECTED: Ears, gastrointestinal system, head, nervous system, stomach

SPECIALTIES AND RELATED FIELDS: Family medicine, neurology, otorhinolaryngology

DEFINITION: A disorder characterized by nausea, vomiting, and vertigo and caused by a combination of repetitive back-and-forth and up-and-down movements.

KEY TERMS:

cranial: pertaining to the bones of the head

medulla oblongata: a continuation of the spinal cord that forms the lower portion of the brain stem; the site of many regulatory centers, as for cardiac rhythm, breathing, and the diameter of blood vessels

transdermal patch: a drug delivery system in which medication is slowly released from a patch and absorbed through the skin over a period of days

vertigo: a specific type of dizziness in which people feel as though either they themselves are spinning around or the room is spinning around them

CAUSES AND SYMPTOMS

Motion sickness appears to be caused by overstimulation of the balance centers of the inner ears by repeated back-and-forth and up-and-down movements. Messages are carried from this area of the inner ear, known as the vestibular apparatus, to the vomiting center in the medulla oblongata. The nerve pathways for this journey are not entirely known, but certainly the cranial nerve, which is responsible for hearing and balance, is involved. Responses in the medulla oblongata set into motion automatic motor reactions in the upper gastrointestinal tract, diaphragm, and abdominal muscles that lead to vomiting.

Individuals vary considerably in their susceptibility to motion sickness, and experts believe that there may be an inherited tendency toward the problem. Shifting visual input (such as watching waves on the horizon), a poorly ventilated environment, and fear and anxiety all seem to play a role in the development and severity of motion sickness.

The diagnosis of motion sickness is usually self-evident. Vertigo, nausea, and vomiting follow exposure to a repetitive and usually irregular rocking motion while in a moving vehicle or on an amusement park ride. The first indication of motion sickness may be yawning, excessive salivation, pale skin, and sweating. The person may begin to breathe deeply or complain of sleepiness. The patient may also develop a need for air, dizziness, or a headache. In most cases, nausea and vomiting occur sooner or later. On an extended trip, patients with motion sickness may eventually develop a tolerance to the motion and feel better, or they may continue to feel sick. If severe rocking motions develop once again, however, patients may also become sick again. Repeated vomiting may lead to dehydration and low blood pressure. Depression is another feature of prolonged motion sickness. As one patient with extreme motion sickness has described it, "First you are afraid you are going to die, and then you are afraid you won't die."

TREATMENT AND THERAPY

This malady is far easier to prevent than to treat. People who suffer from motion sickness should avoid drinking

---

INFORMATION ON MOTION SICKNESS

CAUSES: Overstimulation of balance centers of inner ears, shifting visual input, poorly ventilated environment, fear and anxiety

SYMPTOMS: Yawning, excessive salivation, pale skin, sweating, nausea, vomiting, vertigo

DURATION: Acute

TREATMENTS: Over-the-counter or prescription medications; preventive measures

---

liquids just before and during short trips. On longer trips, they should limit liquids and have only small, easy-to-digest foods at regular intervals. Plenty of fresh air may also help prevent sickness. Those prone to motion sickness should not read in a car or other moving vehicle. Focusing the eyes well above the horizon while riding in a car or on a boat may help. People who are susceptible to motion sickness should also avoid amusement park rides that involve swinging and rocking.

Sufferers may be treated with over-the-counter or prescription medications an hour before travel begins. Medications used for this purpose include diphenhydramine, promethazine, scopolamine, dimenhydrinate, cyclizine, buclizine, and meclizine. They are available in a variety of forms, including tablets, rectal suppositories, and transdermal patches. Many of these drugs cause sleepiness, which may be helpful during a trip but cause drowsiness or lack of alertness on arrival. Another common side effect of some of these drugs is dry mouth. In most cases, these medications are more effective when given before vomiting begins. An extract of ginger root has been recommended as a treatment using a natural substance, and so having fewer side effects. Some objective studies, however, have failed to demonstrate its efficacy.

If the person has already begun vomiting, medications must be given by injection, rectal suppository, or a transdermal patch. In cases of prolonged vomiting, where dehydration is a concern, the patient may require intravenous fluids. Of particular concern is the individual who is already ill with another disease and also suffers from motion sickness. Such patients may have serious complications related to the vomiting and resulting dehydration.

Nonpharmacologic treatments for motion sickness abound. The best known are acupressure wristbands. The autogenic-feedback training (AFT) exercise, designed by the National Aeronautics and Space Administration (NASA), is a self-regulation and biofeedback training scheme that has shown promise in studies of space motion sickness in astronauts. It requires a minimum of six hours of training and so is not the quick fix that drugs promise. NASA scientists have also explored devices for holding the astronaut's head steady, since head movement appears to exacerbate motion sickness. Such an apparatus might be applicable to the civilian population as well.

PERSPECTIVE AND PROSPECTS

Motion sickness is a common problem in children and some adults. New drugs to treat the problem are being explored. A number of chemicals showing promise are related to or interact with serotonin, a chemical that participates in a number of regulatory systems in the body. Drug companies are working on new drug delivery systems to make antinausea medications easier to take. Other advances include drug regimens that will provide antinausea effects without sleepiness.

—*Rebecca Lovell Scott, Ph.D., PA-C;*
updated by Carl W. Hoagstrom, Ph.D.

See also Acupressure; Acupuncture; Audiology; Balance disorders; Biofeedback; Dehydration; Dizziness and fainting; Ear infections and disorders; Ears; Gastrointestinal system; Nausea and vomiting; Nervous system; Neurology; Neurology, pediatric; Over-the-counter medications.

FOR FURTHER INFORMATION:

Canalis, Rinaldo, and Paul R. Lambert, eds. *The Ear: Comprehensive Otology.* Philadelphia: Lippincott Williams & Wilkins, 2000. A text covering all aspects of otology.

Crampton, George H., ed. *Motion and Space Sickness.* Boca Raton, Fla.: CRC Press, 1990. This state-of-the-art compendium, written by active researchers in the field, encompasses anatomical and physiological subjects, such as analyses of stimulus characteristics, prediction of sickness, and consideration of human factors.

Ferrari, Mario. *PDxMD Ear, Nose, and Throat Disorders.* Philadelphia: PDxMD, 2003. A clinical yet accessible reference text that provides a comprehensive list of disorders, with a summary of the condition, background, diagnosis, treatment, outcomes, prevention, and resources.

Litin, Scott C., ed. *Mayo Clinic Family Health Book.* 4th ed. New York: HarperResource, 2009. Perhaps the best general medical text for the layperson, this book covers the entire medical field. While the information is derived from a wide variety of highly technical sources, the articles are written to be easily understood by a general audience.

Mendel, Lisa Lucks, Jeffrey L. Danhauer, and Sadanand Singh. *Singular's Illustrated Dictionary of Audiology.* San Diego, Calif.: Singular, 1999. A comprehensive reference guide to the field that provides numerous photographs, charts, and diagrams, including those of the inner ear. Appendixes cover acronyms, illustrations, topic categories, and physical quantities.

Spock, Benjamin, and Robert Needlman. *Dr. Spock's Baby and Child Care.* 8th ed. New York: Pocket Books, 2004. For more than a half a century, this book has been a virtual bible for parents seeking trustworthy information on child care. Informative, easy to use, and responsive to the changes in society.

Zajonc, Timothy P., and Peter S. Roland. "Vertigo and Motion Sickness, Part 1: Vestibular Anatomy and Physiology." *Ear, Nose, and Throat Journal* 84 (September, 2005): 581-584. Reviews the biological backdrop for motion sickness.

_____. "Vertigo and Motion Sickness, Part 2: Pharmacological Treatment." *Ear, Nose, and Throat Journal* 85 (January, 2006): 25-35. Reviews the drugs available for the treatment of motion sickness and some of the drugs under investigation for that purpose.

MOTOR NEURON DISEASES
DISEASE/DISORDER

ANATOMY OR SYSTEM AFFECTED: Muscles, musculoskeletal system, nerves, nervous system, spine

SPECIALTIES AND RELATED FIELDS: Neurology

DEFINITION: Progressive, debilitating, and eventually fatal diseases affecting nerve cells in muscles.

KEY TERMS:

Babinski's sign: an abnormal response to a neurological test involving a brisk stroke with a sharp object on the bottom of the foot; the normal response is for the toes to bunch together and curve downward, while the abnormal response is for the big toe to pull upward and not in unison with the other toes

corticospinal tracts: neurological pathways descending from the brain to the spinal cord that control and allow voluntary movement

fasciculations: spontaneous electrical impulses from neurons that result in irregular, involuntary muscular contractions; in motor neuron disease, these contractions indicate nerve death

lower motor neuron: a nerve cell whose cell body resides either in the brain stem (to form a cranial nerve) or in the spinal cord (to form a spinal motor neuron)

motor neuron: a nerve that functions either directly or indirectly to control a target organ

muscular atrophy: a wasting of muscle mass; a greatly reduced size of muscle cells caused by the lost innervation (neuron death) or disuse of muscles

spasticity: an abnormal condition in which the limbs demonstrate resistance to passive movement as a result of damage to the corticospinal tracts; the reflexes are hyperactive

tropic factors: chemicals released from nerve cells that have a vital influence on muscle health; in the absence of tropic factors, muscles atrophy

upper motor neuron: a nerve whose cell body resides within the brain but whose axon descends the brain stem and spinal cord to form a corticospinal tract

CAUSES AND SYMPTOMS

In motor neuron diseases, certain nerves die, specifically those that allow any and all body movement. The actual cause of spontaneous motor neuron death is unknown, but genetic defects, neurotoxins, viruses, autoimmune disruptions, and metabolic disorders are contributing factors.

The predominant features of motor neuron disorders are muscular weakness, muscular wasting, and the presence of fasciculations. As a nerve dies, it can no longer effectively innervate its target muscle, but neighboring nerves may sprout to keep the muscle active. A consequence of nerve sprouting is the onset of brief, spontaneous contractions, or twitches. These visible twitches are called fasciculations. Eventually, as increasing numbers of nerves die, fewer healthy nerves are left to sprout until, finally, all muscles are denervated. Dead nerves cannot prompt muscle movement, nor can they release tropic factors as they do in health. This loss of tropic input from the neuron causes muscular atrophy and renders the muscle useless.

Motor neuron diseases are usually first noticed in the hands or upper limbs, where muscle weakness and decreased ability to use arms or hands cause problems. Unlike some disorders, motor neuron diseases fail to show stages of exacerbation or remission. Rather they progress—either rapidly or slowly, but relentlessly—until death, usually as a result of respiratory complications.

Although there are childhood forms, motor neuron diseases are more likely to strike between the ages of fifty and fifty-five, and they are seen in males more than females by a ratio of 1.5 to 1. Motor neuron diseases seem to occur rarely in the obese person and tend to afflict otherwise healthy, thin, and perhaps athletic persons. A famed person afflicted by the debilitating motor neuron disease amyotrophic lateral sclerosis (ALS) was baseball player Lou Gehrig, in whose memory it is often called Lou Gehrig's disease.

Motor neuron diseases are often subgrouped into three categories: ALS, progressive spinal muscular atrophy, and progressive bulbar (brain-stem) palsy. In the plural form, motor neuron diseases refer to all forms of the affliction, whereas the singular form, motor neuron disease, is synonymous with ALS.

Amyotrophic lateral sclerosis is the most familiar of the motor neuron diseases primarily because it accounts for a full 60 percent of all such disorders. The name has clinical meaning: "Amyotrophy" refers to the loss of muscle bulk as a result of missing tropic factors from dying or dead neurons, "lateral" refers to the locations within the spinal cord that are affected, and "sclerosis" refers to the hardened quality of the lateral regions of the diseased spinal cord, which otherwise would be soft tissue. The brain stem may also be sclerotic (hardened). ALS has an incidence of 1 or 2 persons per 100,000, although some Pacific islands, such as Guam, seem to have a higher incidence attributable to undetermined genetic factors. In addition, some populations show an autosomal dominant genetic component. ALS is fatal, and death generally occurs as a result of respiratory failure within three to five years after the onset of symptoms.

ALS is characterized by upper and lower motor neuron signs of neural death; thus the presence of both

---

INFORMATION ON MOTOR NEURON DISEASES

CAUSES: Unknown; possibly genetic defects, neurotoxins, viruses, autoimmune disruptions, metabolic disorders

SYMPTOMS: Muscle weakness or wasting, twitching or spasticity, decreased ability to use arms or hands, increased clumsiness

DURATION: Chronic, sometimes progressive

TREATMENTS: None; management of symptoms and palliative care

fasciculations and spasticity is required for a diagnosis. Spasticity is a medical term that describes a certain kind of muscular resistance (stiffness) to movement. In particular, spastic means a resistance that increases the more rapidly a muscle is extended; tendon reflexes are also hyperactive and Babinski's sign (abnormal reflexes of the toes) must be present. Babinski's sign reveals the death of neurons in the corticospinal tracts, which signals the occurrence of upper motor neuron death. The presence of fasciculations reveals lower motor neuron death.

Progressive spinal muscular atrophy (SMA) will show only lower motor neuron signs—namely, muscular weakness, fasciculations, and atrophy. Babinski's sign or spasticity is not found. The early symptoms may include increased clumsiness in using the fingers for fine movements (including writing or using kitchen utensils), stiffness of the fingers and hands, and cramping of the upper and lower limbs. Once the brain-stem nerves become involved, difficulty in speaking and swallowing occur. Of all persons afflicted with one of the motor neuron diseases, 7 to 15 percent will have lower motor neuron signs only and are presumed to have the progressive spinal muscular atrophy form.

Progressive bulbar palsy literally means progressive brain-stem paralysis. This form of motor neuron disease accounts for 20 to 25 percent of all cases. The tongue is usually the first place to show muscular wasting and fasciculations. As the nerves controlling the tongue die, the tongue shrivels and shrinks so that speaking, chewing, and moving solids or liquids to the back of the mouth for swallowing become difficult or impossible.

Children can be afflicted with spinal muscular atrophy. This disease is believed by many experts to be completely unique from the adult form. The childhood form seems to be more associated with environmental and genetic factors. (This concept is greatly debated, however, since the actual cause of any of the motor neuron diseases is unknown.) Three forms of childhood SMA have been identified: type 1, or acute infantile SMA (also known as Werdnig-Hoffman disease); type 2, or intermediate SMA; and type 3, or juvenile SMA (also known as Kugelberg-Welander disease).

Of children afflicted with SMA, 25 percent have type 1. This form of the disease is an autosomal recessive genetic disorder that occurs in 1 of 15,000 to 25,000 births. In an experienced mother, there may be awareness of minimal fetal movement in the last trimester of pregnancy; the fetus tends to stay still as a result of muscular weakness. Upon birth, the newborn

may be a "floppy" baby of great weakness and may immediately have trouble with nursing and breathing. In other cases, it may take three to six months before symptoms begin. Because of the eventual weakening of the muscles of respiration, the child becomes prone to respiratory infections that cannot be cleared because of a lost cough reflex. Death usually occurs at two to three years of age.

When a child fails to stand or walk between six to twelve months of age, the physician considers the possibility that the child has type 2 SMA. An abnormal curvature of the spine to the forward and sideways position (kyphoscoliosis) is often seen, but rarely is there any problem with feeding or breathing. It is generally the case that very fine tremors of the child's hands can be noticed, and sometimes contractures of the hips and knees can occur. There is no delay in terms of mental health or intellect for these children.

Type 3 SMA is most often seen in the adolescent, but this disease can be observed in some children as early as five years of age. The predominant feature is weakness of the hip muscles. Since these children have been walking for some time, a change in their walking gait to a waddle can be seen over the course of years. Most people with type 3 SMA must use wheelchairs in their mid-thirties, but some may lose their ability to walk earlier. Type 3 SMA has been shown to be an autosomal recessive disorder in many cases, but there are also reported cases of sporadic occurrences within families that have previously been unaffected. Clearly, there are unanswered questions about this disease.

It should be noted that controversy abounds on the assigned classifications of motor neuron diseases. This controversy arises from the fact that the origins of the diseases are not known. Since cause has not been established for any form of motor neuron disease, physicians must use clusters of symptoms to sort the differences in disease manifestation. This sorting is used to plan the best possible treatment programs for the circumstances; nevertheless, these distinctions may seem arbitrary once more is known about the causes of motor neuron death.

TREATMENT AND THERAPY

Perhaps one of the most frustrating attributes of motor neuron diseases is that neither prevention nor effective treatment and cures are available. For a person living with motor neuron disease, physicians and health care professionals must work as a team to manage the symptoms of the diseases and offer palliative care.

In general, patients are encouraged to use and exercise their muscles cautiously in order to avoid disuse atrophy, but activity to the point of fatigue is forbidden since it is believed to aggravate the progression of muscular wasting. In addition, exposure to cold may worsen muscular contractures. Physical therapy facilitates a delay in the total loss of willed body movement by allowing the use of braces, walkers, and wheelchairs as modes of locomotion. Adults are encouraged to continue nonexertive work for as long as possible; it aids both the body and the mind to maintain independence and a sense of wholeness, well-being, and dignity.

As muscular control of the voice wanes, sketch pads, word boards, and computers can aid the ill person in communicating with loved ones, doctors, nurses, and colleagues. In addition, respiratory therapy aids in maintaining healthy breathing in spite of ever-weakening respiratory muscles. Prophylactic immunizations for influenza and pneumococci are given, especially to those who are wheelchair-dependent or bedridden. Forced deep breathing and coughing are needed at least once every four hours to bring up any congestion that may otherwise lead to grave consequences. Almost all persons with motor neuron diseases die from respiratory insufficiency. For this reason, it is imperative that the patient and physician discuss respiratory care early after diagnosis to determine whether the patient wants to be placed on mechanical ventilators in the later stages of the disease. Other issues such as tube feedings should be discussed while the patient is still able to voice an opinion and express any concerns about the dying process associated with the disease.

PERSPECTIVE AND PROSPECTS

Life can be socially difficult for people with motor neuron diseases. Others tend to assume that persons who must use wheelchairs and are unable to control mouth movements (so that speech and swallowing are lost and drooling may occur) are not intelligent, thinking, or aware. This is a sad misperception.

Many persons suffering from a motor neuron disease rise above its physical challenges to conquer in spirit that which the body cannot. For example, former United States senator Jacob Javits labored hard to improve the awareness of and funding for ALS in spite of being on a ventilator and completely immobile because of his battle with the disease. Another example of how well the intellect is preserved in this physically tragic disease can be seen in the life and work of the world-renowned astrophysicist Stephen Hawking.

Until there is an established cause or causes for these diseases, effective treatments or cures are likely to remain hidden. The research continues in the hope of pinning down the ever-elusive motor neuron diseases.

—*Mary C. Fields, M.D.*

See also Amyotrophic lateral sclerosis; Aphasia and dysphasia; Hospice; Huntington's disease; Muscle sprains, spasms, and disorders; Muscles; Nervous system; Neuralgia, neuritis, and neuropathy; Neurology; Neurology, pediatric; Palliative medicine; Palsy; Paralysis; Spinal cord disorders; Spine, vertebrae, and disks; Terminally ill: Extended care.

FOR FURTHER INFORMATION:

Bear, Mark F., Barry W. Connors, and Michael A. Paradiso. *Neuroscience: Exploring the Brain.* 3d ed. Philadelphia: Lippincott Williams & Wilkins, 2007. Undergraduate text that introduces the topics of neuroscience, neurobiology, neurodiseases, and physiological psychology.

Bloom, Floyd E., M. Flint Beal, and David J. Kupfer, eds. *The Dana Guide to Brain Health.* New York: Dana Press, 2006. An easy-to-understand health guide to the brain from neuroscience, neurology, and psychiatry perspectives. More than seventy psychiatric and neurological disorders, their diagnoses, and their treatments are covered.

Calne, Donald B. *Neurodegenerative Diseases.* Philadelphia: W. B. Saunders, 1994. An excellent book with a section devoted to amyotrophic lateral sclerosis and related motor neuron diseases.

Heilman, Kenneth M. *Matter of Mind: A Neurologist's View of Brain-Behavior Relationships.* New York: Oxford University Press, 2002. A leading researcher in behavioral and cognitive neurology uses case studies to explore the knowledge about brain functions such as speaking, reading, writing, emotion, skilled movement, perception, attention, and motivation that has been gained from the study of patients with diseases of or damage to the brain. An excellent, accessible examination of neurological disorders.

Leigh, P. Nigel, and Michael Swash, eds. *Motor Neuron Disease: Biology and Management.* New York: Springer, 1995. This text addresses motor neuron disease from the point of view of health care providers.

National Institute of Neurological Disorders and Stroke (NINDS). *Motor Neuron Diseases Information Page.* http://www.ninds.nih.gov/disorders/

motor_neuron_diseases. A section of the NINDS site that provides a good range of information about motor neuron diseases, scientific research, and organizations.

Parker, James N., and Philip M. Parker, eds. *Official Patient's Sourcebook on Amyotrophic Lateral Sclerosis.* San Diego, Calif.: Icon Health, 2003. Provides comprehensive information drawn from public, academic, government, and peer-reviewed research, and gives myriad sources for basic and advanced information on the disease.

Parsons, Malcolm, and Michael Johnson. *Diagnosis in Color: Neurology.* New York: Mosby, 2001. Impeccably assembled, this atlas shows the most distinguishing clinical features associated with motor neuron diseases, such as muscular wasting of the hands and tongue.

Thompson, Charlotte E. *Raising a Child with a Neuromuscular Disorder: A Guide for Parents, Grandparents, Friends, and Professionals.* New York: Oxford University Press, 2000. Although the field of neuromuscular disorders has grown, many of the guideposts have remained the same. In this rich resource, the author has kept sight of these guideposts, describing them and capturing updated resources, references, and medical help available.

MOTOR SKILL DEVELOPMENT
DEVELOPMENT

ANATOMY OR SYSTEM AFFECTED: Bones, circulatory system, eyes, joints, muscles, musculoskeletal system, nerves, nervous system, psychic-emotional system

SPECIALTIES AND RELATED FIELDS: Exercise physiology, genetics, neonatology, neurology, orthopedics, pathology, pediatrics, perinatology, physical therapy, psychology, sports medicine

DEFINITION: The process of change in motor behavior with advancing age and the numerous physiological and psychological processes that underlie these changes, which describe the adjustments in posture, movement, and skillful manipulation of objects achieved through the coordination of several neurologic control structures.

KEY TERMS:

central nervous system: the brain and spinal cord, which process incoming information from the peripheral nervous system and form the main network of coordination and control in advanced organisms

motor control: the nature and cause of movement, which focuses on stability and movement of the body, and the manipulation of objects, which is achieved through the coordination of many structures organized both hierarchically and in a parallel manner

motor learning: the acquisition and modification of movement as a result of practice and experience, which leads to relatively permanent intrinsic changes in the ability to perform skilled activities; not directly measurable, but inferred from measures of motor performance

motor performance: the directly measurable extent to which the objective of a motor task is met, the scientific study of which originated as a branch of experimental psychology

motor skills: skills in which both movement and the outcome of actions are emphasized

peripheral nervous system: the system of nerves that link the central nervous system to the rest of the body; consists of twelve pairs of cranial nerves, thirty-one pairs of spinal nerves, and the autonomic nervous system

skeletal muscle: striated muscle that contracts voluntarily and involuntarily to carry out the functions of body support, posture, and locomotion

somatosensory system: the system by which muscle, joint, and cutaneous sensory receptors contribute to the perception and control of movement through ascending pathways

PHYSICAL AND PSYCHOLOGICAL FACTORS

Motor skill development, the process of change in motor behavior with increasing age, focuses on adjustments in posture, movement, and the skillful manipulation of objects. Early researchers attributed essentially all developmental changes to modifications occurring within the central nervous system, with increasing motor abilities reflecting increasing neural maturation. Contemporary researchers have determined that the central nervous system works in combination with other body systems (such as the musculoskeletal, cardiovascular, and respiratory systems) and the environment to influence motor development, with all systems interacting in an extremely complex fashion as the individual ages.

Prenatal development of motor behavior takes place between approximately seven weeks after conception and birth, as was first determined during the 1970's using technology to visualize the fetus in utero. Following approximately eight weeks of gestation, the fetus is able to exert reflex and reaction actions, as well as active spontaneous movement. It is currently believed that the ability to self-initiate movements within the womb is an integral part of development, as compared to the traditional view that the fetus is passive and reflexive.

Infancy, the period from birth until the child is able to stand and walk, lasts approximately twelve months. The neonate begins life essentially helpless against the force of gravity and gradually develops the ability to align body segments with respect both to other body segments and to the environment. The Bayley Scales of Infant Development measure the following milestones of motor skill development for the first year of life (with the average age of accomplishment listed in parentheses): erect and steady head holding (0.8 months), side to back turning (1.8 months), supported sitting (2.3 months), back to side turning (4.4 months), momentary independent sitting (5.3 months), rolling from back to stomach (6.4 months), steady independent sitting (6.6 months), early supported stepping movements (7.4 months), arm pull to standing position (8.1 months), assisted walking (9.6 months), independent standing (11.0 months), and independent walking (11.7 months). The transition from helplessness to physical independence during the first twelve months creates many changes for growing children and their caregivers. New areas of exploration open up for the baby as greater body control is gained, the force of gravity is conquered, and less dependence on holding and carrying by caregivers is required.

During the first three months after birth, the infant's motor skill development focuses on getting the head aligned from the predominating posture of flexion. Flexor tone, the tendency to maintain a flexed posture and to rebound back into flexion when the limbs are extended and released, probably results from a combination of the elasticity of soft tissues that were confined to a flexed position while in the womb and of central nervous system activity. As antigravity activity progresses, the infant develops the ability to lift the head. Movements during this period involve brief periods of stretching, kicking, and thrusting of the limbs, in addition to turning and twisting of the trunk and head. Infants tend to be the most active prior to feeding and more quiet and sleepy after feeding.

The third to sixth months after birth are marked by great strides in overcoming the force of gravity by both flexion and extension movements. The infant becomes more competent in head control with respect to sym-

metry and midline orientation with the rest of the body, is able to sit independently for brief periods, and can push up onto hands and knees. These major milestones enable considerably more independence and permit a much greater ability to interact with the rest of the world.

During the sixth to ninth months after birth, the infant is constantly moving and exploring the surrounding environment. As nine months is approached, most babies are able to pull themselves into a standing position using a support such as furniture. The child expends a great deal of energy to stand and often bounces up and down once standing is achieved. The up-and-down bouncing eventually leads to the shifting of body weight from side to side and the taking of first steps, with a caregiver assisting alongside the furniture; this is often called cruising.

The ninth to twelfth months involve forward creeping on hands and knees. This locomotor pattern requires more complicated alternating movements of the opposite arms and legs. Some infants have a preference for creeping even after they are able to walk independently, with many preferring plantigrade creeping (on extended arms and legs) to walking. The ease to which the child moves from sitting to creeping, kneeling, or standing is greatly improved and balance is developed to the point where the child can pivot around in circles while sitting, using the hands and feet for propulsion. The child begins to move efficiently from standing to floor sitting and can initiate rolling from the supine position using flexed legs. Unsupported sitting is accomplished with ease, and weight while sitting can be transferred easily from buttocks to hands.

The early childhood period lasts from infancy until about six years. It involves the child attaining new skills but not necessarily new patterns of movement, with the learning patterns that were acquired during the first year of life being put to use in more meaningful activities. The locomotor pattern of walking is refined, and new motor skills that require increased balance and control of force—such as running, hopping, jumping, and skipping—are mastered.

Running is usually begun between years two and four, as the child learns to master the flight phase and the anticipatory strategies necessary when there is temporarily no body contact with the ground. It is not until about age five or six that control during running with respect to starting, stopping, and changing directions is effectively mastered. Jumping develops at about age 2.5, as the ability and confidence to land after jumping from a height such as a stair is achieved. The ability to jump to reach an overhead object then emerges, with early jumpers revealing a shallow preparatory crouch that progresses to a deeper crouch. Hopping, an extension of the ability to balance while standing on one leg, begins at about age 2.5 but is not performed well until about age six, when a series of about ten hops can be performed consecutively and are incorporated into games such as hopscotch. Skipping, a step and a hop on one leg followed by a step and hop of the other leg, is generally not achieved until about six years, with the opportunity and encouragement for practice being a primary determining factor, as with other locomotor skills.

Throwing is typically acquired during the first year, but advanced throwing, striking (such as with a plastic baseball and bat), kicking (such as with a soccer ball), and catching are not developed until early childhood. Catching develops at approximately age three, with the child initially holding the arms in front of the body and later making anticipatory adjustments to account for the direction, speed, and size of the thrown object. Kicking, which requires balancing on one foot while transferring force to an object with the other foot, begins with little preparatory backswing and eventually develops to involve the knee, hip, and lean of the trunk at about age six.

Fine motor manipulation skills in the upper extremity that are important to normal activities of daily living such as feeding, dressing, grooming, and handwriting are greatly improved in early childhood. The key components include locating a target, which requires the coordination of eye-head movement; reaching, which requires the transportation of the hand and arm in space; and manipulation, which includes grip formation, grasp, and release.

During later childhood (the period from seven years to about eleven years), adolescence, and adult life throughout the remainder of the life span, changes in movement are influenced predominantly by age. Adolescence begins with the onset of the physical changes of puberty, at approximately eleven to twelve years of age in girls and twelve to thirteen years of age in boys, and ends when physical growth is curtailed. Most authorities believe that the growth spurt of adolescence leads to the emergence of new patterns of movement within the skills that have already been acquired. Most adolescents have strong drives to develop self-esteem and become socially acceptable with their peers in school and various recreational activities. Cooperation

and competition become strong components of motor skill development, whereby many skills are stabilized prior to adolescence and preferences for various sports activities emerge. Boys typically demonstrate increased speed and strength as compared to girls, despite recent dramatic changes in available opportunities for girls in recreational and competitive sports activities. Even though age-related changes in motor behavior continue throughout adulthood, the physical skills that permit independence are primarily acquired during the first year of life.

Psychological factors that influence motor skill development include attention level, stimulus-response compatibility, arousal level, and motivation. The level of attention when attempting a motor task is critical, with humans displaying a relatively fixed capacity for concentration during different stages of development. Stimulus identification, response selection, and response programming stages—whereby an individual remembers or determines how to perform a task—affect skill development because the central nervous system takes longer to synthesize and respond to more complex skills. Also important are stimulus-response compatibility—the better the stimulus matches the response, the shorter the reaction time—and arousal, which is described as an "inverted U" by the Yerkes-Dodson model. The inverted U hypothesis implies that there exists an optimal level of psychological arousal to learn or perform a motor skill efficiently, with performance declining when the arousal level at a given moment in time is too great or too small. At a low level of arousal, the scope of perception is broad, and all stimuli (including irrelevant information) are being processed. As arousal level increases, perception narrows so that when the optimal level of arousal is reached and attention is sufficiently focused, concentration on only the stimuli relevant to successful skill learning and performance is enabled. If arousal level surpasses this optimal level, perception narrows to the point of tunnel vision, some relevant stimuli are missed, and learning and skill performance are reduced. The influence of personal motivation during motor skill development encompasses the child's perceived relevance of the activity and also the child's individual ability to recognize the goal of the activity and desire to achieve it.

Three main factors that affect motor skill development in early and later childhood include feedback, amount of practice, and practice conditions. Feedback can be intrinsic, arising from the somatosensory system and senses such as vision and hearing, as information is gathered about a movement and its consequences rather then the actual achievement of the goal. In pathological conditions such as cerebral palsy, intrinsic feedback is often greatly impaired. Feedback can also be extrinsic and is often divided by researchers into knowledge of results, or information about the success of the movement in accomplishing the goal that is available after the skill is completed, and knowledge of performance, or information about skill performance technique or strategy. Knowledge of results provides information about errors as well as successes. True learning occurs by a process of trial and error, with the nervous system serving to detect and correct inappropriate or inefficient movements.

DISORDERS AND EFFECTS

Physical therapists, psychologists, teachers, and other professionals who work with pediatric patients often plan their treatment interventions and instructional lessons based on the normal age-related progression of motor skill development. Motor skill development is often significantly decreased as a consequence of a neurological impairment, however, with the child's resulting movement patterns revealing primary impairments such as inadequate activation of muscle, secondary impairments such as contractures, and compensatory strategies that are adopted to overcome the impairment and achieve mobility. The categories for impairments that have an impact on motor development can generally be divided into musculoskeletal, neuromuscular, sensory, perceptual, and cognitive.

Damage to various nervous system structures somewhat predictably reduces the motor control of movement via both positive symptoms (the presence of abnormal behavior) and negative symptoms (the loss of normal behavior). Positive symptoms include the presence of exaggerated reflexes and abnormalities of muscle tone. Negative symptoms include the loss of muscular strength and the inappropriate selection of muscles during task performance. The broad spectrum of muscle tone abnormalities ranges from flaccidity to rigidity, with muscle spasticity defined as the velocity-dependent increase in tonic stretch reflexes (also called muscle tone), with exaggerated tendon jerks resulting from changes in the threshold of the stretch reflex.

Secondary effects of central nervous system lesions are not directly caused by the lesions themselves but develop as a consequence of the lesions. For example, children with cerebral palsy often exhibit the primary problem of spasticity in muscles of the lower extremities, which causes the secondary problem of muscular and tendon tightness in the ankles, knees, and hips. The secondary problem of limited range of motion in these important areas for movement often impairs motor skills more than the primary problem of spasticity, with the resulting movement strategies reflecting the growing child's best attempt to compensate.

Another common compensatory strategy seen in children with a motor development dysfunction involves standing with the knee hyperextended because of an inability to generate enough muscular force to keep the knee from collapsing. Standing with the knee in hyperextension keeps the line of gravity in front of the knee joint. Contractures of joints are frequent consequences of disordered postural and movement patterns. For example, a habitual crouched sitting posture results in chronic shortening of the hamstring, calf, and hip flexor muscles, and a backward-tipped pelvis accommodates the shortened hamstrings. Chronic shortening of the calf muscles often results in toe walking (in which the heel does not strike the ground) and a reduced walking speed and stride length, because of decreased balance and leg muscle strength. Changes in the availability of sensory information and cognitive factors such as fear of falling and inattention may also contribute strongly to motor skill development in some pediatric patients.

PERSPECTIVE AND PROSPECTS

Interest in the scientific study of motor development was greatly enhanced by Myrtle B. McGraw's *The Neuromuscular Maturation of the Human Infant* (1945). It described four stages of neural maturation: a period in which movement is governed by reflexes as a result of the dominance of lower centers within the central nervous system; a period in which reflex expression declines as a result of maturation of the cerebral cortex and the inhibitory effect of the cortex over lower centers; a period in which an increase in the voluntary quality of activity as a result of increased cortical control produces deliberate or voluntary movement; and a period in which integrative activity of the neural centers takes place, as shown by smooth and coordinated movements.

Arnold Gesell then used cinematography to conduct extensive observations of infants during various stages of growth. He described the maturation of infants based on four behavior categories: motor behavior, adaptive behavior, language development, and personal-social development. Gesell identified six principles of development. The principle of motor priority and fore-reference states that the neuromotor system is laid down before it is voluntarily utilized. The principle of developmental direction states that development proceeds in head-to-foot and proximal-to-distal directions. The principle of reciprocal interweaving states that opposing movements such as extension and flexion show a temporary dominance over one another until they become integrated into mature motor patterns. The principle of functional asymmetry states that humans have a preferred hand, a dominant eye, and a lead foot, with this unilateral dominance being subject to change during development. The principle of self-regulation states that periods of stability and instability culminate into more stable responses as maturity proceeds. The principle of optimal realization states that the human action system has strong growth potential toward normal development if environmental and cultural conditions are favorable and if compensatory and regeneration mechanisms come into play when damage occurs to facilitate attainment of the maximum possible growth.

Esther Thelen suggested the dynamic systems theory. This theory argues that the maturing nervous system interacts with other biomechanical, psychological, and social environment factors to create a dimensional system whereby behavior represents a compression of the degrees of freedom.

A more refined systems theory of motor control developed by Anne Shumway-Cook and Marjorie Woollacott claims that the three main factors that interact in the development of efficient locomotion are progression (ability to generate rhythmic muscular patterns to move the body in the desired direction), stability (the control of balance), and adaptation (the ability to adapt to changing task and environmental requirements). These three factors generally appear sequentially, with muscular patterns appearing first, followed by equilibrium control, and finally adaptive capabilities. Although research on the emergence of human motor skills has primarily concentrated on the developmental milestones of infants and children, it appears that important changes in motor behavior continue throughout the human life span.

—Daniel G. Graetzer, Ph.D.

See also Cerebral palsy; Cognitive development; Developmental stages; Growth; Muscular dystrophy; Muscle sprains, spasms, and disorders; Muscles; Nervous system; Physical examination; Reflexes, primitive; Speech disorders; Well-baby examinations.

FOR FURTHER INFORMATION:

Berk, Laura E. *Child Development*. 8th ed. Boston: Pearson/Allyn & Bacon, 2009. A text that reviews theory and research in child development, cognitive and language development, personality and social development, motor skill development, and the foundations and contexts of development.

Feldman, Robert S. *Development Across the Life Span*. 5th ed. Upper Saddle River, N.J.: Pearson/Prentice Hall, 2008. Traces the physical, cognitive, and social and personality development of one's life span, focusing on basic theories, research findings, and current applications of theory.

Kalverboer, Alex F., Brian Hopkins, and Reint Geuze, eds. *Motor Development in Early and Later Childhood: Longitudinal Approaches*. New York: Cambridge University Press, 1993. An excellent text that reviews motor development in early and later childhood in a longitudinal fashion.

Nathanson, Laura Walther. *The Portable Pediatrician: A Practicing Pediatrician's Guide to Your Child's Growth, Development, Health, and Behavior from Birth to Age Five*. 2d ed. New York: HarperCollins, 2002. An engaging, easy-to-read guide for parents to assess their child's development, medical symptoms, and behavioral problems.

Newell, K. M. "Motor Skill Acquisition." *Annual Review of Psychology* 42 (1991): 213-237. This review focuses on the general laws of motor learning and the specifics of what is learned through repetitive practice.

Shumway-Cook, Anne, and Marjorie Woollacott. *Motor Control: Translating Research into Clinical Practice*. 3d ed. Philadelphia: Lippincott Williams & Wilkins, 2007. This excellent text provides a framework by which the various motor control theories can be incorporated into physical therapy clinical practice for a variety of patient populations.

Thelen, Esther, and Linda B. Smith. *A Dynamic Systems Approach to the Development of Cognition and Action*. 5th ed. Cambridge, Mass.: MIT Press, 2002. This text examines perceptual motor processes, motor abilities, and cognition in infants and children, in addition to describing various points of view of developmental psychobiology.

MOUTH AND THROAT CANCER
DISEASE/DISORDER

ANATOMY OR SYSTEM AFFECTED: Gums, mouth, neck, teeth, throat

SPECIALTIES AND RELATED FIELDS: Dentistry, general surgery, oncology, radiology

DEFINITION: A malignancy of the lips, tongue, gums, salivary glands, or pharynx.

KEY TERMS:

biopsy: the removal and examination of body tissue to determine whether it is cancerous

esophagus: a muscular tube connecting the pharynx and the stomach

pharynx: the area connecting the back of the throat to the esophagus

squamous cells: flat ephithelial cells that resemble scales

CAUSES AND SYMPTOMS

Often, dentists detect cancers of the mouth and throat during routine dental examinations. People who visit their dentists regularly, preferably twice a year, will likely have such cancers detected and diagnosed in their earliest stages when treatment is effective and the cure rate high.

Valid generalizations can be made about the causes of mouth and throat cancers. The most significant cause is the regular use of tobacco products. Cigarette smoking over long periods often results in these cancers or in lung cancer. Males, especially those over forty, have a higher rate of mouth and throat cancer than do females. Pipe and cigar smokers are at greater risk of cancer than are cigarette smokers, and a correlation also exists between the use of chewing tobacco and snuff and the development of mouth cancer. About 90 percent of people suffering from mouth and/or throat cancer have been consistent users of tobacco.

A second causal factor is the regular consumption of substantial quantities of alcoholic beverages, usually over four drinks a day. Some 80 percent of people suffering from mouth and/or throat cancer have used alcohol regularly and in substantial quantities. They are particularly subject to cancers on the floor of the mouth, the tonsils, the lower pharynx, and the tongue.

People who smoke two packs of cigarettes a day and consume over four drinks a day increase the likelihood that they will develop mouth and/or throat cancers by forty times. Other factors in such cancers are poor dental hygiene, ill-fitting dentures, or irregular teeth that cause irritations in the mouth. Those whose work brings them into direct contact with certain toxic chemicals are also at risk.

The most common symptom of lip cancer is the formation of a small, whitish patch (leukoplakia), usually painless, on the lip. It frequently consists of squamous cells. As it develops, it may become ulcerous, causing bleeding and compromising surrounding tissue. If the tongue becomes involved, then it may stiffen. As the malignancy advances, the tongue often becomes painful. Speech, chewing, and swallowing become progressively difficult.

Cancer of the oropharynx, the mid-section of the pharynx, is often accompanied by difficulty in swallowing and hoarseness. Such cancers may also cause patients to expectorate blood-stained sputum. A sore throat frequently accompanies this form of cancer, and earache may also occur, although both of these symptoms frequently result from other causes. People with severe and consistent stomach acid reflux are vulnerable to throat cancer.

TREATMENT AND THERAPY

The usual treatment of mouth and throat cancer is surgery to remove the affected tissue. Such surgery is almost always followed by a course of radiation, which may also precede such surgery to shrink any tumors that might be present. Sometimes, removal of the tongue is indicated, although this is a very drastic treatment because of the problems that it causes for the patient, whose ability to speak and to chew and swallow food will be drastically compromised. Cancer of the tongue is the most aggressive form of mouth cancer, which is justification for using drastic measures to deal with it. Facial disfiguration may also be involved in treating cancers of this sort, so extensive plastic surgery may be necessary following it.

Throat cancers usually require the surgical removal

INFORMATION ON MOUTH AND THROAT CANCER

CAUSES: Tobacco, alcohol, dental problems, toxins, severe acid reflux disease

SYMPTOMS: May include whitish patches on lips, stiff tongue, bloody sputum, sore throat, earache

DURATION: Chronic

TREATMENTS: Surgery, radiation therapy, chemotherapy, plastic surgery of cancerous tissue followed by radiation, but treatment with anticancer medications may also be involved in the management of such cancers. Often, a biopsy is performed in the operating room prior to surgery, usually in conjunction with invasive procedures that permit surgeons and oncologists to view the pharynx, the lungs, and the esophagus using laryngoscopes, bronchoscopes, or esophagoscopes.

PERSPECTIVE AND PROSPECTS

Cancer of the mouth and throat constitute about 8 percent of all the cancers diagnosed in the United States annually. When an early diagnosis is made and is followed by prompt treatment, a cure results in 75 percent of cases. More than half the people diagnosed with mouth cancer, even those for whom late diagnoses are made, survive for at least five years following treatment. As in all cancers, early detection is the key to effective management and desirable outcomes.

Perhaps the most important factor in reducing the incidence of mouth and throat cancer is to convince young people not to develop the habit of using tobacco products and not to abuse alcohol. People who are already smokers and drinkers are well advised to stop smoking and to limit their alcohol intake to two drinks a day or less.

No conclusive correlation has been made between mouth and throat cancer and secondhand smoke. As an increasing number of public venues and workplaces have become smoke-free, however, people who patronize or work in such places have been smoking less.

Most inveterate smokers want to overcome the habit, but nicotine addiction is so powerful that giving it up is difficult. Various methods have proved helpful in enabling people to control their habits, among them hypnosis, acupuncture, laser treatment, psychotherapy, and nicotine replacement through patches or nicotine chewing gum.

—*R. Baird Shuman, Ph.D.*

See also Addiction; Alcoholism; Biopsy; Cancer; Carcinogens; Carcinoma; Cells; Chemotherapy; Dental diseases; Dentistry; Dermatology; Dermatopathology; Esophagus; Glands; Laryngectomy; Malignancy and metastasis; Nasopharyngeal disorders; Oncology; Oral and maxillofacial surgery; Pharyngitis; Pharynx; Plastic surgery; Radiation therapy; Skin cancer; Skin lesion removal; Smoking; Sore throat; Tumor removal; Tumors.

FOR FURTHER INFORMATION:

DeConno, Franco, et al. "Mouth Care." In *Oxford Textbook of Palliative Medicine*, edited by Derek Doyle et al. New York: Oxford University Press, 2004.

Dougherty, Lisa, and Sara E. Lister, eds. *The Royal Marsden Hospital Manual of Clinical Nursing Procedures.* 7th ed. Malden, Mass.: Blackwell, 2008.

Hahn, Michael J., and Anne Jones. *Head and Neck Nursing.* Edinburgh, N.Y.: Churchill Livingstone, 2000.

Lydiatt, William M., and Perry J. Johnson. *Cancers of the Mouth and Throat: A Patient's Guide to Treatment.* Omaha, Nebr.: Addicus Books, 2001.

MRI. *See* MAGNETIC RESONANCE IMAGING (MRI).

MUCOPOLYSACCHARIDOSIS (MPS)
DISEASE/DISORDER

ALSO KNOWN AS: Diferrante syndrome, Hunter syndrome, Hurler's syndrome, Morquio syndrome

ANATOMY OR SYSTEM AFFECTED: All

SPECIALTIES AND RELATED FIELDS: Cardiology, embryology, genetics, pediatrics

DEFINITION: A genetic disorder characterized by accumulations of mucopolysaccharides in tissues.

CAUSES AND SYMPTOMS

Six distinct classes of mucopolysaccharidosis (MPS) have been described, with a number of subclasses. The basis for all mucopolysaccharidosis categories is found in recessive genetic defects of gene products associated with the metabolism of mucopolysaccharides, long chains of sugar molecule that are used to build connective tissue in the body. Specific symptoms are associated with each type, which is a function of which gene locus is at fault. All involve the degradation of specific mucopolysaccharides: dermatan sulfate, heparan sulfate, or keratan sulfate. At least ten enzymes are involved in these metabolic pathways.

The specific syndrome depends upon which enzyme, or which combination, is at fault. For example, MPS I, also called Hurler's syndrome, results from a deficiency of the enzyme alpha-L-iduronidase (IDUA) and is associated with early childhood defects in disparate sites such as the aorta or cornea. Other common symptoms include physical distortion of the face, dwarfism, organ enlargement, mental deficiencies, and shortened life span. MPS IV, also known as Morquio syndrome, is related to reduced activity of galactosamine-6-sulfatase and causes symptoms similar to those in other forms of the disorder.

Diagnosis has generally been based upon laboratory testing for the decreased presence of enzymes involved in the metabolic pathway, as well as the observed accumulation of intermediate polysaccharides such as heparan sulfate in cell lysosomes, reflecting the lack of breakdown. Recent procedures have taken advantage of more accurate laboratory tests, as in use of polymerase chain reaction (PCR) or deoxyribonucleic acid (DNA) blotting techniques for the analysis of specific genes. Fetal cells obtained by means of amniocentesis or chorionic villus sampling and grown in culture can also be tested for defects in the suspected pathways. Generally, symptoms begin to develop after the age of two.

The same tests can be useful for the detection of carriers who do not express the defective traits. The frequency of diagnosis in various populations has ranged from 1 in 25,000 to 1 in 125,000, with significant variation in the specific type.

TREATMENT AND THERAPY

All forms of MPS are progressive, resulting in physical or structural abnormalities of varying severity. Death usually occurs before the age of twenty, though in the most severe types, the child rarely reaches the teenage years. Treatment is primarily symptomatic. Bone marrow transplants have been attempted as a means to replace defective enzymes, with little success. Prospects are currently poor. Most advances have involved improved diagnosis as well as the detection of carriers for the various traits.

—*Richard Adler, Ph.D.*

See also Enzyme therapy; Enzymes; Gaucher's disease; Genetic counseling; Genetic diseases; Glycogen storage diseases; Lipids; Metabolic disorders; Metabolism; Neonatology; Niemann-Pick disease; Screening; Tay-Sachs disease.

FOR FURTHER INFORMATION:

Bach, G., et al. "The Defect in the Hunter Syndrome: Deficiency of Sulfoiduronate Sulfatase." *Proceedings of the National Academy of Sciences* 70 (1973): 2134-2138.

Booth, C., and H. Nadler. "Demonstration of the Heterozygous State in Hunter's Syndrome." *Pediatrics* 53 (1974): 396-399.

Icon Health. *Hunter Syndrome: A Medical Dictionary, Bibliography, and Annotated Research Guide to Internet References.* San Diego, Calif.: Author, 2004.

INFORMATION ON MUCOPOLYSACCHARIDOSIS (MPS)

CAUSES: Genetic enzyme defects
SYMPTOMS: Depends on type; may include defects in aorta or corneas, facial distortion, dwarfism, organ enlargement, mental deficiencies, shortened life span
DURATION: Progressive and fatal
TREATMENTS: None; alleviation of symptoms

_____. *Hurler Syndrome: A Medical Dictionary, Bibliography, and Annotated Research Guide to Internet References.* San Diego, Calif.: Author, 2004.

Porter, Robert S., et al., eds. *The Merck Manual Home Health Handbook.* Whitehouse Station, N.J.: Merck Research Laboratories, 2009.

Scriver, Charles, et al., eds. *The Metabolic and Molecular Basis of Inherited Disease.* 8th ed. New York: McGraw-Hill, 2001.

MULTIPLE BIRTHS

BIOLOGY

ANATOMY OR SYSTEM AFFECTED: All

SPECIALTIES AND RELATED FIELDS: Embryology, genetics, neonatology, obstetrics, pediatrics

DEFINITION: The presence of two or more fetuses in the womb.

KEY TERMS:

chromosomes: the rod-shaped structures in the nucleus of a cell that carry genes

concordance: the condition among twins of having the same physical or psychological trait

dizygotes: fraternal twins; born from two ova separately fertilized by two sperm

embryo: the cells growing after conception until the eighth week of pregnancy

monozygotes: identical twins; born of a single ovum that divides after a single sperm fertilizes it

ovum: the egg cell released from the ovaries during ovulation

placenta: the membrane sac developed from the uterine wall that passes nutrients to the fetus through interconnected blood vessels

ultrasonography: an imaging technique that uses high-frequency sound waves to view fetuses in the womb, as well as other internal structures

zygote: a fertilized ovum before multicellular development begins

INTRODUCTION

Multiple births have historically been rare events, but the incidence is increasing with assisted reproductive technologies. The most common multiple births are twins; this occurs in approximately one of every eighty complete pregnancies. Twins can come from a single egg or from two different eggs. Triplets occur in approximately one in every eight hundred completed pregnancies. Quadruplets occur in one in every eight thousand completed pregnancies. Quintuplets occur naturally in approximately one of every eighty thousand completed pregnancies.

As the number of fetuses increases, the chances that all will survive decreases. Multiple births are most commonly combinations of twins and single eggs. By reviewing the mechanics of twin formation, greater multiples can be understood.

THE DIFFERENT TYPES OF TWINS

Two types of twins are well known: fraternal twins and identical twins. Behind these general terms, however, lies considerable variation. This variation is based on the many changes that a human ovum can undergo after it is released by the ovary, is fertilized, travels along the Fallopian tube to the uterus, and implants there to develop into an embryo.

Fraternal twins are also known as dizygotic or binovular twins. In a normal menstrual cycle, only a single egg is released. When a sperm penetrates an ovum, the fertilized egg releases a chemical that prevents other sperm from penetrating the same egg. If a second egg has been released, however, it can also be fertilized. A newly fertilized egg is called a zygote. If both zygotes succeed in attaching to the uterine walls, a twin pregnancy begins. Usually, this dual insemination occurs during a single release of semen in a single copulation, so that the embryos have the same father. Occasionally, the two eggs may be fertilized in separate copulations during the same ovulation, a phenomenon called superfecundation. It is then possible for dizygotic twins to have different fathers. This possibility seems to have long been recognized. The Greek myth of Leda and the Swan derives from such a pregnancy.

Fraternal twins have separate placentas and membranes in the womb. The placenta comprises maternal and fetal tissues interconnected by blood vessels. Nutrients pass from mother to the fetus through the placenta. Waste products are removed from the fetus by a reverse process. Sometimes, the placentas press against each other in the womb and fuse. Having had separate placentas or one fused together, however, does not affect the nature of the twins after birth. Fraternal twins, even though they share the same birthday, are no more similar in appearance or manner than two siblings from separate births.

Identical twins are the result of different initial events. They are also called monozygotic or monovular twins. Identical or look-alike twins originate when a single egg spontaneously divides after penetration by a sperm cell. Each half develops separately. The reason for this division is not known. One theory holds that sometimes the fertilized ovum does not implant in the uterus right away as is normally the case. During the delay, the chromosomes double and the zygote halves, with each half then implanting and becoming a separate embryo.

Another theory suggests that early in the pregnancy, a genetic mutation occurs in one of the cells. Later, while the embryo is still no more than a few hundred cells, the unmutated cells recognize the genetic difference and reject the mutant cells, much as the immune system rejects substances foreign to it. The rejected group of cells develops separately. If this theory proves to be true, identical twins must not be completely identical after all. Cases in which one identical twin has a genetic disease and the other remains healthy appear to support this theory, although mutation in one twin may occur after splitting rather than causing the splitting.

Variation sometimes appears after birth in monozygotic siblings. Twins can vary in birth weight greatly (one may weigh twice as much), develop at different rates, and die from unrelated natural causes. As a rule, however, identical twins share an overwhelming majority of traits. When two (or more) siblings share a trait, they are considered to be concordant for that trait. Typically, body structures and coloration will be strikingly concordant. Features such as facial shape, hair texture and color, eye color, and height are typical examples of concordance. "Mirror" twins are an uncommon phenomenon. They show mirror-image symmetry in some traits. For example, one may be left-handed while the other is right-handed. Whorls on the scalp may also occur as mirror images. In very rare cases, one mirror twin will have situs inversus: The placement of all internal organs is reversed. An individual with situs inversus will have the liver and appendix on the left side of the abdomen and the spleen on the right.

Genetic variation may account for the subtle variations in even the most concordant of twins. The internal environment of the womb also has an effect. Most identical twin fetuses share the same placenta but have different inner or chorionic sacs. They may have separate placentas (and separate chorions) depending on when the initial splitting of the zygote took place. Usually, those sharing a single placenta have separate chorions. In the rarest variation, the fetuses also share the same amnion. The degree of separation or number of barriers can influence the amount of oxygen or nutrients that each twin receives. Relatively minor differences can affect development.

A third type of twin is theoretically possible. During maturation and before becoming fertilized, the mature ovum could divide into a secondary oocyte (the cell to be fertilized) and a much smaller polar body. It is possible for the ovum to divide into roughly equal portions, both of which are viable and contain the same genetic material. If separate sperm then fertilize these ova, they would become two zygotes. Such twins would have exactly the same maternal genes, but a portion of the paternal genes would differ. They would be less identical

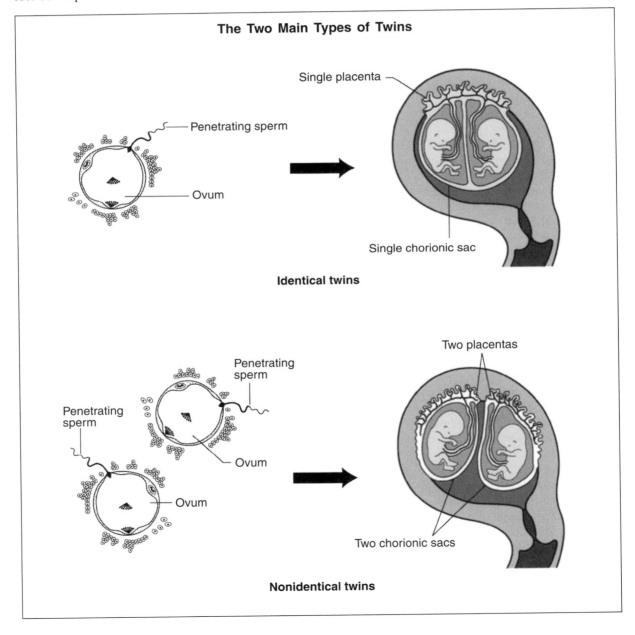

The Two Main Types of Twins

Single placenta

Penetrating sperm

Ovum

Single chorionic sac

Identical twins

Two placentas

Penetrating sperm

Penetrating sperm

Ovum

Ovum

Two chorionic sacs

Nonidentical twins

than monozygotes but more so than dizygotes. Although this type of twinning has been described in rats and mice, no human case has been indisputably identified and reported.

A fourth variant of twinning is conjoined twins, popularly called Siamese twins. Conjoined twins share some tissue. This can range from simple joining of skin on the head or shoulder to having one heart or kidney or two torsos and a single pair of legs. Conjoined twins are identical (or monozygotic) twins created by incomplete cell division during early fetal life. The portion of cells that divide normally continue to develop in a normal fashion. The cells that did not divide completely also develop normally. The result is a portion of the body that is duplicated and a portion that is not. If the incomplete division occurred early in fetal development, the amount of shared tissue is likely to be greater than with an incomplete division that occurred later in fetal development.

About one-third of all twin births result in identical twins. The proportion of males and females is approximately equal. The incidence of identical twins remains constant throughout the world's diverse ethnic populations. Fraternal twins, however, show different proportions and distributions. About half the pairs have the same gender (with a nearly equal number of male-male and female-female pairs); about half are male-female pairs. Fraternal twin births occur most frequently among rural Nigerians (45 pairs per 1,000 births) and least frequently among Chinese and Japanese parents (4 pairs per 1,000 births). European and American rates, for both blacks and whites, are approximately halfway between these extremes.

Evidence suggests that women inherit a tendency to conceive fraternal twins from their mothers. There is little scientific evidence to support the belief that fathers possess a gene for monozygotic twins. Physiological factors can increase the likelihood of a woman having fraternal twins. Women who are tall and heavy and who have previously given birth to children have more twins than small women or those who have not been pregnant before. Women between thirty-five and forty years of age are the most likely to have twins, but the chances decrease thereafter.

Naturally occurring multiple pregnancies (triplets and more) are usually combinations of twins. Identical triplets do rarely occur, but triplets consisting of two identical and one fraternal sibling are the norm. Naturally occurring multiple births of four or more infants are almost always combinations of twins. Physicians can ascertain the status of multiple birth siblings by examining placentas and chorionic sacs.

POSSIBLE COMPLICATIONS

Multiple births create special problems for mothers. Specifically, they are more difficult to carry in the womb and to nurture through infancy than singletons. Multiples are smaller, so that vaginal deliveries are easier. Many physicians, however, recommend birth by cesarean section to manage complications better. Most twins are born healthy, but they must be monitored carefully. As the number of fetuses increases, their size decreases. Because they are not fully mature, this increases the chances for medical problems.

Positively identifying multiple fetuses in the womb is not always an easy task, even though medical science has developed a variety of techniques. The traditional signs of considerable fetal movement, multiple heartbeats, and a large weight gain by the mother can be inaccurate and contradictory. Tests for the human chorionic gonadotropin hormone in the mother's blood or urine or alpha-fetoprotein in the blood may suggest the presence of multiple fetuses if the hormone or protein levels are unusually elevated. Nevertheless, imaging technologies provide the most reliable test. Ultrasonography has supplanted X rays, which declined in use because of the radiation hazard to fetuses. The images produced by ultrasonography can usually resolve multiple fetuses early in the pregnancy.

A multiple pregnancy itself strains the mother's body and is particularly subject to medical complications. Typically, a mother carrying multiple fetuses gains from 30 to 80 pounds, about twice the weight of a single pregnancy. The added weight can cause skeletal and muscular problems. The fetuses' demands on the mother's body may also worsen preexisting medical conditions, such as heart or kidney disease. As the multiple fetuses develop, their size stretches the uterus, which can initiate early labor. For this reason, the premature birth rate is higher for multiple fetuses than for single fetuses. Twins occasionally reach full term; triplets and greater multiples do not.

Similarly, multiple pregnancies miscarry at more than three times the rate of singletons. Occasionally, one fetus will develop at the expense of the other by drawing a disproportionate amount of nutrients from the mother, a condition called twin transfusion syndrome. In cases of identical (monozygotic) twins who share a single placenta, a phenomenon known as a twin-twin transfusion can occur. When this occurs, one twin receives most of the blood, nutrients, and oxygen, in turn becoming much larger than the other twin. In some instances, the smaller twin (the donor) perishes due to lack of these vital substances. In other cases, the larger twin (the recipient) succumbs to heart failure as a result of having to pump the increased blood flow. A new surgical technique (ablation) is currently being used in the third trimester to sever the connection, stopping the twin-twin transfusion. If one fetus dies for any reason, then the mother's body may reabsorb it partially or completely, a phenomenon known as the vanishing twin. Some doctors believe that because of unobserved vanishing twins, miscarriages, and induced abortions, the number of twin conceptions has been underestimated.

Doctors carefully monitor the fetal development of multiple fetuses to ensure their health and, especially, to prepare for delivering them. Amniocentesis and genetic tests detect potential biochemical defects, genetic anomalies, and diseases. Ultrasonography allows doctors to identify defects in shape and the relative position of the fetuses in the womb. Their position is important during labor. Normally, babies are born headfirst. In multiples, one of the fetuses frequently lies crosswise or feetfirst. These positions greatly lengthen and complicate delivery, so that the second fetus runs a higher risk of dying during labor. Moreover, the mother's overdistended uterus, unable to contract properly after delivery, might begin to bleed. The fact that labor lasts too long could result in dangerous maternal exhaustion. Because of such problems, many obstetricians recommend delivery by cesarean section—that is, by cutting a passage through the abdomen into the uterus—at the first sign of trouble to either mother or fetuses.

The prematurity and low birth weight common in multiple infants means that many are placed on life support. Studies have found that multiple infants suffer congenital defects as much as three times more often than singletons. Identical siblings are the most likely of all to have abnormalities. Heart malformations are most common. According to some studies, closed esophagus, clubfeet, excess fingers or toes, and forms of mental retardation such as Down syndrome occur at a slightly higher rate.

Conjoined twins are relatively rare, appearing approximately once in a hundred thousand pregnancies. Most are attached at the back or at the back of the head or neck. In an extreme rarity, one identical twin has a full set of chromosomes while the other has only the X chromosome from the mother and will be a female with a condition called Turner syndrome. Therefore, identical twins will be of opposite gender if the first twin has the XY chromosomes that defines a male and the other is a female with Turner syndrome.

That multiple birth siblings develop in the same environment and from a common origin allows researchers to trace the genetic and environmental influences on human development in general. Most of this research has been conducted on twins because of the relative rarity of triplets or larger groups of siblings. The reasoning is straightforward. In the case of identical twins, either their genetic heritage (nature) or the environment (nurture) dominates in determining how they grow mentally and physically. Researchers have tested the idea by tracking down identical twins who were separated while young, usually at birth, and reared separately. If genetics control development, then the separated twins should still look and behave similarly. If environment predominates, then separated twins should show variations in appearance and temperament.

The reported research results have been mixed. Some separated twins do not look and act any more alike than siblings separately born. Others show an uncanny degree of similarity throughout their lives—dressing the same way, marrying in the same year, having the same number of children, and dying nearly at the same time of the same disease. Their intelligence, which many scientists believe is heavily influenced by environment, nevertheless shows high concordance.

Perspective and Prospects

Worldwide, superstitions and a strong moral overtone have traditionally accompanied multiple births. Some societies viewed one twin as automatically good and the other evil and treated them accordingly as they matured. Others thought twins shameful, a sign of corruption or promiscuity in the mother. These babies might be killed at birth or separated because of it. An African curse reflects the deep suspicion that some societies have held for twins: "May you be the mother of twins." On the other hand, some nations believed that twins have divine origin or power over the elements or special talents for prophecy and telepathy.

Multiple siblings enjoy a special advantage: They are rarely lonely. Some twins even share their own private language, a phenomenon known as idioglossa. Their common development means increased requirements of time and money for their families. It also provides continuous opportunities for sharing and relying on each other. The many national and international organizations created by and for twins and other multiple birth siblings reflect their pride in their status.

Triplets have historically had a reasonable chance for survival. Before the advent of support equipment for premature babies, lung immaturity was the factor that usually determined life or death. Surfactant is a chemical that is secreted in the seventh month of pregnancy. Without surfactant, lung tissues stick together and infants cannot breathe. Because of the combined size of all fetuses, many multiple infants are born before the seventh month of gestation. The Dionne quintuplets, who were born in the 1930's, were unusual in that for the first time in history, all five survived into adulthood. Modern support technology has helped several sets of sextuplets (six infants) to survive. In 1997, the same technology permitted all the McCaughey septuplets (seven infants) to survive. This was the first time such an event had occurred. (The chances of naturally conceiving septuplets are one in eight to ten million conceptions.) In 2009, controversy erupted when Nadya Suleman gave birth to octuplets (eight infants), all of whom survived. A fertility doctor had implanted eight embryos into Suleman, a single mother who already had six children conceived through artificial insemination.

Advances in the field of assisted reproduction have increased the odds of multiple pregnancies. Women who have difficulty conceiving are initially treated with drugs that cause more than one egg to be released during ovulation. This increases the chance of pregnancy but also increases the chance of carrying multiple fetuses. Couples who seek medical assistance to achieve pregnancy routinely use fertility drugs. A woman will have several eggs or zygotes implanted to improve the odds of successfully initiating a pregnancy. The result of this approach is an increased number of multiple births. In 1988, twelve fetuses, which were miscarried, resulted from a fertility drug. Artificially induced pregnancies have posed ethical dilemmas for many who believe that scientists should not manipulate human biological processes.

Multiple births raise other moral and ethical questions as well. Genetic tests can now identify potential fetal defects in the womb early enough that surgeons can remove a defective fetus without harming the healthy fetus, a procedure called selective birth, selective abortion, or selective fetocide. Those who hold abortions to be immoral have reservations about selective fetocide even when the defective fetus has little chance of surviving and may threaten the lives of the remaining healthy fetuses. That selective fetocide may be used simply be-cause a mother does not want to rear more than one child has caused far greater concern. Since the procedure is tricky to perform and can result in the death of all fetuses, most doctors find selective fetocide for nonmedical reasons to be ethically indefensible.

Twin births bear witness to the successes of modern health care. In the United States, incidents of multiple births, both fraternal and identical, have increased since the 1970's, and more multiples are surviving to adulthood. Fertility drugs may account for part of the increase, as does the trend among American women to delay childbearing until their thirties or forties. Nevertheless, prenatal care, better diet, improvements in neonatal intensive care, and education about pregnancy and birth are as important.

—Roger Smith, Ph.D.;
L. Fleming Fallon, Jr., M.D., Ph.D., M.P.H.;
updated by Robin Kamienny Montvilo, R.N., Ph.D.

See also Abortion; Amniocentesis; Assisted reproductive technologies; Birth defects; Cesarean section; Childbirth; Childbirth complications; Chorionic villus sampling; Conception; Embryology; Ethics; Gamete intrafallopian transfer (GIFT); Genetics and inheritance; In vitro fertilization; Miscarriage; Neonatology; Obstetrics; Pregnancy and gestation; Premature birth; Reproductive system; Sibling rivalry; Ultrasonography; Uterus.

For Further Information:

Bowers, Nancy A. *The Multiple Pregnancy Sourcebook.* Chicago: Contemporary Books, 2001. The author, a perinatal nurse specializing in multiple-birth education, provides an excellent guide on topics such as infertility technology, prenatal testing, prenatal development, risk factors and complications, the birth of multiples, and adapting one's life to raise multiples.

Cunningham, F. Gary, et al., eds. *Williams Obstetrics.* 23d ed. New York: McGraw-Hill, 2010. This standard textbook in obstetrics would complement a similar text in gynecology. Provides wide coverage of events related to pregnancy and childbirth. A well-written text for the serious reader who wants detailed information.

Malmstrom, Patricia Maxwell, and Janet Poland. *The Art of Parenting Twins.* New York: Random House International, 2000. Malmstrom and Poland cover the biology and causes of twinning; the emotional terrain of parenting multiples; the differences between twin and single pregnancies; twin development in babyhood, toddlerhood, the preschool and school-age years, and adolescence; and twins' relationships with each other from babyhood to adulthood.

Malone, J. A., S. P. Margevicius, and E. G. Damato. "Multiple Gestation: Side Effects of Antepartum Bed Rest." *Biological Research in Nursing* 8, no. 2 (2006): 115-128. An overview of problems encountered by pregnant women as a result of the bed rest that is often required to deal with multiples.

Moore, Keith L., and T. V. N. Persaud. *The Developing Human.* 8th ed. Philadelphia: Saunders/Elsevier, 2008. An outstanding textbook on human embryonic development, with information about the development of multiple embryos.

Noble, Elizabeth. *Having Twins and More: A Parent's Guide to Pregnancy, Birth, and Early Childhood.* 3d ed. New York: Houghton-Mifflin, 2003. This book is well written and easy to understand. The author is a professional with many years of experience with multiple births.

Novotny, Pamela P. *The Joy of Twins and Other Multiple Births: Having, Raising, and Loving Babies Who Arrive in Groups.* Avenel, N.J.: Crown Books, 1994. The author provides interesting information for parents of multiple infants.

Rand, L., K. A. Eddleman, and J. Stone. "Long-Term Outcomes in Multiple Gestations." *Clinical Perinatology* 32, no. 2 (2005): 495-513. An in-depth look at problems for which multiples are at high risk and their likelihood of occurring.

Rothbart, Betty. *Multiple Blessings: From Pregnancy Through Childhood—A Guide for Parents of Twins, Triplets, or More.* San Francisco: Hearst Books, 1994. In a clear presentation of all the facts, the author helps parents through all stages of pregnancy, providing advice on feeding, home care, juggling hectic schedules, and other critical issues related to the raising of twins and triplets.

MULTIPLE CHEMICAL SENSITIVITY SYNDROME
DISEASE/DISORDER

ANATOMY OR SYSTEM AFFECTED: Eyes, immune system, lungs, muscles, nerves, nervous system, respiratory system, skin

SPECIALTIES AND RELATED FIELDS: Dermatology, environmental health, epidemiology, immunology, neurology, occupational health, public health, toxicology

DEFINITION: An increasing intolerance to commonly encountered chemicals at concentrations well tolerated by other people.

CAUSES AND SYMPTOMS

Multiple chemical sensitivity (MCS) syndrome, idiopathic environmental intolerance (IEI), reactive airway dysfunctions, and the "sick building" syndromes are overlapping disorders caused by intolerance of environmental chemicals. Exactly how many people are affected by MCS is unknown. The onset is often associated with initial acute chemical exposure; patients may report the onset of MCS after moving into a new home, after exposure to chemicals in the workplace, or following the use of pesticides in the home. Patients often describe an increasing intolerance to commonly encountered chemicals at concentrations well tolerated by other people. Diagnosis is made when the following six criteria are met: Repeated exposure reproduces symptoms, the condition is chronic, low chemical exposure levels cause symptoms, symptoms improve with the removal of offending chemicals, responses are triggered by multiple unrelated chemicals, and multiple systems are affected.

Symptoms usually wax and wane with exposure and are more likely to occur in patients with preexisting histories of migraine or classical allergies. Idiosyncratic medication reactions (especially to preservative chemicals) are common in MCS patients, as are dysautonomic symptoms (such as vascular instability), poor temperature regulation, and food intolerance. It is thought that patients with MCS have organ abnormalities involving the liver, the nervous system (including the brain and the limbic, peripheral, and autonomic systems), the immune system, and perhaps porphyrin metabolism, probably reflecting chemical injury to these systems. There is often a substantial overlap of MCS symptoms with fibromyalgia and chronic fatigue syndrome.

The common clinical symptoms may include headaches (often migraine), chronic fatigue, musculoskeletal aching, chronic respiratory inflammation (rhinitis, sinusitis, laryngitis, asthma), attention-deficit disorder, and hyperactivity (affecting younger children). Less common complaints include tremor, seizure, and mitral valve prolapse. Agents associated with the onset of MCS include gasoline, kerosene, natural gas, pesticides (especially chlordane and chlorpyrifos), organic solvents, new carpet and other renovation materials, adhesives and glues, fiberglass, carbonless copy paper, fabric softener, formaldehyde and glutaraldehyde, carpet shampoo (lauryl sulfate) and other cleaning agents, isocyanates, combustion products (poorly vented gas heaters, overheated batteries), and medications (dinitrochlorobenzene for warts, intranasally packed neosynephrine, prolonged antibiotics, and general anesthesia with petrochemicals).

It is believed that the mechanisms that lead to MCS may be multifactorial and include neurogenic inflammation (respiratory, gastrointestinal, and genitourinary symptoms), kindling and time-dependent sensitization (neurologic symptoms), and immune activation or impaired porphyrin metabolism (multiple-organ symptoms). Pathological findings of MCS have rarely been examined. A preliminary study of nasal pathology in these patients indicates that they are characterized by defects in the junctions between cells, desquamation of the respiratory epithelium, glandular hyperplasia, lymphocytic infiltrates, and peripheral nerve fiber proliferation. A consistent physiologic abnormality in these patients has not been established.

Psychiatric, personality, cognitive/neurologic, immunologic, and olfactory studies have been conducted comparing MCS subjects with various control groups. Thus far, the most consistent finding is that patients with MCS have a higher rate of psychiatric disorders across studies and relative to diverse comparison groups. Since these studies are cross-sectional, however, causality cannot be implied. Various working groups have proposed several research questions addressing the relationship between neurogenic inflammation and toxicant-induced loss of tolerance with the development of MCS.

TREATMENT AND THERAPY

The management of patients with MCS at present involves symptomatic and supportive therapy. There is a general consensus among researchers and clinicians that in order to treat patients with MCS effectively, a double-blind, placebo-controlled study performed in an environmentally controlled facility, with rigorous documentation of both objective and subjective responses, is needed to help elucidate the nature and origin of MCS.

—Shih-Wen Huang, M.D.; updated by Sharon W. Stark, R.N., A.P.R.N., D.N.Sc.
See also Allergies; Antihistamines; Asthma; Autoimmune disorders; Chronic fatigue syndrome; Dermatitis; Dermatology; Dizziness and fainting; Environmental diseases; Fatigue; Fibromyalgia; Hay fever; Headaches; Host-defense mechanisms; Immune system; Immunology; Laryngitis; Lungs; Migraine headaches; Mold and mildew; Nasopharyngeal disorders; Nausea and vomiting; Occupational health; Pulmonary medicine; Rashes; Seizures; Sinusitis; Skin; Skin disorders; Sore throat; Wheezing.

FOR FURTHER INFORMATION:

Baron-Faust, Rita, and Jill P. Buyon. *The Autoimmune Connection.* Chicago: Contemporary Books, 2003.

Barrett, Stephen J., and Ronald E. Gots. *Chemical Sensitivity: The Truth About Environmental Illness.* Amherst, N.Y.: Prometheus Books, 1998.

Delves, Peter J., et al. *Roitt's Essential Immunology.* 11th ed. Malden, Mass.: Blackwell, 2006.

Dwyer, John M. *The Body at War: The Miracle of the Immune System.* 2d ed. New York: J. M. Dent, 1993.

Kindt, Thomas J., Richard A. Goldsby, and Barbara A. Osborne. *Kuby Immunology.* 6th ed. New York: W. H. Freeman, 2007.

McCormick, Gail J. *Living with Multiple Chemical Sensitivity: Narratives of Coping.* Jefferson, N.C.: McFarland, 2000.

Morgan, Monroe T. *Environmental Health.* 3d ed. Belmont, Calif.: Thomson/Wadsworth, 2003.

Multiple Chemical Sensitivity, Referral and Resources. http://www.mcsrr.org.

MULTIPLE SCLEROSIS

DISEASE/DISORDER

ANATOMY OR SYSTEM AFFECTED: Muscles, musculoskeletal system, nerves, nervous system, spine

SPECIALTIES AND RELATED FIELDS: Immunology, internal medicine, neurology, pediatrics

DEFINITION: A debilitating chronic inflammatory disease affecting the central nervous system.

KEY TERMS:

autoimmunity: a condition in which the immune system fails to recognize its own tissues as "self" and mounts an immune response against its own cells

demyelination: the destruction of myelin

disseminated sclerosis: another name for multiple sclerosis (MS)

myelin: a fatty substance wrapping nerves as a sheath that accelerates electric impulse propagation

primary progressive MS: the most aggressive form of MS, characterized by the absence of remissions and continual decline

relapsing-remitting MS: the most common form of MS, characterized by unpredictable attacks (relapses) followed by periods free of symptoms (remission)

remyelination: the repair of myelin

sclerosis: a process of hardening of tissues

secondary progressive MS: a form that occurs in patients who initially had relapsing-remitting MS and transition to a more aggressive MS

CAUSES AND SYMPTOMS

Multiple sclerosis (MS) is a chronic and disabling disease of the nervous system. Symptoms can be mild, such as limb numbness, or severe, such as paralysis and loss of vision. How the disease will progress and its severity in specific individuals are difficult to predict because it progresses differently in each of its victims.

Multiple sclerosis is caused by degeneration of the nervous system. A fatty substance called myelin surrounds and protects many nerve fibers of the brain and spinal cord. Myelin is important because it speeds up signals that move along the nerve fibers. In MS, the body attacks its own tissues, termed an autoimmune reaction, and a breakdown in the myelin layer along the nerves occurs. When any part of the myelin sheathing is destroyed, nerve impulses to and from the brain are slowed, distorted, or interrupted. The disease is called "multiple" because it affects many areas of the brain. Scleroids are hardened, scarred patches that form over the damaged areas of myelin.

The initial symptoms of MS may include tingling, numbness, slurred speech, blurred or double vision, loss of coordination, and muscle weakness. Later manifestations include unusual fatigue, muscle tightness, bowel and bladder control difficulties, sexual dysfunction, and paralysis. The most common cognitive functions influenced are short-term memory, abstract reasoning, verbal fluency, and speed of information processing. All the mental and physical symptoms listed may come or go in any combination. The symptoms may also vary from mild to severe in intensity throughout the course of the disease.

The symptoms of MS not only vary from person to person but also may periodically vary within the same person. This makes the prognosis of the disease difficult to foresee. Although the general course of the disease may be anticipated, the symptoms and their severity seem to be quite unpredictable in most individuals. In the "classic" course of MS, as time progresses, chronic problems gradually accumulate over many years, slowly worsening the sufferer's quality of life. The total level of disability will vary from patient to patient.

The typical pattern of MS is marked by active periods of the disease during which the nerves are being ravaged by the immune system. These periods are called attacks, relapses, or exacerbations. The active periods of the disease are followed by calm periods called remissions. The cycle of attack and remission will differ from sufferer to sufferer. Some people have few attacks, and their MS disabilities slowly accumulate over time; in these sufferers, it takes decades to become truly debilitated. Most people with MS have what is known as the relapsing-remitting form of the disease.

INFORMATION ON MULTIPLE SCLEROSIS

CAUSES: Genetic and environmental factors; possibly viral infection

SYMPTOMS: Tingling, numbness, slurring of speech, blurred or double vision, loss of coordination, muscle weakness and/or tightness, fatigue, bowel and bladder control difficulties, sexual dysfunction, paralysis, impaired cognitive functions

DURATION: Chronic with recurrent episodes

TREATMENTS: Steroids, human interferons, regular exercise

They suffer many attacks over time, and these attacks occur unpredictably; the attacks are then followed by complete remission which may last months or years. Again, the injuries may take many years to accumulate to complete disability.

The most aggressive form of the disease is primary progressive MS. In this type of MS, the disease follows a rapid course that steadily worsens from its first onset.

Although there are still attacks and partial remission, the attacks are quite severe and occur more regularly in time. Full paralysis may develop in primary progressive MS in three to five years. Secondary progressive MS occurs in patients who initially have the relapsing-remitting type and later develop the more aggressive form.

Both genetic and environmental factors have been implicated in inducing the onset of MS. Viral infection

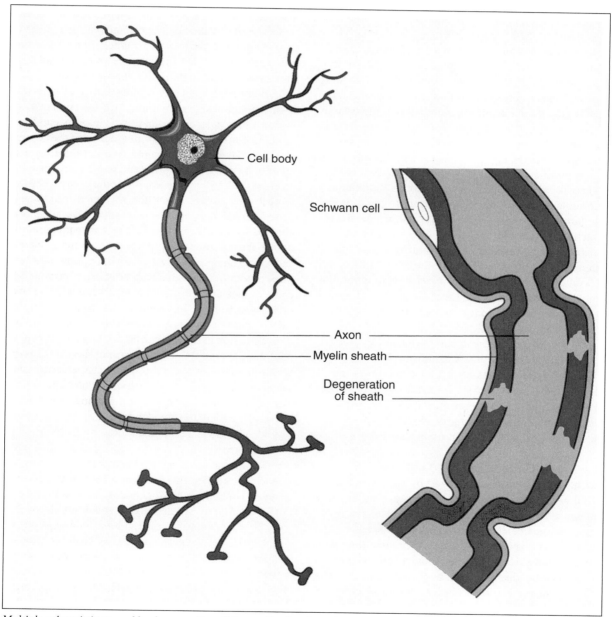

Multiple sclerosis is caused by degeneration of the myelin sheath (right) that insulates the axons of nerve cells; a nerve cell is shown on the left.

has been suggested as a cause, but no single virus has ever been shown to be associated with MS. Although infections such as the common cold, flu, and gastroenteritis increase the risk of relapse, flu vaccination is safe in patients with MS. Risk may be conferred by exposure to a specific environment during adolescence, but that environment and the genetic risk factors have not yet been characterized. The support for the genetic component comes from examining identical twins. The likelihood of MS in the second identical twin, when the first twin has MS, is 30 percent.

Researchers Sharon Lynch and John Rose suggested that certain racial and geographic populations are less susceptible than others to the disease. MS is uncommon in Japanese people as well as among American Indians. The disease is more common among Northern European Caucasians as well as among North Americans of higher latitudes. There is an additional sexual dimorphism in the epidemiology of MS; the disease is found more frequently in women, by a ratio of 2:1.

The disease usually begins its first manifestations in late adolescence (around age eighteen) to early middle age (around age thirty-five). It is not clear how the interaction between the genetics of the sufferer and the environment may trigger onset. The progressive type of MS is more common over the age of forty, so those with late-onset MS often have the quickest deterioration of motor function. The reason that an older age predisposes someone to primary chronic progressive MS is still not clear.

Studies by Swiss researcher Avinoam Safran have shown that occasionally MS manifests after the age of fifty. This condition has been named late-onset multiple sclerosis. Late-onset MS is not rare. Nearly 10 percent of MS patients demonstrate their first symptom after the age of fifty. This type of MS is often not recognized by physicians, who do not expect it in the aged.

TREATMENT AND THERAPY

Scientists have been encouraged by advancements in MS diagnosis using the MRI brain scan. In 2002 they announced that these scans appear to detect damage around nerve fibers in patients with possible early signs of MS. This detection helps doctors predict those who will eventually develop MS and how severe one's experience with the disease might be. In turn, this allows a drug regimen to begin earlier. In the past, doctors did not officially diagnose MS or start treatment until patients had two episodes of nerve problems in different areas of the body—reoccurrences that could come

years apart while damage nonetheless continued silently. New research has found that putting patients on MS drugs at the first sign of nerve inflammation drastically slows the chances of developing MS within a few years, although most will eventually still develop the disease.

While there is no cure for MS, there are many effective treatments. In most cases, steroidal drugs are used to treat relapses or attacks of the disease. Corticotropin was the first steroidal immunosuppressant to be used widely in MS treatment. The primary effect of the drug is to shorten the duration of an attack, although it does not appear to reduce the severity of the attack. Although it is still used with patients who respond well to it, corticotropin has been supplanted by other drugs. Methylprednisolone is an immunosuppressant and steroid that has replaced corticotropin. It has been shown to control the inflammation that accompanies demyelination. These steroids seem to work by sealing leaking blood vessels in the brain and reducing the responsiveness of the white blood cells of the immune system so that they cannot attack the myelin as easily.

Several federally approved drugs can slow the rate of attacks: Avonex, Rebif, and Betaseron are preparations of interferon (proteins regulating the immune system), and Copaxone is a mixture of small peptides that protects myelin. Although these drugs do not stop MS entirely, they actually limit the level of myelin destruction, as observed in magnetic resonance imaging (MRI) scans of the brain. Avonex slows down the rate of progression to disability, and all four slow down the natural course of MS. University of Western Ontario researcher George Ebers was the first to perform experimental treatments on MS patients with interferons. The myelin sheath is actually produced by a special nerve cell called an oligodendrocyte; presumably the oligodendrocytes are stimulated to protect themselves by exposure to interferons. Patients treated with human interferons demonstrated a 34 percent reduction in frequency of attacks; that reduction was sustained over five years of treatment. More impressive was the 80 percent reduction of MS activity detected in their brains. Steroid treatment was rarely required in these patients.

In 2002, researchers announced that preliminary studies using mice and a class of statin drugs used to lower cholesterol in heart patients showed an improvement and some reversal of the debilitating symptoms of MS. The animal data were encouraging because of their demonstration that the statin drugs appear to reprogram the immune cells that attack myelin so they instead pro-

IN THE NEWS: NEW DRUG TREATMENTS FOR MULTIPLE SCLEROSIS

The neurodegeneration that characterizes multiple sclerosis (MS) results from the destruction of myelin that surrounds and protects nerves by the immune system. Myelin-specific T cells are required for this attack. Corticosteroids have been used as therapy because of their known immunosuppressive properties. They have proved to be effective against the symptoms of MS episodes, but they have serious side effects and can be taken only for short times. Because they suppress the immune system in a general, nonspecific way, they inhibit not only the destruction of myelin but also the body's ability to fight infection. This problem has led to the deaths of some MS patients. In addition, corticosteroids do not delay the long-term progression of MS. More recently, interferon-β has been used to treat MS. Although interferon-β therapy can be given for long periods and has been shown to reduce the frequency of relapses and to slow the progression of the disease, why it works is not known. One theory is that it reduces inflammation.

New drugs on the horizon aim to stop the progression of MS and eliminate all relapses. The theory behind them is that a drug should targeted to inhibit only the components of the immune system that destroy myelin. Such drugs, unlike the drugs currently available, would be attacking the underlying cause of MS, rather than its symptoms, and would be expected to cause few or no side effects.

Two of these new drugs, Tovaxin from Opexa Therapeutics and a not-yet named candidate, now called RTL1000, from Artielle Immuno-Therapeutics, act by specifically inactivating the patient's own myelin-specific T cells, while not interacting with other immune system cells. Myelin-specific T cells are required for the destruction of myelin, and when a large number of them are inactivated, myelin destruction slows down.

Another approach is being developed by Immune Response. Their drug NeuroVax acts by specifically stimulating patients' cells that down-regulate myelin-specific T cells. Clinical trials of NeuroVax are underway.

—*Lorraine Lica, Ph.D.*

tect nerve coatings. Also in 2002, another parallel study using MS patients and the drug sold as Zocor—part of the statin class—showed early positive signs of similar anti-inflammatory effects in humans, but potential benefits in MS patients with normal cholesterol are currently under investigation. Another strategy using a monoclonal antibody, Natalizumab, was approved in 2006 for the treatment of the relapsing form of MS. In 2010, the Food and Drug Administration (FDA) approved fingolimod, the first oral drug for MS treatment.

During the 1990's, in a study supported by the National Institutes of Health and conducted at the Mayo Clinic, plasma exchange, also called plasmapheresis, was proven to be an effective treatment for certain patients suffering from severe symptoms of multiple sclerosis who were not responsive to conventional methods of treatment. Plasma exchange involves the removal of the patient's blood; the elimination of the plasma-containing antibodies that target myelin, which is then replaced by a fluid with similar properties, usually containing albumin; and its subsequent return to the patient. This procedure has been used for treatment of other autoimmune diseases such as myasthenia gravis and Guillain-Barré syndrome in the past.

Investigators concluded that plasma exchange might contribute to recovery from an acute attack in people with MS who have not responded to standard steroid treatment. Therefore, they recommended that this treatment only be considered for individuals experiencing a severe, acute attack that is not responding to high-dose steroids. Since the vast majority (90 percent) of people experiencing acute attacks respond well to the standard steroid treatment, plasma exchange would be considered a treatment alternative only for the approximately 10 percent who do not. For those 10 percent, however, plasma exchange may offer an important and beneficial treatment option. Because the exact reasons for the effectiveness of plasmapheresis are not known, researchers feel that further studies are warranted based on the idea that some people may have antibodies in their plasma that are instrumental in certain disease activities that allow disabilities to occur.

As additional therapy, patients with MS should participate in a regular exercise program. Exercise is vital to the maintenance of functional ability in MS sufferers. It strengthens muscles, benefits gait, and generally improves coordination. The best type of exercise is aquatic in nature. Sufferers are often heat-intolerant, and participation in a regular aerobic program would be unpleasant. Also, aquatic exercise is a low-impact activity that puts less stress on chronically sore muscles. Exercise programs also encourage socialization of patients and engender peer support.

PERSPECTIVE AND PROSPECTS

The first written report of MS was published in 1400 when the famed Dutch skater Lydwina of Schieden was diagnosed. It was recognized initially as a wasting disease of unknown origin. The disease was described clinically by Jean-Martin Charcot in 1877. Charcot initially characterized the clinical signs and symptoms of MS. He recognized that the disease affected the nervous system and tried many remedies, without success. In 1890, the cause of MS was thought to be suppression of sweat; the treatment was electrical stimulation and bed rest. At the time, life expectancy for a sufferer was five years after diagnosis. By 1910, MS was thought to be caused by toxins in the blood, and purgatives were alleged the best treatment. In the 1930's, poor circulation was believed to cause MS, and blood-thinning agents became the treatment of choice. In the 1950's through the 1970's, MS was thought to be caused by severe allergies; treatments included antihistamines. Not until the 1980's was the basis of MS understood and effective treatment developed.

By the early twenty-first century, it was estimated that 400,000 Americans had this disorder of the brain and spinal cord, which causes disruption in the smooth flow of electrical messages from brain and nerves to the body. The progress of the disease is slow and may take decades to achieve complete nerve degeneration and paralysis. Although often considered a disease of youth, MS has the potential to become an increasing problem in aging populations. More cases of late-onset MS are coming to light in individuals over forty years of age, including such celebrities as comedian Richard Pryor, entertainer Annette Funicello, and talk-show host Montel Williams.

Several novel therapies are under investigation and include sphingosine receptor modulator (fingolimod), vitamin D, inosine (Axosine), and antimicrobial agents. Various combinations of drugs are also being examined and include mitoxantrone (an immunosuppressant) and Copaxone. Current clinical trials are likely to reveal treatment strategies that will further facilitate controlling symptoms and progression of MS.

—James J. Campanella, Ph.D.;
updated by W. Michael Zawada, Ph.D.

See also Amyotrophic lateral sclerosis; Muscle sprains, spasms, and disorders; Muscles; Nervous system; Neuralgia, neuritis, and neuropathy; Neuroimaging; Neurology; Paralysis; Spinal cord disorders; Spine, vertebrae, and disks.

FOR FURTHER INFORMATION:

Blackstone, Margaret. *The First Year—Multiple Sclerosis: An Essential Guide for the Newly Diagnosed.* 2d ed. New York: Avalon, 2007. Written by an MS patient, guides newly diagnosed patients step-by-step through their first year with MS and sets expectations by providing reliable and updated information on the disease. The second edition includes new research on MS, updated medications, information on support groups, and more.

Halbreich, Uriel. *Multiple Sclerosis: A Neuropsychiatric Disorder.* Boston: American Psychiatric Press, 1993. Describes the psychological conditions that often accompany multiple sclerosis.

Iams, Betty. *From MS to Wellness.* Chicago: Iams House, 1998. An autobiography of an MS sufferer who outlines treatments that have helped her overcome the disease.

Kalb, Rosalind, ed. *Multiple Sclerosis: The Questions You Have, the Answers You Need.* 4th ed. New York: Demos Vermande, 2008. A guide for everyone concerned about multiple sclerosis.

Litin, Scott C., ed. "Multiple Sclerosis." In *Mayo Clinic Family Health Book.* 4th ed. New York: Harper-Resource, 2009. A chapter in a text that discusses both muscles and bones, underscoring the intimate relationship between disorders in the two systems. The text and illustrations are complete and easy to understand.

Matthews, Bryan. *Multiple Sclerosis: The Facts.* 4th ed. New York: Oxford University Press, 2001. Provides information on diagnosis, therapy, medications, and all stages of the disease.

National Multiple Sclerosis Society. http://www.nationalmssociety.org. Provides services to persons with multiple sclerosis through local chapters and promotes research, educates, advocates on critical issues, and organizes a wide range of programs.

Polman, Chris H., et al. *Multiple Sclerosis: The Guide to Treatment and Management.* 6th ed. New York: Demos Vermande, 2006. An updated guide to treatments available for MS and their effectiveness.

Russell, Margot. *When the Road Turns: Inspirational Stories About People with MS.* Deerfield Beach, Fla.:

Health Communications, 2001. Gives the personal stories of seventeen MS patients and details their emotional and physical battles, their struggle to accept the illness, and their courage to create new lives.

Salter, Robert Bruce. *Textbook of Disorders and Injuries of the Musculoskeletal System.* 3d ed. Baltimore: Williams & Wilkins, 1999. Four sections of the book—"Basic Musculoskeletal Science and Its Applications," "Musculoskeletal Disorders: General and Specific," "Musculoskeletal Injuries," and "Research"—examine the diagnosis and treatment principles of disorders and trauma of the musculoskeletal system.

Mumps

Disease/disorder

Also known as: Epidemic parotitis

Anatomy or system affected: Genitals, glands, nervous system, pancreas

Specialties and related fields: Family medicine, pediatrics

Definition: An acute, contagious childhood disease caused by a virus and characterized by swollen salivary glands.

Key terms:

encephalitis: infection and inflammation of the brain

meningitis: infection and inflammation of the covering of the brain

orchitis: infection, inflammation, and swelling of a testicle or ovary; usually occurs only on one side and usually only in adults with mumps infection

parotitis: infection, inflammation, and swelling of the parotid gland, the major salivary gland located near the angle of the jaw; this swelling will often push out the earlobe

Causes and Symptoms

Mumps infection is acquired after contact with infected respiratory secretions. An infected person can spread the disease from twelve to twenty-two days after infection. One case in a family generally means that every family member has been infected. Mumps is most commonly transmitted in the winter and early spring. During the sixteen- to eighteen-day incubation period, the virus grows first in the nose and throat, moves to the regional lymph nodes and then into the bloodstream, and spreads to multiple organs and the central nervous system.

One-third of patients with mumps infection do not have symptoms or have very mild symptoms. Mumps

---

Information on Mumps

Causes: Viral infection

Symptoms: Swollen salivary glands, fever, headache, stomach upset, loss of appetite, mildly congested nose, red rash; occasionally organ infection or joint inflammation

Duration: Sixteen to eighteen days

Treatments: Alleviation of symptoms with mild pain medications, adequate fluid and nutritional intake

---

is more severe after puberty. The first symptoms include fever, headache, stomach upset, loss of appetite, and a mildly congested nose. The most common finding is swelling of the salivary glands. This swelling usually starts on one side and then moves to both sides in three-quarters of cases. Salivary gland pain is most pronounced during the first few days and is associated with discomfort when eating or drinking acidic foods such as orange juice. Rarely, a thin red rash can occur. The fever usually resolves in three to five days, and the salivary gland swelling subsides within seven to ten days.

Between 1 and 10 percent of patients have clinical evidence of central nervous system infection, most commonly meningitis but very rarely encephalitis. Infection of the central nervous system is more common in males than in females. Central nervous system disease typically occurs one to three weeks after the onset of salivary gland swelling, but it can also precede or fol-

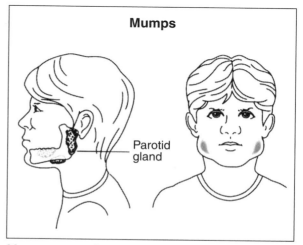

Mumps causes a characteristic swelling of the parotid (salivary) glands.

Orchitis, an infection of the testicles or ovaries, can also occur with mumps. The highest risk for this disease occurs after puberty, usually in males from fifteen to twenty-nine years of age. Between 14 and 35 percent of males with mumps infection develop orchitis. Fever, malaise, vomiting, and stomach pain are common symptoms. Testicular pain, swelling, and tenderness generally last for three to seven days. Involvement is one-sided in most cases. Symptoms usually began four to eight days following the onset of salivary gland swelling, but they can occur in the absence of gland swelling.

Mumps infection can cause other, less common complications. Infection of the kidney is almost always limited, but rare reports of kidney failure with mumps do exist. Multiple joint migratory arthritis with joint fluid has been described and is usually of short duration. Joint complaints are more common in males in their twenties. The usual signs of joint disease occur one to three weeks after the onset of salivary gland swelling. The large joints are more commonly affected.

Inflammation of the heart occurs in 4 to 15 percent of patients with mumps. It is most common in adults and generally resolves itself within two to four weeks. Infection and inflammation of the pancreas can occasionally occur. Pancreatitis can lead to fatty diarrhea and, very rarely, diabetes. Women who have mumps infection during pregnancy do not have an increased risk of delivering an infant with congenital malformation.

Very rarely, mumps will cause death. It is unclear why, prior to the advent of vaccination, mumps infection killed forty persons in the United States each year. More than 50 percent of deaths are of adults.

Not all patients with salivary gland swelling have mumps. Swelling in this area of the face may be attributable to another disease of the salivary gland or another disease affecting other tissues in the face such as lymph nodes or bones. Persistent or recurrent swelling of the parotid gland should be evaluated by a physician.

low this swelling. Symptoms include headache, fever, lethargy, stiff neck, and vomiting. Seizures occur in 20 percent of hospitalized patients. Central nervous system infection is almost always limited, without any lasting effect or complications. Hearing loss occurs during mumps illness in 4 percent of patients but is not higher in those with central nervous system involvement. Higher-tone deficits are noted most frequently. Recovery from hearing loss usually occurs within a few weeks following onset. Persistent hearing loss is usually only one-sided.

TREATMENT AND THERAPY

Conservative therapy is indicated for mumps infection. No antiviral therapy is available. Adequate fluids and nutrition are important. A patient's diet should avoid acidic foods and should be light and generous in fluids. Occasionally, mild pain medications may be necessary for severe headaches or salivary gland discomfort. Stronger pain medications may be needed with testicular involvement. In unusual cases where vomiting is severe, intravenous fluids may be required. A spinal tap (lumbar puncture) is rarely indicated, but patients who have this procedure frequently find that it relieves their headaches.

Exposure to mumps infection may cause anxiety in adult family members or day care employees. A child with mumps should be isolated for nine days after the start of salivary gland swelling. Vaccine administration will probably not prevent infection after exposure, and a history of family exposure to mumps probably indicates past infection. The physician will reassure any adult exposed family members and indicate that it is unlikely that the vaccine will prevent this disease. Nevertheless, exposure may dictate the need to administer the vaccine, as determining immune status is generally not practicable.

Mumps is a self-limited illness and does not require the administration of antiviral medications, antibiotics, or antibody preparations. Mumps vaccine should be given to children to prevent this disease. The combined vaccine containing measles, mumps, and rubella (MMR) vaccines should be given routinely to children from twelve months to eighteen months of age. About 98 percent of children will respond to this vaccine and not acquire mumps infection.

PERSPECTIVE AND PROSPECTS

The term "mumps" is derived from an English dialect meaning "grimace," attributed to the painful parotid gland swelling. The virus was first described in 1934, and a live vaccine was first licensed in 1967. Prior to 1980, the age-group most affected by mumps was five- to nine-year-olds. In the 1980's, this group shifted to children and adolescents aged ten to nineteen. In the 1990's, most cases occurred in adults over twenty. This change was caused by the increased use of the mumps vaccine in children but not in adults.

Vaccination has been very successful, especially when combined with measles and rubella vaccine, given in the second year of life, and repeated prior to school. Side effects from mumps vaccine are extremely rare and can include anything that is seen in mumps infection. Recent research in the area has been directed toward determining whether the vaccine in its present form or in another form should be considered for administration both to decrease adverse reactions and to decrease its cost and improve its applicability to a broader population.

—*Peter D. Reuman, M.D., M.P.H.*

See also Childhood infectious diseases; Encephalitis; Fever; Glands; Immunization and vaccination; Infertility, male; Meningitis; Orchitis; Viral infections.

FOR FURTHER INFORMATION:

American Medical Association. *American Medical Association Family Medical Guide*. 4th rev. ed. Hoboken, N.J.: John Wiley & Sons, 2004. An excellent reference for the beginner. The scientific accuracy of the text is not compromised by its accessibility.

Beers, Mark H., et al., eds. *The Merck Manual of Diagnosis and Therapy*. 18th ed. Whitehouse Station, N.J.: Merck Research Laboratories, 2006. Contains a useful exposition of the characteristics, etiology, diagnosis, and treatment of mumps.

Bellenir, Karen, and Peter D. Dresser, eds. *Contagious and Noncontagious Infectious Diseases Sourcebook*. Detroit, Mich.: Omnigraphics, 1996. A handy reference source on infectious diseases. Includes bibliographical references and an index.

Gorbach, Sherwood L., John G. Bartlett, and Neil R. Blacklow, eds. *Infectious Diseases*. 3d ed. Philadelphia: W. B. Saunders, 2004. A thorough discussion of infectious diseases. Included is a brief history, an account of the mechanisms of disease and immunity, and a concise discussion of a broad range of infectious agents.

Litin, Scott C., ed. *Mayo Clinic Family Health Book*. 4th ed. New York: HarperResource, 2009. Perhaps the best general medical text for the layperson, this book covers the entire medical field. While the information is derived from a wide variety of highly technical sources, the articles are written to be easily understood by a general audience.

Sompayrac, Lauren. *How Pathogenic Viruses Work*. Boston: Jones and Bartlett, 2002. Engaging exploration of the basics of virology. The author uses twelve of the most common viral infections to demonstrate how viruses "devise" various solutions to stay alive.

Woolf, Alan D., et al., eds. *The Children's Hospital Guide to Your Child's Health and Development*.

Cambridge, Mass.: Perseus, 2002. An authoritative and comprehensive guide to children's health, providing a guide to every common illness or condition that affects children and a carefully designed emergency section.

MÜNCHAUSEN SYNDROME BY PROXY
DISEASE/DISORDER

ANATOMY OR SYSTEM AFFECTED: All

SPECIALTIES AND RELATED FIELDS: Ethics, family medicine, pediatrics, psychiatry, psychology

DEFINITION: A disorder in which a parent fabricates, simulates, or induces a medical condition in a child in order to receive attention and acknowledgment as the source of information about the child's health.

KEY TERMS:

covert video surveillance: the monitoring of a child using video equipment in which the parent is unaware of the taping

narcissistic personality disorder: a disorder characterized by maladaptive patterns of behavior that are used to deal with common life situations

CAUSES AND SYMPTOMS

Münchausen syndrome by proxy may occur in different forms. In its least invasive form, this syndrome involves lying about a child's medical problems. For example, a father may claim that his child stopped breathing or had a seizure. The harm to the child comes from the medical studies that are ordered by the physician in an attempt to evaluate and diagnose the condition. A second situation involves the simulation of symptoms in the child. For example, a mother may maintain that her child is experiencing hematuria, and examination of the urine reveals the presence of blood. The blood comes not from the child but from some external source, such as the mother's menstrual blood or animal blood from packaged meat. Again, the child is subjected to needless diagnostic tests, some of which can be invasive.

The most injurious form of Münchausen syndrome by proxy comes when a parent induces the symptoms in the child. This can be done in many ways: The parent can administer syrup of ipecac to induce vomiting, administer substances such as diphtheria-pertussis-tetanus (DPT) vaccine to cause a fever, or inject fecal materials into already existing intravenous lines to induce a bacterial bloodstream infection. Parental induction of an apparent life-threatening event (ALTE) has been documented through the use of covert video surveillance. Parents have been observed placing their hands or other objects over the infant's face. Many of these children demonstrated bleeding from the mouth or gums, a finding not reported in any of the control infants who were experiencing an ALTE.

In addition to being subjected to multiple and invasive diagnostic procedures, some children die as a direct result of their parents' actions. Some families have a history of sudden or unexplained deaths of siblings that may be attributable to Münchausen syndrome by proxy or other types of child abuse.

TREATMENT AND THERAPY

A physician should become concerned about the possibility of Münchausen syndrome by proxy in a child with multiple health care visits in whom an explanation for the problems is elusive. The most common complaints include bleeding, vomiting, apnea, seizures, and fever. In each case, the chronic nature of the problems and the constant switching of health care providers should be clues. Statements by experienced physicians such as "I've never seen anything like this" should also signal that the child may be the victim of Münchausen syndrome by proxy. Some physicians become trapped in the process of ordering multiple studies for fear of missing an exotic disease.

On the other hand, some parents represent the "worried well." These people bring their children in for many minor complaints: every runny nose, low-grade temperature, or nonapparent skin rash. Their motivation is not personal attention. Rather, they are fearful and view their children as vulnerable.

The psychologic profile of the parent helps to distinguish the overly concerned mother from the one with Münchausen syndrome by proxy. The usual perpetrator is the child's mother. The father is often detached, distant, and not involved in the child's care, although cases in which the father is the perpetrator have been documented. Most perpetrators are believed to have borderline personalities and narcissistic personality

---

INFORMATION ON MÜNCHAUSEN SYNDROME BY PROXY

CAUSES: Psychological disorder

SYMPTOMS: Lying about or inducing a child's medical problems

DURATION: Chronic

TREATMENTS: Psychotherapy

disorders. They enjoy the attention that they receive in a medical setting. Medical staff members often characterize these individuals as excellent parents because they are knowledgeable about their child's health, attentive to his or her needs, and cooperative with the staff. Many of the mothers have some type of medical or science background, which facilitates their understanding of medical conditions. Some have worked in physicians' offices, making them knowledgeable about medical terminology or procedures. Psychological assessment is needed to help define parental pathology. Members of the medical staff may be disbelieving of the diagnosis, since they often find the parent to be nice and helpful. Many parents deny the accusations and are resistant to psychiatric intervention.

The task of the medical team is to entertain the diagnosis, obtain evidence, and protect the child. In some institutions, covert video surveillance is used to catch the parent in the act of inflicting the symptoms. Although there is concern about issues of privacy, legal counsel at most institutions has supported the use of covert video surveillance because it assesses the situation of the child.

PERSPECTIVE AND PROSPECTS

Münchausen syndrome by proxy was initially described by Roy Meadow in 1977. In the twenty years after his initial report, more than three hundred cases were reported in the literature. The diversity of ways in which this syndrome is inflicted on children has expanded with each case report. In many cases, the prognosis for affected children is somewhat guarded because of the complexity of establishing the diagnosis on a legal level.

Once the child and the parent are separated, the symptoms resolve. Cases may be difficult to substantiate in court, without the presence of concrete evidence. Some children suffer from long-term sequelae, sometimes behaving like invalids because of the role in which they have been cast since childhood. There are reports of self-destructive behavior and Münchausen syndrome in some survivors. Psychological counseling is critical to ensure the well-being of these children. In most cases, the children cannot be returned to the parental perpetrator because of the intractable nature of the parent's problem.

—*Carol D. Berkowitz, M.D.*

See also Bacterial infections; Critical care; Critical care, pediatric; Domestic violence; Emergency medicine; Emergency medicine, pediatric; Fever; Hypo-

chondriasis; Nausea and vomiting; Physical examination; Psychiatric disorders; Psychiatry; Psychiatry, child and adolescent; Psychosomatic illness.

FOR FURTHER INFORMATION:

Eminson, Mary, and R. J. Postlethwaite, eds. *Münchausen Syndrome by Proxy Abuse: A Practical Approach.* Boston: Butterworth-Heinemann, 2000. Aimed at the health professional, this book brings together a collection of essays discussing different aspects of this syndrome. Chapters deal with confirming factitious illness and the child protection process.

Feldman, Marc D. *Playing Sick? Untangling the Web of Munchausen Syndrome, Munchausen by Proxy, Malingering, and Factitious Disorder.* New York: Brunner-Routledge, 2004. Fascinating case histories of people whose conditions lead them to fake illnesses, in themselves and others, sometimes to the point of death.

Gregory, Julie. *Sickened: The Memoir of a Münchausen by Proxy Childhood.* New York: Bantam, 2003. A personal, engaging story in which the author details years of abuse due to her mother's disorder.

Rosenberg, D. A. "Münchausen Syndrome by Proxy." In *Child Abuse*, edited by Robert M. Reece. 3d ed. Elk Grove, Ill.: American Academy of Pediatrics, 2009. A discussion of the diagnosis and treatment of this abusive syndrome, in a text that includes bibliographical references and an index.

Southall, D. P., M. C. Plunkett, and M. W. Banks, et al. "Covert Video Recordings of Life-Threatening Child Abuse: Lessons for Child Protection." *Pediatrics* 100, no. 5 (November, 1997): 735-760. A descriptive, retrospective, partially controlled case study involving a total of thirty-nine children in whom hospital recordings were used to investigate suspicions of induced illness.

MUSCLE SPRAINS, SPASMS, AND DISORDERS

DISEASE/DISORDER

ALSO KNOWN AS: Myopathies

ANATOMY OR SYSTEM AFFECTED: Legs, ligaments, muscles, musculoskeletal system

SPECIALTIES AND RELATED FIELDS: Exercise physiology, family medicine, osteopathic medicine, physical therapy, sports medicine

DEFINITION: Injuries, defects, or disorders of the muscles of the body.

CAUSES AND SYMPTOMS

There are three kinds of muscle tissue in the human body: smooth muscle, cardiac muscle, and striated muscle. Smooth muscle tissue is found around the intestines, blood vessels, and bronchioles in the lung, among other areas. These muscles are controlled by the autonomic nervous system, which means that their movement is not subject to voluntary action. They have many functions: They maintain the airway in the lungs, regulate the tone of blood vessels, and move foods and other substances through the digestive tract. Cardiac muscle is found only in the heart. Striated muscles are those that move body parts. They are also called voluntary muscles because they must receive a conscious command from the brain in order to work. They supply the force for physical activity, and they also prevent movement and stabilize body parts.

Muscles are subject to many disorders: Muscle sprains, strains, and spasms are common events in everyone's life and, for the most part, they are harmless, if painful, results of overexercise, accidents, falls, bumps, or countless other events. Yet these symptoms can also signal serious myopathies, or disorders within muscle tissue.

Myopathies constitute a wide range of diseases. They are classified as inflammatory myopathies or metabolic myopathies. Inflammatory myopathies include infections by bacteria, viruses, or other microorganisms, as well as other diseases that are possibly autoimmune in origin (that is, resulting from and directed against the body's own tissues). In metabolic myopathies, there is some failure or disturbance in the body's ability to maintain a proper metabolic balance or electrolyte distribution. These conditions include glycogen storage diseases, in which there are errors in glucose processing; disorders of fatty acid metabolism, in which there are derangements in fatty acid oxidation; mitochondrial myopathies, in which there are biochemical and other abnormalities in the mitochondria of muscle cells; endocrine myopathies, in which an endocrine disorder underlies muscular symptoms; and the periodic paralyses, which can be the result of inherited or acquired illnesses. This is only a partial list of the myopathies, the symptoms of which include weakness and pain.

Muscular dystrophies are a group of inherited disorders in which muscle tissue fails to receive nourishment. The results are progressive muscular weakness and the degeneration and destruction of muscle fibers. The symptoms include weakness, loss of coordination,

> **INFORMATION ON MUSCLE SPRAINS, SPASMS, AND DISORDERS**
>
> **CAUSES:** Injury, overexercise, disease, toxin or pesticide exposure, neurological or endocrine disorders, hereditary factors
> **SYMPTOMS:** Vary; can include bruising, pain, inflammation, muscle spasms or cramps, progressive muscle weakness, loss of coordination, impaired gait
> **DURATION:** Acute to chronic
> **TREATMENTS:** Depends on condition; may include physical therapy, surgery, medications (analgesics, steroids and corticosteroids, anti-inflammatory drugs), rest-ice-compression-elevation (R-I-C-E) formula

impaired gait, and impaired muscle extensibility. Over the years, muscle mass decreases and the arms, legs, and spine become deformed.

Neuromuscular disorders include a wide variety of conditions in which muscle function is impaired by faulty transmission of nerve impulses to muscle tissue. These conditions may be inherited; they may be attributable to toxins, such as in food poisoning (for example, botulism) or by pesticide poisoning; or they may be side effects of certain drugs. The most commonly seen neuromuscular disorder is myasthenia gravis.

The muscular disorders most often seen are those that result from overexertion, exercise, athletics, accidents, and trauma. Injuries sustained during sports and games have become so significant that sports medicine has become a recognized medical subspecialty. Besides the muscles, the parts of the body involved in these disorders include tendons (tough, stringy tissue that attaches muscles to bones), ligaments (tissue that attaches bone to bone), synovia (membranes enclosing a joint or other bony structure), and cartilage (soft, resilient tissue between bones). A sprain is an injury in which ligaments are stretched or torn. In a strain, muscles or tendons are stretched or torn. A contusion is a bruise that occurs when the body is subjected to trauma; the skin is not broken, but the capillaries underneath are, causing discoloration. A spasm is a short, abnormal contraction in a muscle or group of muscles. A cramp is a prolonged, painful contraction of one or more muscles.

Sprains can be caused by twisting the joint violently or by forcing it beyond its range of movement. The ligaments that connect the bones of the joint stretch or tear. Sprains occur most often in the knees, ankles, and arches of the feet. There is pain and swelling, and at least some immobilization of the joint.

A strain is also called a pulled muscle. When too great a demand is placed on a muscle, it and the surrounding tendons can stretch and/or tear. The main symptom is pain; swelling and muscle spasm may also occur.

Muscle spasms and cramps are common. Sometimes they occur spontaneously, such as the calf muscle cramps that occur at night. Sometimes they are attributable to muscle strain (the charley horse that tightens thigh muscles in runners and other athletes). Muscles that are used often will go into spasm, such as those in the thumb and fingers of writers (writer's cramp), as can muscles that have remained in one position for too long. Muscle spasms and cramps can also occur as direct consequences of dehydration; they are common in athletes who perspire excessively during hot weather.

Some injuries to muscles and joints occur so regularly that they are named for the activities associated with them. A good example is tennis elbow, a condition that results from repeated, vigorous movement of the arm, such as swinging a tennis racket, using a paintbrush, or pitching a baseball. Runners' knee can afflict joggers and other athletes. It is usually caused by sprains in the knee ligaments; there is pain and there may be partial or total immobilization of the knee. Achilles tendinitis, as the name suggests, is inflammation of the Achilles tendon in the heel. It is usually the result of excessive physical activity that causes small tears in the tendon. Pain and immobility are symptoms. Tendinitis can occur in other joints as well; elbows and shoulders are common sites. Tenosynovitis is inflammation of the synovial membrane that sheathes the tendons in the hand. It may be caused by bacterial infection or may be attributable to overexertion.

Tumors and cancerous growths in muscle tissue are rare. If a lump appears in muscle, it is usually a lipoma, a fatty deposit that is benign. One tumor, called rhabdomyosarcoma, however, is malignant and can be fatal.

TREATMENT AND THERAPY

The myopathies are a wide group of diseases, and treatment varies considerably among them. The muscular dystrophies also vary in their treatment methods. Physical therapy is recommended to prevent contractures, the permanent, disfiguring muscular contractions that are a feature of the disease. Orthopedic appliances and surgery are also used. Because these diseases are genetic, it is sometimes recommended that people with a familial history of muscular dystrophy be tested for certain genetic markers that would suggest the possibility of disease in their children.

Myasthenia gravis is treated with drugs that increase the number of neurotransmitters available where nerves and muscles come together. The drugs help improve the transmission of information from the brain to the muscle tissue. In some cases, a procedure called plasmapheresis is used to eliminate blood-borne substances that may contribute to the disease. Surgical removal of the thymus gland is helpful in alleviating symptoms in some patients.

In treating the many muscle disorders that are caused by athletic activity and excessive wear and tear on the muscle, the R-I-C-E formula is recommended. The acronym stands for rest-ice-compression-elevation: The patient must rest and not use or exercise the limb or muscle involved; an ice pack is applied to the injury; compression is supplied by wrapping a moist bandage snugly over the ice, reducing the flow of fluids to the injured area; and the injured limb is elevated. If there is a fracture involved, the limb must be properly splinted or otherwise immobilized before elevation. The ice pack is held in place for twenty minutes and removed, but the bandage is held in place. Ice therapy can be resumed every twenty minutes.

Heat is also part of the therapy for strains and sprains, but it is not applied until after the initial swelling has gone down, usually after forty-eight to seventy-two hours. Heat raises the metabolic rate in the affected tissue. This brings more blood to the area, carrying nutrients that are needed for tissue repair. Moist heat is preferred, and it can be supplied by an electrical heating pad, a chemical gel in a plastic bag, or hot baths and whirlpools. In using pads and chemical gels, there should be a layer of toweling or other material between the heat source and the body. The temperature for a whirlpool or hot bath should be about 106 degrees Fahrenheit. Only the injured part should be immersed, if possible. As in the ice treatments, heat should be applied for twenty minutes and can be repeated after twenty minutes of rest.

Analgesics are given for pain. Over-the-counter preparations such as aspirin, acetaminophen, or ibuprofen are used most often. Sometimes, when pain is severe, more potent medications are required. Steroids are sometimes prescribed to reduce inflammation, and nonsteroidal anti-inflammatory drugs (NSAIDs) can alleviate both pain and inflammation. If a strained muscle or tendon is seriously torn or otherwise damaged, surgery may be required. Similarly, if a sprain involves torn or detached ligaments, they may have to be surgically repaired.

Muscle spasms and cramps may require both manipulation and the application of heat or cold. The affected limb is gently extended to stretch the contracted muscle. Massage and immersion in a hot bath are useful, as are cold packs.

Tennis elbow, runners' knee, and tendinitis respond to R-I-C-E therapy. Ice is applied to the injured site, and the limb is elevated and allowed to rest. When tenosynovitis is caused by bacterial infection, prompt antibiotic therapy may be necessary to avoid permanent damage. When it is attributable to overexertion, analgesics may help relieve pain and inflammation. Rarely, a corticosteroid is used when other drugs fail.

Often, the injured site requires physical therapy for the full range of motion to be restored. The physical therapist analyzes the patient's capability and develops a regimen to restore strength and mobility to the affected muscles and joints. Physical therapy may involve massage, hot baths, whirlpools, weight training, and/or isometric exercise. Orthotic devices may be required to help the injured area heal.

An important aspect of sports medicine and the treatment of sports-related muscle disorders is prevention. Many painful, debilitating, and immobilizing episodes can be avoided by proper training and conditioning, intelligent exercise practice, and restriction of exertion. Before undertaking any sport or strenuous physical activity, the individual is advised to warm up by gentle stretching, jogging, jumping, and other mild muscular activities. Arms can be rotated in front of the body, over the head, and in circles perpendicular to the ground. Knees can be lifted and pulled up to the chest. Shoulders should be gently rotated to relax upper-back muscles. Neck muscles are toned by gently and slowly moving the head from side to side and in circles. Back muscles are loosened by bending forward and continuing around in slow circles.

If a joint has been injured, it is important to protect it from further damage. Physicians and physical therapists often recommend that athletes tape, brace, or wrap susceptible joints, such as knees, ankles, elbows, or wrists. Sometimes a simple commercial elastic bandage, available in various configurations specific to parts of the body, is all that is required. Neck braces and back braces are used to support these structures.

Benign muscle tumors require no treatment, or may be surgically removed. Malignant tumors may require surgery, radiation, and chemotherapy.

PERSPECTIVE AND PROSPECTS

With the increased interest in physical exercise in the United States has come increasing awareness of the dangers of muscular damage that can arise from improper exercise, as well as of the cardiovascular risks that lie in wait for weekend athletes. Warm-up procedures are universally recommended. Individual exercisers, those in gym classes, professional athletes, and schoolchildren are routinely taken through procedures to stretch and loosen muscles before they start strenuous activity.

Greater attention is being paid to the special needs of young athletes, such as gymnasts. Over the years, new athletic toys and devices have constantly been developed for the young: Skateboards, skates, scooters, and bicycles expose children to a wide range of bumps, falls, bruises, strains, and sprains. Protective equipment and devices have been designed especially for them: Helmets, padding, and special uniforms give children more security in accidents. Similarly, adults should take the time and trouble to outfit themselves correctly for the sports and athletics in which they engage: Joggers should tape, wrap, and brace their joints; and cyclists should wear helmets.

Nevertheless, the incidence of sports- and athletics-related muscular damage is relatively high, pointing to the necessity for increased attention to prevention. The growth of sports medicine as a medical specialty helps considerably in this endeavor. Physicians and nurses in this area are trained to deal with the various problems that arise, and they are often expert commentators on the best means to prevent problems.

—C. Richard Falcon

See also Amyotrophic lateral sclerosis; Ataxia; Back pain; Bell's palsy; Beriberi; Botox; Cerebral palsy; Chronic fatigue syndrome; Electromyography; Exercise physiology; Fibromyalgia; First aid; Guillain-Barré syndrome; Hemiplegia; Hypertrophy; Kinesiology; Motor neuron diseases; Multiple sclerosis; Muscles; Muscular dystrophy; Myasthenia gravis; Neurology; Neurology, pediatric; Numbness and tingling; Osteopathic medicine; Overtraining syndrome; Palsy; Paralysis; Paraplegia; Parkinson's disease; Physical rehabilitation; Poliomyelitis; Ptosis; Quadriplegia; Rabies; Rheumatoid arthritis; Rotator cuff surgery; Seizures; Speech disorders; Sphincterectomy;

Sports medicine; Tendon disorders; Tendon repair; Tetanus; Tics; Torticollis; Weight loss and gain; Whiplash.

FOR FURTHER INFORMATION:

Dragoo, Jason J. *Handbook of Sports Medicine.* Tempe, Ariz.: Renaissance, 1993. Dragoo covers the wide range of sports- and athletics-related disorders with clarity and precision. The text is intended for the general reader, and the illustrations are simple and clear.

Kirkaldy-Willis, William H., and Thomas N. Bernard, Jr., eds. *Managing Low Back Pain.* 4th ed. New York: Churchill Livingstone, 1999. This book covers the anatomy, biomechanics, pathophysiology, diagnosis, and management of low back pain from the perspective of a variety of disciplines. The aim of the book is to "help all those involved in the treatment of patients suffering from low back and leg pain."

Litin, Scott C., ed. *Mayo Clinic Family Health Book.* 4th ed. New York: HarperResource, 2009. Discusses both muscles and bones, underscoring the intimate relationship between disorders in the two systems. The text and illustrations are complete and easy to understand.

McArdle, William, Frank I. Katch, and Victor L. Katch. *Exercise Physiology: Energy, Nutrition, and Human Performance.* 7th ed. Boston: Lippincott Williams & Wilkins, 2010. A wide-ranging text on exercise and the human body, covering topics such as nutrition, energy transfer, exercise training, systems of energy delivery and utilization, enhancement of energy capacity, the effect of environmental stress, and the effect of exercise on successful aging and disease prevention.

Marieb, Elaine N., and Katja Hoehn. *Human Anatomy and Physiology.* 9th ed. San Francisco: Pearson/Benjamin Cummings, 2010. This introductory anatomy and physiology textbook, easily accessible to those with little science background, is richly illustrated with diagrams and photographs, which help to illuminate body systems and processes.

Ryan, Allan J., and Fred L. Allman, eds. *Sports Medicine.* 2d ed. San Diego, Calif.: Academic Press, 1989. Directed to the professional, but the text can be understood by the layperson. Particularly useful in outlining the contemporary status of sports medicine and how it relates to the training and care of the athlete.

Salter, Robert Bruce. *Textbook of Disorders and Injuries of the Musculoskeletal System.* 3d ed. Balti-more: Williams & Wilkins, 1999. Four sections of the book—"Basic Musculoskeletal Science and Its Applications," "Musculoskeletal Disorders: General and Specific," "Musculoskeletal Injuries," and "Research"—examine the diagnosis and treatment principles of disorders and trauma of the musculoskeletal system.

MUSCLES

ANATOMY

ANATOMY OR SYSTEM AFFECTED: Arms, gastrointestinal system, legs, ligaments, musculoskeletal system

SPECIALTIES AND RELATED FIELDS: Cardiology, exercise physiology, orthopedics, osteopathic medicine, physical therapy, sports medicine

DEFINITION: Cardiac muscle, skeletal muscle, and smooth muscle—all of which have the ability to contract, making possible body movement, peristalsis (the movement of food through the gastrointestinal system), and the circulation of blood throughout the body.

KEY TERMS:

cardiac muscle: a type of muscle, found only in the heart, that makes up the major portion of the heart; involved in the movement of blood through the body

muscle contraction: the shortening of a muscle, which may result in the movement of a particular body part

muscle fibers: elongated muscle cells that make up skeletal, cardiac, and smooth muscles

musculature: the arrangement of skeletal muscles in the body

skeletal muscle: a type of muscle that attaches to bone and causes movement of body parts; the only type that is under conscious, voluntary control

smooth muscle: a type of muscle found in the walls of internal organs such as the stomach, intestines, and urinary bladder; involved in the movement of food through the digestive tract

STRUCTURE AND FUNCTIONS

More than half of the body weight of humans is made up of muscle. Three types of muscles are found in the body: skeletal muscle, cardiac muscle, and smooth muscle. These muscles are composed of different types of muscle cells and perform different functions within the body. The characteristics and functions of each of these three muscle types will be discussed separately, starting with skeletal muscle.

Skeletal muscles attach to and cover bones. This type

of muscle is often referred to as voluntary muscle because it is the only muscle type that can be controlled or made to move by consciously thinking about it. Skeletal muscles perform four important functions: bringing about body movement, helping to maintain posture, helping to stabilize joints such as the knee, and generating body heat.

Nearly all body movement is dependent upon skeletal muscle. Skeletal muscle is needed not only to be able to run and jump but also to speak, to write, and to move and blink the eyes. These movements are brought about by the contraction or shortening of skeletal muscles. These muscles are attached to two bones or other structures by tough thin strips or cords of tissue known as tendons. When a muscle contracts or shortens, it pulls the tendons, which then pull on the bones or other structures to which they are connected. In this way, the desired movement is brought about.

Skeletal muscles also aid in the maintenance of posture. Posture is defined as the ability to maintain a position of the body or body parts: for example, the ability to stand or to sit erect. The constant force of gravity must be overcome in order to maintain a standing or seated posture. Small adjustments to the force of gravity are constantly being made through slight contractions of skeletal muscle.

Skeletal muscles—or, more appropriately, their tendons—help to maintain joint stability. Many of the tendons that connect muscles to bones cross movable joints such as the knee and the shoulder. These tendons are kept taut by the constant contraction of the muscles to which they are attached. As a result, they act as walls to prevent the joints from dislocating or shifting out of the normal positions.

More than 40 percent of the human body is composed of skeletal muscle. Skeletal muscles generate heat as they contract. As a result, skeletal muscles are of extreme importance in maintaining normal body temperature. When the body is exposed to cold temperatures, it begins to shiver. This shivering is the result of muscle contractions, which serve to generate body heat and maintain the body's normal temperature.

Skeletal muscles are made up of skeletal muscle cells. These cells are long and tube-shaped and therefore are referred to as skeletal muscle fibers. In some instances, these muscle fibers may be a foot long. When individual skeletal muscle fibers are viewed under a microscope, they display bands that are referred to as striations. For this reason, skeletal muscle is often called striated muscle.

Each skeletal muscle, depending upon its size, is made up of hundreds or thousands of skeletal muscle fibers. These muscle fibers are surrounded by a tough connective tissue that holds the muscle fibers together. These muscle fibers and their surrounding connective tissue form a skeletal muscle. In the human body, there are more than six hundred skeletal muscles. It is the arrangement of these muscles in the body that is referred to as the musculature, or muscle system.

Smooth muscles are often referred to as involuntary muscles because they cannot be made to contract by conscious effort. Smooth muscles are typically found in the walls of internal organs such as the esophagus, stomach, intestines, and urinary bladder. The primary function of smooth muscles in these organs is to enable the passage of material through a tube or tract. For example, the contraction of smooth muscles in the intestines helps to move digested materials through the digestive system.

Smooth muscle is composed of smooth muscle cells. These cells differ from skeletal muscle fibers in that they are short and spindle-shaped. They also differ from skeletal muscle cells in that they are not striated. Furthermore, smooth muscle cells usually are not surrounded by a tough connective tissue to form a muscle; instead, they are arranged in layers.

Cardiac muscle is found only in the heart. Like smooth muscle, cardiac muscle cannot be made to contract by means of conscious effort. Like skeletal muscle, however, cardiac muscle is striated. The contraction of cardiac muscle results in the contraction of the heart. This, in turn, results in the pumping of blood throughout the body.

Although many differences exist among skeletal, smooth, and cardiac muscle, all have one thing in common—their ability to contract. The methods by which this contraction is brought about in skeletal muscle, however, are different from those used by smooth muscle and cardiac muscle.

In order for skeletal muscles to contract, they must first be electrically stimulated. This electrical stimulation is brought about by nerves that are closely associated with the muscle fibers. Each muscle fiber has a branch of a nerve, known as an axon terminal, that lies very close to it. This axon terminal does not touch the muscle fiber, but is separated from it by a tiny space known as the synaptic cleft (or gap). An electrical impulse from the nerve causes the release of a chemical called a neurotransmitter into the synaptic cleft. The specific type of neurotransmitter for skeletal muscle is known as acetylcholine. The neurotransmitter will then pass through the synaptic cleft to the muscle fiber membrane, where it will bind to a special site known as a receptor. When the neurotransmitter binds to the receptor, it causes an electrical impulse to travel down the muscle fiber. This, in turn, causes the contraction of the muscle fiber. When most or all of the muscle fibers contract, the result is the contraction of the entire muscle.

The muscle fibers and muscle will remain in a contracted state as long as the neurotransmitter is bound to the receptor on the muscle fiber membrane. In order for the muscle fiber to relax, the neurotransmitter must be released from the receptor to which it is bound. This is accomplished by the destruction of the neurotransmitter. Another chemical, known as an enzyme, is released into the synaptic cleft. This enzyme destroys the neurotransmitter; thus, the neurotransmitter is no longer bound to the receptor. In skeletal muscle, this enzyme is called acetylcholinesterase, because it destroys the neurotransmitter acetylcholine.

The contraction of cardiac muscle differs from that of skeletal muscle in that each cardiac muscle fiber does not have an axon terminal associated with it. Cardiac muscle is capable of making its own electrical impulse; it does not need a nerve to initiate the electrical impulse for every cardiac muscle fiber. An impulse is started in a particular place in the heart, called the atrioventricular (A-V) node. This impulse spreads from muscle fiber to muscle fiber. Thus, each cardiac muscle fiber stimulates those fibers next to it. The electrical impulse spreads so fast that nearly all the cardiac muscle fibers contract at the same time. As a result, the single impulse that began in the A-V node causes the entire heart to contract.

DISORDERS AND DISEASES

Any type of muscle disorder has the ability to disrupt the normal functions performed by muscles. Skeletal muscle disorders can disrupt body movement and the ability to maintain posture. If these disorders affect the diaphragm, the principal breathing muscle, they can also be fatal.

Perhaps the most common and least detrimental muscle disorder is disuse atrophy. When muscles are not used, the muscle fibers will become smaller, a process called atrophy. As a result of the decrease in the diameter of the muscle fibers, the entire muscle also becomes smaller and therefore weaker.

Disuse atrophy occurs in such circumstances as when an individual is sick or injured and must remain in bed for prolonged periods of time. As a result, the muscles are not used and begin to atrophy. Disuse atrophy is also fairly common in astronauts. This occurs as a result of the lack of gravity against which the muscles must work. If a muscle does not work against a load or force, such as gravity, it will tend to decrease in size.

In general, disuse muscle atrophy is easily treated. The primary treatment is to exercise the unused muscle. Physical activity, particularly those activities in which the muscle must work to lift or pull a weight, will result in an enlargement in the diameter of the skeletal muscle fibers, and thus of the entire muscle. The increase in the diameter of the muscle fibers and muscle is referred to as hypertrophy.

Another common muscle disorder is a muscle cramp. A muscle cramp is a spasm in which the muscle undergoes strong involuntary contractions. These involuntary contractions, which may last for as short a time as a few seconds or as long as a few hours, are extremely painful. Muscle cramps appear to occur more frequently at night or after exercise, but their cause is unknown. Treatment for cramps involves rubbing and massaging the affected muscle.

Muscles are often overused or overstretched. When this is the case, it is possible for the muscle fibers to tear. When the muscle fibers are torn, the result is a muscle strain, more often referred to as a pulled muscle. Although pulled muscles may be painful, they are usually not serious. Treatment for pulled muscles most often involves the resting of the affected muscle. If the muscle fibers are torn completely apart, surgery may be required to reattach the muscle fibers.

Among the more serious skeletal muscle disorders is muscular dystrophy. The term "muscular dystrophy" is used to define those muscle disorders that are genetic or inherited. These diseases most often begin in childhood, but a few cases have been reported to begin during adult life. Muscular dystrophy results in progressive muscle weakness and muscle atrophy. The most common form of muscular dystrophy is known as Duchenne muscular dystrophy. This form of muscular dystrophy primarily affects males. In those affected with Duchenne muscular dystrophy, muscular weakness and atrophy begin to appear at three to five years of age. There is a progressive loss of muscle strength and muscle mass such that, by the age of twelve, those individuals afflicted with the disorder are confined to a wheelchair. Usually between the ages of fourteen and eighteen, the patients develop serious and sometimes fatal respiratory diseases as a result of the impairment of the diaphragm, the primary breathing muscle. The progressive deterioration of the muscles cannot be stopped, but it may be slowed with exercise of the affected muscles.

Myasthenia gravis is also a severe muscle disorder. This disease results in excessive weakness of skeletal muscles, a condition known as muscle fatigue. Those with myasthenia gravis complain of fatigue even after performing normal everyday body movements. Although severe, myasthenia gravis is usually not fatal unless the diaphragm is affected.

Myasthenia results from a decrease in the availability of the receptors for acetylcholine. If fewer acetylcholine receptors are available on the muscle fibers, less acetylcholine binds to the muscle fiber receptors; this binding is needed for contraction to occur. As a result, fewer muscle fibers within the muscle contract. The fewer muscle fibers within the entire muscle that contract, the weaker the muscle.

Myasthenia gravis affects about one in every ten thousand individuals. Unlike Duchenne muscular dystrophy, myasthenia gravis may affect any group, and, overall, women are affected more frequently than men. Myasthenia gravis is usually first detected in the facial muscles, particularly those of the eyes and eyelids. Those afflicted have droopy eyelids and experience difficulty in keeping the eyes open. Other symptoms are weakness in those muscles involved in chewing and difficulty swallowing as a result of weakening of the tongue muscles. In most patients, there is also some weakening of the muscles of the legs and arms.

The prognosis for the treatment of myasthenia gravis is very good. The most important treatment for the disorder is the use of anticholinesterase drugs. These drugs inhibit the breakdown of acetylcholine. As a result, there is a large amount of acetylcholine in the neuromuscular junction to bind with the limited number of acetylcholine receptors. This, in turn, increases the ability and number of the muscle fibers that are able to contract, resulting in an increase in muscle strength and the ability to use the muscles without fatigue.

Also of interest is the effect of pesticides and the way in which they affect muscle function. Some pesticides are classified as organic pesticides that inhibit the enzyme acetylcholinesterase. If acetylcholinesterase is inhibited, it will no longer break down the acetylcholine that is bound to the receptor on the skeletal muscle membrane. If the acetylcholine is not removed from the receptor, the muscle cannot relax and is therefore in a constant state of contraction. As a result, the respiratory muscles are unable to contract and relax, a process required for breathing. Thus, organic pesticides function to prevent the respiratory muscles from working, and an affected animal will die as a result of not being able to breathe.

Muscle fibers also require a blood supply in order to keep them alive. If the blood supply to the muscle fibers is inhibited, death of the muscle fibers can result. If enough muscle fibers are affected, death of the muscle can result. This most commonly occurs in cardiac muscle. If the blood supply to the cardiac muscle making up the heart is reduced or cut off, the result is a decrease in the ability of the cardiac muscle to contract. This, in turn, leads to heart failure.

PERSPECTIVE AND PROSPECTS

The study of muscles and musculature is as old as the study of anatomy itself. The first well-documented study of muscles was done by Galen of Pergamum in the first century. Galen made drawings of muscles and described their functions. In all, Galen described more than three hundred muscles in the human body, almost half of all the muscles now known.

The first refined drawings and descriptions of the skeletal muscles of the body were made in the late fifteenth century. Among those who stood out as muscle anatomists during this period was Leonardo da Vinci. Leonardo's drawings of the skeletal muscles of the body were magnificent. His chief interest in the muscles of the body, like Galen's, was their function. He accurately described, among many other muscles, the muscles involved in the movement of the lips and cheeks.

A major step to the understanding of muscle physiology did not occur until the late eighteenth century. Luigi Galvani in 1791 discovered the relationship between muscle contraction and electricity when he found that an electrical current could cause the contraction of a frog leg. The use of electrical stimulation to study muscle contraction and function was fully utilized in the mid-nineteenth century by Duchenne de Boulogne. The actual measurement of the electrical activity in a muscle came about in 1929, with the invention by Edgar Douglas Adrian and Detlev Wulf Bronk of the needle electrode, which could be placed into the muscle to record the muscle's electrical activity. This recording of the electrical activity of the muscle is known as an electromyogram, or EMG. Electromyograms are important in the evaluation of the electrical activity of resting and contracting muscles. Since the discovery of EMGs, they have been used by anatomists, muscle physiologists, exercise physiologists, and orthopedic surgeons to study and diagnose muscle diseases. Furthermore, the knowledge gained from EMGs has led to the making of artificial limbs that can be controlled by the electrical impulses of the existing muscles.

Knowledge of muscle names, muscle anatomy, and movement, as well as muscle physiology, is needed for many medical fields. These fields include kinesiology, the study of movement; physical and occupational therapy; the treatment and rehabilitation of those who are disabled by injury; exercise physiology and sports medicine, in which the effects of exercise on muscle and the damage of muscle as a result of sports injuries are studied; and, finally, orthopedic surgery, which is the surgical repair of damaged bones, joints, and muscles.

—*David K. Saunders, Ph.D.*

See also Acupressure; Amyotrophic lateral sclerosis; Anesthesia; Anesthesiology; Ataxia; Bed-wetting; Bell's palsy; Botox; Breasts, female; Cells; Cerebral palsy; Chronic fatigue syndrome; Diaphragm; Electromyography; Exercise physiology; Fibromyalgia; Glycolysis; Guillain-Barré syndrome; Head and neck disorders; Hemiplegia; Kinesiology; Lower extremities; Mastectomy and lumpectomy; Motor neuron diseases; Multiple sclerosis; Muscle sprains, spasms, and disorders; Muscular dystrophy; Myasthenia gravis; Myomectomy; Orthopedic surgery; Orthopedics; Orthopedics, pediatric; Osteopathic medicine; Overtraining syndrome; Palsy; Paralysis; Paraplegia; Parkinson's disease; Physical rehabilitation; Poisoning; Poliomyelitis; Ptosis; Quadriplegia; Rabies; Respiration; Rotator cuff surgery; Seizures; Speech disorders; Sphincterectomy; Sports medicine; Steroid abuse; Tendon disorders; Tendon repair; Tetanus; Tics; Torticollis; Tremors; Upper extremities; Weight loss and gain; Whiplash.

FOR FURTHER INFORMATION:

Blakey, Paul. *The Muscle Book*. Honesdale, Pa.: Himalayan Institute, 2000. An accessible guide to the muscles of the human body. Identifies all major muscles, reviews how they work, and discusses common injuries and first aid by massage.

Burke, Edmund. *Optimal Muscle Performance and Recovery*. Rev. ed. New York: Putnam, 2003. A leading exercise physiologist provides a training guide for athletes that details exercise regimens and stresses healthy muscle development and recovery after injury.

Cash, Mel. *Pocket Atlas of the Moving Body*. New York: Crown, 2000. An excellent reference guide that covers information about movement and posture of the human body. Full-page anatomical illustrations; tables of muscles, joints, posture, and movement patterns; definitions of technical terms; and a listing of common types of injury are included.

Guyton, Arthur C., and John E. Hall. *Guyton and Hall Textbook of Medical Physiology*. 12th ed. Philadelphia: Saunders/Elsevier, 2011. This textbook gives many examples of diseases and pathological conditions of skeletal and cardiac muscle. The text does an excellent job of describing how diseases and pathologies affect the normal functioning of the muscle. Although somewhat technical at times, the text is well written and understandable.

Marieb, Elaine N. *Essentials of Human Anatomy and Physiology*. 9th ed. San Francisco: Pearson/Benjamin Cummings, 2009. An excellent place to begin the study of muscles and musculature. This text uses little technical jargon and explains the jargon it does use. Provides good descriptions and drawings of the most important muscles.

Shier, David N., Jackie L. Butler, and Ricki Lewis. *Hole's Essentials of Human Anatomy and Physiology*. 10th ed. Boston: McGraw-Hill, 2009. An introductory college anatomy and physiology book that is easy to read and understand. Provides a good general overview of skeletal, cardiac, and smooth muscle anatomy and function.

Tortora, Gerard J., and Bryan Derrickson. *Principles of Anatomy and Physiology*. 12th ed. Hoboken, N.J.: John Wiley & Sons, 2009. This text clearly explains the functions of many individual muscles. Furthermore, it provides many examples of clinical applications involving muscles, including diseases and the use of medical tests for the diagnosis of muscle disease.

MUSCULAR DYSTROPHY

DISEASE/DISORDER

ANATOMY OR SYSTEM AFFECTED: Legs, muscles, musculoskeletal system

SPECIALTIES AND RELATED FIELDS: Genetics, pediatrics, physical therapy

DEFINITION: A group of related diseases that attack different muscle groups, are progressive and genetically determined, and have no known cure.

KEY TERMS:

disease: an interruption, cessation, or disorder of a body function or system, usually identifiable by a group of signs and symptoms and characterized by consistent anatomical alterations

distal: situated away from the center of the body; the farthest part from the midline of the body

DNA (deoxyribonucleic acid): a type of protein found in the nucleus of a cell comprising chromosomes that contain the genetic instructions of an organism

dystrophin: both the gene and the protein that are defective in Duchenne muscular dystrophy

dystrophy: an improper form of a tissue or group of cells (literally, "bad nourishment")

enzyme: a protein secreted by a cell that acts as a catalyst to induce chemical changes in other substances, remaining apparently unchanged itself in the process

fiber: a slender thread or filament; the elongated, threadlike cells that collectively constitute a muscle

genetic: imparted at conception and incorporated into every cell of an organism

muscle: a bundle of contractile cells that is responsible for the movement of organs and body parts

muscle group: a collection of muscles that work together to accomplish a particular movement

CAUSES AND SYMPTOMS

Muscles, attached to bones through tendons, are responsible for movement in the human body. In muscular dystrophy, muscles become progressively weaker. As individual muscle fibers become so weak that they die, they are replaced by connective tissue, which is fibrous and fatty rather than muscular. These replacement fibers are commonly found in skin and scar tissue and are not capable of movement, and the muscles become progressively weaker. There are several different recognized types of muscular dystrophy. These have in common degeneration of muscle fibers and their replacement with connective tissue. They are distinguished from one another on the basis of the muscle group or groups involved and the age at which individuals are affected.

The most common type is Duchenne muscular dystrophy. In this disease, the muscles involved are in the upper thigh and pelvis. The disease strikes in early childhood, usually between the ages of four and seven. It is known to be genetic and occurs only in boys. Two-thirds of affected individuals are born to mothers who are known to carry a defective gene; one-third are simply new cases whose mothers are genetically normal.

Individuals afflicted with Duchenne muscular dystrophy suffer from weakness in their hips and upper thighs. Initially, they may experience difficulty in sitting up or standing. The disease progresses to involve muscle groups in the shoulder and trunk. Patients lose the ability to walk during their early teens. As the disease progresses, portions of the brain become affected, and intelligence is reduced. Muscle fibers in the heart are also affected, and most individuals die by the age of twenty.

The dystrophin gene normally produces a very large protein called dystrophin that is an integral part of the muscle cell membrane. In Duchenne muscular dystrophy, a defect in the dystrophin gene causes no dystrophin or defective dystrophin to be produced, and the protein will be absent from the cell membrane. As a result, the muscle fiber membrane breaks down and

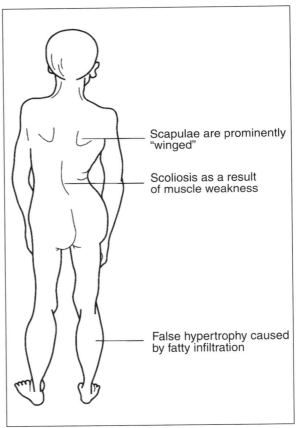

Scapulae are prominently "winged"

Scoliosis as a result of muscle weakness

False hypertrophy caused by fatty infiltration

Duchenne muscular dystrophy, the most common type, is characterized by prominently "winged" scapulae, scoliosis, false hypertrophy of the calves, and other less visible effects; children are the victims, usually not surviving beyond age twenty.

leaks, allowing fluid from outside the cell to enter the muscle cell. In turn, the contents of affected cells are broken down by other chemicals called proteases that are normally stored in the muscle cell. The dead pieces of muscle fiber are removed by scavenging cells called macrophages. The result of this process is a virtually empty and greatly weakened muscle cell.

A second type is Becker's muscular dystrophy, which is similar to the Duchenne form of the disease. Approximately 3 in 200,000 people are affected, and it too is found only among males. The major clinical difference is the age of onset. Becker's muscular dystrophy typically first appears in the early teenage years. The muscles involved are similar to those of Duchenne muscular dystrophy, but the course of the disease is slower. Most individuals require the use of a wheelchair in their early thirties and eventually die in their forties.

Myotonic dystrophy is a form of muscular dystrophy that strikes approximately 5 out of 100,000 people in a population. Myotonia is the inability of a muscle group to relax after contracting. Individuals with myotonic dystrophy experience this difficulty in their hands and feet. On average, the disease first appears at the age of nineteen. The condition is benign, in that it does not shorten an affected person's life span. Rather, it causes inconveniences to the victim. Affected persons also experience a variety of other problems, including baldness at the front of the head and malfunction of the ovaries and testes. The muscles of the stomach and intestines can become involved, leading to a slowing down of intestinal functions and diarrhea.

Another type is limb girdle muscular dystrophy. The muscles of both upper and lower limbs—the shoulders and the pelvis—are involved. The onset of this dystrophy form is variable, from childhood to middle age. While the disorder is not usually fatal, it does progress, and victims experience severe disability about twenty years after the disease first appears. While this variant is also genetically transmitted, men and women are about equally affected.

One type of muscular dystrophy found almost exclusively among individuals of Scandinavian descent is called distal dystrophy. It first appears relatively early in adult life, between the thirties and fifties. The muscles of the forearm and hand become progressively weaker and decrease in size. Eventually, the muscles of the lower leg and foot also become involved. This form of muscular dystrophy is not usually fatal.

Oculopharyngeal muscular dystrophy is a particularly serious form that involves the muscles of the eyes and throat. In this disease, victims are affected in their forties and fifties. There is progressive loss of control of the muscles that move the eyes and loss of the ability to swallow. Death usually results from starvation or from pneumonia acquired when the affected individual accidentally inhales food or drink.

A type of muscular dystrophy for which the location of the genetic abnormality is known is facioscapulohumeral muscular dystrophy; the defect is confined to the tip of the fourth chromosome. This disease initially involves the muscles of the face and later spreads to the muscles of the posterior or back of the shoulder. Eventually, muscles in the upper thigh are involved. The affected person loses the ability to make facial expressions and assumes a permanent pout as a result of loss of muscle function. As the condition advances, the shoulder blades protrude when the arms are raised. Weakness and difficulty walking are eventually experienced. As with other forms of muscular dystrophy, there is some variability in the degree to which individuals are affected. Occasionally, a variety of deafness occurs involving the nerves that connect the inner ear and the brain. Less commonly, victims become blind.

There are other variants of muscular dystrophy that have been recognized and described. These forms of the disease, however, are rare. The main problem facing physicians is differentiating accurately the variety of muscular dystrophy seen in a particular patient so as to arrive at a correct diagnosis.

TREATMENT AND THERAPY

The diagnosis of muscular dystrophy is initially made through observation. Typically, parents notice changes in their affected children and bring these concerns to the attention of a physician. The physician takes a careful family history and then examines a suspected victim to make a tentative or working diagnosis. Frequently, knowledge of other family members with the condition and observations are sufficient to establish a firm diagnosis. Occasionally, a physician may elect to order physiological or genetic tests to confirm the tentative diagnosis. As Duchenne muscular dystrophy is the most common form of muscular dystrophy, it provides a convenient example of this process.

A diagnosis of Duchenne or any other form of muscular dystrophy is rarely made before the age of three. This form of the disease almost always occurs in boys. (Variants, rather than true Duchenne muscular dystrophy, are seen in girls, but this situation is extremely rare.) The reason for this finding is that the genetic defect occurs on the X chromosome, of which males only possess one. Approximately two-thirds of all victims inherit the defective chromosome from their mothers, who are asymptomatic carriers; thus, the condition is recessive and said to be X-linked. The disease occurs in the remaining one-third of victims as a result of a fresh mutation, in which there is no family history of the disease and the parents are not carriers.

Victims usually begin to sit, walk, and run at an older age than normally would be expected. Parents describe walking as waddling rather than the usual upright posture. Victims have difficulty climbing stairs. They also have apparently enlarged calf muscles, a finding called muscular hypertrophy. While the muscles are initially strong, they lose their strength when connective and fatty tissues replace muscle fibers. The weakness of muscles in the pelvis is responsible for difficulties in sitting and the unusual way of walking. Normal children are able to go directly from a sitting position to standing erect. Victims of Duchenne muscular dystrophy first roll onto their stomachs, then kneel and raise themselves up by pushing their hands against their shins, knees, and thighs; they literally climb up themselves in order to stand. These children also have a pronounced curvature of their lower backs, an attempt by the body to compensate for the weakness in the muscles of the hips and pelvis.

There is frequently some weakness in the muscles of the shoulder. This finding can be demonstrated by a physician, but it is not usually seen by parents and is not an early problem for the victim. A physician tests for this weakness by lifting the child under the armpits. Normal children will be able to support themselves using the muscles of the shoulder. Individuals with Du-

chenne muscular dystrophy are unable to hold themselves up and will slip through the physician's hands. Eventually, these children will be unable to lift their arms over their heads. Most victims of Duchenne muscular dystrophy are unable to walk by their teen years. The majority die before the age of twenty, although about one-quarter live for a few more years. Most victims also have an abnormality in the muscles of the heart that leads to decreased efficiency of the heart and decreased ability to be physically active; in some cases, it also causes sudden death. Most victims of Duchenne muscular dystrophy suffer mental impairment. As their muscles deteriorate, their measured intelligence quotient (IQ) drops approximately twenty points below the level that it was at the onset of the disease. Serious mental handicaps are experienced by about one-quarter of victims.

Other forms of muscular dystrophy are similar to Duchenne muscular dystrophy. Their clinical courses are also similar, as are the methods of diagnosis. The critical differences are the muscles involved and the age of onset.

Laboratory procedures used to confirm the diagnosis of muscular dystrophy include microscopic analysis of muscle tissue, measurement of enzymes found in the blood, and measurement of the speed and efficiency of nerve conduction, a process called electromyography. Some cases have been diagnosed at birth by measuring a particular enzyme called creatinine kinase. It is possible to diagnose some types of muscular dystrophy before birth with chorionic villus sampling or amniocentesis.

There is no specific treatment for any of the muscular dystrophies. Physical therapy is frequently ordered and used to prevent the remaining unaffected muscles from losing their tone and mass. In some stages of the disease, braces, appliances, and orthopedic surgery may be used. These measures do not reverse the underlying pathology, but they may improve the quality of life for a victim. The cardiac difficulties associated with myotonic dystrophy may require treatment with a pacemaker. For victims of myotonic dystrophy, some relief is obtained by using drugs; the most commonly used pharmaceuticals are phenytoin and quinine. The inability to relax muscles once they are contracted does not usually present a major problem for sufferers of myotonic dystrophy.

More useful and successful is prevention, which involves screening individuals in families or kinship groups who are potential carriers. Carriers are persons who have some genetic material for a disease or condition but lack sufficient genes to cause an apparent case of a disease or condition; in short, they appear normal. When an individual who is a carrier conceives a child, however, there is an increased risk of the offspring having the disease. Genetic counseling should be provided after screening, so that individuals who have the gene for a disease can make more informed decisions about having children.

Chemical tests are available for use in diagnosing some forms of muscular dystrophy. Carriers of the gene for Duchenne muscular dystrophy can be detected by staining a muscle sample for dystrophin; a cell that is positive for Duchenne muscular dystrophy will have no stained dystrophin molecules. The dystrophin stain test is also used to diagnose Becker's muscular dystrophy, but the results are not quite as consistent or reliable. Approximately two-thirds of carriers and fetuses at risk for both forms of muscular dystrophy can be identified by analyzing DNA. Among individuals at risk for myotonic dystrophy, nine out of ten who carry the gene can be identified with DNA analysis before they experience actual symptoms of the disease.

PERSPECTIVE AND PROSPECTS

Muscular dystrophy has been recognized as a medical entity for several centuries. Initially, it was considered to be a degenerative disease only of adults, and it was not until the nineteenth century that the disease was addressed in children with Guillaume-Benjamin-Amand Duchenne's description of progressive weakness of the hips and upper thighs. An accurate classification of the various forms of muscular dystrophy depended on accurate observation and on the collection of sets of cases. Correct diagnosis had to wait for the development of accurate laboratory methods for staining muscle fibers. The interpretation of laboratory findings depended on the development of biochemical knowledge. Thus, much of the integration of knowledge concerning muscular dystrophy is relatively recent.

Genes play an important role in the understanding of muscular dystrophy. All forms of muscular dystrophy

---

IN THE NEWS: THE PATH TOWARD GENE THERAPY FOR MUSCULAR DYSTROPHY

Gene therapy in the treatment of Duchenne muscular dystrophy (DMD), the gravest and most common form of muscular dystrophy, has been a subject of intensive research. The goal of such therapy is to introduce the normal gene for dystrophin, which is defective in DMD, into diseased muscle cells so that their ability to withstand the wear and tear of contractile activity is restored. Significant progress in this effort was reported in the October, 2002, issue of the *Proceedings of the National Academy of Science of the United States of America* by collaborating groups at the University of Washington in Seattle and the University of Michigan in Ann Arbor.

The researchers used as their model system the transgenic *mdx* mouse, which carries a truncated dystrophin gene and therefore produces virtually no dystrophin protein. The leg muscles of such mice are susceptible to contraction-induced injury and subsequent deterioration, much as in human DMD.

To deliver functionally effective levels of normal full-length dystrophin, the gene was engineered into an adenovirus, which was then injected directly into the *mdx* leg muscles. This viral vector, which is related to the family of viruses that cause the common cold, is an excellent choice as a genetic vehicle because of its efficiency at infecting muscle cells. However, the researchers needed to make significant changes to the adenoviral deoxyribonucleic acid (DNA) in order to overcome two major problems. First, the dystrophin gene is extremely large and therefore is not amenable to being inserted into a viral DNA sequence. Second, the immune systems of the mice tend to reject the adenoviral DNA. To solve both of these problems, the viral vector was stripped of all unnecessary DNA ("gutted") so that it would accommodate the entire cDNA sequence of dystrophin while not being rejected.

The gutted adenoviral vector made it possible for the first time to introduce full-length dystrophin into adult *mdx* leg muscles without eliciting an immune response. One month later, the muscle tissue near the injection sites was making 25 to 30 percent of normal dystrophin levels; furthermore, there was a 40 percent improvement in contraction-induced injury. These findings constitute an important step toward the use of adenoviral vector-based gene therapy to treat DMD. For the therapy to be truly effective, it will be necessary to develop systemic techniques for delivering the normal gene to all muscles.

—*Mary A. Nastuk, Ph.D.*

are hereditary, although different chromosomes are involved in different forms of the disease. The development of techniques for routine testing and diagnosis has also occurred relatively recently. Specific chromosomes for all forms of muscular dystrophy have not yet been discovered. Considering initial successes of the Human Genome Project, an effort to identify all human genes, it seems likely that more precise genetic information related to muscular dystrophy will emerge.

There still are no cures for muscular dystrophies, and many forms are relentlessly fatal. Cures for many communicable diseases caused by bacteria or viruses have been discovered, and advances have been made in the treatment of cancer and other degenerative diseases by identifying chemicals that cause the conditions or by persuading people to change their lifestyles. Muscular dystrophy, however, is a group of purely genetic conditions. Many of the particular chromosomes involved are known, but no techniques are yet available to cure the disease once it is identified.

The availability of both a mouse model and a dog model of Duchenne muscular dystrophy, however, has facilitated the testing of gene therapy for this disease. Dystrophic mouse early embryos have been cured by injection of a functional copy of the dystrophin gene; however, this technique must be performed in embryos and is not useful for human therapy. Two avenues of research under way in these animal models are the introduction of normal muscle-precursor cells into dystrophic muscle cells and the direct delivery of a functional dystrophin gene into dystrophic muscle cells. It is hoped that these studies will lead to a cure for the disease.

In the meantime, muscular dystrophy continues to cause human suffering and to cost victims, their families, and society large sums of money. The disease is publicized on an annual basis via efforts to raise money for research and treatment, but there is little publicity on an ongoing basis. For these reasons, muscular dystrophy remains an important medical problem in contemporary society.

—L. Fleming Fallon, Jr., M.D., Ph.D., M.P.H.;
updated by Karen E. Kalumuck, Ph.D.

See also Connective tissue; Genetic counseling; Genetic diseases; Genetics and inheritance; Hypertrophy; Muscle sprains, spasms, and disorders; Muscles; Pediatrics; Physical rehabilitation; Screening.

FOR FURTHER INFORMATION:

Beers, Mark H., et al., eds. *The Merck Manual of Diagnosis and Therapy.* 18th ed. Whitehouse Station, N.J.: Merck Research Laboratories, 2006. The more common forms of muscular dystrophy are discussed in clear, relatively nontechnical language. The entries are brief and succinct. This work is useful for an overview of muscular dystrophy; the more unusual and rarer forms of muscular dystrophy are not included.

Behrman, Richard E., Robert M. Kliegman, and Hal B. Jenson, eds. *Nelson Textbook of Pediatrics.* 18th ed. Philadelphia: Saunders/Elsevier, 2007. The forms of muscular dystrophy found in children are discussed in a logical and complete format. Pictures clearly depict the difficulties in movement experienced by victims of Duchenne muscular dystrophy.

Brown, Susan S., and Jack A. Lucy, eds. *Dystrophin: Gene, Protein, and Cell Biology.* New York: Cambridge University Press, 1997. This compilation of the latest research into the causes of muscular dystrophy at the molecular level is suitable for the nonspecialist with an introductory background in biology, as well as the specialist and clinician dealing with patients and their families affected by the disorder.

Emery, Alan E. H. *Muscular Dystrophy: The Facts.* 2d ed. New York: Oxford University Press, 2000. Covers all aspects of the disease in a question-answer format.

Goldman, Lee, and Dennis Ausiello, eds. *Cecil Textbook of Medicine.* 23d ed. Philadelphia: Saunders/Elsevier, 2007. The descriptions of muscular dystrophy are clear and detailed. The language used in the book is precise. Using multiple authors, each section is written by an internationally recognized expert.

Kumar, Vinay, Abul K. Abbas, and Nelson Fausto, eds. *Robbins and Cotran Pathologic Basis of Disease.* 8th ed. Philadelphia: Saunders/Elsevier, 2010. A complete discussion about the pathology of several forms of muscular dystrophy. Technical language is employed, but the book is well written. Photographs of microscopic sections of muscle are included, as well as descriptions of the clinical course of muscular dystrophy.

Tierney, Lawrence M., Stephen J. McPhee, and Maxine A. Papadakis, eds. *Current Medical Diagnosis and Treatment 2007.* New York: McGraw-Hill Medical, 2006. In a brief and concise format, the diagnosis and management of muscular dystrophy are discussed. The section authors are recognized experts in their fields. Treatment protocols are included.

Wolfson, Penny. *Moonrise: One Family, Genetic Identity, and Muscular Dystrophy.* New York: St. Martin's Press, 2003. A personal memoir of a mother and her son, who suffers from Duchenne muscular dystrophy, which details the early days of her son's life, the diagnosis, and the impact on her family. Questions about scientific advances and their implications, special education, giftedness, prenatal testing, and familial genetic links are covered in the narrative.

MUTATION

BIOLOGY

ANATOMY OR SYSTEM INVOLVED: Cells, immune system

SPECIALTIES AND RELATED FIELDS: Cytology, genetics, pathology

DEFINITION: An error in the process that copies genetic information for each new generation, resulting in an alteration in the organism that can be beneficial, harmful, or neutral.

KEY TERMS:

alleles: alternate forms of a gene; each person has two alleles of each gene, and these alleles may be the same or different; a person inherits one allele from each parent

chromosomes: the parts of a cell that contain genetic information, made of DNA covered with protein; each human cell has twenty-three pairs of chromosomes

deoxyribonucleic acid (DNA): a long, spiral-shaped molecule that makes up the bulk of chromosomes; the sequence of subunits contains the genetic information of the cell and organism

gene: the basic unit of inheritance; at the molecular level, a gene consists of a segment of DNA that codes for a particular protein

genotype: the genetic makeup of an individual; it is usually expressed as a list of alleles

heterozygous: having two different alleles for a particular gene

homozygous: having two identical alleles of a particular gene

meiosis: a special kind of cell division whereby four cells are produced; each cell has only half of the original number of chromosomes; meiosis produces the sex cells (eggs and sperm)

nucleotides: the subunits from which DNA is made

THE FUNCTION OF GENES

An individual is not a random assortment of characteristics. The way individuals look, their physiological makeup, their susceptibility to disease, and even how long they may live are determined by information re-

ceived from their parents. The smallest unit of information for inherited characteristics is the gene. For each characteristic, an individual has two copies of the gene controlling that characteristic. The gene can have two forms, called alleles. For example, the alleles for eye color can be designated using the letters B and b, with the B allele carrying the information for brown eyes and the b allele specifying blue eyes. Thus the genotype, or genetic makeup, of an individual can be one of three types: BB, bb, or Bb. A BB individual will have brown eyes. A bb person will have blue eyes. A Bb individual will have brown eyes since the brown allele is dominant over the blue one. The dominant allele will always be expressed, whether present as two copies or only one. For a recessive allele to be expressed, an individual must have two recessive alleles (bb).

When a person reproduces, he or she passes on one allele for each gene to the child. Therefore, the child also has two alleles for each gene, one from each parent. A person with two identical alleles for a given gene is said to be homozygous for that trait and can pass on only one kind of allele. Someone with two different alleles for a particular gene is said to be heterozygous. A heterozygous person will pass on the dominant allele to 50 percent of his or her children, on average; the other 50 percent will receive the recessive allele. Alleles are passed on in the sex cells—the eggs and sperm. Eggs and sperm are produced by a special type of cell division, meiosis, that reduces by half the amount of genetic information carried by the cell. When an egg is fertilized by a sperm cell, the amount of genetic information is once again doubled. In "normal" cell division, called mitosis, the amount of genetic material in each cell is kept constant. After fertilization, the egg cell divides repeatedly by mitosis to produce the millions of cells that make up the embryo and later the adult organism.

If the genetic makeup of a couple for a given trait is known, the probable characteristics of their children for this trait can be predicted. For example, one can predict the eye color for children of a brown-eyed husband and blue-eyed wife. Assuming that the husband comes from a family of only brown-eyed people, one can be fairly certain that he is homozygous for this trait (BB). Since his wife has blue eyes, and blue is recessive, she must be homozygous for the other allele (bb). Their children will each have a brown allele from their father and a blue allele from their mother; they will all be heterozygous (Bb). Since brown is dominant, they will all have brown eyes.

FIGURE 1. A PUNNETT SQUARE SHOWING ALLELES FOR EYE COLOR

Father's Sperm Cells

		B	b
Mother's Egg Cells	b	Bb	bb
	b	Bb	bb

FIGURE 2. A PUNNETT SQUARE SHOWING ALLELES FOR HEIGHT

Father's Sperm Cells

		T	t
Mother's Egg Cells	T	TT	Tt
	t	Tt	tt

One can take this example a step further and predict the outcome for the next generation. If one of this couple's brown-eyed sons marries a blue-eyed woman, then one can predict the eye colors of their children using a simple diagram called a Punnett square. (Reginald Crundall Punnett contributed much to the early study of genetics.)

Using this simple tool, with the possible alleles in the sperm cells along the top and those from the eggs down the side, one can show all the possible combinations of inherited alleles (see figure 1). These boxes represent the genotypes of the fertilized eggs. In this case, one would expect about half of their children to have brown eyes (the Bb boxes) and half to have blue eyes (the bb boxes). Since chance determines exactly which sperm actually fertilizes the egg in every conception event, however, such a prediction is not always accurate. Nevertheless, the more children they have, the closer the actual percentage of brown-eyed or blue-eyed children will come to half.

Actually, the inheritance of eye color is somewhat more complicated than it is described above. Several genes contribute to eye color. Depending on the mix of dominant and recessive alleles for each gene involved, eye color can range from pale blue to dark brown. Other combinations produce green eyes.

In addition, many genes do not show complete dominance. For example, evidence shows that height is controlled by several genes that exhibit incomplete dominance. One homozygous individual (TT) will be tall, the other (tt) will be short, and the heterozygous individual (Tt) will be of medium height. The laws that determine how the alleles may be passed on from generation to generation, however, are exactly the same. One can use a simplified example of two people who are heterozygous for a hypothetical height gene (see figure 2).

Since both parents are heterozygous, each will be able to produce two kinds of sex cells, those with "tall" alleles and those with "short" alleles. From all the possible outcomes shown in the boxes of the Punnett square, one would predict 25 percent tall (TT), 25 percent short (tt), and 50 percent medium-height (Tt) children.

If several genes are involved, a wide range of heights is possible. A person who is homozygous for the "tall" alleles in most of the height genes will be very tall. Someone homozygous for most of the "short" alleles will be short. Someone who is heterozygous in most of these genes will be of medium height. Since even relatively short people will have some "tall" alleles, and since chance determines which sex cells are actually used, it is possible for two short people to have a tall child: By chance, the egg and sperm that united had more than the usual share of "tall" alleles.

The preceding examples have used genes that have only two alleles: brown or blue, tall or short. There are genes, however, for which more than two alleles are possible—although any one individual may have only two alleles in his or her genetic makeup. A good example of such a gene is the one that controls human blood type. There are three blood type alleles: A, B, and O. The A and B alleles are dominant, while the O allele is recessive. This allows for the various types of blood (see table on the following page).

This table allows one to see the mechanism of dominance. A person with an A allele produces a particular chemical in the blood. Similarly, the B allele causes the production of a different chemical. The O allele produces no chemical at all. If a chemical not already present in the blood is introduced, such as in a blood transfusion, the body will react against it, destroying the new blood. Since people with type O blood produce

THE RELATIONSHIP BETWEEN GENOTYPE AND BLOOD TYPE

Genotype	Blood Type	Comments
AA AO	A A	These two genotypes produce identical blood types.
BB BO	B B	These two genotypes produce identical blood types.
AB	AB	Both dominant alleles are expressed.
OO	O	With no dominant alleles, the recessive allele is expressed.

neither chemical, they are sometimes referred to as "universal donors." Their blood can be given safely to anyone. Similarly, people with AB blood can receive any other blood type because their bodies already contain both types of chemical.

One can also use a blood type example to show how parents can produce children who are genetically unlike both parents. The mother has type A blood and is heterozygous (AO), while the father has type B blood and is also heterozygous (BO). Their child could have any of the four blood types (see figure 3).

Although blood type is not an obvious visible feature, many genes that express themselves in an individual's appearance behave in a similar manner. Therefore, one should not be surprised to see two parents with a child who resembles neither of them.

FIGURE 3. A PUNNETT SQUARE SHOWING ALLELES FOR BLOOD TYPE

		Father's Sperm Cells	
		B	O
Mother's Egg Cells	A	AB (AB blood)	AO (A blood)
	O	BO (B blood)	OO (O blood)

The genes that control heredity actually consist of strands of deoxyribonucleic acid (DNA) that make up the chromosomes. Humans have twenty-three pairs of chromosomes in each cell. This explains how an individual can have two alleles for each gene, one on each chromosome of a pair. The exception is the sex chromosomes, which are different in males and females. Sex chromosomes come in two kinds, a relatively large X and a small Y. The X chromosomes can carry many more genes than the Y. Females have two X chromosomes and thus have two alleles for every gene found on the X chromosome. Males have only one X chromosome; therefore, they only have one allele for those genes carried on the X. The Y chromosome of the male has been shown to carry very little, although important, genetic information. Genes carried on the X chromosome are called sex-linked, since they typically are expressed in only one sex—the male. Females may be merely carriers of a sex-linked trait.

One sex-linked trait is the disorder called hemophilia. A hemophiliac fails to produce a chemical that allows the blood to clot. This disorder is usually fatal if the hemophiliac is not constantly supplied with the clotting factor. Such an individual would simply bleed to death following even the slightest injury. Suppose that a woman who carries the trait for hemophilia marries a man who does not have the disorder. Hemophilia is a recessive condition; therefore, the woman has one normal X chromosome and one bearing the recessive allele (denoted by Xh). Since the normal allele directs the production of the clotting factor, her blood can clot and she is perfectly normal. Since her husband is not a hemophiliac, his one X chromosome must bear the normal allele. One can use a Punnett square to predict the likelihood of their children inheriting the disease (see figure 4 on the following page). From this figure, one can see that their daughters should all be normal. About half of them will be carriers for the trait, but there is no way of knowing which ones they are. Of the sons, one half will be normal and the other half will suffer from hemophilia.

HOW MUTATIONS OCCUR

There is a variety of genetic information in the human population, leading to a diversity of internal and external features. The process of sexual reproduction randomly selects among that variety for each new individ-

FIGURE 4. A PUNNETT SQUARE SHOWING ALLELES FOR HEMOPHILIA

		Father's Sperm Cells	
		X	Y
Mother's Egg Cells	X	XX Normal Girl	XY Normal Boy
	X_h	XX_h Normal Girl (carrier)	X_hY Hemophiliac Boy

ual who is born. Mutation is the process that created the variety originally, and it can continue to add to it today.

A human being begins as a single fertilized cell. That cell contains two copies of the genetic information in its twenty-three pairs of chromosomes. The cell divides constantly during growth and development to produce the millions of cells that make up an adult. Each one of those cells, with very few exceptions, also has twenty-three pairs of chromosomes. In order for each cell to have its own double copy of information, the DNA that makes up the chromosomes must replicate, once for each cell division. This process of replication must ensure that the information contained in the DNA is copied exactly, and for the most part, it is.

To understand how a mistake can occur, one must look at the structure of DNA, the genetic blueprint. The DNA molecule resembles a spiral staircase. The outside rails are strings of sugar molecules hooked together by phosphate groups. The steps are made of bases that project from each sugar-phosphate backbone toward the middle. The information is contained in the sequence of base pairs that make up the steps of the staircase. The bases that can form such a pair are determined by their shape and bonding properties. Of the four bases, only two pairs are possible. Adenine (A) always pairs with thymine (T), leaving cytosine (C) and guanine (G) to form the other pair. This structure explains the accuracy with which DNA replicates. During replication, the original molecule unwinds from its spiral structure. The two strands separate, and a new complementary strand forms on each of the original strands. The order of bases on the new strand is determined by the original strand and the base-pairing rules. Where

there is an A in the old strand, there must be a T in the new one. The other bases will not fit because they do not have the correct shape or bonding properties. Similarly, where the old strand has a C, the new one must have a G. Each base is attached to a deoxyribose sugar and a phosphate group, all three forming a nucleotide. Once all proper nucleotides are linked together, the new strand is complete, the original DNA is rewound, and there are two molecules where there once was one.

The accuracy with which the DNA template is copied is impressive. It has been estimated that an error occurs only once for every 100,000 nucleotides copied. The replication of DNA is a chemical process that relies on random movements of molecules to put the correct ones together. There are enzymatic systems to make sure that only the correct nucleotides end up as part of the new DNA strand. There are also error detection and correction mechanisms that can remove an incorrect nucleotide and replace it with the correct one. This correction process reduces the error rate to one in 10 billion. Nevertheless, with the amount of DNA that has to be copied, mistakes do occur. If a mistake is made in a gamete (sperm or egg cell), the mutated DNA can be passed on to future generations.

The mistake will not be detected until the section of DNA that contains it is actually used by the cell to make a specific protein molecule. At the molecular level, a gene is a section of DNA that has the information necessary to make a particular protein molecule. Proteins are the working molecules of the body: They make up flesh and bone and the enzymes that speed up chemical reactions. The sequence of bases on a DNA molecule codes for the sequence of amino acids that makes up a protein molecule. Since there are twenty commonly used amino acids, and a protein can contain thousands of amino acids, there is an almost infinite number of different protein molecules. A mutation on a DNA molecule will usually mean that one amino acid in the protein for which it codes is changed.

Changing one unit in a thousand may not seem very significant, and usually it is not. Such a small change in a protein molecule generally has very little effect on the functioning of that molecule. Perhaps this mutation will make the molecule able to withstand a slightly higher temperature before breaking down. If the protein is an enzyme, the change may speed or slow its reaction time by a little bit. During human evolution, an individual may have been able to live slightly longer if the mutated protein was slightly improved in function. The longer that he or she lived, the greater was the chance that the individual could produce offspring—who would also have the mutated gene. In this way, positive, useful mutations became more common in the population. A change that made the protein less functional was less likely to be reproduced since the individual possessing the mutation may not have lived long enough to have children.

A slight change in a protein can make a very big difference. The hemoglobin (the oxygen-carrying protein in red blood cells) of a person with sickle cell disease differs from normal hemoglobin by one amino acid. The amino acid, however, is in a critical position. With the changed amino acid, the hemoglobin clumps uselessly in the cell and does not carry oxygen. This is a lethal mutation, as a person afflicted with sickle cell disease cannot live very long. One would assume that this mutation would not survive in the human population. Yet, in some parts of Africa, the mutant allele is carried by as much as 20 percent of the black population. To understand how this can be, one must consider the heterozygous individual. With one normal allele and one mutant one, such an individual makes both kinds of hemoglobin, including enough normal hemoglobin to be able to live comfortably under normal conditions. Moreover, the presence of the altered hemoglobin confers significant resistance to malaria. Because the heterozygous individual has a selective advantage over the other two genotypes, this mutant allele not only has been maintained but even has increased in the black population in Africa.

PERSPECTIVE AND PROSPECTS

The modern study of genetics is conducted mostly at the molecular level. One project has identified every human gene and its location on a specific chromosome. Dubbed the Human Genome Project, it was a cooperative venture among scientists worldwide. This map tells researchers where each gene is located, and it is hoped that the defective copies in people with genetic diseases can be repaired using this knowledge. Genetic engineering techniques have already isolated many genes. For example, the gene for the production of insulin has been identified and extracted from human cells in culture. The gene has been inserted into the chromosomes of bacteria, and the bacteria are then grown in large quantities in commercial cultures. The insulin that they produce is harvested, purified, and made available to diabetics. This genuine human insulin is more potent than the insulin extracted from animals. In addition, such a process is essential for diabetics who suffer adverse reactions to the inevitable impurities that are found in insulin extracted from animals.

Ultimately, it should be possible to insert a functioning gene, like the one for insulin, directly into an afflicted person's chromosomes—thus curing the genetic disease. The cured individual, however, would still be able to pass the defective allele on to his or her children. The possibility of splicing genes into the chromosomes of sex cells does not seem likely in the near future.

More traditional genetics is also of value to prospective parents. A woman with a history of hemophilia in her family would want to know the chances that her children could inherit the disease. A genetic counselor would analyze the family tree of the woman and calculate a statistical probability. Some other genetic diseases can be detected in a fetus still in the womb. For example, a condition called phenylketonuria (PKU) can cause severe mental retardation and other medical problems. A genetic analysis of prospective parents with a family history of the condition could indicate the likelihood of PKU occurring in their children. If the chances are high, cells of the couple's child can be extracted and tested early in pregnancy. In the case of PKU, early detection can be used to prevent the effects of the disease. If the diet of the mother and then the newborn are carefully regulated, the toxic chemical that causes the disease will not accumulate in the fetus or newborn.

Genetic mutations have not stopped occurring in modern society. In fact, they are more likely. Many environmental factors have been shown to increase the mutation rate in animals. Several types of radiation and many chemicals can increase the mutation rate. This is why an X-ray technician will place a lead apron over the abdomen of a patient being X-rayed. Lead prevents the X rays from penetrating to the genital organs, where actively dividing DNA is particularly sensitive to the radiation. Such care should always be taken to protect the genetic makeup of future generations.

—*James Waddell, Ph.D.*

See also Bacteriology; Biostatistics; Cancer; Carcinogens; DNA and RNA; Embryology; Environmental diseases; Environmental health; Genetic counseling; Genetic diseases; Genetic engineering; Genetics and inheritance; Genomics; Microbiology; Oncology; Pathology; Radiation sickness; Screening.

FOR FURTHER INFORMATION:

Campbell, Neil A., et al. *Biology: Concepts and Connections.* 6th ed. San Francisco: Pearson/Benjamin Cummings, 2008. Chapters cover classical and molecular genetics, respectively. The text is accessible, and the many diagrams are useful.

Lewin, Benjamin. *Genes IX*. 9th rev. ed. Sudbury, Mass.: Jones and Bartlett, 2008. A college textbook that discusses the entire field of molecular biology and genetics, with many references to the structure and activity of the cell nucleus. Although written at the college level, it is readable and accessible to a general audience. Many highly informative illustrations and diagrams are included.

Lewis, Ricki. *Human Genetics: Concepts and Applications*. 9th ed. Dubuque, Iowa: McGraw-Hill, 2009. A very accessible undergraduate text that covers the fundamentals, transmission genetics, DNA and chromosomes, and the latest genetic technology, among other topics.

Radman, Mirislav, and Robert Wagner. "The High Fidelity of DNA Duplication." *Scientific American* 259 (August, 1988): 40-46. Provides a readable account of the "proofreading" and error-correcting mechanisms that make mutations so rare. The author is careful to point out what is fact and what is speculation. The bibliography refers the reader to more technical articles on the subject.

Rusting, Ricki L. "Why Do We Age?" *Scientific American* 267 (December, 1992): 130-135. A review of contemporary research into the genetics of aging. Evidence is presented for the presence of genes that determine how long animals and humans may expect to live.

Stahl, Franklin W. "Genetic Recombination." *Scientific American* 256 (February, 1987): 90-101. This article describes how genes are constantly shuffled to make new genetic combinations for each generation. This process occurs when chromosomes exchange pieces during the cell divisions that produce the sex cells.

MYASTHENIA GRAVIS

DISEASE/DISORDER

ANATOMY OR SYSTEM AFFECTED: Immune system, musculoskeletal system, nervous system

SPECIALTIES AND RELATED FIELDS: Immunology, neurology

DEFINITION: A disorder characterized by selective muscle fatigue following repeated use; it is caused by an abnormal immune reaction to specific receptors on the muscle surface.

KEY TERMS:

acetylcholine: a chemical released by motor neuron terminals; it causes muscle contraction

acetylcholine receptor: a protein on the surface of muscle cells; binding of acetylcholine to this receptor causes muscle cells to contract

acetylcholinesterase: an enzyme that degrades acetylcholine

antibody: a protein produced by the immune system to inactivate substances detected as foreign

autoimmune disease: a disorder in which the immune system targets proteins that are normal components of body tissues

thymus: a gland located at the base of the neck; part of the immune system

CAUSES AND SYMPTOMS

Myasthenia gravis is a neuromuscular disorder characterized by weakness of skeletal muscles following repeated use. The prevalence of the disease in the United States is approximately 14 in 100,000. It occurs in both genders of all ethnic groups, and the average age of onset is under forty for women and over sixty for men.

Normally, body movements result from the contraction of skeletal muscles, which are voluntary muscles attached to bone. These muscles are stimulated to contract by motor neurons in the brain and spinal cord. Nerve impulses travel down the motor neurons to their terminals, where a small amount of a substance known as a neurotransmitter is released onto the muscle's surface. In this case, the neurotransmitter is the chemical acetylcholine. When acetylcholine binds to specific receptors on the muscle surface, contraction results.

In myasthenia gravis, an autoimmune disease, the patient's immune system fails to recognize the acetylcholine receptors on skeletal muscle as part of "self"; thus, antibodies are erroneously produced against these receptors. Antibody binding to acetylcholine receptors causes the total number of functional receptors to be reduced because they are internalized and degraded by the muscle cells. With fewer remaining receptors, the muscle's contractile response is weakened.

The root cause of this aberrant immune response remains unknown. The thymus, a gland involved in immune function, is abnormal in about 75 percent of patients with the disease. Two distinct thymic anomalies may occur in myasthenia gravis: One of these is thymic hyperplasia (an increase in the number of certain immune cells in the thymus) or thymoma (a thymic tumor). In some late-onset cases of myasthenia gravis, however, the thymus appears normal or even shrunken—yet these cases are also accompanied by elevated levels of antibodies recognizing acetylcholine

Information on Myasthenia Gravis

Causes: Autoimmune disorder in which immune system fails to recognize muscle receptors as "self"

Symptoms: Weakness of muscles following repeated use, resulting in visual disorders, difficulty chewing and swallowing, slurred speech, limb weakness, breathing difficulties; in most cases, abnormal thymus gland

Duration: Chronic, usually progressive

Treatments: Alleviation of symptoms; may include medications (neostigmine, prednisone, azathioprine), surgery (removal of thymus), plasma exchange

receptors. Such inconsistencies are part of the reason that the relationship between the thymus and myasthenia gravis is not fully understood.

Skeletal muscle weakness is a symptom common to all forms of myasthenia gravis. Because this weakness is exacerbated with muscle use, it is not surprising that the first muscles to be affected are those used most often. Thus, the earliest signs of the disease often involve the muscles of the eye, including drooping of the eyelids and double vision. As other muscle groups become affected, advancing symptoms may include difficulty in chewing and swallowing, slurred speech, limb weakness, and breathing difficulties. Although symptoms are highly variable from patient to patient, they often fluctuate in severity with a similar daily pattern: Weakness is usually more pronounced in the evening than in the morning. Factors other than exertion that can provoke symptoms include viral illness, excitement, elevated temperature, menses, and pregnancy.

Although the long-term course of the disease can vary, it is usually progressive. In a minority of patients, weakness affects only the eye muscles. In other cases, progression is often most rapid within the first three years and may be punctuated with spontaneous temporary remissions. Treatment can help keep the symptoms under control.

Early symptoms are not always recognized as being linked to myasthenia gravis. A definitive diagnosis includes testing for the presence of antibodies that bind acetylcholine receptors. In addition, impaired nerve-muscle communication should be demonstrated in the form of specific muscle weakness elicited by repetitive

nerve stimulation. Finally, it should be shown that muscle weakness is briefly relieved following the administration of edrophonium. This drug blocks the breakdown of acetylcholine, temporarily increasing the amount of the neurotransmitter available to act on muscle receptors.

Treatment and Therapy

Several treatment options have been developed with the goal of symptomatic control of myasthenia gravis. Treatment must be individually tailored depending on disease history and severity. Therapies include medications, surgery, and plasma exchange.

To improve neuromuscular transmission, drugs can be given to inhibit the action of acetylcholinesterase, the naturally occurring enzyme that degrades acetylcholine, thus prolonging the availability of acetylcholine so that its contractile effect is enhanced. Such drugs include neostigmine. Another pharmacological approach is to suppress the immune system with drugs such as prednisone and azathioprine; as a result, the production of abnormal antibodies is reduced.

Thymectomy, the surgical removal of the thymus, is commonly recommended as a treatment for myasthenia gravis. In general, this procedure is considered the most effective approach for obtaining sustained relief or remission. Maximum postsurgical improvement may take several years to occur, and results are usually best in younger patients early in their disease.

Plasma exchange is used as an immediate intervention to combat the sudden onset of severe symptoms such as respiratory failure, or in cases where the patient has not responded to other treatments. In this procedure, abnormal antibodies are removed from the blood plasma.

Perspective and Prospects

Myasthenia gravis was first described by the British physician Thomas Willis in 1685. Although relatively rare, it was the first neurological disease to be identified as having an autoimmune basis. The understanding of the disease was aided by converging research among neurophysiologists, neurologists, and immunologists; as such, these combined approaches have helped to elucidate other autoimmune diseases.

Although patients undergoing treatment for myasthenia gravis can expect a normal life span marked by significant improvement of their symptoms, as of 2003 there was no cure for the disease. Research is aimed at gaining a better understanding of the factors triggering the autoimmune response in myasthenia gravis, elucidating the relationship between the thymus and the disease, and fully understanding the molecular basis of normal and aberrant nerve-muscle transmission. This research should guide developments in treatment strategy, with a key goal being to cure the immune abnormality that underlies the disease.

—*Mary A. Nastuk, Ph.D.*

See also Autoimuune disorders; Electromyography; Glands; Immune system; Immunology; Immunopathology; Muscle sprains, spasms, and disorders; Muscles; Muscular dystrophy; Thymus gland.

FOR FURTHER INFORMATION:

Icon Health. *Myasthenia Gravis: A Medical Dictionary, Bibliography, and Annotated Research Guide to Internet References.* San Diego, Calif.: Author, 2004.

Kaminski, Henry J., ed. *Myasthenia Gravis and Related Disorders.* Totowa, N.J.: Humana Press, 2003.

Kasper, Dennis L., et al., eds. *Harrison's Principles of Internal Medicine.* 16th ed. New York: McGraw-Hill, 2005.

Vincent, Angela. "Unravelling the Pathogenesis of Myasthenia Gravis." *Nature Reviews Immunology* 2 (October, 2002): 797-804.

MYOCARDIAL INFARCTION. *See* HEART ATTACK.

MYOMECTOMY
PROCEDURE

ANATOMY OR SYSTEM AFFECTED: Reproductive system, uterus

SPECIALTIES AND RELATED FIELDS: Gynecology

DEFINITION: The removal of a uterine myoma, also known as a fibroid or leiomyoma.

INDICATIONS AND PROCEDURES

The most common indication for a myomectomy is the need to remove a symptomatic fibroid. In many cases, these fibroids are large (greater than 8 centimeters). A myomectomy is chosen over a hysterectomy (removal of the uterus) if the patient desires future childbearing and if there is no evidence of malignancy of the uterus. A myomectomy can be performed using abdominal, laparoscopic, vaginal, or hysteroscopic approaches. The choice of approach depends on the location and size of the fibroids, as well as on the experience of the surgeon.

The most common type is abdominal myomectomy. This procedure is performed in the operating room with the patient under general anesthesia. The abdomen is incised and entry into the pelvic cavity is obtained. The uterus is then identified and inspected for fibroids. Some surgeons apply a tourniquet to the uterine arteries for hemostasis. A vasocontrictive agent is injected into the myometrium surrounding the fibroid to minimize blood loss. The myometrium over the fibroid is then incised, and the fibroid is dissected out. Finally, the myometrial defect is closed with a suture to stop blood flow. In patients desiring fertility, care is taken to minimize entry into the endometrial cavity, as the procedure may increase the risk of uterine rupture with pregnancy.

In laparoscopic and vaginal myomectomies, access to the fibroids is obtained using endoscopic instruments and through an incision in the vagina, respectively. In hysteroscopic myomectomies, access to fibroids in the endometrial cavity is obtained using a hysteroscope inserted through the cervical canal. The hysteroscope holds an instrument that shaves away fibroids in the endometrial cavity.

USES AND COMPLICATIONS

The primary use of myomectomy is the relief of symptoms caused by fibroids. These symptoms can be any of the following: pressure sensation, pelvic pain, dyspareunia (painful intercourse), menorrhagia (excessive menstruation), dysmenorrhea (painful menstruation), urinary urgency or frequency, urinary incontinence, and constipation.

The short-term risks of abdominal myomectomies are the same as those for most pelvic surgeries. These risks are small but include infection, damage to internal organs such as the bowel or bladder, blood loss requiring transfusion, and complications from anesthesia. Long-term consequences include an increased risk of uterine rupture with future pregnancy, the recurrence of fibroid growth, and pelvic adhesion (scar tissue) formation. Laparoscopic myomectomies are less invasive than abdominal myomectomies, but the same short-term and long-term risks are present. Hysteroscopic myomectomies carry less risks than abdominal procedures, since no incision is made on the abdomen and there is no entry into the pelvic cavity, but the risks unique to hysteroscopy exist, such as uterine perforation and fluid overload.

—*Anne Lynn S. Chang, M.D.*

See also Dysmenorrhea; Genital disorders, female; Gynecology; Hysterectomy; Menorrhagia; Menstruation; Muscles; Reproductive system; Tumor removal; Tumors; Uterus; Women's health.

FOR FURTHER INFORMATION:

Bieber, Eric J., and Victoria M. Maclin, eds. *Myomectomy*. Malden, Mass.: Blackwell Science, 1998.

Falcone, T., and M. A. Bedaiwy. "Minimally Invasive Management of Uterine Fibroids." *Current Opinion in Obstetrics and Gynecology* 14, no. 4 (August, 2002): 401-407.

Rock, John A., and Howard W. Jones III, eds. *Te Linde's Operative Gynecology*. 10th ed. Philadelphia: Wolters Kluwer/Lippincott Williams & Wilkins, 2008.

Stenchever, Morton A., et al. *Comprehensive Gynecology*. 4th ed. St. Louis, Mo.: Mosby/Elsevier, 2006.

Tulandi, Togas, ed. *Uterine Fibroids: Embolization and Other Treatments*. New York: Cambridge University Press, 2003.

MYOPIA

DISEASE/DISORDER

ALSO KNOWN AS: Nearsightedness
ANATOMY OR SYSTEM AFFECTED: Eyes
SPECIALTIES AND RELATED FIELDS: Ophthalmology, optometry
DEFINITION: A visual defect that impairs the perception of distant objects.

CAUSES AND SYMPTOMS

Nearsightedness (myopia) occurs when light from distant objects reaches a focal point in front of the retina, the photoreceptive tissue of the eye. Consequently, vision of distant objects is blurred on the retina. The primary cause of myopia is an eyeball that is too long from front to back. Higher testosterone levels in the womb and a genetic predisposition have been advanced as possible causes of this condition. Research has also found that prolonged eyestrain, especially that which often accompanies long periods of reading, can distort the shape of the eye. This is one reason why well-educated people manifest higher rates of nearsightedness than less-educated individuals.

All children are born nearsighted; by the age of six months, however, vision begins to improve. Myopia is an uncommon problem in younger school-age children but begins to increase in prevalence as children move into their teenage years. From the twenties until the late sixties, the rate of visual deterioration tends to slow down. By the time people reach their seventies, however, the rate of visual decline accelerates again. People past the age of seventy are fourteen times as likely to experience myopia resulting in legal blindness as those in their twenties.

INFORMATION ON MYOPIA

CAUSES: Unknown; possibly higher testosterone levels in womb, genetic predisposition, prolonged eyestrain
SYMPTOMS: Impaired perception of distant objects
DURATION: Varies
TREATMENTS: Wearing concave lenses, correction through laser surgery

---

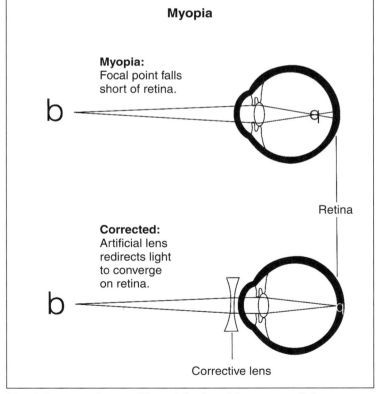

Myopia is commonly termed "nearsightedness" because most light rays entering the eye will not resolve, or focus, on the retina unless they are coming from a very near distance; corrective lenses or surgery can solve this problem.

Treatment and Therapy

For several centuries, nearsightedness has been corrected by the use of a concave lens, which moves the focal point of light in myopic eyes closer to the retina. The first evidence for the use of concave lenses is found in a 1517 painting of Pope Leo X by Italian artist Raphael. As the twentieth century drew to a close, innovative surgical approaches were developed. Most of these procedures, such as laser surgery, move the focal point of light closer to the retina by changing the shape of the cornea.

—*Paul J. Chara, Jr., Ph.D.*

See also Aging; Blurred vision; Cataracts; Glaucoma; Eye infections and disorders; Eye surgery; Eyes; Laser use in surgery; Ophthalmology; Optometry; Optometry, pediatric; Sense organs; Vision; Vision disorders.

For Further Information:

Buettner, Helmut, ed. *Mayo Clinic on Vision and Eye Health: Practical Answers on Glaucoma, Cataracts, Macular Degeneration, and Other Conditions.* Rochester, Minn.: Mayo Foundation for Medical Education and Research, 2002.

Icon Health. *Myopia: A Medical Dictionary, Bibliography, and Annotated Research Guide to Internet References.* San Diego, Calif.: Author, 2004.

National Foundation for Eye Research. http://www.nfer.org.

Riordan-Eva, Paul, and John P. Whitcher. *Vaughan and Asbury's General Ophthalmology.* 17th ed. New York: Lange Medical Books/McGraw-Hill, 2007.

Sutton, Amy L., ed. *Eye Care Sourcebook: Basic Consumer Health Information About Eye Care and Eye Disorders.* 3d ed. Detroit, Mich.: Omnigraphics, 2008.

Myringotomy

Procedure

Anatomy or system affected: Ears

Specialties and related fields: Family medicine, otorhinolaryngology

Definition: The creation of an opening in the eardrum (tympanic membrane) to allow drainage of accumulated fluid in the middle ear.

Indications and Procedures

Fluid can collect in the middle ear as a result of infection or allergy; this fluid consists of blood, pus, water, and debris. An ear, nose, and throat specialist may surgically insert small tubes into the middle ear to facilitate drainage. Usually, local anesthesia is administered, particularly if the patient is a young child.

This procedure, called myringotomy, is used to relieve pain caused by pressure and to prevent temporary or permanent hearing loss. Physiologically, the problem involves blockage of the Eustachian tube, a narrow canal that connects the middle ear to the back of the nasal cavity. This tube regulates air pressure in the middle-ear cavity, allowing the hearing mechanism to function properly and helping to maintain a sense of balance.

Prior to performing a myringotomy, medical treatment may involve the prescription of antihistamines, decongestants, and perhaps steroids, which usually reduce the swelling of the Eustachian tube and sometimes preclude a myringotomy. After the procedure, improvement in hearing is usually immediate, and the middle-ear infection should heal. Antibiotic eardrops may be prescribed; three or four drops should be placed in each ear twice a day for five days. In approximately six to twelve months, the myringotomy tube will be expelled into the outer ear canal automatically and can be removed by a physician. Treatment may include follow-up visits every two months.

Uses and Complications

Postoperatively, it is not unusual for the patient to experience a certain amount of pulsation, popping, clicking, and other sounds in the ear. It is important during the postoperative period to make certain that the patient does not get water in his or her ear, especially when the tube is in place. When washing the hair or face, cotton covered with petroleum jelly may be placed in the outer part of the ear. For long-term protection, earplugs may be used during showering, bathing, and swimming. Diving, deep swimming, and any other activities that may place pressure on the eardrum are not recommended.

—*John Alan Ross, Ph.D.*

See also Deafness; Ear infections and disorders; Ear surgery; Ears; Hearing; Hearing loss; Otorhinolaryngology; Surgery, pediatric.

For Further Information:

American Medical Association. *American Medical Association Family Medical Guide.* 4th rev. ed. Hoboken, N.J.: John Wiley & Sons, 2004.

Canalis, Rinaldo, and Paul R. Lambert, eds. *The Ear: Comprehensive Otology.* Philadelphia: Lippincott Williams & Wilkins, 2000.

Ferrari, Mario. *PDxMD Ear, Nose, and Throat Disorders*. Philadelphia: PDxMD, 2003.

Pender, Daniel J. *Practical Otology*. Philadelphia: J. B. Lippincott, 1992.

Sataloff, Robert T., and Joseph Sataloff. *Hearing Loss*. 4th ed. New York: Taylor & Francis, 2005.

Turkington, Carol, and Allen E. Sussman. *The Encyclopedia of Deafness and Hearing Disorders*. Rev. 2d ed. New York: Facts On File, 2004.

Woolf, Alan D., et al., eds. *The Children's Hospital Guide to Your Child's Health and Development*. Cambridge, Mass.: Perseus, 2002.

NAIL REMOVAL

PROCEDURE

ANATOMY OR SYSTEM AFFECTED: Feet, hands, nails

SPECIALTIES AND RELATED FIELDS: Emergency medicine, family medicine, internal medicine, pediatrics, podiatry, sports medicine

DEFINITION: The partial or total removal of either fingernails or toenails.

INDICATIONS AND PROCEDURES

Nail removal is one of the most common office procedures seen in primary care. Nail disorders leading to removal occur most often in toenails, but they can also occur in fingernails. Common reasons for removal are infection, ingrown nail, or trauma. Patients usually experience pain and inability to function in their normal activities. Rarely are there any systemic signs or symptoms such as fever, chills, or nausea, unless the cause is serious infection.

The patient's foot or hand is first cleansed and draped. Sterile techniques are used throughout the procedure. Patients undergoing partial or total nail removal require adequate anesthesia, which is usually done through a digital block. A digital block is performed at the base of the digit with lidocaine or similar anesthetic to numb the entire finger or toe. The provider should wait five minutes for the anesthesia to become effective. A tourniquet may be applied to minimize bleeding and enhance anesthesia. An instrument is then used to separate the nail from the nailbed with the least trauma possible. In a complete removal, the nail is then gently pulled away from the nailbed. In a partial removal, scissors are used to cut the desired amount of nail away from the intact nail. Some providers will also chemically destroy the nail matrix in the area of the partial removal to prevent recurrent ingrown nails, if clinically indicated. Compression for a few minutes may be needed to slow any bleeding from the nail removal. Topical antibiotic ointment may be applied with gauze and a compression dressing. When a toenail is removed, patients may walk immediately after the procedure and resume any activity as tolerated. Local wound care instructions are given, and, if the procedure is performed secondary to an infected digit, oral antibiotics may be ordered. The procedure usually takes approximately fifteen minutes to complete.

USES AND COMPLICATIONS

Partial nail removal or trimming may also be performed in diabetic patients or those unable to perform routine nail care. Fungal infections cannot be cured with nail removal.

Nail removal has few complications if performed properly. Pain is one of the most common complications of the procedure, especially if the digit was already infected. Bacterial infection may also occur after the procedure without proper wound care management. Bleeding may occur, as epinephrine is not used in digital blocks. Adequate compression or cautery usually stops any continued bleeding after the procedure. Patients must also be warned that the nail may not grow back with the same shape prior to removal. Nails should be cut straight across without curvature to prevent any ingrown nail recurrence.

—*Jeffrey R. Bytomski, D.O.*

See also Bacterial infections; Diabetes mellitus; Feet; Lower extremities; Nails; Podiatry; Upper extremities; Wounds.

FOR FURTHER INFORMATION:

Clark, Robert E., and Whitney D. Tope. "Nail Surgery." In *Cutaneous Surgery*, edited by Roland G. Wheeland. Philadelphia: W. B. Saunders, 1994.

Zuber, Thomas J. "Ingrown Toenail Removal." *American Family Physician* 65, no. 12 (June 15, 2002): 2547.

NAILS

ANATOMY

ANATOMY OR SYSTEM AFFECTED: Hands, feet, skin

SPECIALTIES AND RELATED FIELDS: Dermatology, histology

DEFINITION: The thin, horny plates covering the dorsal ends of the fingers or toes.

KEY TERMS:

cuticle: cutaneous or skin tissue that surrounds the nail plate on its proximal sides and provides a protective barrier to the nail bed; it is attached to the proximal nail fold and to the nail plate

hyponychium: cutaneous tissue underlying the free nail at its point of separation from the nail bed; structurally similar to the cuticle

keratinocytes: matrix basal epithelial cells that differentiate, fill with keratin, and form the dead horny substance making up the nail plate

lunula: a whitish, crescent-shaped area at the end of the proximal nail fold that marks the end of the nail matrix and is the site of mitosis and nail growth

onychomycosis: common nail disorder in which fungal organisms invade the nail bed causing progressive changes in the color, texture, and structure of the nail

STRUCTURE AND FUNCTIONS

Nails function to protect fingers and toes against bumps and trauma. Fine touch is amplified and skillful manipulation of small objects with the fingers is enabled by the presence of nails. Nails also provide the ability to scratch, both as a temporary relief of an itch or in personal defense. Nails are important social communicators of beauty and sexuality and hence are the focus of a major cosmetic industry.

Biologically, nails are characterized as plates of tightly packed, hard epidermis cells filled with a protein called keratin. Nails are normally seen on the dorsal side (the side opposite the palm or sole) of all fingers and toes. The anatomy of the normal nail consists of a nail plate, proximal nail fold, nail bed, matrix, and hyponychium. These components are epithelial derived structures, like skin and hair, which emerge from the live germinative zone of the epidermis. These cells differentiate and form the horny layer, which is considered to be dead.

The nail plate is a relatively hard and flat, transparent, horny structure that is rectangular in shape. It rests on the underlying nail bed but typically extends beyond the bed as an unattached, free-growing edge reaching beyond the tip of the finger or toe. In the fingers, the thickness of the plate in adults increases from the proximal edge to the distal edge from about 0.7 millimeter to 1.6 millimeters. The terminal tip thickness varies considerably between persons.

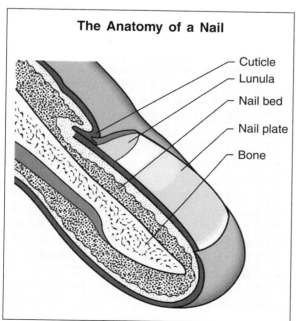

The Anatomy of a Nail

Cuticle

Lunula

Nail bed

Nail plate

Bone

Normally, a pinkish nail bed is seen through the transparent nail plate. Frequently in the thumb nail and sometimes in the other fingers, a whitish, semimoon-shaped structure called the lunula is seen that extends under the proximal nail fold. The borders of the nail plate are covered by skin structures: two lateral folds and a single proximal fold.

The proximal nail fold or the cuticle is the cutaneous or skin structure that is in continuity with the visible proximal border of the nail but overlies part of the nail root. The ventral side (underside) of the proximal nail fold provides physical protection to the germinative zone of the nail and aids in the physical attachment of the nail plate. About a fourth of the total surface area of the nail plate is located under the proximal fold. The cuticle is a layer of epidermis extending from the proximal nail fold and attached to the dorsal side of the nail. The cuticle functions to provide a physical seal against microbes and chemical irritants, which may otherwise enter the matrix and affect nail production.

The nail bed is the portion of the digit upon which the nail rests. The nail bed is highly vascular, with numerous capillaries, consists of epithelial tissue, and extends from the lunula to the point where the bed separates from the nail. A series of fine longitudinal folds in the nail bed corresponds to the undersurface structure of the nail. This arrangement enhances the adherence of the nail plate to the nail bed.

The nail matrix generally is considered the most proximal part of the nail bed and is bordered by the proximal nail fold. On the distal end it is bordered by the distal margin of the lunula. The nail matrix epithelium cells consist predominantly of keratinocytes in both a basal and spinous layer. Melanocytes and Langerhans' cells are intermingled with keratinocytes. It is within the matrix that the germinating center of nail growth is found. Basal epithelial cells increase in number through mitosis or division and then differentiate into keratinocytes, which are epithelial cells filled with keratin protein. These keratinocytes condense their cytoplasm, lose their nucleus, and form flat, horny-looking cells that are dead. As further cell division occurs in the nail matrix, the more distal keratinocytes are pushed out to form the nail plate.

The hyponychium consists of epidermis tissue that underlies the edge of the nail plate and extends from the nail bed to the distal groove. It functions to provide a defense against entry of bacteria under the free edge of the nail plate. Excessively vigorous cleaning may damage the hyponychium and allow for bacteria to enter more readily under the nail plate.

The turnover rate of matrix cells determines the growth rate of the nail. This rate varies with age, environmental conditions, nutritional status, and the specific digit. The growth rate proportionately increases with the length of the digit; thus the middle finger nail grows the fastest while the growth rate in the little finger is the slowest. Fingernails grow three times as rapidly as toenails. The growth rate is more rapid in the winter than in the summer. Furthermore, nails grow faster in young children than in older adults. It takes about six months for a fingernail to completely grow in. Male nails grow faster than female nails. Nails on the dominant hand grow faster than those on the other hand.

If nails are protected and untrimmed, they can grow to considerable lengths. Such long nails were prized by the wealthy classes in imperial Chinese culture as an indication of status. The practice of painting toenails red may have originated in the Ottoman seraglio, where it was a signal of menstrual status.

Nails continue to grow throughout life without a resting phase. Contrary to folk belief, nails cease growing when an individual dies. The matrix cells stop producing deoxyribonucleic acid (DNA) and dividing soon after death and thus the nail bed cannot grow longer. The appearance of nail growth after death is due to a retraction or shrinkage of nail matrix tissue, resulting in the apparent lengthening of the nail plate.

Professional grooming of the nails for both men and women is termed a manicure. Manicure procedures include cutting the nails according to fashion standards to improve their cosmetic appearance. A pedicure is the term applied to grooming the toenails. Typically, the nails are first soaked in a soapy solution to soften the nail plate and to remove dirt and debris. Currently it is fashionable to trim the nails to a delicate arc at the middle of the fingertip. The corners of the nail are typically filed. While this shape is attractive in creating the illusion of longer, slender fingers, it heightens the probability of nail plate fractures, hangnails, or ingrown nails. The cuticle, considered to be unattractive by manicurists, is typically minimized, partially removed, or traumatized. This may increase the incidence of fungal invasion and disease. Most of the problems associated with a manicure arise from excessive manipulation of the cuticle.

Nail polish typically consists of pigments suspended in a volatile solvent that also contains a film-forming agent. When the polish is applied to the finger, a covering film develops over the nail. The film is permeable to oxygen, which allows gas exchange to occur between the atmosphere and the nail plate. Resins and plasticizers are added to the polish to increase the flexibility of the film and to minimize chipping. The variety in nail polish color is due to the addition of coloring agents. Deep red nail polishes can cause a temporary yellowish staining of the nail plate.

Nail adornments are sometimes used. Frequently, small nail jewels or ribbons are applied to the fingernails immediately before the nail polish dries, allowing the decoration to adhere to the nail plate. Since some people frequently develop contact dermatitis to nickel, gold or nickel-free jewels should be selected. Artificial nail tips made of plastic also are glued to the nail tip to create the illusion of an elongated natural nail tip. The gluing may cause nail problems, since a portion of the natural nail is occluded by the glue. This occlusion inhibits oxygen transfer and stresses the nail plate. Frequently, the nail may thin and be unable to support its own weight after the plastic tip is removed. Removal of the plastic tip may result in nail pitting.

DISORDERS AND DISEASES

Nails are useful indicators of skin disease as well as of internal disorders. An abnormally pigmented band in the nail may indicate a malignant melanoma. A yellow nail may indicate psoriasis or a fungal infection. Pulmonary disease or smoking may also cause yellow or brownish nails. Antimalarial drugs may cause the nail to darken in appearance. Frequently, psoriasis causes pitting of nails and an acceleration in their growth rate. Chronic chest disease or a cyanotic congenital heart disorder is frequently associated with club-shaped deformity of the nail plate. Beau's lines, which are transverse depressions in the nail plates, are associated with illnesses such as coronary thrombosis, pneumonia, and severe injuries. Drug treatment may cause nail breakdown or destruction or complete shedding of the nail plate.

An unexplained aspect of nail physiology is its relationship to lung physiology. Hippocrates first described a connection between lung parenchymal disorders and an edema in the connective tissue beneath the lunula that results in clubbing. The relationship has long been recognized, but the causal link is still unexplained.

An ingrown nail results when a deformed nail grows improperly into the skin, or when the skin around the nails engulfs part of the nail. Wearing narrow, tight shoes can cause or worsen this pathology. Initially, symptoms may be slight or mild, but with time may come increasing pain. The affected area becomes reddish and, if not treated, may become infected. If infected, the area becomes swollen, inflamed, and painful. Blisters may develop. Treatment involves trimming away the nail from the infected area, allowing the inflammation to decline and the area to heal.

Clubbing is a disorder characterized by a bulblike enlargement of the nail with increased horizontal and longitudinal curvatures. Clubbing involves both fingers and toes and commonly begins at puberty. The disorder may be genetically inherited or acquired. Clubbed nails often have a spongy feel when pressure is placed on the proximal nail fold. This is due to the expanded soft tissue that underlies the nail. Acquired clubbing is often associated with another clinical pathology, most commonly pulmonary or cardiovascular disease. However, at times it is also associated with gastrointestinal inflammatory disease or cystic fibrosis.

A fungal infection is the cause of onychomycosis, which is the most common nail disorder. About half of all nail problems can be linked to this disease, which affects as many as 15 to 20 percent of people in North America. It is uncommon in children but more frequently seen in aged adults.

Several fungi may be the causal agents, although most belong to the group called dermatophytes. The fungi are present in soil, and indirect transmission to humans frequently occurs through public swimming pools and shower floors. Some yeasts and molds are also thought to cause this clinical condition. Alternatively, this infection is associated with athlete's foot infection. Typically this condition is found in toenails more frequently than fingernails. The presence of the fungus is furthered evidenced by scaling on the plantar surface of the foot, where it is often harbored.

In onychomycosis, the fungal organism invades the nail bed, causing a progressive change in the color, texture, and structure of the nail. The nail may turn white, thicken, and even detach from the nail bed. Debris from the infected nail often collects under its free edge. If untreated, the pathology may involve the entire nail plate, and rarely will the nail unit spontaneously heal itself.

Since several organisms may induce the pathology, effective treatment depends on matching the curative with the causal agent. Topically applied antifungals seldom are effective because most cannot penetrate the nail plate barrier to reach the causal organism. Systemically (orally) administered antifungal therapy frequently uses one of several drugs such as griseofulvin, thiabendazole, or ketoconazole. These drugs are generally effective in halting further invasion of the fungus. While treatment continues the new growing nail is usually normal. Thus treatment typically continues until the old nail is replaced by new nail, and then the treatment is discontinued.

More than seventy tumors associated with parts of the nail have been found. Their origins may be from the epidermis, dermis, subcutaneous tissues, or the bone. The tumors may be found in the nail bed, nail matrix, hyponychium, or nail fold. The tumors may take various forms such as warts, erosion or ulceration of the nail bed, malignant neoplasms from underlying melanocytes, benign fibromas of the connective tissue, or squamous cell carcinomas. Diagnosis usually is made by taking a biopsy of the affected area. Treatment typically involves surgical removal of the tumor.

Perspective and Prospects

The earliest cellular growth leading to nail formation can be seen histologically at eight weeks of human development, the end of the embryonic period. Microscopically, the cells forming the proximal edge of the nail field and the future matrix can be distinguished at this time. The earliest gross anatomical appearance of nails is seen on the finger digit surface at about nine weeks of development, the very early fetal stage. By eleven weeks of age, the nail field is seen clearly on the hand digits of the fetus. By twenty weeks of age, the fetus shows a nail plate and bed and a proximal cuticle. By thirty-two weeks, the third trimester of pregnancy, adult-type nail structures are visible in the fetus, including a nail plate, matrix, and bed and a forming hyponychium.

Aging results in changes and disorders in nails. When people get older the color, contour, growth rate, surface texture, and thickness of the nail plate change. Some disorders are more prevalent with aging, such as brittle nails, splitting or fissuring of the nail plate, and increased infections. Aged nails appear dull and opaque, with a color varying from yellow to gray. Frequently in older persons, the lunula is decreased in size or is absent. The growth rate of nails decreases with aging. The most rapid period of growth is during the first thirty years; thereafter the rate steadily declines. With older persons, the nail plate thickness frequently increases, paralleled with discoloration and a loss of translucency of the nail plate.

For many years, blood and urine specimens have been used to detect and measure body concentrations of therapeutic drugs or drugs of abuse. During the past decade, alternative biological specimens, nails and hair, have been frequently used as the basis for drug detection. The basis for drug detection in nail clippings is that the dividing epidermal cells that form the nail plate also incorporate drugs from the systemic circulation. The subsequent cornification of these cells traps the drug within the forming nail plate. Drug detection methods involve taking a sample of nail clippings, and extracting and identifying drug molecules by using immunochemical or chromatographic techniques that are extremely sensitive and capable of detecting minute quantities of drug in the samples. As little as ten milligrams of nail clippings is required to detect the presence of drugs. Twenty-first century drug screening methods have detected amphetamines and cocaine in nail clippings. Using nail clippings for drug analysis and screening provides a long-term measure of drug exposure that potentially may represent months of drug use. Furthermore, nail clippings are relatively easy to collect and involve a noninvasive procedure; samples are easily stored, and once incorporated in the nail tissue most of the drugs are presumably stable.

Modern medicine in the early twenty-first century still lacks adequate descriptive science as well as understanding of the molecular mechanisms that control nail development and growth. To date, the specific genes or gene products that initiate nail growth have not been identified. The molecular basis for brittle nails, clubbing, and other nail pathologies is not known. Is onychomycosis affected by a systemic immune deficit? What causes yellow nail syndrome? Answers to these questions as well as additional information about the molecular control of nail physiology will greatly increase understanding and lead to better treatments for nail disorders.

—*Roman J. Miller, Ph.D.*

See also Feet; Fungal infections; Lower extremities; Nail removal; Pulmonary diseases; Skin; Skin disorders; Upper extremities.

FOR FURTHER INFORMATION:

Baran, R., et al., eds. *Baran and Dawber's Diseases of the Nails and Their Management.* 3d ed. Malden, Mass.: Blackwell Science, 2001. Describes the normal physiology and pathology of nails. Superb color photographs vividly illustrate various nail diseases.

Du Vivier, Anthony. *Atlas of Clinical Dermatology.* 3d ed. Edinburgh: Churchill Livingstone, 2002. Along with a comprehensive survey of skin pathologies, this atlas also covers nail disorders.

Hordinsky, Maria K., Marty E. Sawaya, and Richard K. Scher, eds. *Atlas of Hair and Nails.* Philadelphia: Churchill Livingstone, 2000. This vividly illustrated atlas emphasizes nail disorders and special issues affecting nail physiology. Numerous colored photographs.

Mix, Godfrey F. *Salon Professional's Guide to Foot Care.* Clifton Park, N.Y.: Delmar, 1999. Written by a podiatrist for those in the beauty profession, making this an accessible guide to foot care and foot anatomy, including toenails.

Porter, Robert S., et al., eds. *The Merck Manual Home Health Handbook.* Whitehouse Station, N.J.: Merck Research Laboratories, 2009. This manual, written for home use, describes several common nail disorders. Symptoms, characteristics, and possible treatments are given.

Standring, Susan, et al., eds. *Gray's Anatomy.* 40th ed. New York: Churchill Livingstone/Elsevier, 2008. This classic anatomy text uses simple line drawings to illustrate the parts of a nail. The accompanying text accurately describes the parts of a nail and is well recognized as authoritative by health care professionals.

Zaias, Nardo. *The Nail in Health and Disease.* 2d ed. Norwalk, Conn.: Appleton & Lange, 1992. Describes in detail the anatomy and physiology of nails, specific disorders, and cosmetic care. Written for the health care professional, this well-illustrated text is also understandable for the average reader.

NARCOLEPSY

DISEASE/DISORDER

ANATOMY OR SYSTEM AFFECTED: Brain, nervous system, psychic-emotional system

SPECIALTIES AND RELATED FIELDS: Neurology

DEFINITION: An apparently inherited disorder of the nervous system characterized by brief, numerous, and overwhelming attacks of sleepiness throughout the day.

KEY TERMS:

cataplexy: brief periods of partial or total loss of skeletal muscle tone, usually triggered by emotional stimuli, which can cause the person to collapse

electroencephalogram (EEG): a recording of brain wave activity using electrodes attached to the scalp

excessive daytime sleepiness: a strong tendency to fall asleep, accompanied by reduced energy and lack of alertness during the entire day

hypnogogic hallucination: a bizarre, sometimes frightening, dreamlike occurrence just as one is falling asleep or just after waking

maintenance of wakefulness test: a polysomnographic technique to measure a person's ability to remain awake during repeated trials throughout the day

multiple sleep latency test: a polysomnographic technique to measure how quickly one falls asleep during repeated trials throughout the day

polysomnography: the continuous recording of brain waves, eye movements, skeletal muscle movements, and other body functions to determine bodily changes during the stages of sleep

REM sleep: a period of intense brain activity, often associated with dreams; named for the rapid eye movements that typically occur during this time

sleep paralysis: an inability to move voluntarily, occurring just at the beginning of sleep or upon awakening

---

INFORMATION ON NARCOLEPSY

CAUSES: Genetic factors

SYMPTOMS: Attacks of irresistible sleepiness in daytime, episodes of cataplexy, hypnogogic hallucinations, sleep paralysis, memory difficulties, eye fatigue, sleep apnea

DURATION: Chronic with acute episodes

TREATMENTS: Stimulant medications (dextroamphetamine, pemoline, Ritalin), tricyclic antidepressants, supportive counseling

---

CAUSES AND SYMPTOMS

Narcolepsy (*narco* meaning "numbness" and *lepsy* meaning "seizure") consists primarily of attacks of irresistible sleepiness in the daytime. The sleepiness is extreme; it has been described as the feeling that most people would experience if they tried to add columns of numbers in the middle of the night after forty-eight hours without sleep.

The narcoleptic's day is broken up by a series of brief and repetitive sleep attacks, perhaps even two hundred attacks in a single day. These transient, overpowering attacks of sleepiness may last from a few seconds to thirty minutes, with an average spell lasting two minutes. It is excruciatingly difficult, and frequently impossible, to ignore the urge to sleep, no matter how inconvenient or inappropriate. Narcoleptics typically fall asleep suddenly, on the job, in conversation, standing up, and even while eating, driving, or making love.

These sleep attacks result from an abrupt failure in resisting sleep, as opposed to a sudden surge in sleepiness, because narcoleptics are actually sleepy all day. The misconception that their daytime sleepiness is caused by insufficient nighttime sleep prompts undiagnosed patients to spend inordinately long hours in bed. Narcoleptics will be sleepy during the day regardless of how much sleep they get at night.

One of the most prominent and troubling features of narcolepsy is cataplexy, a sudden loss of muscle tone that causes the person to collapse. Cataplexy occurs during the daytime while the person is awake. It may involve all the muscles at once or only a select few, so the severity may range from total collapse to the ground to partial collapse of a limb or the jaw. The cataplectic sometimes remains conscious, able to think, hear, and see, although vision may be blurred. At other times, there is a brief loss of consciousness, associated with an experience of dreaming. Although most attacks of cataplexy last less than a minute, occasionally they go on for as long as twenty minutes. Cataplexy is often triggered by enjoyable feelings, laughter, or excitement during which the person suddenly crumples into a heap. For other patients, a strong negative emotion, such as fear or anger, precipitates an attack.

Many narcoleptics notice the symptom of excessive daytime sleepiness for as much as a year before the onset of cataplexy. After many years of experiencing cataplexy, some patients find that less emotional stimulus is required to induce the muscle collapse and that increasingly more muscles are involved. Others find that this symptom diminishes, possibly because they have become adept at anticipating and avoiding the situations that trigger attacks. It has been noted that other hypersomnias—that is, other diseases of excessive sleepiness—do not include cataplexy; only narcoleptics suffer from this embarrassing and troubling symptom of muscle collapse.

Many narcoleptics also experience hypnogogic hallucinations, dreams that intrude into the waking state. In normal sleep, dreaming generally occurs approximately ninety minutes after falling asleep; narcoleptics begin their sleeping episodes with vivid dreams. These hallucinations are extremely realistic and often violent. The patient sees someone else in the room or hears someone calling his or her name, for the hallucinations are nearly always visual and are usually auditory. The vivid sights, sounds, and feelings characteristic of hypnogogic hallucinations are thought to occur while the person is awake, both during the day and just at the edges of nighttime sleep. Since narcoleptics typically fall asleep dozens if not hundreds of times a day, they can experience these disturbing hallucinations with great frequency. Somewhat more than 50 percent of daytime sleep attacks include hallucinations, while only about 7 percent are usually marked by cataplexy.

Approximately 40 to 60 percent of narcoleptics suffer another frightening symptom: sleep paralysis. This condition occurs at the beginning or end of sleep and renders immobile virtually every voluntary muscle, except those around the eyes. During sleep paralysis, the mind is awake and one is aware of the external surroundings, but the muscles refuse to move. The paralysis usually lasts only a few seconds, but it may continue for as long as twenty minutes. Sleep researchers find that almost everyone has an episode of sleep paralysis that lasts a few seconds some time during his or her lifetime. When the paralysis continues for more than a few seconds, however, it is usually a sign of narcolepsy. Although either sleep paralysis or hypnogogic hallucinations alone are distressing enough, they often happen simultaneously.

Because of their frequent, irresistible sleep attacks, narcoleptics often wobble back and forth between sleep and wakefulness in a state that has been likened to sleepwalking and is termed automatic behavior. When in this state, the person seems to behave normally but later does not remember extended periods of time. For example, narcoleptics might find themselves in a different building or several exits farther down a highway than they last remembered. Obviously, automatic behavior is very anxiety-producing; it is very troubling to narcoleptics to be unable to remember what they have done in the minutes or hours that have just passed.

In addition to these memory difficulties, some narcoleptics experience constant eye fatigue, difficulty focusing, and double vision. They also have a higher incidence of the heart abnormality called mitral valve prolapse, which affects blood flow to the left ventricle. The reason for this association is not clear.

Although narcolepsy is an illness of excessive daytime sleepiness, the nighttime sleep of those afflicted is far from normal as well. It is often troubled by restlessness and frequent awakenings, which are brief or may last for hours. Patients also experience many nightmares about murder and persecution. Many narcolep-

tics talk, cry out, or thrash about periodically during the night.

One narcoleptic in ten has the added complication of suffering from sleep apnea. This sleep disorder consists of recurrent interruptions in breathing during sleep. This further disturbance of nighttime sleep aggravates the narcoleptic's tendency to excessive daytime sleepiness.

Narcolepsy was once thought to be extremely rare. By the late twentieth century, however, the United States Department of Health estimated that 250,000 Americans suffer from this disease, which is more than the number afflicted by multiple sclerosis. The American Medical Association considers 250,000 to be a very conservative estimate and believes the number to be between 400,000 and 600,000.

Males and females are equally affected by narcolepsy. Although the disorder has been diagnosed in a five-year-old, its symptoms most frequently appear for the first time during adolescence. In about 75 percent of cases, the attacks begin between the ages of fifteen and twenty-five; only 5 percent of cases begin before the age of ten. Onset is rare after the age of forty; if narcolepsy seems to appear in an older person, it has probably existed undiagnosed for years. Sleep researchers believe that the extra need for sleep characteristic of adolescence may make this stage of development particularly vulnerable for the onset of narcolepsy. Thus, this disorder may typically begin in adolescence because it is somehow triggered by the brain changes associated with sexual maturation.

Between two and five persons in one thousand in the general population of the United States have scattered episodes of excessive daytime sleepiness but are not considered narcoleptics. It is not until a person has one to several attacks each day that narcolepsy is suspected.

TREATMENT AND THERAPY

Narcolepsy is now known to be a disease of the nervous system. Although incurable, it can be successfully treated with various medications once it has been diagnosed. The diagnosis of narcolepsy, however, is often slow to occur. The average interval between the first appearance of symptoms and diagnosis is often as long as thirteen years. Because early symptoms are usually mild, narcoleptics typically spend years wondering whether they are sick or whether they merely lack initiative. They are often called lazy because they repeatedly nap during the day and are lethargic even when awake. Diagnosis is made more difficult by the wide range of severity of symptoms. For example, excessive daytime sleepiness may trouble a person for ten or twenty years before cataplexy appears. Patients may even occasionally experience a temporary or partial remission in their condition. Narcoleptics often fight off their sleep attacks by ingesting large amounts of caffeine and never realize that they have an actual disease until years later.

If narcolepsy is suspected, a polysomnographic study is done at a sleep disorders center to confirm the diagnosis. The most reliable confirmation of narcolepsy can be obtained by what is called the multiple sleep latency test (MSLT). The MSLT is easy, convenient, inexpensive, and very informative. The person is given four or five opportunities to lie down and fall asleep during the daytime. Normal individuals take fifteen to thirty minutes to fall asleep. In the MSLT, falling asleep in less than five minutes is considered abnormal. Those afflicted with narcolepsy always fall asleep in less than five minutes and often within a minute. The maintenance of wakefulness test (MOWT) is also used in the confirmation of narcolepsy. In the MOWT, the person is kept all day in a comfortable reclining position. Polysomnography is used to measure the patient's ability to stay awake and how many times he or she falls asleep.

Along with the MSLT and the MOWT, a thorough physical examination is needed to discover if the person has some other disorder that can mimic narcolepsy; an underactive thyroid gland, diabetes, chronic low blood sugar, anemia, and a malfunctioning liver can each cause excessive daytime sleepiness. Similarly, drug use, poor nutrition, emotional frustration, dissatisfaction, or poor motivation can also result in the type of sleepiness that a narcoleptic experiences.

When the diagnosis of narcolepsy is confirmed, treatment usually consists of stimulant medications such as dextroamphetamine, pemoline, or methylphenidate (Ritalin) during the daytime. These stimulant drugs can increase alertness and cut down the number of sleep attacks from perhaps several per day to several per month. Unfortunately, patients can quickly develop tolerance to these medications.

Even on low doses, some patients become irritable, aggressive, or nervous, or they may develop obesity and sexual problems. It is very important, therefore, to monitor a narcoleptic carefully, determining the lowest effective dose and the best times of day to take it. It may be months before the positive effects of drug therapy are fully experienced. The MSLT will often be given on

a day that one takes the medication and on another when it is not taken, in order to evaluate the success of a given treatment.

Because specific drug and dosage schedules may have to be altered frequently, patients may repeatedly have to face drug withdrawal symptoms such as intensified sleepiness and disturbing dreams. To prevent adverse reactions, narcoleptics must often avoid certain foods and common medications. Their use of stimulant drugs may even be viewed as morally wrong, in these days of widespread drug abuse, by neighbors or co-workers who do not comprehend that narcolepsy is a disabling disease.

If cataplexy is present, medications other than amphetamines or Ritalin are required and useful. The class of drugs called tricyclic antidepressants, including protriptyline and imipramine, or the class of drugs called monoamine oxidase inhibitors may alleviate cataplexy. These medicines can often reduce attacks—for example, from three a day to three a month. In addition, effective treatment for cataplexy usually also relieves sleep paralysis and hypnogogic hallucinations.

Since the development of tolerance is common and these drugs can aggravate the symptom of sleepiness, determining the best timing and dose is critical. Another side effect of cataplexy drugs is impaired sexual function in males. Some men even discontinue these medications periodically for a day or two in order to sustain sexual relations. In addition, none of the drugs used for any symptoms of narcolepsy are safe to take during pregnancy.

In some cases, narcoleptics can be treated without medication if they carefully space naps during the day to relieve excessive sleepiness. Patients keep nap diaries to rate their alertness at regular intervals during the day. They then schedule short, strategically timed naps during those daytime periods when their sleep attacks are most likely to occur.

Naps are particularly valuable in treating children with narcolepsy because the consequences of a lifetime of medication on their development or on the course of their illness is unknown. Some children who show hyperactive behavior actually have narcolepsy; they are working frantically to overcome their persistent sleepiness and to keep themselves awake. Children with narcolepsy may also justifiably fear falling asleep, day or night, because of hallucinations and sleep paralysis.

It is evident that supportive counseling must be a strong component of treatment, whatever the patient's age. Sensitive medical monitoring can offer narcoleptics a measure of satisfactory daily living, but the use of stimulants to improve alertness may also make them more aware of their limitations and, therefore, more frustrated. Depression is not the cause of narcolepsy but may result primarily from the disruption in their lives and the feeling that they are denied the right to a "normal" life. Their constant sleepiness engenders feelings of inferiority and inadequacy. Narcoleptics usually refrain from mentioning their hallucinations and try to hide their automatic behavior for fear of being labeled insane. Loss of work, broken marriages, and social isolation are often witnesses to the crippling effects of narcolepsy.

Of all the people with narcolepsy seen at major sleep disorders centers, more than one-half have been completely disabled with respect to regular employment by the age of forty. With part-time, homebound, or self-employment, however, most narcoleptics can gain self-respect and help support themselves through work that is safe and tailored to their needs. They must be given tasks that can be divided into parts performed in relatively short time periods.

Drug and nap therapy can do little for narcoleptics without education of their families, friends, acquaintances, employers, and coworkers about the reality of this neurological disease. Most people find it hard to accept the notion that sleepiness cannot be controlled and insist that narcoleptics could be more alert if they tried harder. Narcoleptics are often stigmatized as slackers or incompetents, or assumed to be drug abusers or closet drinkers. It is most important that patients and all the people in their lives comprehend that excessive daytime sleepiness is not the patients' "fault."

Further help for narcoleptics seems to lie in animal studies, which may fill in many important pieces of the narcolepsy puzzle. The effects of the disease on behavior, the way in which it is inherited, and the benefits and risks of specific drugs continue to be evaluated in narcoleptic dogs.

PERSPECTIVE AND PROSPECTS

Once viewed as "all in the mind," narcolepsy is now recognized as a neurological disorder. Its origin is unknown, but research has already discovered evidence of possible causes. An understanding of narcolepsy both depended on and advanced the understanding of normal sleep and of other sleep disorders. Scientists define sleep as a reduction in awareness of and interaction with the environment, lowered movement and muscle activity, and partial or complete suspension of voluntary behavior and consciousness.

Although narcolepsy was named and described in 1880, it could not be genuinely studied until the 1930's, when the electroencephalograph (EEG) was developed to record brain activity during the various stages of sleep. By the 1940's, this advancement led to a description of the narcoleptic tetrad, the four usual symptoms of narcolepsy: excessive daytime sleepiness, cataplexy, sleep paralysis, and hypnogogic hallucinations.

In the 1950's, narcolepsy still only rated a paragraph in one neurology textbook, which mistakenly called it a rare variety of epilepsy. A major discovery occurred in 1960: Narcoleptics bypass the normal stages of light and deep sleep and fall directly into rapid eye movement (REM) sleep. Thus, sudden-onset REM period (or SOREMP) became the major distinguishing feature of this brain disorder.

It was soon noted that relatives of narcoleptics are sixty times more likely to have the disease than members of the general population. Clearly, there is a hereditary factor involved, and geneticists have joined the hunt for narcolepsy's cause. The hereditary aspects of the disease are particularly important to counselors because parents with narcolepsy may feel guilty if their child develops it. (Indeed, some patients abandon plans to have children.) Geneticists have found a gene that may be responsible for narcolepsy. Since the gene produces an antigen called DR2 on patients' white blood cells, which is not found in nonnarcoleptics, immunologists have also begun to search for the origins of narcolepsy.

Rapid advances have been made in the last few years in determining the cause of narcolepsy. The disease is thought to arise from a biochemical imbalance in the brain that disturbs the mechanism that activates the on/off cycle of sleep. Biochemists are studying the possible relationship of various brain chemicals called neurotransmitters to narcolepsy. A defect in the way in which the body produces or uses dopamine, acetylcholine, or some other neurotransmitter is suspected to precipitate narcolepsy, which never spontaneously disappears once it is developed. The newest discovery has been the finding of abnormalities in the structure and function of a particular group of nerve cells, called hypocretin neurons, in the brains of patients with narcolepsy. The molecules implicated in narcolepsy are neuropeptides known as orexins (originally described as hypocretins). Researchers discovered that changes in the hypocretin receptor 2 and preprohypocretin genes are able to produce narcolepsy in animals. In one study involving nine human subjects, hypocretin could not be detected in seven of the subjects. Other studies have produced hypocretin knockout mice, which have symptoms that are quite similar to those found in human narcoleptics. Hypocretins have been found to occur normally in the regions of the central nervous system that appear to be involved in the regulation of sleep. An autosomal recessive mutation has been discovered in narcoleptic dogs that alters the hypocretin receptor 2 gene. In humans, a similar disruption or deficiency in hypocretin is associated with most cases of narcolepsy, although it is still unclear as to what underlies the exact genetic predisposition to the disease. Scientists speculate that they one day may cure narcolepsy or reduce its effects with drugs mimicking secretions of the missing nerve cells or even with brain-cell transplants.

Two interesting discoveries may help in the diagnosis of narcolepsy even before the classical clinical symptoms develop. There is some evidence that REM sleep is entered with abnormal rapidity years before the disorder develops. The drug physostigmine salicylate has no effect on normal dogs but elicits cataplexy in puppies with narcolepsy. Both these discoveries may be useful in screening the children of narcoleptics.

Because narcolepsy involves the fundamental processes of sleep, the combined efforts of neuroscientists, geneticists, biochemists, immunologists, and other scientists to unravel its mysteries will continue to yield important information about the basic mechanism of sleep—that state in which humans spend almost one-third of their lives.

—*Grace D. Matzen*

See also Apnea; Brain; Electroencephalography (EEG); Hallucinations; Memory loss; Nervous system; Neurology; Neurology, pediatric; Paralysis; Sleep; Sleep disorders; Sleeping sickness; Unconsciousness.

FOR FURTHER INFORMATION:

Bassetti, Claudio L., Michel Billiard, and Emmanuel Mignot, eds. *Narcolepsy and Hypersomnia*. New York: Informa Healthcare, 2007. Discusses narcolepsy as an autoimmune disease. Covers diagnostic procedures, criteria, genetics, and epidemiological surveys.

Caldwell, J. Paul. *Sleep: The Complete Guide to Sleep Disorders and a Better Night's Sleep*. Rev. ed. Toronto, Ont.: Firefly Books, 2003. A thorough examination of sleep disorders constitutes a good portion of this book, including such topics as what causes sleep apnea, sleep disorders in children and seniors, what drugs interfere and help with sleep, and treatment guidelines.

Dement, William C. *The Sleepwatchers*. Stanford, Calif.: Stanford Alumni Association, 1992. A lively and often amusing book by the chair of the National Commission on Sleep Disorders Research. Traces the story of such research since the 1950's, when Dement first studied narcolepsy. Solid science that reads like a novel.

Hartmann, Ernest. *The Sleep Book: Understanding and Preventing Sleep Problems in People over Fifty*. Glenview, Ill.: Scott, Foresman, 1987. An easily understood discussion by a well-known pioneer in normal sleep and sleep disorders research. Contains a forty-page appendix of sleep disorders classification, centers, and specialists.

Kryger, Meir H., Thomas Roth, and William C. Dement, eds. *Principles and Practices of Sleep Medicine*. 4th ed. Philadelphia: Saunders/Elsevier, 2005. Covers normal sleep and abnormal sleep, including narcolepsy and the diagnostic and therapeutic aspects of sleep problems.

Narcolepsy Network. http://www.narcolepsynetwork .org. Provides referral service, support group meetings, and communication among members.

Poceta, J. Steven, and Merrill Mitler, eds. *Sleep Disorders: Diagnosis and Treatment*. Totowa, N.J.: Humana Press, 1998. This volume fills an important need by making this field accessible to primary care physicians and giving them the tools and confidence to diagnose and treat those cases that do not need specialized help. It also makes clear which patients should be referred to a sleep disorder service and when.

Reite, Martin, John Ruddy, and Kim E. Nagel. *Concise Guide to Evaluation and Management of Sleep Disorders*. 3d ed. Washington, D.C.: American Psychiatric Press, 2002. Goals of this book are to provide a portable and practical approach to the diagnosis and treatment of sleep problems and a current summary of the classification of sleep disorders.

Walsleben, Joyce A., and Rita Baron-Faust. *A Woman's Guide to Sleep: Guaranteed Solutions for a Good Night's Rest*. New York: Crown, 2001. Writing in an informal, easily comprehensible style, Walsleben, director of the Sleep Disorders Center at New York University School of Medicine, and freelancer Baron-Faust cover nearly every sleep disorder suffered by women.

NARCOTICS

TREATMENT

ANATOMY OR SYSTEM AFFECTED: Brain, nervous system, psychic-emotional system

SPECIALTIES AND RELATED FIELDS: Pharmacology

DEFINITION: The use of drugs from the opiate family, which mimic the action of the body's own painkilling substances, to treat pain, anxiety, coughing, diarrhea, and insomnia.

KEY TERMS:

agonist: a drug that acts in a fashion similar to that of a hormone or neurotransmitter normally found in the body

analgesia: the absence of pain; analgesics are compounds that stop the neurotransmission of pain messages

antagonist: a drug that acts to block the effects of a hormone or neurotransmitter normally found in the body

brain stem: the region between the brain and spinal cord that controls such functions as respiration and heart rate

central nervous system: the brain and spinal cord

dependence: a craving for a drug

endogenous: something naturally found in the body, such as neurotransmitters

exogenous: something originating outside the body and administered orally or by injection

neuron: a nerve cell that can conduct electrical impulses from one region of the body to another; it is capable of releasing neurotransmitters

neurotransmitter: a chemical substance released by one nerve cell to stimulate or inhibit the function of an adjacent nerve cell; a chemical message released from a neuron

opioids: drugs derived from opium; also known as narcotics or opiates

tolerance: the ability to endure ever-increasing amounts of a drug

THE EFFECTS OF NARCOTICS

Narcotics are drugs commonly used to treat pain (analgesics), suppress coughing, control diarrhea, and aid in anesthesia. These drugs are some of the oldest and most used agents. Most drugs are able to alter the effects of body functions by mimicking naturally occurring chemicals (as with agonists) or by blocking the physiological effects of these chemicals (as with antagonists).

Researchers have examined the many effects of the substances derived from the opium poppy, including morphine, codeine, and heroin. They have identified endogenous opioid-like chemicals called endorphins, dynorphins, and enkephalins that act as neurotransmitters; that is, some opioid compounds are normally found in the human nervous system as substances that allow nerve cells to communicate with one another. The synthetic opioid morphine mimics the actions of endorphins, dynorphins, and enkephalins by taking the place of these neurotransmitters. Scientists and physicians now know that morphine and related compounds produce their major effects by acting on the central nervous system, which includes the brain and spinal cord. To understand how opioids affect the body's response to pain, one must first understand the physiology of pain.

Any time tissues are damaged, they release chemical substances into the space outside the damaged cell, known as the extracellular space. Sensory neurons that have the ability to detect these chemicals are known as pain neurons. Once the chemicals bind to receptors on a pain neuron, the neuron is stimulated to send an electrical message to the spinal cord. Two actions occur once this message arrives. The first is an immediate initiation of a reflex which attempts to remove the tissue from the source of injury. For example, when one accidentally places an arm on a hot stove, a neural reflex causes the muscles of the limb to retract the arm from the burner. This is accomplished when the pain neuron releases a chemical message (neurotransmitter) in the spinal cord to stimulate neurons that control the muscles of the affected limb. This neurotransmitter is known as substance P. The second action of the sensory pain neuron is to inform the brain of the tissue damage, so that appropriate behavioral modification can take place. For example, one may become more cautious around the kitchen after burning one's arm on the stove. Notification of the brain is also accomplished by activating a second neuron using the neurotransmitter substance P, which will carry this electrical message toward the brain. Morphine and related opioids are very effective analgesics that seem to alter this pathway, thus dampening the transmission of pain messages.

Morphinelike drugs act at several sites in the nervous system. One of the most clinically important places is within the spinal cord at the region where the pain neurons release substance P. Opioids are known to reduce the amount of substance P that is released and thereby to decrease the stimulatory message in the neural pathway to the brain. If the pain impulses traveling to the brain are reduced, so is one's perception of pain. The second area of the nervous system known to be involved in regulating the perception of pain is a diffuse area of neurons located between the brain and spinal cord referred to as the brain stem. When researchers stimulate a region of the brain stem, the pain impulses traveling to the brain are reduced. Opioid peptides have been identified in this area which, as in the spinal cord, are probably responsible for reducing the pain message.

Because exogenous opioids must act to mimic endogenous opioids, one may wonder why there is a need for narcotic drugs if the body already produces the opioid-like endorphins and enkephalins. The reason is that every individual has a different degree of pain tolerance. How much pain one can endure also changes with certain circumstances. For example, one hardly notices the pain of a cut when participating in an exciting outdoor game. If the same wound occurs while one's attention is focused on it, however, the cut becomes noticeably painful. Perhaps the best explanation for the differing interpretation of pain during these activities and among different people is the endogenous opioid system. It is likely that the acupuncture pins used to block pain messages cause neurons to release increasing amounts of endorphins, enkephalins, and dynorphins. In the same way, with the administration of narcotics, one artificially increases the amount of opioids in the body in order to block pain impulses.

Opioids act on the brain stem to affect several systems other than the one associated with pain. They suppress coughing in a way that is similar to their effect on neural signals to decrease pain messages to the brain. Narcotics seem to inhibit release of the neurotransmitters responsible for the cough reflex. Unfortunately, opioids can activate another area in the brain stem to produce nausea and vomiting. This unwanted effect is related to the dose and type of drug used. Therefore, physicians can usually diminish the vomiting response with appropriate treatment selections. Perhaps the most dangerous problem with opioid usage is the effect that opioids have on the brain stem's regulation of respiration. When the brain stem senses that the level of carbon dioxide is too high, breathing is increased to rid the body of this excess waste gas. Narcotics decrease the responsiveness of the brain stem to carbon dioxide. Therefore, breathing rates tend to be inappropriately low, causing a buildup of carbon dioxide.

Constriction of the pupils of the eyes is a very common effect of opioids on the visual system. In fact, this constriction serves as an important diagnostic clue in examining a patient who has taken an overdose of a narcotic.

Opioids have a constipating effect, indirectly through the central nervous system and directly through their influence on the intestines. Opioids cause a decrease in peristalsis, the series of muscular contractions of the intestinal wall that would normally move food toward the anus.

Most opioid analgesics have no direct effect on the heart and blood vessels. Thus, they do not alter heart rate or rhythm or blood pressure to any significant degree. The only noticeable effect of narcotics on the cardiovascular system is a flushing and warming of the skin because of a slight increase in blood flow to the skin. Occasionally, this is accompanied by sweating. Kidney function tends to be depressed by opioids, which may be attributable to a decrease in the amount of blood that is filtered through the kidneys. There is also a decrease in the ability to urinate, as these drugs increase contraction of the muscle that prevents urine from leaving the bladder.

USES AND COMPLICATIONS

Medical personnel use this knowledge of how narcotics alter the body to the patient's advantage. Narcotics are used in the relief of pain and anxiety, as sedatives and anesthetics, to reduce coughing, and as a way to control diarrhea.

Opioid analgesics are among the most effective and valuable medications for the treatment of serious pain. Morphinelike drugs dampen the pain response but do not affect to a great extent other senses such as vision and hearing. They are often used to treat pain in the postoperative period, in which they effectively reduce or eliminate the short-term pain from tissue trauma that is caused by surgery. When pain is reduced, patients tend to eat, sleep, and recover much more rapidly. Physicians often prescribe narcotics such as meperidine (Demerol) or codeine on an as-needed basis. In this way, the patient, who knows firsthand the effectiveness of the drug, can control the frequency of analgesic administration. In fact, patients are usually advised to administer a small dose before the pain becomes too intense, thus decreasing the pain message before it reaches a high level and requires a relatively high dose to make the patient comfortable again.

A painful sensation consists of the neural response to

the tissue damage and the patient's reaction to the stimulus. The analgesic properties of narcotics are related to their ability to diminish both pain perception and the reaction of the patient to pain. These drugs effectively raise the threshold for pain, perhaps because of the euphoria experienced by patients given opioids. For example, a patient in pain who is given morphine experiences a pleasant floating sensation with a great reduction in distress and anxiety. It is interesting to note, however, that some subjects do not experience euphoria when given morphine. In fact, they tend to have an unpleasant response known as dysphoria, which often includes restlessness and a feeling of general discomfort.

Physicians and other health care workers must achieve a delicate balance between alleviating pain from known causes and masking pain as a warning signal from unexpected sources. For example, a patient having abdominal surgery would likely require relatively high doses of narcotic analgesics to reduce the postoperative pain. Yet the administration of an analgesic could mask the pain from an unexpected abdominal infection. Therefore, if used excessively, narcotics may prevent the early recognition of complications.

In addition to their analgesic effects, opioids tend to have a sedative effect and are often used as a preanesthetic drug or as an anesthetic. Potent opioids are used in relatively large doses to achieve general anesthesia, particularly in patients undergoing heart surgery. These narcotics are also commonly used during other surgeries in which it is important that heart function be affected only minimally. Examples of narcotic agents used in anesthesia include fentanyl (Sublimaze), sufentanil, alfentanil, and propafol.

Suppression of the cough reflex is a clinically useful effect of narcotics. The therapeutic doses of opioids needed to reduce coughing are much lower than the doses to achieve analgesia. The opioid derivatives most commonly used to suppress the cough reflex are codeine, dextromethorphan, and noscapine. How these agents work to reduce coughing is not known, but they are thought to act on the brain stem.

Diarrhea from almost any cause can be controlled with opioids. Diphenoxylate (Lomotil) and loperamide (Imodium), narcotics commonly used to treat diarrhea, do not possess analgesic properties. These drugs appear to act on the nerves within the intestinal tract to decrease muscular activity.

Like all drugs, narcotics have both beneficial and undesired effects. The toxic effects of an opioid depend on the dosage, the agent used, the clinical condition in which it is used, and an individual patient's response to the drug. Some of the more common unwanted effects include restlessness and hyperactivity instead of sedation, respiratory depression, nausea and vomiting, increased pressure within the brain, low blood pressure, constipation, urinary retention, and itching around the nose. Most of these conditions are of short duration and resolve themselves after the drug has been discontinued.

Patients, or more often narcotic drug abusers, may become tolerant and dependent upon these agents. These individuals, such as heroin abusers, have a strong craving for the drugs. These agents are abused for their euphoric effect at relatively high doses. The human body is very efficient in tolerating the effects of opioids. Their effects lessen somewhat with each succeeding dose, so that a higher dose must be taken to achieve the same effect. Physiological adaptation to the long-term use of opioids (two to three weeks) causes the development of tolerance for these drugs.

Exogenous opioids take the place of endogenous ones. Therefore, the nervous system and other physiological systems attempt to bring the levels of these neurotransmitters back to normal. First, the liver speeds up its metabolism of the drugs to eliminate them from the system more rapidly. Second, the regions of the nervous system that respond to opioids become desensitized by reducing the number of neural receptors that are available. Finally, after a few weeks of high levels of opioids, changes in other areas of the brain attempt to compensate for the rising opioid levels. Individuals who abruptly stop taking the drugs enter a period of withdrawal in which the symptoms are similar to a bad case of influenza. Morphine and heroine withdrawal symptoms usually start within twelve hours of the last dose. Peak symptoms of narcotic withdrawal occur after one to two days. Most symptoms gradually subside and are usually gone after one week. It should be emphasized that, under a physician's direction, the abuse potential of narcotics is very low.

There are certain clinical conditions in which opioid drugs should not be used or should be used with extreme caution. Because of the potential for respiratory depression with opioid treatment, these drugs should not be administered to patients with head injuries or impaired lung function. Most opioid drugs can cross the placenta and therefore should be avoided during pregnancy; with long-term use, the infant can be born addicted to narcotics.

Fortunately, some drugs can reverse the effects of narcotics. Three opioid antagonists are nalmefene, naloxone (Narcan), and naltrexone (Trexan). When these agents are given in the absence of an opioid agonist, they have no noticeable effect. When administered to a morphine-treated patient, however, they completely reverse the opioid effects almost immediately. These narcotic antagonists are particularly useful in treating patients who have taken an overdose of opioids. Such patients often arrive in the hospital emergency room not breathing and in a coma. These antagonists will normalize respiration, restore consciousness, and counteract other opioid effects. Interestingly, individuals who have become tolerant to and dependent upon opioids will immediately experience withdrawal symptoms when given naloxone or naltrexone.

PERSPECTIVE AND PROSPECTS

Narcotic drugs were originally found in the opium poppy five thousand years ago. Opium is obtained from the milky fluid of the unripe seed capsules of the poppy plant. The juice is dried in the air and forms a brown, sticky substance. With continued drying, the mass can be pulverized into powder. It is this powder that contains opioids. Morphine, codeine, and papaverine are the natural opioids that are used clinically. Most other narcotics are chemically derived.

The opium poppy, *Papaver somniferum*, was named after the Roman god of sleep, Somnis. Ancient Egyptian medical texts listed opium as a cure for illness and as a poison. Although opium was used extensively, the abuse potential was low because the poppy has a very bitter taste. Smoking opium became popular in eighteenth century China as a treatment for severe diarrhea and was also used as a socially acceptable drug mainly for its euphoric effects.

The opium poppy contains more than twenty distinct agents with a variety of potencies and unwanted effects. In 1806, a pharmacist refined opium into one active substance, morphine, which was found to be ten times as potent. Morphine was named after Morpheus, the Greek god of dreams, because the drug has powerful sedative effects. The discovery of other medically active agents quickly followed. Codeine and papaverine were identified next and found to be slightly less potent than morphine. At this time, clinicians used these purified products rather than the crude opium juice.

Shortly after purified narcotics became available, so did the widespread use of hypodermic needles. This allowed physicians to administer narcotics directly into the bloodstream. The injected opioids would travel via the blood to the brain in as short a time as twenty seconds. In the United States, morphine found widespread use as an analgesic for wounded soldiers during the Civil War. It was one of the most powerful painkillers available to physicians, but its unrestricted availability created great potential for addiction with long-term use.

Opioids became so popular that hundreds of medications became available to the public. These tonics promised to cure everything from "tired blood" to common aches and pains. Their widespread, unregulated use produced a large number of addicts. At the beginning of the twentieth century, the U.S. government attempted to reduce the number of addicts by making it illegal to buy any opioid-containing compound without a prescription. Medical scientists tried to synthesize compounds with morphinelike characteristics but without the addictive effects.

Physicians now have available to them a wide range of narcotics with different pharmacological properties. For example, there are drugs without addictive, euphoric, or sedative properties that can treat coughing or diarrhea. Some of these are available without a prescription for the treatment of occasional coughing and diarrhea. Narcotic analgesics, however, are given only under the direction of a physician. For example, morphine is still used as a potent pain reliever; when it is used appropriately, there is little chance of addiction. It is likely that other clinical uses will be found for narcotic drugs as researchers learn more about the human body's own endogenous narcotics, the endorphins.

—*Matthew Berria, Ph.D.*

See also Addiction; Anesthesia; Anesthesiology; Coughing; Diarrhea and dysentery; Marijuana; Over-the-counter medications; Pain; Pain management; Pharmacology; Prescription drug abuse; Self-medication; Substance abuse.

FOR FURTHER INFORMATION:

Acker, Caroline Jean. *Creating the American Junkie: Addiction Research in the Classic Era of Narcotic Control.* Baltimore: Johns Hopkins University Press, 2002. A fascinating examination of how the construction of addiction in the early twentieth century was influenced by a nexus of actors and events: psychiatrists, pharmacologists, and the American Medical Association's campaign to reduce prescriptions of opiates.

Davenport-Hines, J. P. *The Pursuit of Oblivion: A*

Global History of Narcotics. New York: W. W. Norton, 2002. Blends social, political, and cultural history to trace the evolution of drugs, their role in society, and addiction.

Griffith, H. Winter. *Complete Guide to Prescription and Nonprescription Drugs.* Revised and updated by Stephen Moore. New York: Penguin Group, 2010. A complete guide to both prescription and nonprescription drugs, including major uses, unwanted effects, precautions, and interactions with other drugs. A highly organized, useful tool for the nonscientist.

Inaba, Darryl S., William E. Cohen, and Michael E. Holstein. *Uppers, Downers, All Arounders: Physical and Mental Effects of Psychoactive Drugs.* 6th ed. Ashland, Oreg.: CNS, 2007. Mainly covers drug abuse, but also contains brief descriptions of the history and medical uses for drugs with abuse potential. A reader-friendly book that offers numerous statements from drug addicts regarding their addiction and, in some cases, their recovery.

Ling, W., and D. R. Wesson. "Drugs of Abuse: Opiates." *Western Journal of Medicine* 152 (May, 1990): 565-572. This article reviews the ways that addiction can be treated. Also addresses the use of narcotic antagonists in the treatment of drug overdose.

Liska, Ken. *Drugs and the Human Body, with Implications for Society.* 8th ed. Upper Saddle River, N.J.: Pearson/Prentice Hall, 2009. Examines the use of drugs in the North American culture by discussing such topics as what constitutes a drug and where drugs come from, federal laws, drug metabolism, and the different classifications of drugs.

Voth, Eric A., Robert L. Dupont, and Harold M. Voth. "Responsible Prescribing of Controlled Substances." *American Family Physician* 44 (November, 1991): 1673-1680. This article details some of the important problems in prescribing narcotics. Gives a description of characteristics that both health care workers and nonprofessionals can watch for in their attempts to identify drug abusers.

Nasal polyp removal

Procedure

Anatomy or system affected: Head, nose

Specialties and related fields: Family medicine, general surgery, otorhinolaryngology

Definition: The excision of benign growths that project from the mucous membrane lining the nasal cavity.

Indications and Procedures

Nasal polyps are swollen masses that project from the nasal wall. These benign structures are commonly found in patients with allergies. They may cause chronic nasal obstruction, which results in diminished air flow through the nasal cavity.

Once a polyp is detected, the physician may prescribe a nasal spray to reduce its size, such as the corticosteroids beclomethasone or flunisolide. This treatment is usually effective for small nasal polyps that cause only minor symptoms. When pharmacological management is not successful, however, the polyps should be removed surgically.

Surgical removal of nasal polyps (nasal polypectomy) is typically done as an outpatient procedure. It requires either general anesthesia or local anesthesia with sedation. After the patient is asleep or sedated, the lining of the nasal cavity is injected with a combination of local anesthesia and epinephrine to control pain and bleeding. The surgeon (usually an otorhinolaryngologist) visualizes the polyps with a head-

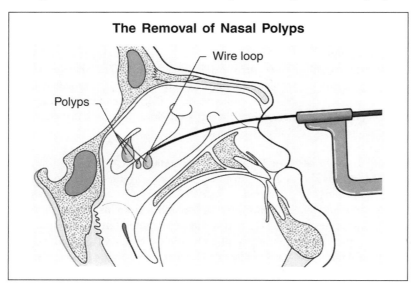

The Removal of Nasal Polyps

Allergies or chronic sinus infections can lead to the development of nasal polyps, distended areas of the nasal lining. If they interfere with breathing or the sense of smell or if they cause frequent nosebleeds, the polyps may be removed with a wire loop.

light, and the polyps are removed with specialized, long surgical instruments inserted into the nasal cavity. After the polyps are removed, the nasal passages are packed with ointment-coated gauze to help control bleeding and aid in the healing of the nasal mucosa. The gauze is removed in the physician's office a few days after the surgery. Once the packing is removed, the patient enjoys improved breathing through the nasal passages.

USES AND COMPLICATIONS

There are relatively few complications associated with nasal polyp removal. Some of the more common complications include bleeding from the surgical site, nasal and ear discomfort or anxiety as a result of the packing, and nausea from the anesthesia. The recurrence of nasal polyps after polypectomy is not unusual. Patients with cystic fibrosis have a high rate of occurrence of nasal polyps and often have recurrent problems.

*—Matthew Berria, Ph.D.,
and Douglas Reinhart, M.D.*

See also Allergies; Nasopharyngeal disorders; Oral and maxillofacial surgery; Otorhinolaryngology; Polyps; Sense organs; Sinusitis; Smell.

FOR FURTHER INFORMATION:

Adelman, Daniel C., et al., eds. *Manual of Allergy and Immunology.* 4th ed. Philadelphia: Lippincott Williams & Wilkins, 2002.

Benjamin, Bruce, et al. *A Color Atlas of Otorhinolaryngology.* Edited by Michael Hawke. Philadelphia: J. B. Lippincott, 1995.

Bull, P. D. *Lecture Notes on Diseases of the Ear, Nose, and Throat.* 10th ed. Malden, Mass.: Blackwell Science, 2007.

Ferrari, Mario. *PDxMD Ear, Nose, and Throat Disorders.* Philadelphia: PDxMD, 2003.

Icon Health. *Nasal Polyps: A Medical Dictionary, Bibliography, and Annotated Research Guide to Internet References.* San Diego, Calif.: Author, 2004.

Kimball, Chad T. *Colds, Flu, and Other Common Ailments Sourcebook.* Detroit, Mich.: Omnigraphics, 2001.

Morelock, Michael, and J. B. Vap. *Your Guide to Problems of the Ear, Nose, and Throat.* Philadelphia: Lippincott Williams & Wilkins, 1985.

Settipane, Guy A., et al., eds. *Nasal Polyps: Epidemiology, Pathogenesis, and Treatment.* Providence, R.I.: OceanSide, 1997.

NASOPHARYNGEAL DISORDERS
DISEASE/DISORDER

ANATOMY OR SYSTEM AFFECTED: Nose, respiratory system, throat

SPECIALTIES AND RELATED FIELDS: Family medicine, occupational health, otorhinolaryngology

DEFINITION: Disorders of the nose, nasal passages (sinuses), and pharynx (mouth, throat, and esophagus).

KEY TERMS:

acute disease: a short and sharp disease process

chronic disease: a lingering illness

esophagus: the tube that leads from the pharynx to the stomach

larynx: the organ that produces the voice, which lies between the pharynx and the trachea; commonly called the voice box

nasopharyngeal: referring to the nose and pharynx (the upper part of the throat that leads from the mouth to the esophagus)

trachea: a tube that leads from the throat to the lungs; commonly called the windpipe

CAUSES AND SYMPTOMS

Nasopharyngeal disorders include all the diseases that can be present in the nasal cavity and the pharynx. These include the common cold, pharyngitis (sore throat), laryngitis (inflammation of the larynx), epiglottitis (inflammation of the lid over the larynx), tonsillitis (inflammation of the lymph nodes at the rear of the mouth), sinusitis (inflammation of the sinus cavities that surround the nose), otitis media (earache that is often associated with nasopharyngeal infection), nosebleed, nasal obstruction, halitosis (bad breath), and various other disorders.

The common cold is one of the most prevalent diseases that afflict humankind. Pharyngitis, or sore throat, often accompanies the common cold, or it may appear by itself. Acute infections can be caused by viruses or bacteria, often by certain streptococcus strains—hence the common term for the disorder, strep throat. Acute pharyngitis can also be caused by chemicals or radiation. As a chronic disorder, pharyngitis can be caused by lingering infection in other organs such as the lungs and sinuses, or it can be attributable to constant irritation from smoking, drinking alcohol, or breathing polluted air. The usual symptoms of pharyngitis include sore throat, difficulty in swallowing, and fever. The infected area appears red and swollen. Ordinarily, pharyngitis is not serious. If certain strains of streptococcus are the cause, however, then the infection may progress to rheumatic fever. This disease appears to be the result of an immune system reaction to some streptococcus bacteria. It can have painful effects in many parts of the body, such as in joints, and can do permanent damage to parts of the heart. In rare cases, rheumatic fever can be fatal.

Acute laryngitis is usually caused by a viral infection, but bacteria, outside irritants, or misuse of the voice are other causes. Ordinarily, the vocal cords produce sounds by vibrating in response to the air passing over them. When inflamed or irritated, they swell, causing distortion in the sounds produced. The voice becomes hoarse and raspy and may even diminish to a soft whisper. This distortion of sound is the main symptom of laryngitis, but there may also be a sore throat and congestion that causes constant coughing. The condition generally resolves itself and requires no treatment. Chronic laryngitis has the same symptoms but does not go away spontaneously. It may be caused by an infectious agent but more likely is attributable to some irritant activity, such as constantly misusing the voice, smoking, drinking alcohol, or breathing contaminated air.

The epiglottis is a waferlike tissue covered by a mucous membrane that sits on top of the larynx. It can become infected by such microorganisms as the bacteria *Haemophilus influenzae* type b in a condition called epiglottitis. Although the symptoms of epiglottitis can resemble those of pharyngitis, the infection can quickly progress to a very serious, life-threatening disorder. Epiglottitis usually afflicts children from two to four years of age, but adults can also be affected. The infection can begin rapidly, causing the epiglottis to swell and obstruct the airway to the lungs, creating a major medical emergency. Within twelve hours of the onset of symptoms, 50 percent of patients require hospitalization and intubation (insertion of a breathing tube into the trachea). The symptoms are high fever, severe sore throat, difficulty in breathing, difficulty in swallowing, and general malaise. As the airway becomes more and more occluded, the patient begins to gasp for air. The lack of oxygen may cause cyanosis (blue color in the lips, fingers, and skin), exhaustion, and shock.

Another disease associated with the larynx is croup, or laryngotracheobronchitis. As the medical name indicates, croup involves the larynx, the trachea, and the bronchi (the large branches of the lung). It is usually caused by a virus, but some cases are attributable to bacterial infection. Children from three to five years of age are the usual victims. This disease causes the airways to narrow because of inflammation of the inner mucosal surfaces. Inflammation causes coughing, but the narrowed airway causes the cough to be sharp and brassy, like the barking of a seal. Croup is usually relatively benign, but sometimes it progresses to a severe disease requiring hospitalization.

Various other disorders can afflict the larynx, such as damage to the vocal cords because of infection by bacteria, fungi, or other microorganisms. The vocal cords can also be damaged by misusing the voice, smoking, or breathing contaminated air. Polyps (masses of tissue growing on the surface), nodes (little knots of tissue), or "singers' nodules" may develop. Sores called contact ulcers may form on the vocal cords.

Tonsillitis is an inflammation of two large lymph nodes located at the back of the throat, the tonsils. It may also involve the adenoids, lymph nodes located at the top of the throat. The function of these lymph nodes is to remove harmful pathogens (disease-causing organisms) from the nasopharyngeal cavity. At times, the load of microorganisms that they absorb becomes more than they can handle, and they become infected. The tonsils and adenoids may then become enlarged. A sore throat develops, along with a headache, fever, and chills. Glands of the neck and throat feel sore and may become enlarged. Young adults can also suffer from quinsy, or peritonsillar abscess. In this condition, one of the tonsils becomes infected and pus forms between the tonsil and the soft tissue surrounding it. Quinsy is characterized by pain in the throat and/or the soft palate, pain on swallowing, fever, and a tendency to lean the head toward the affected side.

The nasal sinuses are four pairs of cavities in the

bone around the nose. There are two maxillary sinuses, so called because they are found in the maxilla, or upper jaw. Slightly above and behind them are the ethmoid sinuses, and behind them are the sphenoid sinuses. Sitting over the nose in the lower part of the forehead are the two frontal sinuses. All these sinuses are lined with a mucous membrane and have small openings that lead into the nasal passages. Air moves in and out of the sinuses and allows mucus to drain into the nose. In acute sinusitis, infection builds up in the mucous membrane of any or all of the sinuses. The membrane lining the sinus swells and shuts the opening into the nasal passages. At the same time, membranes of the nose swell and become congested. Mucus and pus build up inside the sinuses, causing pain and pressure. Most often, sinusitis accompanies the common cold: The mucous membrane that lines the nose extends into the sinuses, so the infection of a cold can readily spread into the sinuses. The various viruses responsible for the common cold may be involved, as well as a wide group of bacteria. Chronic sinusitis can be caused by repeated infections that have allowed scar tissue to build up, closing the sinus openings and impeding mucus drainage, or may be the result of allergies.

According to the Centers for Disease Control and Prevention, chronic sinusitis is the most common long-term illness in the United States, surpassing the rates for asthma, arthritis, and congestive heart disease and causing nearly 14 million doctor office visits per year. For reasons that are not yet understood, sinusitis sufferers are often beset with inflammation of the ducts, trapping mucus, bacteria, and viruses inside. Nasal polyps can then develop. Thus, researchers have been very interested in finding causes and effective treatments for sinusitis. In the late twentieth century, most chronic cases of sinusitis were treated with fiber optic surgery that allowed access to the cramped sinus passageways. However, patients often returned within weeks or months with ongoing problems. This fact recently has prompted a reconsideration of the problem and its underlying causes as well as a struggle to redefine sinusitis. Some medical experts suspect that inflammation or the responses of the immune system are the culprit but note that additional research must be completed before any definitive answers are found.

Tissues in the nasopharyngeal cavity may be affected by conditions occurring in other parts of the body. For example, vocal cord paralysis may be caused by vascular accidents, certain cancers, tissue trauma, and other events.

Some infections in the nasopharyngeal cavity can spread to the ear through the Eustachian tubes that connect the two areas. Chief among the diseases of the ear that can be associated with nasopharyngeal disorders are the various forms of acute otitis media, an earache occurring in the central part of the ear. There are four basic types of otitis media. With the first type, serous otitis media, there is usually no infection, but fluid accumulates inside the middle ear because of the blockage of the Eustachian tube or the overproduction of fluid; the condition is usually mild, with some pain and temporary loss of hearing. The second type is otitis media with effusion; with this condition comes both infection and accumulation of fluid. The third form is acute purulent otitis media, the most serious type. Pus builds up inside the middle ear, and its pressure may rupture the eardrum, allowing discharge of blood and pus. The fourth type is secretory otitis media, which usually occurs after several bouts of otitis media. Cells within the middle ear start producing a fluid that is thicker than normal and produced in greater amounts.

Chronic otitis media is bacterial in origin. It is characterized by a perforation of the eardrum and chronic pus discharge. The eardrum is a flat, pliable disk of tissue that vibrates to conduct sounds from the outside to the inner-ear structures. The perforation that occurs in chronic otitis media can be one of two types: a relatively benign perforation occurring in the central part of the eardrum or a potentially dangerous perforation occurring near the edges of the eardrum. The latter perforation can be associated with loss of hearing, increased discharge of pus and other fluids, facial paralysis, and the spread of infection to other tissues. When the perforation of chronic otitis media is near the edges of the eardrum, something called a cholesteatoma develops. This accumulation of matter grows in the inner ear and can be destructive to bone and other tissue.

The same organisms that cause otitis media can be responsible for a condition called mastoiditis. The mastoid process is a bone structure lined with a mucous membrane. Infection from otitis media can spread to this area and in severe cases can destroy the bone. Mastoiditis used to be a leading cause of death in children.

Nosebleeds are common and most often result from a blow to the nose, but they can also be caused by colds, sinusitis, and breathing dry air. The septum (the cartilaginous tissue that separates the nostrils) and the surrounding intranasal mucous membrane contain many tiny blood vessels that are easily ruptured. If an individual receives a blow to the nose, these vessels can break and bleed. They can also rupture because of irritation from a cold or other condition. Breathing very dry air sometimes causes the nasal mucous membrane to crust over, and bleeding can follow. Nosebleeds are not usually serious, but sometimes they are indicative of an underlying condition, such as hypertension (high blood pressure), a tumor, or another disease.

Nasal obstruction is common during colds and allergy attacks, but it can also be caused by a deviated septum, a malformation in the cartilage between the nostrils that can be congenital or caused by a blow to the nose. Also, nasal obstruction can be attributable to nasal polyps, nasal tumors, or swollen adenoids. A common source of nasal obstruction is overuse of nasal decongestants. These agents relieve nasal congestion by reducing intranasal inflammation and swelling. If used too often or too long, however, they can cause the very problem that they were intended to cure: Intranasal blood vessels dilate, the area swells, secretions increase, and the nose becomes blocked. This is known as rebound congestion, or in medical terminology, rhinitis medicamentosa (nasal inflammation that is caused by a medication).

Halitosis, or bad breath, can be considered a nasopharyngeal disorder in the sense that it can originate in the mouth. It can be caused by diseases of the teeth and/or gums, but the most common causes are smoking or eating aromatic foods such as onions and garlic. Bad breath may also be a sign of disease conditions in other parts of the body, such as certain lung disorders or cancer of the esophagus. Hepatic failure, a liver dysfunction, may be accompanied by a fishy odor on the breath. Azotemia, the retention of nitrogen in the blood, may give rise to an ammonia-like odor. A sweet, fruity odor on the breath of diabetic patients may accompany ketoacidosis, a condition that occurs when there are high levels of glucose in the blood. Sometimes, young children stick foreign objects or other materials into their noses; it has been reported that these materials can fester, causing severe halitosis. Bad breath is rarely apparent to the individual who has it, however offensive it may be to others. A good way to check one's breath is to lick the back of one's hand and smell the spot; malodor, if it exists, will usually be apparent.

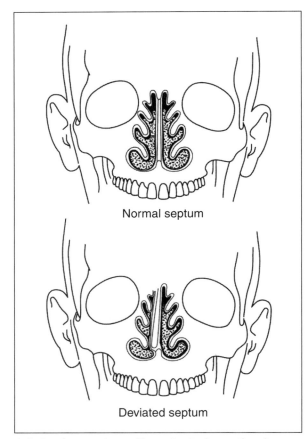

A deviated septum is a malformation in the cartilage between the nostrils, either present at birth or caused by a blow to the nose.

TREATMENT AND THERAPY

Nasopharyngeal disorders are most often mild illnesses that can be treated at home. For example, acute pharyngitis or sore throat is easily managed most of the time. The patient is advised to rest, gargle with warm salt water several times a day, and soothe the pain with lozenges or anesthetic gargles. If the infection is caused by a virus, it usually will clear without further treatment. If the physician suspects, however, that the infection is bacterial in origin, throat smears may be taken so that the organism can be identified. If bacteria are discovered, antibiotic therapy will be undertaken to eradicate the pathogens. This is particularly important if the infection is caused by certain strains of streptococcus bacteria. In this case, it is vital to destroy the organism in order to avoid the development of rheumatic fever.

In acute laryngitis caused by viral infection, the patient is advised to rest the voice, inhale steam, and drink warm liquids. If bacteria are the cause of the laryngitis, antibiotic therapy is undertaken. In treating chronic laryngitis, the physician must discover the cause and remove it. If allergy is the cause, antihistamine therapy could help. If the cause is bacterial, antibiotic therapy is used. If smoking or drinking alcohol is the problem, the patient should be counseled to stop. The simple palliative measures used for acute laryngitis—resting the voice, drinking warm liquids, and breathing steam—are also useful for chronic laryngitis.

Symptoms of epiglottitis are often similar to those of sore throat. If there is any evidence of difficulty in breathing, however, the patient should be seen by a physician quickly because an emergency situation may be developing. If epiglottitis is obstructing the airway, the patient should be treated in an intensive care setting. Antibiotics must be given to the patient to treat the infection. It is important, as well, to make an airway for the patient, and it may be necessary to insert a tube into the trachea to allow the patient to breathe.

Before the age of antibiotics, tonsillitis was often treated surgically, with both tonsils and adenoids removed. This procedure is now rare because the infection usually responds to antibiotic therapy. Similarly, in peritonsillar abscess or quinsy, antibiotics usually clear the condition satisfactorily. In some cases, accumulations of pus may be removed surgically. If the abscesses return, it may be advisable to remove the tonsils.

As a rule, the child with croup is treated at home. Because the disease is usually caused by viruses, antibiotics are not used unless bacteria are known to be involved. Steam is often used to help liquefy mucus deposits on the interior walls of the trachea, the larynx, and the bronchi. The patient is given warm liquids to drink and is closely watched so that any signs that the condition is getting worse will be detected. The following symptoms should alert the caregiver to the possibility that an emergency situation is developing and that medical help is needed quickly: drooling, difficulty in swallowing, difficulty in breathing, inability to bend the neck forward, blue or dark color in the lips, high-pitched sounds when inhaling, rapid heartbeat, and loss of consciousness.

The main goals of therapy for sinusitis are to control infection, relieve the blockage of the sinus openings to permit drainage, and relieve pain. When sinusitis is known to be of bacterial origin, an appropriate antibiotic will be used to eradicate the organism. Often, however, sinusitis is attributable to viral infection, and other procedures are used to treat it. Inhaling steam is useful for thinning secretions and promoting drainage, as are mucolytic agents such as guaifenesin. Decongestant sprays and oral decongestants reduce swelling and open passages. Analgesics can be given for pain. In certain circumstances, the sinuses are drained surgically.

Acute otitis media is most often diagnosed with the aid of an otoscope, an instrument that the doctor uses to look at the eardrum and surrounding tissues. The eardrum will be a dull red color, bulging, and perhaps perforated. While a viral infection may precede otitis media, the causative microorganisms for this and related ear infections, such as mastoiditis, are usually bacteria. Antibiotics are used both to treat the infections and to prevent the spread of disease to other areas. The drugs are usually taken orally. Penicillin and its derivatives are used, as are erythromycin and sulfisoxazole. Antibiotic therapy for acute otitis media is usually continued for ten days to two weeks. Sometimes, pus and other fluids and solid matter build up in the inner ear. It may be necessary to pierce the eardrum in order to remove these deposits. To help relieve blockage of the Eustachian tubes, a topical vasoconstrictor may be used in the nose to reduce the swelling of blood vessels. Antihistamines could be helpful to patients with allergies, but otherwise they are not indicated.

For chronic otitis media, it is necessary to clean both the outer ear canal and the middle ear thoroughly. A mild acetic acid solution with a corticosteroid is used for a week to ten days. Meanwhile, aggressive oral antibiotic therapy is undertaken to eradicate the pathogen. The perforated eardrum associated with chronic otitis media can usually be repaired surgically with little or no loss of function, and the cholesteatoma must be surgically removed.

Simple nosebleed can be treated by pinching the nose with the fingers and breathing through the mouth for five or ten minutes, to allow the blood to clot. Also, a plug of absorbent paper or cloth can be inserted into the bleeding nostril. A nosebleed that does not stop easily should be seen by a physician.

Nasal obstruction resulting from colds or allergies is treated by appropriate medications, decongestants for colds, and antihistamines for allergies. A deviated septum may require surgery. The only therapy for rhinitis medicamentosa, or rebound congestion caused by overuse of nasal decongestants, is to stop the medication and endure the congestion for as long as it takes the condition to clear. Sometimes, it is necessary to consult a physician.

For simple halitosis caused by smoking or food, breath fresheners (with or without "odor-fighting" chemicals) are often used, even though they usually simply replace a "bad" odor with a "good" one. Some people firmly believe that chewing parsley or other leaves rich in chlorophyll will counteract the smell of garlic. When halitosis is attributable to tooth or gum disease, it will persist until the condition is cured. Halitosis may be of diagnostic value in certain situations where a characteristic odor could alert the physician to the possibility of a disease condition.

Perspective and Prospects

Diseases and infections of the nasal cavity and throat have always been common among human populations, as have therapies to deal with them. Until the advent of antibiotics, some of these disorders were quite serious, especially in young children, but modern medications and surgeries, where appropriate, have greatly lessened the danger. The widespread use of a vaccine against *Hemophilus influenzae*, the most common causative organism of epiglottitis, has made this life-threatening disease a rarity. Many over-the-counter drugs are used to combat sore throats, sinus congestion, and other nasopharyngeal symptoms of the common cold, although colds themselves remain incurable because of the hundreds or thousands of different microorganisms that may be responsible.

Despite the numerous medications that can be taken, however, more serious infections or diseases, such as chronic tonsillitis or laryngitis, require a doctor's care, with more potent, prescription drugs and surgery if needed. The treatments available to physicians and patients for the symptoms of nasopharyngeal disorders are many, but the search continues for better drugs and perhaps preventive measures such as vaccinations to address the causes of these conditions.

—*C. Richard Falcon*

See also Allergies; Antihistamines; Choking; Common cold; Decongestants; Ear infections and disorders; Ears; Earwax; Esophagus; Halitosis; Hearing; Hearing loss; Laryngectomy; Laryngitis; Mouth and throat cancer; Multiple chemical sensitivity syndrome; Nasal polyp removal; Nosebleeds; Oral and maxillofacial surgery; Otorhinolaryngology; Pharyngitis; Pharynx; Plastic surgery; Respiration; Rhinitis; Rhinoplasty and submucous resection; Sinusitis; Smell; Sore throat; Strep throat; Taste; Tonsillectomy and adenoid removal; Tonsillitis; Tonsils; Voice and vocal cord disorders.

For Further Information:

Ferrari, Mario. *PDxMD Ear, Nose, and Throat Disorders*. Philadelphia: PDxMD, 2003. A clinical yet accessible reference text that provides a comprehensive list of disorders, with a summary of the condition, background, diagnosis, treatment, outcomes, prevention, and resources.

Friedman, Ellen M., and James M. Barassi. *My Ear Hurts! A Complete Guide to Understanding and Treating Your Child's Ear Infections*. Darby, Pa.: Diane, 2004. Reviews current research on ear infections and reviews a range of treatment approaches from both conventional and alternative medicine.

Greene, Alan R. *The Parent's Complete Guide to Ear Infections*. Reprint. Allentown, Pa.: People's Medical Society, 2004. Every parent who has ever had a child with recurrent otitis will appreciate this book. It explains the anatomy of normal ears, causes of infections, prevention, symptoms, evaluation, initial and ongoing treatment, antibiotics, the pros and cons of surgical intervention, hearing loss, tubes, and complications.

Kimball, Chad T. *Colds, Flu, and Other Common Ailments Sourcebook*. Detroit, Mich.: Omnigraphics, 2001. A comprehensive guide for general readers covering treatment issues and controversies surrounding common ailments and injuries. Includes discussions on ailments of the nose, throat, lungs, ears, eyes, and head.

Litin, Scott C., ed. *Mayo Clinic Family Health Book*. 4th ed. New York: HarperResource, 2009. A thorough, updated medical text for the layperson. The section on nasopharyngeal diseases is quite complete and offers excellent anatomic illustrations.

Wagman, Richard J., ed. *The New Complete Medical and Health Encyclopedia*. 4 vols. Chicago: J. G. Ferguson, 2002. The chapters on upper respiratory diseases in this work are thorough and clear, with good illustrations.

National Cancer Institute (NCI)

Organization

Definition: A federal agency devoted to the study of cancer, as well as communication and education about this condition.

Key terms:

carcinogenesis: the biological process of the initiation, promotion, and progression of cancer

epidemiology: the study of the relationships between a host, an agent, and an environment that lead to a condition or disease

Overview

The U.S. Department of Health and Human Services (DHHS) is the federal agency responsible for public health. The DHHS includes twelve divisions, one of which is the National Institutes of Health (NIH). The

National Cancer Institute (NCI) is one of seventeen institutes within NIH. The NCI was established under the National Cancer Act of 1937 and is the principal federal agency for cancer research and training. Following special legislation in 1971, the scope of the NCI has continued to broaden through new initiatives and legislation.

The purpose of the NCI is to eliminate cancer as far as possible and to discover treatment for those cancers which cannot be eradicated. The NCI approaches these goals by supporting research, coordinating efforts in prevention and treatment, facilitating the movement of research findings into medicine, and providing education and resources for patients and their families, health educators, and scientists. The NCI conducts research in its own laboratories and clinics in Bethesda, Maryland, but also supports and coordinates research projects conducted by universities, hospitals, research foundations, and businesses throughout the United States and many other countries.

THE ORGANIZATION AND FOCUS OF THE NCI

The NCI is organized into the Office of the Director of NCI and eight divisions. Each division specializes in a different aspect of cancer research, although there is overlap among them. The divisions include the Division of Basic Sciences, the Division of Cancer Biology, the Division of Cancer Control and Population Sciences, the Division of Cancer Epidemiology and Genetics, the Division of Cancer Prevention, the Division of Cancer Treatment and Diagnosis, the Division of Clinical Sciences, and the Division of Extramural Activities.

The Division of Basic Sciences focuses on research relating to cellular, molecular, genetic, biochemical, and immunological mechanisms critical to the understanding, diagnosis, and treatment of cancer. Research in cancer cell biology, such as carcinogenesis and cancer immunology, falls within the realm of the Division of Cancer Biology. This division also examines the biological and health effects of exposures to ionizing and nonionizing radiation. The Division of Cancer Epidemiology and Genetics focuses on the special interests of genetic predisposition, lifestyle factors, environmental contaminants, occupational exposures, medications, radiation, and infectious agents, as well as epidemiological methods development. The efforts of the Division of Cancer Prevention center on early detection methods and the efficacy of nutritional or lifestyle changes on cancer prevention. The results of research in this area led to the 5 a Day for Better Health program. Initiated in 1991, this program is a collaborative effort

between the food industry and the NCI, which encourages Americans to eat five or more servings of vegetables and fruits each day as part of a low-fat, high-fiber diet. The Division of Cancer Treatment and Diagnosis includes programs in biomedical imaging, cancer diagnosis, cancer therapy evaluation, developmental therapeutics, and radiation research.

The mission of the Division of Clinical Sciences is to take the scientific discoveries to the medical clinic. It has five major research areas: cancer genetics, cancer vaccines and immunotherapy, molecular therapeutics, experimental transplantation, and advanced technology. The clinical cancer genetics program integrates all aspects of clinical and laboratory medicine, particularly in studies of breast, colon, renal, and prostate cancer. Processes include molecular diagnostics, novel imaging techniques, and the molecular assessment of normal tissues in at-risk populations. The cancer vaccines and immunotherapy program investigates the clinical feasibility of using vaccines against known conditions associated with cancer, such as the human papillomavirus and human immunodeficiency virus (HIV), as well as with cancer-specific products, such as in melanoma and in lymphomas. The molecular therapeutics program is concerned with most clinical trial experiments. Important recent discoveries include the development of Taxol as an effective anticancer agent, the development of AZT as an important anti-HIV drug, and the use of adoptive immunotherapy in the treatment of malignant melanoma. The scientific thrust of the molecular therapeutics program is the belief that the analysis of the molecular profile of individual cancers will help determine the most effective chemotherapeutic approaches. The experimental transplantation program examines bone marrow biology in order to advance transplantation techniques and the effectiveness of this approach.

Integrating many programs and divisions is the advanced technology program. New technology is an essential key to identifying genetic elements involved in cancer initiation and progression, as well as in drug efficacy and drug resistance. Although many drugs have been discovered that inhibit the growth of cancer cells successfully, they also affect healthy cells. This causes side effects that have a negative impact on patients' health and quality of life. New therapeutics and technology are being investigated to minimize or eliminate these side effects and enhance the effectiveness of therapy.

The eighth division of the NCI is the Division of Extramural Activities, which is responsible for handling all applications for funding and for monitoring research that has received funding from the NCI. Extramural activities also include the oversight of scientific communications. To enhance communication, the NCI has a number of advisory boards and groups that provide the institute with input from the public, medical, and research communities.

In 1998, the Office of Cancer Complementary and Alternative Medicine was established to coordinate research and communication activities in the arena of complementary and alternative medicine, both within the NCI and with other agencies.

The NCI is strengthening the information base for cancer care decision making. Researchers, medical providers, and patients seek to understand better what constitutes quality cancer care. The NCI is concerned with both geographic and racial or ethnic disparities in who receives quality care. The Cancer Information Service, established in 1976, is the section of the NCI that is the link to the public, attempting to explain research findings in a clear, timely, and understandable manner. To this end, the Cancer Information Service helps develop education efforts targeting minority audiences and people with limited access to health care information or services.

PERSPECTIVE AND PROSPECTS

To be successful in managing this range of responsibilities and breadth of mission, the NCI has a budget in the billions of dollars. Through the years, the work of the NCI has led to a decline in deaths due to cancer, even though advances in the treatment of infectious diseases have made cancer the second leading cause of death in the United States. Creative and dedicated scientists at the NCI have goals to lower its numbers even further in the near future. The NCI will enhance collaborations among institutions and researchers so that priorities are targeted and goals are achieved. An important path to achieving these goals is a program to increase access to clinical trials. Achievement of research goals may also be expedited through a program of extraordinary opportunities for scientific areas of recent importance and promise.

—*Karen Chapman-Novakofski, R.D., L.D.N., Ph.D.*

See also Cancer; Chemotherapy; Clinical trials; Department of Health and Human Services; Environmental diseases; Environmental health; Epidemiology; Genetics and inheritance; National Institutes of Health (NIH); Nutrition; Oncology; Preventive medicine; Radiation therapy.

FOR FURTHER INFORMATION:

Hewitt, Maria Elizabeth, et al., eds. *Ensuring Quality Cancer Care.* Washington, D.C.: National Academy Press, 1999.

Lerner, Barron H. *The Breast Cancer Wars: Fear, Hope, and the Pursuit of a Cure in Twentieth-century America.* New York: Oxford University Press, 2003.

National Cancer Institute. *The Cancer Information Service: A Fifteen-Year History of Service and Research.* Bethesda, Md.: Author, 1993.

_____. *National Cancer Institute's Research Programs: Pursuing the Central Questions of Cancer Research.* Bethesda, Md.: Author, 1999.

_____. *NCI Fact Book.* Bethesda, Md.: Author, 1979-   .

Reuben, Suzanne H. *Assessing Progress, Advancing Change: 2005-2006 Annual Report.* Bethesda, Md.: National Institutes of Health, National Cancer Institute, 2006.

NATIONAL INSTITUTES OF HEALTH (NIH)

ORGANIZATION

DEFINITION: The National Institutes of Health (NIH), composed of more than twenty-five separate institutes, centers, and offices, is one of eight agencies constituting the U.S. Department of Health and Human Services.

KEY TERMS:

AIDSLINE: a database that is part of the National Library of Medicine (NLM) and is devoted to the topic of research on acquired immunodeficiency syndrome (AIDS)

CATLINE: the online catalog of books and manuscripts in the NLM

grant proposals: research plans that outline scientific methods to pursue new knowledge, the required budget, and the resulting products and significance of that work

institute: a specific subagency of the NIH that has the charge of advancing scientific discovery and clinical practice in a specific area of medical science

MEDLINE: a database that is available via the Internet featuring current and historical medical literature, research articles, monographs, presentations, and abstracts

HISTORY AND MISSION

The National Institutes of Health (NIH) is a U.S. federal agency that occupies a multibuilding campus in

Bethesda, Maryland. It consists of a variety of offices, institutes focused on specific medical problems, research laboratories and centers, a center for scientific review, and a national medical library. Its main goal is to discover knowledge that will improve the state of public health for all persons, especially those in the United States. This goal extends to all medical conditions afflicting men, women, and children of all ethnic backgrounds. It also extends to seeking knowledge in areas of basic biological research, clinical research, and research on policy and practice in health care.

The National Institute of Health (precursor to the NIH) was formally established by the Ransdell Act of 1930, which bestowed the name on what was formerly called the Hygienic Laboratory (HL) of the Marine Hospital Service (MHS) in New York. The Ransdell Act also allowed for the establishment of fellowships for basic medical and biological research. The very beginnings of the NIH extend back to 1887, however, when basic laboratory work into medical problems was pursued by the MHS, the founding body of the United States Public Health Service (PHS). The MHS was formed in 1798 to provide hospital care for seamen, but by the 1880's it had shifted its focus to screening ship passengers for infectious diseases capable of starting epidemics.

New European research in the 1880's suggesting that microorganisms caused such diseases spurred American interest in medical research and helped form the original HL. Work by the HL continued, with the laboratory eventually moving from the MHS to its own Washington, D.C., campus. The study of microorganisms continued, extending from study of individual persons to studying the effects of bacteria on water and air pollution. Progress for such work was rewarded in 1901 with governmental money for the construction of a building (completed in 1904) to house the HL and further foster work focused on advancing the public health. Because the value of such work was not well established, however, no permanent funding was provided, leaving the organization subject to ongoing evaluation and supplemental funding.

In 1902 the MHS was reorganized and renamed the Public Health and Marine Hospital Service (PH-MHS); in 1912 it adopted the shortened name of the Public Health Service (PHS). During the intervening time, the HL continued its work and expanded to work in chemistry, pharmacology, zoology, immunology, and the regulation and production of vaccines and antitoxins. Additionally, new scientific staff were added to the staff of medical doctors already on board. Changes in the mission of the organization in 1912 also opened the door for the pursuit of research on noncontagious diseases and water pollution. This work continued during World War I in the form of examining sanitation, anthrax outbreaks, smallpox, tetanus, influenza, and other combat-related conditions. The success of the PHS's work in these areas caught the attention of legislators and resulted in the Ransdell Act of 1930, which established both the National Institute of Health and the practice of setting aside public monies for funding medical research. In 1937, the National Cancer Institute (NCI) was created. In 1944, the PHS formally designated the NCI as a component of the NIH, setting the pattern of a problem-focused structure within the NIH that continues to the present.

World War II led the NIH to focus almost exclusively on war-related problems. This involved examinations of fitness for military service and issues such as dental problems and syphilis. The effects of hazardous substances and conditions on workers in war industries; risks armed service professionals faced from lack of oxygen, cold temperatures, and blood clots while flying; burns, shock, bacterial infections, and fever; and the development of vaccines and therapies for tropical diseases such as malaria also composed much of its work during this time.

Successes established during the wars by such medical research led the PHS to take the 1944 Public Health Service Act to Congress. This act led to grant-funding mechanisms being extended from the NCI alone to the entire National Institute of Health. Additionally, an increasing public interest in health organizations caused Congress to create additional institutes for research on mental health, dental diseases, and heart disease between 1946 and 1949. In 1948, the National Heart Act allowed for the formal pluralization of the National Institutes of Health, rather than a singular institute with the NCI as a subinstitute. The Public Health Service Act of 1944 also provided funding for the Warren Grant Magnuson Clinical Center, which opened in 1953 to focus exclusively on clinical research on health.

From this point forward, each of the individual institutes now composing the NIH came into being. By 1960 there were ten institutes, by 1970 there were fifteen, and by 1998 there were twenty-four institutes and centers. As different health interests develop and advances in medical knowledge are needed, the NIH has responded by allocating its resources to pursue goals in those areas. This has been done both by developing institutes and also by creating specialized offices to pursue contemporary medical problems.

Illness and medicine know no boundaries, however, so the NIH has also maintained an interest in global public health issues. Such interest was formally shown in 1947, when grants were first awarded to investigators abroad. Similarly, in 1968, the John E. Fogarty International Center (FIC) was created to coordinate international research efforts, involving liaisons with the World Health Organization and a variety of international research organizations. The FIC also supports language translation, documentation, and reviews of new health findings. It facilitates biomedical communications through its maintenance of the National Library of Medicine (NLM), MEDLINE, CATLINE, AIDSLINE, and numerous other databases for researchers, physicians, and the public at large. Similarly, focused consensus development conferences, where investigators and clinicians from around the world can meet to evaluate new and existing therapies, are another way that international interests are pursued. Since these conferences were initiated in 1977, more than one hundred such conferences have been held.

In keeping with its practical focus, the NIH has strived to seek out knowledge that yields new drugs, devices, and procedures that are useful not just for the government but for the public at large as well. In 1986, the Technology Transfer Act allowed for a partnership between NIH-funded research and the private sector. Encouraging researchers to examine possible commercial and practical applications of basic medical research to wide-reaching clinical or research use benefits overall scientific and health progress. Partnering with business allows private industries to take over the process of marketing and developing products in a manner more affordable to them than to the government, allowing the government to focus on development while benefiting through the use of the eventual marketed products.

ORGANIZATIONAL STRUCTURE AND METHOD

The NIH is organized to accomplish its goals by using its offices, institutes, and research centers. Research is conducted on the NIH campus in its own funded laboratories, as well as in the labs of scientists supported by NIH funding, who are stationed in institutes of higher education, teaching hospitals, and free-standing research institutions in the United States and other countries. In addition to supporting ongoing research, the NIH also supports research infrastructure by maintaining a library and a variety of printed and electronic resources to facilitate communication among its researchers, the larger scientific community, policymakers, and the public. Scientific research also is supported by developing one of the most valuable resources known to medicine: new researchers. The NIH sponsors a variety of training programs focusing on medical training and research in order to keep a large body of high-quality scholars and investigators in development. Such programs extend from career development for postdoctoral researchers and predoctoral training, to high school level learning in the sponsoring of internships and other learning experiences for teenagers interested in medical science careers.

Funding for research and training programs outside the NIH campus and research centers is facilitated through grant proposal programs that distribute federal tax monies devoted to such endeavors. Applicants to such programs are able to submit independent proposals for work related to the goals of the NIH that they believe is demanded by the state of science and knowledge. They are also able to submit proposals in response to program announcements and calls for proposals on specific topics as outlined by the institutes and offices of the NIH. Many different grant mechanisms exist for such proposals, including grants supporting the work of individual trainees, training programs for cohorts of researchers at different stages of career development, the ongoing work of career scientists, small grants for new or experimental work, focused projects, and even centers of research excellence where many researchers focus on the same topic of study. In addition, grant support is offered to sponsor conferences and academic meetings on special topics in health research and training.

To receive this funding, those wishing to be considered for receiving such grant monies need to submit proposals for confidential peer review through the Center for Scientific Review (CSR), which is part of the NIH structure. Proposals are reviewed by panels of experts who evaluate the research plans, goals, staff, environment, and overall innovation and merit of the work proposed. In addition, ethical considerations about the proposed research are reviewed and considered for both animal welfare and the welfare of human research participants. Emphasis on ethical issues has been a long-standing issue for medical research. It was, however, highlighted in the 1960's, when grantees receiving NIH grant monies were required to state the ethical principles guiding their research on humans, and in

1979, when written guidelines for research on human subjects were established. Once through peer review, proposals are reviewed again by a national advisory council to determine the priority of the work in addressing the goals of the NIH and its institutes and offices. After the proposals are approved by this council for advancement, the individual institutes (sometimes cooperating with specific NIH offices) work to fund them with the monies allotted. Unfortunately, not all proposals can be funded. It should be noted that even after funding, the work of the NIH Office for Protection from Research Risks continues so as to ensure that proper research ethics are followed through the life of the research.

Each year the CSR reviews more than thirty-eight thousand applications, while the NIH supports nearly thirty-five thousand grants nationally and internationally. Such work is facilitated by the various institutions and research offices that fall under the organizational umbrella of the NIH, each focusing on a discrete area of health interest. Some of the institutions involved include the NCI; the National Eye Institute; the National Heart, Lung, and Blood Institute; and the National Human Genome Research Institute. Also included are the National Institutes on Aging, Alcohol Abuse and Alcoholism, Allergy and Infectious Diseases, Arthritis and Musculoskeletal and Skin Diseases, Child Health and Human Development, Deafness and Other Communication Disorders, Dental and Craniofacial Research, Diabetes and Digestive and Kidney Diseases, Drug Abuse, Environmental Health Sciences, Mental Health, and Neurological Disorders and Stroke.

In addition to these institutes, the NIH has numerous offices focusing on specific issues or populations that need to be addressed in health research. These offices focus on contemporary issues of importance for research and include the Offices of Technology Transfer, AIDS Research, Research on Minority Health, Research on Women's Health, Behavioral and Social Sciences Research, Dietary Supplements, Medical Applications of Research, Rare Diseases, Science Policy, Biotechnology Activities, Science Education, and Information Technology. There are also offices that focus on the management of research, specific organizational issues at the NIH, or the communication of information from the NIH to members of the public. These include the Offices of Intramural Research, Extramural Research, Evaluation, Equal Opportunity, Human Resource Management, Financial Management, Procurement Management, Logistics Management, Contracts Management, Management Assessment, Communications and Public Liaison, and General Counsel, as well as the NIH Legal Advisor, and the Freedom of Information Act Office.

PERSPECTIVE AND PROSPECTS

The NIH has been responsible for supporting some very influential research for more than one hundred years, garnering more than eighty Nobel Prizes for NIH-supported work. More vaccines against infectious diseases are available than ever before. The successful mapping of the human genome has set the stage for enhanced genetic testing and the development of gene therapies. Substantial decreases in mortality rates have been achieved for heart disease and strokes. Survival rates for individuals afflicted by cancer have increased, as have survival rates for infants with respiratory distress syndrome. Recovery from spinal cord injuries has been enhanced so as to lessen the probability of long-term disability. Advances in the pharmacological and behavioral treatment of mental health problems such as depression, anxiety, bipolar disorders, and schizophrenia have been achieved. Preventive approaches in dentistry have been highly successful in stopping and slowing dental problems.

Given such successes, billions of dollars of federal tax monies continue to be devoted to the NIH budget to foster continued scientific advances. New work focused on improving prevention, screening, assessment, diagnosis, and treatment for conditions such as AIDS, alcoholism and drug dependence, Alzheimer's disease, arthritis, blindness, communication disorders, diabetes, heart disease, kidney disease, lung cancer, lupus, mental illnesses, Parkinson's disease, stroke, and other persisting conditions continues on a daily basis. While great successes have been achieved to date with the majority of the population, new research is needed that will focus on specialized approaches that may enhance health for women, minorities, youth, and the elderly. The combination of these needs, past successes, and governmental commitment to improving the state of the public health ensures that the NIH will continue onward with its mission for the foreseeable future.

—*Nancy A. Piotrowski, Ph.D.*

See also Childhood infectious diseases; Department of Health and Human Services; Disease; Environmental diseases; Environmental health; Epidemics and pandemics; Epidemiology; Health Canada; Immunization and vaccination; National Cancer Institute (NCI); Occupational health; World Health Organization.

FOR FURTHER INFORMATION:

Desalle, Rob. *Epidemic! The World of Infectious Disease.* New York: New Press, 1999. A book designed to accompany the American Museum of Natural History's exhibit of the same title, an accessible book that details the world of infectious disease from the perspective of science and medicine. Examines what is understood about bacteria, viruses, parasites, and their remedies.

Eberhart-Philips, Jason. *Outbreak Alert: Responding to the Increasing Threat of Infectious Diseases.* Oakland, Calif.: New Harbinger, 2000. Emphasizes the importance of public health to national health; defines and identifies infectious diseases posing a public health threat and how the current way that society functions relates to this threat.

Garrett, Laurie. *Betrayal of Trust: The Collapse of Global Public Health.* New York: Hyperion, 2001. Discusses global public health, putting the status of health in the United States in perspective on some very basic matters related to public health.

Institute of Medicine. *Scientific Opportunities and Public Needs: Improving Priority Setting and Public Input at the National Institutes of Health.* Washington, D.C.: National Academy Press, 1998. Provides an overview of scientific and popular perceptions of the needed long-term health interests of the United States, as well as other global health concerns.

Lee, Philip R., and Carroll L. Estes, eds. *The Nation's Health.* 7th ed. Sudbury, Mass.: Jones and Bartlett, 2003. A compendium of articles compiled by two preeminent American health policy analysts. Chapters discuss the complex web of issues, policies, controversies, and proposed solutions that surround health policy, public health, community health, and health care in the United States.

Shnayerson, Michael, and Mark J. Plotkin. *The Killers Within: The Deadly Rise of Drug Resistant Bacteria.* Boston: Little, Brown, 2003. Traces the evolution of drug-resistant bacteria and how physicians are trying to combat it.

Tulchinsky, Theodore H., and Elena A. Varavikova. *The New Public Health: An Introduction for the Twenty-first Century.* San Diego, Calif.: Academic Press, 2000. Discusses global perspectives on how organizational structures of health care and other public activities affect the state of public health and health care service delivery.

NATIVE AMERICAN HEALTH. *See* **AMERICAN INDIAN HEALTH.**

NAUSEA AND VOMITING
DISEASE/DISORDER

ANATOMY OR SYSTEM AFFECTED: Brain, gastrointestinal system, nervous system, stomach

SPECIALTIES AND RELATED FIELDS: Gastroenterology, otorhinolaryngology

DEFINITION: Nausea is an unpleasant subjective sensation, accompanied by epigastric and duodenal discomfort, which often culminates in vomiting, the regurgitation of the contents of the stomach.

KEY TERMS:

affect: the emotional reactions associated with experience

antiemetics: drugs that prevent or relieve the symptoms of nausea and/or vomiting

chemoreceptor trigger zone: a sensory nerve ending in the brain that is stimulated by and reacts to certain chemical stimulation localized outside the central nervous system

emesis: the act of vomiting

psychogenic: of mental origin

psychotropics: drugs that affect psychic function, behavior, or experience

CAUSES AND SYMPTOMS

Nausea is defined as a subjectively unpleasant sensation associated with awareness of the urge to vomit. It is usually felt in the back of the throat and epigastrium and is accompanied by the loss of gastric tone, duodenal contractions, and reflux of the intestinal contents into the stomach. Retching is defined as labored, spasmodic, rhythmic contractions of the respiratory muscles (including the diaphragm, chest wall, and abdominal wall muscles) without the expulsion of gastric contents. Vomiting, or emesis, is the forceful expulsion of gastric contents from the mouth and is brought about by the powerful sustained contraction of the abdominal muscles, the descent of the diaphragm, and the opening of the gastric cardia (the cardiac orifice of the stomach).

Nausea and vomiting are important defense mechanisms against the ingestion of toxins. The act of emesis involves a sequence of events that can be divided into three phases: preejection, ejection, and postejection. The preejection phase includes the symptoms of nausea, along with salivation, swallowing, pallor, and tachycardia (an abnormally fast heartbeat). The ejection phase comprises retching and vomiting. Retching is characterized by rhythmic, synchronous, inspiratory movements of the diaphragm, abdominal, and external intercostal muscles, while the mouth and the glottis are kept closed. As the antral (cavity) portion of the stomach contracts, the proximal (nearest the center) portion relaxes and the gastric contents oscillate between the stomach and the esophagus. During retching, the hiatal portion of the diaphragm does not relax, and intra-abdominal pressure increases are associated with a decrease in intrathoracic pressure.

In contrast, relaxation of the hiatal portion of the diaphragm (near the esophagus) permits a transfer of intra-abdominal pressure to the thorax during the act of vomiting. Contraction of the muscles of the anterior abdominal wall, relaxation of the esophageal sphincter, an increase in intrathoracic and intragastric pressure, reverse peristalsis (movement of the contents of the alimentary canal), and an open glottis and mouth result in the expulsion of gastric contents. The postejection phase consists of autonomic and visceral responses that return the body to a quiescent phase, with or without residual nausea.

The complex act of vomiting, involving coordination of the respiratory, gastrointestinal, and abdominal musculature, is controlled by what researchers label the emetic center. This center in the brain stem has access to the motor pathways responsible for the visceral and somatic output involved in vomiting, and stimuli from several areas within the central nervous system can affect this center. These include afferent (inward-directed) nerves from the pharynx and gastrointestinal tract, as well as afferents from the higher cortical centers (including the visual center) and the chemore-

ceptor trigger zone (CTZ) in the area postrema (a highly vascularized area of the brain stem). The CTZ can be activated by chemical stimuli received through the blood or the cerebrospinal fluid. Direct electrical stimulation of the CTZ, however, does not result in emesis.

Clinical assessment of nausea and vomiting usually focuses on the occurrence of vomiting, that is, the frequency and number of episodes. Nausea, however, is a subjective phenomenon unobservable by another. Few data collection instruments that measure separately the patient's experience of nausea and vomiting and his or her symptom distress have been reported in the literature. In fact, the Rhodes Index of Nausea and Vomiting (INV) Form 2 is the only available tool that measures the individual components of nausea, vomiting, and retching. This index measures the patient's perception of the duration, frequency, and distress from nausea; the frequency, amount, and distress from vomiting; and the frequency, amount, and distress from retching (dry heaves). The INV score provides a measurement of the total symptom experience of the patient.

While the causes of nausea and vomiting are numerous—they include gastrointestinal diseases, infections, intracranial disease, toxins, radiation sickness, psychological trauma, migraines, and circulatory syncope—three of the most common causes are motion sickness (air, sea, land, or space), pregnancy, and anesthesia administered during operative procedures.

The sequence of symptoms and signs that constitute motion sickness is fairly characteristic. Premonitory symptoms often include yawning or sighing, lethargy, somnolence, and a loss of enthusiasm and concern for the task at hand. Increasing malaise is directed toward the epigastrium, a sensation best described as "stomach awareness," which progresses to nausea. Diversion of the blood flow from the skin toward the muscles results in pallor. A feeling of warmth and a desire for cool air is often accompanied by sweating. Frontal headache and a sensation of disorientation, dizziness, or light-headedness may also occur. As symptoms progress, vomiting occurs early in the sequence of symptoms for some; in others, malaise is severe and prolonged and vomiting is delayed. After vomiting, there is often a temporary improvement in well-being; however, with continued provocative motion, symptoms build again and vomiting recurs. The symptoms may last for minutes, hours, or even days.

The most coherent explanation for the development of motion sickness is provided by sensory conflict the-

---

INFORMATION ON NAUSEA AND VOMITING

CAUSES: May include gastrointestinal diseases, infections, intracranial disease, toxins, radiation sickness, migraines, motion sickness, pregnancy, anesthesia, psychological trauma

SYMPTOMS: Increased salivation and swallowing, pallor, rapid heartbeat, sweating

DURATION: Typically acute; can be recurrent with acute episodes

TREATMENTS: Depends on cause; may include drug therapy, diet regulation, lifestyle change, emotional support

ory. Motion sickness is generally thought to occur as the result of a "sensory conflict" between information arising from the semicircular canals and organs of the vestibular system, visual and other sensory input, and the input that is expected on the basis of past experience or exposure history. It is argued that conflicts between current sensory inputs are by themselves insufficient to produce motion sickness since adaptation occurs even though the conflicting inputs continue to be present. Visual input alone, however, can produce symptoms of motion sickness, such as watching motion pictures shot from a moving vehicle or looking out of the side window (as opposed to the front window) of a moving vehicle.

Nausea and/or vomiting in the early morning during pregnancy, so-called morning sickness, is so common that it is accepted as a symptom of normal pregnancy. Occurring soon after waking, it is often retching rather than actual vomiting and usually does not disturb the woman's health or her pregnancy. The symptoms nearly always cease before the fourteenth week of pregnancy. In a much smaller proportion of cases, approximately 1 in 1,000 births, the vomiting becomes more serious and persistent, occurring throughout the day and even during the night. The term "hyperemesis gravidarum" is given to this serious form of vomiting. Theories on the etiology of morning sickness have tended to be grouped under four main areas: endocrine (caused by estrogen and progesterone levels), psychosomatic (a conscious or unconscious wish not to be pregnant), allergic (a histamine reaction), and metabolic (a lack of potassium).

Nausea and vomiting occur frequently as unpleasant side effects of the administration of anesthesia in many clinical procedures. Most postoperative vomiting is mild, and only in a few cases will the problem persist so as to cause electrolyte disturbances and dehydration. The factors affecting postoperative nausea and vomiting may be divided into two categories: by the type of patient and surgery, and by the anesthetic and preoperative and postoperative medication uses. Patients with a history of motion sickness have a predisposition to postoperative vomiting. Nearly 43 percent of patients who vomited following previous surgery vomited again, whereas slightly more than 14 percent of those who did not vomit previously had an emetic episode at their next operation. Patients undergoing their first anesthetic procedure had an incidence of vomiting of approximately 30 percent.

No direct association between vomiting and age has been found. That vomiting may be hormonally related, however, is suggested by the higher incidence of nausea and vomiting in the latter half of the menstrual cycle. Other factors that may affect nausea and vomiting associated with anesthesia include patient weight (female obese patients being particularly more vulnerable), amount of hydration, metabolic status, and psychological state.

With regard to the type of surgery performed, the highest incidence of nausea and vomiting appears to be associated with abdominal surgery, as well as ear, nose, and throat surgery, with middle-ear surgery being the major category. The length of surgery, and therefore the duration of anesthesia, also has a direct effect on nausea and vomiting. Short (thirty-minute to sixty-minute) operations using cyclopropane had an emetic incidence of 17.5 percent, while operations lasting one and a half to three and a half hours had an incidence of 46.4 percent.

Most of the causes of vomiting associated with general anesthesia are expected to be eliminated with regional or spinal anesthesia. The type of anesthesia used also has an effect on nausea and vomiting. Research indicates that cyclopropane, ether, and nitrous oxide are potent emetics.

TREATMENT AND THERAPY

Since the generation of sensory conflict underlies all motion environments that give rise to motion sickness, practical measures that reduce conflict are likely to reduce motion sickness incidence. Motion sickness can be minimized if the subject has the widest possible view of a visual reference in which the earth is stable. Passengers aboard ships are less likely to be seasick if they remain on deck at midship, where vertical motion is minimized, and view the horizon. In a car or bus, individuals should be in a position to see the road directly ahead, since the movement of this visual scene will correlate with the changes in the direction of the vehicle. While head movements in a rotating environment are known to precipitate motion sickness, there is no clear experimental evidence that they elicit nausea in mild linear oscillation. Thus, some nonpharmacologic remedies for motion sickness are restricting head movements, lying in a supine position, or closing the eyes. In addition, the use of acupressure wrist bands has proven effective in combating motion sickness.

Pharmacologically, the drug hyoscine hydrobromide (also called hyoscine or scopolamine) emerged as a valuable prophylactic drug following extensive research during World War II into the problems of motion sickness in troops transported in aircraft, ships, and landing craft. It remains one of the most effective drugs for short-duration exposures to provocative motion. Doses in excess of 0.6 milligram, however, are very likely to lead to drowsiness, and there is much experimental evidence that hyoscine impairs short-term memory. Hyoscine can be absorbed transdermally, and in order to extend the duration of action, a controlled-release patch was developed to deliver 1.2 milligrams on application and 0.01 milligram hourly thereafter. There is substantial evidence of its sustained effectiveness, but, perhaps as a result of variable absorption rates, there is an increased risk of blurred vision after more than twenty-four hours of use.

Amphetamines, ephedrine, and a number of antihistamines (such as dimenhydrinate) have been found to be clinically useful in motion sickness. Following oral administration, these drugs are generally slower than hyoscine in reaching their peak efficacy, but they have a longer duration of action.

For most susceptible subjects whose exposure to motion sickness-inducing stimuli is infrequent, prophylactic drugs offer the only useful treatment. When exposure to provocative stimuli is more frequent, as for example in professional aircraft pilots, spontaneous adaption occurs during training and an initially high incidence of motion sickness decreases with time.

In medical conditions in which the cause is relatively unknown, it is usual to find a wide variety of suggested therapies; nausea and vomiting during pregnancy and hyperemesis gravidarum (the serious, persistent form of vomiting in pregnancy) are no exception. Prior to 1968, treatments numbered approximately thirty. In subsequent years, however, suggested therapy has been mainly drugs of the antiemetic variety. Yet since the thalidomide tragedy (in which severe deformities occurred in the children of women who took this drug), there has been a reluctance to use drugs of any kind during early pregnancy. Probably the only value of drug therapy is at the stage of morning sickness, when antiemetics or mild sedatives may counter the feeling of nausea and prevent women from experiencing excessive vomiting and entering the vicious cycle of dehydration, starvation, and electrolyte imbalance. Once the patient has reached the stage of hyperemesis gravidarum, much more basic therapy is required, and the regimen calls for correction of dehydration, carbohydrate deficiency, and ionic deficiencies. This program is best managed by intravenous therapy, with or without the addition of vitamin supplements and sedative agents.

Nonpharmacologic self-care actions for morning sickness fall into the three broad categories of manipulating diet, adjusting behavior, and seeking emotional support. Some of the most effective self-care actions are getting rest, eating several small meals rather than three large ones, avoiding bad smells, avoiding greasy or fried foods, avoiding cooking, and receiving extra attention and support.

In terms of postoperative nausea and vomiting caused by anesthesia, it has been found that routine antiemetic prophylaxis of patients undergoing elective surgical procedures is not indicated, since fewer than 30 percent of patients experience postoperative nausea and vomiting. Of those who develop these symptoms, many have transient nausea or only one or two bouts of emesis and do not require antiemetic therapy. In addition, commonly used antiemetic drugs can produce significant side effects, such as sedation. Nevertheless, antiemetic prophylaxis may be justified in those patients who are at greater risk for developing postoperative nausea and/or vomiting. Such therapy is often given to patients with a history of motion sickness or to those undergoing gynecologic procedures, inner-ear procedures, oral surgery (in which the jaws are occluded by wires, causing a high risk of breathing in vomitus), and operations on the ear or eye and plastic surgery operations (in order to avoid disruption of delicate surgical work).

Many different antiemetic drugs are available for the treatment of postoperative nausea and vomiting. Researchers have found it difficult to interpret the results of antiemetic drug studies because the severity of postoperative vomiting and the response to therapeutic agents can be influenced by many variables in addition to the antiemetic drug being studied. Even with the use of the same drugs in a homogeneous population undergoing the same procedure, the severity of emesis varies from individual to individual.

Because antiemetic drugs have differing sites of action, better results can be obtained by using a multidrug approach. If a combination of drugs with a similar site of action is used, however, the incidence of side effects may be increased. There are few data regarding combination antiemetic prophylaxis or therapy for postoperative nausea and emesis. Drug combinations have been avoided in postsurgical patients because of concerns about additive central nervous system toxicity. An exception is the combination of low-dose droperidol and metoclopramide, which appears to be more effective than droperidol alone for outpatient gynecologic procedures.

Although a full stomach is best avoided before any operative procedure, with situations such as emergencies, in which danger from vomiting is acute, a rapid sequence of administering anesthesia (induction) and clearing the air passage (intubation) remains the method of choice to avoid nausea and vomiting in patients with a full stomach. After the procedure, it is recommended that the patient minimize movement in order to avoid nausea and vomiting. Also, it has been found that avoiding eating solid food for at least eight hours after a surgical procedure is helpful in preventing postoperative nausea and vomiting.

Perspective and Prospects

Though it has existed for as long as there have been human beings, the symptom of nausea has never received much attention in health care practice or research. In fact, until the early 1970's the sensation of nausea was frequently dismissed as merely a passing phenomenon. The rationale for this dismissal was most likely the understanding that nausea is self-limiting (it always passes with time), is never life-threatening in itself, is probably psychogenic in nature (at least to some degree), and, being subjective, is very difficult to measure. In addition, in the past the most predictable nausea was related to pregnancy, which may also explain the lack of attention given to nausea.

Until the late 1980's, there was still little research being conducted on the nausea associated with pregnancy, although it is a common symptom. The historical lack of interest in nausea and vomiting during pregnancy may be traced to the fact that, since the symptoms generally persist only through the first trimester, health care professionals have viewed the problem as relatively insignificant. As more pregnant women work outside the home in demanding positions, however, these women have exhibited less tolerance for illness. Demands upon the health care industry and upon personal physicians for more research and effective treatment have become more widespread.

While it is surprising that nausea has received scant attention in the history of clinical research, it is even more astonishing that vomiting, an observable behavior, has received so little attention as well. Although vomiting is a primitive neurologic process that has remained almost unchanged in the evolution of animals, the mechanisms that regulate the behavior remain virtually unknown.

One reason for the paucity of information on the subject of nausea in particular stems from the lack of a reliable animal model. This fact has hampered research aimed at establishing the etiological basis for nausea and its relationship to vomiting. While some species of lower animals, for example rats, cannot vomit, it is not known whether rats experience the phenomenon of nausea. Thus no effective means of measuring nausea in lower animals has been devised.

Since the early 1970's, there has been a noticeable increase in research on nausea as a drug side effect because it was so frequently seen in cancer chemotherapy clinical trials sponsored by the National Cancer Institute and the American Cancer Society. As more powerful chemotherapy agents and aggressive combinations were clinically investigated, patients began to experience severe, potentially life-threatening nausea and vomiting. Older drugs such as antihistamines, phenothiazines, and benzodiazepines are still used for their antiemetic characteristics, but they are augmented by newer agents such as benzamides, neurokinin-1-receptor antagonists, and serotonin antagonists.

Aside from the pharmacological investigations of new drugs and drug combinations in the treatment of nausea and vomiting, an interesting branch of scientific investigation has begun the process of exploring alternative ways of managing these symptoms. Behavioral interventions, such as progressive muscle relaxation, biofeedback, imagery, or music therapy, have been used to alleviate postchemotherapy anxiety. These methods may also be used to treat other patients suffering from the symptoms of nausea and vomiting, such as pregnant women.

Another noninvasive, nonpharmacologic measure that has been considered in the relief of nausea and vomiting is transcutaneous electrical nerve stimulation (TENS). Several research studies indicate that TENS may be useful in alleviating chemotherapy-related nausea and vomiting, including delayed nausea and vomiting. Side effects from using TENS units are negligible, and with further study they may prove to be an acceptable, helpful relief measure.

—*Genevieve Slomski, Ph.D.*

See also Acid reflux disease; Anesthesia; Appetite loss; Botulism; Bulimia; Chemotherapy; Colitis; Crohn's disease; Diaphragm; Digestion; Eating disorders; Esophagus; Food biochemistry; Food poisoning; Gastroenteritis; Gastroenterology; Gastroenterology, pediatric; Gastrointestinal disorders; Gastrointestinal system; Heartburn; Indigestion; Influenza; Lactose intolerance; Motion sickness; Multiple chemical sensitivity syndrome; Noroviruses; Poisoning; Poisonous plants; Pregnancy and gestation; Radiation sickness; Rotavirus; Salmonella infection; Stomach, intestinal, and pancreatic cancers; Ulcer surgery; Ulcers; Vagotomy.

FOR FURTHER INFORMATION:

Blum, Richard H., and W. LeRoy Heinrichs. *Nausea and Vomiting: Overview, Challenges, Practical Treatments, and New Perspectives*. Philadelphia: Whurr, 2000. Discusses such topics as drugs to prevent and control nausea and vomiting, pregnancy nausea and vomiting, allergy and immunology, anesthesiology, and gastroenterology.

Edmundowicz, Steven A., ed. *Twenty Common Problems in Gastroenterology*. New York: McGraw-Hill, 2002. Surveys common problems with the gastrointestinal tract, examining nausea and vomiting as both symptom and disorder.

Funk, Sandra G., et al., eds. *Key Aspects of Comfort: Management of Pain, Fatigue, and Nausea*. New York: Springer, 1989. This work, which discusses the management of pain, fatigue, and nausea, functions both as an introduction to these topics and as a sourcebook for treatment.

Hesketh, Paul J., ed. *Management of Nausea and Vomiting in Cancer and Cancer Treatment*. Sudbury, Mass.: Jones and Bartlett, 2005. Reviews the therapies available to prevent nausea and vomiting in cancer patients.

Kucharczyk, John, David J. Stewart, and Alan D. Miller, eds. *Nausea and Vomiting: Recent Research and Clinical Advances*. Boca Raton, Fla.: CRC Press, 1991. After an introductory chapter on pioneers in emesis research, discusses the mechanisms of emesis, including respiratory muscle control, digestive tract activity, and neural mechanisms; the clinical characteristics and consequences of vomiting; and antiemetic therapies.

Litin, Scott C., ed. *Mayo Clinic Family Health Book*. 4th ed. New York: HarperResource, 2009. Perhaps the best general medical text for the layperson, this book covers the entire medical field. While the information is derived from a wide variety of highly technical sources, the articles are written to be easily understood by a general audience.

Sleisenger, Marvin H., ed. *The Handbook of Nausea and Vomiting*. New York: Caduceus Medical/Parthenon, 1993. A short manual for dealing with the symptoms and causes of nausea and vomiting. Includes a bibliography and an index.

NECK INJURIES AND DISORDERS. *See* **HEAD AND NECK DISORDERS.**

NECROSIS
DISEASE/DISORDER
ALSO KNOWN AS: Gangrene, mortification
ANATOMY OR SYSTEM AFFECTED: Bones, cells
SPECIALTIES AND RELATED FIELDS: Oncology, orthopedics
DEFINITION: Tissue damage occurring as a result of cell death.

CAUSES AND SYMPTOMS
"Necrosis" refers to the degeneration of cells or tissues after cell death occurs for any reason, generally in localized regions of the body. Thus, necrosis is tissue degeneration, which occurs secondary to cell death from any cause. Necrosis is most commonly the result of ischemia, traumatic injury, bacterial infection, or toxins (including excessive steroids or alcohol).

In its earliest stage, there are often no symptoms of necrosis. Tissue damage begins to occur within twelve hours of cell death. When symptoms do begin to occur, they range from atrophy through decreased range of motion and pain to the development of gangrenous tissue.

TREATMENT AND THERAPY
The damage done to the tissue resulting from cell death is permanent. Any treatment of necrosis is aimed at minimizing further cell death and tissue injury. In the case of heart disease, treatment of the underlying condition to alleviate hypoxia prevents further cell death from ischemia. In the case of bacterial infection, antibiotics are used to treat the infection and prevent cell death and tissue damage. In the case of necrosis of bone tissue from decreased blood supply, the aim of treatment is to minimize further bone loss. This type of necrosis, known as avascular necrosis, is treated with nonsteroidal anti-inflammatory drugs (NSAIDs) to re-

---

INFORMATION ON NECROSIS

CAUSES: Cell death leading to degeneration of tissue over time
SYMPTOMS: Pain, tissue decay
DURATION: Permanent, irreversible
TREATMENTS: Pain relievers (NSAIDs), surgery

lieve pain, exercise to improve range of motion, electrical treatment to stimulate bone growth, or surgery to reshape bone, graft bone, or replace joints.

PERSPECTIVE AND PROSPECTS

The term "necrosis" was used nearly two thousand years ago in ancient Greek textbooks to refer to changes within tissue, long after cell death had occurred, that were visible to the naked eye. With the advent of light microscopy, the tissue damage following cell death became visible within twelve to twenty-four hours.

In 1859, Rudolf Virchow, in his renowned text *Cellular Pathology as Based upon Physiological and Pathological Histology*, discussed degeneration, necrosis, mortification, and gangrene, using these terms more or less synonymously. It should be noted that he used the term "necrosis" to refer to an advanced stage of tissue breakdown. At this point, the breakdown had to be visible to the naked eye, since light microscopy had not yet been developed. Today, using the microscope, tissue damage resulting from cell death is obvious and often identical whether caused by ischemia, traumatic injury, bacteria, or toxins.

—*Robin Kamienny Montvilo, R.N., Ph.D.*

See also Cells; Circulation; Gangrene; Ischemia; Necrotizing fasciitis; Osteonecrosis; Pathology; Vascular medicine; Vascular system.

FOR FURTHER INFORMATION:

Majno, G., and I. Joris. "Apoptosis, Oncosis, and Necrosis: An Overview of Cell Death." *American Journal of Pathology* 146, no. 1 (1995): 3-15.

Parker, J. N., and P. M. Parker. *The Official Patient's Sourcebook on Avascular Necrosis.* San Diego, Calif.: Icon Health, 2002.

NECROTIZING FASCIITIS
DISEASE/DISORDER

ANATOMY OR SYSTEM AFFECTED: Blood vessels, muscles, skin

SPECIALTIES AND RELATED FIELDS: Bacteriology, critical care, dermatology, emergency medicine, epidemiology, histology, plastic surgery, vascular medicine

DEFINITION: An invasive bacterial infection that occurs in the connective tissue between the skin and muscle known as the fascia, cutting off blood flow; it must be urgently treated surgically and, even in the best circumstances, has a high mortality rate.

CAUSES AND SYMPTOMS

Although it had been identified in the past, in 1994 there were numerous headline newspaper reports describing a new "flesh-eating bacteria." These articles detailed the devastating effect of seemingly minor wounds infected with streptococcal bacteria. Patients quickly become very sick, with a rapidly progressive downward course, even from trauma resulting in a deep muscle bruise or muscle strain or in "minor" cuts and scrapes.

In the former nonpenetrating injuries, it is likely that the bacteria were already present in the blood and then seeded the site of damage. Most of these patients, however, did not recall any prior recent infection that may have made them susceptible. Penetrating injuries, where the normally protective barrier of the skin has been broken, were often minor and not originally treated as contaminated or infected. Other cases of necrotizing fasciitis are caused by surgical infections and bowel contamination. These cases are more rare and often found to have a mixture of bacteria, such as staphylococci or *Escherichia coli* (*E. coli*).

Patients with necrotizing fasciitis have fever, inflammation, severe pain, and blistering at the site of infection. If this cellulitis is not recognized and urgently treated, the infection will quickly spread in the layers of connective tissue just under the skin known as the fascia. As the bacteria multiply, they cause blood vessels supplying the skin to form clots and thus cut off blood flow to the skin. Without nutrients, oxygen, and the ability to remove waste products, the skin dies. Once this occurs, the nerves are destroyed and the patient no longer has the excruciating pain. The skin at this point appears to be "eaten away." The possibility exists that the underlying muscle adjacent to the fascia will become infected. Thus, the potential for muscle death as well as skin death is of great concern, particularly if the infection begins in the arms, legs, abdomen, or back, as

---

INFORMATION ON NECROTIZING FASCIITIS

CAUSES: Bacterial infection

SYMPTOMS: Fever, inflammation, severe pain, blistering at site of infection, tissue death

DURATION: Acute

TREATMENTS: Emergency care, extensive surgical debridement, antibiotics

these areas have large muscle groups directly underlying the skin. In necrotizing fasciitis, the extremities and the area around the genitals and anus (perineum) are most commonly and extensively involved. Multiplication and movement of these streptococcal bacteria and their toxins into the bloodstream produces a shocklike state.

TREATMENT AND THERAPY

The patient with necrotizing fasciitis must be stabilized quickly in an intensive care unit, where fluids can be administered and heart and lung condition can be closely monitored. The only lifesaving treatment available is extensive surgical debridement to remove the necrotic (dead) tissue and slow the spread of the bacteria. Antibiotics including penicillins, clindamycin, and gentamicin are given to help eradicate the pathogen. Because the infection spreads so rapidly, death often results even with heroic surgical and drug therapy unless the condition is diagnosed and treated early. Fortunately, these infections remain relatively rare.

—*Matthew Berria, Ph.D.*

See also Antibiotics; Bacterial infections; Bacteriology; Connective tissue; Dermatology; Epidemiology; Fascia; Necrosis; Shock; Skin; Skin disorders; Streptococcal infections; Toxic shock syndrome; Wounds.

FOR FURTHER INFORMATION:

Biddle, Wayne. *A Field Guide to Germs.* 2d ed. New York: Anchor Books, 2002.

Forbes, Betty A., Daniel F. Sahm, and Alice S. Weissfeld. *Bailey and Scott's Diagnostic Microbiology.* 12th ed. St. Louis, Mo.: Mosby/Elsevier, 2007.

Roemmele, Jacqueline A., and Donna Batdorff. *Surviving the Flesh-Eating Bacteria: Understanding, Preventing, Treating, and Living with the Effects of Necrotizing Fasciitis.* Garden City Park, N.Y.: Avery, 2000.

Salyers, Abigail, and Dixie D. Whitt. *Bacterial Pathogenesis: A Molecular Approach.* 2d ed. Washington, D.C.: ASM Press, 2002.

Snyder, Larry, and Wendy Champness. *Molecular Genetics of Bacteria.* 3d ed. Washington, D.C.: ASM Press, 2007.

Wilson, Michael, Brian Henderson, and Rod McNab. *Bacterial Disease Mechanisms: An Introduction to Cellular Microbiology.* New York: Cambridge University Press, 2002.

NEONATOLOGY

SPECIALTY

ANATOMY OR SYSTEM AFFECTED: All

SPECIALTIES AND RELATED FIELDS: Cardiology, critical care, embryology, genetics, obstetrics, pediatrics, perinatology

DEFINITION: A subspecialty of pediatrics that involves the care of newborn infants from birth through the first month of life, especially those infants with life-threatening conditions such as prematurity, genetic defects, and serious illnesses.

KEY TERMS:

congenital disorders: abnormalities present at birth that occurred during fetal development as a result of genetic errors, exposure to toxins and microorganisms, or maternal illness

incubator: in the nursery, a plexiglass unit that encloses the premature or sick infant to allow strict temperature regulation

intrauterine growth retardation: the condition of infants who are born significantly smaller than the standard for the number of weeks that they have spent in the uterus

neonatal intensive care unit: a hospital nursery with advanced equipment and specially trained staff to maintain the vital functions of sick newborns and to monitor their progress closely

neonatal period: the first month of life; derived from the Greek *neo* (meaning "new") and the Latin *natum* (meaning "birth")

prematurity: strictly defined, birth before a full-term pregnancy (thirty-eight weeks); more commonly associated with birth before thirty-five weeks

respirator: a machine that inflates and deflates the lungs, imitating normal breathing; connected to the patient through a tube placed into the windpipe (endotracheal tube)

respiratory distress syndrome: a life-threatening illness primarily of premature infants; immature lungs lack surfactant, a vital substance that keeps the tiny air sacs (alveoli) from collapsing upon exhalation

SCIENCE AND PROFESSION

Neonatology has grown dramatically since its beginnings in the late 1960's, and neonatologists have become an integral part of the obstetric-pediatric team at major medical centers throughout the world. In addition to being cared for by physicians who specialize in neonatology, some neonatal infants, in particular those who are critically ill or premature, are cared for by nurse practitioners with the specialty certification of neonatal nurse practitioner (N.N.P.). In large part because of an ever-expanding technological base and marked advances in scientific research, these health care professionals have changed the outlook for premature and sick newborns.

As a subspecialty of pediatrics, neonatology is concerned with the most critical time of transition and adjustment—the first four weeks of life, or the neonatal period—whether the infant is healthy (a normal birth) or sick (as a result of genetic problems, obstetric complications, or medical illness). By the early 1970's, it became increasingly clear to health administrators that hospitals throughout the United States had varying abilities to care for medical and pediatric cases requiring the most sophisticated staff and equipment. Consequently, they developed a system that designated hospitals as either level I (small, community hospitals), level II (larger hospitals), or level III (major regional medical centers, also called tertiary care centers). It was in the last group that the most advanced neonatal care could be delivered. In these major centers, there are two types of nurseries, separating the normal healthy infant from the sick or high-risk infant: the routine nursery and the neonatal intensive care unit (NICU).

Routine nurseries are the temporary home of the vast majority of newborns. The services of the neonatologist are rarely needed here, and the general pediatrician or family practitioner observes and examines the infant for twenty-four to forty-eight hours to be sure that it has made a smooth transition from intrauterine to extrauterine life. These babies soon leave the hospital for their homes. Those neonates with minor problems arising from multiple births, difficult deliveries, mild prematurity, and minor illness are easily managed by their primary care physician in consultation with a neonatologist, perhaps at another hospital. It is in the neonatal intensive care unit, however, that the most difficult situations present themselves. Here several teams of pediatric subspecialists—surgeons, cardiologists, anesthesiologists, and highly trained nurses, along with many other health professionals—are led by a neonatologist, who coordinates the team's efforts. These newborns have life-threatening conditions, often as a result of extreme prematurity (more than six weeks earlier than the expected date of delivery), major birth defects (genetic or developmental), severe illness (such as overwhelming infections), or being born to drug- or alcohol-addicted mothers. They require the most advanced technological and medical interventions, often

to sustain life artificially until the underlying problem is corrected. It is in this setting that the most dramatic successes of neonatology are found.

After hours of being inside a forcefully contracting uterus and sustaining the stress of passing through a narrow birth canal, the newborn emerges into a dry, cold, and hostile environment. The umbilical cord, which has provided oxygen and nutrients, is clamped and cut; the fluid-filled lungs must now exchange air instead, and the respiratory center of the infant's brain begins a lifetime of spontaneous breathing, usually heralded by crying. The vast majority of neonates make this extraordinary adjustment to extrauterine life without difficulty. At one minute and again at five minutes, the newborn is evaluated and scored on five physical signs: heart rate, breathing, muscle tone, reflexes, and skin tone. The healthy infant is vigorously moving, crying, and pink regardless of race. These Apgar scores, named for founder Virginia Apgar, evaluate the need for immediate resuscitation. A brief physical examination follows, which can identify other life-threatening abnormalities.

It is essential to remember that the medical history of a neonate is in fact the medical and obstetric history of its mother, and seemingly normal infants may develop problems shortly after birth. Risk factors include very young or middle-aged mothers; difficult deliveries; babies with Rh-negative blood types; mothers with diabetes mellitus, kidney disease, or heart disease; and concurrent infections in either the mother or the baby. Anticipating these problems of the healthy newborn by using the Apgar scores and the results of the physical examination allows the proper assignment of the infant to the nursery or NICU.

The NICU is a daunting place containing high-tech equipment, a tangle of wires and tubes, the sounds of beeps and alarms, and tiny, fragile infants. All this technology serves two simple purposes: to monitor vital functions and to sustain malfunctioning or nonfunctioning organ systems. Looked at individually, however, the machines and attachments become much more understandable. The incubator, perhaps the most common device, maintains a warm, moist environment of constant temperature at 37 degrees Celsius. Small portholes with rubber gloves allow people to stroke the child safely. Generally, the infants will have small electrodes taped on their chests, connected to video monitors that record the heart and breathing rates and that will sound alarms if significant deviations occur. These monitors will also record blood pressure through an

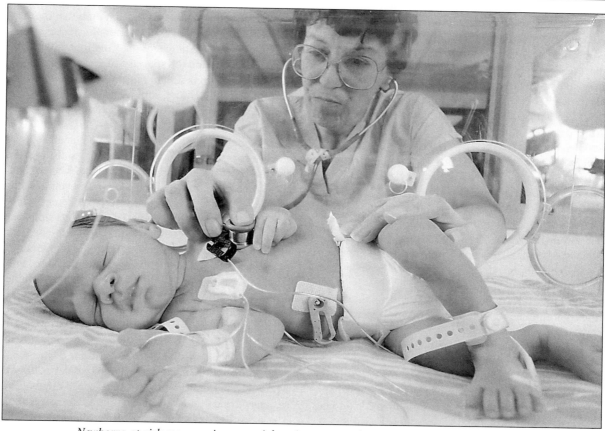

Newborns at risk may require a special environment such as an incubator. (Digital Stock)

arm or thigh cuff. To ensure immediate access to the blood, for delivering medications and taking blood for testing, catheters (plastic tubes) are placed into larger arteries or veins near the umbilicus, neck, or thigh (in adults, intravenous access is found in the arms).

The remaining equipment is used for the very serious business of life support, in particular the support of the respiratory system. Maintaining adequate oxygenation is critical and can be accomplished in several ways, depending on the baby's needs. The least stressful are tubes placed in the nostrils or a face mask, but these methods require that breathing be spontaneous although inadequate. More often, unfortunately, neonates with the types of problems that bring them to an intensive care unit cannot breathe on their own. In these cases, a tube must be connected from the artificial respirator into the windpipe (the endotracheal tube). Warm, moistened, oxygen-rich air is delivered under pressure and removed from the lungs rhythmically to simulate breathing. Tranquilizers and paralytic agents are used to calm and immobilize the infant. Sick or pre-

mature infants are also generally unable to feed or nurse naturally, by mouth. Again, several methods of feeding can be employed, depending on the problems and the length of time that such feedings will be needed. For the first few days, simple solutions of water, sugar, and protein can be given through the intravenous catheters. These lines, because of the very small, fragile blood vessels of the newborn, are seldom able to carry more complex solutions. A second method, known as gavage feeding, employs tubing that is inserted through the nose directly into the stomach. Through that tube, infant formula (water, sugar, protein, fat, vitamins, and minerals) and, if available, breast milk can be given.

As the underlying problems are resolved, the infant is slowly weaned, first feeding orally and then breathing naturally. Next, the infant will be placed in an open crib, and gradually the tangled web of tubes and wires will clear. With approval from the neonatologist, the baby is transferred to the routine nursery, a transitional home until discharge from the hospital is advisable.

DIAGNOSTIC AND TREATMENT TECHNIQUES

Neonatology has amassed an enormous body of knowledge about normal neonatal anatomy and physiology, disease processes, and, most important, how to manage the wide variety of complications that can occur. Specific treatment protocols have been developed that are practiced uniformly in all neonatal intensive care units. Approximately 12 percent of all neonates in the United States require admission to the NICU. Short-term stays (twenty-four to forty-eight hours) are meant to observe and monitor the infant with respiratory distress at birth that required immediate intervention. Long-term stays, lasting from several weeks to months, are the case for the sickest newborns, most commonly those with severe prematurity and low birth weight (less than 1,500 grams), respiratory distress syndrome (also known as hyaline membrane disease), congenital defects, and drug or alcohol addictions.

Infants born prematurely make up the major proportion of all infants at high risk for disability and death, and each passing decade has seen younger and younger babies being kept alive. While many maternal factors can lead to preterm delivery, often no explanation can be found. The main problem of prematurity lies in the functional and structural immaturity of vital organs. Weak sucking, swallowing, and coughing reflexes lead to an inability to feed and to the danger of choking. Lungs that lack surfactant, a substance that coats the millions of tiny air sacs (alveoli) in each lung to keep them from collapsing and sticking together after air is exhaled, cause severe breathing difficulty as the infant struggles to reinflate the lungs. When premature delivery is inevitable but not immediate, lung maturity can be increased by administration of steroids to the mother. An immature immune system cannot protect the newborn from the many viruses, bacteria, and other microorganisms that exist. Inadequate metabolism causes low body temperature and inadequate use of food or medications. Neurological immaturity can lead to mental retardation, blindness, and deafness.

Aggressive management of the preterm baby begins in the delivery room, with close cooperation between the obstetrician and the neonatologist. Severely preterm infants, some born after only twenty weeks of pregnancy, require immediate respiratory and cardiac support. Placement of the endotracheal tube, assisted ventilation with a handheld bag, and delicate chest compressions similar to the cardiopulmonary resuscitation (CPR) done on adults to stimulate the heartbeat are each accomplished quickly. Once the respiratory and circulatory systems have been stabilized, excess fluid will be suctioned, while a brief physical examination is performed to note any abnormalities that require immediate attention. As soon as transport is considered safe, the newborn is sent to the NICU. If the infant has been delivered at a small, community hospital, this may involve ambulance or even helicopter transport to the nearest tertiary care center.

Once in the unit, the neonate will be placed in an incubator and attached to video monitors that record heart rate, breathing, and blood pressure. The endotracheal tube can now be attached to the respirator machine, and intravenous or intra-arterial catheters will be placed to allow the fluid and medication infusions and the blood drawing for the battery of tests that the neonatologist requires. Feeding methods can be set up as soon as the infant has stabilized. Within a short time after delivery, the premature newborn has had a flurry of activity about it and is surrounded by the most sophisticated equipment and staff available. Supporting the immature organs becomes the first priority, although the ethical issues of saving very sick infants must soon be addressed as complications begin to occur. Nearly 15 percent of surviving preterm infants whose birth weights were less than 2,000 grams have serious physical and mental disabilities after discharge. The majority, however, grow to lead normal, healthy lives.

Congenital defects are common, with nearly 7 percent of the American population having some physical or cosmetic deformity, although most are not serious. Unfortunately, nearly 2 percent of all newborns have life-threatening abnormalities that require immediate attention and admission to the NICU. It is estimated that the majority of miscarriages are a direct result of congenital defects that are incompatible with life. Many infants that do survive development and delivery die shortly after birth despite the most sophisticated and heroic attempts to intervene. The causes of such defects are arbitrarily assigned to two broad categories, although a combination of these factors is the most likely explanation: genetic errors (such as breaks, doubling, and mutations) and environmental insults (such as chemicals, drugs, viruses, radiation, and malnutrition). In the United States, among the most common birth defects that require immediate intervention are heart problems, spina bifida (an open spine), and tracheo-esophageal fistulas and esophageal atresias (wrongly connected or incomplete wind and food pipes).

The birth of a malformed infant is rarely expected,

and the neonatologist's team plays a key role in its survival. Congenital heart disease is the most prevalent life-threatening defect. During development in utero, the umbilical cord supplies the necessary oxygen; it is not until birth, when that lifeline is cut, that the neonate's circulatory and respiratory systems acquire full responsibility. At delivery, all may appear normal, and the one-minute Apgar score may be high. Several minutes later, however, the pink skin color may begin to darken to a purplish blue (cyanosis), indicating that insufficient oxygen is being extracted from the air. Immediately, the infant receives rescue breathing from the bag mask. Upon admission to the neonatal unit, the source of the cyanosis must be determined. A chest X ray may provide significant information about the anatomy of the heart and lungs, but special tests are usually needed to pinpoint the problem. Catheters that are threaded from neck or leg vessels into the heart can reveal the pressure and oxygen content of each chamber in the heart and across its four valves. Echocardiograms, video pictures similar to sonograms generated by sound waves passing through the chest, enhance the data provided by the X rays and catheterizations, and a diagnosis is made. Based on the physical signs and symptoms of the newborn, a treatment plan is devised.

Because of the nature of congenital defects and structural abnormalities, their correction generally requires surgery. Openings between the heart's chambers (septal defects), valves that are too narrow or do not close properly, and blood vessels that leave or enter the heart incorrectly are all common defects treated by the pediatric heart surgeon. Because of the delicacy of the operation and the vulnerability of the newborn, surgery may be postponed until the baby is larger and stronger while it is provided with supplemental oxygen and nutrients. The risk of such operations is high, and depending on the degree of abnormality, several operations may be required.

Another group of infants who have benefited from advances in neonatology are those born to drug-addicted women. The lives of these infants are often complicated by congenital defects and life-threatening withdrawal symptoms. For example, heroin-addicted babies are quite small, are extremely irritable and hyperactive, and develop tremors, vomiting, diarrhea, and seizures. The newborn must be carefully monitored in the unit, and sedatives and antiseizure medications are given, sometimes for as long as six weeks. Cocaine and its derivatives frequently cause premature labor, fetal death, and maternal hemorrhaging during delivery. Infants that do survive often have serious congenital defects and suffer withdrawal symptoms. The risk of acquired immunodeficiency syndrome (AIDS) adds another dimension to an already complicated picture.

NUMBER OF INFANT DEATHS IN THE UNITED STATES, 2004

Cause of Death

Congenital malformations, deformations, and chromosomal abnormalities	5,622
Disorders related to short gestation and low birth weight	4,642
Sudden infant death syndrome (SIDS)	2,246
Newborn affected by maternal complications of pregnancy	1,715
Accidents (unintentional injuries)	1,052
Newborn affected by complications of placenta, cord, and membranes	1,042
Respiratory distress	875
Bacterial sepsis	827
Neonatal hemorrhage	616
Diseases of the circulatory system	593
All other causes	8,706
Total	**27,936**

Source: National Center for Health Statistics.

PERSPECTIVE AND PROSPECTS

Throughout human history, maternal and neonatal deaths have been staggering in number. Ignorance and unsanitary conditions frequently resulted in uterine hemorrhaging and overwhelming infection, killing both mother and baby. Highly inaccurate records at the beginning of the twentieth century in New York City show maternal death averaging 2 percent; in fact, the rate was probably greater, since most births occurred at home. Neonatal deaths from respiratory failure, congenital defects, prematurity, and infection loom large in these medical records. The expansion of medical, obstetric, and pediatric knowledge and technology that began after World War II has dramatically lowered maternal and infant mortality. It should not be forgotten, however, that nonindustrialized nations, the majority in the world, remain devastated by the neonatal problems that have plagued civilization for thousands of years.

Ironically, the problems associated with neonatology in Western nations are now at the other end of the spectrum: saving and prolonging life beyond what is natural or "reasonable." As neonatology advanced scientifically and technically, saving life took precedence over ethical issues. The famous and poignant story of "Baby Doe" in the early 1980's illustrates the dilemmas that occur daily in neonatal intensive care units. Baby Doe was a six-pound, full-term male born with Down syndrome and three severe congenital defects of the heart, trachea, and esophagus. These malformations were deemed surgically correctable, although the underlying problem of Down syndrome, a disease characterized by mental retardation and particular facial and body features, would remain. The parents would not agree to any operations and requested that all treatment be withheld. He was given only medication for sedation and died within a few days. The case was related by the attending physician in a letter to *The New England Journal of Medicine*. Enormous controversy was sparked. On July 5, 1983, a law was passed in effect stating that all handicapped newborns, no matter how seriously afflicted, should receive all possible life-sustaining treatment, unless it is unequivocally clear that imminent death is inevitable or that the risks of treatment cannot be justified by its benefit. The legislators believed that Baby Doe had been allowed to die because of his underlying condition (Down syndrome).

Since then, attorneys, ethicists, juries, and the courts have used the example of Baby Doe, and the law that grew from it, to interpret many cases that have come to light. Life-and-death decisions are made on a daily basis in the neonatal care unit. They are always difficult, but they usually remain a private matter between the parents and the neonatologist. These cases become public matters, however, when the family disagrees with the medical staff. Then the question of what is in the best interest of the child is compounded by who will pay for the treatments and who will care for the baby after it is discharged.

Such ethical dilemmas will continue as expertise and technology grow. A multitude of questions, previously relegated to philosophy and religion, will arise, and the benefits of saving a life will have to be weighed against its quality and the resources necessary to maintain it.

—*Connie Rizzo, M.D., Ph.D.;*
updated by Alexander Sandra, M.D.

See also Apgar score; Birth defects; Blue baby syndrome; Bonding; Cardiology, pediatric; Cesarean section; Childbirth; Childbirth complications; Chlamydia; Circumcision, male; Cleft lip and palate; Cleft lip and palate repair; Cognitive development; Colic; Congenital disorders; Congenital heart disease; Craniosynostosis; Critical care, pediatric; Cystic fibrosis; Developmental disorders; Developmental stages; Down syndrome; Embryology; Endocrinology, pediatric; Failure to thrive; Fetal alcohol syndrome; Fetal surgery; Gastroenterology, pediatric; Genetic diseases; Genetics and inheritance; Hematology, pediatric; Hemolytic disease of the newborn; Hydrocephalus; Intraventricular hemorrhage; Jaundice, neonatal; Metabolic disorders; Motor skill development; Multiple births; Nephrology, pediatric; Neurology, pediatric; Obstetrics; Orthopedics, pediatric; Pediatrics; Perinatology; Phenylketonuria (PKU); Polydactyly and syndactyly; Premature birth; Pulmonary medicine, pediatric; Rh factor; Shunts; Sudden infant death syndrome (SIDS); Surgery, pediatric; Tay-Sachs disease; Teratogens; Toxoplasmosis; Urology, pediatric; Well-baby examinations.

FOR FURTHER INFORMATION:

Behrman, Richard E., Robert M. Kliegman, and Hal B. Jenson, eds. *Nelson Textbook of Pediatrics*. 18th ed. Philadelphia: Saunders/Elsevier, 2007. This bible of pediatrics is notable not only for its breadth and scope but also for its clarity and accessibility. The several chapters devoted to neonatology, intensive care, prematurity, and congenital defects provide a good overview in the context of pediatrics as a whole.

Bradford, Nikki. *Your Premature Baby: The First Five Years*. Toronto, Ont.: Firefly Books, 2003. Guides the logistics of care for premature infants from birth into the preschool years and sets expectations for hospital care by describing hospital terms, procedures, treatments, and equipment.

Cunningham, Nicholas, ed. *Columbia University College of Physicians and Surgeons: Complete Guide to Early Child Care.* New York: Crown, 1990. A very well written and organized book meant for health professionals as well as parents; the finest of this type. Its material is thorough but not too technical, so it is accessible to a wider audience. A good place to start for an overview before turning to more difficult texts.

Levin, Daniel L., and Frances C. Morriss, eds. *Essentials of Pediatric Intensive Care.* 2d ed. New York: Churchill Livingstone, 1997. This superb paperback focuses on the daily routine of the neonatal intensive care unit. Good photographs and diagrams explain the technology and the procedures used. Often used as a supplement to hardcover neonatology texts, but it can be used alone.

MacDonald, Mhairi G., Mary M. K. Seshia, and Martha D. Mullett, eds. *Avery's Neonatology: Pathophysiology and Management of the Newborn.* 6th ed. Philadelphia: Lippincott Williams & Wilkins, 2005. This excellent text, used as a main reference for neonatologists, provides a thorough scientific background, including the anatomy, physiology, and biochemistry of all known abnormal conditions. As one of the most respected sources in the field, it can be technical and involved at times, but it is well worth the effort.

Martin, Richard J., Avroy A. Fanaroff, and Michele C. Walsh, eds. *Fanaroff and Martin's Neonatal-Perinatal Medicine: Diseases of the Fetus and Infant.* 2 vols. 8th ed. Philadelphia: Mosby/Elsevier, 2006. This classic reference work is one of the most comprehensive to date and features discussions on the diverse practice of neonatal-perinatal medicine, pregnancy disorders and their impact on the fetus, delivery room care, provisions for neonatal care, and the development and disorder of organ systems.

Moore, Keith L., and T. V. N. Persaud. *The Developing Human.* 8th ed. Philadelphia: Saunders/Elsevier, 2008. An outstanding textbook on human embryonic development, with specific information about the causes of congenital malformations and common defects occurring in each of the body's systems.

Ruhlman, Michael. *Walk on Water: Inside an Elite Pediatric Surgery Unit.* New York: Viking-Penguin, 2003. A fascinating foray into life in a pediatric heart center—Cleveland Clinic—specializing in neonatal open-heart surgery, focusing on the daily experiences of world-renowned surgeon Roger Mee.

Sadler, T. W. *Langman's Medical Embryology.* 11th ed. Philadelphia: Lippincott Williams & Wilkins, 2009. Text that covers the fundamentals of embryology, with a chapter devoted to birth defects.

Woolf, Alan D., et al., eds. *The Children's Hospital Guide to Your Child's Health and Development.* Cambridge, Mass.: Perseus, 2002. An authoritative and comprehensive guide to children's health, providing a guide to every common illness or condition that affects children and a carefully designed emergency section.

NEPHRECTOMY

PROCEDURE

ANATOMY OR SYSTEM AFFECTED: Abdomen, kidneys, urinary system

SPECIALTIES AND RELATED FIELDS: General surgery, nephrology, oncology, urology

DEFINITION: The removal of the kidney, which may be performed to treat disorders and disease or for the purpose of transplantation.

KEY TERMS:

adrenal gland: a small hormone-producing gland which is adjacent to the upper pole of the kidney

donor nephrectomy: a procedure in which a kidney is removed for transplantation into another patient; the kidney can be removed from a person who is brain-dead but whose heart is still beating (cadaveric donor nephrectomy) or from a relative of the recipient (a living related donor)

nephroureterectomy: a procedure similar to a radical nephrectomy, with the additional removal of the ureter and a cuff of the bladder; performed to treat transitional cell carcinomas of the ureters and the pelvis of the kidneys

radical nephrectomy: a procedure in which a kidney is removed along with the covering layers of tissue and the adjacent adrenal gland; performed with cancerous conditions

renal cell carcinoma (RCC): cancer of the small tubules of the kidney; generally known as kidney cancer

simple nephrectomy: a procedure in which a kidney is removed but the covering layers of tissue and the adjacent adrenal gland are left intact; usually performed to treat benign (noncancerous) conditions

transitional cell carcinoma (TCC): cancer arising from the lining of the urine-collecting system of the kidneys, ureters, and bladder

ureters: the tubes that drain urine from the kidneys to the bladder

Indications and Procedures

A kidney may be removed for several reasons, including congenital defects, trauma, cancer, inflammation, and transplantation. Congenital problems, or birth defects, associated with the kidneys include abnormal development, nonfunctional cysts, blockage, tumors, and cysts that are functional but which cause difficulty in breathing because of their large size. A kidney may be removed if the organ or its main blood vessels have been damaged beyond repair by trauma, such as a gunshot wound. Cancer is one of the most common reasons for nephrectomy; kidney cancers include renal cell carcinomas, transitional cell carcinomas, and tumors in the capsules of the kidneys or in surrounding layers of tissue. Infections or abscesses in the kidney that are beyond medical treatment and that become life-threatening also necessitate a nephrectomy. Finally, a kidney may be removed from a donor for transplantation.

Depending on the underlying disease and the surgeon's preference and experience, the kidney can be approached from the front, side, or back. In certain situations, the chest is also opened. The incisions used to reach the kidney are similar for simple, radical, and donor nephrectomies, but the steps that follow differ once the abdomen has been entered. For nephroureterectomy, in which the kidney, the connecting ureter, and a part of the bladder are removed, the surgeon makes either one long, S-shaped incision starting in the flank and ending near the bladder, or two separate incisions.

In the frontal approach to nephrectomy, the patient lies on his or her back and the abdomen and peritoneal cavity are opened. The intestines near the kidney are pushed to the side, and the kidney is approached from the front. The advantage of this approach includes better evaluation of the liver and the structures surrounding the kidney, better control of the blood vessels, and easy removal of clots from veins if necessary. The disadvantages of this approach are the possibility of adhesions developing in the intestines and lung complications after the surgery.

In the side approach, the patient is placed on his or her side and the incision is made through the eleventh or twelfth ribs. The kidney is approached from behind. This type of incision involves cutting into muscle and results in significant postoperative pain. The main advantage is that the peritoneal cavity is not entered.

In the back approach, known as dorsal lumbotomy, the patient is placed facedown and a muscle-splitting incision is used. The kidney is approached from behind. This method is usually used for simple nephrectomy. Its primary advantages are less postoperative pain and avoidance of the peritoneal cavity. Its main disadvantage is a limited view of the surgery site.

In simple nephrectomy, after the kidney has been exposed, Gerota's fascia (the covering envelope of the kidney) is opened, and the fat around the kidney is dissected. The adjacent blood vessels and the connecting ureter are tied and cut, and the kidney is removed. In radical nephrectomy, the adjacent adrenal gland and

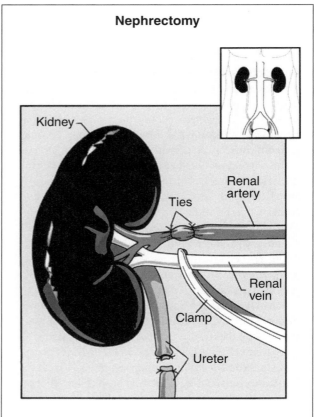

Nephrectomy

Kidney

Ties

Renal artery

Clamp

Renal vein

Ureter

The removal of a kidney may be necessary because of disease or because the kidney is intended for transplantation into another patient; the inset shows the location of the kidneys.

surrounding lymph glands are also removed in the one block. For nephroureterectomy, the ureter is not cut close to the kidney but is dissected all the way down to the bladder. A 2-centimeter cuff of bladder is cut off, the entire specimen is removed, and the hole in the bladder is closed.

The techniques used with kidney transplantation differ for cadaveric donor nephrectomy and living related donor (LRD) nephrectomy. For cadaveric donor nephrectomy, the abdominal aorta (the main artery bringing blood to the kidney) and the inferior vena cava (the main vein taking blood away from the kidney) are isolated above and below the kidneys and cannulated with pipes to irrigate both kidneys with cold preservation fluid. Both kidneys and ureters, along with their related blood vessels, are removed. For LRD nephrectomy, the kidney is dissected along with its blood vessels and ureter. Great care is taken to obtain the maximum length of ureter and blood vessels without causing damage to the donor.

USES AND COMPLICATIONS

The major complications of nephrectomy during surgery are bleeding, damage to surrounding structures, and problems related to anesthesia. Therefore, there is significant evaluation of the patient before surgery. A battery of tests may be performed, including blood testing, urinalysis, electrocardiography, and X rays. A thorough medical examination is done to determine whether the patient can be placed under anesthesia safely. The patient's blood is also typed and cross-matched in the event that a transfusion is required. Good surgical skills, the availability of blood for transfusion, and proper anesthesia techniques usually ensure that any complications that occur are not life-threatening. Nevertheless, the patient may also experience complications during the procedure that are not directly related to the surgery, such as a heart attack.

After a nephrectomy, the patient is at some risk for other problems. These complications may include bleeding, infection, intestinal obstruction, blood clots in the legs or lungs, or a heart attack.

PERSPECTIVE AND PROSPECTS

Significant advances have been made in nephrectomy since the first such procedure was performed by Gustav Simmons in 1869. Thorough preoperative evaluation; improved anesthesia techniques; a greater understanding of anatomy, physiology, and pathology (including the nature of infections and microorganisms); and the

discovery of antibiotics have all led to better surgical techniques. As a result, the death rate for nephrectomy operations is only 1 percent.

—*Saeed Akhter, M.D.*

See also Adrenalectomy; Dialysis; Hemolytic uremic syndrome; Kidney cancer; Kidney disorders; Kidney transplantation; Kidneys; Nephritis; Nephrology; Nephrology, pediatric; Transplantation.

FOR FURTHER INFORMATION:

Brenner, Barry M., ed. *Brenner and Rector's The Kidney.* 8th ed. Philadelphia: Saunders/Elsevier, 2008. This treatise, at more than two thousand pages, is a comprehensive and authoritative source on the normal and diseased human kidney.

Danovitch, Gabriel, ed. *Handbook of Kidney Transplantation.* 5th ed. Philadelphia: Lippincott Williams & Wilkins, 2010. A clinical handbook that gives a practical overview of renal transplantation and includes coverage of topics such as immunosuppressive drugs, short- and long-term post-transplant management, complications, and ethical/legal issues.

Hinman, Frank, Jr. *Atlas of Urologic Surgery.* 2d ed. Philadelphia: W. B. Saunders, 1998. This is an excellent book with very useful diagrammatic and graphic details of operations and good descriptions of both old and new procedures.

Marshall, Fray F., ed. *Textbook of Operative Urology.* Philadelphia: W. B. Saunders, 1996. This book presents updated information on indications for operation, preoperative management, operative technique, postoperative management, and complications specific to each procedure.

Novick, Andrew C., and Stevan B. Streem. "Surgery of the Kidney." In *Campbell-Walsh Urology*, edited by Patrick Walsh et al. 9th ed. 4 vols. Philadelphia: Saunders/Elsevier, 2007. A chapter in a classic urology text, which maintains its encyclopedic approach while following a new organ systems orientation. Halftone illustrations and contributions by multiple authors.

Schrier, Robert W., ed. *Diseases of the Kidney and Urinary Tract.* 8th ed. Philadelphia: Wolters Kluwer Health/Lippincott Williams & Wilkins, 2007. Covers full range of the biochemical, structural, and functional correlations in the kidney, as well as hereditary diseases, urological diseases and neoplasms of the genitourinary tract, acute renal failure, and nutrition, drugs and the kidney, among many additional topics.

Nephritis

Disease/disorder

Anatomy or system affected: Blood vessels, immune system, kidneys

Specialties and related fields: Immunology, internal medicine, nephrology

Definition: An inflammatory response of the kidneys, particularly of the glomeruli, to infectious agents or immunological challenges.

Key terms:

albuminuria: excretion in the urine of the protein albumin, usually as a result of changes occurring in the glomeruli

amyloidosis: the deposition of immunoglobulin fibrils in various tissues, including the kidneys

dialysis: the use of artificial membranes to remove metabolites from the blood when the kidneys fail; the peritoneum can also be used (peritoneal dialysis)

filtration rate: the amount of fluid passing per minute from blood across the glomerular capillaries to form glomerular fluid

glomeruli: structures consisting mainly of capillary blood vessels contained in a capsule, across whose walls water and solutes pass (filter) to form glomerular fluid

glomerulonephritis: inflammation of glomeruli

hematuria: the presence of red blood cells or red blood cell casts in the urine

immunoglobulins: proteins associated with immune responses

nephrotic syndrome: a condition involving edema, the retention of water and of sodium and chloride ions, urinary protein losses greater than 3 grams per day, and hypoalbuminemia

proteinuria: the presence of proteins, including globulins, in the urine; usually considered a sign of changes in the glomerular structures

renal blood flow: the amount of whole blood entering the renal arteries per minute; a fraction of water and solutes is removed to form urine

renal failure: severe kidney insufficiency requiring the use of dialysis or transplantation to return and maintain composition of body fluids at or near normal values

renal insufficiency: the inability of the kidneys to maintain a normal internal environment of the body and its fluids

streptococci: bacteria responsible for the development of some cases of acute glomerulonephritis, but without infection of the kidneys

tubules: hollow structures conducting glomerular fluid to the collecting ducts and the renal pelvis; they produce composition and volume changes of glomerular fluid passing through them and may reabsorb some of the protein that crosses the glomerular capillaries

Causes and Symptoms

Nephritis means any inflammatory responses of the kidney, whether the cause is infectious or immunological. Generally, it involves mainly the glomeruli, where the initial formation of urine takes place. The term is therefore equivalent in meaning to glomerulonephritis. Pathological changes may also occur in the interstitium (the extravascular, extracellular domain in which the tubules are embedded) and affect tubular functions. This condition, referred to as tubulointerstitial nephritis, is associated with localized cellular infiltrates and the accumulation of fluid.

The classic cause of acute glomerulonephritis is an infection in the throat or of the skin by a nephritogenic strain of Group A streptococci. The clinical presentation can be dramatic and can be associated not only with a sore throat but also with headaches, shortness of breath, and swelling of the ankles. Physical examination may find hypertension, rales in the lungs, peripheral pitting edema, and changes in the retinal vessels. In the chronic form, the onset is usually insidious; an infection may have been forgotten or ignored, without specific complaints except for some ankle edema, tiredness, and perhaps pallor. The physical findings for chronic glomerulonephritis are similar to but less striking than in the acute form.

The diagnosis in each type of nephritis is presumed on the basis of urinalysis, with a finding of blood (hematuria) in the acute form; proteinuria (actually mainly albuminuria, although globulins may also be present); and a decreased glomerular filtration rate. Diagnosis is established on the basis of renal biopsy with examination by both light and electron microscopy. Throat cultures and streptococcal group determination are appropriate if an infection is suspected.

Both conditions may be followed by the development of nephrotic syndrome, which is characterized by major losses of albumin in the urine, decreased serum albumin concentrations (hypoalbuminemia), the retention of water and of sodium and chloride ions, and massive edema and ascites (fluid leakage from blood vessels into the abdomen). Nephrotic syndrome may also appear without any history or evidence of a preceding

---

INFORMATION ON NEPHRITIS

CAUSES: Inflammation of kidney from bacterial infection (often streptococcal) or immune disorder

SYMPTOMS: In acute form, sore throat, headache, shortness of breath, ankle swelling, hypertension, edema; in chronic form, ankle swelling, fatigue, pallor; either may lead to nephrotic syndrome (loss of albumin in urine, decreased serum albumin, water retention, sodium and chloride ion retention, massive edema and ascites)

DURATION: Acute or chronic

TREATMENTS: Usually none needed for acute form; for nonresolving or chronic form, dietary control (decreased protein and potassium), steroids, hemodialysis or peritoneal dialysis, kidney transplantation

---

episode of acute glomerulonephritis. On renal biopsy, essentially no changes or only minimal changes may be noted on inspection by light microscopy (minimal change disease), although characteristic changes are found with electron microscopy affecting particularly the foot processes (podocytes) of the glomeruli.

Acute glomerulonephritis resolves spontaneously and rapidly in about 95 percent of cases, without detectable residual damage to kidney functions. Apart from control of hypertension, no specific treatment is available. The edema is rarely sufficient to warrant the use of diuretics. Antibiotics are not indicated unless there is evidence of an infection. Patients can be considered to be cured but should nonetheless be followed in the event of a reappearance of symptoms or manifestations.

In nonresolving acute glomerulonephritis and in chronic glomerulonephritis, there can be progression of damage to the glomeruli so that the number of functioning glomeruli (normally, about one million in each kidney) diminishes. This process may be gradual or may occur as a part of acute exacerbations that subside but leave the patient with diminished renal functions. As a result, glomerular filtration is decreased and the accumulation of metabolic end-products, particularly urea, occurs in the blood and tissue fluids. Abnormalities of acid-base regulation appear with decreased blood pH (acidemia), decreased serum bicarbonate concentration, and increased potassium concentration.

Generally, a significant anemia exists, and renal blood flow is decreased so that the metabolic activities of the renal tubule cells are affected. Renal insufficiency is established, and dietary control is instituted, with decreased intakes of protein and potassium. Paradoxically, with decreased glomerular function, proteinuria decreases, serum albumin increases, and edema decreases or disappears.

Unfortunately, the progression of glomerular dysfunction continues, and dietary measures provide insufficient control of metabolic abnormalities. Resort is then made to hemodialysis or peritoneal dialysis to control the metabolic abnormalities and lift dietary restrictions to some degree while the patient awaits kidney transplantation. During this waiting period, stimulants of the bone marrow, such as erythropoietin, are administered in the expectation of maintaining the red cell count and the hematocrit at a satisfactory level. Transplants will require the use of immunosuppressive agents to prevent rejection unless an identical twin is the donor.

Other diseases in which glomerular damage can occur include diabetes mellitus, amyloidosis, systemic lupus erythematosus (SLE), Wegener'sgranulomatosis, Goodpasture's syndrome, syphilis, and human immunodeficiency virus (HIV) infection. Common problems associated with glomerular damage of any etiology are hypertension, strokes, heart failure, pulmonary edema, arteriolar vasoconstriction and sclerosis, impaired vision from exudates, pericarditis, and pericardial effusions.

TREATMENT AND THERAPY

Acute glomerulonephritis is characterized by the disappearance of signs and symptoms, or at least their marked reduction, in most patients. In 90 to 95 percent of cases, there is no progression and no recurrence. In some patients, the problems may reappear after apparent complete remission, while in others the disease progresses, often to nephrotic syndrome. This phase, too, disappears as the disease worsens, reaching the stage where hemodialysis or peritoneal dialysis becomes necessary. A renal biopsy can aid in determining the appropriate treatment. For example, if the biopsy confirms that poststreptococcal nephritis is present, then no specific treatment is available. If progressive glomerulonephritis is the diagnosis, then steroids may be indicated.

Hemodialysis depends on an arteriovenous shunt being created, usually in the forearm, so that the patient's blood can pass through a dialysis machine, which functions in a manner similar to glomeruli. Usually, several sessions, two or three times per week for several hours at a time, are required. Peritoneal dialysis involves the introduction of large amounts of fluid into the peritoneal cavity and its withdrawal after adequate exchanges with body fluids across the peritoneal surfaces have occurred. Hemodialysis requires going to a hospital or specialized facility, while pertoneal dialysis can be performed at home. Both procedures require careful and frequent monitoring of the patient's acid-base, electrolyte, and metabolic statuses.

While arrangements can usually be made for local dialysis, patients on dialysis lose a significant degree of mobility and independence. This independence can be regained to a considerable degree through kidney transplantation. Kidneys may be obtained from cadavers, unrelated living donors, and related living donors, such as identical twins. Except with the latter group, rejection phenomena may occur. Infections can occur with the use of immunosuppressive agents. Rarely, malignancies can be introduced with transplanted kidneys.

A low protein intake is recommended in the later stages of glomerulonephritis because too high a protein intake may accelerate the progression of the disease. Lack of control of water intake may lead to edema. Anemia is common in the later stages and may require the administration of erythropoietin.

In the nephrotic phase and in minimal change disease, control of edema is sought through one or more of the following measures: salt restriction, diuretics, intravenous (IV) administration of concentrated human serum albumin, corticosteroids (such as prednisone, which is more likely to be effective in minimal change disease), and other immunosuppressive agents. Nephrotic syndrome may occur in the presence of other underlying diseases, such as lupus, diabetes mellitus, HIV infection, syphilis, amyloidosis, and microvascular angiopathies. Specific treatments should be used when applicable.

PERSPECTIVE AND PROSPECTS

The monograph *Reports of Medical Cases* by Richard Bright, published in 1827, marks the first clear description of nephritis through clinical findings (edema), laboratory assessment (proteinuria), and gross structural changes in the kidneys at postmortem. For many years, nephritis was referred to as Bright's disease. Apart from the measurement of blood constituents such as urea and creatinine, functional assessment was limited until the development, by Donald D. Van Slyke, of the clearance concept, defined as the amount of a given substance excreted in the urine per unit time relative to its concentration in plasma or blood. Van Slyke focused on the clearance of urea, while P. B. Rehberg in Denmark proposed that the clearance of creatinine could be used as a measure of the glomerular filtration rate. Glomerular fluid had been shown by Newton Richards to have the same composition as an ultrafiltrate of plasma. Accordingly, if creatinine was neither secreted nor reabsorbed by the tubules, then its clearance would be equivalent to the glomerular filtration rate.

The assumptions with respect to creatinine were shown to be incorrect, and inulin, a polyfructoside studied by Homer Smith, was found to be a reliable and correct indicator for measuring the glomerular filtration rate. Smith and his collaborators systematized and advanced knowledge of the kidney as a whole organ in a quantitative manner. Detailed understanding of the components of the whole organ progressed rapidly with the discovery of the significance of countercirculation in establishing the solute concentration gradient from cortex to medulla reported by H. Wirz and B. Hargitay. Functions of limited segments of the tubules (and later of individual cells) have provided additional important information on transport and metabolic processes in the kidneys.

On the clinical side, the introduction of renal biopsies and of hemodialysis (and later peritoneal dialysis) by way of an arteriovenous shunt made for more accurate diagnoses and longer life expectancies for patients with chronic renal disease. Further encouragement was provided by the development of techniques for successful renal transplants, first from identical twins, then from living donors and cadavers. Problems of rejection remain. Another major challenge is to find the means of delaying or arresting the progression of chronic renal disease before dialysis and transplants become necessary.

—Francis P. Chinard, M.D.

See also Bacterial infection; End-stage renal disease; Hemolytic uremic syndrome; Kidney cancer; Kidney disorders; Kidneys; Nephrectomy; Nephrology; Nephrology, pediatric; Proteinuria; Pyelonephritis; Renal failure; Stone removal; Stones; Streptococcal infection; Systemic lupus erythematosus (SLE); Transplantation.

FOR FURTHER INFORMATION:

Brenner, Barry M. "Retarding the Progression of Renal Disease." *Kidney International* 64 (2003): 370-378.

Addresses the control of various manifestations of renal disease (proteinuria, hyperlipidemia) through dietary and pharmacologic approaches. The goal is to prevent progression to end-stage renal disease (ESRD) when dialysis or a transplant is required.

_____, ed. *Brenner and Rector's The Kidney.* 8th ed. Philadelphia: Saunders/Elsevier, 2008. A multiauthored text reviewing the anatomy, physiology, and responses to injury of the kidneys.

Cameron, J. Stewart, and Richard J. Glassock, eds. *The Nephrotic Syndrome.* New York: Marcel Dekker, 1988. Reviews clinical aspects as well as pathophysiology. Contains an excellent historical account.

D'Amico, G., and C. Bazzi. "Pathophysiology of Proteinuria." *Kidney International* 63 (2003): 809-825. A critical review of the roles of the glomerular capillary walls and of the tubule cells in determining the identities and quantities of the proteins excreted in the final urine.

Eddy, A. A., and J. M. Symons. "Nephrotic Syndrome in Children." *The Lancet* 362 (2003): 629-639. Nephrotic syndrome is trying for children, their families, and their physicians. Steroids are successful in reversing the problem in many but not all patients. The underlying pathogenesis, clinical presentations, treatment, and possible outcomes are well and critically addressed.

Hricik, D. E., M. Chung-Park, and J. R. Sedor. "Glomerulonephritis." *New England Journal of Medicine* 339 (1998): 888-899. Focuses on immunological and cellular responses, risk factors for progression, genetic factors, and absence of specific therapies.

NEPHROLOGY

SPECIALTY

ANATOMY OR SYSTEM AFFECTED: Abdomen, blood, kidneys, urinary system

SPECIALTIES AND RELATED FIELDS: Biochemistry, biotechnology, endocrinology, genetics, hematology, internal medicine, urology

DEFINITION: The field of medicine that deals with the anatomy and physiology of the kidneys.

KEY TERMS:

analyte: any chemical substance undergoing measurement; includes charged electrolytes found in the blood, such as sodium or potassium

creatinine: a nitrogen-containing by-product of metabolism; levels of creatinine may be indicative of kidney function

endocrine: referring to a process in which cells from an organ or gland secrete substances into the blood; these substances in turn act on cells elsewhere in the body

glomerulonephritis: inflammation of the glomeruli, the clusters of blood vessels and nerves found throughout the kidney

nephritis: any disease or pathology of the kidney that results in inflammation

nephron: the structural and functional unit of the kidney; composed of the renal corpuscle, the loop of Henle, and renal tubules

nephrotic syndrome: an abnormal condition of the kidneys characterized by a variety of conditions, including edema and proteinuria; often accompanies glomerular dysfunction and diabetes

renal: pertaining to the kidney

urea: a waste product of protein metabolism that represents the form in which nitrogen is eliminated from the body

SCIENCE AND PROFESSION

Nephrology is the branch of medicine that deals with the function of the kidneys. As a consequence, a nephrologist frequently deals with problems related to homeostasis, that is, the maintenance of the internal environment of the body. The most obvious function of the kidneys is their ability to regulate the excretion of water and minerals from the body, at the same time serving to eliminate nitrogenous wastes in the form of urea. While such waste material, produced as byproducts of cell metabolism, is removed from the circulation, essential nutrients from body fluids are retained within the renal apparatus. These nutrients include proteins, carbohydrates, and electrolytes, some of which help maintain the proper acid-base balance within the blood. In addition, cells in the kidneys regulate red blood cell production through the release of the hormone erythropoietin.

The human excretory system includes two kidneys, which lie in the rear of the abdominal cavity on opposite sides of the spinal column. Urine is produced by the kidneys through a filtration network composed of 2 million nephrons, the actual functional units within each kidney. Two ureters, one for each kidney, serve to remove the collected urine and transport this liquid to the urinary bladder. The urethra drains urine from the bladder, voiding the liquid from the body.

Each adult human kidney is approximately 11 centimeters in length, with a shape resembling a bean. When the kidney is sectioned, three anatomical regions are visible: a light-colored outer cortex; a darker inner region, called the medulla; and the renal pelvis, the lowest portion of the kidney. The cortex consists primarily of a network of nephrons and associated blood capillaries. Tubules extending from each nephron pass into the medulla. The medulla, in turn, is visibly divided into about a dozen conical masses, or pyramids, with the base of the pyramid at the junction between the cortex and medulla and the apex of the pyramid extending into the renal pelvis. The loops (such as the loop of Henle) and tubules within the medulla carry out the reabsorption of nutrients and fluids that have passed through the capsular network of the nephron. The tubules extend through the medulla and return to the cortical region.

There are approximately 1 million nephrons in each kidney. Within each nephron, the actual filtration of blood is carried out within a bulb-shaped region, Bowman's capsule, which surrounds a capillary network, the glomerulus. In most individuals, a single renal artery brings the blood supply to the kidney. Since the renal artery originates from a branch of the aorta, the body's largest artery, the blood pressure within this region of the kidney is high. Consequently, hypotension, a significant lowering of blood pressure, may also result in kidney failure.

The renal artery enters the kidney through the renal pelvis, branching into progressively smaller arterioles and capillaries. The capillary network serves both to supply nutrition to the cells that make up the kidney and to collect nutrients or fluids reabsorbed from the loops and tubules of the nephrons. Renal capillaries also enter the Bowman's capsules in the form of balls or coils, the glomeruli. Since blood pressure remains high, the force filtration in a nephron pushes about 20 percent of the fluid volume of the glomerulus into the cavity portion of the capsule. Most small materials dissolved in the blood, including proteins, sugars, electrolytes, and the nitrogenous waste product urea, pass along within the fluid into the capsule. As the filtrate passes through the series of convoluted tubules extending from the Bowman's capsule, most nutrients and salts are reabsorbed and reenter the capillary network. Approximately 99 percent of the water that has passed through the capsule is also reabsorbed. The material which remains, much of it waste such as urea, is excreted from the body.

Nephrology is the branch of medicine that deals with these functions of the kidney. Loss of kidney function can quickly result in a buildup of waste material in the blood; hence kidney failure, if untreated, can result in serious illness or death. Within the purview of nephrology, however, is more than the function of the kidneys as filters for the excretion of wastes. The kidneys are also endocrine organs, structures that secrete hormones into the bloodstream to act on other, distal organs. The major endocrine functions of the kidneys involve the secretion of the hormones renin and erythropoietin.

Renin functions within the renin-angiotensin system in the regulation of blood pressure. It is produced within the juxtaglomerular complex, the region around Bowman's capsule in which the arteriole enters the structure. Cells within the tubules of the nephron closely monitor the blood pressure within the incoming arterioles. When blood pressure drops, these cells stimulate the release of renin directly into the blood circulation.

Renin does not act directly on the nephrons. Rather, it serves as a proteolytic enzyme that activates another protein, angiotensin, the precursor of which is found in the blood. The activated angiotensin, called angiotensin II, has several effects on kidney function that involve the regulation of blood pressure. First, by decreasing the glomerular filtration rate, it allows more water to be retained. Second, angiotensin II stimulates the release of the steroid hormone aldosterone from the adrenal glands, located in close association with the kidneys. Aldosterone acts to increase sodium retention and transport by cells within the tubules of the nephron, resulting in increased water reabsorption. The result of this complex series of hormone interactions within the kidney is a close monitoring of both salt retention and blood pressure and volume. In this manner, nephrology also relates to the pathophysiology of hypertension—high blood pressure.

The kidneys also regulate the production of erythrocytes, red blood cells, through the production of the hormone erythropoietin. Erythropoietin is secreted by the peritubular cells associated with regions outside the nephrons in response to lowered oxygen levels in the blood, also monitored by cells within the kidney. The hormone serves to stimulate red cell production within the bone marrow. Approximately 85 percent of the erythropoietin in blood fluids is synthesized within the kidneys, the remainder by the liver.

Since proper kidney function is related to a wide variety of body processes, from the regulation of nitrogenous waste disposal to the monitoring and control of blood pressure, nephrology may deal with a number of disparate syndromes. The kidney may represent the primary site of a disease or pathology, an example being the autoimmune phenomenon of glomerulonephritis. Renal failure may also result from the indirect action of a more general systemic syndrome, as is the case with diabetes mellitus. In many cases, the decrease in kidney function may result from any number of disorders, which poses many problems for the nephrologist.

Proper function of the kidney is central to numerous homeostatic processes within the body. Thus nephrology by necessity deals with a variety of pathophysiological disorders. Renal dysfunction may involve disorders of the organ itself or pathology associated with individual structures within the kidneys, the glomeruli or tubules. Likewise, the disorder within the body may be of a more general type, with the kidney being a secondary site of damage. This is particularly true of immune disorders such as lupus (systemic lupus erythematosus) or diabetes. Conditions that affect proper kidney function may result from infection or inflammation, the obstruction of tubules or the vascular system, or neoplastic disorders (cancers).

Immune disorders are among the more common processes that result in kidney disease. They may be of two types: glomerulonephritis or the more general nephrotic syndrome. Glomerulonephritis can result either from a direct attack on basement membrane tissue by host antibodies, such as with Goodpasture's syndrome, or indirectly through deposits of immune (antigen-antibody) complexes, such as with lupus. Nephritis may also be secondary to high blood pressure. In any of these situations, inflammation resulting from the infiltration of immune complexes and/or from the activation of the complement system may result in a decreased ability of the glomeruli to function. Treatment of such disorders often involves the use of corticosteroids or other immunosuppressive drugs to dampen the immune response. Continued recurrence of the disease may result in renal failure, requiring dialysis treatment or even kidney transplantation.

Activation of the complement system as a result of immune complex deposition along the glomeruli is a frequent source of inflammation. Complement consists of a series of some dozen serum proteins, many of which are pharmacologically active. Intermediates in the complement pathway include enzymes that activate subsequent components in a cascade fashion. The terminal proteins in the pathway form a "membrane attack complex," capable of significantly damaging a target (such as the basement membrane of a Bowman's capsule). Activation of the initial steps in the pathway begins with either the deposition of immune complexes along basement membranes or the direct binding of antibodies on glomerular surfaces. The end result can be extensive nephrotic destruction.

Nephrotic syndrome, which can also result in extensive damage to the glomeruli, is often secondary to other disease. Diabetes is a frequent primary disorder in its development; approximately one-third of insulin-dependent diabetics are at risk for significant renal failure. Other causes of nephrotic syndrome may include cancer or infectious agents and toxins.

DIAGNOSTIC AND TREATMENT TECHNIQUES

Nephrologists can measure glomerular function using a variety of tests. These tests are based on the ability of the basement membranes associated with the glomeruli to act as filters. Blood cells and large materials such as proteins dissolved in the blood are unable to pass through these filters. Plasma, the liquid portion of the blood containing dissolved factors involved in blood-clotting mechanisms, is able to pass through the basement membrane, the driving force for filtration being the hydrostatic pressure of the blood (blood pressure).

The glomerular filtration rate (GFR) is defined as the rate by which the glomeruli filter the plasma during a fixed period of time. Generally, the rate is determined by measuring either the time of clearance of the carbohydrate inulin from the blood or the rate of clearance of creatinine, a nitrogenous by-product of metabolism. Though the rate may vary with age, it generally is about 125 to 130 milliliters of plasma filtered per minute.

Any significant decrease in the GFR is indicative of renal failure and can result in significant disruptions of acid-base or electrolyte balance in the blood. A decrease in the GFR can sometimes be observed through measurements of urine output. Healthy individuals usually excrete from 1 to 2 liters of urine per day. If the urine output drops to less than 500 milliliters (0.5 liter) per day, a condition known as oliguria, the body suffers a diminished capacity to remove metabolic waste products (urea, creatinine, or acids). Taken to an extreme, in which the filtering capacity is completely shut down and urine formation drops below 100 milliliters per day (anuria), the resulting uremia may cause death in a matter of days.

Anuria may have a variety of causes: kidney failure; hypotension, in which blood pressure is insufficient to maintain glomerular filtration; or a blockage in the urinary tract. As waste products, fluids, and electrolytes (especially sodium and potassium) build up, the person may appear puffy, be feverish, and exhibit muscle weakness. Heart arrhythmia or failure may also occur. Mediation of the problem, in addition to attempts to alleviate the reasons for kidney dysfunction, include regulation of fluid, protein, and electrolyte uptake. Medications are also used to increase the excretion of potassium and tissue fluids, assuming that the cause is not a urinary blockage.

The nephrologist or other physician may also monitor kidney function through measurements of serum analytes or through observation of certain chemicals within the urine. The levels of blood, urea, and nitrogen (BUN), nitrogenous substances in the blood, present a rough measure of kidney function. Generally, BUN levels change significantly only after glomerular filtration has been significantly disrupted. The levels are also dependent on the amount of protein intake in the diet. When changes occur as a result of renal dysfunction, BUN levels can be a useful marker for the progression of the disease. A more specific indicator of renal function can be the creatinine concentration within the blood. Serum creatinine, unlike BUN levels, is not related to the diet. In the event of renal failure, however, changes in BUN levels usually can be detected earlier than those of creatinine.

As the glomeruli lose their ability to distinguish large from small molecules during filtration, protein can begin to appear in the urine, the condition known as proteinuria. Usually, the level of protein in the urine is negligible (less than 250 milligrams per day). A transient proteinuria can result from heavy exercise or minor illness, but persistent levels of more than 1 gram per day may be indicative of renal dysfunction or even complications of hypertension. Generally, if the problem resides in the loss of tubular reabsorption, levels of protein generally are below 1 to 2 grams per day, with that amount usually consisting of small proteins. If the problem is a result of increased glomerular permeability caused by inflammation, levels may reach greater than 2 grams per day. In cases of nephrotic syndrome, excretion of protein in the urine may exceed 5 grams per day.

Measurement of urine protein is a relatively easy process. A urine sample is placed on a plastic stick with an indicator pad capable of turning colors, depending on the protein concentration. Analogous strips may be used for detection of other materials in urine, including acid, blood, or sugars. The presence of either red or white blood cells in urine can be indicative of infection or glomerulonephritis.

In addition to the filtration of blood fluids through the nephrons, the reabsorption of materials within the tubules results in increased urine concentration. A normal GFR within a healthy kidney produces a urine concentration three or four times as great as that found within serum. As kidney failure progresses, the concentration of urine begins to decrease, with the urine becoming more dilute. The kidneys compensate for the decreased concentration by increasing the amount of urine output: The frequency of urination may increase, as well as the volume excreted (polyuria). In time, if renal failure continues, the GFR will decrease, resulting in the retention of both analytes and water.

Determination of urine concentration is carried out following a brief period of dehydration: deprivation of fluids for about fifteen hours prior to the test. This dehydration will result in increased production by the hypothalamus of antidiuretic hormone (ADH), or vasopressin, a chemical that decreases the production of urine through increased renal tubule reabsorption of water. The result is a more concentrated urine. Following the dehydration period, the patient's urine is collected over a period of three hours and assessed for concentration. Significantly low values may be indicative of kidney disease.

A battery of tests in addition to those already described may be utilized in the diagnosis of kidney disease. These may include intravenous pyelography (in which a contrast medium is injected into the blood and followed as it passes through the kidneys), kidney biopsy, and ultrasound examinations. Diagnosis and course of treatment depend on an evaluation of these tests.

PERSPECTIVE AND PROSPECTS

The roots of modern nephrology date from the seventeenth century. In the early decades of that century, the English physician William Harvey demonstrated the principles of blood circulation and the role of the heart in that process. Harvey's theories opened the door for more extensive analysis of organ systems, both in humans and in other animals. As a result, in 1666, Italian anatomist Marcello Malpighi, while exploring organ structure with the newly developed microscope, discovered the presence of glomeruli (what he called Malpighian corpuscles) within the kidneys. Malpighi thought that these structures were in some way connected with collecting ducts in the kidneys that had recently been found by Lorenzo Bellini. Malpighi also suspected that these structures played a role in urine formation.

Sir William Bowman, in 1832, was the first to describe the true relationship of the corpuscles discovered by Malpighi to urine secretion through the tubules. Bowman's capsule, as it is now called, is a filter that allows only the liquid of the blood, as well as dissolved salts and urea within the blood, into the tubules, from which the urine is secreted. It remained for Carl Ludwig, in 1842, to complete the story. Ludwig suggested that the corpuscles function in a passive manner, in that the filtrate is filtered by means of hydrostatic pressure through the capsule into the tubules and from there concentrated as water and solutes that are reabsorbed.

The first definitive work on urine formation, *The Secretion of the Urine*, was published by Arthur Robertson Cushny in 1917. In the monograph, Cushny offered a thorough analysis of the data published on kidney function. Though Cushny was incorrect in some of his conclusions, the work catalyzed intensive research activity on the functions of the kidney. A colleague of Cushny, E. Brice Mayrs, made the first attempt to determine the glomerular filtration rate, measuring the clearance of sulfate in rabbits. In 1926, the Danish physiologist Poul Brandt Rehberg demonstrated the superiority of creatinine as a marker for glomerular filtration; the "guinea pig" for the experiment was Rehberg himself.

A pioneer in renal physiology, Homer William Smith, began his research while serving in the United States Army during World War I. Until he retired in 1961, Smith was involved in much of the research related to renal excretion. It was Smith who developed inulin clearance as a measure of the GFR; his later years dealt with studies on mechanisms of solute excretion.

With the newer technology of the late twentieth century, more accurate methods for analysis became available. These have included ultrasound scanning, intravenous pyelography, and angiography. In addition, better understanding of immediate causes of many kidney problems has served to control or prevent some forms of renal failure.

—*Richard Adler, Ph.D.*

See also Abdomen; Abdominal disorders; Adrenalectomy; Blood and blood disorders; Cysts; Diabetes mellitus; Dialysis; Edema; End-stage renal disease; Hemolytic uremic syndrome; Internal medicine; Kidney cancer; Kidney disorders; Kidney transplantation; Kidneys; Lithotripsy; Nephrectomy; Nephritis; Nephrology, pediatric; Polycystic kidney disease; Pyelonephritis; Renal failure; Stone removal; Stones; Systemic lupus erythematosus (SLE); Terminally ill: Extended care; Transplantation; Urinalysis; Urinary system; Urology; Urology, pediatric.

FOR FURTHER INFORMATION:

Brenner, Barry M., ed. *Brenner and Rector's The Kidney.* 8th ed. Philadelphia: Saunders/Elsevier, 2008. This treatise, at more than two thousand pages, is a comprehensive and authoritative source on the normal and diseased human kidney.

Cameron, Stewart. *Kidney Disease: The Facts.* 2d ed. New York: Oxford University Press, 1990. A brief but thorough discussion of types of kidney disease. Written in a style that falls between detailed analysis and cursory treatment. Some knowledge of biology is helpful.

Hricik, Donald E., R. Tyler Miller, and John R. Sedor, eds. *Nephrology Secrets.* 2d ed. Philadelphia: Hanley & Belfus, 2003. Written by leading nephrology clinicians, covers "the seventy most important topics in nephrology" in a question-answer format.

Legrain, Marcel, et al. *Nephrology.* Translated by M. Cavaillé-Coll. New York: Masson, 1987. A basic text on the function of the kidney. The book provides an overview of kidney structure, diseases of the kidney, and their treatment. Also included is a chapter dealing with appropriate diets for the prevention or alleviation of kidney disease.

Marieb, Elaine N. *Essentials of Human Anatomy and Physiology.* 9th ed. San Francisco: Pearson/Benjamin Cummings, 2009. This introductory anatomy and physiology textbook, easily accessible to those with little science background, is richly illustrated with diagrams and photographs, which help to illuminate body systems and processes.

O'Callaghan, Chris A., and Barry M. Brenner. *The Kidney at a Glance.* Boston: Blackwell Scientific, 2000. Covers a range of topics related to the kidneys, presenting text on one page and accompanying illustrations on the facing page. Covers basic anatomy and physiology and the pathologies and presentations of renal and urinary tract disease.

Tanagho, Emil A., and Jack W. McAninich, eds. *Smith's General Urology.* 17th ed. New York: McGraw-Hill, 2008. A text within the Appleton and Lange series of medical publications. An outstanding overview of kidney structure and function. Written at a level appropriate for readers with a basic knowledge of biology, but contains enough detail that it can also serve as a reference work.

Wallace, Robert A., Gerald P. Sanders, and Robert J. Ferl. *Biology: The Science of Life.* 4th ed. New York: HarperCollins, 1996. Included in the chapter on excretion is a fine description of the human excretory system. Written on a basic level, the section includes useful diagrams and a concise discussion of kidney function written for those with only rudimentary knowledge of the field.

Whitworth, Judith A., and J. R. Lawrence, eds. *Textbook of Renal Disease.* 2d ed. New York: Churchill Livingstone, 1994. A detailed analysis of kidney anatomy and function, with an emphasis on types of disease. The book provides a fine description of the effects of systemic problems on renal dysfunction. Also included are sections on imaging and diagnosis.

NEPHROLOGY, PEDIATRIC

SPECIALTY

ANATOMY OR SYSTEM AFFECTED: Abdomen, blood, kidneys, urinary system

SPECIALTIES AND RELATED FIELDS: Biochemistry, biotechnology, endocrinology, genetics, hematology, internal medicine, neonatology, pediatrics, urology

DEFINITION: The specialty involving the diagnosis and treatment of kidney disorders and diseases in children and adolescents.

KEY TERMS:

dialysis: the process of separating crystalloid molecules in solution by diffusion through a semipermeable membrane (essentially, a machine performing the function of the nephrons in the kidney)

glomerulus: one of the very small units in the kidney, where blood is filtered through a membrane

immunology: the science concerned with various phenomena of immunity, increased sensitivity, and allergy

nephrology: the medical science of the kidneys and their function

nephron: the basic functioning unit of the kidney, consisting of the glomerulus plus a series of collecting and transport tubules; there are approximately one million nephrons in each kidney

renal: referring to the kidneys

urea: a nitrogenous molecule found in the blood and urine; the largest component of urine besides water

SCIENCE AND PROFESSION

Pediatric nephrology is a major subspecialty limited to children and adolescents that involves the study of normal and abnormal kidney (renal) function. This discipline not only relates to kidney diseases and renal dysfunction but also places heavy emphasis on the kidneys' adaptive role in many diseases and disorders of nonrenal origin. Pediatric nephrologists are doctors of medicine or osteopathy who have completed three years of pediatric residency training, followed by two or three years in a pediatric nephrology fellowship.

The kidneys are among the most interesting and complex organs in the human body. Kidney diseases often involve the fields of immunology, oncology, genetics, chemistry, physiology, biotechnology, and both gross anatomy and microanatomy (histology). While the cognitive aspects of nephrology dominate the day-to-day work of its specialists, hands-on procedures such as renal biopsies and renal dialysis add variety and interest. Pediatric nephrologists spend approximately 60 percent of their time dealing with primary renal disease, while 40 percent of their time is spent with diseases and conditions of nonrenal origin, especially in critically ill children.

While the kidneys have many functions, their main role is filtering metabolic wastes from the blood and eliminating them via the urinary tract. The process of filtering blood, concentrating its wastes, and reabsorbing water and useful metabolic components (such as protein, sodium, and potassium salts) is accomplished with an elaborate system of passive and active mechanisms in the nephrons in each kidney. The kidneys respond to many factors, including blood volume, blood pressure, the salt and acid content of the blood, nitrogenous wastes (urea), and even hormonal and neural (nerve) stimuli. The kidneys deliver feedback to other vital organs with chemical messengers via the bloodstream and also through the nervous system.

Several key areas in pediatric nephrology make it unique from adult nephrology: immature renal function in infancy, growth retardation in chronic renal disease, and the role of genetics.

DIAGNOSTIC AND TREATMENT TECHNIQUES

The patient's history, a physical examination, and routine urinalysis are the cornerstones of diagnosis in nephrology. Urinalysis is one of the most available, fastest, and least expensive tests in clinical medicine. Frequently, diagnosis is made or suspected from a routine urinalysis done in screening or as part of a routine physical. The test can reveal evidence of infection; microscopic traces of blood, protein, or sugar; and many other abnormalities. Often, early diagnosis of silent renal disease will aid in early intervention, treatment, and the prevention of advanced disease and morbidity. In addition to blood chemistry tests—such as for sodium, potassium, glucose (sugar), and blood, urea, and nitrogen (BUN)—many quantitative tests are available to measure other aspects of renal function.

Dramatic advances in imaging techniques have been made. X rays, ultrasound, computed tomography (CT) scans, magnetic resonance imaging (MRI), and nuclear scans are making detailed anatomical diagnosis possible in noninvasive ways. Very small tumors and structural abnormalities can be identified. Some scans can provide useful information on renal function.

Renal biopsy with a percutaneous (through-the-skin) technique, using a large-bore needle, was developed in the 1960's. The samples allow detailed examination at microscopic and submicroscopic (electron microscopy) levels. Since many renal diseases reveal a characteristic thickening from immunoglobulin deposits and inflammation of membranes in the glomerulus, exact diagnoses are often made by biopsy alone or in conjunction with immunological tests.

In the early part of the twentieth century, the treatment of renal diseases was limited to symptomatic and supportive measures. By the 1940's and 1950's, the advent of antibiotics allowed definitive treatment of kidney and urinary tract infections. Since that era, chemotherapy and immunotherapy have developed rapidly, and many primary renal diseases are now being treated successfully by such methods. Immunotherapy also plays a major role in renal transplantation.

In chronic renal disease, in which the total renal function becomes inadequate to sustain life, children can be treated successfully with renal dialysis. Evolving from pioneer efforts in the 1960's and early 1970's, dialysis is now done routinely for such children, including infants. The effectiveness, safety, and efficiency of the procedure have improved dramatically. Now infants and toddlers usually have peritoneal (abdominal cavity) dialysis conducted at home. Older children usually have hemodialysis about three times a week at a dialysis center. The dialysis machine is connected to a cannula (tubing) that is placed in the patient's arm.

Severe growth retardation is a major problem associated with chronic renal disease in children, often compounded by psychological problems such as severe depression. A combination of improved aggressive nutritional and metabolic support plus treatment with growth hormone has improved the health and mental well-being of these children.

By the early 1970's, kidney transplantation was being done on children. This operation is performed by urologists and pediatric surgeons. Originally, rejection rates and other complications were very high. Results have improved dramatically, and in the United States a national collaborative database reported in 1993 that five years after live donor grafts, 75 percent of the kidneys had not been rejected. This procedure allows thousands of children to lead healthy, normal lives.

The study of renal function in newborns, especially premature ones, has led to sophisticated intensive care for critically ill infants. Pediatric nephrologists may also act as consultants for older children with critical illnesses, injuries, poisonings, and even trauma. Such cases often involve sophisticated intravenous (IV) fluid therapy. Because of temporary renal failure, some of these cases require dialysis.

PERSPECTIVE AND PROSPECTS

The progress in renal dialysis and transplantation has been remarkable. Continued advances in effectiveness, success rates, safety, and convenience are certain. The gene that causes familial polycystic kidney disease has been identified. Such discoveries, coupled with advances in genetics, may revolutionize therapy and even prevent some renal diseases through genetic engineering.

—*C. Mervyn Rasmussen, M.D.*

See also Abdomen; Abdominal disorders; Adrenalectomy; Blood and blood disorders; Diabetes mellitus; Dialysis; Edema; End-stage renal disease; Hemolytic uremic syndrome; Internal medicine; Kidney disorders; Kidney transplantation; Kidneys; Nephrectomy; Nephritis; Nephrology; Pediatrics; Polycystic kidney disease; Pyelonephritis; Renal failure; Systems and organs; Transplantation; Urinalysis; Urinary system; Urology; Urology, pediatric.

FOR FURTHER INFORMATION:

Bock, Glenn H., Edward J. Ruley, and Michael P. Moore. *A Parent's Guide to Kidney Disorders.* Minneapolis: University of Minnesota Press, 1993. A good overview. Nicely organized, with a glossary.

Faris, Mickie Hall. *When Your Kidneys Fail: A Handbook for Patients and Their Families.* 3d ed. Los Angeles: National Kidney Foundation of Southern California, 1994. A handbook for patients and their families. Easy to read and contains an excellent glossary.

Frank, J. David, John P. Gearhart, and Howard M.

Snyder, eds. *Operative Pediatric Urology.* 2d ed. New York: Churchill Livingstone, 2002. A technical clinical text that documents open reconstructive urologic procedures for congenital anomalies of the genitourinary tract.

O'Callaghan, Chris A., and Barry M. Brenner. *The Kidney at a Glance.* Boston: Blackwell Scientific, 2000. Covers a range of topics related to the kidneys, presenting text on one page and accompanying illustrations on the facing page. Covers basic anatomy and physiology and the pathologies and presentations of renal and urinary tract disease.

Orsini, Jenoveva. "Comprehensive Care for Children with Renal Disease." *Exceptional Parent* 29, no. 9 (September, 1999): 36, 38. With commitment, patience, and the support of an outstanding pediatric nephrology team, parents of children with kidney disease and renal failure can provide the care and attention that will enhance the health of their children. Topics such as nutrition, medication, dialysis, and transplantation are addressed.

Webb, Nicholas J. A., and Robert J. Postlethwaite, eds. *Clinical Paediatric Nephrology.* 3d ed. New York: Oxford University Press, 2003. Discusses kidney diseases in infants and children. Includes a bibliography and an index.

NERVOUS SYSTEM

ANATOMY

ANATOMY OR SYSTEM AFFECTED: Ears, nerves, spine
SPECIALTIES AND RELATED FIELDS: Neurology
DEFINITION: The major control system of the body, which synchronizes physiologic activity by interpreting incoming stimuli and which is responsible for memory and reasoning; it is composed of the central nervous system (the brain and spinal cord) and the peripheral nervous system (nerve processes, sensory receptors, and ganglia).

KEY TERMS:

cerebrospinal fluid (CSF): the extracellular fluid of the central nervous system; it flows through the ventricles of the brain and the central canal of the spinal cord, circulating nutrients and providing a cushion for the brain

effector: a general term referring to skeletal, smooth, and cardiac muscles or glands that respond to impulses produced by the nervous system

glial cells: nonexcitable cells of the nervous system; they include astrocytes, microglial cells, oligodendrocytes, and Schwann cells

receptors: membrane-bound proteins with specific binding sites for neurotransmitters

synapse: a juncture between neurons or between neurons and muscle

STRUCTURE AND FUNCTIONS

The nervous system serves as the major control system of the human body. It is responsible for the synchronization of body parts, the integration of physiologic activity, the interpretation of incoming stimuli, and all intellectual activity, including memory and abstract reasoning. The nervous system regulates these activities by communication between various nerve cells; by controlling the actions of skeletal, smooth, and cardiac muscle; and by stimulating the secretion of products from various glands of the body.

Anatomically, the nervous system is divided into the central nervous system, which is composed of the brain and the spinal cord, and the peripheral nervous system, which includes all nervous structures outside the central nervous system—primarily, nerve processes, sensory receptors, and a limited number of cells of the nervous system that are located in special structures known as ganglia. Ganglia are found at various locations throughout the body. They are the only locations of neurons outside the central nervous system. Information from incoming cells can be transmitted to the ganglion cells, which in turn can transmit that information to other locations.

Although the brain and the spinal cord contain several different types of cells that are morphologically unique, there is only one functional cell present, which by convention is always referred to as the neuron. The neuron is one of the few cells in the body that cannot reproduce; a fixed number of these cells develop in infancy, and the number never increases. The number of neurons can, however, decrease in the event of injury or disease.

The neuron consists of a cell body that is similar to that of the typical animal cell familiar to most people. In addition, the neuron has extensions called processes. In the typical neuron, there are two types of processes: dendrites and axons.

Usually a neuron has many dendrites. Dendrites are very short, receive information from nearby cells, and relay that information to the cell body. Each cell has only a single axon, which may be very long, extending up and down the spinal cord or from the spinal cord to the ends of the fingers or toes. The axons conduct information from the cell bodies to the effectors—that is, the muscles and glands—or to other neurons.

Functionally, the nervous system is divided into two areas: the somatic nervous system and the autonomic nervous system. The somatic system controls posture and locomotion by stimulating the skeletal muscles. It is responsible for knowing where the body is in space and for ensuring that there is sufficient muscle contraction (tone) to maintain posture. Responses of the somatic system occur through the motor neurons.

The autonomic nervous system regulates the internal activities through the innervation, or nerve stimulation, of the smooth muscles or the glands. It is anatomically different from the somatic nervous system in that the stimulation of body parts always involves two neurons. The cell body of the second neuron in the sequence is located in a ganglion outside the central nervous system.

The autonomic nervous system is broken down further into two divisions: the sympathetic and the parasympathetic. The sympathetic system is also known as the "fight or flight" reaction, since it evolved from the mechanism in lower animals by which an animal would prepare to fight a predator or run from it. More commonly, it is referred to in humans as the adrenaline response, which is active during stressful situations, strenuous physical activity, public performance, or competition.

The parasympathetic system, which is responsible for the digestive functions of the body, controls stimulation of salivary gland secretions, increased blood flow to digestive organs, and movement of materials through the digestive system. The sympathetic and parasympathetic systems usually function in balance; the parasympathetic system predominates after meals, and the sympathetic system predominates during periods of stress or physical activity.

Neurons communicate with other neurons or effectors through the release of chemical messengers known as neurotransmitters. At the termination of the axon, there is a widened area known as the synaptic knob. It produces and/or stores neurotransmitters. The effects of neurotransmitters are always localized and of short duration. There are many types of neurotransmitters, some of which are well known, such as acetylcholine and norepinephrine.

Neurotransmitters are released in response to an electrical impulse that is conducted along the axon. Once released, a neurotransmitter binds to cells that have appropriate receptors on their dendrites. Neurotransmitters may either stimulate or inhibit the activity of the second cell. If there is significant stimulation of the second cell, it will conduct the information along its axon and release a neurotransmitter from the axon terminal, which will in turn stimulate or inhibit the next neuron or effector. There must be a mechanism for the immediate removal of neurotransmitters from the synaptic cleft if the stimulation of the second neuron is to cease and if other impulses are to be conducted.

Neurotransmitters can influence only those cells that have the appropriate receptors on their surfaces. It is through the neurotransmitter-

The Nervous System

- Cerebrum
- Cerebellum
- Brachial plexus
- Spinal cord
- Medulla oblongata (behind cerebellum)
- Spinal nerves
- Sciatic nerves

receptor complex that neurotransmitters are able to influence cells, and any alteration of the number of receptors or type of receptors on a cell membrane will lead to an alteration of cellular functioning.

The axons of some neurons are covered with multiple layers of a cell membrane known as myelin. The myelin is produced by specialized cells in the brain known as oligodendrocytes and by cells in the peripheral axons known as Schwann cells. Myelin serves as an insulator for axons and is effective in speeding up the conduction of nerve impulses. It is essential for the normal functioning of the nervous system.

The brain and spinal cord are enclosed by three membranes of dense connective tissue called the meninges. The meninges separate the nervous system from other tissue and from the skull and spinal cord. The meninges are, from the outside inward, the dura mater, the arachnoid mater, and the pia mater. Many of the blood vessels of the brain travel through the meninges; therefore, the surface of the brain is very vascular and is subject to bleeding or clotting after trauma.

DISORDERS AND DISEASES

Diseases of the nervous system can be arranged into several general categories: infections, congenital diseases, seizure disorders, circulatory diseases, traumatic injury, demyelinating diseases, degenerative diseases, mental diseases, and neoplasms.

Infections of the nervous system are described according to the tissues infected. If the meninges are infected, the disease is known as meningitis; if the brain tissue is infected, the disease is referred to as encephalitis. The development of abscesses in the nervous tissue can also occur. The conditions described can be caused by viruses, bacteria, protozoa, or other parasites.

In most cases, the organism that causes meningitis is spread via the bloodstream. It is also possible, however, for infections to be spread from an infected middle ear or paranasal sinus, a skull fracture, brain surgery, or a lumbar puncture. The infectious agent can usually be determined by analyzing the spinal fluid. Bacterial infections are treated with antibiotics, while viral infections receive only supportive treatment.

An abscess of nervous tissue is usually a complication resulting from an infection at some other anatomical site, particularly from middle-ear infections or sinus infections. Abscesses may also occur following penetrating injuries. The abscess can create pressure inside the skull, and, if left untreated, it may rupture and lead to death.

Viral encephalitis is an acute disease that is often spread to humans by arthropods from animal hosts. After a carrier insect bites a human, the virus is spread to the brain of the human via the bloodstream. The specific causative agent often goes undiagnosed. Some well-known forms of encephalitis are herpes simplex encephalitis, poliomyelitis, rabies, and cytomegalovirus encephalitis. In addition, some forms of encephalitis fall into the category of slow virus infections, which have latent periods as long as several years between the time of infection and the development of encephalitis.

Other serious infections include neurosyphilis, which occurs in the late stages of untreated syphilis infections; toxoplasmosis, a protozoan infection that is extremely dangerous to fetuses but rarely causes serious problems in adults; cerebral malaria; and African trypanosomiasis, which is also known as sleeping sickness.

Congenital diseases of the brain vary in the degree of malfunction they produce. Spina bifida is a general term for a group of disorders in which the vertebrae do not develop as they should. As a result, the spinal cord may protrude from the lower back. In some cases, the effects may be so minimal as to produce no symptoms; in other cases, however, these malformations may lead to major neurologic impairment.

Hydrocephalus is another congenital malformation. It may lead to an increase in the size of the ventricles of the brain. It may be caused by blockage of the flow of spinal fluid, which in the fetus may lead to expanded brain size. In some cases, the spinal fluid produced by the nervous system fills the ventricles and limits the space available for the growing brain and nervous tissue. The result under these conditions is the presence of larger-than-normal ventricles and a smaller-than-normal amount of nervous tissue.

A seizure disorder is any sudden burst of excess electrical activity in the neurons of the brain. Epilepsy is a general term for seizure disorders. The condition may be mild and have only minimal effects, or it may be severe, leading to convulsions. The cause is often unknown, but epilepsy may result from infection, trauma, or neoplasms.

Cerebrovascular accident (CVA) is the term used to describe a variety of malfunctions of the blood circulation in the nervous system that are not a result of trauma. More commonly, the term "stroke" is used to describe the condition. Strokes have many causes that generally fall into two categories: ischemic and hemorrhagic.

Ischemic strokes are those in which the nervous tissue is deprived of oxygen as a result of an impairment of blood flow to the area. An ischemic stroke is often the result of a blood clot that blocks the blood vessels leading to the brain or the blood vessels in the brain itself. Although there are other causes, these are the most common. Since the cells can live for only a few minutes without oxygen, the consequence of an ischemic stroke can be neurological impairment or even death.

In hemorrhagic strokes, there is bleeding in the brain itself. It may be caused by hypertension or by the rupture of a weakened blood vessel, which is known as an aneurysm. Both ischemic and hemorrhagic strokes lead to the death of neurons in the affected area. The degree of damage to the brain is determined by the number of cells destroyed by the oxygen deprivation.

Traumatic injury to the brain can generally be classified as penetrating or nonpenetrating. Penetrating injuries produce a risk of infection as well as bleeding at the site of the wound. Since many large blood vessels are located in the meninges, even injuries that penetrate only into the meninges may be sufficient to cause serious injury. Nonpenetrating injuries may also cause bleeding of the meninges, which can limit blood flow to the nervous tissue or put excessive pressure on the tissue.

Injury to the spinal cord may result in severing the spinal cord from the brain. If this should occur, communications between the brain and any structures below the area of the injury are lost, as is all sensory and motor function in those areas. Since neurons are unable to regenerate and axon repair is limited, there is little hope for reversal of this condition, although extensive research is being conducted in this area.

Demyelinating diseases are those that result in changes in the myelin sheaths of neurons. The most common example is multiple sclerosis, which affects myelin in the central nervous system but not in the peripheral nervous system. Although there are varying degrees of severity, the condition causes limb weakness, impaired perception, and optic neuritis, among other things. Some cases present only mild symptoms, while others are degenerative and can lead to death—in some patients, within months. Many patients, however, survive for more than twenty years. The cause of the disease is not yet clear, although viral infections have been associated with some demyelinating diseases.

Degenerative diseases are those in which there is a gradual decline in nervous function. The disease may be hereditary, as in the case of Huntington's disease, or may occur without any apparent genetic basis, as in the case of Parkinson's disease. Parkinson's disease involves the death of certain neurons in the brain and a decreased concentration of neurotransmitters. As the disease progresses, there is a gradual loss of motor ability and, ultimately, a complete loss of motor function. Not much is known about neurotransmitter replacement or mechanisms to stop degenerative diseases.

Little is known about mental diseases such as schizophrenia and manic depression. They appear to involve abnormal levels of neurotransmitters or errors in the membrane receptors associated with those neurotransmitters. Success in localizing the causes of these diseases has been slow in coming; there has been much more success in the development of medications to treat them.

Cancer of the brain can be primary or metastatic. Metastatic tumors, the more common variety, can arise from any source. Of the primary neoplasms, the most common are those derived from glial cells, which are responsible for more than 65 percent of all primary neoplasms. The second most common are neoplasms resulting from transformation of cells of the meninges. Since neurons cannot divide, neuron tumors are almost nonexistent except in children.

PERSPECTIVE AND PROSPECTS

When the control system of the body experiences a malfunction, the effects are wide ranging. Since the nervous system has the responsibility of regulating so many diverse activities, nervous system injury or disease must be treated immediately if the patient is to survive. This problem is further complicated by the fact that the brain is a difficult organ to study, because of its location within the skull and because its cells are vital and can be studied only after they have died.

Disease or injury of the cells of the nervous system—especially the brain—creates problems that are unique to that organ for several reasons, including the facts that those cells cannot repair themselves and cannot divide. In addition, the cells of the brain are restricted to a limited area. The cells of the nervous system are unique in that they are so highly specialized that they are not capable of cell division. As a result, humans have the greatest number of neurons during early childhood. Any neural injury or disease that kills cells results in a decreased number of neurons. In addition, neurons are not very good at repairing themselves. Furthermore, the space in the skull is tightly packed with cells and cerebrospinal fluid. There is no room for the blood that might appear as the result of an injury or the fluid accumulation that might be caused by tissue infection or tumors. Any of these conditions will increase the pressure within the skull and will also increase the extent of the injury to the nervous tissue.

Although there is no mechanism for replacing cells that have died, the prognosis is not totally bleak. There are cells in the brain that can, in the event of disease or injury, assume the responsibilities of the dead cells. For example, a person who has lost the capacity to speak following a stroke may be retaught to speak using cells that previously did not perform that function.

Among the problems with which the nervous system must cope, there are many things that can go wrong at the synapse of a neuron. The cell may produce too little or too much neurotransmitter. It is possible that the neurotransmitter may not be released on cue or that, if it is released, the postsynaptic cells will not have the appropriate receptors. There also may be no mechanism for removal of the neurotransmitter from the synaptic cleft. These are only a few of the problems that can interfere with communication between neurons and between neurons and other effectors. As science learns more about the communication system of neurons, efforts to correct these problems will intensify. Already there are many drugs available that can alter activity at the synapse. Correcting these errors can lead to methods for the treatment of mental diseases.

Someday it may be possible to transplant healthy neurons from one person to another. This procedure may permit physicians to prevent total paralysis in a person who has suffered a broken neck or total loss of motor function in an individual who suffers from Parkinson's disease. In 1990, normal neurons were grown in tissue culture for the first time. Such scientific breakthroughs will lead to more and better treatments for individuals who suffer from diseases of the nervous system.

—*Annette O'Connor, Ph.D.*

See also Acupressure; Acupuncture; Alzheimer's disease; Amnesia; Amputation; Anesthesia; Anesthesiology; Aneurysmectomy; Aneurysms; Anxiety; Aphasia and dysphasia; Apnea; Aromatherapy; Ataxia; Autism; Balance disorders; Behçet's disease; Bell's palsy; Biofeedback; Botox; Brain; Brain damage; Brain disorders; Brain tumors; Caffeine; Carpal tunnel syndrome; Cells; Cerebral palsy; Cluster headaches; Coma; Computed tomography (CT) scanning; Concussion; Craniotomy; Cysts; Deafness; Dementias; Disk removal; Dizziness and fainting; Dyslexia; Ear infec-

tions and disorders; Ear surgery; Ears; Electrical shock; Electroencephalography (EEG); Electromyography; Encephalitis; Epilepsy; Fetal alcohol syndrome; Fetal tissue transplantation; Ganglion removal; Guillain-Barré syndrome; Hallucinations; Head and neck disorders; Headaches; Hearing loss; Hemiplegia; Huntington's disease; Hydrocephalus; Hypothalamus; Intraventricular hemorrhage; Laminectomy and spinal fusion; Lead poisoning; Learning disabilities; Leprosy; Leukodystrophy; Lower extremities; Lumbar puncture; Memory loss; Meningitis; Mental retardation; Migraine headaches; Motor neuron diseases; Motor skill development; Multiple sclerosis; Narcolepsy; Neuralgia, neuritis, and neuropathy; Neurofibromatosis; Neuroimaging; Neurology; Neurology, pediatric; Neurosurgery; Numbness and tingling; Paget's disease; Palsy; Paralysis; Paraplegia; Parkinson's disease; Physical rehabilitation; Poisoning; Poliomyelitis; Porphyria; Premenstrual syndrome (PMS); Quadriplegia; Rabies; Reflexes, primitive; Restless legs syndrome; Sciatica; Seizures; Sense organs; Shingles; Shock therapy; Skin; Sleep disorders; Snakebites; Spina bifida; Spinal cord disorders; Spine, vertebrae, and disks; Strokes; Sympathectomy; Systems and organs; Tetanus; Tics; Touch; Toxicology; Transient ischemic attacks (TIAs); Tremors; Unconsciousness; Upper extremities; Vagotomy; Vagus nerve.

FOR FURTHER INFORMATION:

Afifi, Adel K., and Ronald A. Bergman. *Functional Neuroanatomy: Text and Atlas.* 2d ed. New York: Lange Medical Books/McGraw-Hill, 2005. Written by a physician and an anatomist, this book is designed to be an integrated neuroscience textbook and atlas covering the regions of the central nervous system. The peripheral nervous system, however, is not covered.

Barondes, Samuel H. *Molecules and Mental Illness.* New York: Scientific American, 1999. A well-written book that describes the chemistry and physiology of mental illness. Provides a good background for understanding the pathology of mental illness.

Bear, Mark F., Barry W. Connors, and Michael A. Paradiso. *Neuroscience: Exploring the Brain.* 3d ed. Philadelphia: Lippincott Williams & Wilkins, 2007. Undergraduate text that introduces the topics of neuroscience, neurobiology, neurodiseases, and physiological psychology.

Bloom, Floyd E., M. Flint Beal, and David J. Kupfer, eds. *The Dana Guide to Brain Health.* New York:

Dana Press, 2006. An easy-to-understand health guide to the brain from neuroscience, neurology, and psychiatry perspectives. More than seventy psychiatric and neurological disorders, their diagnoses, and their treatments are covered.

McCance, Kathryn L., and Sue M. Huether. *Pathophysiology: The Biologic Basis for Disease in Adults and Children*. 6th ed. St. Louis, Mo.: Mosby/Elsevier, 2010. This book, which was written for nurses, describes the physiologic basis of diseases. There is an extensive section on diseases of the nervous system.

McLendon, Roger E., Marc K. Rosenblum, and Darell D. Bigner, eds. *Russell and Rubinstein's Pathology of Tumors of the Nervous System*. 7th ed. 2 vols. London: Hodder Arnold, 2006. This classic work of neuroscience has been completely redesigned from its previous edition. Collected together are the writings of thirty different authors, who approach neuro-oncology from a number of different perspectives.

Nicholls, John G., A. Robert Martin, and Bruce G. Wallace. *From Neuron to Brain*. 4th ed. Sunderland, Mass.: Sinauer, 2007. An excellent and detailed undergraduate neurobiology text that describes how nerve cells transmit signals, how signals are put together, and how higher functions emerge from this integration.

Underwood, J. C. E., ed. *General and Systematic Pathology*. 4th ed. New York: Churchill Livingstone/ Elsevier, 2004. A well-developed pathology book written for students that contains illustrations and tables. Although some terms will be unfamiliar to the layperson, most of the material is presented in a straightforward manner.

Woolsey, Thomas A., Joseph Hanaway, and Mokhtar Gado. *Brain Atlas: A Visual Guide to the Human Central Nervous System*. 2d ed. New York: Wiley, 2002. This book provides an overview of modern neuroimaging. Particularly helpful is the display of magnetic resonance images and photographs of sections of fixed brain on facing pages.

Neuralgia, neuritis, and neuropathy

Disease/disorder

Anatomy or system affected: Nerves, nervous system, spine

Specialties and related fields: Neurology

Definition: Pathological conditions affecting the peripheral nerves of the body and interfering with the proper functioning of those nerves.

Key terms:

autonomic neuropathy: a disorder involving the nerves that work independently of conscious control, and including those nerves that go to small blood vessels, sweat glands, the urinary bladder, the gastrointestinal tract, and the genital organs

axon: the portion of a neuron that carries electrical impulses away from the nerve cell body

mononeuropathy: a neuropathy involving only one peripheral nerve

nerve: a bundle of sensory and motor neurons held together by layers of connective tissue

neuralgia: pain associated with a nerve, often caused by inflammation or injury

neuritis: inflammation of a nerve

neuron: a nerve cell that is capable of conducting electrical impulses; several different types of neurons exist, including motor neurons, sensory neurons, and interneurons

neuropathy: a disorder that causes a functional disturbance of a peripheral nerve, brought about by any cause

peripheral nervous system: the portion of the nervous system found outside the brain and spinal cord

polyneuropathy: a disease that involves a disturbance in the function of several peripheral nerves

Causes and Symptoms

Peripheral nerves, those nerves found outside the brain and spinal cord, function to carry information between the central nervous system and the other portions of the body. These peripheral nerves consist of a bundle of nerve cells, also called neurons, which are wrapped in a protective sheath of connective tissue. A nerve consisting only of neurons that carry impulses toward the central nervous system is termed a sensory nerve. Nerves that contain only neurons that carry information from the central nervous system to the periphery of the body are called motor nerves, because they usually carry information telling a particular body part to move. Most nerves, however, consist of both sensory and motor neurons and are thus called mixed nerves.

The nerves of the peripheral nervous system can be divided into two different categories, cranial nerves and spinal nerves. Cranial nerves come directly out of the brain and supply information to and about the head and neck. There are twelve pairs of cranial nerves. Spinal nerves come directly out of the spinal cord and provide information to and from the arms, legs, chest, gut, and all other parts of the body not supplied by cranial nerves. In humans, there are usually thirty-one pairs of spinal nerves. Both cranial and spinal nerves can be affected by neuropathies.

Neurons (nerve cells) are highly specialized structures designed to convey information from one part of the body to another. This information is passed along in the form of electrical impulses. Neurons consist of three main parts: a cell body, which contains the nucleus and is the control center of the entire neuron; dendrites, which are slender, fingerlike extensions that convey electrical impulses toward the cell body; and an axon, which is a slender extension that carries electrical impulses away from the cell body.

Most of the dendrites and axons of peripheral nerves are covered with a white, fatty substance called myelin. Myelin acts to protect and insulate axons and dendrites. By insulating the axons and dendrites, myelin actually speeds up the rate at which an electrical impulse can be carried along these two structures. Damage to the myelin sheath surrounding axons and dendrites can greatly impair the function of a nerve.

Often, when a nerve becomes pinched, damaged, or inflamed, the result is excessive electrical stimulation of the nerve, which will be registered as pain. The pain associated with the damaged nerve is referred to as neuralgia. One of the most common forms of neuralgia occurs upon the striking of the "funny bone." This area around the elbow is the spot where the ulnar nerve is easily accessible. The ulnar nerve runs from just under the shoulder to the little finger, and when the ulnar nerve is struck near the elbow it is compressed or pinched, leading to pain or a tingling sensation from the elbow down to the little finger.

Compression of nerves for prolonged periods can also lead to neuralgia. The most common example of compression neuralgia is carpal tunnel syndrome. In this syndrome, the median nerve becomes compressed at the wrist, usually as a result of an inflammation of the sheaths of the tendons located on either side of the median nerve. The swelling of these tendon sheaths causes the compression of the median nerve, which may initially lead to neuralgia. As this condition progresses, it can lead to a loss of feeling along the palm side of the thumb and the index and middle fingers. This condition is most common in people who use their fingers for rigorous work over prolonged periods of time, such as operators of computer terminals.

Sciatica is another common form of neuralgia, in which pain is associated with the sciatic nerve. The sciatic nerve is the longest nerve in the human body, running from the pelvis down the back of the thigh to the lower leg and then down to the soles of the feet. The symptoms of sciatica include sharp pains along the sciatic nerve. The pain may involve the buttocks, hip, back, posterior thigh, leg, ankle, and foot. Sciatica can result from many different causes, but the most common cause is from a ruptured intervertebral disk that puts pressure on, or causes a pinching of, the sciatic nerve.

Neuritis is defined as the inflammation of a nerve or of the connective tissue that surrounds the nerve. Many diseases can lead to the inflammation of peripheral nerves. Perhaps the most common disease leading to neuritis is shingles. Shingles are caused by the occurrence of herpes zoster, a virus that attacks the dorsal root ganglion, a place near the spinal cord that houses the cell bodies of neurons. A rash, swelling, and pain progress from the dorsal root ganglion along one or more spinal nerves. The rash along the course of the spinal nerves usually disappears within two or three days, but the pain along this path can persist for months.

Leprosy is another disease that leads to the inflammation of nerves. Leprosy is a bacterial disease caused by *Mycobacterium leprae*. These bacteria invade the cells that make up the myelin sheath that surrounds the nerve. The result is a noticeable swelling of the nerves affected, primarily those that are close to the skin. Many times, this swelling will lead to neuralgia and, if left untreated, to muscle wasting.

"Neuropathy" is a general term used to describe a decrease in the function of peripheral nerves, which may be caused by many factors. The first signs of a neuropathy are usually a tingling, prickling, or burning sensation in some part of the body. This is followed by a sensory loss; the inability to perceive touch, heat, cold, or pressure; and a weakness in the muscles in the area affected. This weakness may eventually lead to a loss of muscle termed muscular atrophy. Neuropathies may affect sensory neurons, motor neurons, or both and can occur in both spinal and cranial nerves. A neuropathy may develop over a few days or many years. Neuropathies can be caused by a number of factors, including toxic exposure to solvents, pesticides, or heavy metals; viral illness; certain medications; metabolic disturbances such as diabetes mellitus; excessive use of alcohol; vitamin deficiency; loss of blood to the nerve; or cold exposure.

Neuropathies can be categorized based on the number of nerves that they affect, whether it is the myelin sheath surrounding the axon that is affected or the axon itself is destroyed, and the amount of time before symptoms of the neuropathy occur and progress. Thus, neuropathies are usually broken down into four different types: polyneuropathy, in which more than one nerve is affected; mononeuropathy, in which only one nerve is affected; axonal neuropathy, in which the axon is affected and degenerates; and demyelinating neuropathy, in which the myelin sheath surrounding the nerve is destroyed. Each of the four categories can be further subdivided based on the time frame in which the symptoms occur. Those neuropathies that appear over days are termed acute, those that appear over weeks are termed subacute, and those neuropathies whose symptoms slowly appear over months or years are termed chronic.

Another type of neuropathy is autonomic neuropathy, a condition which affects the nerves of the autonomic nervous system. These are the peripheral nerves that go to the sweat glands, small blood vessels, gastrointestinal tract, urinary bladder, and genital organs. These nerves are referred to as autonomic since they automatically provide information between these organs and the central nervous system without the individual's conscious effort. The symptoms associated with this form of neuropathy include loss of control over urination, difficulty swallowing food, occasional stomach upset, diarrhea, impotence, and excessive sweating.

The most common cause of neuropathies in the Western world is diabetes mellitus, while leprosy is the more common cause of neuropathies elsewhere. It is estimated that at least 70 percent of all diabetics have some degree of peripheral neuropathy. In most of these cases, the neuropathy is very slight and causes the patient no noticeable symptoms. In about 10 percent of those diabetics with a neuropathy, however, the symptoms will be serious.

TREATMENT AND THERAPY

Often, the first notable feature of a neuropathy that prompts a patient to seek medical attention is a tingling, prickling, or burning sensation in a particular area of the body. The occurrence of these sensations without any external stimuli is termed paresthesias. Since diabetes is the most common cause of neuropathy in the Western world, the sensations experienced by a diabetic patient can serve as an example of the symptoms that are associated with common neuropathies. These patients may first notice the above-mentioned symptoms in the balls of the feet or tips of the toes. As the neuropathy progresses, patients may lose feeling in their feet and experience a weakness in the muscles of the feet, leading to a difficulty in flexing the toes upward. This makes walking difficult, and many patients remark that they feel as if they are walking on stumps. This condition may lead to difficulties in maintaining balance. The neuropathy will begin to affect the legs above the ankles and then travel up the legs, eventually leading to atrophy of the leg muscles.

As the neuropathy worsens, it is critical that patients seek help because they can no longer feel pain. This situation is dangerous, as the patient may no longer sense the pain that can be caused by injuries from sharp objects or even a pebble in the shoe. If unnoticed, these injuries lead to ulcers that can easily become infected.

The first step in treating a neuropathy is to diagnose the type of neuropathy affecting the patient. A patient's medical history is taken to identify any recent viral or bacterial illness, any exposure to toxic substances such as pesticides or heavy metals, the patient's habits concerning alcohol use, or any other illness or injury that might have brought about a possible neuropathy. Next, a physical exam will be performed to determine if the patient's sensations regarding touch, pain, pressure, or temperature have been affected, as well as the ability of the patient to react to these stimuli. The physician may also feel the affected area to determine if the nerve or nerves are inflamed and enlarged.

If the patient's history and the physical examination point toward a neuropathy, further testing using electrodiagnostic tests will be performed. These tests measure the speed at which an electrical impulse travels down a nerve, which is called the nerve conduction velocity. Motor nerve conduction velocity is measured by stimulating the nerve with electrodes placed on the skin above the nerve. Stimulation of the nerve is typically done at two different sites. Using the arm as an example, one electrode would be placed on the inside of the arm at the elbow. The time that it takes for the impulse to reach a recording electrode on the thumb would be measured. A second site at the wrist would be tested to determine the time that it takes for the electrical impulse to reach the recording electrode on the thumb. The time that it took for the impulse to travel from the wrist to thumb would be subtracted from the amount of time that it took for the impulse to go from the inside of the arm at the elbow to the thumb. The resulting value would then be divided by the distance between the site at the wrist and the site at the elbow, giving a nerve conduction velocity value measured in meters per second.

The typical nerve conduction velocity for the motor and sensory peripheral nerves of adults is approximately 40 to 80 meters per second. If a neuropathy is the result of demyelination, the affected nerve will have a much slower nerve conduction velocity. If the neuropathy is a result of axonal damage, then the nerve conduction velocity is usually not altered from normal. Thus, electrodiagnostic testing helps to determine if the neuropathy is a demyelination neuropathy or an axonal neuropathy. Such a determination is important because the different neuropathies are caused by different diseases and are thus treated differently. Electrodiagnostic tests can also provide useful information regarding the site of the neuropathy and whether the neuropathy is affecting sensory neurons, motor neurons, or both.

The last diagnostic test to be performed, if other methods are inconclusive, is a biopsy of the affected nerve. This procedure involves the surgical removal of a portion of the afflicted nerve. The small sample of nerve will be placed under a microscope and examined for specific changes in the nerve. The nerve sample may also be subjected to various biochemical studies to determine if metabolic disturbances have occurred. Nerve biopsies are rarely performed, however, and are usually not recommended.

Once the type of neuropathy afflicting the patient has been determined, treatment can begin. Unlike axons in the central nervous system, axons in the peripheral nervous system are capable of regenerating under certain conditions. If the neuropathy is the result of exposure to toxic substances such as pesticides or heavy metals, removal of the patient from the exposure to such substances is the simple cure. If the neuropathy is the result of viral or bacterial infections, the treatment and recovery from these infections will also usually correct the neuropathy. The same principle applies to neuropathies caused by metabolic diseases and vitamin deficiencies: Corrections of these problems will lead to the correction of the neuropathy.

Should the neuropathy be of the mononeuropathy type and caused by trauma, anti-inflammatory drugs such as corticosteroids may be used or surgery may be performed to repair the nerve. If the mononeuropathy is caused by compression, as in carpal tunnel syndrome, surgery may also be needed to increase the space around the nerve and thus relieve the compression. Surgery is also used to remove tumors on the nerve that might be causing a neuropathy.

The time required to recover from a neuropathy is dependent on the severity and type of neuropathy. Recovery from demyelination is typically quicker than recovery from axonal neuropathies. If only the myelin surrounding the axon is damaged, and not the axon itself, the axon can quickly replace the damaged myelin. Demyelinating neuropathies usually require three to four weeks for recovery. In contrast, recovery from axonal neuropathies may take from two months to more than a year, depending on the severity of the neuropathy.

PERSPECTIVE AND PROSPECTS

Perhaps the earliest documentation of peripheral neuropathies occurred during biblical times, when the term "leprosy" was coined. It is likely, however, that this term was employed rather loosely, as it was used to describe not only the disease leprosy but also a number of skin diseases not involving neuropathies, such as psoriasis.

The actual diagnosis of neuropathies and their subsequent categorization did not occur until the advent of electrical diagnostic testing. The earliest use of electricity to study nerve function occurred in 1876 when German neurologist Wilhelm Erb noted that the electrical stimulation of a damaged peripheral nerve below the site of injury resulted in muscular contraction. In contrast, electrical stimulation at a site above the injured nerve brought about no activity in the muscle. Erb concluded that the injury blocked the flow of electrical impulses down the nerve.

The actual use of electrical diagnostic testing did not take place until the late 1940's, when electrodes and an oscilloscope, an instrument that measures electrical activity, were used to measure the rate at which an electrical impulse could travel down a nerve. This discovery allowed the testing of nerve function and would become useful in the discrimination between axonal and demyelinating neuropathies. During this period, the invention of the electron microscope and the discovery of better nerve-staining techniques enhanced the ability of scientists to study the physiological and anatomical changes that occur in nerves with the onset of neuropathies.

Neuropathies received considerable attention in 1976 when approximately five hundred cases of the neuropathy called Guillain-Barré syndrome occurred in the United States following a national vaccination program for swine flu. The reason that the swine flu vaccine caused this neuropathy has never been discovered, but this syndrome often occurs after an upper respiratory tract or gastrointestinal infection.

Those suffering from neuropathies that result from exposure to toxic substances, viral or bacterial infections, or metabolic diseases have a good prognosis of recovery if the underlying cause of the neuropathy is treated. The prognosis of recovery is not as good for those who suffer neuropathies as a result of hereditary diseases. Advances made in genetic research and continued research in gene therapy may someday greatly increase the prognosis of recovery for those suffering from hereditary neuropathies.

—*David K. Saunders, Ph.D.*

See also Batten's disease; Botox; Carpal tunnel syndrome; Cerebral palsy; Chiari malformations; Cluster headaches; Diabetes mellitus; Electromyography; Encephalitis; Epilepsy; Guillain-Barré syndrome; Hallucinations; Headaches; Hemiplegia; Huntington's disease; Lead poisoning; Leprosy; Leukodystrophy; Meningitis; Migraine headaches; Motor neuron diseases; Multiple sclerosis; Nervous system; Neuroimaging; Neurology; Neurology, pediatric; Neurosurgery; Numbness and tingling; Pain; Palsy; Paralysis; Paraplegia; Parkinson's disease; Quadriplegia; Radiculopathy; Restless legs syndrome; Sciatica; Seizures; Shingles; Sympathectomy; Tics; Vagotomy; Vagus nerve.

FOR FURTHER INFORMATION:

Facial Neuralgia Resources. http://facial-neuralgia .org. Covers a range of information about facial neuralgias and other cranial neuralgias and neuralgialike disorders.

Kandel, Eric R., James H. Schwartz, and Thomas M. Jessell, eds. *Principles of Neural Science*. 5th ed. Norwalk, Conn.: Appleton and Lange, 2006. Although this book is used in many college graduate courses, the discussion involving peripheral neuropathies should be understandable to the general reader. Provides examples of neuropathies, their syndromes, causes, diagnosis, and history.

Margolis, Simeon, and Hamilton Moses III, eds. *The Johns Hopkins Medical Handbook: The One Hundred Major Medical Disorders of People over the Age of Fifty*. Rev. ed. Garden City, N.Y.: Random House, 1999. This book deals primarily with neuropathies associated with diabetes mellitus, discussing the symptoms and dangers of neuropathies in diabetic patients.

Marieb, Elaine N. *Essentials of Human Anatomy and Physiology*. 9th ed. San Francisco: Pearson/Benjamin Cummings, 2009. An excellent book to begin the study of the peripheral nervous system. This text is easy to understand, as it uses little technical jargon and explains the jargon that it does use. Provides good descriptions and drawings of most parts of the peripheral nervous system.

Parker, James N., and Philip M. Parker, eds. *The Official Patient's Sourcebook on Peripheral Neuropathy*. San Diego, Calif.: Icon Health, 2002. Guides patients in using the Web to educate themselves about neuropathies and draws from public, academic, government, and peer-reviewed research to provide information on virtually all topics related to neuropathic diseases, from the essentials to the most advanced areas of research.

Senneff, John A. *Numb Toes and Other Woes: More on Peripheral Neuropathy*. San Antonio, Tex.: MedPress, 2001. A guide for both patients and care providers, covers research on peripheral neuropathy, treatments for the pain it causes, new drugs, and nutrient supplements. Also details unusual neuropathies, drug causes, neuropathic pain, selecting a doctor, and patient assistance.

Trigeminal Neuralgia Association. http://www.tna support.org. A group that serves as an advocate for patients suffering from trigeminal neuralgia and related facial pain conditions by providing information, encouraging research, and offering support.

NEUROFIBROMATOSIS

DISEASE/DISORDER

ALSO KNOWN AS: Von Recklinghausen disease

ANATOMY OR SYSTEM AFFECTED: Bones, nervous system, skin

SPECIALTIES AND RELATED FIELDS: Dermatology, genetics, neurology, orthopedics, plastic surgery

DEFINITION: A genetic disease affecting the nervous system, skin, and bones that produces multiple nerve tumors (neurofibromas), deeply pigmented areas of skin (café-au-lait spots), and bone deformities.

CAUSES AND SYMPTOMS

Most infants born with neurofibromatosis, which is also known as Von Recklinghausen disease, have few symptoms until puberty. Disease progression and signs and symptoms vary from mild (in about one-third of affected children) to moderate and severe disfigurement and organ failure. The disease causes abnormal growths of nerve tissue along the peripheral nerve tracts of the head, neck, trunk, and extremities, usually involving the brain and spinal cord (the central nervous system) later. These so-called neurofibromas appear as multiple, visible growths lying beneath the skin. Also typical are the many areas of deeply pigmented skin, known as café-au-lait (coffee-and-milk) spots. In addition, severely disfiguring bone defects of the skull and spine can be caused by neurofibromas.

Some patients lead nearly normal lives, with only cosmetic problems from the café-au-lait spots and visible neurofibromas. Most patients, however, experience serious consequences from deep growths and skeletal deformities. Depending on the size and location of these tumors, they can cause blindness, deafness, mental retardation, seizures, pain, and paralysis. Other organs, especially the kidneys and glands, are frequently damaged as well. The most feared complication is the transformation of these benign tumors into cancerous ones.

TREATMENT AND THERAPY

No cure exists for neurofibromatosis. Supportive therapy includes surgical removal of the neurofibromas and reconstructive plastic surgery for the sometimes severe disfigurement that can result from deep tumors and bone deformities. The skull, spine, and eye sockets

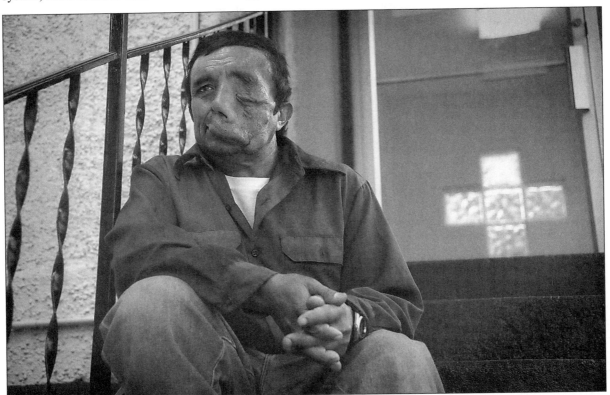

Manuel Raya was born with neurofibromatosis, a genetic disease that causes tumors to grow on nerves. (AP/Wide World Photos)

INFORMATION ON NEUROFIBROMATOSIS

CAUSES: Genetic factors
SYMPTOMS: Multiple nerve tumors, deeply pigmented areas of skin (café-au-lait spots), bone deformities
DURATION: Chronic
TREATMENTS: Supportive therapy, including surgical removal of neurofibromas, reconstructive plastic surgery to correct disfigurement, counseling

---

are particularly affected. Social isolation and embarrassment are serious problems with neurofibromatosis, and counseling is essential. The prognosis is variable depending on the size and location of the tumors. Both cancer and organ failure can shorten the patient's life.

Because neurofibromatosis is genetic, occurring in one in three thousand births, genetic analysis of the parents is essential if there is a family history of the disease. Prenatal testing can determine if the fetus has inherited the defect. Research is now focusing on correcting the genetic error in the developing fetus.

—*Connie Rizzo, M.D., Ph.D.*

See also Bone disorders; Bones and the skeleton; Dermatology; Dermatopathology; Genetic diseases; Genetics and inheritance; Nervous system; Neuralgia, neuritis, and neuropathy; Neurology; Neurology, pediatric; Skin; Skin cancer; Skin disorders; Skin lesion removal; Tumor removal; Tumors.

FOR FURTHER INFORMATION:

Ablon, Joan. *Living with Genetic Disorder: The Impact of Neurofibromatosis*. Westport, Conn.: Auburn House, 2001.

Children's Tumor Foundation. http://www.ctf.org.

Currey, John D. *Bones: Structures and Mechanics*. 2d ed. Princeton, N.J.: Princeton University Press, 2006.

Daube, Jasper R., ed. *Clinical Neurophysiology*. 3d ed. New York: Oxford University Press, 2009.

Korf, Bruce R., and Allan E. Rubenstein. *Neurofibromatosis: A Handbook for Patients, Families, and Health Care Professionals*. 2d ed. New York: Thieme Medical, 2005.

Nicholls, John G., A. Robert Martin, and Bruce G. Wallace. *From Neuron to Brain*. 4th ed. Sunderland, Mass.: Sinauer, 2007.

Victor, Maurice, and Allan H. Ropper. *Adams and Victor's Principles of Neurology*. 9th ed. New York: McGraw-Hill, 2009.

NEUROIMAGING

PROCEDURE

ALSO KNOWN AS: Neuroradiology
ANATOMY OR SYSTEM AFFECTED: Back, blood vessels, brain, head, neck, nerves, nervous system, spine
SPECIALTIES AND RELATED FIELDS: All
DEFINITION: The art and science of photographing living brain or nervous system tissue.
KEY TERMS:

cerebral angiography: X-ray photography of blood vessels inside the skull

computed tomography (CT): originally computed axial tomography (CAT) scan; any of several techniques, with or without contrast media, for creating images of internal body structures by means of the mathematical reconstruction of a large series of parallel sectional X rays

contrast medium: any substance or chemical that is inserted, ingested, or injected into the body to improve the visibility of certain parts seen by X-ray or other medical imaging technique

echoencephalography: a technique of using reflected ultrasound to create a graphic representation of brain structures

electroencephalography (EEG): electronic measurement and graphic depiction of brain waves

magnetic resonance imaging (MRI): a technique of creating images by resonating hydrogen nuclei inside the body

magnetoencephalography (MEG): a type of MRI, designed to measure brain activity directly rather than infer it from other data

positron emission tomography (PET): a type of CT using a short-lived radioactive isotope as a contrast medium

single photon emission computed tomography (SPECT): a type of CT using a gamma camera to record the pattern of gamma rays emitted from a radioactive drug given to the patient

INDICATIONS AND PROCEDURES

Images of the living brain or other part of the central nervous system are indicated for any disorder anywhere in the body that may have neurological involvement or complications. Psychiatrists may also order neurological images for their patients whose mental disorders may have physical causes. Typical indications for neuroradiologic diagnosis include cancer, stroke, and head trauma, especially closed head injury.

Depending on what tissue is involved and what condition is suspected, the physician may order any of dozens of neuroimaging methods. The two most common in the early twenty-first century are computed tomography (CT), including positron emission tomography (PET) and single photon emission computed tomography (SPECT), and magnetic resonance imaging (MRI), including magnetoencephalography (MEG). Additional methods include plain film X rays, cerebral angiography, electroencephalography (EEG), echoencephalography, and other ultrasound applications.

USES AND COMPLICATIONS

Besides clinical uses in diagnosing disease in individual patients, neuroimaging is also valuable as a research tool for studying Alzheimer's disease, Parkinson's disease, multiple sclerosis, epilepsy, and other degenerative and acute conditions that affect the central nervous system. It can also increase the understanding of drug effects on the brain, natural aging processes, brain function localization, autism, psychiatric disorders, and many other kinds of physiological events. Well-funded initiatives exist for "brain mapping," to create precise, molecular-level, function-specific atlases of the human brain, as well as the brains of mice, rats, and many other animals. The Laboratory of Neuro Imaging (LONI) at the University of California, Los Angeles (UCLA) is the world leader in these kinds of research.

Risks are minimal for patients undergoing brain scans. Usually the worst that can happen is that the scan may provide inadequate diagnosis. The physical dangers are generally the same as for CT or MRI scans on other parts of the body. Occasionally, CT brain scans trigger seizures, especially in children. The chance of these inadvertent seizures is much less with MRI. Another safety advantage of MRI over CT is that MRI does not use radioactive materials.

PERSPECTIVE AND PROSPECTS

Neuroimaging began almost immediately after German physicist Wilhelm Conrad Röntgen discovered X rays in 1895. The limits of using plain film X rays to diagnose nervous system diseases and other soft tissue disorders soon became apparent. Nevertheless, because of its simplicity and thanks to the pioneering

work of Austrian neurologist Artur Schüller and Swedish radiologist Erik Lysholm, physicians until the early 1970's generally preferred plain film to the three other methods available for intracranial and spinal diagnosis: pneumography, radiopaque myelography, and cerebral angiography. These other three all involved using contrast media to improve the detail in the X ray.

American physician Walter Dandy invented pneumography at Johns Hopkins University in 1918. After observing that X rays show air as black, soft tissue as gray, and bone as white, Dandy developed techniques to inject air into the central nervous system to serve as a contrast medium. The resulting X rays clearly highlighted abnormalities such as tumors, but the technique was very dangerous. French scientists Jean Athanase Sicard and Jacques Forestier developed radiopaque myelography, the use of contrast media in spinal X rays, in the early 1920's.

In the 1920's, Portuguese physician António Egas Moniz developed cerebral angiography, a technique in which a rapid series of skull X rays were taken immediately after injecting a radioactive contrast medium into both carotid arteries. This proved to be an excellent method of showing abnormalities and displacements caused by tumors but was disfavored because of its significant danger to the patient and the ugly surgical scars left on the patient's neck.

British physicist Godfrey Newbold Hounsfield and his team of radiologists built the first practical clinical CT scanning machine in 1971. Between 1971 and 1977, several scientists developed practical MRI from facts about the magnetic properties of atomic nuclei that had been known since the 1950's. These two methods soon superseded both plain film and cerebral angiography as the preferred methods of neuroimaging.

—*Eric v. d. Luft, Ph.D., M.L.S.*

See also Angiography; Brain; Computed tomography (CT) scanning; Echocardiography; Imaging and radiology; Magnetic resonance imaging (MRI); Mammography; Nervous system; Noninvasive tests; Nuclear medicine; Nuclear radiology; Positron emission tomography (PET) scanning; Radiation sickness; Radiation therapy; Radiopharmaceuticals; Single photon emission computed tomograph (SPECT); Ultrasonography.

FOR FURTHER INFORMATION:

Cabeza, Roberto, and Alan Kingstone, eds. *Handbook of Functional Neuroimaging of Cognition.* 2d ed. Cambridge, Mass.: MIT Press, 2006.

Carter, Rita, and Christopher D. Frith. *Mapping the Mind*. Berkeley: University of California Press, 1998.

Clarke, Edwin, and Kenneth Dewhurst. *An Illustrated History of Brain Function: Imaging the Brain from Antiquity to the Present*. 2d rev. ed. San Francisco: Norman, 1996.

Damasio, Hanna. *Human Brain Anatomy in Computerized Images*. 2d ed. New York: Oxford University Press, 2005.

D'Esposito, Mark. *Functional MRI: Applications in Clinical Neurology and Psychiatry*. Boca Raton, Fla.: Taylor & Francis, 2006.

Dumit, Joseph. *Picturing Personhood: Brain Scans and Biomedical Identity*. Princeton, N.J.: Princeton University Press, 2004.

Mori, Susumu, et al. *MRI Atlas of Human White Matter*. Boston: Elsevier, 2005.

Taveras, Juan M. "Diamond Jubilee Lecture: Neuroradiology—Past, Present, and Future." *Radiology* 175 (1990): 593-602.

Toga, Arthur W., and John C. Mazziotta, eds. *Brain Mapping: The Methods*. 2d ed. Boston: Academic Press, 2002.

_____. *Brain Mapping: The Systems*. San Diego, Calif.: Academic Press, 2000.

Toga, Arthur W., John C. Mazziotta, and Richard S. J. Frackowiak, eds. *Brain Mapping: The Disorders*. San Diego, Calif.: Academic Press, 2000.

Van Bruggen, Nick, and Timothy P. L. Roberts, eds. *Biomedical Imaging in Experimental Neuroscience*. Boca Raton, Fla.: CRC Press, 2003.

NEUROLOGY

SPECIALTY

ANATOMY OR SYSTEM AFFECTED: Brain, ears, hands, head, muscles, musculoskeletal system, nerves, nervous system, psychic-emotional system, spine

SPECIALTIES AND RELATED FIELDS: Audiology, endocrinology, genetics, physical therapy

DEFINITION: The study of the structure and function of the nervous system.

KEY TERMS:

axon: the cellular extension of the neuron that conducts electrical information, transmitting it to the dendrite of the next neuron through the synaptic gap between them

cellular automaton: a self-reproducing entity and mathematical model for complex systems, including animal nervous systems

dendrite: the extension of the neuron that receives electrical information from neurotransmitters moving across the synaptic gap from the axon of a preceding neuron

neuroglial cell: a supportive cell for neurons within the central nervous system of animals

neuron: the principal nervous system cell that conducts electrical information from its dendritic extensions, through its cell body, to its axonic extensions, and on to other cells

neurotransmitter: a chemical messenger or hormone that relays electrical information across a synapse from the axon of one neuron to the dendrite of another neuron

plasticity: a phenomenon of many animal nervous systems, particularly those in higher vertebrates, in which central nervous system neurons grow in patterns based upon input information

Schwann cell: a supportive cell for neurons in the peripheral nervous systems of vertebrate animals that wraps around and insulates axons using the protein myelin

synapse: the gap between the transmitting axon of one neuron and the receiving dendrite of another neuron

von Neumann machine: a cellular automaton or machine that can think and self-replicate; based on the attempts of the physicist John von Neumann to duplicate the human nervous system in computers

THE PHYSIOLOGY OF THE NERVOUS SYSTEM

Neurology is the study of the nervous system, an intricate arrangement of electrically conducting nerve cells that permeate the entire animal body. Nervous tissue, which represents a principal means of cell-to-cell communication within animals, is one of four adult tissues found within the organs of most animals. The remaining three adult tissues—epithelia, connective tissue, and muscle—rely heavily on nervous tissue for their proper functioning, particularly muscle tissue.

Nervous tissue is a primary characteristic of most animal species, the exceptions including thousands of species of the animal phyla Porifera (sponges) and Coelenterata (consisting of hydra, sea anemones, and jellyfish). Nervous tissue is a prominent tissue in every other major animal phylum, including the primitive platyhelminths (flatworms) and nematodes (roundworms).

Evolutionarily, nerve tissue arose from cells that primarily were endocrine in origin. Endocrine cells are hormone producers that secrete hormones for distribu-

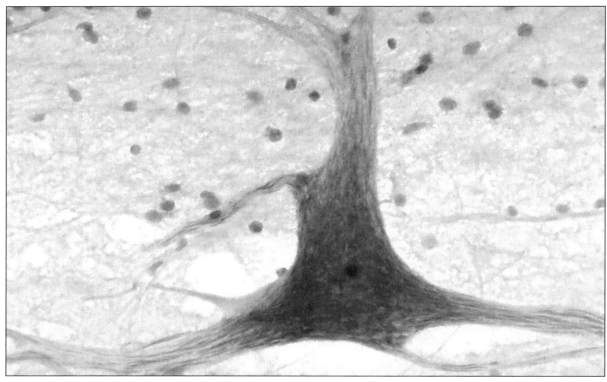

A nerve cell. (Digital Stock)

tion through the organism via the organism's bodily fluids and circulatory systems. Hormones and closely related chemical messengers called neurotransmitters are molecules that are produced in one part of the organism (such as by an endocrine cell or gland), travel through the organism, and target cells in another part of the organism. Hormones or neurotransmitters usually are composed of proteins (long chains of amino acids, or polypeptides) or of fats such as steroids. These chemical messengers affect gene expression within their target cells. Hormones and neurotransmitters determine whether genes are active or inactive. In active genes, the deoxyribonucleic acid (DNA) of the gene encodes messenger ribonucleic acid (mRNA), which encodes protein. An inactive gene does not encode protein. All events within the target cell are influenced by the presence or absence of gene-encoded proteins.

Hormones are effective cell-to-cell communicative and control molecules within all organisms, including animals. In animals, however, hormones and neurotransmitters have become elaborated as parts of extensive nervous systems. The nervous systems of animals have developed according to the evolution of a specialized nervous cell type called a neuron.

The neuron, a specialized, electrically conducting cell, is the basic unit of the nervous system. A neuron is unlike many other cells because it can assume diverse shapes and can assume (relatively) great lengths, sometimes spanning many centimeters. A neuron consists of a cell body containing a nucleus, where the genetic information resides, and numerous organelles, including the energy-producing mitochondria and protein-synthesizing ribosomes. There may be a few or many cellular extensions of its cytoplasm and membrane that twist the neuron into a very distorted appearance. The two principal types of extensions are axons and dendrites.

A dendrite is an electrically receiving extension of a neuron; it receives electrical information from another neuron. An axon is an electrically transmitting extension of a neuron; it transmits electrical information to another neuron. An axon of one neuron transmits electrical information to the dendrite of another neuron. Yet the two neurons are not in direct contact; the axon does not touch the dendrite. A gap called a synapse separates the axon from the receiving dendrite.

Electrical information crosses the synapse via a special type of hormone called a neurotransmitter, a protein encoded by the genes and synthesized by the ribosomes of the neuron. Electrical information traveling along the axon of a neuron triggers the release of a specified quantity of neurotransmitter proteins at the synapse. The neurotransmitters diffuse across the synapse where, upon making contact with the dendritic membrane of the next neuron, they depolarize the dendrite and allow the electrical information transmission to continue unabated.

Actual electrical conduction in a neuron involves membrane depolarization and the influx of sodium ions and the efflux of potassium ions. Electrical conduction along a neuronal segment involves the depolarization of the membrane with the movement of sodium cations into the neuron. Electrical conduction for a particular neuronal segment ends with repolarization of the neuronal membrane as potassium cations move across the neuronal membrane and out of the neuron. The passing electrical action potential, which is measured in millivolts, involves simultaneous depolarization and repolarization in successive regions of the neuron. The initial depolarization is triggered by neurotransmitters contacting the dendritic membrane. Sodium and potassium ion pumps continue the successive stages of depolarization and repolarization along the dendrites, cell body, and axons of the neuron until neurotransmitters are released from a terminal axon across a synaptic gap to depolarize the membrane of the next neuron.

Within animal nervous systems, neurons are very plastic: They grow in specified patterns, much like crystals, in response to stimuli and contacts with other neurons. A neuron may have one or many axonic and dendritic extensions. A neuron with one dendrite and one axon is termed bipolar. A neuron with many dendrites and many axons is termed multipolar; such a neuron makes many contacts with other neurons for the transmission of electrical information along many different neural pathways.

Animal nervous systems usually consist of centralized, concentrated neurons that form the center of nervous control, called the central nervous system. In vertebrate animals, the central nervous system consists of the billions of neurons composing the brain and spinal cord. Additionally, peripheral neurons extend throughout the animal body, permeating virtually every cell and tissue region and thus forming the peripheral nervous system, composed of billions of dispersed neurons.

Functionally, neurons are of three principal types: sensory, motor, and internuncial neurons. Sensory neurons detect stimuli and transmit the electrical infor-

mation from the stimulus toward the central nervous system. The sensory neurons are arranged one after another, transmitting the electrical action potential from axon to neurotransmitter to dendrite, and so on. The central nervous system processes this information, usually utilizing an intricate array of connected internuncial neurons and specialized neuronal regions devoted to specific bodily functions. Once the central nervous system has processed a response to the stimulus, the response is effected by motor neurons, which transmit electrical information back to the body. Motor neurons will transmit electrical information between each other in the same fashion as sensory neurons. The motor neurons, however, often will terminate at some effector tissue, usually a muscle. Neurotransmitters released from the last motor neuron will depolarize the muscle membranes and trigger the biochemical and physical contraction of muscle. The muscle responds to the stimulus.

The primary purpose of nervous systems in animals is to respond to stimuli, both internal and external. Sensory neurons detect stimuli and direct this information to the central nervous system, where internuncial neurons process the information to appropriate decision centers, which direct a response along a chain of motor neurons to a muscle or muscles that physically respond to the initial stimulus. This chain of nervous communication is called a reflex arc. Virtually every activity in the body requires reflex arcs involving central and peripheral nervous system sensory, internuncial, and motor neurons.

The neurons of vertebrate animal nervous systems are very plastic and make trillions of neuron-to-neuron interconnections for the accurate processing of information, the reception of stimuli information, and the direction of response information along reflex arcs. Within the central and peripheral nervous systems of the human body, millions of information transfer processes occur by reflex arcs every second along trillions of neuronal interconnections. The number of such electrical information transfers that must occur accurately every moment within the body is staggering, yet the human nervous system accomplishes these amazingly intricate tasks with ease. No supercomputer yet devised even comes close to the complexity and efficiency of the vertebrate animal nervous system.

SCIENCE AND PROFESSION

Neurologists attempt to understand the structure of the nervous system, including the functioning of the neuron, neuronal plasticity, supporting nerve cells (neuroglia and Schwann cells), neurotransmitters, neuronal patterning in learning, how vision and hearing occur, nerve disorders, and the embryological development of the nervous system.

Neurons are among the most flexibly specialized cells in animal tissues. Animal nerve tissue is derived from embryonic ectodermal tissue. The ectoderm is a tissue layer of cells formed very early in animal development. Very early in development following conception, all animals undergo a blastula stage, in which the embryo is a hollow sphere of roughly five hundred cells. A region of the blastula called the blastopore folds to form a channel of cells through the blastula, thus initiating the gastrula stage.

The gastrula has three embryonic tissues: ectoderm, mesoderm, and endoderm. The ectoderm and endoderm continue to divide and differentiate into epithelial cells. Mesodermal cells multiply and differentiate into muscle and connective tissue cells. Dorsal ectodermal cells (cells that will become the back side of the organism) fold inward to form a nerve cord. The neurons of this nerve cord multiply and differentiate into central and peripheral nervous tissue.

In humans, the dorsal nerve cord becomes the billions of centralized neurons composing the spinal cord. The neurons in the anterior region of the spinal cord will fold, multiply, and differentiate into the various brain regions. The complete, fully functional human brain has approximately one hundred billion neurons that grow plastically and form trillions of interconnections for the accurate processing of electrical information.

The embryonic brain consists of three principal enfolded regions: the prosencephalon (forebrain), the mesencephalon (midbrain), and the rhombencephalon (hindbrain). Each of these three embryonic regions folds and differentiates further. The prosencephalon neurons multiply and differentiate to become the cerebrum, thalamus, and hypothalamus. The mesencephalon region becomes the corpora quadrigemina and cerebral peduncles, areas that connect other brain regions and coordinate sensory and motor impulses for basic reflexes. The rhombencephalon becomes the cerebellum, pons, and medulla oblongata; these are brain regions that control basic bodily processes such as coordination, prediction of movements, and maintenance of heart rate and respiration.

Furthermore, special regions of brain tissue develop into external sensory apparatuses: eyes for vision, ears for hearing and balance, nasal and tongue chemoreceptors for smell and taste. Millions of sensory neurons flow from these special sense organs to highly complicated brain regions that analyze, interpret, learn from, and react to these sensory stimuli. Neurophysiologists attempt to decipher the mechanisms by which the brain processes information. For example, the hundreds of thousands of retinal neurons in the eye collect light images reflected from objects, convert these diverse stimuli into thousands of bits of electrical information, and combine this information along an optic nerve. The optic nerve then transmits the electrical information of vision to the posterior occipital region of the cerebrum within the brain, where millions of visual processing neurons position the inverted, reversed visual image and interpret it.

How the brain neurons process such information is poorly understood and is the subject of intense study. While neurophysiologists have a fairly good understanding of nervous system structure, nervous system function represents a tremendous challenge to investigating scientists.

Structurally, neurons are supported by nerve cells called neuroglia in the central nervous system and Schwann cells in the peripheral nervous system. Neuroglia include four cell types: astrocytes, ependyma, microglia, and oligodendrocytes. Astrocytes stabilize neurons, ependyma allow cerebrospinal fluid exchange between brain ventricles and neurons, microglia clean up dead and foreign tissue, and oligodendrocytes insulate neurons by wrapping around them and secreting an electrically insulating protein called myelin. In the peripheral nervous system, Schwann cells behave much like oligodendrocytes; they wrap around axons and electrically insulate the axons with myelin for the efficient conduction of electrical information.

Specific neurological research is focused on neuronal plasticity in learning, the effects of various neurotransmitters upon neural activity, and diseases of the central nervous system. Various models of neuronal plasticity have been proposed to explain how learning occurs in higher vertebrates, including humans and other mammals. Most of these neuronal processing models involve the spatial patterning of neural bundles, which orient information in space and time. The plastic growth of these neurons in specified directions and locking patterns contributes to memory, learning, and intelligence in higher mammals such as primates (which include humans and chimpanzees) and cetaceans (dolphins and whales).

Neurotransmission can be affected by a variety of physical states and chemical influences. The extensive use and misuse of pharmaceuticals and drugs can have serious effects upon the nervous system. Furthermore, developmental errors of the nervous system and aging can contribute to various diseases and disorders.

PERSPECTIVE AND PROSPECTS

The nervous system of humans and higher vertebrate animals presents a tremendous variety of exciting research possibilities. The brain, the seat of human consciousness, represents a mystery to scientists even with the intense scientific scrutiny devoted to this organ. The brain is studied to understand how humans learn and how they might accelerate this exceptional ability. The intricate connections between billions of very plastic cerebral cortical neurons enable millions of electrical information impulses to direct millions of simultaneous activities every second. Brain structure, neural pathways, and techniques of learning and cognition are studied indirectly in human subjects and more directly in other intelligent mammals such as chimpanzees, gorillas, dolphins, and whales. These studies include analyses of the senses as well as poorly understood extrasensory perceptions that no doubt are linked to exceptional nervous system activity.

Researchers in the field of artificial intelligence attempt to generate cellular automatons, machines that can think and self-replicate. Artificial intelligence research began with the work of the brilliant physicist and computer pioneer John von Neumann, who attempted to mimic the human nervous system within computer systems—systems that have been called von Neumann machines. Yet no true thinking machines have been developed. The best supercomputers yet devised by humans may process data far more rapidly than the human brain, but they are no match for the human brain's capacity to process millions of data items simultaneously.

While the basic physical and chemical mechanisms of neuronal function have been deciphered by neurological scientists, research into neurotransmission across synaptic gaps continues. One principal neurotransmitter at muscular junctions is acetylcholine, which triggers muscle contractions following a motor neural impulse. When acetylcholine is not needed, it is destroyed by a molecule called acetylcholinesterase. Two types of molecular poisons can affect neuromuscular activity: acetylcholine inhibitors, which compete with acetylcholine; and antiacetylcholinesterases, which inhibit acetylcholinesterase and, therefore, accelerate acetylcholine activity. Acetylcholine competitors (such as at-

ropine, nicotine, caffeine, morphine, cocaine, and valium) block acetylcholine at neuromuscular junctions, thereby stopping muscular contractions and producing flaccid paralysis; death can result if the heart or respiratory muscles are affected. Antiacetylcholinesterases, such as the pesticides sevin and malathion, leave acetylcholine free to contract muscles endlessly, thereby causing convulsions.

Neurology also is devoted to understanding the biochemical and genetic basis for various neurological disorders, including Alzheimer's disease, parkinsonism, seizures, abnormal brain wave patterns, paralysis, and coma. Neurological research also is concerned with the nature of pain, the sense organs, and viral diseases of the nervous system, such as meningitis, encephalitis, herpes simplex virus 2, and shingles. The complexity of the human nervous system has inspired an enormous variety and quantity of research.

—*David Wason Hollar, Jr., Ph.D.*

See also Alzheimer's disease; Amnesia; Anesthesia; Anesthesiology; Aneurysmectomy; Aneurysms; Aphasia and dysphasia; Apnea; Ataxia; Attention-deficit disorder (ADD); Audiology; Balance disorders; Batten's disease; Behçet's disease; Bell's palsy; Biofeedback; Biophysics; Botox; Brain; Brain damage; Brain disorders; Brain tumors; Carpal tunnel syndrome; Cerebral palsy; Chiari malformations; Cluster headaches; Concussion; Craniotomy; Creutzfeldt-Jakob disease (CJD); Critical care; Critical care, pediatric; Cysts; Dementias; Disk removal; Dizziness and fainting; Dyslexia; Ear infections and disorders; Ear surgery; Ears; Electrical shock; Electroencephalography (EEG); Electromyography; Emergency medicine; Encephalitis; Epilepsy; Fetal tissue transplantation; Ganglion removal; Grafts and grafting; Guillain-Barré syndrome; Hallucinations; Head and neck disorders; Headaches; Hearing loss; Hemiplegia; Huntington's disease; Hypothalamus; Intraventricular hemorrhage; Laminectomy and spinal fusion; Learning disabilities; Leukodystrophy; Lower extremities; Lumbar puncture; Memory loss; Ménière's disease; Meningitis; Migraine headaches; Motor neuron diseases; Motor skill development; Multiple sclerosis; Narcolepsy; Nervous system; Neuralgia, neuritis, and neuropathy; Neurofibromatosis; Neuroimaging; Neurology, pediatric; Neurosurgery; Numbness and tingling; Otorhinolaryngology; Palsy; Paralysis; Paraplegia; Parkinson's disease; Physical examination; Poliomyelitis; Porphyria; Prion diseases; Psychiatry; Psychiatry, child and adolescent; Psychiatry, geriatric; Quadriplegia; Rabies;

Radiculopathy; Reflexes, primitive; Restless legs syndrome; Sciatica; Seizures; Sense organs; Shock therapy; Skin; Sleep disorders; Smell; Snakebites; Spina bifida; Spinal cord disorders; Spine, vertebrae, and disks; Strokes; Subdural hematoma; Sympathectomy; Taste; Tay-Sachs disease; Tetanus; Tics; Touch; Transient ischemic attacks (TIAs); Tremors; Unconsciousness; Upper extremities; Vagotomy; Vagus nerve.

FOR FURTHER INFORMATION:

Alberts, Bruce, et al. *Molecular Biology of the Cell*. 5th ed. New York: Garland, 2008. Leading molecular biologists have collaborated to produce this valuable textbook describing the genetics, biochemistry, and developmental biology of eukaryotic cells.

Bear, Mark F., Barry W. Connors, and Michael A. Paradiso. *Neuroscience: Exploring the Brain*. 3d ed. Philadelphia: Lippincott Williams & Wilkins, 2007. Undergraduate text that introduces the topics of neuroscience, neurobiology, neurodiseases, and physiological psychology.

Bloom, Floyd E., M. Flint Beal, and David J. Kupfer, eds. *The Dana Guide to Brain Health*. New York: Dana Press, 2006. An easy-to-understand health guide to the brain from neuroscience, neurology, and psychiatry perspectives. More than seventy psychiatric and neurological disorders, their diagnoses, and their treatments are covered.

Chiras, Daniel D. *Biology: The Web of Life*. St. Paul, Minn.: West, 1993. Chiras's outstanding biology textbook is an excellent introduction to the subject. Chapter 17, "The Nervous System: Integration, Coordination, and Control," is an excellent presentation of neurons, the brain, and the senses for the beginning biology student.

Daube, Jasper R., ed. *Clinical Neurophysiology*. 3d ed. New York: Oxford University Press, 2009. Covers the basics of clinical neurophysiology, considers the assessment of disease by anatomical system, and explains how clinical neurophysiologic techniques are used in the clinical assessment of diseases of the nervous system.

Lilly, John C. *Programming and Metaprogramming in the Human Biocomputer*. Rev. 4th ed. New York: Julian Press, 2000. Lilly, a controversial and pioneering neurophysiologist, presents the results of a five-year study of the effects of LSD on cognitive abilities in humans and dolphins in this work.

Marieb, Elaine N. *Essentials of Human Anatomy and Physiology*. 9th ed. San Francisco: Pearson/Benjamin Cummings, 2009. This introductory anatomy and physiology textbook, easily accessible to those with little science background, is richly illustrated with diagrams and photographs, which help to illuminate body systems and processes.

Nicholls, John G., A. Robert Martin, and Bruce G. Wallace. *From Neuron to Brain*. 4th ed. Sunderland, Mass.: Sinauer, 2007. In this comprehensive work, three leading neurophysiologists describe contemporary knowledge of the neuron: its structure, its function, and its roles in the central and peripheral nervous systems.

Snyder, Solomon H. "The Molecular Basis of Communication Between Cells." *Scientific American* 253, no. 4 (October, 1985): 132-141. In this scientific survey article, Snyder describes the structures and functions of neurotransmitters and related hormones. This article is one of several in a *Scientific American* edition devoted to "The Molecules of Life."

NEUROLOGY, PEDIATRIC
SPECIALTY

ANATOMY OR SYSTEM AFFECTED: Brain, ears, hands, head, muscles, musculoskeletal system, nerves, nervous system, psychic-emotional system, spine

SPECIALTIES AND RELATED FIELDS: Audiology, endocrinology, genetics, neonatology, pediatrics, perinatology, physical therapy

DEFINITION: The treatment of nervous system disorders in infants and children.

KEY TERMS:

autonomic nervous system: the body system that regulates involuntary vital functions and is divided into sympathetic and parasympathetic divisions

brain stem: the medulla oblongata, pons, and mesencephalon portions of the brain, which perform motor, sensory, and reflex functions and contain the corticospinal and reticulospinal tracts

cerebrum: the largest and uppermost section of the brain that integrates memory, speech, writing, and emotional response

lesion: a visible local tissue abnormality such as a wound, sore, rash, or boil, which can be benign, cancerous, gross, occult, or primary

neurologic: dealing with the nervous system and its disorders

paralysis: the loss of muscle function or sensation as a result of trauma or disease

pediatric: pertaining to neonates, infants, and children up to the age of twelve

SCIENCE AND PROFESSION

Neurologic illness and injury are principal causes of chronic disability when they occur in children because they result in the development of abnormal motor and mental behaviors and/or in the loss of previously existing capabilities, with a common problem in children being musculoskeletal dysfunction. Pediatric neurology involves the ongoing assessment of an infant's or child's neurologic function, which requires the pediatric neurologist to identify problems; set goals; use appropriate interventions, including physical therapy, teaching, and counseling; and evaluate the outcome of treatment.

The pediatric neurologist looks for certain positive or negative signs of dysfunction in the nervous system. Positive signs of neurologic dysfunction include the presence of sensory deficits; pain; involuntary motor events such as tremor, chorea, or convulsions; the display of bizarre behavior or mental confusion; and muscle weakness and difficulty controlling movement. Negative signs are those which represent the loss of function, such as paralysis, imperception of external stimuli, lack of speaking ability, and/or loss of consciousness.

The major manifestations of neurologic disease include disorders of motility, such as motor paralysis, abnormalities of movement and posture caused by extrapyramidal motor system dysfunction, cerebellum dysfunction, tremor, myoclonus, spasms, tics, and disorders of stance and gait; pain and other disorders of somatic sensation, headache, and backache, such as general pain and localized pain in the craniofacial area, back, neck, and extremities; disorders of the special senses, such as smell, taste, hearing, vision, ocular movement, and pupillary function, as well as dizziness and equilibrium disorders; epilepsy and disorders of consciousness, such as seizures and related disorders, coma and related disorders, syncope, and sleep abnormalities; derangements of intellect, behavior, and language as a result of diffuse and focal cerebral disease (such as delirium and other confusional states, dementia, and Korsakoff's syndrome), lesions in the cerebrum, and disorders of speech and language; and anxiety and disorders of energy, mood, emotion, and autonomic and endocrine functions, such as lassitude and fatigue, nervousness, irritability, anxiety, depression, disorders of the limbic lobes and autonomic nervous system, and hypothalamus and neuroendocrine dysfunction.

DIAGNOSTIC AND TREATMENT TECHNIQUES

The pediatric neurologist begins with a medical history of the infant or child to determine if the problem is congenital or acquired, chronic or episodic, and static or progressive. The focus of the pediatric neurologist in taking the patient's history is on genetic disorders, the medical history of family members, and perinatal events, with an emphasis on the mother's health, nutrition, medications, and tobacco, alcohol, or drug use during pregnancy. Considerable information about a child's or infant's behavior or neuromuscular function can be obtained by observation of the child's alertness and curiosity, trust or apprehension, facial and eye movements, limb function, and body posture and balance during simple motor activities. If possible, the pediatric neurologist will ask the child about instances of weakness, numbness, headaches, pain, tremors, nervousness, irritability, drowsiness, loss of memory, confusion, hallucinations, and loss of consciousness. Headaches, abdominal pain, or reluctance to attend school are often associated with neurologic disturbances, with contributing factors including subtle mental retardation, specific learning disabilities, and depression. Disorders of movement include tics, developmental clumsiness, ataxia, chorea, myoclonus, or dystonia.

A complete neurologic examination includes an evaluation of mental status, craniospinal inspection, cranial nerve testing, sensory testing, musculature evaluation, an assessment of coordination, and autonomic function testing. Mental status evaluation involves the assessment of orientation, memory, intellect, judgment, and affect. Craniospinal inspection includes the palpation, percussion, and auscultation of the cranium and spine. Cranial nerve testing assesses the motor and sensory function of the head and neck. Sensory testing measures peripheral sensations, including responses to pinprick, light touch, vibration, and fine movement of the joints. In musculature evaluation, weakness is associated with altered tendon reflexes, indicating lower motor neuron lesions, whereas exaggerated tendon reflexes are associated with an extensor response of the big toe following plantar stimulation (Babinski's sign). In coordination assessment, smooth fine and gross motor movements demand integrated function of the pyramidal and extrapyramidal systems, whereas hyperreflexia, increased muscle stiffness, and problems with muscle coordination reflect spasticity. The evaluation of autonomic function involves bowel and bladder function, emotional state, and symmetry of reflex activity, particularly resting muscle tone and positioning of the head. Additional diagnostic aids include lumbar puncture (spinal tap), complete blood count (CBC), myelography, electroencephalography (EEG), and computed tomography (CT) scanning.

Perspective and Prospects

Pediatric neurologists have been greatly assisted in their recognition of neurologic disease in infants and children by recently developed brain-imaging techniques, such as CT scanning and magnetic resonance imaging (MRI). Event-mediated evoked potentials are also used to assess the conduction and processing of information within specific sensory pathways. These advances have enabled an accurate evaluation of the integrity of the visual, auditory, and somatosensory pathways and the uncovering of single and multiple lesions within the brain stem and cerebrum. Particularly noteworthy are CT scanning and sonographic detection of clinically silent intracranial hemorrhages in premature infants.

Recent success in assisting premature infants has produced a population of patients at risk for developing cerebral palsy, mental retardation, epilepsy, and various learning disorders. The recent higher incidence of neurologic disease in the pediatric age group probably results from the increased ability of medical science to detect nervous system disturbances and from the increased survival rate of premature infants. Neurologic patients are compromised in nearly every aspect of living and have a high incidence of psychiatric problems, and their recovery is often slow and unpredictable. Because medical advances have resulted in an increased survival rate following serious neurological insult, more individuals are in need of long-term rehabilitation. The financial cost associated with this care presents an ongoing challenge to health care systems and to researchers examining effective means to restore function.

—*Daniel G. Graetzer, Ph.D., and Charles T. Leonard, Ph.D., P.T.*

See also Amnesia; Anesthesia; Anesthesiology; Aphasia and dysphasia; Apnea; Ataxia; Attention-deficit disorder (ADD); Audiology; Batten's disease; Biofeedback; Biophysics; Brain; Brain damage; Brain disorders; Brain tumors; Carpal tunnel syndrome; Cerebral palsy; Chiari malformations; Cluster headaches; Concussion; Craniotomy; Creutzfeldt-Jakob disease (CJD); Critical care, pediatric; Dizziness and fainting; Dyslexia; Ear infections and disorders; Ear surgery; Ears; Electrical shock; Electroencephalography (EEG); Emergency medicine; Encephalitis; Epilepsy; Ganglion removal; Grafts and grafting; Guillain-Barré syndrome; Hallucinations; Head and neck disorders; Headaches; Hearing loss; Huntington's disease; Hydrocephalus; Intraventricular hemorrhage; Laminectomy and spinal fusion; Learning disabilities; Leukodystrophy; Lower extremities; Lumbar puncture; Memory loss; Ménière's disease; Meningitis; Migraine headaches; Motor neuron diseases; Motor skill development; Multiple sclerosis; Narcolepsy; Nervous system; Neuralgia, neuritis, and neuropathy; Neurofibromatosis; Neuroimaging; Neurology; Neurosurgery; Numbness and tingling; Otorhinolaryngology; Palsy; Paralysis; Paraplegia; Pediatrics; Physical examination; Poliomyelitis; Porphyria; Prion diseases; Psychiatry, child and adolescent; Quadriplegia; Rabies; Reflexes, primitive; Seizures; Sense organs; Skin; Sleep disorders; Smell; Snakebites; Spina bifida; Spinal cord disorders; Spine, vertebrae, and disks; Sympathectomy; Taste; Tay-Sachs disease; Tetanus; Tics; Touch; Tremors; Unconsciousness; Upper extremities.

For Further Information:

Behrman, Richard E., Robert M. Kliegman, and Hal B. Jenson, eds. *Nelson Textbook of Pediatrics*. 18th ed. Philadelphia: Saunders/Elsevier, 2007. This standard pediatric textbook has been around for years and deservedly so. Minimal medical jargon makes it readable by laypersons.

Fenichel, Gerald M. *Clinical Pediatric Neurology: A Signs and Symptoms Approach*. 6th ed. Philadelphia: Saunders/Elsevier, 2009. Thoroughly revised and updated. The main neurological disorders of childhood are uniquely organized by presenting signs, which offers a practical approach to diagnosis and management.

Hay, William W., Jr., et al., eds. *Current Diagnosis and Treatment in Pediatrics*. 19th ed. New York: Lange Medical Books/McGraw-Hill, 2009. Easy-to-read and comprehensive general pediatrics book aimed at a wide audience, ranging from the medical student to the practicing pediatrician. Chapters are organized by pediatric subspecialty.

Victor, Maurice, and Allan H. Ropper. *Adams and Victor's Principles of Neurology*. 9th ed. New York: McGraw-Hill, 2009. This classic "teaching text" in neurology is completely revised and features a new art program and the latest advances in diagnosis and treatment. Includes new coverage of papillary function, sleep, syncope, inherited metabolic disease, degenerative disease, epilepsy, and cerebellar disease.

Volpe, Joseph. *Neurology of the Newborn.* 5th ed. Philadelphia: Saunders/Elsevier, 2008. A scholarly, thorough, single-author reference for pediatricians, obstetricians, or neurologists on diagnosis and treatment of neurological disorders in the newborn. Well-referenced and illustrated.

NEUROSIS

DISEASE/DISORDER

ANATOMY OR SYSTEM AFFECTED: Brain, nerves, nervous system, psychic-emotional system

SPECIALTIES AND RELATED FIELDS: Ethics, family medicine, neurology, psychiatry, psychology, public health

DEFINITION: A psychiatric disorder in which the patient continues to be rational and in touch with reality.

KEY TERMS:

agoraphobia: the fear of being in crowds

anxiety disorder: an emotional state that ranges from mild concern to disabling fear

bipolar disorders: disorders characterized by periods of depressed and elevated mood

hysterical amnesia: a dissociative disorder in which patients, capable of reading and writing, cannot remember simple things like their names

obsessive-compulsive disorder: a condition characterized by the ritualistic performance of repetitive actions

somatization disorder: a persistent condition in which patients complain about physical problems for which no cause is apparent

CAUSES AND SYMPTOMS

The distinction between neurosis and psychosis is that those suffering from neuroses are in touch with reality and usually realize that they have a problem. In contrast, psychotics frequently lose touch with reality and do not recognize that they are sick and in need of immediate professional help.

The most common neurosis is depression. Those with major depression experience, for no overt reason, a persistent and overwhelming sadness coupled with an all-encompassing sense of despair. It is normal for people who suffer such ills as the death of a loved one, the loss of a job, or severe financial reverses to be de-

pressed. In such cases, their depression is usually mitigated when the cause is removed or when they distance themselves from it. On the other hand, those who suffer from major depression cannot attribute their suffering to an immediate cause. They are frequently sad and usually do not know why. Depression is also a major component of bipolar disorders, in which episodes of major depression are followed by periods of mania, or elevated mood.

Other common forms of neurosis are obsessive-compulsive disorder (OCD), somatization disorder, hypochondria, various phobias or fears, anxiety disorders, psychosexual disorders, and hysterical amnesia. All these problems occur less frequently than major depression.

An example of obsessive-compulsive disorder may be the compulsion of its victims to wash their hands thirty or forty times a day. Those who have a somatization disorder complain of largely imagined illnesses for which no physical cause can be detected. Often termed hypochondria, this disorder is more frequent in women, especially middle-aged women, than in men.

Most people suffer from one or more phobias that do not disable them. Fear of heights (acrophobia) and abnormal fear of public or open areas (agoraphobia) are quite common, as are the fear of some living things such as spiders or scorpions (arachnophobia) or the fear of closed places (claustrophobia). Many of those suffering from such phobias can usually control them by confronting them rationally, although some phobias may be so intense that they result in panic.

Hysterical amnesia, a dissociative disorder, is relatively rare. Often it is connected with anxiety disorder. Victims tend to panic to the point that they suffer temporary memory loss. Although they remain in touch with reality, they may not be able to remember their names, addresses, telephone numbers, and other obvious bits of information.

INFORMATION ON NEUROSIS

CAUSES: Psychological disorder

SYMPTOMS: Distressing and unacceptable anxiety, impaired daily functioning, depression, abnormal fear

DURATION: Often chronic; may involve acute episodes

TREATMENTS: Counseling, psychoactive medications

Post-traumatic stress disorder (PTSD) has become increasingly common. In extreme cases, it may result in psychotic behavior, although it is more often neurotic in its manifestation. PTSD usually occurs in people who have been subjected to combat situations or to life-threatening natural disasters such as earthquakes, hurricanes, floods, and fires.

TREATMENT AND THERAPY

The usual treatment in persistent cases of neurosis is psychotherapy rendered by a clinical psychologist or psychiatrist, frequently over an extended period. Severe cases may require meetings with a professional three or four times a week in order to be effective. Mild cases can sometimes be dealt with in only two or three visits, especially if the patient is cooperative and committed to dealing with the problem.

Neuroses usually do not require such drastic treatment as electric shock therapy or brain surgery, although such treatment was sometimes prescribed in the past. Currently, more than twenty prescription drugs exist to treat such neuroses as bipolar and somatization disorders. Often, patients need to try several of these medications before finding the one that suits them best. Patients must be cautioned, however, not to expect immediate results. When they find a medication that works well for them, they are advised to continue taking it even after their initial symptoms disappear.

PERSPECTIVE AND PROSPECTS

Substantial biochemical advances during the early years of the twenty-first century have resulted in improved understanding of the relationship between body chemistry and both neuroses and psychoses. Such advances have also been accompanied by changes in the way psychiatric therapy is delivered. Group therapy reduces the cost of treatment. In many situations, because it is so interactive, it proves superior to the one-on-one therapy that psychotherapy and psychoanalysis provide.

The public at large has become more sophisticated than past generations in dealing with neuroses. Nevertheless, the management of the most common neurosis, depression, remains challenging. Most suicides are committed by those suffering from the depths of depression, a condition that gives them a sense of hopelessness.

—*R. Baird Shuman, Ph.D.*

See also Antianxiety drugs; Anxiety; Bipolar disorders; Depression; Hypochondriasis; Midlife crisis;

Obsessive-compulsive disorder; Panic attacks; Paranoia; Phobias; Postpartum depression; Post-traumatic stress disorder; Psychiatric disorders; Psychiatry; Psychiatry, child and adolescent; Psychiatry, geriatric; Psychoanalysis; Psychosis; Psychosomatic disorders; Stress.

FOR FURTHER INFORMATION:

Craske, Michelle G. *Origins of Phobias and Anxiety Disorders: Why More Women than Men?* New York: Elsevier, 2003.

Frankl, Victor E. *On the Theory and Therapy of Mental Disorders: An Introduction to Logotherapy and Existential Analysis.* New York: Brunner-Routledge, 2004.

Gossop, Michael. *Theories of Neurosis.* New York: Springer, 1981.

Rapee, Ronald M., and David H. Barlow, eds. *Chronic Anxiety: Generalized Anxiety Disorder and Mixed Anxiety-Depression.* New York: Guilford Press, 1991.

Russon, John. *Human Experience: Philosophy, Neurosis, and Elements of Everyday Life.* Albany: State University of New York Press, 2003.

NEUROSURGERY

PROCEDURE

ANATOMY OR SYSTEM AFFECTED: Bones, brain, glands, head, nerves, nervous system, psychic-emotional system, spine

SPECIALTIES AND RELATED FIELDS: General surgery, neurology, psychiatry

DEFINITION: Surgery involving the brain, spinal cord, or peripheral nerves, including craniotomy, lobotomy, laminectomy, and sympathectomy.

KEY TERMS:

aneurysm: the swelling of a blood vessel, which occurs with the stretching of a weak place in the vessel wall

cannula: a tube or hypodermic needle implanted in the body to introduce or extract substances

commissurotomy: the severing of the corpus callosum, the fiber tract joining the two cerebral hemispheres

hematoma: a localized collection of clotted blood in an organ or tissue as a result of internal bleeding

lesion: a wound or tumor of the brain or spinal cord

lobectomy: the removal of a lobe of the brain, or a major part of a lobe

lobotomy: the separation of either an entire lobe or a major part of a lobe from the rest of the brain

trephination: the opening of a hole in the skull with an instrument called a trephine

INDICATIONS AND PROCEDURES

Neurosurgery refers to any surgery performed on a part of the nervous system. Brain surgery may be used to remove a tumor or foreign body, relieve the pressure caused by an intracranial hemorrhage, excise an abscess, treat parkinsonism, or relieve pain. In cases of severe mental depression or untreatable epilepsy, psychosurgery (such as lobotomy) may alleviate the worst symptoms. Surgery may be performed on the spine to correct a defect, remove a tumor, repair a ruptured intervertebral disk, or relieve pain. Surgery may be performed on nerves to remove a tumor, relieve pain, or reconnect a severed nerve.

Most brain operations share some common procedures. Bleeding from the numerous tiny blood vessels in the brain is controlled by use of an electric needle, a finely pointed instrument that shoots a minute electric current into the vessel and seals it. (This same instrument can be used as an electric knife for bloodless cutting.) Brain tissue is kept moist by continued washing with a dilute salt solution. The brain tissue itself is handled with damp cotton pads attached to the end of forceps.

If the brain is swollen, it may be treated by intravenous injections of urea. The resulting increase in the salt concentration of the blood draws the water away from the brain. In addition to drawing off excess water, the brain's size is temporarily reduced, giving the surgeon extra room to maneuver. To help reduce bleeding within the brain, the patient's blood pressure can be lowered by half temporarily through an injection of a drug into the blood. The patient's temperature is also reduced, which lowers the brain's need for oxygen and ensures that the reduced blood flow will not be deleterious.

An operation in which a hole is cut into the skull is called a craniotomy. The instrument used is called a trephine (trepan); it resembles a corkscrew with a short, nail-like tip and a threaded cutting disk. The size of the opening that is made ranges from 1.5 centimeters (0.6 inches) to 3.8 centimeters (1.5 inches) in diameter and, if necessary, may be enlarged with an instrument called a rongeur. This type of surgery is performed to insert needles or cannulas and to remove subdural hematomas. If too much of the bony skull has to be removed (or is fractured by accidental means), a substitute for the bone is inserted. The substitute is usually made of plastic, such as acrylic.

A depressed fracture of the skull, especially if it is a compound fracture (involving an open laceration), is surgically treated as soon as possible. Because an open wound is an easy way for bacteria to enter the body and cause infection, disinfection and closure are done quickly. The patient is often conscious and requires local anesthesia, so that consciousness is maintained. The surgeon drills burr holes at the edges of the depression, lifts the bone fragments, and places them in their original positions. Some pieces of bone may be too damaged to be used, and they are discarded. If the hole is large, a later surgery may close the hole with a metal or plastic plate or with a graft from a rib. Another method of filling large holes is the use of metal or fabric mesh; these materials suffice because scalp tissue and heavy muscle are protective as well.

Surgery for parkinsonism will not cure the disease but will help alleviate some of its symptoms. The major symptoms are tremor, stiffness, weakness, and slowed movements. Neurosurgery can be used to reduce or stop the shaking. Surgery to the directly affected areas, however, is all but prohibited by their unavailability: The sites are so deep in the brain that the knife would damage or destroy other vital brain tissue.

When pain becomes unbearable, such as the pain associated with cancer, the nerves carrying these pain messages can be interrupted anywhere between the brain and the cancerous region. The nerve to the affected organ can be severed, the nerve roots of the spinal cord can be cut, or the cut can be made within the spinal cord.

Hypophysectomy is the surgical removal of the pituitary gland. It is usually performed to slow the growth and spread of endocrine-dependent malignant tumors of the breast, ovary, or prostate gland. It may also be used to stop the deterioration of the retina that may come with diabetes mellitus or to remove a pituitary tumor. Hypophysectomy is considered only as a last resort when cryosurgery or radioactive implants fail to destroy the pituitary tissue. There are two ways to reach a diseased pituitary gland by surgery. One way is to go through the nose. The skull is entered through the sphenoid sinus, and the floor of the bony saddle of the middle of the skull is cut to reach the gland. The second means is by craniotomy. The skull is opened through an incision in the hairline above the forehead. A flap of bone, hinged at eyebrow level, is brought forward so that the surgeon can see the entire affected area clearly. The gland is completely excised.

Psychosurgery is now considered only as a last resort, when nothing else can possibly work. It is rarely undertaken because of the availability of so many drugs to control mental illnesses. In the cases when a lobotomy is performed, it can be done under local anesthesia through tiny holes drilled in the roof of the eyes' orbits. An instrument is then inserted to separate the lobes of the brain.

A laminectomy is performed to relieve compression of the spinal cord caused by injury (the displacement of a bone) or by the degeneration of a disk; it may also be used to find and remove a displaced intervertebral disk. A laminectomy is performed under general anesthesia. The surgeon makes an incision in the back, vertically over the tips of the vertebral bones. The large, thick muscles that lie on either side are peeled back from the surface of the bones. The lamina itself is the part of a vertebral bone that forms the back wall of the spinal canal. When the laminae are cut away, the spinal canal is opened so that the spinal cord covering can be cut. Once the cord is exposed, a particular condition can be treated. It may then be necessary to fuse the vertebrae. The removal of the laminae causes little interference with support or motion of the spine, although recovery from the surgery requires that the patient remain prone for several days to keep the spine in alignment.

Fusion of the vertebrae is the surgical joining of two or more spinal vertebrae to stabilize a segment of the spinal column following severe trauma, a herniated (ruptured) disk, or a degenerative disease. The surgery is performed under general anesthesia. The cartilage pads are removed from between the posterior portions of the affected vertebrae. Bone chips are cut from the vertebral ridges and inserted as a replacement for the removed cartilage. Postoperative motion must be limited until the articulating bones heal.

Severe pain that cannot be controlled by analgesics (painkillers) may be treated by surgery. One procedure, a cordotomy, removes a section of the spinal cord so that most of the nerve fibers that transmit pain messages to the brain are destroyed. At first, the patient does experience less pain, but after a few months, the pain recurs and is worse than before. The recurrence of pain is likely attributable to the reconstruction of some axons that carry ascending messages. Other painful conditions can be treated with surgery. Trigeminal neuralgia (or tic douloureux) is one such condition. These severe attacks of stabbing pain in the face may last a minute or more. The trigeminal nerve can be injected with a concentrated alcohol solution, which will prevent it from working for a year or two. This condition is usually treated surgically by drilling a burr hole in the temple and cutting across the lower two-thirds of the nerve trunk at the site.

A sympathectomy surgically interrupts a part of the sympathetic nerve pathways. It is used to relieve the pain of vascular disease. The surgery involves removing the sheath from around an artery. This sheath carries the sympathetic nerve fibers that control vasoconstriction. Once the sheath is removed, the vessel relaxes and expands so that more blood travels through it.

USES AND COMPLICATIONS

While neurosurgery offers the hope of recovery to sufferers of tumors, aneurysms, and brain injuries, it may result in complications that can bring disability, coma, or even death. Therefore, three considerations must be taken into account before neurosurgery is performed. First, these surgeries involve more high-risk procedures than most other types. Second, diseases that necessitate neurosurgical treatment often render patients wholly or partially incompetent to understand the implications of their surgery. Third, sometimes matching the appropriate surgery to the patient's condition is an uncertain process. Even standard neurosurgical procedures have not been proven in every event.

Because the diagnosis of a brain tumor is often seen as fatal, many believe that surgery has little value as therapy, especially for malignant tumors. Others suggest, however, that the more radical the surgery, the greater the chance of survival for the patient. The problem arises when a tumor is found within the center area of the brain, where the primary sensory and motor cortices are situated. Surgical methods of the past tended to exacerbate the problems of the patient. The use of lasers and microscopy, however, may increase the chance of successful treatment. Using these tools, incisions of no longer than 2 centimeters can be made. Using the microscope, the surgeon can guide the laser to the tumor, which is gently melted and vaporized—all without disturbing the brain. This method is especially useful for reaching deep-seated tumors.

Stereotaxic surgery is a means by which monitoring devices are inserted into the brain cortex. These devices can detect lesions, stimulate or record areas within the cortex, or in some other way study the brain. The two things necessary to perform this surgery are a stereotaxic atlas (or map) of the brain and the instrumentation for the procedure. The atlas is a series of individual maps, each representing a slice of the brain. The stereotaxic instrument consists of two parts: a head holder, which maintains the patient's head in a particular position and orientation, and an electrode holder, which holds the device that is to be inserted.

The purpose of the lesion method of stereotaxic surgery is to remove, damage, or destroy a part of the brain in such a way that the behavior of the patient can be monitored to determine the functions of the affected area, or lesion. Surgery to produce lesions is an extremely precise, and therefore dangerous, surgery. Structures within the brain are tiny, convoluted, and tightly packed; it is likely that any surgery performed on an area will damage adjacent areas. There are four different methods of producing lesions.

Aspiration lesions are performed when the lesion is in a more accessible area of the brain, where the surgeon can see it clearly and can use the proper instruments. The cortical tissue is aspirated by a handheld pipette, and then the tougher white matter layers are peeled away. Deeper lesions are cut away with high-frequency (radiofrequency) currents passed through carefully placed electrodes. The heat of the current destroys the tissue. The amount of tissue to be removed is regulated through control of the current's duration and intensity. In the third method, a nerve or tract to be removed can be cut with a scalpel. A tiny incision severing the nerve does not have to do damage to surrounding tissues, so the lesion is small.

The fourth method is cryogenic blockade. Blockade is a preferable alternative because virtually no structural damage results and a return to normal temperature causes neural activity to resume. In this method, a coolant is pumped through the tip of an implanted cryoprobe to cool the area. When the tissue is cooled, the neurons do not fire. The temperature must remain above freezing, however, to prevent destruction of the tissue. Although the result is not a true lesion, since function returns, this cooled area acts as a lesion because the behavior that it governs is interrupted. Consequently, cryogenic blockade is said to produce a reversible lesion.

A commissurotomy, or cutting apart of the two cerebral hemispheres, may be performed in cases of severe epilepsy if no other treatment is successful. After the two halves are separated (the brain stem is left intact), each hemisphere maintains all the centers that mediate its functions, except that each cortex sees only half the world. For example, visual messages are crossed so that the opposite hemisphere is stimulated by only one eye's input. If both eyes and both hemispheres are working, however, vision should be unaffected. In fact, no real deficits should occur in these patients' behavior. They retain the same verbal intelligence, reasoning, perception, motor coordination, and personality because of the brain's extraordinary ability to preserve unity, or oneness.

Commissurotomies were first performed in the hope of reducing the severity of convulsions and seizures associated with epilepsy. The rationale was that the severity of the convulsions would be reduced if discharges could be limited to the hemisphere from which they originated. The benefits far surpassed expectations; many patients never experience another convulsion.

Studies of lobotomized patients, especially those who have undergone a frontal lobotomy, have provided insight into the importance of these lobes. Frontal lobotomies are generally performed to lessen psychoses that cannot be treated successfully by any other means or to relieve unbearable pain, such as that induced in the latter stages of cancer.

Lobotomies are somewhat controversial. It has been shown that the surgery results in diminished anxiety and concern in the patient, but in some patients this reaction is extreme, causing them to lose their ethical standards. Their judgment and planning ability are decreased. Actions and behavior are not necessarily matched to stimuli; they may be inappropriate or badly timed: For example, crying may be a response to a comic situation. One patient may plan a meal but forget how to cook, and another may urinate in public while dressed for a formal occasion. Thus, although a lobotomy does not diminish intellect, memory, or consciousness to the extent that injury to other parts of the brain does, it is debasing. Perseverance or the ability to continue some activity is decreased, and patients often cannot deal with or overcome challenges.

PERSPECTIVE AND PROSPECTS

People living in the Stone Age often performed trephination. This operation consisted of boring or making holes in the skull and removing pieces or disks of bone. Trephination was likely performed to release evil spirits or demons: There is little evidence of fractures of the skulls that have been found, and the pieces of skulls that were excised were preserved and worn as talismans. Today, surgeons in some tribal cultures perform the same surgery; in some cases, some are done for ritual purposes, while others are performed for head injuries as well as headache, dizziness, and epilepsy. Trephination provided the groundwork for brain surgery as it is still practiced.

Perhaps the most intriguing possibility for future research is transplanting brains or brain tissue. Brain transplants have come a long way from their portrayal in science fiction. In 1971, the first real evidence that transplanted tissue could survive was found. These successful attempts were made in rats. Further studies have shown that transplants have a higher survival rate in tissue richly vascularized with sufficient room to grow. It is hoped that neurotransplant surgery can be used to treat brain damage. One approach would be to develop procedures of implantation that would stimulate the regeneration of the patient's own tissue. A second approach would be to replace damaged tissue with healthy tissue of the same type.

The major question that will have to be answered before successful regeneration is accomplished is why neurons of the peripheral nervous system (PNS) regenerate but the neurons of the central nervous system (CNS) do not. One hypothesis would be that they are too structurally different. This theory is disputed by studies that show CNS neuron regeneration in the peripheral nervous system, while PNS neurons do not regenerate in the central nervous system. Other evidence to refute the hypothesis is that peripheral sensory neurons regenerate until they reach the spinal cord, then regeneration ceases. Therefore, perhaps there is an environmental factor within the central nervous system that prohibits regeneration, such as scar tissue that forms only in the area of CNS damage. Experiments to prove or disprove this theory are inconclusive. The other possibility is that the insulating cells wrapped around CNS neurons are different enough from the Schwann cells of PNS neurons that regeneration is discouraged.

Attempts to replace damaged tissue with healthy tissue have been most useful in treating Parkinson's disease (with its rigidity, tremors, and lack of spontaneous movement). One type of tissue used for replacement is fetal neural tissue. It not only survives but also innervates adjacent tissue, releases neurotransmitters (in this case dopamine), and alleviates the symptoms of parkinsonism. Even though this procedure is highly successful, it is unlikely that fetal tissue transplantation will become common. The use of fetal tissue raises serious ethical questions regarding the harvesting of donor tissue from human fetuses. A possible substitute for neural tissue is autotransplantation with some of the patient's own adrenal medulla. This tissue could be used because it too releases dopamine. Investigations thus far have been controversial, but the operation is being performed worldwide.

—*Iona C. Baldridge*

See also Aneurysmectomy; Brain; Brain damage; Brain disorders; Brain tumors; Chiari malformations; Craniotomy; Cysts; Electroencephalography (EEG);

Fetal tissue transplantation; Ganglion removal; Laminectomy and spinal fusion; Laser use in surgery; Lumbar puncture; Nervous system; Neuroimaging; Neurology; Neurology, pediatric; Pain; Pain management; Parkinson's disease; Positron emission tomography (PET) scanning; Psychiatric disorders; Psychiatry; Radiculopathy; Spina bifida; Spinal cord disorders; Spine, vertebrae, and disks; Stem cells; Subdural hematoma; Tics; Tumor removal; Tumors.

FOR FURTHER INFORMATION:

Bear, Mark F., Barry W. Connors, and Michael A. Paradiso. *Neuroscience: Exploring the Brain*. 3d ed. Philadelphia: Lippincott Williams & Wilkins, 2007. Undergraduate text that introduces the topics of neuroscience, neurobiology, neurodiseases, and physiological psychology.

Bloom, Floyd E., M. Flint Beal, and David J. Kupfer, eds. *The Dana Guide to Brain Health*. New York: Dana Press, 2006. An easy-to-understand health guide to the brain from neuroscience, neurology, and psychiatry perspectives. More than seventy psychiatric and neurological disorders, their diagnoses, and their treatments are covered.

Daube, Jasper R., ed. *Clinical Neurophysiology*. 3d ed. New York: Oxford University Press, 2009. Covers the basics of clinical neurophysiology, considers the assessment of disease by anatomical system, and explains how clinical neurophysiologic techniques are used in the clinical assessment of diseases of the nervous system.

Pinel, John P. J. *Biopsychology*. 7th ed. Boston: Pearson Allyn & Bacon, 2009. A textbook for introductory courses in biopsychology, which studies a combination of neurology and behavior. The chapters are rich in case studies and illustrations, and they conclude with key word definitions and references.

Post, Kalman, et al., eds. *Acute, Chronic, and Terminal Care in Neurosurgery*. Springfield, Ill.: Charles C Thomas, 1987. An interesting compilation of chapters written by various health care workers on the various aspects of neurosurgery. The procedures themselves are not the focus of the pieces, but medical care, ethics, and facing death are addressed.

Zollinger, Robert M., Jr., and Robert M. Zollinger, Sr. *Zollinger's Atlas of Surgical Operations*. 8th ed. New York: McGraw-Hill, 2003. A comprehensive examination of surgery. Covers basic surgical anatomy and vascular, gynecologic, neurologic, gastrointestinal, and miscellaneous abdominal procedures.

NICOTINE

DISEASE/DISORDER

ANATOMY OR SYSTEM AFFECTED: Brain, gums, heart, immune system, lungs, mouth, nose, psychic-emotional system, reproductive system, respiratory system, skin, teeth, throat

SPECIALTIES AND RELATED FIELDS: Cardiology, dentistry, embryology, immunology, neonatology, obstetrics, oncology, orthodontics, otorhinolaryngology, pathology, pharmacology, psychiatry, public health, pulmonary medicine, toxicology, vascular medicine

DEFINITION: A colorless, poisonous alkaloid derived from tobacco plants.

CAUSES AND SYMPTOMS

Nicotine is an addictive substance found in cigarettes, cigars, and chewing snuff. Nicotine dependence is a diagnosis given to a person who continues to use the drug despite negative consequences resulting from its use. Problems can include tolerance, withdrawal, uncontrolled use, unsuccessful efforts to quit, considerable time spent getting or using the drug, a decrease in other important activities because of use, and health problems caused or worsened by use. These health problems include cardiovascular problems, such as blood clots, high blood pressure, and strokes; cancers of the bladder, head, lungs, neck, pancreas, and throat; and chronic lung problems, such as emphysema. Studies have shown lower birth weight in the babies of mothers who smoke; higher rates of allergies, asthma, bronchitis, and colds in children of parents who smoke; and higher death rates from cancer in individuals regularly exposed to secondhand smoke.

TREATMENT AND THERAPY

In primary prevention, an entire population is provided with a form of treatment. Examples are antismoking campaigns focused on the dangers of smoking. Laws prohibiting individuals from smoking in airplanes are also a good example of primary prevention. In secondary prevention, interventions are applied to individuals at greater-than-average risk for smoking. Children of smokers would be such a group. An appropriate intervention might be giving these children health information to encourage them to avoid starting tobacco use. In smoking cessation programs, also known as tertiary prevention, people with nicotine dependence are provided with self-help materials or the use of professional services. With professional service providers, interventions may include combinations of treatments such as nicotine replacement patches, nicotine gum, prescription drugs, and psychological therapy.

PERSPECTIVE AND PROSPECTS

Nicotine was identified chemically in the nineteenth century, but tobacco had been used by Native Americans to celebrate religious rituals and sacred rites for many years. In contrast, in contemporary society, the use of nicotine is habitual and seldom attached to rituals of religious significance. From 1970 to 2000, smoking rates decreased in the United States. It appears, however, that this decline was more apparent in men than in women. As such, it is likely that treatment and prevention approaches will need to address such gender differences.

—*Nancy A. Piotrowski, Ph.D.*

See also Addiction; Bronchitis; Chronic obstructive pulmonary disease (COPD); Emphysema; Lung cancer; Lungs; Pulmonary diseases; Pulmonary medicine; Respiration; Smoking; Substance abuse; Wheezing.

FOR FURTHER INFORMATION:

Carlson-Berne, Emma, ed. *Nicotine*. Detroit: Greenhaven Press/Thomson Gale, 2006.

Dodgen, Charles E. *Nicotine Dependence: Understanding and Applying the Most Effective Treatment Interventions*. Washington, D.C.: American Psychological Association, 2005.

INFORMATION ON NICOTINE

CAUSES: Addictive properties of drug, exposure to secondhand smoke

SYMPTOMS: Dependence possibly leading to such health problems as cardiovascular disease (blood clots, hypertension, stroke); cancer of bladder, head, lungs, neck, pancreas, and throat; chronic lung problems (emphysema)

DURATION: Often chronic

TREATMENTS: Primary prevention (antismoking campaigns, regulations); secondary prevention (interventions with at-risk individuals); tertiary prevention (smoking cessation programs, which may include nicotine replacement patches, nicotine gum, prescription drugs, psychological therapy)

George, Tony P., ed. *Medication Treatments for Nicotine Dependence.* Boca Raton, Fla.: CRC/Taylor & Francis, 2007.

Julien, Robert M. *A Primer of Drug Action: A Concise, Nontechnical Guide to the Actions, Uses, and Side Effects of Psychoactive Drugs.* 11th ed. New York: Freeman, 2008.

Kozlowski, Lynn T., Jack E. Henningfield, and Janet Brigham. *Cigarettes, Nicotine, and Health: A Biobehavioral Approach.* Thousand Oaks, Calif.: Sage Publications, 2001.

Weil, Andrew, and Winifred Rosen. *From Chocolate to Morphine: Everything You Need to Know About Mind-Altering Drugs.* Rev. ed. Boston: Houghton Mifflin, 2004.

NIEMANN-PICK DISEASE

DISEASE/DISORDER

ANATOMY OR SYSTEM AFFECTED: Bones, brain, liver, lungs, nervous system, respiratory system, spleen

SPECIALTIES AND RELATED FIELDS: Biochemistry, endocrinology, family medicine, genetics, hematology, internal medicine, neurology, pathology, pediatrics, public health

DEFINITION: This lipid disease group, resulting from inactive sphingomyelinase and cholesterol-modifying enzymes, causes lipid buildup in the brain and other organs, mental and physical debilitation, and a short life span.

KEY TERMS:

enzyme: a protein biocatalyst that speeds up a biochemical reaction

foam cell: a large, foamy-appearing, lipid-rich cell, usually a white blood cell

lipid: a fatlike substance

CAUSES AND SYMPTOMS

Niemann-Pick disease (NPD), which consists of several lipid storage diseases, is characterized by an enlarged liver and spleen and the accumulation of fatlike sphingomyelin and cholesterol. Many patients have enlarged spleens and livers soon after birth and develop severe mental damage. In others, symptoms lag; mental damage may not occur, or organ enlargement and mental damage may be postponed. The main forms, types A through C, are attributable to low levels of sphingomyelinase, which normally alters sphingomyelin for use and excretion.

Type A, or infantile NPD, is the most common type. The abdominal organs enlarge, and nervous system damage occurs in early infancy. The spleen and liver enlarge by the age of six months, motor function and intellectual capabilities are then lost, and death occurs by four years of age. Patients are emaciated, jaundiced, and have swollen abdomens and cherry-red spots in the macular region of the eye. Large histiocytes (foam cells) abound in the bone marrow, spleen, lymph nodes, adrenal glands, and lungs.

Type B, or juvenile nonneuropathic NPD, is also common. Enlarged abdominal organs develop as quickly as in type A, but no neurological impairment occurs. An enlarged spleen appears first, followed by liver enlargement. Lungs are often so damaged that frequent breathlessness occurs. Abdominal pain is caused by the huge size of the liver, and the patient is susceptible to respiratory infections. Nevertheless, patients with this type of disease reach adulthood in fair health.

Type C, a rarer chronic form, is asymptomatic for approximately two years. Symptoms then develop gradually, accompanied by lost speech and motor coordination and epilepsy. The liver and spleen are smaller than in types A and B. These patients die in their teens.

The pathology of Niemann-Pick disease includes abundant foam cells in the spleen, bone marrow, liver, lungs, and lymph nodes. Nervous tissue may be altered similarly. Foam cells contain brown lipofuscin pigment. This and blue to blue-green stained intracellular material leads to an alternate name, sea-blue histiocytes.

The spleen of a patient with NPD is large, pale, and filled with foam cells, though few hematologic changes occur except for anemia late in the disease. The liver of a type A patient is usually about 50 percent larger than normal, while the liver of a type B patient grows so large that it deforms and causes abdominal pain. Foam cells soon fill the liver, although it usually functions ad-

---

INFORMATION ON NIEMANN-PICK DISEASE

CAUSES: Genetic enzyme deficiency

SYMPTOMS: Liver and spleen enlargement; sometimes severe mental damage, loss of motor function, emaciation, jaundice, swollen abdomen, red spots in eyes, breathlessness

DURATION: Chronic and progressive

TREATMENTS: None; enzyme and genetic testing of prospective parents, symptom alleviation through spleen removal or antibiotics

equately. They also fill the lymph nodes, spleen, lungs, and bone marrow. Their number varies with NPD type and duration. In most types, the foam cell-filled adrenal glands, gonads, thyroid, pituitary, and pancreas function adequately. However, the brains of type A and C patients drop in weight by 25 to 50 percent and are severely damaged.

The predominant lipid accumulant is sphingomyelin, made of fatty acids joined to substances called sphingosine and phosphocholine. Sphingomyelin content in the spleens of type A, B, and C patients is twenty-five, eighteen, and two to twelve times normal, respectively. A thirtyfold increase of liver sphingomyelin occurs in types A and B. Smaller increases, approximately ten times normal, occur in type C. Also, sphingomyelin levels increase threefold to sevenfold in the lymph nodes of all NPD patients. Cholesterol and other sphingolipids also increase in the tissues of NPD patients. It is believed that lipid increases are causative.

Sphingomyelinase deficiency is greatest in types A and C, in which 4 to 20 percent of normal levels occur. In type C, they are about 50 to 90 percent normal levels. The NPD defect is genetic alteration of sphingomyelinase, yielding mutant enzyme less able to break down sphingomyelin.

TREATMENT AND THERAPY

Niemann-Pick disease can be prevented only through the enzymatic and genetic testing of prospective parents. Members of at-risk ethnic groups can be tested for sphingomyelinase in their lymphocytes and muscle cells. Genetic counseling can also be used. The disease is transmitted through an autosomal recessive gene, so both parents must carry the gene to transmit disease. If both parents are carriers of a defective NPD gene, each of their children has a 25 percent chance of having the disease and a 50 percent chance of being an asymptomatic carrier.

There is no cure for Niemann-Pick disease. Therapeutic approaches include spleen removal, which diminishes abdominal pain, but it is not widely used. Patients with lung damage who experience frequent respiratory infections and pneumonia are treated with antibiotics, but long courses and high doses are required. Bone marrow transplantation has been done, with mildly encouraging results, but it is not a common treatment. Some children or teenagers with type C disease have been helped by low-cholesterol diets. However, the life expectancy of patients with NPD has not been prolonged much.

PERSPECTIVE AND PROSPECTS

In 1914, Albert Niemann, a German pediatrician, reported an eighteen-month-old Jewish child with huge liver and spleen, swollen lymph glands, and jaundice. The child had poor motor control, could not suckle, and died before age two. Postmortem examination showed large lipid deposits in the liver, spleen, lymph nodes, kidneys, and adrenal glands. The overall symptoms and rapid death suggested a new illness. In the 1920's, Ludwig Pick studied other cases and named Niemann-Pick disease. NPD, seen in all ethnic groups, is most common in Ashkenazic Jews. Type B patients are often of Spanish ancestry. Type C, which is less common, occurs most in Nova Scotians.

It is believed that enzyme replacement therapy (mostly sphingomyelinase) may ease the lives of NPD victims when an effective methodology for the frequent delivery of purified enzymes is developed and the enzymes are available in sufficient amounts. Recombinant deoxyribonucleic acid (DNA) research should contribute greatly. However, such treatment of severe NPD (types A and C) will be difficult because of the need to deliver enzymes to the brain.

Another avenue is transplanting healthy livers and spleens, which is presently done to treat other diseases. The problems are scarce donated organs and difficulty placing them in debilitated NPD patients. Transplantation may prove more promising in the future. Also, researchers have identified animal models and genes that, when defective, contribute to NPD. Understanding these issues may produce successful NPD treatments.

—Sanford S. Singer, Ph.D.;
updated by LeAnna DeAngelo, Ph.D.

See also Brain damage; Enzyme therapy; Enzymes; Gaucher's disease; Genetic counseling; Genetic diseases; Glycogen storage diseases; Lipids; Metabolic disorders; Metabolism; Mucopolysaccharidosis (MPS); Screening; Tay-Sachs disease.

FOR FURTHER INFORMATION:

Lichtman, Marshall A., et al., eds. *Williams Hematology.* 7th ed. New York: McGraw-Hill, 2006. Contains information on foam cells and Niemann-Pick disease. Includes illustrations, references, and an index.

National Institute of Neurological Disorders and Strokes. "Niemann-Pick Disease Information Page." http://www.ninds.nih.gov/disorders/niemann. A U.S. government Web site devoted to this disease.

National Niemann-Pick Disease Foundation. http://

www.nnpdf.org. A group that promotes advocacy, research, support, and awareness.

Parker, James, and Phillip Parker, eds. *Official Parent's Sourcebook on Niemann-Pick Disease: A Revised and Updated Directory for the Internet Age.* San Diego, Calif.: Icon Health, 2002. Useful in helping laypersons understand the scientific concepts associated with Niemann-Pick disease. Includes good references for research foundations and support groups.

Raddidadi, Ali A., and Abdulazix Al Twaim. "Type A-Niemann-Pick Disease." *Journal of European Academy of Dermatology and Veneriology* 14 (July, 2000): 301-303. A case study showing the disease course. Good illustrations and references.

NIGHTMARES
DISEASE/DISORDER

ANATOMY OR SYSTEM AFFECTED: Psychic-emotional system

SPECIALTIES AND RELATED FIELDS: Family medicine, pediatrics, psychiatry, psychology

DEFINITION: Anxiety-provoking, scary, unpleasant, and frightening dreams that disturb sleep, causing children to cry in their sleep or awake in an emotionally upset, typically anxious state.

KEY TERMS:

dream sleep: sleep during which dreaming occurs and rapid eye movements are produced

night terrors: episodes characterized by screaming and rapid awakening from deep sleep; sometimes confused with nightmares

rapid eye movement (REM) sleep: the stage of sleep in which dreaming occurs; in addition to rapid eye movements, which are easily visible through closed eyelids, it is characterized by facial and body movements, changes in heart and breathing rates, inhibition of certain (deep) reflexes, and increased blood flow to the brain

CAUSES AND SYMPTOMS

Nightmares have intrigued people for centuries, inspiring a range of explanations about what causes them. It is now known that they occur in all children shortly after the developmental stage of the "terrible two's," which overlaps but is not the same as the chronological age of two.

Two concurrent developments mark this period of growth. The first is intellectual and cognitive. Children develop the ability to conceptualize, process, and recall information in ways that they could not before and begin

---

INFORMATION ON NIGHTMARES

CAUSES: Unknown; related to developmental stages in children

SYMPTOMS: Disturbed sleep, anxiety

DURATION: Vary; children most affected between ages two and four; in adults, may be temporary or related to a chronic psychological disorder

TREATMENTS: Reassurance, possible counseling

---

reporting that they had dreams the previous night. These dreams usually involve things they wish for, playful fantasies, and daytime activities. The second development is emotional. At this stage, children are growing beyond the autonomy and individuation issues that characterize the infamous "terrible two's." They start involuntarily to experience strong aggressive feelings and desires to control, and they direct these emotions toward those with whom they have the most trouble in establishing their autonomy: parents and siblings. At the same time, children also experience anxiety from speculating about what would happen if their feelings were ever directly expressed. This intellectual and emotional combination gives rise to vividly intense nightmares, what children commonly refer to as "bad dreams."

In addition to aggressive impulses, nightmares may involve big dogs, snakes, insects, or other dangerous animals; monsters; giants; a "bad man"; or harm coming to them or someone in their family. During nightmares, children sense their own helplessness and vulnerability, which adds to the awful feelings experienced afterward. Children who dream that they are victorious over the threat—for example, they beat up the monster—usually report that they have had "good dreams" and are not frightened.

Nightmares affect boys and girls equally, although individually children experience, or recall the experience, with wide-ranging frequency. Some will have few nightmares throughout this preschool period; others will have many. Regardless of the baseline, all children will experience an increase in frequency during times of worsening stress. Both a marked increase in the frequency of nightmares and the experience of having a single frequently recurring nightmare have psychological significance and causes. Rapid awakening after any dream is associated with good recall, which is also true with nightmares.

Night terrors also begin around this time, although,

unlike nightmares, not all children experience them. They occur with regularity only between the ages of two and six. Night terrors are characterized by screaming and rapid awakening from deep sleep during the first third of the night, with vague or no recollection of the scary dream or image that presumably caused them. The child is terrified, hard to comfort, and difficult to awaken fully. Episodes last from ten to twenty minutes. It is often more upsetting for parents to witness a child thrashing and screaming than it is for the children who experience night terrors, as there is usually no recollection of the episodes the next morning.

Electroencephalogram (EEG) testing during night terrors shows the electrical activity in the brain as similar to that which occurs during small seizures, although night terrors are neither seizures nor caused by seizures and should not be treated as such. Usually, when night terrors occur, either the preceding day or the period right before bedtime has been particularly challenging or difficult. Night terrors may be a way in which children work off the psychological steam that they have built up as a result.

Treatment and Therapy

Nightmares are often problematic because parents are uncertain about what to do. Do they look under the bed or in the closet for the "bogeyman"? Do they keep the lights on all night? Do they let the child sleep with them after having a nightmare? Parents can help a child who has had a bad dream and who is afraid of monsters by looking under the bed or opening the closet together, while reassuring the child that they both know nothing is there.

All children experience imagined fears like monsters or spiders. These fears need to be taken seriously because they are real to the children having them. It is important that parents not scold or embarrass already frightened children or tell them that they should not feel the way they do. Parents should not discount or dismiss fears of imaginary and fantasized threats. Children need to feel that when their fantasies and worries get out of control, as in nightmares, someone can take charge and provide safety, security, and reassurance. Children must know that their worries and fears are important to their parents and caregivers.

When nightmare frequency begins to signal an underlying adjustment problem, nightmares should be thought of as an expression of intense anxiety caused by something or someone. In such cases, professional help in the form of a child therapist should be sought.

Night terrors, as disturbing as they can be, usually do not require professional intervention. In most cases, a calm, reassuring parent is all that a child needs to be comforted, to settle down, and to resume the sleep cycle. When the frequency of night terrors becomes problematic, parents should consult a sleep disorder specialist, whose professional discipline is usually medicine or psychology. In both disciplines, sleep disorders constitute a specialized area of clinical practice, and most physicians and psychologists are not trained to treat them.

—*Paul Moglia, Ph.D.*

See also Anxiety; Cognitive development; Developmental stages; Emotions: Biomedical causes and effects; Phobias; Psychiatry, child and adolescent; Sleep; Sleep disorders; Sleepwalking.

For Further Information:

Brazelton, T. Berry, and Joshua D. Sparrow. *Sleep: The Brazelton Way.* Cambridge, Mass.: Perseus, 2003. A thorough exploration of children's sleep troubles, including nightmares.

_____. *Touchpoints: Your Child's Emotional and Behavioral Development.* New York: Addison-Wesley, 1994. Brazelton is a knowledgeable physician with years of experience with thousands of children, and he brings that experience to bear on virtually every issue faced by families with kids, from birth through age six.

Caldwell, J. Paul. *Sleep: The Complete Guide to Sleep Disorders and a Better Night's Sleep.* Rev. ed. Toronto, Ont.: Firefly Books, 2003. A thorough examination of sleep disorders constitutes a good portion of this book, including such topics as what causes sleep apnea, sleep disorders in children and seniors, what drugs interfere and help with sleep, and treatment guidelines.

Cohen, George J., ed. *American Academy of Pediatrics Guide to Your Child's Sleep: Birth Through Adolescence.* New York: Villard Books, 1999. A compendium of advice on getting newborns, toddlers, and school-age children to sleep. Topics include preventing sudden infant death syndrome, getting your baby to sleep through the night, and solving sleep-wake problems such as night terrors.

Ferber, Richard. *Solve Your Child's Sleep Problems.* Rev. ed. New York: Simon & Schuster, 2006. Based on Ferber's research as the director of Boston's Center for Pediatric Sleep Disorders at Children's Hospital, this book is a practical, easy-to-understand guide to common sleeping problems for children ages one to six. Detailed case histories on night waking, difficulty sleeping, and more serious disorders such as sleep apnea and sleepwalking help illustrate a wide variety of problems and their solutions.

Nathanson, Laura Walther. *The Portable Pediatrician: A Practicing Pediatrician's Guide to Your Child's Growth, Development, Health, and Behavior from Birth to Age Five*. 2d ed. New York: HarperCollins, 2002. An engaging, easy-to-read guide for parents to assess their child's development, medical symptoms, and behavioral problems.

Spurr, Pam. *Understanding Your Child's Dreams*. New York: Sterling, 1999. Illuminating real-life case histories show just how much youthful dreams reveal, and a dictionary of common images will help the reader with interpretation. Includes extraordinary color drawings to help children visualize and focus on their dreams.

NONALCOHOLIC STEATOHEPATITIS (NASH)

DISEASE/DISORDER

ALSO KNOWN AS: Fatty liver, nonalcoholic fatty liver disease (NAFLD)

ANATOMY OR SYSTEM AFFECTED: Endocrine system, gastrointestinal system, liver

SPECIALTIES AND RELATED FIELDS: Endocrinology, family medicine, gastroenterology, internal medicine, pediatrics

DEFINITION: Fatty inflammation of the liver that is not caused by alcohol.

KEY TERMS:

central obesity: excessive abdominal fat

hyperlipidemia: an excess of fat or lipids in the blood

insulin resistance syndrome: a condition characterized by the decreased sensitivity to insulin that is associated with central obesity, metabolic syndrome, and diabetes

metabolic syndrome: a condition defined by the presence of three or more of high blood pressure, abdominal obesity, high triglycerides, low high-density lipoproteins (HDL) cholesterol, and abnormal fasting blood sugar

nonsteroidal anti-inflammatory drugs (NSAIDs): a class of medications for inflammation that do not contain steroids; includes aspirin and ibuprofen

CAUSES AND SYMPTOMS

The liver is a complex organ located in the right upper abdomen. It is responsible for converting carbohydrates, fats, and proteins from food into usable forms for the body. It also manufactures cholesterol, stores sugar, and metabolizes certain medications and chemicals. Nonalcoholic steatohepatitis (NASH) is characterized by the storage of excess fat in the liver with associated inflammation. The cause of this disorder is not completely understood. The accumulation of excess fat in the liver is related to the body's inability to use its own insulin, a common problem found in adults and children with central obesity. NASH is also found in individuals with other medical conditions, such as diabetes, metabolic syndrome, high blood pressure, and hyperlipidemia. Other causes of excess fat storage are certain medications, exposure to occupational toxins, and some surgical procedures. The excess fat causes damage to the cells of the liver that is similar to the damage caused by excess alcohol intake.

The majority of people with NASH have no symptoms, and the disorder is suspected from liver function tests. Studies have shown, however, that elevated liver enzymes do not always occur in individuals with NASH. If symptoms are present, then they may include fatigue or mild discomfort in the upper right side of the abdomen. The liver may be enlarged. Fatty liver may be identified on ultrasound, but a biopsy of the liver must be performed in order to determine the extent of the disorder. A liver biopsy is a minor surgical procedure that is performed by inserting a large needle into the liver through a small incision and removing cells for evaluation under the microscope. The disorder may range from inflammation of the liver to cirrhosis, a chronic, progressive disease with extensive scarring of the liver that causes destruction of liver cells. If the destruction advances, then the liver loses the ability to function. Severe liver disease occurs in approximately 20 percent of those with NASH.

TREATMENT AND THERAPY

Treatment goals include the identification and treatment of associated conditions and the reduction of insulin resistance. Adopting a healthy lifestyle is the primary treatment for NASH. Those who are overweight are encouraged to lose weight gradually and to exercise. Triglyceride and cholesterol levels should be kept within normal limits. Strict blood sugar control is indicated for diabetics with NASH. A small study of children with NASH found that daily vitamin E reduced abnormal liver enzymes. Another small study found that daily treatment for one year with a natural bile acid, ursodeoxycholic acid (Actigall or Urso), improved liver

function tests and seemed to have a protective effect on
the liver. Follow-up studies, however, did not show these
improvements. Two insulin-sensitizing drugs have had
mixed results in small studies. Liver inflammation was
significantly improved in one study, but both drug studies had subjects withdrawn as a result of liver toxicity.
Lipid-lowering drug studies have also shown some improvement in blood liver function tests, but not in the
follow-up biopsy tests for inflammation and damage.

It is generally recommended that individuals with
NASH avoid alcohol and certain medications, such
as acetaminophen and nonsteroidal anti-inflammatory
drugs (NSAIDs), that may further damage the liver. If
the individual develops severe cirrhosis, then a liver
transplant may be necessary to avoid death.

PERSPECTIVE AND PROSPECTS

In 1958, fatty liver disease was first identified in a small
group of obese individuals. It was not until the 1970's,
when surgeons were performing gastric bypass surgeries for the treatment of obesity, that the disorder was reported. In 1980, the term nonalcoholic steatohepatitis
was coined to describe a small group of patients at
Mayo Clinic who had liver biopsy findings similar to
those with alcoholic liver disease. Since 2000, pediatricians have reported the presence of NASH in obese
children, as well as in children with other endocrine
disorders. The increase in obesity and diabetes in the
United States has been linked to the increasing numbers of individuals diagnosed with NASH.

Diagnosis is confirmed with a liver biopsy, but controversy over this procedure exists, given the possible
risks and the lack of treatment options available for the
disorder. Recently, efforts to establish a noninvasive
method for diagnosis have been made. Ultrasound and
abdominal computed tomography (CT) scans are often

used but have not been able to distinguish the extent of
the disease process adequately. Newer X-ray techniques and more specific laboratory blood analyses are
being investigated as diagnostic methods.

Drug therapy continues to be investigated after
promising pilot studies. Further study is also needed in
the area of the disease process and its potential for progression in some individuals.

—*Amy Webb Bull, D.S.N., A.P.N.*

See also Abdomen; Abdominal disorders; Alcoholism; Cholesterol; Cirrhosis; Diabetes mellitus;
Gastroenterology; Gastroenterology, pediatric; Gastrointestinal disorders; Gastrointestinal system; Hypercholesterolemia; Hyperlipidemia; Inflammation;
Insulin resistance syndrome; Internal medicine; Liver;
Liver disorders; Liver transplantation; Metabolic syndrome; Metabolism; Obesity; Obesity, childhood;
Transplantation.

FOR FURTHER INFORMATION:

Adams, L. A., and P. Angulo. "Treatment of Non-
alcoholic Fatty Liver Disease." *Postgraduate Medi-
cine Journal*, 82 (May, 2006): 315-322.
Harrison, Stephen A., and Adrian M. Di Bisceglie.
"Advances in the Understanding and Treatment of
Nonalcoholic Fatty Liver Disease." *Drugs* 63, no. 22
(2003): 2379-2394.
"Liver Disease: Fat Inflames the Liver." *Harvard
Health Letter* 26 (February, 2001): 4.
Nakajima, Kenichirou, et al. "Pediatric Nonalcoholic
Steatohepatitis Associated with Hypopituitarism."
Journal of Gastroenterology 40, no. 3 (March,
2005): 312-315.
Porth, Carol M. "Disorders of Hepatobiliary and Exo-
crine Pancreas Function." In *Pathophysiology: Con-
cepts of Altered Health States*. 8th ed. Philadelphia:
Wolters Kluwer/Lippincott Williams & Wilkins,
2010.

NONINVASIVE TESTS

PROCEDURES

ANATOMY OR SYSTEM AFFECTED: All
SPECIALTIES AND RELATED FIELDS: Cardiology,
emergency medicine, nuclear medicine, obstetrics,
pathology, preventive medicine, radiology
DEFINITION: Diagnostic techniques that do not involve the collection of tissue or fluid samples or the
introduction of any instrument into the body; most
noninvasive tests involve imaging or the measurement of electrical activity.

KEY TERMS:

computed tomography (CT) scanning: a method of producing images of cross sections of the body

diagnosis: recognition of diseases based on physical examination, the microscopic and chemical results of laboratory findings, and an analysis of imaging results

Doppler shift: the increase in frequency of sound waves as the source of the waves approaches the observer or instrument; Doppler techniques are often used to assess blood flow in body channels such as veins

echocardiogram (EC): a graph of cardiac motion and heart valve closure produced by sending sound waves to the heart and recording their deflections

electrocardiogram (EKG or ECG): a diagnostic tool used to detect disturbances in the electrical activity of the heart

magnetic resonance imaging (MRI): a procedure using magnetic fields to determine blood vessel condition, fluid flow, and tissue contours and to detect abnormal masses

signal-averaged electrocardiogram (SAECG): a sophisticated EKG which detects subtle and potentially lethal cardiac conduction defects

sonography: the use of sound waves deflected from internal body organs to find growing masses (including fetuses) and abnormal lesions; also called ultrasound

X radiology: the use of ionizing radiation of short wavelength to detect abnormalities in primarily dense portions of the body

INDICATIONS AND PROCEDURES

Noninvasive tests are used in the initial diagnosis of a disease or abnormality and for the monitoring of certain conditions and body processes. Most such tests involve imaging techniques. Primary among them are X radiology, computed tomography (CT) scanning, magnetic resonance imaging (MRI), electrocardiography (EKG or ECG), and ultrasound.

Diagnostic X-ray examinations are often the first step in complex technological solutions to medical diagnoses and health problems. New uses for diagnostic X rays are constantly being devised. It is common practice for hospitals to require chest X rays for all outpatients visiting X-ray departments, and hospital inpatients are usually given chest X rays before admission or surgery.

Computed tomography (CT) scanning, also known as computed axial tomography (CAT) scanning, uses a computer to interpret multiple X-ray images in order to reconstruct a cross-sectional image of any area of the body. The inventors of the procedure for CT scanning were awarded a Nobel Prize in 1979.

After the patient is placed in the CT scanner, an X-ray source rapidly rotates around it, taking hundreds of pictures. The pictures are electronically recorded and stored by a computer. The computer then integrates the data into cross-sectional "slices." The CT scanner can assess the composition of internal structures, which it is able to discriminate from fat, fluid, and gas. The scanner can show the shape and size of various organs and lesions and has the capability of detecting abnormal lesions as small as 1 or 2 millimeters in diameter.

Magnetic resonance imaging (MRI), unlike CT scanning (which uses X rays), uses magnetic fields passing through the body to detect details of anatomy and physiology.

MRI equipment consists of a tunnel-like magnet that creates a magnetic field around the patient. This magnetic field causes the hydrogen atoms found in the body—water has two hydrogen atoms and one oxygen atom in the molecule—to line up. At the same time, a radio frequency signal is quickly transmitted to upset the uniformity of the formation. When the radio frequency signal is turned off, the hydrogen atoms return to their proper lineup, and a small current is generated. By detecting the speed and volume with which the atoms return, the computer can display a diagnostic image on a monitor.

MRI is noninvasive, and no pain or radiation is involved. The procedure takes from fifteen to forty-five minutes, depending on the number of views needed. Diagnostic X rays rely on variations of density on film, and areas of soft tissue, for example, produce little or no shadow and are difficult to distinguish in any detail. MRI images, on the other hand, allow tumors, muscles, arteries, and vertebrae to be seen with great clarity.

Monitoring and providing electrical support to the heart constitute other useful noninvasive techniques. A healthy heart generates electrical impulses rhythmically and spontaneously; this activity is controlled by the sinoatrial (S-A) node, the heart's natural pacemaker. From there, the impulses pass through specialized conduction tissues in the atria and into the atrioventricular (A-V) node. Then the electrical impulses enter the ventricular conduction system, the bundle of His, and the right and left bundle branches. From the bundle branches, the impulses spread into the ventricles through the network of Purkinje fibers. The spread of electrical stimulation through the atria and the ventricles is known as depolarization. The standard electrocardiogram (ECG or EKG) records this activity from twelve different angles. The EKG records the heart's electrical activity and provides vital information concerning its rate, rhythm, and conduction system status. Detecting changes in the EKG can help to diagnose ventricular conduction problems and ventricular hypertrophy.

The signal-averaged electrocardiogram (SAECG) is another noninvasive procedure that is a promising diagnostic tool for many cardiac patients. Unlike the standard twelve-lead EKG, the SAECG can detect conduction abnormalities that often precede sustained ventricular tachycardia—which is second only to myocardial infarction (heart attack) as the leading cause of sudden death. The SAECG records the heart's electrical activity via six electrodes applied to the frontal and posterior chest walls. The SAECG can often pick up repolarization delays that occur when ischemic (damaged) tissue impedes the passage of electrical impulses through a portion of the myocardium, a condition that can lead to ventricular tachycardia.

A valuable weapon in the battle against sudden cardiac death is the temporary pacemaker, that provides support for the heart's electrical conduction system. Four types of temporary devices are available to manage cardiac arrhythmias. One of these is a noninvasive temporary pacemaker, known as Zoll NTP, a transcutaneous pacemaker that can provide vital support when there is no time to prepare for an invasive procedure. Such pacemakers are also used when invasive procedures are contraindicated.

Another method for diagnosing heart problems is echocardiography, a technique for recording echoes of ultrasonic waves when these waves are directed at areas of the heart. The principle is similar to that used in the sonar detection of submarines and other underwater objects. In this very simple and painless procedure, the patient lies on a table while a small, high-frequency generator (transducer) is moved across the chest. The instrument projects ultrasonic waves and receives the returning echoes. As the waves pass through the heart, their behavior differs, depending on whether there is any calcification present, whether there is a blood clot or any other mass in the cavity of the heart, whether certain heart chambers are enlarged, whether the valves within the heart open and close in the proper fashion, and whether any part of the heart is thicker than it should be.

Sonography, or ultrasound, imaging and the images produced are unique: Patients can hear their blood flowing through the carotid arteries of the neck, and physicians can see a brain tumor or watch a human fetus suck its thumb. This simple and inexpensive imaging technique has aided in the development of fetal medicine as a subspecialty. Sonography uses sound waves to look within the body by using a piezoelectric crystal to convert electric pulses into vibrations that penetrate the body. These sound waves are reflected back to the crystal, which reconverts them into electric signals. Many doctors foresee much growth in the use of ultrasound as a noninvasive procedure.

USES AND COMPLICATIONS

Historically, diagnostic X rays have been used for the detection of metal objects, cavities in teeth, and broken bones. Films of various parts of the body, such as the abdomen, skull, and chest, have been taken ever since X rays were first discovered in the late nineteenth century. Dentists and orthodontists use X rays to check for jaw fractures, tooth misalignment, gum disease, tartar deposits, impacted teeth, and bone cancer. Chronic illnesses that can be detected by X rays include arthritis, tuberculosis, osteoporosis, emphysema, ulcers, pneumonia, and urinary tract infections.

The CT scanner uses a series of narrow, pencil-like X-ray beams to scan the section of the body under investigation. CT scans allow the rapid diagnosis of brain abnormalities, cysts, tumors, and blood clots. Newly developed body scanners assist in the early detection of cancers and other diseases of the internal organs.

Magnetic resonance imaging has undergone an explosive growth in applications. In 1982, there were only six machines in operation. Hospitals often used a portable MRI device, which can be driven from place to place with a tractor-trailer truck. As the cost for MRI machines decreases, however, more hospitals are purchasing this equipment instead of sharing it.

The MRI machine is able to differentiate the brain's gray matter (nerve cells) from the brain's white matter (nerve fibers). Gray matter contains 87 percent water, and white matter contains 72 percent water. Thus, since MRI detects the protons in the hydrogen in water, a great difference in contrast between the two types of brain material is seen on the resulting scan. MRI is also useful in detecting and monitoring the progression of multiple sclerosis because the fatty tissue that normally exists around nerve fibers deteriorates, and these abnormal, fat-free areas can be clearly imaged.

MRI research seeks ways of analyzing the numerous chemical elements found in the body and aids in the study, diagnosis, treatment, and cure of a host of human diseases.

EKGs are useful in the detection of irregularities in the heart's electrical conduction system. This technology can also help in the diagnosis of ventricular hypertrophy, pulmonary emboli, and intraventricular conduction problems.

Echocardiograms, based on sound waves, are used to detect infarcts (areas of necrosis, or tissue death), valve closure between heart chambers, and abnormal thickening of myocardial muscle. Sonography is perhaps best known for its contribution to diagnostic medicine in the study of human fetal development. Determining the age of a developing embryo is now standard procedure, and clear images can be obtained at five weeks of gestation, when the embryo is only 5 millimeters long. Fetal weight can be determined by volume, and fetal anatomy can also be studied. Congenital heart defects can be spotted very early, and neural brain defects can be discovered as well.

The great advantage of ultrasound is that it emits no ionizing radiation and thus can be used on pregnant women without danger to the fetus. Ultrasound can detect gallstones, kidney stones, and tumors and can monitor blood flow. Its applications have grown exponentially since its discovery.

The American Cancer Society estimates that one in every four people in the United States will develop cancer at some point in his or her life. These statistics suggest the enormous problem that cancer presents to American society. Cancer detection, as early as possible, can be of primary importance because aggressive treatment can be initiated to deter further progression of the disease. The roles of X rays, MRI, and CT scanning in determining the source and extent of the malignancy are vital in the treatment of cancer.

Mammography is a subset of X-ray imaging which is useful in detecting breast cancer. The equipment used in mammography is designed to image breast tissue, which is usually soft and of uniform density. Very small changes in density can be identified in fine detail, including small areas of calcification. Radiation doses must also be kept to a minimum. The film interpretation of mammograms is difficult, but early detection of breast cancer is often possible.

In the United States, the Public Health Service, in a memo dated June 1, 1993, delegated authority for implementing the Mammography Quality Standards Act (MQSA) of 1992 to the Food and Drug Administration (FDA). The MQSA is intended to ensure that mammography is reliable and safe. The act makes it unlawful for any facility to provide services unless it is accredited by an approved private nonprofit or state body and it has received federal certification indicating that it meets standards for quality. Each facility must also pass an annual inspection conducted by approved federal personnel. The law was enacted in response to the need for safe, early detection of breast cancer. Mammography is the most effective technique for early detection of this type of cancer.

Given a choice, most persons would prefer a noninvasive diagnostic tool. The earliest used diagnostic tool was the X ray. X rays were discovered in 1895 by a German professor named Wilhelm Conrad Röntgen. The first X rays were produced in a Crookes tube, a pear-shaped, glass tube in which two electrodes, the cathode (negative electrode) and anode (positive electrode), were placed at right angles to each other. The tube was then evacuated of gas. In Röntgen's first experiment, the cathode was "excited" with an electrical current, producing a beam of cathode rays, or electrons. These electrons were directed across the tube from the cathode and struck the glass, causing it to glow and, at the same time, producing X rays, which excited a fluorescent screen. In a modern X-ray tube, the cathode ray strikes a target in the anode rather than the glass. Modern equipment also uses high-energy electricity in order to energize the tube at the high voltages necessary for producing X rays.

Radiology has come far. From a medical discipline with a limited but vital function (that of aiding diagnosis), it has become interventional. It is a field that has moved into therapy—repairing a growing variety of abnormalities, averting surgery, and sometimes achieving results beyond the reach of surgery.

In addition to the simple X ray, physicians now have more powerful diagnostic devices: MRI, CT scanning, and sonography. Cardiac conditions and abnormalities are quite easily analyzed via the ECG or echocardiogram. Where once the diagnosis of gallstones required a two-day X-ray test and 12 grams of diarrhea-causing pills, now ultrasound allows a diagnosis to be made painlessly and noninvasively, in ten to fifteen minutes.

The computer has been the core in the revolution in imaging. As more information becomes available and the density of information grows exponentially, larger and faster computers have been developed to assimilate this information. Computer visualization both interprets data and generates images from data in order to provide new insight into disease states through visual methods. Visualization and computation promise to play a key role in diagnostic medicine.

—Jane A. Slezak, Ph.D.

See also Computed tomography (CT) scanning; Diagnosis; Echocardiography; Electrocardiography (ECG or EKG); Electroencephalography (EEG); Imaging and radiology; Magnetic resonance imaging (MRI); Mammography; Neuroimaging; Physical examination; Prognosis; Radiation therapy; Screening; Single photon emission computed tomography (SPECT); Ultrasonography; Urinalysis.

FOR FURTHER INFORMATION:

Chopra, Sanjiv. *The Liver Book: A Comprehensive Guide to Diagnosis, Treatment, and Recovery.* New York: Simon & Schuster, 2002. Although expressly about the liver, covers the tests used to diagnose liver ailments and what to expect from tests and screening.

Crawford, Michael, ed. *Current Diagnosis and Treatment—Cardiology.* 3d ed. New York: McGraw-Hill Medical, 2009. Discusses advances in cardiac diagnostics, treatments, and prognostic indicators.

Galton, Lawrence. *Med Tech.* New York: Harper & Row, 1985. A book for laypeople which explains, in simple terms, advanced therapies and techniques used in medicine. Elucidates the controversies, dangers, and costs of treatment and answers specific questions regarding medical research.

Griffith, H. Winter. *Complete Guide to Symptoms, Illness, and Surgery.* Revised and updated by Stephen Moore and Kenneth Yoder. 5th ed. New York: Perigee, 2006. Covers more than five hundred diseases and disorders and their diagnostic tests.

Merva, Jean. "SAECG: A Closer Look at the Heart." *RN* 56 (May, 1993): 51-53. Describes the use of signal-averaged EKGs.

Pagana, Kathleen Deska, and Timothy J. Pagana. *Mosby's Diagnostic and Laboratory Test Reference.* 9th ed. St. Louis, Mo.: Mosby/Elsevier, 2009. A clinical handbook that gives alphabetically organized laboratory and diagnostic tests for easy reference. Each listing includes such things as alternate or abbreviated test names, type of test, normal findings, possible critical values, test explanation and related physiology, and potential complications.

Sochurek, Howard. *Medicine's New Vision.* Easton, Pa.: Mack, 1988. The many forms of radiology are described, with illustrative images of several diagnostic modalities including MRI, CT scanning, ultrasound, and radiation therapy.

Solomon, Jacqueline. "Take the EKG One Step Further." *RN* 55 (May, 1992): 56-60. Discusses the diagnostic use of EKGs.

Wolbarst, Anthony Brinton. *Looking Within: How X-Ray, CT, MRI, Ultrasound, and Other Medical Images Are Created.* Berkeley: University of California Press, 1999. Modern medical imaging has changed perceptions of the overall workings of the human body. The author explains how imaging tools work and what noninvasive imaging procedures do to and for the patient.

NOROVIRUSES

DISEASE/DISORDER

ALSO KNOWN AS: Norwalk-like viruses

ANATOMY OR SYSTEM AFFECTED: Gastrointestinal system, immune system

SPECIALTIES AND RELATED FIELDS: Gastroenterology, immunology, virology

DEFINITION: A family of viruses that cause acute gastroenteritis.

KEY TERMS:

gastroenteritis: an inflammation of the stomach and large intestines

Norwalk virus: a virus named for a 1968 outbreak of acute gastroenteritis in Norwalk, Ohio; it is the prototype strain for a group of single-stranded ribonucleic acid (RNA) viruses now called noroviruses

CAUSES AND SYMPTOMS

Noroviruses, also known as Norwalk-like viruses (NLV), are members of the family Caliciviridae and are the leading cause of nonbacterial acute gastroenteritis outbreaks in the United States. Noroviruses are suspected of causing twenty-three million cases of acute gastroenteritis annually. Often, norovirus-caused gastroenteritis is thought to be "stomach flu," but it is not related to influenza, a respiratory illness caused by the influenza virus. Norovirus infection is also commonly referred to as "food poisoning," although there are other numerous causes of food poisoning. Noroviruses are not related to bacteria or parasites that can cause gastroenteritis.

The illness associated with a norovirus infection lasts twelve to sixty hours and is characterized by a sudden onset of nausea, vomiting, abdominal cramps, and wa-

INFORMATION ON NOROVIRUSES

CAUSES: Viral infection transmitted through contaminated food or water, fecal-hand-oral contamination, direct person-to-person contact, or direct contact with contaminated surface

SYMPTOMS: Sudden onset of nausea, vomiting, abdominal cramps, and watery diarrhea; may also include headache, fever, chills, and muscle pain

DURATION: Twelve to sixty hours

TREATMENTS: None; prevention through food safety measures (proper handing) and good hygiene (frequent hand-washing, germicides)

tery diarrhea. Vomiting is more prevalent among children, whereas adults tend to experience diarrhea. Additional symptoms, including headache, fever, chills, and myalgia (muscle pain), are also reported. Although NLV causes a self-limited acute gastroenteritis, the elderly, children, and those with severe underlying medical conditions are at increased risk for complications as a result of volume depletion, dehydration, and electrolyte disturbances. Although rare, severe dehydration caused by NLV gastroenteritis can be fatal. Hospitalization of otherwise healthy adults infected with NLV is rare.

The incubation period after exposure to a norovirus is twelve to forty-eight hours. The virus is transmitted by a fecal-hand-oral contamination route, directly from person to person, through contaminated food or water, or by direct contact with a contaminated surface. One of the main transmission sources is the diapers of infants with diarrhea. Aerosolized vomit has also been implicated as a transmission mode. Noroviruses are very contagious and can spread rapidly throughout closely populated environments: Schools, hospitals, restaurants, amusement parks, fairgrounds, summer camps, and cruise ships are especially susceptible to mass infections. However, any place that food or drink is served, including the home environment, is susceptible to NLV infection. Because of high rates of infection and the persistence of noroviruses in the environment, transmission is difficult to control through routine sanitary procedures. People infected with NLV are contagious from the moment that they begin feeling symptoms to at least three days after recovery. In some cases, infected individuals have been contagious two weeks after recovery.

Most people infected with noroviruses recover in twenty-four to forty-eight hours, with no long-term health effects related to their infection. No evidence suggests that infected persons can become long-term carriers of the virus, but it is essential for those recovering from an infection to use good hand-washing and other hygienic practices.

TREATMENT AND THERAPY

Outbreaks of norovirus gastroenteritis can occur in multiple settings. Between January, 1996, and November, 2000, a total of 39 percent occurred in restaurants or at catered events; 29 percent in nursing homes, residential institutions, and hospitals; 12 percent in schools and day care centers; 10 percent in vacation settings, including camps and cruise ships; and the rest in other settings. While person-to-person spread extends NLV outbreaks, the initial event is often the contamination of a common source such as food or water. As a result, efforts to prevent an initial contamination and subsequent transmission help to prevent the occurrence and spread of norovirus gastroenteritis outbreaks.

Food contamination by food handlers is the most frequent transmission agent. Any food item has the potential to be infected with norovirus through fecal contamination, and certain foods show a higher concentration of infections. Shellfish tend to concentrate NLVs in their tissues if they live in contaminated waters, in which fecal waste is either dumped overboard from ships or released from shoreline sewage systems. Ready-to-eat foods that require handling but no subsequent cooking pose a risk. Noroviruses are relatively resistant to environmental change and can survive temperatures as high as 60 degrees Celsius and can survive in up to 10 parts per million of chlorine, well in excess of levels in public water systems. NLV infection can occur as a result of the ingestion of contaminated water, including municipal water, well water, stream water, commercial ice, lake water, and swimming pools.

Noroviruses can be spread person-to-person by direct fecal-oral contact and airborne transmission. This is the most effective way that the virus spreads in populations in close proximity, such as people in nursing homes and on cruise ships. The most effective means of stopping the transmission of NLV is by frequent hand-washing with soap and hot water. It is recommended that all surfaces be lathered with soap vigorously for ten seconds, then rinsed thoroughly under moving water. A mask should be worn by anyone cleaning areas contaminated with feces or vomitus. Soiled linen and clothes should be handled carefully, with a minimum of agitation.

Soiled surfaces should be cleaned with a germicidal product containing at least 10 percent bleach.

Neither a specific antiviral treatment nor a vaccine has been developed for noroviruses. NLV infection cannot be treated with antibiotics because it is not caused by bacteria. Because there are many different strains of norovirus, developing an individual long-lasting immunity is difficult. As a result, NLV infections can recur throughout a person's lifetime. As a result of genetic factors, some people are more likely than others to be infected and to develop severe symptoms.

—*Randall L. Milstein, Ph.D.*

See also Childhood infectious diseases; Common cold; Diarrhea and dysentery; Epidemics and pandemics; Epidemiology; Fever; Food poisoning; Gastroenteritis; Gastroenterology; Gastroenterology, pediatric; Gastrointestinal disorders; Influenza; Nausea and vomiting; Rotavirus; Viral infections.

FOR FURTHER INFORMATION:

Centers for Disease Control and Prevention. "Outbreaks of Gastroenteritis Associated with Noroviruses on Cruise Ships—United States, 2002." *Morbidity and Mortality Weekly Report* 51 (2002): 1112-1115.

Dolan, Raphael. "Noroviruses—Challenges to Control." *New England Journal of Medicine* 357 (2007): 1072-1073.

Fankhauser, R. L., S. S. Monroe, J. S. Noel, et al. "Epidemiologic and Molecular Trends of 'Norwalk-Like Viruses' Associated with Outbreaks of Gastroenteritis in the United States." *Journal of Infectious Disease*, no. 186 (2002): 1-7.

Meyers, H. "Norwalk Virus, Noroviruses, and Viral Gastroenteritis." *Public Health Bulletin, County of Orange Health Care Agency* 52, no. 2 (2003): 1-8.

Umesh, D. P., E. S. Wuiroz, A. W. Mounts, et al. "Norwalk-Like Viruses: Public Health Consequences and Outbreak Management." *Morbidity and Mortality Weekly Report* 50, no. RR-9 (2001): 1-13.

NOSEBLEEDS

DISEASE/DISORDER

ALSO KNOWN AS: Epistaxis

ANATOMY OR SYSTEM AFFECTED: Blood, blood vessels, circulatory system, nose, throat

SPECIALTIES AND RELATED FIELDS: Emergency medicine, family medicine, general surgery, hematology, internal medicine, otorhinolaryngology, pediatrics

DEFINITION: Bleeding from the nose.

KEY TERMS:

mucosa: the moist membrane covering the internal nose, mouth, sinuses, respiratory tract, gastrointestinal tract, and other sites in the body

nasal polyp: a small growth, usually benign, on the nasal mucosa

nasal septum: the midline wall inside the front of the nose that separates the nostrils

CAUSES AND SYMPTOMS

The nose is a highly vascular area and is therefore a common site of bleeding. Most nosebleeds are benign. They may result from local causes that affect the mucosa of the nose directly. They can also result from systemic causes, which affect the body as a whole.

The major cause of nosebleeds is irritation of the nasal mucosa. Simple trauma from nose picking is the most common in children. Chronic irritation can be associated with allergies, a dry environment or changes in the weather, smoking or the inhalation of smoke, or the inhalation of caustic substances, such as cocaine. Sneezing as a result of recurrent colds or infections of the nose and throat can be associated with nosebleeds. The use of medications such as decongestants, antihistamines, and allergy/cold nasal sprays may also result in nosebleeds because of local irritation.

Trauma to the nose may result from blunt injury, such as associated with sports or other accidents. Occasionally, children may place small objects high in the nose; these objects may go undetected for periods of time before eventually causing infection and bleeding. Rarely, bleeding may be caused by structural problems, such as nasal polyps, malignant growths, or deviation of the midline nasal septum.

Systemic causes of nosebleeds include underlying bleeding disorders, fevers, bacterial or viral infections,

---

INFORMATION ON NOSEBLEEDS

CAUSES: Injury, exposure to dry air or environmental toxins, disease (e.g., leukemia), allergies, certain medications, anatomical problems (e.g., polyps), infection, high blood pressure

SYMPTOMS: Bleeding from nose

DURATION: Typically acute; chronic when related to disease

TREATMENTS: Sitting upright with gentle pressure to nose; moisturizing agents; nasal packing

high blood pressure, cancer, and liver or kidney problems. Bleeding disorders should be considered in cases where the bleeding is recurrent and/or prolonged or if there is a significant family history of bleeding problems. Medications such as aspirin, ibuprofen (or other anti-inflammatory agents), anticoagulants, or steroids may produce a transient or short-lived coagulation defect that may cause nosebleeds.

TREATMENT AND THERAPY

Most nosebleeds can be stopped by sitting upright (or by holding a young child on one's lap) and gently squeezing the front or anterior of the nose closed for five to ten minutes. It is important to seek medical attention if the bleeding does not stop or if there is continued bleeding or oozing of blood. Occasionally, nasal packing (placement of gauze inside the nose) or other procedures may be required to control severe bleeding. People with coagulation problems need special consideration and require specific medical treatment.

Efforts to keep the nasal mucosa from becoming too dry may be helpful in preventing recurrent nosebleeds. Applying petroleum jelly or other moisturizing agents inside the nose or using a humidifier in the home to keep the air moist may also be helpful.

Most nosebleeds are not life-threatening, but they can be very frightening for patients, especially children and their parents or caregivers. When caring for a child who is bleeding, it is important to remain calm to help decrease the child's anxiety and to assess and begin to treat the bleeding.

—*Frank E. Shafer, M.D.*

See also Allergies; Bleeding; Blood and blood disorders; Common cold; Nasopharyngeal disorders; Otorhinolaryngology; Respiration; Sneezing.

FOR FURTHER INFORMATION:

Ferrari, Mario. *PDxMD Ear, Nose, and Throat Disorders.* Philadelphia: PDxMD, 2003.

Kimball, Chad T. *Childhood Diseases and Disorders Sourcebook: Basic Consumer Health Information About Medical Problems Often Encountered in Preadolescent Children.* Detroit, Mich.: Omnigraphics, 2003.

_____. *Colds, Flu, and Other Common Ailments Sourcebook.* Detroit, Mich.: Omnigraphics, 2001.

Lichtman, Marshall A., et al., eds. *Williams Hematology.* 7th ed. New York: McGraw-Hill, 2006.

Litin, Scott C., ed. *Mayo Clinic Family Health Book.* 4th ed. New York: HarperResource, 2009.

Ratnoff, Oscar D., and Charles D. Forbes, eds. *Disorders of Hemostasis.* 3d ed. Philadelphia: W. B. Saunders, 1996.

Rodak, Bernadette, ed. *Hematology: Clinical Principles and Applications.* 3d ed. St. Louis, Mo.: Saunders/Elsevier, 2007.

Thompson, Arthur R., and Laurence A. Harker. *Manual of Hemostasis and Thrombosis.* 3d ed. Philadelphia: F. A. Davis, 1983.

Woolf, Alan D., et al., eds. *The Children's Hospital Guide to Your Child's Health and Development.* Cambridge, Mass.: Perseus, 2002.

NUCLEAR MEDICINE

SPECIALTY

ANATOMY OR SYSTEM AFFECTED: Bones, gallbladder, glands, kidneys, musculoskeletal system

SPECIALTIES AND RELATED FIELDS: Cardiology, endocrinology, internal medicine, radiology

DEFINITION: The field of medicine that employs radioactivity for both diagnostic and therapeutic purposes; the former involves imaging techniques, while the latter uses large amounts of radioactive material to destroy cells.

KEY TERMS:

cathode-ray tube: a display device used for the presentation of nuclear medicine data; it displays images in real time

collimator: a device used for restricting and directing gamma rays by passing them through a grid made of metal, which absorbs the rays

gamma radiation: electromagnetic radiation of a short wavelength that is emitted by the nucleus of a radionuclide during radioactive decay

half-life: a unique characteristic of a radionuclide defined by the time during which its initial activity is reduced to one-half; this period varies among radionucleotides from less than one-millionth of a second to millions of years

pharmacological stress testing: a procedure wherein a pharmacological agent is administered to a patient to increase blood flow to the heart, thereby enabling coronary artery disease, if present, to manifest itself

radionuclide: a species of atom (of natural or artificial origin) that exhibits radioactivity

radiopharmaceutical: a sterile, radioactively tagged compound that is administered to a patient for diagnostic or therapeutic purposes

scintillation: the production of flashes emitted by luminescent substances when excited by high-energy radiation

tomography: the term that describes all types of body-section imaging techniques, in which a visual representation is restricted to a specified section or "cut" of tissue within an organ

tracer: a radioactive substance introduced into the body, the progress of which may be followed by means of an external radioactivity detector; it must not affect the process that it is used to measure

SCIENCE AND PROFESSION

Nuclear medicine is the branch of medicine that uses radioactive substances in the diagnosis and treatment of diseases. A discussion of such technology requires an understanding of the nature of radioactivity and the tools employed by specialists in this medical field.

Radioactivity is the spontaneous emission of particles from the nucleus of an atom. Several kinds of emissions are possible. Gamma-ray emission is the type with which nuclear medicine imaging is concerned. The activity of radionuclides is measured in terms of the number of atoms disintegrating per unit time. The basic unit of measurement is the curie. Radiopharmaceuticals that are administered are in the microcurie or millicurie range of activity. Most radionuclides used in nuclear medicine are produced from accelerators, reactors, or generators. Accelerators are devices that accelerate charged particles (ions) to bombard a target. Cyclotron-produced radionuclides that are used frequently in nuclear medicine include gallium 67, thallium 201, and indium 111. The core of a nuclear reactor consists of material undergoing nuclear fission. Nuclides of interest in nuclear medicine that are formed from reactors include molybdenum 99, iodine 131, and xenon 133.

In generator systems, a "parent" isotope decays spontaneously to a "daughter" isotope in which the half-life of the parent is longer than that of the daughter. The parent is used to generate a continuous supply of the relatively short-lived daughter radionuclides and is therefore called a generator. The most commonly used generator system is molybdenum 99 (with a half-life of sixty-seven hours) and technetium 99m (with a half-life of six hours). The daughter, technetium 99m, is the most widely used radioisotope in nuclear medicine. It is obtained from the generator in a physiologic sodium chloride solution as the pertechnetate ion. It can be used alone to image the thyroid, salivary glands, or gastric mucosa, or it can be labeled to a wide variety of complexes that are picked up physiologically by various organ systems.

The scintillation camera, or Anger camera (named for its inventor, Hal O. Anger), is the most commonly used static imaging device in nuclear medicine. The scintillation camera produces a picture on a cathode-ray tube of the distribution of an administered radionuclide within the target organ of a patient. It uses the gamma rays emitted by the nuclide and a collimator to create the image as a series of light flashes on a disk-shaped sodium iodide crystal. The system determines the location of each scintillation and then produces a finely focused dot of light on the face of the cathode-ray tube in a corresponding position. The complete picture is then produced on photographic film. The camera normally contains two parts, the head and the computer console. The head serves as the gamma-ray detector. It absorbs incoming gamma rays and generates electrical signals that correspond to the positions where the absorptions took place. These signals are sent to a computer to be processed and to produce a picture that can be displayed on film or stored on disk for video display.

The collimator normally consists of a large piece of lead with many small holes in it. There are many types of collimators. The most commonly used are parallel-hole types. The holes are of equal, constant cross section, and their axes form a set of closely spaced, vertical, parallel lines. The materials between the holes are called septa.

Putting this all together, the radioisotope, once injected or ingested, travels to the target organ. Gamma rays from the target organ are emitted in all directions. The collimator allows only those gamma rays traveling in a direction essentially parallel to the axis of its holes to pass through to the crystal. The crystal is made of sodium iodide, with a small amount of thallium impurity. The thallium is transparent and emits light photons whenever it absorbs a gamma ray. This action by the collimator causes the light flashes in the crystal to form an image of the nuclide distribution located below it. This image will preserve gray-scale information, since the number of gamma rays received by any given region of the crystal will be directly proportional to the amount of nuclide located directly below that region.

Single photon emission computed tomography (SPECT) is a tomographic imaging technique employing scintillation cameras to display the information at a given depth in sharp focus, while blurring information above and below that depth. There are two distinct methods of SPECT, each based on the type of images produced. The first, longitudinal section tomography, provides images of planes parallel to the long axis of the body. The second method, transverse section tomography, is perpendicular to the long axis of the body. Transverse section tomography with a rotating gamma camera has received wide clinical acceptance, partly because of the information that it provides and its multiple-use capability, since these systems can perform routine planar imaging as well as SPECT imaging. In this system, the gamma camera is a device mounted to a gantry and capable of rotating 360 degrees around the patient. These systems must be interfaced with a computer. The orbit around the patient is circular, and from 32 to 180 equiangular images are acquired over a 360-degree arc. Image acquisition is by computer. The images are stored digitally, and image reconstruction is achieved by filtering each projection, with geometric correction for photon attenuation. Noise reduction is generally accomplished by the application of filters. The efficiency of rotating systems can be improved by incorporating additional detectors (most often two or three), which rotate around the patient. Virtually any organ in the body for which an appropriate radiopharmaceutical exists can be studied with SPECT techniques.

No overview of nuclear medicine would be complete without a brief description of positron emission tomography (PET) scanning. Positron-emitting radionuclides, such as carbon 11, nitrogen 13, oxygen 15, and fluorine 8 (a bioisosteric substitution for hydrogen), are isotopes of elements that occur naturally in organic compounds. These tracers enter into the biochemical processes in the body so that blood flow; oxygen, glucose, and free fatty acid metabolism; amino acid transport; pH; and neuroreceptor densities can be measured. A positron is an antimatter electron. This positron-emitting radiopharmaceutical is distributed in a patient's system. As a positron is emitted, it travels several millimeters in tissue until it meets a free electron and annihilation occurs. Two gamma rays appear and are emitted 180 degrees apart from each other. A scintillation camera could be used to detect these gamma rays, but a collimator is not needed. Instead, the patient is surrounded by a ring of detectors. By electronically coupling opposing detectors to identify the pair of gamma rays simultaneously, the location where the annihilation event must have occurred (the coincidence) can be determined. The raw PET scan consists of a number of coincidence lines. Reconstruction could simply be the drawing of these lines as they would cross and superimpose wherever there is activity in the patient. In practice, the data set is reorganized into projections.

DIAGNOSTIC AND TREATMENT TECHNIQUES

Nuclear medicine is widely used in the diagnosis and prognosis of coronary artery disease, especially in conjunction with either physical stress testing (treadmill or bicycle exercise) or pharmacological stress testing. The patient is instructed to exercise on the treadmill until his or her heart rate has significantly increased. At peak exercise, a radioisotope, usually thallium 201 or technetium 99m, is injected into a vein. Stress images are obtained. Because the injected tracer corresponds to the blood flow through the arteries that supply oxygen to the heart muscle, those vessels that have a blockage exhibit decreased flow, or decreased tracer delivered to that area of the heart. Rest images are also obtained. Rest and stress images are compared, and differences in the intensity of the tracer, analyzed by a computer, help to identify blocked arteries and the extent of the blockage. This technique is also used in follow-up of patients who have undergone bypass surgery or angioplasty to determine if blockage has recurred.

Nuclear cardiology is also used to measure the ejection fraction (the amount of blood ejected by the left ventricle to all parts of the body) and motion of the heart. Patients with cardiomyopathy, coronary artery disease, or congenital heart disease often have decreased function of the heart. Certain medications used in cancer therapy can also damage the heart muscle. These patients are followed closely to determine if they are developing toxicity from their drug therapy. In these studies, commonly called MUGA scans, a small portion of the patient's blood is extracted. A radioactive tracer is tagged to this blood, which is then reinjected. The gamma camera takes motion pictures of the beating heart and, through the aid of computers, calculates the ejection fraction.

Nuclear medicine can be very helpful in locating primary or metastatic tumors throughout the body, and it is unique in its ability to assess the viability of a known lesion and its response to radiation or chemotherapy. Breast cancer, lymphomas (especially low-grade), differentiated thyroid cancer, and most sarcomas (both bone and soft tissue) are tumors that will metabolize the appropriate injected radiopharmaceutical. The resulting images will show increased localization in an active tumor but none in those masses that have been destroyed by treatment.

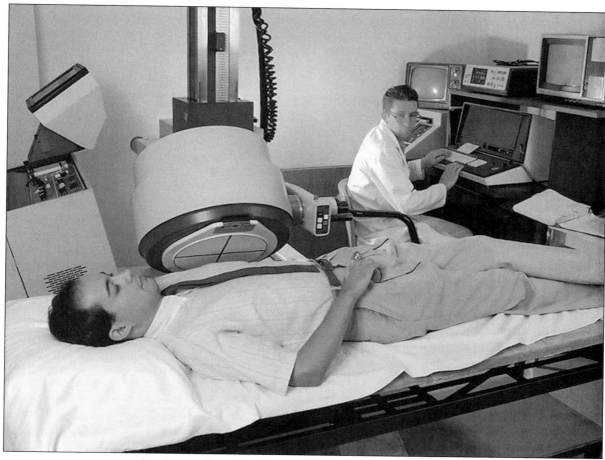

A patient undergoes a nuclear medical procedure. (Digital Stock)

By injecting a radioisotope that has been tagged by bone-seeking agents, doctors can view images of an entire skeleton. Multiple fractures, metastatic disease, osteomyelitis, osteoporosis, and Paget's disease are but a few of the diseases that can be identified quickly and with minimal exposure of the patient to radiation.

Functional as well as anatomical information can be obtained by using nuclear medicine techniques to image the genitourinary tract, especially the kidneys. A perfusion study may be performed as the first phase of structural imaging. This study is done primarily to evaluate the vascularity (amount of blood vessels) of renal (kidney) masses. Cystic lesions and abscesses are usually avascular (having few or no blood vessels), and tumors are usually moderately or highly vascular. Uncommonly occurring arteriovenous (A-V) malformations show high vascularity. An evaluation of blood flow may also be important in patients who have received a kidney transplant. Anatomical renal imaging

is performed to evaluate the position, size, and shape of the kidneys. Renal function studies have proven to be very sensitive in the diagnosis of both bilateral and unilateral kidney disease. By following specific tracers through the kidneys, doctors are able to evaluate the filtration by the glomeruli (capillary tufts) and the function of the tubules. Radionuclide cystography (imaging of the bladder), although not performed routinely, is extremely useful in diagnosing vesicoureteral reflux (urine reflux from the bladder back to the ureters), a relatively common problem in children.

Radionuclide imaging plays a significant role in the diagnosis of disease involving the gastrointestinal tract. Swallowing function, esophageal transit, gastroesophageal reflux, gastric emptying, gallbladder function, pulmonary aspiration of liver disease, and gastrointestinal bleeding can all be evaluated with nuclear medicine. The application of radioactive materials in the endocrine system provides historical benchmarks in the field of nuclear medicine with the use of radioiodine to assess the dynamic function of the thyroid gland. Radioiodine uptake testing is important and useful in the diagnosis of thyroid disease, specifically hyperthyroidism and hypothyroidism, thyroiditis, and goiters. Thyroid imaging is employed for the detection and functional evaluation of solitary or multiple thyroid nodules and the evaluation of aberrant thyroid tissue, metastases of thyroid cancer, and other tumors containing thyroid tissue.

The therapeutic value of nuclear medicine is best demonstrated in its role in the treatment of Graves' disease, toxic adenoma, toxic multinodular goiter, and metastatic thyroid carcinoma. The purpose of the therapeutic application of radioiodine to hyperthyroidism (an overactive thyroid) is to control the disease and return the patient to a normal state. The accumulation and retention of radioiodine, with the subsequent radiation effects upon the thyroid cells, underlie the basic principle behind radionuclide therapy. The treatment of thyroid carcinoma with radioiodine is directed toward the control of metastatic foci and palliation of patients with thyroid carcinoma. Not all thyroid tumors localize radioiodine; therefore, care must be taken for proper patient selection by assuring a tumor's response to iodine.

Monoclonal antibody imaging has become important not only diagnostically but therapeutically as well. Antibodies with perfect specificity for antigens of interest—in this case, malignancies—are produced. These antibodies are labeled with a large dose of radioactivity and injected into the patient. This "magic bullet" is then directed only to the antigen-producing areas. As in thyroid treatment, the radiation effect destroys only those cells to which the radioactivity is attached, leaving the noncancerous cells undamaged. Although this treatment is primarily a research protocol, the future role of radioactive monoclonal antibodies in the treatment of malignant disorders could be significant.

Clinical applications of PET scanning have focused on three areas: cardiology, oncology, and neurology/psychiatry. The principal clinical utility of PET in cardiology lies primarily in accurately differentiating infarcted, scarred tissue from myocardium, which is viable but not contracting because of a reduced blood supply. PET offers a noninvasive procedure to distinguish tissue viability, which allows more accurate patient selection for surgery and angioplasty than conventional approaches. In cancer cases, PET can determine cellular viability and the growth of tumor tissue. It can directly measure the effectiveness of a given radiation or chemotherapy regimen on the metabolic process within the tumor. PET can differentiate tumor regrowth from radiation necrosis.

Because of the unique ability of PET scanning to assess metabolic function, it can aid in the diagnosis of dementia and other psychoses as well as offer possible effective treatment of these disorders. PET is also helpful in detecting the origin of seizures in patients with complex epilepsy and can be used to locate the lesion prior to surgical intervention. Strokes are the third most common cause of death in the United States. A total of 1.6 million people are affected, 40 percent of whom are in need of special services. PET can determine the viability of brain tissue, permitting the clinician to select the most effective (and least invasive and expensive) form of treatment.

Nuclear imaging techniques are quite safe. Allergic reactions to isotopes are essentially nonexistent. In fact, the few that have been reported can be traced back to a contaminant in the injected dose. The radiation burden is far less than that of fluoroscopic radiographic examination and is equal to that of one chest X ray, regardless of the picture produced.

PERSPECTIVE AND PROSPECTS

Natural radioactivity was discovered in the late nineteenth century. The first medical success with a radioisotope was Robert Abbe's treatment of an exophthalmic goiter with radon in 1904. In 1934, the Joliot-Curies produced artificial radioisotopes, specifically phosphorus 32. In 1938, Glenn T. Seaborg synthesized iodine 131. Phosphorus 32 was used to treat chronic leukemia and iodine 131 to treat thyroid cancer. Both treatments fell victim to radiation hysteria fueled by the aftermath of World War II and the dropping of the atomic bomb on Hiroshima. For a decade, nuclear medicine was equated with the "atomic cocktail" and was used only sporadically as a therapeutic modality. In 1949, the first gamma camera was introduced by Benjamin Cassen. It was called a "tap scanner" because as it measured radioactivity, it would tap ink on a piece of paper. The intensity of the ink mark was directly proportional to the radioactivity that was being scanned. The first nuclear medicine image was that of a thyroid gland.

Although discovered in the late 1930's, the imaging properties of the short-lived technetium 99m were not understood until the early 1960's. Its six-hour half-life and its chemical properties were ideally suited to imaging with the scintillation camera newly introduced in 1965. From that time on, nuclear medicine grew in its role as a diagnostic tool, with technetium agents becoming the primary radiopharmaceuticals employed in the detection of disease.

With the addition of computers and array processors to the technology, tomographic imaging became increasingly useful in the localization and quantification of disease states. Improved body attenuation correction and computerized three-dimensional imaging enable physicians to quantify the size and extent of abnormalities quite accurately. When one examines the relative role and costs of transmission computed tomography (CT) scanning versus SPECT, a number of factors must be kept in mind. On the side of advantage of SPECT are the low costs compared to CT scanning. Additionally, no contrast is required in the SPECT study, which lessens the chance of adverse patient reaction. CT scanning is still primarily an anatomic diagnostic tool, while SPECT, by employing physiological radiopharmaceuticals, demonstrates the functional features of organs. By repeated imaging during the course of treatment, minute changes in the physiologic biochemical process can be detected and appropriately addressed.

Because of the physiologic nature of nuclear medicine, the development of radiopharmaceuticals to detect other disease states is essential for further growth in this field. It is interesting that much activity in this area is now centered on the treatment of diseases, primarily malignant ones. It seems as if radiation phobia has run its course and researchers will be permitted to develop the "magic bullet" that will target only those cells that it has been programmed to destroy. As PET scanning becomes more frequently used, new positron radiopharmaceuticals will be introduced. Theoretically, all biochemical reactions in the body can be imaged, if the proper radiopharmaceutical is produced.

Much of the human body can now be visualized employing anatomic, physiologic, or biochemical modalities. Nuclear medicine minimized its original emphasis on therapy and developed a new form of physician diagnosis, a physiological radiology now called imaging. This all goes back to an offhand remark made by Hippocrates to a student: "You really ought to look at a patient before making a diagnosis."

—*Lynne T. Roy*

See also Biophysics; Imaging and radiology; Invasive tests; Magnetic resonance imaging (MRI); Noninvasive tests; Nuclear radiology; Positron emission tomography (PET) scanning; Radiation therapy; Radiopharmaceuticals; Single photon emission computed tomography (SPECT).

FOR FURTHER INFORMATION:
Brown, G. I. *Invisible Rays: A History of Radioactivity.* Stroud, England: Sutton, 2002. Traces the history of radioactivity with the use of biographical information on Marie Curie and other nuclear medicine pioneers.

Brucer, Marshall. *A Chronology of Nuclear Medicine, 1600-1989.* St. Louis, Mo.: Heritage, 1990. In an immensely enjoyable book, the author traces the history of nuclear medicine from the seventeenth century, when Robert Boyle defined a new intellectual discipline that would eventually be called "science," through the April 28, 1986, Chernobyl nuclear accident in the Soviet Union.

Christian, Paul E., Donald Bernier, and James K. Langan, eds. *Nuclear Medicine and PET: Technology and Techniques.* 5th ed. St. Louis, Mo.: Mosby, 2004. A comprehensive text that encompasses the spectrum of nuclear medicine technology from basic and applied mathematics, physics, chemistry, and biology to the details of performance and principles of interpretation of individual nuclear medicine procedures, regulations, and patient care.

Iskandrian, Ami E., and Mario S. Verani, eds. *Nuclear Cardiac Imaging: Principles and Applications.* 4th ed. New York: Oxford University Press, 2008. Many strides have occurred in the field of nuclear cardiology since the 1970's. These developments have had considerable impact on reshaping the entire field of cardiovascular medicine. This book provides an indepth analysis of relevant pathophysiologic concepts and the results of the most commonly available cardiac imaging modalities.

Iturralde, Mario P. *Dictionary and Handbook of Nuclear Medicine and Clinical Imaging.* 2d ed. Boca Raton, Fla.: CRC Press, 2002. This medical dictionary provides overview information to those readers unfamiliar with the field of nuclear medicine science and clinical imaging. Clear definitions of terms are provided in an easy-to-use reference.

Taylor, Andrew, David M. Schuster, and Naomi P. Alazraki. *A Clinician's Guide to Nuclear Medicine.* 2d ed. Reston, Va.: Society of Nuclear Medicine, 2006. Aimed at the medical professional, this handy guide covers many aspects of nuclear medicine. Includes bibliographical references and an index.

NUCLEAR RADIOLOGY

PROCEDURE

ALSO KNOWN AS: Nuclear medicine

ANATOMY OR SYSTEM AFFECTED: Bones, brain, glands, kidneys, musculoskeletal system, nervous system

SPECIALTIES AND RELATED FIELDS: Nuclear medicine, radiology

DEFINITION: The use of radiopharmaceuticals for the diagnosis of disease and the assessment of organ function.

KEY TERMS:

collimator: a device that directs photons into a crystal for their detection

gamma camera: a system composed of a cesium-iodide crystal, collimator, and computer which is used to detect radioactivity and create an image of its distribution

radioisotope: a radioactive atom

radiopharmaceutical: the combined form of a pharmaceutical labeled with a radioisotope

INDICATIONS AND PROCEDURES

Nuclear radiology, also known as nuclear medicine, is similar to conventional radiology in that radiation is used to look inside the patient's body. Unlike conventional radiology, however, nuclear radiology looks not only at the anatomy of the patient but also at the functioning of the organ of interest. In conventional radiology (X rays), the radiation or X-ray photon is produced by accelerating electrons, elemental negative charges, up to 50,000 to 125,000 volts and then ramming them into a metal anode. The physical act of stopping the electrons causes about 0.2 percent of the electrons to give off the accelerating energy as packets of energy called photons. This radiation is then directed by the lead housing of the X-ray tube toward the patient. The radiation transmitted through the patient is then recorded on either film or an image-intensifying tube.

Nuclear radiology differs from conventional radiology because there is no X-ray tube generating the radiation. The radiation comes from the pharmaceuticals injected into the patient. The source of the radiation is from a radioactive atom attached to a pharmaceutical (therapeutic drug). The physiological action and distribution of the pharmaceutical determines the diagnostic ability of the radiation given to the patient. The radiation can be emitted in any direction from the atom. The radiation, which travels in the direction of a piece of cesium-iodine crystal and through a collimator, or set of lead holes, is detected. The cesium-iodine crystal with the accompanying computer is known as a gamma camera.

The radioactive atom currently used in most nuclear radiology departments is an isotope of technetium. The isotope is in a semistable state known as a metastable state. When it becomes unstable and decays, it emits a single photon with the energy equivalent of an electron accelerated in a 140,000 volt potential (140 keV). After the emission of this single photon, the technetium atom is nonradioactive. The number of photons given off is dependent on the number of technetium atoms present in the metastable state. The time required for half of those present to emit the photons is called its half-life. The half-life of technetium is 6.02 hours. Because of its ease of production and reasonable half-life, technetium is used in many pharmaceuticals.

Specialty isotopes are also used. A gaseous isotope of xenon 133 is used for some lung studies. Xenon has a more complicated decay than does technetium. Xenon decays by release of an energetic electron to unstable states of cesium 133. Cesium 133 gives off six gamma rays, with the predominant one being 80.9 keV. The half-life of xenon is 5.31 days. Xenon, being a noble gas, is chemically inert.

An isotope that can be used without being attached to a pharmaceutical is thallium 201. Thallium can be used in cardiac studies since it is readily taken up in the cardiac tissue. When thallium 201 decays, it becomes mercury 201. As mercury 201 becomes stable, it gives off high-energy X rays and gamma rays with the predominant energy being between 68.8 and 80 keV. Iodine is another isotope that does not necessarily need to be attached to a pharmaceutical. The three isotopes of iodine used are iodine 123, 125, or 131. All give off gamma rays that can be detected, predominant being 159.1, 35.4, and 364.4 keV, respectively. Iodine 131 also gives off energetic electrons when it decays and as such is used when energetic electrons are desired for therapy purposes. The emission of energetic electrons can damage surrounding tissues. Iodine 123 and iodine 125 decay by absorbing an electron from the atom and only emit gamma rays. The use of one over the other depends on the cost, with iodine 123 more costly because of its 13-hour half-life. Iodine 125 has a half-life of 60.2 days. Iodine 131 has a half-life of 8.06 days. Other isotopes are used for specialty purposes, such as chromium 51, which can be used to attach to red blood cells. Chromium has a half-life of 27.7 days, with a predominant gamma emission of 320 keV.

A collimator is employed to force only the radiation from the front of the crystal through a known path to be detected. A collimator can consist of a piece of metal, usually lead, with one or multiple holes. The size and length of the hole determine the number of photons that will reach the crystal. The collimator works because it absorbs the photons that are not directed along the axis of the hole. The higher the energy of the photon being directed, the thicker the sides of the holes, known as septa, must be. The smaller the hole, the better the spatial resolution and ease of detecting small concentrations of the isotope of interest. The longer the hole, the better defined the path will be from the crystal face out through the hole to the patient. The limitations of the size and length are dictated by the need to detect a sufficient number of photons to give a diagnostic result. Unlike conventional radiology, in which the films are acquired in a short time (usually a fraction of a second), nuclear radiology can require fifteen to thirty minutes or more to acquire enough photons for a clinician to make a diagnostic determination.

PERSPECTIVE AND PROSPECTS

The main structures that nuclear medicine studies are blood, brain, heart, thyroid gland, parathyroid glands, liver, kidneys, lungs, and bones. Blood studies use several different pharmaceuticals and radioisotopes depending on what is being measured. These studies involve the measurement of the blood volume or blood filtration. Brain studies use technetium with several different pharmaceuticals. Some pharmaceuticals will not pass the blood-brain barrier and can be used to detect bleeding in the cranial compartment. Others pass easily through the blood-brain barrier and can be used to detect sections of the brain that are either hyperactive or hypoactive. Heart studies are involved in determining the health of the cardiac muscles. By the use of thallium and new, additional technetium-labeled pharmaceuticals, the viability of heart tissue after a heart attack can be assessed, along with the thickness of cardiac structures such as the septa between the right and left ventricles. Other properties such as the filling and ejection fractions can be determined in this study. Thyroid studies look at the size and location and are easiest to use with iodine isotopes. A different thallium-labeled radiopharmaceutical can be used to look at the same properties of the parathyroid glands. Liver studies involve the determination of areas that are not function-

ing and that are revealed as voids on a scan. These pharmaceuticals use technetium as the labeled isotope. Kidney studies, which determine whether the kidneys are filtering the blood properly and in sufficient quantities, use technetium as the labeled isotope. Lung studies determine if all the lobes of the lungs are filling properly by using an inhalation isotope of xenon or aerosol compounds labeled with technetium. The health of the alveoli can be determined by introduction of a radiopharmaceutical that congregates in the alveolar space. Bone studies are involved in determining whether new bone is being formed.

—*Anthony J. Wagner, Ph.D.*

See also Biophysics; Imaging and radiology; Invasive tests; Magnetic resonance imaging (MRI); Nuclear medicine; Positron emission tomography (PET) scanning; Radiation therapy; Radiopharmaceuticals.

FOR FURTHER INFORMATION:

Bontrager, Kenneth, and John P. Lampignano. *Textbook of Radiographic Positioning and Related Anatomy.* 7th ed. St. Louis, Mo.: Mosby/Elsevier, 2010. A clinical text for student radiographers but nonetheless helpful in its coverage of basic radiologic procedures and the sections on special procedures, including CT scanning and MRI, and digital imaging.

Cherry, Simon R., James A. Sorenson, and Michael E. Phelps. *Physics in Nuclear Medicine.* 3d ed. Philadelphia: W. B. Saunders, 2003. This excellent book covers in detail the physical principles necessary for an understanding of radionuclide properties and the nuclear medicine instrumentation techniques for imaging. The authors have considerable experience in this field.

Saha, Gopal B. *Physics and Radiobiology of Nuclear Medicine.* 3d ed. New York: Springer, 2006. A textbook and study guide for medical residents preparing to take the American Board of Radiology examination, especially those specializing in nuclear radiology. Reviews the fundamental physics of radiology, the instrumentation, radiobiology, dosimetry, and safety regulations.

Sandler, Martin P., R. Edward Coleman, and James A. Patton, eds. *Diagnostic Nuclear Medicine.* 4th ed. Philadelphia: Lippincott Williams & Wilkins, 2003. A clinical text with an encyclopedic focus that covers clinically relevant developments in nuclear medicine, including instrumentation, radiopharmaceuticals, and applications.

Numbness and Tingling

Disease/disorder

Also known as: Paresthesias, dysesthesias, hypesthesias

Anatomy or system affected: Legs, muscles, musculoskeletal system, nerves, nervous system, skin

Specialties and related fields: Neurology, physical therapy

Definition: Abnormalities of sensation that are attributable to nerve damage or disorders.

Symptoms. Patients commonly report various sensory aberrations that are often described as "pins and needles," tingling, prickling, burning of varying severity, or sensations resembling electric shock. The accepted term for these symptoms is "paresthesias" or "dysesthesias." When severe enough to be painful, they can be referred to as painful paresthesias.

The other major sensory symptom is a reduction or loss of feeling in an area of skin. Most patients use the relatively unambiguous term "numbness"; however, the more formal medical term is "hypesthesia." Paresthesias and hypesthesias are usually restricted to a part rather than all of the cutaneous territory of a damaged root or nerve.

The distribution of nonparesthetic pain is seldom as anatomically specific as the paresthesias themselves. Patients with carpal tunnel syndrome, for example, often have arm and shoulder pain that suggests compression of a cervical root rather than of the distal median nerve (a combined motor and sensory nerve). The paresthesias, by contrast, are usually localized to the tips of the fingers innervated by the median nerve. Similarly, in patients with cervical or lumbosacral radiculopathies (any diseased condition of the roots of spinal nerves), the distribution of pain in the upper or lower limbs often correlates poorly with the root involved. The paresthesias, however, are felt usually either along the entire area or, more commonly, in the distal part of the skin area innervated by the damaged root (the dermatome).

Examination. In attempting to localize the site of a lesion, the physician innervates major muscles from the spinal nerve roots (myotomes) through the plexuses, the individual peripheral nerves and their branches, and also the cutaneous areas supplied by each of these components of the peripheral nervous system. Traditionally, the site of the lesion can be deduced from which muscles and nerves are involved and from where the various branches of the peripheral nerves arise.

In motor examination, the muscles and tendon reflexes are examined first because weakness and reflex changes are often easier to elicit than are sensory signs. The muscles are first examined for atrophy. Since muscles become atrophic when denervated, the focal atrophy can sometimes identify accurately a nerve lesion. The lack of atrophy in a weak muscle either indicates an upper motor neuron lesion or raises the suspicion of spurious weakness. A systematic examination of individual muscles is then performed.

In sensory examination, the patient describes the area of sensory abnormality, which often tells as much as a formal examination. Testing light touch with the examiner's finger is frequently all that is required for confirmation. If this reveals no abnormality, retesting with a pin may disclose an area of sensory deficit. Pinpricks in normal and abnormal areas are compared.

It is important to examine the entire course of an affected nerve for bone, joint, or other abnormalities that may be causing the nerve damage. Local tenderness of the nerve and/or a positive Tinel's sign (paresthesias produced in the area of the nerve when the nerve is tapped or palpated) may also help to identify the site. Many normal persons experience mild tingling when nerves such as the ulnar at the elbow or the median at the wrist are tapped lightly, so this finding is significant only when the nerve is very sensitive to light percussion. Conversely, a badly damaged nerve may be totally insensitive to percussion or palpation.

Nerve conduction studies and the electromyographic examination of muscles evaluate the function of large-diameter, rapidly conducting motor and sensory nerve fibers. These two complementary techniques are valuable tools in the accurate assessment of focal peripheral

---

Information on Numbness and Tingling

Causes: May include neurological damage or disease, exposure to environmental toxins, infection, carpal tunnel syndrome, injury or trauma, metabolic disturbances

Symptoms: Prickling or burning sensations; pain and inflammation; impaired mobility

Duration: Acute to chronic

Treatments: Varies; may include physical therapy, use of ergonomic or corrective devices, surgery, drug therapy

neuropathies, helping in the localization of the nerve lesion and the assessment of its severity.

Diagnosis. Peripheral nerves causing sensory symptoms may be damaged anywhere along their course from the spinal cord to the muscles and skin that they innervate. The site of a focal neuropathy (the focus of neurologic disease) may therefore be in the nerve roots, the spinal nerves, the ventral or dorsal rami (branches), the plexuses (network of nerves), the major nerve trunks, or their individual branches. The character, site, mode of onset, spread, and temporal profile of sensory symptoms must be established and precipitating or relieving factors identified. These features—and the presence of any associated symptoms—help identify the origin of sensory disturbances, as do the physical signs. Sensory symptoms or signs may conform to the territory of individual peripheral nerves or nerve roots. Involvement of one side of the body, or of one limb in its entirety, suggests a central lesion. Distal involvement of all four extremities suggests polyneuropathy (several neurologic disorders), a cervical cord or brainstem lesion, or, when symptoms are transient, a metabolic disturbance such as hyperventilation syndrome. Short-lived sensory complaints may be indicative of sensory seizures or cerebral ischemic phenomena (local and temporal deficiency of blood supply caused by obstruction of the circulation to a part) as well as metabolic disturbances. In patients with cord lesions, there may be a transverse sensory level. Dissociated sensory loss is characterized by the loss of some sensory modalities and the preservation of others. Such findings may be encountered in patients with either peripheral or central disease and must therefore be interpreted in the clinical context in which they are found.

The absence of sensory signs in patients with sensory symptoms does not mean that symptoms have a nonorganic basis. Symptoms are often troublesome before signs of sensory dysfunction have had time to develop.

—*Genevieve Slomski, Ph.D.*

See also Carpal tunnel syndrome; Nervous system; Neuralgia, neuritis, and neuropathy; Neurology; Neurology, pediatric; Pain; Sense organs; Spinal cord disorders; Spine, vertebrae, and disks.

FOR FURTHER INFORMATION:

Bellenir, Karen, ed. *Back and Neck Disorders Sourcebook*. Detroit, Mich.: Omnigraphics, 1997. A reference for lay readers on the causes and consequences of spinal cord disorders, recognizing symptoms, current treatment options, prevention strategies, and sources of help.

Herkowitz, Harry N., et al. *Rothman-Simeone The Spine*. 5th ed. Philadelphia: Saunders/Elsevier, 2006. Discusses diseases and abnormalities of the spine and evaluates surgical remedies. Includes bibliographical references and an index.

Mathers, Lawrence H., Jr. *The Peripheral Nervous System: Structure, Function, and Clinical Correlations*. Menlo Park, Calif.: Addison-Wesley, 1985. Discusses diseases of the peripheral nervous system. Includes bibliographical references and an index.

Rosenbaum, Richard B., and José L. Ochoa. *Carpal Tunnel Syndrome and Other Disorders of the Median Nerve*. 2d ed. Boston: Butterworth-Heinemann, 2002. A thorough examination of carpal tunnel syndrome and related problems. Includes chapters on anatomy of the median nerve, historical perspectives, clinical presentation and diagnosis, electrodiagnostic evaluation, occupational issues, and treatment.

Senneff, John A. *Numb Toes and Other Woes: More on Peripheral Neuropathy*. San Antonio, Tex.: MedPress, 2001. A guide for both patients and care providers, covers research on peripheral neuropathy, treatments for the pain it causes, new drugs, and nutrient supplements. Also details unusual neuropathies, drug causes, neuropathic pain, selecting a doctor, and patient assistance.

NURSING

SPECIALTY

ANATOMY OR SYSTEM AFFECTED: All

SPECIALTIES AND RELATED FIELDS: Critical care, emergency medicine, geriatrics and gerontology, neonatology, nutrition, pediatrics, perinatology, preventive medicine, public health

DEFINITION: A helping profession that focuses on the care of the sick and disabled and on the maintenance of the health and well-being of all individuals.

KEY TERMS:

assessment: the systematic process of collecting, validating, and communicating patient data; these data will include information gathered from the patient's history and from physical examination and laboratory test results

healing: the restoration to a normal physical, mental, or spiritual condition

health: a condition in which all functions of the body, mind, and spirit are normally active

holistic: the philosophy that individuals function as complete units or integrated systems and are not understood merely through their parts

illness: the condition of being sick or diseased

nurture: the act or process of raising or promoting development and well-being

service: work done or duty performed for another or others

treatment: any specific procedure used for the cure or improvement of a disease or pathological condition

THE ROLE OF NURSING

It is difficult at times to distinguish nursing from medicine, since there are so many ways in which they interrelate. Whereas some people think that nursing began with Florence Nightingale (1820-1910), nursing is as old as medicine itself. Throughout history, there have been periods when the two fields functioned interdependently and times when they were practiced separately from each other. It seems likely that the role of the mother-nurse would have preceded the magician-priest or medicine man. Even the seeds of medical knowledge were sown by the natural remedies used by the mother.

Over the course of human history, the words "nurse" and "nursing" have had many meanings, and the connotations have changed as tribes became highly developed and sophisticated nations. The word "nurse" comes from the Latin *nutrix,* which means "nursing mother." The word "nursing" originated from the Latin *nutrire,* meaning "to nourish." The word "nurse" as a noun was first used in the English language in the thirteenth century, being spelled "norrice," then evolving to "nurice" or "nourice," and finally to the present "nurse." The word "nurse" as a verb meant to suckle and to nourish. The meanings of both the noun and the verb have expanded to include more and more functions related to the care of all human beings. In the sixteenth century, the meaning of the noun included "a person, but usually a woman, who waits upon or tends the sick." By the nineteenth century, the meaning of the verb included "the training of those who tend the sick and the carrying out of such duties under the supervision of a physician."

With the origin of nursing as mother care came the idea that nursing was a woman's role. Suckling and nurturing were associated with maternal instincts. Ill or helpless children were also cared for by their mothers. The image of the nurse as a loving and caring mother remains popular. The true spirit of nursing, however, has no gender barriers. History has seen both men and women respond to the needs of the sick.

The role of the nurse has certainly expanded from that of the mother in the home, nourishing infants and caring for young children. Care of the sick, infirm, helpless, elderly, and handicapped and the promotion of health have become vital aspects of nursing as a whole. In history, the role of nursing developed with the culture and society of a given age. Tribal women practiced nursing as they cared for the members of their own tribes. As tribes developed into civilizations, nursing began to be practiced outside the home. As cultures developed, nursing care became more complex, and qualities other than a nurturing instinct were needed to do the work of a nurse. Members of religious orders, primarily those composed of women, responded by devoting their lives to study, service, and self-sacrifice in caring for the needs of the sick. These individuals were among the educated people of their time, and they helped set the stage for nursing to become an art and a science.

It was not until the nineteenth century that the basis of nursing as a profession was established. The beliefs and examples of Florence Nightingale laid that foundation. Nightingale was born in Italy in 1820, but she grew up in England. Unlike many of the children of her time, she was educated by governesses and by her father. Against the wishes of her family, she trained to be a nurse at the age of thirty-one. Amid enormous difficulties and prejudices, she organized and managed the nursing care for a military hospital in Turkey during the Crimean War. She returned to England after the war, where she established a school, the Nightingale Training School for Nurses, to train nurses. Again, she encountered great opposition, as nurses were considered little more than housemaids by the physicians of the time. Because of her efforts, the status of nurses was raised to a respected occupation, and the basis for professional nursing in general was established.

Nightingale's contributions are noteworthy. She recognized that nutrition is an important part of nursing care. She instituted occupational and recreational therapy for the sick and identified the personal needs of the patient and the role of the nurse in meeting those needs. Nightingale established standards for hospital management and a system of nursing education, making nursing a respected occupation for women. She recognized the two components of nursing: promoting health and treating illness. Nightingale believed that nursing is separate and distinct from medicine as a profession.

Nightingale's methods and the response of nursing to American Civil War casualties in the 1860's pointed out the need for nursing education in the United States. Schools of nursing were established, based on the values of Nightingale, but they operated more like apprenticeships than educational programs. The schools were also controlled by hospital administrators and physicians.

In 1896, nurses in the United States banded together to seek standardization of educational programs, to establish laws to ensure the competency of nurses, and to promote the general welfare of nurses. The outcome of their efforts was the American Nurses Association. In 1900, the first nursing journal, the *American Journal of Nursing*, was founded.

The effects of World War II also made clear the need to base schools of nursing on educational objectives. Many women had responded to the need for nurses during the war. A great expansion in medical knowledge and technology had taken place, and the roles of nurses were expanding as well. Nursing programs developed in colleges and universities and offered degrees in nursing to both women and men.

While there were impressive changes in the expectations and styles with which nursing care has been delivered from ancient times into the twenty-first century, the role and function of the nurse have been and continue to be diverse.

The nurse is a caregiver, providing care to patients based on knowledge and skill. Consideration is given to physical, emotional, psychological, socioeconomic, and spiritual needs. The role of the nurse-caregiver is holistic and integrated into all other roles that the nurse fulfills, thus maintaining and promoting health and well-being.

The nurse is a communicator. Using effective and therapeutic communication skills, the nurse strives to establish relationships to assist patients of all ages to manage and become responsible for their own health needs. In this way, the nurse is also a teacher who assists patients and families to meet their learning needs. Individualized teaching plans are developed and used to accomplish set goals.

The nurse is a leader. Based on the self-confidence gained from a nursing education and experience, the nurse is able to be assertive in meeting the needs of patients. The nurse facilitates change to improve care for patients, whether individually or in general. The nurse is also an advocate. Based on the belief that patients have a right to make their own decisions about health

and life, the nurse strives to protect their human and legal rights in making those choices.

The nurse is a counselor. By effectively using communication skills, the nurse provides information, listens, facilitates problem-solving and decision-making abilities, and makes appropriate referrals for patients.

Finally, the nurse is a planner, a task that calls forth qualities far beyond nurturing and caring. In an age confronted with controversial topics such as abortion, organ transplants, the allocation of limited resources, and medical research, the role of nurses will continue to expand to meet these challenges in the spirit that allowed nursing to evolve and become a respected profession.

SCIENCE AND PROFESSION

While the nurse-mother of ancient times functioned within a very limited framework, the modern nurse has the choice of many careers within the nursing role. The knowledge explosion of the last century created many job specialties from which nurses can choose a career. The clinical nurse specialist is a nurse with experience, education, or an advanced degree in a specialized area of nursing. Some examples are enterostomal therapy, geriatrics, infection control, oncology, orthopedics, emergency room care, operating room care, intensive and coronary care, quality assurance, and community health. Nurses who function in such specialties carry out direct patient care; teach patients, families, and staff members; act as consultants; and sometimes conduct research to improve methods of care.

The nurse practitioner is a nurse with an advanced degree who is certified to work in a specific aspect of patient care. Nurse practitioners work in a variety of settings or in independent practice. They perform health assessments and give primary care to their patients.

The nurse anesthetist is a nurse who has also successfully completed a course of study in anesthesia. Nurse anesthetists make preoperative visits and assess patients prior to surgery, administer and monitor anesthesia during surgery, and evaluate the postoperative condition of patients.

The nurse midwife is a nurse who has successfully completed a midwifery program. The nurse midwife provides prenatal care to expectant mothers, delivers babies, and provides postnatal care after the birth.

The nurse administrator functions at various levels of management in the health care field. Depending on the position held, advanced education may be in busi-

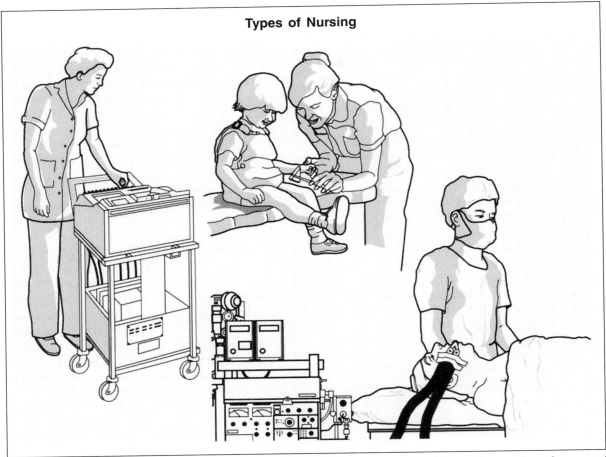

Types of Nursing

Nurses may become involved in many areas of health care, including the administration of diagnostic tests, the performance of physical examinations, and assistance during surgical procedures.

ness or hospital administration. The administrator is directly responsible for the operation and management of resources and is indirectly responsible for the personnel who give patient care.

The nurse educator is a nurse, usually with a master's degree, who teaches or instructs in clinical or educational settings. This nurse can teach both theory and clinical skills.

The nurse researcher usually has an advanced degree and conducts special studies that involve the collection and evaluation of data in order to report on and promote the improvement of nursing care and education.

DUTIES AND PROCEDURES

Creativity and education are the keys to keeping pace with continued changes and progress in the nursing profession. Nurses are expected to play many roles, function in a variety of settings, and strive for excel-

lence in the performance of their duties. A service must be provided that contributes to the health and well-being of people. The following examples of nursing—an operating room nurse and a home health nurse—provide a limited portrait of how nurses function and what roles they play in medical care.

Operating room nurses function both directly and indirectly in patient care and render services in a number of ways. Operating room nurses, usually known as circulating nurses, briefly interview patients upon their arrival at the operating room. They accompany patients to specific surgery rooms and assist in preparing them for surgical procedures. They are responsible for seeing that surgeons correctly identify patients prior to anesthesia. They are also directly attentive to patients when anesthesia is first administered.

Circulating nurses perform the presurgical scrub, which is a cleansing of the skin with a specified solution for a given number of minutes. It is their overall responsibility to monitor aseptic (sterile) techniques in certain areas of the operating room and to deal with the situation immediately if aseptic techniques are broken. They count the surgical sponges with surgical technologists before the first incision is made, throughout the procedure as necessary, and again before the incision is closed. They secure needed items requested by surgical technologists, surgeons, or anesthesia personnel: medications, blood, additional sterile instruments, or more sponges. At times, they prepare and assist with the operation of equipment used for surgeries, such as lasers, insufflators (used for laparoscopic surgery), and blood saver and reinfuser machines. They arrange for the transportation of specimens to the laboratory. They may also be instrumental in sending communications to waiting family members when the surgery takes longer than anticipated. When the surgery is completed, they accompany patients to the recovery room with the anesthesia personnel.

Home health nurses, on the other hand, function in a very different manner. This type of nurse usually works for a private home health services agency, or as part of an outreach program for home services through a hospital. Referrals come to the agency or program via the physician, through the physician's office, by way of the social services department in a hospital, or by an individual requesting skilled services through the physician.

The following scenario is an example of a patient whom a home health nurse may be requested to see: a seventy-six-year-old man who was hospitalized with a recent diagnosis of diabetes mellitus, for which he is now insulin-dependent. He also has an open wound on his right ankle. The number of days allowed for hospitalization for his diagnosis has expired, but he still needs help using a glucometer to take his blood sugar readings and assistance with drawing up his insulin. He still has questions about how to manage his diabetes, especially the dietary parameters. He is unable to manage the wound care on his right ankle. His wife is willing to assist him, but she has no knowledge about diabetes or wound care.

The home health nurse performs the following assessments on the initial visit: general physical condition, the patient's level of knowledge and understanding and his ability to manage his diabetic condition, all medications used, and the patient's understanding of the actions, side effects, and interactions of these medications. An assessment is made of the home setting in general: the patient's safety, the support system, and any special needs, such as assistive devices. If services such as physical therapy, occupational therapy, or speech therapy are needed, the nurse makes these referrals. If the patient requires additional in-home services, a referral to a medical social worker is made. Wound care is performed, and the nurse will then set up a plan of care, with the patient's input, for follow-up visits. Guidelines requested by the physician, as well as approval needed by health insurance companies covering the cost for home health services, will be taken into consideration when planning ongoing visits. If the home health agency has a nurse who is a diabetic specialist, the nurse can either consult with that specialist about the care of this patient or have the diabetic specialist make a home visit.

PERSPECTIVE AND PROSPECTS

From the beginning of time, nursing and the role of the nurse have been defined by the people and the society of a particular age. Nursing as it is known today is still influenced by what occurred over the centuries.

In primitive times, people believed that illness was supernatural, caused by evil gods. The roles of the physician and the nurse were separate and unrelated. The physician was a medicine man, sometimes called a shaman or a witch doctor, who treated disease by ritualistic chants, by fear or shock techniques, or by boring holes into a person's skull with a sharp stone to allow the evil spirit or demon an escape. The nurse, on the other hand, was usually the mother who tended to family members and provided for their physical needs, using herbal remedies when they were ill.

As tribes evolved, the centers for medical care were temples. Some tribes believed that illness was caused by sin and the displeasure of gods. The physician of this age was a priest and was held in high regard. The nurse was a woman, seen as a slave, who performed menial tasks ordered by the priest-physician.

Living in the same era were Hebrew tribes who used the Ten Commandments and the Mosaic Health Code to develop standards for ethical human relationships, mental health treatment, and disease control. Nurses visited the sick in their homes, practiced as midwives, and provided for the physical and spiritual needs of family members who cared for the ill. These nurses provided a family-centered approach to care.

With the advent of Christianity, the value of the individual was emphasized, and the responsibility for recognizing the needs of each individual emerged. Nursing gained an elevated position in society. A spiritual foundation for nursing was established as well. The first organized visiting of the sick was done by deaconesses and Christian Roman matrons of the time. Members of male religious orders also cared for the sick and buried the dead.

During the time of the Crusades, there were both male and female nursing orders, and nursing at this time was a respected vocation. Men usually belonged to military nursing orders, who cared for the sick, on one hand, and defended the hospital when it was under attack, on the other. In medieval times, hospitals became a place to keep, not cure, patients. There were no methods of infection control. Nursing care was largely custodial, and the practice of accepting individuals of low character to supplement inadequate nursing staffs became common.

The worst era in nursing history was probably from 1500 to 1860. Nursing at this time was not a respected profession. Women who had committed a crime were sent into nursing as an alternative to serving a jail term. Nurses received poor wages and worked long hours under deplorable conditions. Changes in the Reformation and the Renaissance did little or nothing to improve the care of the sick. The attitude prevailed that nursing was a religious and not an intellectual occupation. Charles Dickens quite aptly portrayed the nurse and nursing conditions of the time through his immortal caricatures of Sairey Gamp and Betsey Prig in *Martin Chuzzlewit* (1843-1844).

It was not until the middle of the nineteenth century that this situation began to change. Through Nightingale's efforts, nursing became a respected occupation once more, the quality of nursing care improved tremendously, and the foundation was laid for modern nursing education.

As innovations in health care have an impact on nursing, nurses' roles will continue to expand in the future. Nursing can also be a background from which both men and women begin to bridge gaps of service where other affiliations are needed: computer science, medical-legal issues, health insurance agencies, and bioethics, to name a few. The words of Florence Nightingale still echo as a challenge to the nursing profession:

> May the methods by which every infant, every human being will have the best chance of health, the methods by which every sick person will have the best chance of recovery, be learned and practiced! Hospitals are only

an intermediate state of civilization never intended, at all events, to take in the whole sick population.

Nursing will continue to meet this challenge to improve the quality of health care around the world.

—*Karen A. Mattern*

See also Aging: Extended care; Allied health; Anesthesiology; Cardiac rehabilitation; Critical care; Critical care, pediatric; Emergency medicine; Geriatrics and gerontology; Holistic medicine; Hospitals; Immunization and vaccination; Intensive care unit (ICU); Neonatology; Nutrition; Pediatrics; Physical examination; Physician assistants; Preventive medicine; Surgical procedures; Surgical technologists; Terminally ill: Extended care.

FOR FURTHER INFORMATION:

Berman, Audrey, et al. *Kozier and Erb's Fundamentals of Nursing: Concepts, Process, and Practice.* 8th ed. Upper Saddle River, N.J.: Pearson/Prentice Hall, 2008. An accessible text for the undergraduate that explores the fundamentals of nursing care within the framework of the nursing process. Using case studies and real-world examples, covers the nature of nursing, contemporary health care, health beliefs and practices, life-span development issues, assessing health, and promoting psychosocial and physiologic health.

Delaune, Sue C., and Patricia K. Ladner, eds. *Fundamentals of Nursing: Standards and Practices.* 4th ed. Clifton Park, N.Y.: Cengage Learning, 2010. Presents fundamental nursing concepts and covers step-by-step clinical procedures, while also including such contemporary topics as family and community health issues, legal frameworks, home health care, and alternative and complementary treatment.

Dolan, Josephine A., M. Louise Fitzpatrick, and Eleanor K. Herrmann. *Nursing in Society: A Historical Perspective.* 15th ed. Philadelphia: W. B. Saunders, 1983. A concise yet systematic history of nursing for those who wish to orient themselves in this field without having to explore extensive and detailed documents.

Donahue, M. Patricia. *Nursing: The Finest Art.* 2d ed. St. Louis, Mo.: Mosby, 1996. A presentation of the proud heritage of nursing. Describes the emergence of nursing using a global approach. The text is accompanied by reprints of paintings, photographs, and other illustrations pertinent to nursing, making it a breathtaking photojournalistic work.

NUTRITION

BIOLOGY

ANATOMY OR SYSTEM AFFECTED: All

SPECIALTIES AND RELATED FIELDS: Biochemistry, preventive medicine, public health

DEFINITION: The science of food and beverage analysis, metabolism, physical needs for health and disease prevention.

KEY TERMS:

calorie: a measure of the energy in food or of the energy used by the body

carbohydrate: one of three macronutrients; foods that provide carbohydrates are starches, sugars, fruit, vegetables, and milk products

fat: one of three macronutrients; foods that provide fat are oils, margarine, butter, meat, and dairy

macronutrient: carbohydrate, protein, or fat

minerals: inorganic substances that are essential for body processes; the major minerals include calcium, phosphorus, magnesium, sodium, chloride, and potassium

protein: one of three macronutrients; foods that provide protein are meat and dairy, with smaller amounts of protein found in starches

vitamins: organic (carbon-containing) substances found in plants and animals that are essential for body processes; examples include vitamins A, C, and D and the B vitamins

STRUCTURE AND FUNCTIONS

Nutrients are necessary for all aspects of living, including cellular metabolism, individual organ function, and multiple organ systems function. Breathing, moving, thinking, playing, and working all rely on the availability of nutrients. The study of nutrition has revolved around either healthy growth and development or nutrition in relation to the prevention and treatment of disease. Periods of noticeable growth, such as pregnancy, infancy, childhood, and adolescence, are particular areas of study in nutrition because nutrient needs change during these periods.

The amount of calories required to maintain a healthy weight during each stage of the life cycle depends upon the amount of energy expended. Higher caloric requirements are found when body mass is relatively large and energy output is relatively high, as seen in later adolescence and young adulthood. Because men generally have a larger body mass than women, they usually have a larger caloric requirement.

Macronutrients. Carbohydrates are an important source of energy. The recommended range of intake is 45 to 65 percent of the total caloric intake. Each gram of carbohydrate contributes 4 calories to the diet. Carbohydrates are found in starchy foods such as potatoes or corn, in vegetables and fruits, and in milk and yogurt. Carbohydrates are not found in meats or fats unless the food is a mixed dish, such as a hamburger casserole or a candy bar. Simple carbohydrates are those that require little digestion, such as sucrose or sugar. Complex carbohydrates include those that require more digestion, such as starches and fiber. General dietary guidelines suggest an increase in the higher fiber foods. The recommendation is to consume 25 to 35 grams of fiber each day; Americans generally consume 5 to 10 grams. In addition to fruits and vegetables, nuts and seeds, whole wheat bread, and cereal are higher fiber foods.

Dietary protein is required to supply essential amino acids so that the body can synthesize new proteins such as enzymes or hormones, or structural proteins to build muscle. Meats (including pork, beef, chicken, or turkey), fish, eggs, and nuts contain substantial amounts of protein. Protein is also found in dairy products such as milk, cheese, and yogurt. Some protein can be found in most foods, including starches and vegetables, the exception being those foods that are all fat, such as oil, or all simple carbohydrates, such as sugar. Each gram of protein contributes 4 calories to the diet. Protein requirements are closely related to caloric intake. With adequate or excess calories, protein is pared, meaning that less can be consumed while still meeting all body demands for protein. In these cases, protein does not need to be used for energy. With inadequate caloric intake, however, higher levels of protein are required to meet the body's needs because some protein will also be converted to calories for energy needs. The recommended intake assumes that adequate calorie needs are consumed. Protein requirements may be higher than the recommend levels in cases of stress. Although both psychological and physical stress can increase protein requirements, physical stress (including surgery and burns) usually causes a more substantial increase in requirements.

Dietary fat is a risk factor in the development of atherosclerosis or heart disease. Because of this, dietary fat intake recommendations are restricted both in total intake and type of fat ingested. Saturated fat is solid at room temperature and is derived from animals. Lard, shortening, and bacon fat are examples. Unsaturated fat can either have many unsaturated bonds (polyunsaturated) in the structure or one (monounsaturated).

Polyunsaturated fat is liquid at room temperature and derived from plants such as corn or soybeans. Monounsaturated fat is derived from plants such as canola or olive oil. Whereas recommendations had previously specified levels of intake for both polyunsaturated and monounsaturated fats, current recommendations reflect only a limited total fat intake with a restriction on transfats in particular. Transfat is an unsaturated fat that has been partially hydrogenated. This process causes a liquid fat to become more solid and is sometimes desirable in baked products. Transfats are linked to cardiovascular disease and should be limited. Foods that have higher values of transfat should be labeled as such and are most often processed baked goods, such as cookies, cakes, or pies, or snack foods, such as chips. Regardless of the type of fat, each gram of fat contributes 9 calories to the diet.

Minerals. The major minerals include calcium, phosphorus, magnesium, sodium, chloride, and potassium. These minerals are at times referred to as electrolytes, meaning that they can have a negative or positive charge, thus conducting electricity. In the body, these anions (negatively charged) and cations (positively charged) are important for the action potentials of cells, nerve conduction, and the excitation of muscles. The trace minerals are so called because only very small amounts are needed on a daily basis. One of the most common trace minerals is iron. The amounts of minerals in a particular food often vary depending on the soil in which a plant is grown or the feed that an animal consumes. Minerals are inorganic and cannot be destroyed with cooking or processing.

Calcium is required for normal growth and development of bone as well as nervous and muscular activity, enzyme regulation, and blood clotting. Food labels may designate a food as an excellent source (at least 200 milligrams of calcium) or a good source (100 to 199 milligrams of calcium). Poor intake of calcium is associated with the development of porous bones, or osteoporosis.

Most phosphorus is in bone as hydroxyapatite, although phosphorus also occurs as phospholipids in most cell membranes and is a component of nucleic acids. Phosphorus functions as an acid-base buffer, in enzymatic reactions, and in energy transfer. Phosphorus is found in nearly all foods, but good sources include meat, milk products, eggs, grains and legumes, and soft drinks.

About half of the body magnesium is found in bone, but magnesium is essential for hundreds of enzymatic reactions as well as muscle contraction. Green leafy vegetables, fruits, grains, and nuts as well as milk, meat, shellfish, and eggs are good sources of magnesium.

Potassium is found in many foods, including milk, meat, fruit, and vegetables. Together with sodium, potassium is involved with maintaining fluid balance. A diet high in sodium and low in potassium may be involved in the development of high blood pressure, or hypertension. The major source of sodium in the diet is salt, which is sodium chloride. Foods high in sodium include any food with visible salt (such as crackers and snack foods), pickled foods, processed foods such as lunch meat, canned soup, canned meat, and cured foods such as bacon and ham. A diet high in potassium and calcium and low in sodium is recommended to prevent hypertension.

Most of the body's iron is found in hemoglobin in red blood cells, where its function is to transport oxygen in the blood. Food sources of iron are either heme (from meat) or nonheme (from plant sources or iron-fortified foods). Very little iron is excreted from the body, with most of the iron from degraded hemoglobin being reabsorbed in the gastrointestinal tract. A deficiency of iron occurs gradually with chronic poor intake of iron-rich foods. Other causes of iron deficiency include excess blood loss and malabsorption. Chronic iron deficiency will cause anemia.

Vitamins. Vitamin A food sources include both animal sources (retinoids) and plant sources (carotenoids). Good animal food sources of vitamin A include liver, egg yolks, milk fat, and fish oils. Carotenoids can be converted to retinol in the intestinal mucosa and will then have the same metabolic role as retinoids from animal sources. The most common of these is beta carotene, but there are more than five hundred carotenoids. Vitamin A is required for optimal vision, with most of its effects found in the maintenance of night vision. Vitamin A also has a role in maintaining epithelial tissues, mucus production, and bone health. Vitamin A appears to have a role in fertility and in maintaining immune function as well.

Vitamin C is an important antioxidant with the biochemical ability to neutralize free radicals. Free radicals are metabolites of oxygen used in the cell and are believed to promote aging and several chronic diseases. Good sources of vitamin C include citrus fruits, broccoli, kiwi, potatoes, strawberries, and tomatoes, as well as most other fruits and vegetables. Heat, alkalinity, and exposure to air will destroy vitamin C. Therefore, certain cooking, processing, and storage practices can greatly reduce the vitamin C content of food.

Another antioxidant is vitamin E. Vitamin E is really a group of compounds, the most common of which is α-tocopherol. Good sources of vitamin E include vegetable oils, margarines, and nuts. Vitamin E is not destroyed by exposure to air, primarily because it is protected in dietary fat. Vitamin E can be destroyed by high temperatures such as in frying.

Vitamin D food sources are very limited. While milk is fortified with vitamin D, other dairy products, such as cheese and yogurt, generally are not. Some new products are being fortified with both calcium and vitamin D, such as yogurt, margarine, and juice. Exposure of the skin to sunlight converts a pre-vitamin D compounds to vitamin D_3 (cholecalciferol). Cholecalciferol will be hydroxylated in the liver and the kidney before it becomes active vitamin D. Vitamin D is required for calcium regulation and bone health, but emerging areas of research suggest that vitamin D may have a role in autoimmune diseases as well.

The B vitamins are water soluble and include thiamin, niacin, riboflavin, pantothenic acid, vitamin B_6, biotin, folate, and vitamin B_{12}. As a group, the B vitamins are essential for the metabolism of macronutrients, as well as cell growth and division and all organ functions. The B vitamins are found in a variety of foods, although vitamin B_{12} is primarily found in animal products. Once a concern for vegetarians, vitamin B_{12} is now fortified in many cereals and nonmeat breakfast foods.

DISORDERS AND DISEASES

Most chronic diseases result as a complex interaction between genetics and environmental factors. Diet is an important environmental factor that is potentially modifiable, and it has received much attention in the prevention of chronic disease. Most chronic disease prevention or treatment includes a nutritional component. The most prevalent chronic diseases in the United States are cancer, cardiovascular disease, diabetes, obesity, and osteoporosis.

Cancer. Although overall rates are declining in the United States, cancer continues to be a major cause of mortality. In general, cancer involves three phases: initiation, promotion, and progression. During the initiation step, there is a genetic alteration that may remain quiescent or continue though the second step of promotion. During promotion, cellular proliferation is stimulated and the abnormal cells begin to grow without regulation. The third phase is progression, when the neoplastic cells become invasive and spread or metastasize to other parts of the body. Dietary components may be involved in the initiation and promotion of certain cancers as well as their inhibition. The dietary components that have been linked to the development of cancer include dietary fat, total calories, and alcohol, as well as salted, cured foods and molds that may grow in certain foods.

Antioxidants have been investigated as inhibitors of cancer. Fruits and vegetables are rich sources of antioxidants, and high fruit and vegetable intake has been linked to a lower incidence of certain cancers. The results of many studies, however, are inconclusive. Although high intake of dietary fat and red meat has been associated with an increased risk of colon cancer, lower fat diets have not proved to be an effective intervention in decreasing colon cancer incidence. Nevertheless, a diet high in fruits and vegetables, at least five servings each day, and lower in fat and alcohol is recommended as a preventive measure against cancer. Some of the benefit of high fruit and vegetable intake may be attributable to the fiber content of these foods. Higher fiber diets increase fecal bulk, thereby diluting any carcinogens that enter the gastrointestinal tract. By increasing intestinal motility, fiber also decreases the amount of time that fecal material is in the gastrointestinal tract, thereby limiting exposure of the mucosa to potential toxins.

Cardiovascular disease. Cardiovascular diseases are the leading cause of death in the United States. They include arrhythmias, congestive heart failure, and valvular diseases, but most of the morbidity and mortality is related to coronary heart disease, or atherosclerosis. Hyperlipidemia is a risk factor for atherosclerosis, and dietary fat has influence on the level of blood lipids. The recommended intake of fat is 25 to 35 percent of total calories per day. Of that dietary fat, less than 7 percent of total calories should be saturated fat and less than 1 percent should be transfat. Lower fat meats and dairy are recommended, as well as replacement of some meat with vegetable alternatives. Sources of transfat should be limited. The effects of various levels of polyunsaturated and monounsaturated fats are debated. While limited intake of cholesterol is recommended, cholesterol intake has had less of an effect on blood lipids than total fat and transfat.

Eating fish, especially oily fish, is recommended as a source of omega-3 fatty acids, which are long-chain polyunsaturated fatty acids associated with a decreased risk of certain heart diseases. The two omega-3 fatty acids are eicosapentaenoic acid (EPA) and docosahexaenoic acid (DHA). Although fish may contain contaminants known to be hazardous to health, the benefits of eating it are believed to outweigh the risks for adults. Restricted intake may be recommended for children and pregnant women. Supplements of DHA and EPA are not recommended for the prevention of heart disease, although they may be prescribed as treatment under a physician's supervision.

Higher intakes of fruits, vegetables, and whole grains are recommended to prevent heart disease. In addition to fiber, these foods may contain antioxidants or other bioactive compounds that are beneficial to health. In addition, these foods may displace other, higher calorie foods from the diet, thus promoting a healthy weight. Limiting foods high in added sugars is recommended because of the association of these foods with weight gain and obesity. Obesity is a significant risk factor for cardiovascular disease, and achieving a healthy weight through diet and physical activity is important.

A healthy weight is also significant in the maintenance of optimal blood pressure. Because sodium intake is associated with increases in blood pressure on average, limiting sodium intake is also recommended for heart health. Limited amounts of alcohol, if alcohol is consumed at all, is also included as a healthy lifestyle measure for the prevention of heart disease. Moderate alcohol intake is generally considered to be two drinks for men and one drink for women each day.

Foods that are being investigated concerning their role in the prevention of cardiovascular disease include soy and plant stanols. Supplements of antioxidants and fish oils for their DHA and EPA are generally not recommended, but foods containing these compounds may be beneficial.

Diabetes. The incidence of diabetes continues to grow in parallel to the incidence of obesity. Diabetes mellitus has been categorized as either insulin-dependent diabetes mellitus (IDDM), which is also called type 1 diabetes, and non-insulin-dependent diabetes mellitus (NIDDM), also known as type 2 diabetes. Nutrition is an important component of both the prevention and treatment of diabetes, regardless of type.

Obesity enhances insulin resistance. Therefore, a main goal in type 2 diabetes is to prevent or reduce obesity. Weight loss in obese persons with type 2 diabetes improves glycemic control and blood lipid profile. Because carbohydrates are the main determinant of postprandial plasma glucose, the amount of carbohydrates

and timing of foods eaten may need to be regulated. The total amount of carbohydrates in the diet or meal is more important than the type of carbohydrate, with certain exceptions. Liquid carbohydrates are more easily digested and absorbed than those from solid foods. Beverages such as milk and orange juice may cause a more rapid rise in blood glucose. Sucrose and sucrose-containing foods do not need to be eliminated, but these foods do need to be included in the total carbohydrates and calories consumed for meal planning and coverage with medication. Restriction of sucrose and sucrose-containing foods usually relates to the restriction of total calories. The glycemic response to carbohydrates depends on many components, including the type of carbohydrate, the cooking or processing, prior food intake, other macronutrients in the food, and glycemic control of the individual. Because dietary modifications need to be individualized, people with diabetes should receive individualized medical nutrition therapy, preferably by a registered dietitian or certified diabetes educator.

Obesity. Obesity occurs when caloric intake exceeds the needs of the individual and is therefore stored in adipose tissue. Although normal weight varies with age, gender, and height, for each group there are indicators of obesity. Usual indicators of obesity are based on the assumption that variations in weight at various heights are attributable to body fat and are often calculated as the body mass index (BMI). A BMI of between 25 and 30 is considered overweight, and above 30 is considered obese. The optimal macronutrient distribution to facilitate weight loss is not known. Higher and lower amounts of protein, fat, and carbohydrates have been investigated, without clear conclusions. Consuming fewer calories while increasing the amount of calories used through physical activity remains the cornerstone of obesity prevention and treatment.

Osteoporosis. As with other chronic diseases, the incidence of osteoporosis continues to rise. Osteoporosis is asymptomatic until the condition produces deformity or contributes to fractures. While genetics play an important role in the development of osteoporosis, modifying risk factors include diet and physical activity. Optimal levels of calcium have been shown to be beneficial in maintaining high bone mineral density, which is critical in preventing osteoporosis. Most calcium is obtained from dairy products, although increasingly grain-based foods and juices are being fortified with calcium. Vitamin D plays a critical role in regulating calcium balance. Therefore, adequate vitamin D status is important in preventing osteoporosis. Vitamin D deficiency can be a contributing factor to osteoporosis in older individuals secondary to poor skin synthesis, lower hydroxylation of vitamin D in the kidneys, and inadequate nutritional intake. As with calcium, more food products are being fortified with vitamin D with an increasing awareness of osteoporosis.

PERSPECTIVE AND PROSPECTS

Although the science of nutrition began as a branch of biochemistry, early discoveries of the health properties of food date to the eighteenth century and the discovery that limes could prevent the painful bleeding disorder scurvy. Since then, the knowledge of nutrition has progressed beyond identifying deficiency diseases toward an understanding and appreciation of the complexity of nutrition in optimal health. In addition to further investigations into macronutrients, vitamins, and minerals, many bioactive substances in foods are being identified, such as bioflavinoids and probiotics. The interactions of these and more traditional nutrients are being investigated as potential modifiers of chronic disease and promoters of longevity.

—*Karen Chapman-Novakofski, R.D., L.D.N., Ph.D.*

See also Acid reflux disease; Aging: Extended care; Anorexia nervosa; Antioxidants; Appetite loss; Arteriosclerosis; Beriberi; Breast-feeding; Bulimia; Caffeine; Cancer; Carbohydrates; Carcinogens; Cholesterol; Diabetes mellitus; Dietary reference intakes (DRIs); Digestion; Eating disorders; Enzyme therapy; Enzymes; Failure to thrive; Fiber; Food biochemistry; Food Guide Pyramid; Gastroenterology; Gastroenterology, pediatric; Gastrointestinal system; Gastrostomy; Geriatrics and gerontology; Heart disease; Hirschsprung's disease; Hypercholesterolemia; Hyperlipidemia; Kwashiorkor; Lactose intolerance; Lipids; Macronutrients; Malabsorption; Malnutrition; Mercury poisoning; Metabolic disorders; Metabolism; Obesity; Obesity, childhood; Osteoporosis; Phenylketonuria (PKU); Phytochemicals; Pinworms; Protein; Roundworms; Scurvy; Sports medicine; Supplements; Tapeworms; Taste; Tropical medicine; Vitamins and minerals; Weaning; Weight loss and gain; Weight loss medications; Worms.

FOR FURTHER INFORMATION:

American Diabetes Association. *American Diabetes Association Complete Guide to Diabetes*. 4th rev. ed. New York: Bantam Books, 2006. Provides a comprehensive guide to self-management of diabetes, including practical advice for living and how to interact with the health care team.

Duyff, Roberta Larson. *American Dietetic Association Complete Food and Nutrition Guide*. 3d ed. Hoboken, N.J.: John Wiley & Sons, 2007. Provides an overview of nutritional needs through the life cycle, including food choices for healthy diets, vitamins, minerals, and macronutrients, as well as suggestions for meal planning and shopping.

Lichtenstein, Alice H., et al. "Diet and Lifestyle Recommendations Revision 2006: A Scientific Statement from the American Heart Association Nutrition Committee." *Circulation* 114, no. 1 (July 4, 2006): 82-96. Provides an overview of the dietary recommendations for cardiovascular health and summary of the rationale for these recommendations.

U.S. Department of Health and Human Services and U.S. Department of Agriculture. *Dietary Guidelines for Americans 2005*. 6th ed. Washington, D.C.: Government Printing Office, 2005. Provides guidelines for healthy eating as well as food sources of nutrients and dietary patterns to prevent hypertension.

OBESITY

DISEASE/DISORDER

ANATOMY OR SYSTEM AFFECTED: Abdomen, blood vessels, circulatory system, endocrine system, gastrointestinal system, heart, intestines, joints, psychic-emotional system, respiratory system, stomach

SPECIALTIES AND RELATED FIELDS: Endocrinology, family medicine, internal medicine, nutrition, psychiatry, psychology, public health

DEFINITION: A condition in which the body carries abnormal or unhealthy amounts of fat tissue, leading the individual to weigh in excess of 20 percent more than his or her ideal weight.

KEY TERMS:

adipose tissue: fat; a soft tissue of the body composed of cells (adipocytes) that contain triglyceride, a compound consisting of glycerol and fatty acids; in obesity, there may be increased numbers of adipocytes, and the cells may contain an increased amount of triglyceride

basal metabolic rate (BMR): the minimal energy expended for maintenance of the vegetative functions of the body (respiration, heat production, and so on), expressed as calories per hour per square meter of body surface

body mass index (BMI): weight in kilograms divided by height in meters, squared (kg/m^2); since this value is relatively independent of height and sex, the same standard values can be used for all adults, both men and women

calorie: 1 kilocalorie, which is the amount of heat (energy) needed to raise the temperature of 1 kilogram of water by 1 degree Celsius

metabolism: the sum of the physical and chemical processes by which living matter is produced, maintained, and transformed

resting metabolic rate (RMR): similar to the BMR, but more easily measured (the subject is resting rather than in a truly basal state)

CAUSES AND SYMPTOMS

Obesity is a condition in which the body accumulates an abnormally large amount of adipose tissue, or fat. It is a multifactorial, chronic disease that is rapidly increasing and having devastating effects on health, especially in the United States. The disease has social, cultural, genetic, metabolic, behavioral, and psychological components. People who are obese also face stigma and discrimination in work and social settings. Obesity is the second leading cause of preventable

deaths in the United States, resulting in an estimated 300,000 deaths each year.

Because it is not practical to measure body fat content directly but it is easy to measure weight and height, the body mass index (BMI), which correlates closely with body fat, is often used to identify and quantify obesity.

Being overweight and being obese are not the same condition. A BMI of 25 to 29.9 is considered to be overweight, a BMI of 30 or more is obese, and a BMI of 40 or more is severely obese. Approximately 127 million adults in the United States are overweight, 60 million are obese, and 9 million are severely obese. More men than women are overweight (67 versus 62 percent). In 2006, it was estimated that 64.5 percent of adults in the United States were overweight, 30.5 percent were obese, and 4.7 percent were severely obese. This latter figure increased from only 2.9 percent in a 1994 survey done by the National Health and Nutrition Examination Survey, which also found that 46.6 percent of adults were overweight and 14.4 percent were obese.

Each year, health care costs for obese persons exceed $100 billion. Little money is available, however, to counter this condition. The National Institutes of Health spends only 1 percent of its budget on obesity research, and all research organizations are impeded by a shortage of funds. Moreover, health insurance companies rarely pay for obesity treatment.

An important function of adipose tissue is to store energy. If the intake of energy, in the form of food calories (usually measured in kilocalories, or calories), is greater than the expenditure of energy, then the excess calories are stored, mainly in the adipose tissue, with a resulting gain in weight. Expenditure of energy de-

---

INFORMATION ON OBESITY

CAUSES: May include endocrine disorders, poor diet, lack of exercise, psychic-emotional disorders, genetic factors

SYMPTOMS: Excessive weight possibly leading to such health problems as strain on weight-bearing body parts leading to arthritis, hypertension, arteriosclerosis, difficulty breathing, sleepiness from inadequate oxygen delivery to tissues

DURATION: Often chronic

TREATMENTS: Diet and lifestyle regulation, medications, surgery

pends largely on the resting metabolic rate or resting energy expenditure, defined as the calories used each day to maintain normal body metabolism. Additional calories are expended by exercise or other activity, by the digestion and metabolism of food, and by other metabolic processes. Because of this simple relationship between energy intake, energy utilization, and energy storage, weight gain can occur only when there is increased caloric intake, decreased caloric expenditure, or both.

Genetic factors appear to be very important in determining the presence or absence of obesity. Body weight tends to be similar in close relatives, especially in identical twins, who share the same genetic makeup. The extent to which genetic factors affect food intake, activity level, or metabolic processes is not known.

One theory holds that each individual has a "set point" that determines body weight. When food intake is decreased, experiments have shown less weight loss than predicted by the caloric deficit, suggesting that the body has slowed its metabolic rate, thus minimizing the deviation from the original weight. Many believe that physiologic regulation of body weight, which tends to maintain a preferred weight for each individual, explains some of the difficulty in treating obesity. The discovery and role of leptin in regulating weight helps to explain this apparent set point of weight for each individual.

There are other causes of obesity as well. Producing lesions in the hypothalamus, a part of the brain, can make animals eat excessively and become obese, and rare cases of obesity in humans are attributable to disease of the hypothalamus. In hypothyroidism, a condition in which the thyroid gland produces too little thyroid hormone, the metabolic rate is slowed, which may cause a mild gain in weight. In Cushing's syndrome, which is caused by excessive amounts of the adrenal hormone cortisol or by drugs that act like cortisol, there is an accumulation of excessive fat in the face and trunk, which disappears when the disease is cured or the drug is stopped. Weight gain has also occurred with the use of other drugs, including some antidepressants and tranquilizers.

While most physicians and the public assume that the main factor causing obesity is excessive food intake in relation to physical activity, it has not been possible to prove that overweight people eat more than slender people do. This may be the case because it is very difficult to measure food intake under normal conditions, or perhaps because obese individuals tend to underesti-

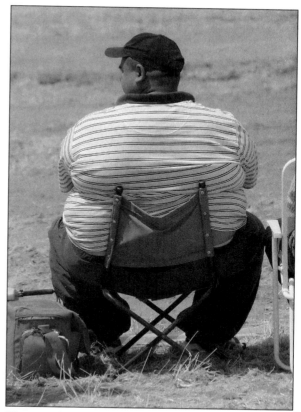

The rates of severe obesity are increasing in the United States. (© Armand Upton/Dreamstime.com)

mate their food intake when dietary histories are taken. Some experts believe, however, that differences in metabolic efficiency and the physiologic set point for body weight are the principal causes of obesity in some people, rather than excessive food intake. The basal metabolic rate (BMR) varies fairly widely among persons of the same age, sex, and body size, and studies have shown large differences in the daily caloric intake needed to maintain a constant body weight in normal people; these observations support the possibility that metabolic differences could contribute to obesity.

Many health problems are associated with obesity. The majority of people who develop non-insulin-dependent diabetes mellitus are overweight, and manifestations of the disease commonly improve or disappear if the individual succeeds in losing weight. Hypertension (high blood pressure) is more common with obesity, and weight loss may lower the blood pressure enough to lessen or avoid the need for medication. Arteriosclerosis, or "hardening of the arteries," is more prevalent in obese persons and causes an increased risk for heart attacks and strokes. Certain forms of cancer are more prevalent with obesity: cancer of the colon, rectum, and prostate in men and cancer of the uterus, gallbladder, ovary, and breast in women. Severe obesity can cause difficulties in breathing, with sleepiness resulting from inadequate oxygen delivery to the tissues and sometimes from interruption of sleep at night. In addition, conditions such as arthritis may be worsened by the additional strain that obesity places on weight-bearing parts of the body.

The distribution of excess adipose tissue differs among individuals. Two main patterns have been described: android obesity (more commonly affecting men), in which fat accumulates mainly in the abdomen and upper body; and gynoid obesity (more common in women), in which fat accumulates mainly in the hips, thighs, and lower body. This distinction has received much attention because persons with android obesity are more likely to suffer from diabetes, hypertension, and cardiovascular disease. The closest association with these diseases is seen when sensitive measurements of abdominal visceral fat mass are made with computed tomography (CT) scanning, a special X-ray technique. A simple measurement of the waist circumference compared with the hip circumference—the waist-to-hip ratio—can also be used to identify those obese individuals at greater risk for diabetes and cardiovascular disease.

Treatment and Therapy

Many obese people are highly motivated to lose weight because of the common perception that a slim body build is more attractive than an obese one. Many other overweight individuals desire to lose weight because of health problems related to obesity. As a result, the human and financial resources devoted to weight loss efforts are extensive. Unfortunately, the long-term results of the treatment of obesity are successful in only a minority of cases.

The only measures useful in the treatment of obesity are those that decrease the intake or absorption of calories or those that increase the expenditure of calories. The basis for any long-term weight reduction program is a low-calorie diet. The average daily calorie requirement in the United States is approximately 1,600 calories for women and 2,300 calories for men; decreasing an individual's intake, usually to between 800 and 1,500 calories, will result in weight loss, provided that energy expenditure does not decrease. A balanced diet, with 20 percent to 30 percent of the calories derived

from fat (considerably less fat than is found in the typical American diet) is usually recommended. Many unbalanced diets, or "fad diets," have enjoyed periods of popularity. Rice diets, low carbohydrate diets, vegetable diets, and other special diets may produce rapid weight loss, but long-term persistence with an unbalanced diet is rare and the lost weight is often regained.

Many patients fail to lose weight with low-calorie diets. More severe calorie restriction can be achieved with very-low-calorie diets that provide only 400 to 800 calories daily. This level of caloric restriction is unsafe unless a very high proportion of the diet consists of high-quality protein, with correct amounts of other nutrients such as vitamins and minerals. These requirements can be met with special formula diets under careful medical supervision. Such a program is recommended for severely obese patients who are otherwise healthy enough to tolerate this degree of caloric restriction.

Because most people find it difficult to lower their calorie intake, behavioral management programs may be combined with dietary restrictions. Dieters can be taught techniques for self-monitoring of food intake, such as keeping a daily log of meals and exercise, which will increase the awareness of eating behavior as well as point out ways in which that behavior can be modified. There are techniques for reducing exposure to food and the stimuli associated with eating, such as keeping food out of sight, keeping food handling and preparation to a minimum, and eliminating the occasions when food is eaten out of habit or as part of a social routine. Ways can be sought to increase the social support of friends and family for weight-losing behavior and for reinforcement of compliance with dietary restrictions. Interestingly, the "diet merry-go-round" which many mildly obese individuals experience—restricting their caloric intake until a weight goal is achieved, ending the diet only to resume overeating and regain the weight lost—often results in higher weight. Over time, such a pattern can "cycle" the individual to a dangerously high weight. Such individuals tend to experience more success if they can adjust their long-range eating behavior to moderate, rather than restrictive, intake of food. Many physicians would prefer to see their obese patients remain relatively stable in weight, reducing slowly over time, to avoid physical stress and ensure success.

Because obesity is caused by an excess of calorie intake over calorie expenditure, another approach to weight loss is to increase energy utilization by increasing physical activity. Some studies have shown that overweight individuals are less active than their non-obese counterparts. This fact could contribute to their obesity, since less energy utilization results in more energy available for storage as fat. Decreased activity could also be a result of obesity, since a heavier person must do more work, by carrying more pounds, than a nonobese person who walks or climbs the same distance.

Each pound of fat contains energy equal to about 4,000 calories. If an obese person expends 400 extra calories each day by walking briskly for one hour, it will take ten days for this activity to result in the loss of one pound. In a year, this increased calorie expenditure would result in a thirty-six-pound weight loss. More vigorous exercise, such as running, swimming, or calisthenics, would lead to more rapid weight loss, but might not be advisable for every person because of the increased prevalence of certain health problems in obese individuals, such as heart disease, hypertension, and musculoskeletal disorders. For this reason, any exercise program that involves vigorous physical activity should be undertaken with medical supervision.

Exercise as part of a weight-loss program has additional benefits. The function of the cardiovascular system may be improved, and muscles may be strengthened. Exercise will lead to loss of adipose tissue and gain in lean body mass as weight is lost, a change in body composition that is beneficial to overall health. Although some fear that physical activity will lead to an increase in appetite, studies show that any increase in food intake that occurs after exercise is usually not great enough to match the calories expended by the exercise.

Medications that decrease appetite are occasionally used to help people comply with a low-calorie diet. Some appetite suppressants act like adrenaline and may cause such side effects as nervousness, irritability, and increased heart rate and blood pressure. Other drugs may stimulate serotonin, a chemical transmitter in the central nervous system that decreases appetite, and may cause drowsiness as a side effect. The use of these medications is controversial because of their side effects and their limited effectiveness in promoting weight loss.

Several surgical procedures, collectively referred to as bariatric surgery, have been used to treat severe obesity that has impaired the patient's health and has resisted other treatment. The operation now most commonly performed is gastroplasty, which creates a small pouch in the stomach with a narrow outlet through which all food must pass. This procedure decreases the effective volume of the stomach, causing fullness and nausea if more than small amounts of solid food are eaten. Patients have lost about half of their excess weight after one and one-half to two years, but some weight may be regained after this period. Gastroplasty has produced fewer serious complications than an older form of treatment, no longer done, called intestinal bypass. Care must be taken to avoid certain foods that might cause blockage of the narrowed opening from the surgically created stomach pouch, and the benefit of the operation can be overcome by eating soft or liquid foods, which can be consumed in large quantities. The long-term benefit of this procedure is being evaluated.

PERSPECTIVE AND PROSPECTS

Fat has several important functions in the human body. It serves as a cushion for the body frame and internal organs, it provides insulation against heat loss, and it is a storage site for energy. Fat stores energy very efficiently since it contains approximately 9 calories per gram, compared with approximately 4 calories per gram in protein and carbohydrate. The presence of reserve stores of energy in the form of fat is particularly important when regular food intake is interrupted and the body becomes dependent on its fat deposits to maintain a source of fuel for daily metabolism and physical activity.

In affluent, culturally advanced societies, however, where food is abundant and modern conveniences greatly reduce the need for physical exertion, many people tend to accumulate excessive amounts of fat, since energy that is taken in but not utilized is stored in the adipose tissue. In the early twenty-first century, health officials were concerned by new findings that showed one in every fifty Americans were "extremely obese," meaning their BMI measured at least 50 and they were at least 100 pounds overweight. This number had quadrupled since the 1980's. Obesity is a critical public health problem because it increases the risk of diabetes, hypertension, cardiovascular disease, and other illnesses. Also, many overweight men and women are distressed by the effects of their weight on their social interactions and self-image, and, despite laws, face discrimination in workplace settings. Therefore, many obese individuals desire to lose weight.

Unfortunately, the results of weight-loss programs and countless individual efforts at dieting to achieve this goal have often been disappointing. Short-term weight loss can often be achieved; programs utilizing low-calorie diets, behavior modification, exercise, and sometimes appetite-suppressing drugs usually lead to a weight loss of ten to thirty pounds or more over a period of several weeks or months. The problem is that after a year or more, the great majority of these dieters have regained the lost weight. It appears that the maintenance of a low-calorie diet and an increase in physical activity require a degree of commitment and willingness to endure inconvenience, self-deprivation, and sometimes even physical discomfort that most people can accept for short periods of time but not indefinitely. There are exceptions—some people do succeed in maintaining long-term weight loss—but more commonly dieters return to or surpass their original weight. It is as if the body's set point can be overcome temporarily by intense effort, but not permanently.

Because of the poor prognosis for long-term weight loss, some experts now question the extent to which efforts should be devoted to the treatment of obesity. Nevertheless, because one cannot predict which obese individuals will succeed in achieving long-term weight reduction and because of the important health benefits of maintaining a normal body weight, most physicians agree that serious efforts should be made to treat obesity. Overweight individuals should identify the modifications in their diet and lifestyle that would be most beneficial and should attempt, with medical supervision, to initiate and maintain the behavior needed to bring about permanent weight loss.

In 2006, in an effort to reduce the incidence rate of obesity in the United States, the Alliance for a Healthier Generation, the William J. Clinton Foundation, and the American Heart Association announced an agreement to fight childhood obesity. The five leading food manufacturers—Campbell's Soup, Dannon, Kraft, Mars, and PepsiCo—vowed to reformulate their products in order to provide more nutritious choices for children in schools.

—E. Victor Adlin, M.D.;
Karen E. Kalumuck, Ph.D.;
updated by LeAnna DeAngelo, Ph.D.

See also Arteriosclerosis; Bariatric surgery; Cholesterol; Cushing's syndrome; Diabetes mellitus; Eating disorders; Endocrine disorders; Endocrinology; Exercise physiology; Glands; Heart disease; Hormones; Hyperadiposis; Hypercholesterolemia; Hyperlipidemia; Hypertension; Malnutrition; Metabolic syndrome; Metabolism; Nutrition; Obesity, childhood; Prader-Willi syndrome; Sleep apnea; Thyroid disorders; Weight loss and gain; Weight loss medications.

FOR FURTHER INFORMATION:

American Academy of Pediatrics. *A Parent's Guide to Childhood Obesity: A Roadmap to Health.* Edited by Sandra G. Hassink. Elk Grove Village, Ill.: Author, 2006. A research-based book that gives parents an authoritative yet practical guide to understanding and preventing obesity, including self-assessment inventories, preparing nutritious meals, and coping with challenges.

American Obesity Association. http://www.obesity .org. A comprehensive Web site with information on the disease, research resources, advocacy, disability issues, community action, and personal stories, among many other topics.

Björntorp, Per, ed. *International Textbook of Obesity.* New York: Wiley, 2001. Text that examines all aspects of obesity, from basic considerations of metabolism, body composition, and etiology, to practical questions of the psychological and medical consequences and the various methods of treatment.

Brownell, Kelly D., and Katherine Battle Horgen. *Food Fight: The Inside Story of America's Obesity Crisis and What We Can Do About It.* New York: McGraw-Hill, 2004. A critical examination of the United States' "toxic environment" of obesity. Explores the roots of the obesity epidemic and its impact on the country's health and productivity.

Koplan, Jeffrey P., Catharyn T. Liverman, and Vivica I. Kraak, eds. *Preventing Childhood Obesity: Health in the Balance.* Washington, D.C.: National Academies Press, 2005. Examines the factors that contribute to childhood obesity and outlines a prevention program.

Ravussin, Eric, and Albert J. Stunkard. *Handbook of Obesity Treatment.* New York: Guilford Press, 2004. A comprehensive text that examines the epidemiology, prevalence, and health consequences of obesity. Topics include binge-eating disorder and night-eating syndrome, energy metabolism, genetics, exercise, behavioral weight control, drug and surgical treatment, and treatment in minorities and children.

Wadden, Thomas A., and Albert J. Stunkard, eds. *Handbook of Obesity Treatment.* Rev. ed. New York: Guilford Press, 2004. Designed for nonspecialist clinicians. Discusses the basic science aspects and treatment of obesity. Includes psychological aspects, an analysis of popular diets, possible obstetrical problems, and cultural issues.

Obesity, childhood

Disease/disorder

Anatomy or system affected: Abdomen, blood vessels, circulatory system, endocrine system, gastrointestinal system, heart, intestines, joints, psychic-emotional system, respiratory system, stomach

Specialties and related fields: Endocrinology, family medicine, internal medicine, nutrition, pediatrics, psychiatry, psychology, public health

Definition: Having a body mass index (BMI) at or above the 95th percentile for children of the same age and sex. Rapid changes from infancy through adolescence are part of normal and expected development, and the norm used to identify childhood obesity must be correct for that child's age and sex.

Key terms:

adipose tissue: a type of fat storage cell constellation that is also involved in energy regulation and hormone release

body mass index (BMI): a formula that estimates the percentage of body fat compared to overall weight; usually expressed in metrics, a person's weight in kilograms divided by height in meters, squared (kg/m^2)

hormones: chemical signaling substances in the bloodstream that foster communication between individual organs and the rest of the body

metabolic syndrome: a cluster of traits that can include obesity, high blood pressure, abnormal lipid levels, and high insulin levels in blood; their presence often marks the first phase of more serious diseases

Causes and Symptoms

A chronic or recurrent imbalance between energy expended (how active one is) and energy ingested (how much one eats and drinks) will promote ill health. When ingestion regularly exceeds expenditure, the unused energy is stored in adipose tissue, or body fat. Animal species that developed the capacity to store fat had a better chance of surviving times of scarcity. Chronic storage of excessive energy, as commonly occurs when high levels of physical activity are less and less necessary for survival, produces its own physical pathology. Almost every person who eats and drinks more than he or she uses in energy (usually calculated in calories) will produce adipose tissue to store the excess energy.

Peptide hormones such as leptin and adiponectin regulate and balance energy expended with energy ingested. When leptin is absent (leptin deficiency), massive obesity is present; this condition improves when

people are given leptin. Adiponectin, the most abundant hormone in fat cells, is also an insulin sensitizer and an anti-inflammatory signaler. Leptin and adiponectin, along with other peptide hormones, initiate a series of signaling processes that eventually lead to signaling hormones that turn on the food-seeking abilities of organs and muscles.

The formal definition of obesity in children is a BMI greater than or equal to the 95th percentile. Children between the 85th and 95th percentiles are at risk for obesity; those less than the 85th percentile are generally considered to have normal weight when correlated with their height.

Childhood obesity has many detrimental effects and comorbidities (other diseases and disorders) that often extend into adolescence and adulthood. It is simplistic to say that obese children will become obese adults. Still, childhood obesity often produces a metabolic syndrome that children easily bring into adolescence and adulthood. This syndrome has serious implications for quality of life and life expectancy. Metabolic syndrome is a combination of high insulin levels (hyperinsulinemia), obesity, high blood pressure (hypertension), and abnormal lipid levels (dyslipidemia). More than one million American adolescents have it. Metabolic syndrome initiates a process that leads to an excess of insulin production that, in turn, promotes high blood pressure and dyslipidemia. Together, these produce aortic and coronary atherosclerosis (hardening of the arteries) and clogging of the arteries by fatty deposits in the blood.

Genetic factors play a fundamental role in childhood obesity, as genetically obese families illustrate. People cannot exchange the genes that they have inherited, but environmental factors are also important, as they are the only ones where management is possible.

The psychosocial impact of childhood obesity is no

Information on Childhood Obesity

Causes: May include poor diet, lack of exercise, genetic factors

Symptoms: Excessive weight relative to age and height, possibly leading to health problems and adult obesity

Duration: Often chronic

Treatments: Improved diet and increased activity

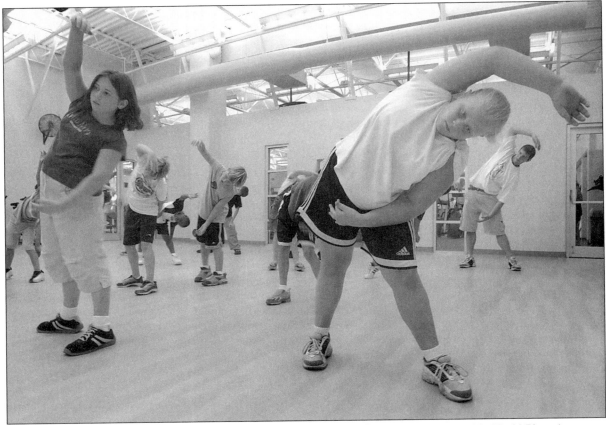

Children take part in a summer program designed to fight childhood obesity. (AP/Wide World Photos)

less serious than physical syndromes, leading to poor body image, low self-confidence, social isolation, recurrent anger, early forms of eating disorders, clinical depression, and negatively acting-out in school and other social settings. Obese children are more likely to become underachievers who are underactive, less popular, and unhappy. Promoting physical activity is an important intervention to lessen the psychological harm of obesity as much as is controlling the amount and type of food and drink.

TREATMENT AND THERAPY

The most effective treatment for child obesity is prevention, and it can begin shortly after birth. Research shows that breast-fed children have significantly lower rates of obesity in later years. All children must gain weight as they grow, and having an adequate amount of fat cells during early antenatal development is critically important for maximal growth of key organs. Baby fat is important; its absence is problematic. As infants become toddlers and toddlers become children, the differ-ence between healthy weight gains and weight gains that suggest the onset of obesity often require the expert eye of a pediatrician or family physician. A healthy five-pound weight gain in one five-year-old child may not be healthy in another child of the same age.

It is not until adolescence that children play a signifi-cant role in choosing and purchasing food. Until then, whatever children eat is most likely what adults have purchased or provided. Preventing obesity and correct-ing it when it occurs requires thoughtful selection of food and beverage items at home and school. Fast and take-out foods are always an easy solution to busy, hectic family schedules, but they are almost always obesity-promoting. Junk food snacks, also a quick so-lution to the transient hunger pangs of youth, are simi-larly harmful.

Prevention and treatment are almost one and the same in dealing with child obesity. Parents control the food world of children, and making available a vari-ety of healthy choices becomes an important part of achieving and maintaining healthy bodies that have modest amounts of adipose tissue, as children with a BMI of less than 20 are also unhealthy. Obesity is much less likely to occur in families and schools that support healthy lifestyles: balanced nutritional consumption, physical activity and exercise, and sufficient sleep. (As a group, children who consistently get less sleep than they need are more likely to be obese than are children who sleep enough. The specific number of hours any child might need is a function of several factors, including age.)

Successful school-based interventions in the management of obesity include a prioritization of physical education classes, healthy choices on the student menu and in vending machines, proportional servings, encouraging water as the main beverage, and the ready availability of after-school activities that involve physical activity, such as intramural sports. When these elements are not present, effective obesity management for school-age children is difficult.

The key to successful long-term obesity prevention and treatment involves awareness of and respect for the individual child's personal preferences and enjoyments—nothing will enhance motivation more. Decreasing sitting time and the active encouragement of free play is far more effective than mandates to exercise or reduce food intake. Even in families where genetics play a major role in obesity, a healthy lifestyle will decrease the negative impact that obesity can have on the children's overall health.

PERSPECTIVE AND PROSPECTS

Childhood obesity is a still-growing epidemic that has achieved the status of a public health crisis. Obesity has profound impacts on children's long-term physical and psychological health and, more often than not, leads to serious comorbidities in adulthood that are costly to treat and difficult to control. Focused strategies on modifying behavior and the slow but steady acquisition of healthy habits are the only ways that children will reliably manage the balance between calories consumed and calories burned. Adult habits, good and bad, are usually fostered during childhood. They reflect the level of care, attention, and perseverance of caregivers. Childhood obesity can be a problem of adults' mismanagement much more than it is a problem of children's choices. Parents and teachers make a major contribution to children when they provide a health-oriented environment in which children are more likely to acquire the habits that promote wellness throughout their lives.

—Paul Moglia, Ph.D., and Kenneth Dill, M.D.

See also Bariatric surgery; Cholesterol; Diabetes mellitus; Eating disorders; Endocrine disorders; Endocrinology; Exercise physiology; Glands; Heart disease; Hormones; Hyperadiposis; Hypercholesterolemia; Hyperlipidemia; Hypertension; Malnutrition; Metabolic syndrome; Metabolism; Nutrition; Obesity; Thyroid disorders; Weight loss and gain; Weight loss medications.

FOR FURTHER INFORMATION:

Berg, Frances. *Underage and Overweight: America's Childhood Obesity Epidemic—What Every Parent Needs to Know.* New York: Random House, 2005.

Okie, Susan. *Fed Up! Winning the War Against Childhood Obesity.* Washington, D.C.: National Academies Press, 2005.

Sothern, Melinda S., Heidi Schumacher, and T. Kristian von Almen. *Trim Kids: The Proven Twelve-Week Plan That Has Helped Thousands of Children Achieve a Healthier Weight.* New York: HarperCollins, 2003.

OBSESSIVE-COMPULSIVE DISORDER

DISEASE/DISORDER

ANATOMY OR SYSTEM AFFECTED: Psychic-emotional system

SPECIALTIES AND RELATED FIELDS: Psychiatry, psychology

DEFINITION: An anxiety disorder characterized by intrusive and unwanted but uncontrollable thoughts, by the need to perform ritualized behavior patterns, or both; the obsessions and/or compulsions cause severe stress, consume an excessive amount of time, and greatly interfere with a person's normal routine, activities, or relationships.

KEY TERMS:

anal stage: the stage of psychosexual development in which a child derives pleasure from activities associated with elimination

anxiety: an unpleasant feeling of fear and apprehension

biogenic model: the theory that every mental disorder is based on a physical or physiological problem

major affective disorder: a personality disorder characterized by mood disturbances

monoamine oxidase inhibitors: antidepressant compounds used to restore the balance of normal neurotransmitters in the brain

phobia: a strong, persistent, and unwarranted fear of a specific object or situation

selective serotonin reuptake inhibitors (SSRIs): primary medications used for obsessive-compulsive disorder

Tourette's syndrome: a childhood disorder characterized by several motor and verbal tics that may develop into the compulsion to shout obscenities

tricyclics: medications used to relieve the symptoms of depression

Causes and Symptoms

Obsessive-compulsive disorder (OCD) is an anxiety disorder characterized by intrusive and uncontrollable thoughts and/or by the need to perform specific acts repeatedly. Obsessive-compulsive behavior is highly distressing because one's behavior or thoughts are no longer voluntarily controlled. The more frequently these uncontrolled alien and perhaps unacceptable thoughts or actions are performed, the more distress is induced. A disturbed individual may have either obsessions (which are thought-related) or compulsions (which are action-related), or both. At various stages of the disorder, one of the symptoms may replace the other.

OCD affects 1 to 2 percent of the population; most of those afflicted begin suffering from the disorder in early adulthood, and it is often preceded by a particularly stressful event such as pregnancy, childbirth, or family conflict. It may be closely associated with depression, with the disorder developing soon after a bout of depression or the depression developing as a result of the disorder. OCD affects men and women equally.

Obsessions generally fall into one of five recognized categories. Obsessive doubts are persistent doubts that a task has been completed; the individual is unwilling to accept and believe that the work is done satisfactorily. Obsessive thinking is an almost infinite chain of thought, targeting future events. Obsessive impulses are very strong urges to perform certain actions, whether they be trivial or serious, that would likely be harmful to the obsessive person or someone else and that are socially unacceptable. Obsessive fears are thoughts that the person has lost control and will act in some way that will cause public embarrassment. Obsessive images are continued visual pictures of either a real or an imagined event.

Four factors are commonly associated with obsessive characteristics, not only in people with OCD but in the general population as well. First, obsessive individuals are unable to control their mental processes completely. Practically, this means the loss of control over thinking processes, such as intrusive thoughts of a loved one dying or worries about hurting someone unintentionally. Second, there may be thoughts and worries over the potential loss of motor control, perhaps causing impulses such as shouting obscenities in church or school or performing inappropriate sexual acts. Third, many obsessive individuals may be afraid of contamination and suffer irrational fear and worry over exposure to germs, dirt, or diseases. The last factor is checking behavior, or backtracking previous actions to ensure that the behavior was done properly, such as checking that doors and windows are shut, faucets are turned off, and so on. Some common obsessions are fear of having decaying teeth or food particles between the teeth, worry about whether the sufferer has touched germs, and fear of contracting a sexually transmitted disease.

Compulsions may be either mild or severe and debilitating. Mild compulsions might be superstitions, such as refusing to walk under a ladder or throwing salt over one's shoulder. Severe compulsions become fixed, unvaried ritualized behaviors; if they are not practiced precisely in a particular manner or a prescribed number of times, then intense anxiety may result. These strange behaviors may be rooted in superstition; many of those suffering from the disorder believe that performing the behavior may ward off danger. Compulsive acts are not ends in themselves but are "necessary" to produce or prevent a future event from occurring. Although the enactment of the ritual may assuage tension, the act does not give the compulsive pleasure.

Several kinds of rituals are typically enacted. A common ritual is repeating; these sufferers must do everything by numbers. Checking is another compulsive act; a compulsive checker believes that it is necessary to check and recheck that everything is in order. Cleaning is a behavior in which many compulsives must engage; they may wash and scrub repeatedly, especially if they think that they have touched something dirty. A fourth common compulsive action is avoidance; for certain superstitious or magical reasons, certain objects must be avoided. Some individuals with compulsions experience compelling urges for perfection in even the most trivial of tasks; often the task is repeated to ensure that it has been done correctly. Some determine that objects must be in a particular arrangement; these individuals are considered "meticulous." A few sufferers are hoarders; they are unable to throw away trash or rubbish. All these individuals have a constant need for reassurance; for example, they want to be told repeatedly that they have not been contaminated.

No single cause for OCD has been isolated. Several theories provide some examples of attempts to explain the basis of OCD psychologically. They involve guilt, anxiety, and superstition. Sigmund Freud first proposed that obsessive thoughts are a replacement for more disturbing thoughts or actions that induce guilt in the sufferer. These thoughts or behaviors, according to Freud, are usually sexual in nature. Freud based his ideas on the cases of some of his young patients. In the case of a teenage girl, for example, he determined that she exchanged obsessive thoughts of stealing for the act of masturbation. The thoughts of stealing produced far fewer guilt feelings than masturbation did. Replacing guilt feelings with less threatening thoughts prevents one's personal defenses from being overwhelmed. Other defense mechanisms may be parlayed into OCD. Undoing, one of these behaviors, is obliterating guilt-producing urges by undergoing repetitive rituals, such as handwashing. Since the forbidden urges continue to recur, the behavior to replace those urges must continue. These behaviors are then negatively reinforced because anxiety decreases when the behavior is performed, thereby maintaining the behavior. Another mechanism is reaction formation. When an unacceptable thought or urge is present, the sufferer replaces it with an exactly opposite behavior. Many theorists believe that both obsessive and compulsive behaviors arise as a consequence of overly harsh toilet training. Thus the person is fixated at the anal stage and, by reaction formation, resists the urge to soil by becoming overly neat and clean. A third mechanism is isolation, the separation of a thought or action from its effect. Detachment or aloofness may isolate an individual from aggressive or sexual thoughts.

The superstition hypothesis proposes a connection between a chance association and a reinforcer that induces a continuation of the behavior. Many theorists believe that the same sequence is involved in the formation of many superstitions. A particular obsessive-compulsive ritual may be reinforced when a positive outcome follows the behavior; anxiety results when the ritual is interrupted. An example would be a student who only uses one special pencil or pen to take exams, based on a previous good grade. In actuality, there is seldom a real relationship between the behavior and the outcome. This hypothesis, too, fails to explain the development of obsessions.

Another theory is accepted by those who believe that mental disorders are the result of something physically or physiologically amiss in the sufferer, employing data from brain structure studies, genetics, and biochemistry. Indeed, brain activity is altered in those suffering from OCD, and they experience increased metabolic activity. Whether the activity is a cause or an effect, however, is unclear. Studies of genetics in families, at least in twins, reinforce the idea that genetics may play a small role in OCD because there appears to be a higher incidence of the disorder in identical twins than in other siblings. Yet these results may be misleading: Because all the studies were carried out on twins who were reared together, environment must also be considered as a contributing cause. It should be noted, however, that relatives of OCD sufferers are twice as likely as unrelated individuals to develop the same disorder, indicating that the tendency for the behavior could be heritable.

Treatment and Therapy

Obsessional symptoms are not uncommon in the general population, and approximately 2.2 million Americans have been diagnosed with OCD. Many people, however, are too horrified to admit to their symptoms, or they do not realize that their behavior is abnormal and do not seek treatment.

Diagnostic techniques evaluating OCD usually involve psychological evaluation. It is important to determine whether an individual is actually suffering from OCD or other potential problems such as schizophrenia or a mood disorder. Additionally, it is important to determine whether more than one disorder is present. OCD may occur in conjunction with other disorders, such as substance use disorders, eating disorders, and mood disorders. When this occurs, treatment must be adjusted. For example, when depression is also noted, both disorders must be treated.

In cases where differentiation is required between OCD and schizophrenia, the concern is to understand the nature of the dysfunctional thoughts and behaviors. For instance, a distinction can be made by determining the motive behind the ritualized behavior. Stereotyped behaviors are symptomatic of both disorders. In the person with schizophrenia, however, the behavior is triggered by delusions rather than by true compulsions. People suffering from true delusions cannot be shaken from them. They do not resist the ideas inundating their minds, and ritualized behavior does not necessarily decrease the feelings associated with the intrusive ideas. On the other hand, obsessive people usually experience decreases in anxiety when they perform their rituals and may be absolutely certain of the need to perform their rituals, though other aspects of their thinking and logic are perfectly clear. They generally resist the ideas that enter their minds and realize the absurdity or abnormality of the thoughts to some extent. As thoughts and images intrude into the obsessive person's mind, the person may sometimes appear to have symptoms that mimic schizophrenia.

Other problems having symptoms in common with OCD are Tourette's syndrome and stimulant use. What seems to separate the symptoms of these disorders from those experienced with OCD is that the former are organically induced. Thus, the actions of a sufferer from Tourette's syndrome may be mechanical since they are not intellectually dictated or purposely enacted. In the case of the stimulant user, the acts may bring pleasure and are not resisted, but reinforced by the drug effects.

"Normal" people also have obsessive thoughts; in fact, the obsessions of normal individuals are not significantly different from the obsessions of those with OCD. The major difference is that those with the disorder have longer-lasting, more intense, and less easily dismissed obsessive thoughts. The importance of this overlap is that mere symptoms are not a reliable tool to diagnose OCD, since some of the same symptoms are experienced by the general population.

Assessment of OCD separates the obsessive from the compulsive components so that each can be examined. Obsession assessment should determine the triggering fears of the disorder, both internal and external, including thoughts of unpleasant consequences. The amount of anxiety that these obsessions produce should be monitored. The compulsive behaviors then should be examined in the same light.

The greatest chance for successful treatment occurs with individuals who experience mild symptoms that are usually obsessive but not compulsive in nature, who seek help soon after the onset of symptoms, and who had few problems before the disorder began. While OCD can be challenging to treat, many valuable and successful treatment strategies are available. Types of treatment fall into four categories: psychotherapy, behavioral therapy, drug therapy, and psychosurgery. The treatments of choice tend to be behavioral and drug therapies.

When psychotherapy is attempted, it usually begins with some type of analysis. The degree of dysfunction, the stressor triggering the symptoms, and the psychological makeup of the individual often determine whether the analysis will be successful. The major goal of a more psychoanalytical approach is to find and then remove an assumed repression so that the individual can deal with whatever they fear in an open and honest fashion. Some analysts believe that focusing on the present is most beneficial, since delving into the past may strengthen the defensive mechanism (the compulsive behavior). If the patient attempts to "return" to the mitigating event, then the analyst usually intervenes directly and actively and brings the individual back to the present by encouraging, pressuring, and guiding him or her.

The most effective treatment for controlling OCD is the behavioral approach. Behavioral therapy focuses on breaking the connection between the stimulus (what induces the compulsion or obsession) and the compulsions and obsessions. Response prevention involves two stages. First, the individual is subject to flooding, the act of exposing the individual to the real and/or imagined stimuli that cause anxiety. This process begins with brief exposure to the stressors while the therapist assesses the individuals's thoughts, feelings, and behaviors during the stimulus period. In the second stage, the individual is flooded with the stimuli but restrained from acting on those stressors. Although flooding may produce intense discomfort at first, patients are gradually desensitized to the stimuli, causing the resulting anxiety to decrease. The therapist must expend considerable time preventing the response, discussing the anxiety as it appears, and supporting the person as the anxiety abates. To be more effective, treatment may also occur in the home with the guidance and support of family members who have been informed about how best to interact with the person needing treatment. Therapists may also help the person break the connection between triggers and responses by aiding the individual in replacing the symptoms of the obsession or compulsion with healthier preventive or replacement actions. Similarly, aversive methods may be used to break the chain of behavior. They might include a nonvocal, internal shout of "Stop!" The action of snapping a rubber band on the wrist when the obsessive thoughts enter the mind or physically restraining oneself if the compulsive action begins may also be helpful. This latter approach may be so uncomfortable and disconcerting to the patient that it may work only under the supervision supplied by a hospital. With any of these approaches, however, if the individual is also depressed or has other complicating conditions, then successful treatment will require additional steps.

Drugs commonly used to treat OCD that have met with some success include selective serotonin reuptake inhibitors (SSRIs), antidepressants, tricyclics, monoamine oxidase inhibitors, LSD, and tryptophan. SSRIs often have remarkable effects on OCD, helping individuals to experience a change in their thinking and behavior, as well as relief. They are usually the first line of treatment in addressing OCD through drug therapy. Psychiatrists also may prescribe tranquilizers to reduce the client's anxiety; however, these drugs are usually not adequate to depress the frequent obsessive thoughts or compulsive actions and so are not a treatment of choice. More general antidepressants may benefit those suffering from depression as well as OCD. It has also been observed that as depression lifts, some of the compulsive behavior may also decrease. Monoamine oxidase inhibitors (MAOIs), another form of antidepressants, are used in treating OCD associated with panic attacks, phobias, and severe anxiety. When medication is halted, however, the patient often relapses into the previous obsessive-compulsive state, so these too are not necessarily a treatment of choice. Drugs such as tryptophan may provide some relief through its affects on melatonin. Similarly, LSD and other hallucinogenic drugs have been tested as potential treatments for this condition because of their effects on serotonin receptors; however, their status as illicit drugs and the significant side effects from other aspects of the actions of these substances do not make them practically useful.

Some psychosurgeons may resort to psychosurgery to relieve a patient's symptoms. The improvement noted after surgery may simply be attributable to the loss of emotion and dulling of behavioral patterns found in any patient who has undergone a lobotomy. Because such surgery may result in a change in the patient's intellect and emotional response, it should be considered only in extreme, debilitating cases. Newer surgical techniques

do not destroy as much of the cerebral cortex. These procedures separate the frontal cortex from lower brain areas in only an 8-centimeter square area.

PERSPECTIVE AND PROSPECTS

Descriptions of OCD-like behavior go back to medieval times; a young man who could not control his urge to stick out his tongue or blurt out obscenities during prayer was reported in the fifteenth century. Medical accounts of the disorder and the term "obsessive-compulsive" originated in the mid-nineteenth century. At that time, obsessions were believed to occur when mental energy ran low. Later, Freud stated that OCD was accompanied by stubbornness, stinginess, and tidiness. He attributed the characteristics to a regression to early childhood, when there are perhaps strong urges to be violent and/or to dirty and mess one's surroundings. To avoid acting on these tendencies, he theorized, an avoidance mechanism is employed, and the symptoms of obsession and/or compulsion appear. Other features related to this regression are ambivalence, magical thinking, and a harsh, punitive conscience.

An unpleasant consequence of OCD behavior is the effect that the behavior has on the people who interact with the sufferer. The relationships with an obsessive person's family, schoolmates, or coworkers all suffer when a person with OCD takes up time with uncontrollable and lengthy rituals. These people may feel not only a justifiable concern but also resentment. Some may feel guilt over the resentful feelings because they know the obsessive-compulsive cannot control these actions. An obsessive-compulsive observing these conflicting feelings in others may respond by developing depression or other anxious feelings, which may cause further alienation.

Although not totally disabling, OCD behaviors can be strongly incapacitating. A famous figure who suffered from OCD was millionaire and aviator Howard Hughes (1905-1976). A recluse after 1950, he became so withdrawn from the public that he communicated only via telephone and intermediaries. His obsession-compulsion was the irrational fear of germs and contamination. It began with his refusal to shake hands with people. If he had to hold a glass or open a door, he covered his hand with a tissue. He would not abide any of his aides eating foods that gave them bad breath. He disallowed air conditioners, believing that they collected germs. Because Hughes acted on his obsessions, they became compulsions.

Most parents will agree that children commonly

have rituals to which they must adhere or compulsive actions they carry out. A particular bedtime story may be read every night for months on end, and children's games involve counting or checking rituals. It is also not atypical for adults without psychiatric disorders to experience some mild obsessive thoughts or compulsive actions, as seen in an overly tidy person or in group rituals performed in some religious sects. Excessively stressful events may trigger obsessions as well.

Further research into the biopsychosocial causes of OCD will be important in developing future treatment approaches. Such causes and treatment may also be useful for understanding other behaviors that have compulsive features, such as problems related to substance use, gambling, eating, and sexual behavior.

—Iona C. Baldridge;
updated by Nancy A. Piotrowski, Ph.D.

See also Addiction; Anorexia nervosa; Antianxiety drugs; Anxiety; Bipolar disorders; Bulimia; Depression; Eating disorders; Grief and guilt; Neurosis; Panic attacks; Paranoia; Phobias; Post-traumatic stress disorder; Psychiatric disorders; Psychiatry; Psychiatry, child and adolescent; Psychiatry, geriatric; Psychoanalysis; Schizophrenia; Stress; Tics.

FOR FURTHER INFORMATION:

American Psychiatric Association. *Diagnostic and Statistical Manual of Mental Disorders: DSM-IV-TR.* 4th ed. Arlington, Va.: Author, 2000. The bible of the psychiatric community, this is a compendium of descriptions of disorders and diagnostic criteria widely embraced by clinicians. Included is an extensive glossary of technical terms, making this volume easy to understand.

Barlow, David H. *Anxiety and Its Disorders.* 2d ed. New York: Guilford Press, 2004. Examines the subject in the context of recent developments in emotion theory, cognitive science, and neuroscience. Reviews the implications for treatment and integrates them into newly developed treatment protocols for the various anxiety disorders.

_____, ed. *Clinical Handbook of Psychological Disorders.* 3d ed. New York: Guilford Press, 2001. This collection defines and describes psychological disorders and uses case histories as illustrations for treatment. The chapter on OCD provides a series of tests that can be given to determine the presence and severity of this disorder.

Kring, Ann M., et al. *Abnormal Psychology.* 11th ed. Hoboken, N.J.: John Wiley & Sons, 2010. This college text addresses the causes of psychopathology and treatments commonly used to treat various disorders. The book is well organized, readable, and interesting. An extensive reference list and a glossary are included.

Menzies, Ross, and Padmal de Silva, eds. *Obsessive Compulsive Disorder: Theory, Research, and Treatment.* New York: Wiley, 2003. Authored by international experts on OCD, this text covers recent research and theories; treatment, focusing mainly on cognitive therapy methods; and the nature of a wide range of subtypes of OCD.

Obsessive-Compulsive Foundation (OCD). http://www.ocfoundation.org. A group that educates the public and professional communities about OCD and related disorders, provides assistance to individuals with OCD and their family and friends, and funds research into causes and effective treatments.

Oltmanns, Thomas F., et al. *Case Studies in Abnormal Psychology.* 8th ed. Hoboken, N.J.: John Wiley & Sons, 2009. A sample of clinical case histories of abnormal psychology. Included are descriptions of a given disorder, ways to view and treat the disease, and the origin and causes of the disease.

OBSTETRICS

SPECIALTY

ANATOMY OR SYSTEM AFFECTED: Reproductive system, uterus

SPECIALTIES AND RELATED FIELDS: Embryology, genetics, gynecology, neonatology, perinatology

DEFINITION: The medical science dealing with pregnancy and childbirth, including the health of both mother and unborn infant and the delivery of the child and the placenta at the time of birth.

KEY TERMS:

amniocentesis: a technique by which a fine needle is inserted through a pregnant woman's abdomen and into the uterus and amniotic sac in order to collect fetal amniotic cells for biochemical and genetic analysis

birth defect: a genetic or developmental abnormality which occurs in utero that leads to anatomic or functional problems after birth; the defect can be serious, with potentially significant consequences for the fetus or mother, or the defect can be minor

cesarean section: a surgical procedure whereby the infant is delivered through an incision on the mother's abdomen

forceps: curved metal blades that are carefully placed

around the fetal head through the vagina to facilitate delivery

gestation: the period from conception to birth, in which the fetus reaches full development in order to survive outside the mother's body

placenta: an organ in the uterus through which the fetus receives its oxygen and nutrients and removes its waste products; it serves as a blood barrier between the mother's circulatory system and the fetal circulatory system

Rh0(D) immune globulin: also known as RhoGAM; a type of gamma globulin protein injected into Rh-negative mothers who may have an Rh-positive fetus to protect the fetus from an immune reaction called isoimmunization

trimester: one of three periods of time in pregnancy, each period lasting three months; the first trimester is zero to twelve weeks of gestational age, the second trimester is thirteen to twenty-four weeks of gestational age, and the third trimester is twenty-five to thirty-seven weeks of gestational age

ultrasonography: an imaging modality in which sound waves penetrate bodily tissues in order to generate an image; in obstetrics, this technique is commonly used to assess the fetus, amniotic fluid, and uterus and ovaries

vacuum: a device with a suction cup that is applied to the fetal head through the vagina to assist in delivery of the infant

SCIENCE AND PROFESSION

Obstetrics is the branch of medical science dealing with pregnancy and childbirth in women. Once conception has occurred and a woman is pregnant, major physiological changes occur within her body as well as within the body of the developing embryo or fetus. Obstetrics deals with these changes leading up to and including childbirth. As such, obstetrics is a critical branch of medicine, for it involves the complex physiological events by which every person comes into existence.

The professional obstetrician is a licensed medical doctor whose area of expertise is pregnancy and childbirth. Often, the obstetrician is also a specialist in the closely related science of gynecology, the study of diseases and conditions that specifically affect women, particularly nonpregnant women. The obstetrician is especially knowledgeable in female anatomy and physiology, including the major bodily changes that occur during and following pregnancies. Obstetricians also have a detailed understanding of the necessary diag-

nostic procedures for monitoring fetal and maternal health, and they are educated in the latest technologies for facilitating a successful pregnancy and childbirth with minimal complications. Obstetrical care is also provided by certified nurse midwives (C.N.M.'s) and by nurse practitioners, particularly those with certification in women's health (women's health care nurse practitioners).

Broadly, the diseases and conditions managed by the clinicians in this field include preconception counseling, normal prenatal care, and the management of pregnancy-specific problems such as preeclampsia, gestational diabetes, premature labor, premature rupture of membranes, multiple gestations, fetal growth problems, and isoimmunization. In addition, obstetricians manage medical problems that can occur in any woman but that take on special importance in pregnancy, such as thyroid disorders or infections. Obstetricians make assessments and decisions regarding when a baby is best delivered, particularly if there are in utero conditions that make it safer for the baby to be born immediately, even if prematurely. Obstetricians manage both normal and abnormal labors. They are able to assess the progress and position of the infant as it makes its way down the birth canal. They are knowledgeable about pain control options during labor and make decisions regarding when a cesarean section is indicated. Obstetricians assist with normal vaginal deliveries, either spontaneous or induced, and sometimes use special instruments such as forceps or vacuum-suction devices. They also perform cesarean sections. Obstetricians are trained in appropriate postpartum care for the mother and infant.

In natural, spontaneous fertilization, pregnancy begins with the fertilization of a woman's egg by a man's sperm following sexual intercourse, the chances of which are highest if intercourse takes place during a two-day period following ovulation. Ovulation is the release of an unfertilized egg from the woman's ovarian follicle, which occurs roughly halfway between successive periods during her menstrual cycle. Fertilization usually occurs in the upper one-third of one of the woman's Fallopian tubes connecting the ovary to the uterus; upon entering the woman's vagina, sperm must travel through her cervix to the uterus and up the Fallopian tubes, only one of which contains a released egg following ovulation.

Once fertilization has occurred, the first cell of the new individual, called a zygote, is slowly pushed by cilia down the Fallopian tube and into the uterus. Along the way, the zygote undergoes several mitotic cellular divisions to begin the newly formed embryo, which at this point is a bundle of undifferentiated cells. Upon reaching the uterus, the embryo implants in the lining of the uterus. Hormonal changes occur in the woman's body to maintain the pregnancy. One of these hormones is human chorionic gonadotropin, which is the chemical detected by most pregnancy tests. Failure of the embryo to be implanted in the endometrium and subsequent lack of hormone production (specifically the hormone progesterone) will cause release of the endometrium as a bloody discharge; the woman will menstruate, and there will be no pregnancy. Therefore, menstrual cycles do not occur during a pregnancy.

The embryo will grow and develop over the next nine to ten months of gestation. The heart forms and begins beating at roughly five and one-half weeks following conception. Over the next several weeks and months, major organ systems begin to organize and develop. By the end of the first three months of the pregnancy, the developing human is considered to be a fetus. All the major organ systems have formed, although not all systems can function yet. The fetus is surrounded by a watery amniotic fluid within an amniotic sac. The fetus receives oxygen and nutrients from the mother and excretes waste products into the maternal circulation through the placenta. The fetus is connected to the placenta via the umbilical cord. During the second and third trimesters, full organ system development; massive cell divisions of certain tissues such as nervous, circulatory, and skeletal tissue; and preparation of the fetus for survival as an independent organism occur. The fetus cannot survive outside the mother's body, however, until the third trimester.

Changes also occur in the mother. Increased levels of the female steroid hormone estrogen create increased skin vascularization (that is, more blood vessels near the skin) and the deposition of fat throughout her body, especially in the breasts and the buttocks. The growing fetus and stretching uterus press on surrounding abdominal muscles, often creating abdominal and back discomfort. Reasonable exercise is important for the mother to stay healthy and to deliver the baby with relative ease. A balanced diet also is important for the nourishment of her body and that of the fetus.

Late in the pregnancy, the protein hormones prolactin and oxytocin will be produced by the woman's pituitary gland. Prolactin activates milk production in the breasts. Oxytocin causes muscular contractions, particularly in the breasts and in the uterus during labor.

Near the time of birth, drastically elevated levels of the hormones estrogen and oxytocin will cause progressively stronger contractions (labor pains) until the baby is forced through the vagina and out of the woman's body to begin its independent physical existence. The placenta, or afterbirth, is discharged shortly thereafter.

DIAGNOSTIC AND TREATMENT TECHNIQUES

The role of the obstetrician is to monitor the health of the mother and unborn fetus during the course of the pregnancy and to deliver the baby successfully at the time of birth. Once the fact of the pregnancy is established, the obstetrician is trained to identify specific developmental changes in the fetus over time in order to ensure that the pregnancy is proceeding smoothly.

The mainstay of diagnosis is the physical examination during prenatal visits. Early in the pregnancy, prenatal visits occur monthly, but they become more frequent as the pregnancy progresses. During these visits, the woman may receive counseling regarding a balanced diet, folic acid and iron supplementation, and substances or foods to avoid that may pose a risk to the pregnancy. The woman's growing uterus is measured to confirm proper growth, and, if indicated, a vaginal or cervical examination may be performed. After ten weeks of gestational age, fetal heart tones are also assessed at every prenatal visit using a simplified ultrasonic technique, to ensure that they are within the normal number of beats per minute. Fetal heart tones that are abnormally slow may indicate a fetus in jeopardy.

The other main component of diagnosis is through laboratory tests. Early in the pregnancy, the woman will receive a Pap test to screen for cervical cancer. Blood tests will be ordered to determine whether the mother is a carrier of the human immunodeficiency virus (HIV) or hepatitis B or C viruses, which can be transmitted to the fetus. In addition, the mother is checked for anemia, and the blood type of the mother is assessed. If the mother's blood type indicates that she is Rh negative, she will receive RhoGAM in the third trimester to prevent the development of a disease called isoimmunization, a condition that could be fatal to the fetus. An additional diagnostic test performed routinely during pregnancy is a screening test for diabetes, which pregnant women are at increased risk for.

Another important method of diagnosis in obstetrics is ultrasonography. Ultrasonography early in pregnancy can determine the gestational age of a pregnancy in cases in which a woman's last menstrual period is unverified. The correct development of the fetus and the presence of any birth defects can be assessed using this procedure. Ultrasound can also determine whether the placenta is growing in a safe location and whether the proper amount of amniotic fluid is found in the amniotic sac. Toward the end of pregnancy, ultrasound is an invaluable diagnostic tool for determining fetal well-being and the position of the infant in the uterus in preparation for delivery. Ultrasound is also a useful tool in guiding diagnostic procedures. For instance, amniocentesis can be extremely safe when performed under ultrasound guidance. Finally, one of the main methods of diagnosis in the third trimester is fetal heart monitor-

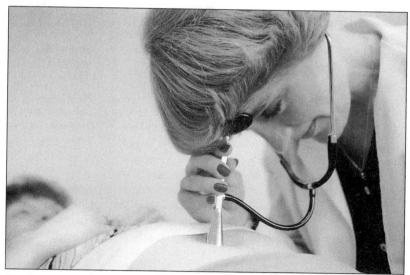

Starting at around twenty weeks of gestation, an obstetrician can usually hear the fetal heartbeat using a special stethoscope called a fetoscope. (PhotoDisc)

ing. This technique involves following the heartbeat of the infant while in utero. The heart rate of the infant is typically followed for twenty to thirty minutes. Any concerning dips in the heart rate may be indicative of a poor fetal state and a cause for increased monitoring or, in extreme cases, delivery of the infant.

Obstetricians have at their disposal a variety of treatment modalities. They are trained to turn manually fetuses that are in a breech (feet-first) position, a procedure called external cephalic version. In cases where the artificial induction of labor is desirable, the obstetrician may employ mechanical or hormonal means of cervical dilation, followed by infusions of a hormone called pitocin to stimulate contractions or the artificial rupture of the amniotic sac to promote natural contractions. When immediate delivery of the infant is needed and the chances of it emerging via the vaginal route are remote, then the obstetrician may perform a cesarean section. Common indications for cesarean section include fetal distress and lack of progress in labor.

Other treatments commonly used by obstetricians include the use of medications such as magnesium to relax the uterus in cases of premature labor and maternal steroid injections to induce fetal lung maturity when the fetus is premature but delivery is anticipated. When a woman experiences difficulty in the final stages of labor and the fetal head has descended almost to the vaginal opening, the obstetrician may employ forceps or vacuum devices to facilitate the delivery, particularly in cases of fetal distress. Obstetricians also treat

the complications associated with childbirth, including postsurgical care after a cesarean section and repair of any lacerations of the vagina, cervix, or rectum after vaginal delivery.

PERSPECTIVE AND PROSPECTS

Obstetrics is central to medicine because it deals with the very process by which all humans come to exist. The health of the fetus and its mother in pregnancy is of primary concern to these doctors. The field of obstetrics has blossomed as a sophisticated specialty, more likely to be practiced by obstetricians, certified nurse midwives, and specially trained and certified nurse practitioners, rather than the general practitioners who used to provide this care.

Advances in medical technology have enabled more precise analysis and monitoring of the fetus inside the mother's uterus, and obstetrics has therefore become a complex specialty in its own right. Technology such as ultrasonography and fetal heart rate monitoring, among other techniques, allows the obstetrician to collect a much larger supply of fetal data than was available to the general practitioner of the 1960's. Increased data availability enables the obstetrician to monitor the pregnancy closely and to identify any problems earlier.

New advances in product development continue to improve the diagnostic ability of obstetricians. One example is the development of a test for fetal fibronection, which enables obstetricians to predict which patients are at low risk of premature delivery. This test involves a simple swab of the upper vagina. When negative, this test is highly reliable and allows the pregnant patient to leave the hospital and avoid prolonged and unnecessary hospitalization.

Advances in prenatal diagnosis and basic science have made it possible for parents to obtain information about their fetuses down to the molecular level. Through techniques such as amniocentesis and chorionic villus sampling (in which a small sample of placental cells is obtained early in pregnancy), genetic analysis has enabled the detection of chromosomal defects responsible for mental retardation and single-gene defects responsible for inherited diseases (such as cystic fibrosis). Amniocentesis has also made it possible to detect biochemical changes that may be indicative of major structural defects in the fetus, as well as to assess the developmental maturity of organs such as the lungs.

Advances in medical practice have dramatically decreased the morbidity and mortality of premature birth. For instance, with the introduction and widespread use of maternal steroid injections, the severity of serious diseases of prematurity, such as respiratory distress syndrome, has been dramatically reduced. The development of drugs against HIV has prevented the transmission of the virus from mother to infant in many cases.

The medical science of obstetrics continues to advance. There is ongoing research into the physiology and basic science of preeclampsia and eclampsia, common and potentially dangerous diseases peculiar to pregnancy. Fetal surgery programs at academic centers open the possibility that serious birth defects may be correctable while the fetus is in utero. Although many controversies currently exist in the field of obstetrics, an increased push toward medical practice grounded in scientific evidence promises many exciting advances in the future. It is hoped that many of these advances will result in improved outcomes and quality of life for patients.

—*David Wason Hollar, Jr., Ph.D.;*
updated by Anne Lynn S. Chang, M.D.

See also Amniocentesis; Assisted reproductive technologies; Birth defects; Breast-feeding; Breasts, female; Cesarean section; Childbirth; Childbirth complications; Chorionic villus sampling; Conception; Congenital disorders; Critical care; Down syndrome; Ectopic pregnancy; Embryology; Emergency medicine; Episiotomy; Family medicine; Fetal alcohol syndrome; Fetal surgery; Gamete intrafallopian transfer

(GIFT); Genetic counseling; Genetic diseases; Genital disorders, female; Gestational diabetes; Gonorrhea; Growth; Gynecology; In vitro fertilization; Incontinence; Miscarriage; Multiple births; Neonatology; Ovaries; Pap test; Perinatology; Placenta; Postpartum depression; Preeclampsia and eclampsia; Pregnancy and gestation; Premature birth; Reproductive system; Rh factor; Rubella; Spina bifida; Stillbirth; Teratogens; Toxoplasmosis; Ultrasonography; Urology; Uterus; Women's health.

FOR FURTHER INFORMATION:

Cohen, Barbara J. *Memmler's The Human Body in Health and Disease.* 11th ed. Philadelphia: Wolters Kluwer Health/Lippincott Williams & Wilkins, 2009. This short but thorough work is an excellent introduction to human anatomy and physiology for the layperson. Chapter 20, "Reproduction," is a concise survey of human reproductive anatomy and processes and of the major events of pregnancy and childbirth.

Gabbe, Steven G., Jennifer R. Niebyl, and Joe Leigh Simpson, eds. *Obstetrics: Normal and Problem Pregnancies.* 5th ed. Philadelphia: Churchill Livingstone/Elsevier, 2007. One of the definitive textbooks on obstetrics. Surveys the entirety of pregnancy, from conception to following childbirth, including sections on female anatomy and physiology. Also describes common and uncommon problems of pregnancy in an easy-to-read, yet complete manner.

Gaudin, Anthony J., and Kenneth C. Jones. *Human Anatomy and Physiology.* New York: Harcourt Brace Jovanovich, 1997. Gaudin and Jones's introductory textbook in human anatomy and physiology is geared toward health science majors, both premedical and prenursing. They describe the subject matter in appropriate detail, with excellent illustrations and supporting material. Chapter 28, "Development and Inheritance," offers a good discussion of the issues confronting obstetricians in their practices.

Harkness, Gail, ed. *Medical-Surgical Nursing: Total Patient Care.* 10th ed. St. Louis, Mo.: Mosby, 1999. A comprehensive introduction to nursing care for various types of patients, ranging from the aged to pregnant women. Covers human reproductive anatomy, diagnostic procedures, ultrasonography, and other important aspects of reproduction and obstetrics.

Limmer, Daniel, et al. *Emergency Care.* 11th ed. Upper Saddle River, N.J.: Pearson/Prentice Hall Health,

2009. A detailed survey of patient care for the training of emergency medical technicians (EMTs) and paramedics. A chapter on childbirth deals with the basics of the birthing process, obstetrics, and problems that may arise during a pregnancy or during birth. An excellent source of basic medical information.

Wallace, Robert A., Gerald P. Sanders, and Robert J. Ferl. *Biology: The Science of Life.* 4th ed. New York: HarperCollins, 1996. Chapter 11, "Going Beyond Mendel," discusses the genetics of Rh incompatibility and RhoGAM. Chapter 43, "Animal Development," describes fetal development in mammals, with an emphasis on human development during the three trimesters.

OBSTRUCTION

DISEASE/DISORDER

ANATOMY OR SYSTEM AFFECTED: Abdomen, gastrointestinal system, intestines

SPECIALTIES AND RELATED FIELDS: Gastroenterology

DEFINITION: Partial or complete closure of the channels through which food normally passes; it may be silent, or it may cause either acute and life-threatening or chronic and debilitating illness.

KEY TERMS:

biliary tract: the series of ducts that drain bile from the liver and gallbladder into the intestine; also called the biliary tree

colon: the large intestine except for the cecum and rectum; includes the ascending colon, transverse colon, descending colon, and sigmoid colon

distal: away from the point of origin; for example, the stomach is distal to the esophagus

endoscopic retrograde cholangiopancreatography: an endoscopic procedure in which dye is injected into the common bile duct and pancreatic ducts for visualization with X rays

endoscopy: the process of passing a fiber-optic instrument into the gastrointestinal tract for visualization; upper endoscopy is also called esophagogastroduodenoscopy, whereas lower endoscopy is called sigmoidoscopy or colonoscopy, depending on how far the scope is inserted

esophagus: the tube that extends from the pharynx to the stomach

gut: the gastrointestinal tract; includes the esophagus, stomach, and small and large intestines

peristalsis: the series of involuntary muscular contractions that propel material along the gastrointestinal tract

proximal: toward the point of origin; for example, the small intestine is proximal to the large intestine

small intestine: the organ that extends from the stomach to the large intestine; its three regions are the duodenum, jejunum, and ileum

CAUSES AND SYMPTOMS

The gastrointestinal (GI) tract runs from the mouth to the anus and includes the throat, esophagus, stomach, small intestine, large intestine, and rectum. Accessory glands whose secretions drain into the GI tract include the liver, gallbladder, and pancreas. Because the GI tract is essentially a hollow tube, its inner channel being called its lumen, it is susceptible to being closed off. The same holds true for the biliary tree, which is a series of ducts draining bile from the liver and gallbladder into the duodenum, and the pancreatic duct, which drains secretions from the pancreas into the duodenum.

Obstruction of the gastrointestinal tract is a blockage severe enough to impair the transit of materials through the lumen. Although often caused by narrowing, that term differs from obstruction in that a narrowing may be without consequences. A partial obstruction is one in which there is still some flow through the narrowing; in complete obstruction, there is no flow.

Obstruction of these organs or ducts may be mechanical or functional. Mechanical obstructions result when a problem arises from within the bowel lumen (intraluminal), from within the wall of the organ (mural), or from something outside the organ causing its lumen to be narrowed (extrinsic). Functional obstructions are caused by some motor abnormality, such as spasm or lack of peristalsis, causing impaired transit of materials.

An example of an intraluminal obstruction is a gallstone occluding the cystic duct. The liver produces bile, a fluid that has various functions including excretion of bilirubin, which is a breakdown product of hemoglobin, the protein inside red blood cells that carries oxygen. Bile also contains bile salts and cholesterol, substances that help break down large fat globules in the duodenum into smaller droplets, initiating fat digestion. Bile from the liver flows through tiny ducts that eventually unite to form the common hepatic duct. The gallbladder, a hollow sac that stores bile, joins the common hepatic duct via the cystic duct; these two ducts unite to form the common bile duct, which drains bile into the duodenum.

If there is excess cholesterol in bile, it tends to form gallstones. These stones most often form in the gallbladder, but they may form in other areas of the biliary tree such as in the common bile duct. If the stones are formed in the gallbladder but do not occlude the cystic duct, bile may still flow in and out of the organ. If the stones become impacted in the cystic duct, however, they cause obstruction to the flow of bile, leading to inflammation of the gallbladder, called acute cholecystitis.

With cystic duct obstruction, the impacted stone and some of the components of bile cause the gallbladder to become inflamed. The inflamed lining secretes fluid into the gallbladder; this fluid cannot escape because the cystic duct is occluded by the gallstone. The accumulating fluid causes the gallbladder to become distended.

This inflamed gallbladder causes abdominal pain that often lasts several hours. It is also associated with nausea, vomiting, and a fever. The fever may be attributable to a bacterial infection of the bile: When not flowing well, bile tends to be a good place for bacteria to multiply. The stones may pass through the cystic duct and occlude the common bile duct. In this situation, there is no route for bile to flow into the duodenum. Therefore it backs up, dilating the common bile duct, and is reabsorbed into the bloodstream. This causes jaundice, or a yellowish pigmentation of the skin; it may be associated with dark-colored urine.

There are ways to distinguish between acute cholecystitis caused by cystic duct obstruction and biliary tract infection (cholangitis) caused by obstruction of the common bile duct. Ultrasonography is excellent for detecting stones in the gallbladder and dilated bile ducts, but it is not as good at detecting stones in the common duct. To detect such stones, endoscopic retrograde cholangiopancreatography (ERCP) may be performed. In this study, an endoscope is passed through the mouth, esophagus, and stomach and into the duodenum. A catheter is inserted into the opening of the common bile duct, and dye is injected. The dye outlines stones in the common bile duct.

An example of a mechanical obstruction caused by a mural process is an esophageal obstruction caused by a cancer which grows from the walls of the esophagus into its lumen. The most common symptom of esophageal obstruction is dysphagia, or a sensation of food sticking in the throat after being swallowed. If food becomes impacted in the narrowed region, it may cause an aching sensation in the chest wall.

INFORMATION ON OBSTRUCTION

CAUSES: Gastrointestinal blockage resulting from disease (e.g., stones) or anatomical defect

SYMPTOMS: Depends on location; may include nausea, pain, vomiting, fever, heartburn

DURATION: Acute or chronic

TREATMENTS: Depends on cause; may include surgery, radiation therapy

---

The obstruction is evaluated with a barium esophagram, in which barium is swallowed and an X ray of the esophagus is taken. It may show findings such as severe narrowing of the lumen of the esophagus. Endoscopy is then performed, which can be used to visualize the area, looking for evidence of cancer, and to take a piece of the lining of the esophagus for evaluation under the microscope.

An example of an extrinsic mechanical obstruction is one caused by scar tissue, or adhesions, compressing a portion of the small intestine. Adhesions may be caused by previous abdominal surgery. If they cause obstruction, the bowel proximal to the obstruction dilates to a diameter that is larger than normal. Its function changes: Normally the small intestine absorbs fluid, whereas in obstruction it secretes fluid. Since intestinal contents cannot pass through the narrowing, vomiting occurs.

Normally, the bacterial content of the small intestinal lumen is kept low because of the continuous flow of contents through it. During small bowel obstruction, this flow is partially or completely diminished, enabling bacteria to overgrow in the small intestine. These bacteria may pass through the wall of the small intestine into the bloodstream, causing a systemic infection or even death.

An example of a functional obstruction is a disorder called chronic intestinal pseudo-obstruction (CIP). The prefix "pseudo" means "false": A pseudo-obstruction is a disorder in gastrointestinal motility that results in diminished peristalsis through the diseased segment of gut, creating an illness similar to a mechanical obstruction but without any occlusion of the lumen. There are a variety of causes of CIP, which can involve the different regions of the gastrointestinal tract. It may occur as part of the spectrum of some systemic diseases, or it may be of unknown cause (idiopathic).

If the esophagus is involved, dysphagia and heartburn are predominant symptoms, resulting from decreased esophageal peristalsis. Everyone experiences occasional reflux, or the backward flow of stomach acid into the esophagus. Normal esophageal peristalsis keeps this acid in the stomach; if peristalsis is diminished, then the acid may cause heartburn. If the stomach and small intestine are involved, symptoms include nausea, vomiting, bloating, and abdominal discomfort. The abdomen may become extremely distended. Since the flow of small intestinal contents is slowed, overgrowth of bacteria that are normally present only in the colon occurs. These bacteria may take up so much vitamin B_{12} in the gut that a deficiency results. Bacterial overgrowth may also cause diarrhea. If the colon is extensively involved and exhibits markedly diminished peristalsis, abdominal distension and constipation result. An abdominal X ray may show that the colon has become very dilated, a condition called megacolon.

TREATMENT AND THERAPY

Obstructions caused by gallstones can be treated in several ways. If the stones are in the gallbladder and are obstructing the cystic duct, surgery is often performed within a day or two. One technique for removing the gallbladder is laparoscopic cholecystectomy, which involves making a small incision in the abdominal wall and inserting an instrument called a laparoscope. The structures of the biliary tree are identified, and dye is injected into the cystic duct to obtain a cholangiogram, an X ray that helps identify where the stones are located. After cholangiography, clips are placed along the cystic duct, and the duct is cut between the clips (similar to cutting the umbilical cord between the ties). Bile and stones are evacuated from the gallbladder, which is then removed. The advantages of laparoscopic cholecystectomy over other surgical approaches are that the laparoscopic approach is less invasive, causes less scarring and less pain, and allows a more rapid recovery.

If the stones are in the common bile duct, one way to remove them is endoscopically. The endoscope is advanced into the duodenum, and the opening of the common bile duct is visualized. An instrument is passed through the endoscope into the opening of the common bile duct. Electrical current is applied, creating a small incision in the opening of the common bile duct. This enlarges the opening, and sometimes bile and stones come gushing out into the duodenum. If the stone is still in the common duct, a balloon-tipped catheter is passed into the common bile duct and advanced up above the stone. The balloon is inflated, and the cathe-

ter is pulled out of the common duct, bringing the stone with it. If this procedure fails, other options include surgery or extracorporeal shock-wave lithotripsy. This involves generating shock waves and focusing them onto the stone, causing it to break into tiny fragments.

Despite progress made in the care of esophageal cancer patients, the overall five-year cure rate did not change from the 1950's to the 1990's. A main treatment goal is to relieve the symptom of dysphagia. This can be done by passing dilators down through the narrowed area, stretching it so that food, saliva, and liquids can pass. Because the tumor is undoubtedly growing, repeated dilations are necessary. This treatment obviously does nothing to reduce the mass of the tumor, but it helps relieve the symptom of dysphagia.

Two treatments aimed at reducing the tumor mass are surgical removal of the tumor and radiation therapy. Before deciding that surgery is a viable option, several factors need to be taken into consideration, including the potential risks of surgery. For example, surgery performed on patients with advanced heart or lung disease has a very high mortality risk. If the tumor involves the lower esophagus, that area can be removed and the stomach can be sewn to the remaining end of the esophagus. This surgery can be dangerous: Mortality rates from the operation range from 2.8 to 17 percent.

Another treatment, which is effective if the tumor is of a specific cell type called a squamous cell carcinoma, is to irradiate the tumor, attempting to kill tumor cells by focusing beams of radiation onto the mass. This procedure produces survival rates that are roughly equal to surgical survival rates and avoids the risk of surgery. The most common way to apply radiation is to focus it onto the chest wall using an external source. The radiation energy penetrates into the area on which it is focused—the esophageal tumor. One complication of radiation therapy is that the radiation, which kills rapidly dividing cells, cannot distinguish between cancer cells and those lining the wall of the esophagus. Therefore the lining of the esophagus may become very inflamed, a condition called radiation esophagitis. Another approach for applying radiation is with a delivery system such as a specialized radioactive device which fits inside the lumen of the esophagus and delivers radiation locally.

Small bowel obstructions can be fatal. Their treatment first consists of generalized care, such as correcting fluid deficits. All oral intake is stopped, and a nasogastric tube, which is a tube inserted into the nose and passed into the stomach, is hooked up to suction to try to decompress the dilated loops of bowel. Since surgery may be imminent, it is important to optimize the functions of various organ systems so that the mortality risk of surgery is minimized. The likelihood of needing surgery depends on whether the obstruction is partial or complete: About 81 percent of partial small bowel obstructions and about 16 percent of complete obstructions resolve without surgery. This likelihood also depends on the cause of obstruction. For example, many partial obstructions resulting from adhesions resolve with conservative treatment, whereas obstructions caused by a loop of intestine twisting at its base, called a volvulus, carry a high probability of needing surgery.

The treatment of CIP is difficult: Nothing is curative, and nothing slows the progression of the diseases causing pseudo-obstruction. The most effective drug for increasing intestinal motility is probably cisapride. Some studies show that it improves symptoms and hastens the transit of material through the gut. Antibiotics to treat bacterial overgrowth in the small intestine are sometimes used in CIP, especially in cases where diarrhea is present. Dietary measures may be somewhat helpful, including lowering fat, lactose, and fiber. Vitamin supplementation may be necessary, especially with injectable vitamin B_{12}.

Occasionally, surgery is helpful in CIP, especially for a localized problem. Because the disease often causes widespread gut involvement, however, surgery will not cure the problem. Nevertheless, when the problem is caused by the lower esophageal sphincter (LES) failing to open properly, creating a distal esophageal obstruction, a myotomy (or cutting of the circular smooth muscle in the LES) may improve dysphagia symptoms. If the stomach or colon is massively dilated, it may need to be removed. Sometimes removal of portions of the small intestine may be helpful. Once abdominal surgery has been performed, it may be difficult to distinguish future attacks of CIP from mechanical bowel obstruction caused by adhesions.

Alternative forms of nutrition may need to be considered. For example, if the disease mainly affects the esophagus and stomach, a feeding tube could be placed into the small intestine. If the gut has such widespread involvement that jejunal feeding would be fruitless, parenteral nutrition, which is the administration of nutrition intravenously, may be necessary.

PERSPECTIVE AND PROSPECTS

Since obstructions of various areas in the gastrointestinal tract can be life-threatening, they served as the sources of some of the most exciting diagnostic and therapeutic advances in medicine during the twentieth century.

The earliest way to diagnose mechanical obstruction, such as small bowel obstruction, was by exploratory surgery. Then came X-ray studies, which were initially able to outline the gastrointestinal tract first by plain-film studies that showed various findings such as loops of small intestine dilated with air that suggested obstruction. Later, the addition of contrast dyes, given either by mouth or by rectum, increased the ability to outline the anatomy of the GI tract and to diagnose obstructions.

Endoscopy has revolutionized the ability to diagnose mechanical obstructions that are attributable to various causes. Developed initially using a rigid endoscope, which was difficult to position and required that the patient be put under general anesthesia, endoscopes now are flexible, only about one centimeter in diameter, and easily passed well into the duodenum. The instruments passed through the endoscope have also been greatly improved. There are instruments for removing coins lodged in the esophagus, inserting feeding tubes through the stomach wall, injecting drugs to stop the bleeding in ulcers, and cutting the opening of the common bile duct for removing stones impacted in it.

Surgical techniques have improved. Crohn's disease can cause inflammation and segments of narrowing of the intestine called strictures; these strictures can cause problems such as mechanical small bowel obstructions. Surgeons used to remove the strictured areas, plus a significant margin of small intestine on either side of the stricture, in the belief that such removal would eliminate the diseased segments of the small intestine. The disease tends to recur, however, and a patient needing repeated operations to remove strictures might end up with a small intestine so short that it would be unable to absorb fluids and nutrients. Therefore, the individual could have massive diarrhea and malabsorption of nutrients and need to be fed intravenously. By the 1990's, surgical treatment for Crohn's disease sought to relieve the stricture but preserve as much small intestine as possible.

In the 1970's, therapy for biliary stones began to move away from traditional surgery and toward the use of stone-dissolving medications, endoscopic techniques, lithotripsy, and laparoscopy.

Manometry, which involves the measurement of pressure inside the GI tract, has been especially useful in helping scientists understand the physiology of functional obstruction and its relationship to emotions. For example, in 1987, L. D. Young and coworkers published an article describing how exposing research subjects to experimental noise and complicated thinking problems would increase the pressure inside the esophagus, in effect concluding that it increased the strength and speed of esophageal muscle contractions.

—*Marc H. Walters, M.D.*

See also Abdomen; Abdominal disorders; Bile; Cancer; Cholecystectomy; Cholecystitis; Cholesterol; Colon; Colon therapy; Colonoscopy and sigmoidoscopy; Colorectal polyp removal; Colorectal surgery; Colorectal cancer; Constipation; Crohn's disease; Diarrhea and dysentery; Endoscopic retrograde cholangiopancreatography (ERCP); Endoscopy; Esophagus; Gallbladder; Gallbladder diseases; Gastroenterology; Gastroenterology, pediatric; Gastrointestinal disorders; Gastrointestinal system; Heartburn; Intestinal disorders; Intestines; Laparoscopy; Lithotripsy; Nausea and vomiting; Peristalsis; Pyloric stenosis; Radiation therapy; Stone removal; Stones; Tumor removal; Tumors.

FOR FURTHER INFORMATION:

Classen, Meinhard, G. N. J. Tytgat, and C. J. Lightdale, eds. *Gastroenterological Endoscopy.* 2d ed. New York: Thieme Medical, 2010. Text that examines such topics as the impact of endoscopy, its history of use, diagnostic procedures and techniques, therapeutic procedures, descriptions of diseases involving the upper and lower intestine, endoscopic features of infectious diseases of the GI tract, and pediatric endoscopy.

Feldman, Mark, Lawrence S. Friedman, and Lawrence J. Brandt, eds. *Sleisenger and Fordtran's Gastrointestinal and Liver Disease: Pathophysiology, Diagnosis, Management.* New ed. 2 vols. Philadelphia: Saunders/Elsevier, 2010. A comprehensive textbook of gastrointestinal diseases and physiology. Contains excellent chapters on all disorders mentioned in the text, as well as some beautiful endoscopic photographs.

Ganong, William F. *Review of Medical Physiology.* 23d ed. New York: Lange Medical Books/McGraw-Hill Medical, 2009. This classic text has a good section emphasizing normal gastrointestinal physiology that provides a solid background for understanding obstruction.

Kapadia, Cyrus R., James M. Crawford, and Caroline Taylor. *An Atlas of Gastroenterology: A Guide to Diagnosis and Differential Diagnosis.* Boca Raton,

Fla.: Pantheon, 2003. Provides a fully illustrated, nonspecialist understanding of myriad gastrointestinal diseases and disorders, including heartburn, dyspepsia, diarrhea, irritable bowel syndrome, and obstruction. Includes bibliographic references and an index.

Kumar, Vinay, Abul K. Abbas, and Nelson Fausto, eds. *Robbins and Cotran Pathologic Basis of Disease.* 8th ed. Philadelphia: Saunders/Elsevier, 2010. An introductory pathology textbook that is less detailed than that used by physicians, but it still contains a wealth of information on the various disorders that can cause obstruction of the GI tract.

Peikin, Steven R. *Gastrointestinal Health.* Rev. ed. New York: Quill, 2001. Concerned almost completely with the effect of nutrition on GI maladies, the author offers a self-help guide for the afflicted. After explaining the GI tract's workings and describing common symptoms, Peikin specifies diets that he argues will relieve symptoms.

OCCUPATIONAL HEALTH

SPECIALTY

ANATOMY OR SYSTEM AFFECTED: All

SPECIALTIES AND RELATED FIELDS: Environmental health, epidemiology, internal medicine, preventive medicine, psychology, public health, pulmonary medicine, toxicology

DEFINITION: The application of health care that focuses on injury and illness prevention and the treatment of injuries that can occur in the workplace or that result from a person's employment.

SCIENCE AND PROFESSION

The discovery that eighteenth century chimney sweeps were prone to developing testicular cancer is often cited as the first example of an acknowledged occupational illness. In fact, physicians and other health care professionals had been aware for many centuries that certain jobs were linked to particular medical disorders: Millers developed coughs, and hatmakers became mentally unbalanced. Textbooks urged physicians to consider a patient's occupation both in diagnosing and in treating illness. The emergence of occupational health as a distinct specialty within the medical professions is, however, a relatively recent phenomenon.

The Industrial Revolution brought with it not only the separation of one's home life from one's work life but also an increased risk of injury from factory machinery. Spinning jennies, power looms, mill wheels and belts, and early assembly line processes all carried the risk of accidental amputations, mangled limbs, and other permanently crippling injuries. Not surprisingly, much of the early emphasis of occupational health focused on safety. While company doctors treated the injured workers, engineers sought ways to reduce the job hazards.

By the twentieth century, several different but related specialties had evolved that focused on different aspects of occupational health. Industrial hygienists combine training in engineering and public health and attempt to improve safety in the workplace by providing education and training for workers and by redesigning the work area to eliminate hazards. Doctors of occupational medicine are employed by both government and industry to diagnose and to treat occupational illnesses and work-related disabilities. In addition to diagnosing and treating work-related injuries and illnesses, occupational health care providers may provide preemployment physical examinations, health screenings, and health promotion education and risk management programs based on occupational hazards and outcomes of trends of injuries or risks identified in the workplace. Public awareness of occupational health issues has led to the passage of legislation creating such agencies as the United States Occupational Safety and Health Administration (OSHA). All occupational health specialists in the United States must work within guidelines established by OSHA. There is a high cost to society from such disabilities as the black lung disease suffered by coal miners and the toxic or radioactive exposure experienced by workers ranging from hospital laboratory technicians to pipefitters and welders. As a result, occupational health has become an ever-expanding, complex, and important medical specialty.

DIAGNOSTIC AND TREATMENT TECHNIQUES

Because occupational health problems can affect any part of the human anatomy, their diagnostic and treatment techniques are drawn from all areas of medical science. If a worker is injured on the job or suffers from an easily recognizable problem, such as a repetitive motion disorder, diagnosis and treatment can be quite straightforward. In the case of repetitive motion, problems such as carpal tunnel syndrome, which is sometimes experienced by word processing operators, might be treated by advising patients to change their work posture, providing them with splints to align the wrists and hands properly, employing corrective surgery to alleviate pain, and redesigning the work site to prevent future problems. The treatment for many on-the-job injuries will also include an extensive course of physical and rehabilitative therapy to allow the worker to return to work eventually, either at the old job or at a new one.

Many occupational health problems, however, are not as readily diagnosed as carpal tunnel syndrome. The industrial hygienist and the doctor of occupational medicine often must rely on the expertise of epidemiologists and toxicologists to determine the substances to which occupational exposure may be responsible for a worker's ill health. In cases where workers complain of vague symptoms such as chronic fatigue, nausea, or neuropathy (loss of nerve function), an accurate diagnosis can prove elusive. The medical literature contains numerous examples of occupational illnesses that mimicked other common disorders. For example, doctors misdiagnosed a cosmetologist as suffering from multiple sclerosis (a degenerative disease of the central nervous system) when she was actually experiencing nerve damage caused by many years of exposure to the chemical solvents used to apply and remove artificial fingernails. Because many occupational illnesses can take years or even decades to appear, in some cases an accurate diagnosis may never be achieved. Once a diagnosis is made, treatment for an occupational illness caused by exposure to chemicals, for example, can be as simple as assigning the worker to tasks that eliminate exposure or as technologically sophisticated as using dialysis or chemical chelation to remove toxins from a patient's blood.

PERSPECTIVE AND PROSPECTS

Occupational health is one of the most challenging specialties in modern medicine. Practitioners must combine skills and knowledge gleaned from a wide spectrum of related skills. The proliferation of technologically complex methods and materials in the workplace has resulted in occupational exposures and illnesses that were unknown until the twentieth century. At the time that occupational health first emerged as a distinct concern in the medical community, industrial hygiene focused almost exclusively on safety in the workplace. If the factory could be designed so that workers did not risk losing a limb whenever they operated machinery, the hygienist could feel a sense of accomplishment.

Workplace safety remains a concern in occupational health, but obvious hazards such as poorly lit work areas or exposed moving parts on machines have been joined by a host of subtler threats to workers' well-being. Epidemiologists and toxicologists have linked on-the-job exposure to dust, heavy metals, radiation, solvents and other chemicals, and even blood-borne pathogens to a host of cancers, disabling diseases, reproductive problems, and other concerns. Yet, not only must the industrial hygienist and doctor of occupational medicine worry about protecting workers from these physical hazards, but the modern occupational health specialist must also be concerned with the long-term effects of repetitive motions, noise exposures, and even emotional stress. As the influence of workers' jobs on those workers' health and on the health of their families is recognized as a major factor in a family's overall well-being, the importance of the occupational health specialist becomes increasingly obvious within modern society. Occupational health specialists employed in government, industry, and private practice, each approaching the question of worker wellness from a slightly different perspective, all fill a vital and expanding niche in modern medical practice.

The regulatory agency OSHA was created by Congress in 1970 to ensure safe work environments free of hazards that could cause death or serious physical harm to employees. It has the authority to fine and/or charge employers who do not follow safety regulations. The National Institute of Occupational Safety and Health (NIOSH), also created in 1970, conducts research and advise OSHA on issues related to hazards in the workplace.

—*Nancy Farm Mannikko, Ph.D.; updated by Sharon W. Stark, R.N., A.P.R.N., D.N.Sc.*

See also Allied health; Altitude sickness; Asbestos exposure; Asphyxiation; Biofeedback; Carcinogens; Cardiac rehabilitation; Carpal tunnel syndrome; Chronic obstructive pulmonary disease (COPD); Environmental diseases; Environmental health; Hearing loss; Interstitial pulmonary fibrosis (IPF); Law and medicine; Lead poisoning; Lung cancer; Lungs; Mesothelioma; Multiple chemical sensitivity syndrome; Nasopharyngeal disorders; Preventive medicine; Pulmonary diseases; Pulmonary medicine; Pulmonary medicine, pediatric; Radiation sickness; Skin disorders; Stress; Stress reduction; Tendon disorders; Tendon repair; Teratogens; Toxicology.

For Further Information:

Caplan, Robert D., et al. *Job Demands and Worker Health: Main Effects and Occupational Differences.* Ann Arbor: University of Michigan Press, 1980. Discusses such topics as job stress, occupational diseases, psychological occupational medicine, and industrial hygiene. Includes bibliographical references.

Cralley, Lester V., and Patrick R. Atkins, eds. *Industrial Environmental Health: The Worker and the Community.* 2d ed. New York: Academic Press, 1975. An older but still-valuable book that details known workplace hazards, including toxic materials, radiation, and noise. The emphasis is on monitoring techniques and a thorough survey of the literature.

Koren, Herman. *Illustrated Dictionary and Resource Directory of Environmental and Occupational Health.* 2d ed. Boca Raton, Fla.: CRC Press, 2005. Detailed illustrations enhance the definitions and provide visual tools for understanding. Definitions are supplemented with synonyms, acronyms, and abbreviations, all of which are cross-referenced.

Levy, Barry S., et al., eds. *Occupational Health: Recognizing and Preventing Disease and Injury.* 5th ed. Philadelphia: Lippincott Williams & Wilkins, 2006. Text that focuses on the organization of occupational health systems, hazardous exposures, and occupational injuries specific to organ systems and selected groups of workers.

Morgan, Monroe T. *Environmental Health.* 3d ed. Belmont, Calif.: Thomson/Wadsworth, 2003. Examines the links between environmental sciences and human population, focusing on the practices that support human life as well as the need to control factors that are harmful to human life.

Sadhra, Steven S., and Krishna G. Rampal, eds. *Occupational Health: Risk Assessment and Management.* Malden, Mass.: Blackwell Scientific, 1999. This textbook is divided into four sections with three appendixes. Each of the twenty-eight chapters, written by recognized specialists in the field, contains a list of references to original material.

Sellers, Christopher C. *Hazards of the Job: From Industrial Disease to Environmental Health Science.* Chapel Hill: University of North Carolina Press, 1999. Traces the evolution of modern environmentalism in the early twentieth century United States in the context of industrial hygiene expertise and its concerns with lead and other poisonings among workers.

World Health Organization. "Occupational Health." http://www.who.int/occupational_health/en. This Web site provides an overview of global definitions of occupational health, strategies for protecting the health of workers, and links to resources related to topics in occupational health.

ONCOLOGY

SPECIALTY

ANATOMY OR SYSTEM AFFECTED: All

SPECIALTIES AND RELATED FIELDS: Critical care, cytology, general surgery, genetics, immunology, pathology, pharmacology, radiology

DEFINITION: The study of cancer—its causes, its possible spread throughout and destruction of the body, and its medical treatment.

KEY TERMS:

cancer: a tumorous growth of abnormal cells that invade other tissues, choke off available resources, and eventually destroy major organs and the organism

carcinogen: a chemical or radiation mutagen that causes changes in genes, leading to the cancerous state in a cell

cellular transformation: the process in which a cell becomes cancerous, which begins with abnormal changes in gene expression and cell differentiation

hormone: a chemical messenger, usually composed of protein or steroid, that controls the gene expression within target cells and thereby affects cellular development

mutagen: a chemical or an ionizing radiation that causes a change in the nucleotide sequence of the DNA of a gene, possibly affecting the gene's normal expression

mutation: a change in the nucleotide sequence of the DNA (that is, the genetic information) of a gene

oncogene: a gene within the chromosomes of all the cells of an individual organism that triggers cancerous cellular transformation when it is expressed incorrectly

protein kinase: an enzyme type that often is encoded by oncogenes; this enzyme attaches phosphate molecules to certain amino acids on specifically targeted proteins

tumor: an uncontrollable growth of cells within a tissue region that may be benign (noninvasive) or malignant (invasive cancer)

virus: an obligate intracellular parasite, composed of nucleic acid protected by a protein capsid, which reproduces inside cells

SCIENCE AND PROFESSION

Oncology is the scientific study and treatment of cancers, tumors, and other abnormal tissue growths. This field is an important part of medical science because of the prevalence of cancer within the human population, particularly in the progressively older populations of Western societies, in which people enjoy life-prolonging medical advances. Cancer ranks second only to heart disease as a killer of people in Western nations. Its victims number in the hundreds of thousands each year.

The study of cancer and its various physiological manifestations involves an understanding of several diverse biological disciplines, including genetics, developmental biology, embryology, neurology, endocrinology, and general physiology. The oncologist must synthesize information from these scientific fields in diagnosing, monitoring, and treating the disease. The oncologist works closely with the cancer patient's physician, surgeons, laboratory technicians, radiation therapists and chemotherapists, and pharmacists in treating cancerous tumors.

A tumor is an abnormal growth of cells within a specific tissue or organ beyond that tissue or organ's normal developmental pattern. Tumors may be either benign or malignant. Benign tumors are noninvasive; benign tumor cells multiply more rapidly than normal cells within a single, localized region that grows larger and larger. A benign tumor does not spread to other body regions. A malignant tumor, however, is invasive; it grows rapidly and uncontrollably. A malignant tumor is a cancer that consists of grotesquely aberrant cells that break off and are carried through the affected individual's bloodstream to other body regions, where they lodge and overcrowd or outcompete normal body cells.

Cells function normally as a result of the hormonal control of thousands of protein-encoding genes located on twenty-three pairs of chromosomes. The order of nucleotide nitrogen bases on a gene's deoxyribonucleic acid (DNA) polynucleotide chain serves as the genetic code. A change in the nucleotide sequence of DNA is called a mutation. A substance causing a mutation, which is called a mutagen, may be ionizing radiation (for example, ultraviolet light, X rays, gamma radiation) or a chemical. The DNA of a gene encodes ribonucleic acid (RNA), which encodes protein. Thus, an alteration in the nucleotide sequence of DNA, such as the replacement of a cytosine by an adenine nitrogen base, affects the messenger RNA nucleotide information sequence and, subsequently, the protein amino acid sequence. Proteins serve important structural, enzymatic, and hormonal roles within and between cells. A mutation within the DNA nucleotide sequence of a particular cellular gene affects the resulting protein encoded by that gene. Consequently, a variety of cellular functions are affected in sequence. In some cases, the cell is transformed into a cancerous state.

Mutagens that alter certain genes and then trigger cellular transformation into a cancerous state are called carcinogens. Only certain mutagens are carcinogens. An altered gene encodes a protein that has an incorrect amino acid sequence, thereby altering the normal functioning of the protein. An aberrant protein enzymatically or hormonally alters the functioning of other molecules within the cell, thereby directing the cell into the cancerous state.

The precise genes and proteins that are affected in transformed cells have not been identified completely. It appears that certain cancer-causing genes called oncogenes are involved, as well as certain oncogene-encoded enzymes called protein kinases. Protein kinases attach phosphate molecules to certain amino acids on certain cellular proteins, thereby altering the functioning of the proteins and triggering developmental changes within the cell. Certain viruses can also trigger these changes by activating oncogenes and protein kinases. The cell becomes cancerous as a result of these influences.

DIAGNOSTIC AND TREATMENT TECHNIQUES

Oncologists must confront a variety of cancers that affect many different tissues. The six most common cancers affecting American women are breast, colon, lung, uterine, ovarian, and lymphatic cancers, whereas the five most prevalent cancers affecting American men are prostate, lung, colon, bladder, and lymphatic cancers, according to the American Cancer Society. Oncologists must identify and treat these tumors as rapidly and as efficiently as possible.

The successful treatment of cancer begins with its early detection. The classic seven warning signs of cancer are a sore that does not heal, a lump on the body, a persistent cough, difficulty in swallowing, unusual bleeding, a change in a wart or mole, and a change in bladder or bowel movements. The presence of cancer in a patient can be identified by an oncologist by means of several techniques, including cytological (cellular) analysis, biopsy, and direct observation. Cytological techniques employ the microscopic examination of discarded cells from the suspected cancerous region. Biopsy involves the surgical removal of suspected cancerous tissue from an individual and the subsequent chemical and microscopic analysis of the removed tissue cells. Cancer cells are morphologically and chemically distinct from normal body cells.

Cancerous cell masses can be directly observed within the body by means of probing tubes that contain fiber-optic imaging devices and that can be inserted into body cavities. Such medical technology can visualize directly the trachea, bronchi, and larger bronchioles of the lungs; the esophagus and stomach; the colon and rectum; and the reproductive organ passageways, such as the vagina and cervix. Cancerous tumors also can be located via more elaborate techniques, such as computed tomography, magnetic resonance imaging, mammography, radioactive isotopes, X rays, and ultrasound.

Computed tomography (CT) scanning is an enhanced X-ray survey of selected regions of the patient's body. The patient lies within the device, which rotates and X rays around the patient, thereby generating a three-dimensional, computer-enhanced image of the tumor. Conventional X rays can identify many tumors; however, computed tomography can penetrate deeper tissues with greater sensitivity. Mammography is an example of a regular X-ray treatment that utilizes low-energy X rays beamed at a woman's breasts. Mammography is recommended every two years for women of age fifty or older with an average risk for breast cancer.

Similarly, the ingestion of certain radioactive isotopes such as iodine can be used to localize tumors. Certain elemental isotopes concentrate in specific body tissues and organs. The radioactive isotope concentrates in a particular tissue, the tissue is imaged, and any abnormal growths can be detected. Magnetic resonance imaging and ultrasound utilize magnetic fields and sound waves, respectively, to image interior tissues and abnormalities in tissue growth.

Once the presence of cancer and the type of cancer have been established, prompt treatment must ensue. The oncologist must determine the appropriate course of treatment. Surgical removal of the tumor may be possible. Radiotherapy and chemotherapy can be used in conjunction with, or instead of, surgery. Radiotherapy, or radiation therapy, involves the killing of the cancerous tumor by using a concentrated beam of ionizing radiation such as X rays or gamma rays, or by using an ingested radioactive isotope (such as cobalt 60) that will concentrate in the target cancerous tissue. Chemotherapy involves the internal administration of cytotoxic (cell-killing) chemicals to the patient; cancer cells are particularly susceptible to these chemicals.

Treatment for all forms of cancer involves combinations of chemotherapy and radiation therapy. Cancer cells are more sensitive to these treatments than are normal body cells, and they are killed more easily as a result. Early detection of cancer is critical to the success of such treatments. Accessible cancers, such as skin cancers, can be removed surgically or frozen.

Common chemicals used in cancer chemotherapy include alkylating agents, antimetabolites, antibiotics, plant alkaloids, human and synthetic hormones, and enzymes. All these chemicals kill cells, especially cancer cells. Examples of alkylating agents are cisplatin for the treatment of testicular and ovarian cancers, cyclophosphamide for the treatment of breast and lymphatic cancers, and mechlorethamine for the treatment of Hodgkin's disease. A typical antimetabolite is 5-fluorouracil, which is used for the treatment of breast and colon cancer. Examples of antibiotics are mitomycin-C and actinomycin-D. Vincristine is a plant alkaloid that is used to treat leukemia. The human male hormone testosterone and the female hormone progesterone are both used to treat breast cancer, while the female hormone estrogen is used to treat prostate cancer.

Radiation therapies include concentrated beams of X rays or gamma rays aimed at target cancerous tissues or the ingestion of specific radioactive isotopes that concentrate in target cancerous tissues. Both radiation and chemical therapies for cancer have numerous side effects, because normal cells are damaged as well as cancerous cells in both treatments. Such side effects include nausea, weakness, vomiting, diarrhea, loss of hair, and anemia.

In cases of certain tissue tumors and cancers, such as leukemia and bone cancer, tissue transplants from carefully matched individuals have been very effective in saving the lives of these cancer patients. The advent of molecular cloning and the use of tissue-specific viral gene vectors provide another avenue by which the oncologist will treat cancer in the future.

The oncologist's goals are to remove and/or kill the cancerous growth and to arrest its spread (metastasis) to other body tissues. The prevention of metastatic spreading is of critical importance, because the establishment of tumors in multiple body regions makes treatment much more difficult and patient death much more likely. Also, the oncologist must help the patient to cope psychologically with the disease and the possibility of dying.

Oncological research and the treatment of neoplastic (cancerous) tissues represent formidable tasks for medical science. Cancer is the number-two killer of Americans, and tumors are responsible for countless other ailments and millions of dollars of medical expenses. The use of surgery, cytotoxic chemical agents, and radiation to destroy or remove cancers has proven to be effective in saving thousands of lives. The incidence of cancer is increasing, however, and hundreds of thousands of people die from cancer each year.

PERSPECTIVE AND PROSPECTS

Cancer is an increasing problem in Western societies, where medical science is increasing longevity and where industry and business place extraordinary levels of stress upon individuals. Most theories of aging maintain that accumulated genetic mutations in somatic cells during organismal development contribute to the breakdown of body systems, particularly the immune system. Aging is contained for much of an individual's life. Aging accelerates, however, following the end of an individual's period of reproduction. Although cancer can occur at any age, its probability of occurrence accelerates with aging.

Cancer cells are present in the bodies of all humans. Out of approximately 1,000 trillion cells within the human body, it is inevitable that mistakes will occur frequently within the gene regulation mechanisms of certain cells. Humans and other life-forms are exposed continuously to radiation and carcinogenic chemicals of varying types. A critical gene within a critical cell eventually will mutate so that the cell follows a cancerous pathway.

A healthy person with a strong immune system, however, quickly will destroy these mutated, transformed cancers. Individuals having weakened immune systems as a result of stress, aging, illness, and so forth are more susceptible to cancer because the mutated cells have the opportunity to multiply and spread rapidly throughout the body before the person's immune system can respond. Many scientists are beginning to identify aging and stress as diseases, and cancer as a symptom of these diseases.

As the body ages, more and more mutations accumulate, thereby increasing the probability that cancer cells will develop, survive, and multiply. At the same time, the aging immune system cannot respond to abnormal cells and infections as rapidly. Consequently, cancer cells elude the victim's immune system and spread to other body regions.

Evidence is implicating stress as a contributor to incidences of disease, illness, cancer, aging, and premature death in the human population. Stress causes abnormal elevations in nerve and endocrine (hormonal) systems that affect a tremendous variety of cellular and tissue-specific processes within the human body. Elevated levels of hormones for prolonged periods of time can permanently alter the gene expression of certain body tissues, causing these tissues to develop abnormally. Stress is a major problem in fast-paced, technological societies, and it is probably no coincidence that heart disease and cancer are the two principal killers of people in such societies.

Additionally, certain cancers may be infectious. In 1910, Peyton Rous determined that the Rous sarcoma virus, which infects chickens, can trigger cancerous tumors. Subsequent investigators corroborated Rous's findings, and nearly two dozen viruses have been identified that are capable of initiating cellular transformation in animals. Such oncogenic viruses either carry an oncogene or activate oncogenes in their host cells when they infect cells. All viruses must infect cells in order to reproduce. Some viruses can insert their genetic material into the host cell's DNA, thereby affecting the expression of host-cell genes at the viral insertion point; this may be one method of oncogenic viral cellular transformation into cancer. Among the oncogenic viruses that infect humans are hepatitis B; the papillomavirus, which also causes warts; and the Epstein-Barr virus. The Epstein-Barr virus usually causes infectious mononucleosis. In a region of western central Africa, however, humans develop a deadly lymph node cancer called Burkitt's lymphoma when exposed to the virus—a phenomenon that has baffled oncologists.

Genetic damage caused by chemicals and radiation to which humans are exposed has a substantial effect upon the incidences of tumors and cancer. The link between ionizing radiation (for example, ultraviolet light, X radiation, gamma radiation) and cancer has been established. The links between various chemicals and cancer are more difficult to sustain, however, often leading to controversies over the banning of certain substances and the health risks associated with contact with such substances (for example, saccharin or motor oil). The Ames test for chemical mutagens is a very effective assessment of whether a chemical is mutagenic; it was developed by biochemist Bruce Ames and his colleagues at the University of California, Berkeley in the 1970's.

The problems posed by cancer are immense and will require decades of intense medical research. Advances in oncological research are saving many lives each year. Understanding gene regulation within living cells and developing more effective diagnostic techniques and cancer-inhibiting treatments are important steps in conquering this dreaded disease.

—*David Wason Hollar, Jr., Ph.D.*

See also Amputation; Anal cancer; Biopsy; Bladder cancer; Bladder removal; Blood testing; Bone cancer; Bone grafting; Bone marrow transplantation; Breast biopsy; Breast cancer; Breasts, female; Burkitt's lymphoma; Cancer; Carcinogens; Carcinoma; Cells; Cervical, ovarian, and uterine cancers; Chemotherapy; Colorectal cancer; Colorectal polyp removal; Cytology; Cytopathology; Dermatology; Dermatopathology; Endometrial biopsy; Gallbladder cancer; Gene therapy; Genital disorders, female; Genital disorders, male; Gynecology; Hematology; Histology; Hodgkin's disease; Hysterectomy; Imaging and radiology; Immunology; Immunopathology; Kaposi's sarcoma; Kidney cancer; Laboratory tests; Laryngectomy; Liver cancer; Lung cancer; Lymphadenopathy and lymphoma; Malignancy and metastasis; Mammography; Mastectomy and lumpectomy; Melanoma; Mouth and throat cancer; National Cancer Institute (NCI); Nephrectomy; Parathyroidectomy; Pathology; Plastic surgery; Proctology; Prostate cancer; Prostate gland removal; Radiation therapy; Sarcoma; Screening; Serology; Skin cancer; Skin lesion removal; Stomach, intestinal, and pancreatic cancers; Stress; Terminally ill: Extended care; Testicular cancer; Thyroidectomy; Tumor removal; Tumors.

FOR FURTHER INFORMATION:

Alberts, Bruce, et al. *Molecular Biology of the Cell.* 5th ed. New York: Garland, 2008. Leading molecular biologists collaborated to produce this valuable textbook describing the genetics, biochemistry, and developmental biology of eukaryotic cells. Discusses tumorigenesis, cancer cells, and viral-induced cancers. Numerous other chapters are devoted to gene regulation and hormones.

Dollinger, Malin, et al. *Everyone's Guide to Cancer Therapy.* 5th ed. Kansas City, Mo.: Andrews McMeel, 2008. An excellent source of medical information about cancer, written for the general public. Describes various cancer sites in the body. Includes a helpful glossary of medical terminology.

Eyre, Harmon J., Dianne Partie Lange, and Lois B. Morris. *Informed Decisions: The Complete Book of Cancer Diagnosis, Treatment, and Recovery.* 2d ed. Atlanta: American Cancer Society, 2002. This text from the American Cancer Society is intended for the layperson. It is exemplary in its discussion of cancer.

Harnett, Paul, John Cartmill, and Paul Glare, eds. *Oncology: A Case-Based Manual.* New York: Oxford

University Press, 1999. More than eighty cases are used to illustrate and discuss management of patients with cancer. The editors introduce this slim text with an emphasis on data that the practicing physician should know but might have difficulty finding elsewhere in a digestible form.

Joesten, Melvin D., Mary E. Castellion, and John L. Hogg. *The World of Chemistry: Essentials.* 4th ed. New York: Brooks Cole, 2007. This textbook is both a valuable reference and an excellent introduction to environmental chemistry for anyone who has had no prior exposure to the subject. Chapters describe mutagens, carcinogens, and teratogens in detail.

Jorde, Lynn B., et al. *Medical Genetics.* 3d ed. St. Louis, Mo.: Mosby/Elsevier, 2006. An introductory text that covers basic molecular genetics, chromosomal and single gene disorders, immunogenetics, and cancer genetics.

Ophthalmology

Specialty

Anatomy or system affected: Eyes

Specialties and related fields: General surgery, optometry

Definition: The study of the anatomy and physiology of the eye, as well as treatment of vision problems or diseases, ranging from corrective lenses to delicate surgery.

Key terms:

ciliary body: a ring of tissue that surrounds the eye; the uveal portion of this tissue contains the ciliary muscle that adjusts the degree of curvature of the lens

cornea: the transparent portion of the first layer of the eye

keratitis: a state of inflammation of the cornea that may cause partial or total opacity, leading to loss of vision

retina: the key sensory element located in the eye's inner layer

sclera: the opaque portion of the outer layer of the eye; commonly referred to as the "white of the eye"

Science and Profession

Among the sense organs and functions in the body, probably the most complex are the eye and the process of vision that it supports. Ophthalmologists study both the anatomy and the physiology of the eye in order to understand and treat common and rare eye diseases.

The principal anatomical element of vision is the eyeball, or eye globe, located in the right and left orbital openings of the skull. It is embedded in a complex system of tissues surrounded by ocular muscles that control its movement. Adjacent to the eye and also within the bony orbit is the lacrimal gland, which is responsible for keeping the eye moist. Only the front one-third of the globe is exposed. This exposed area is made up of the central transparent portion, the cornea, and a surrounding white portion, which is only part of the sclera, the main component mass of the globe itself. The sclera is a very dense collagenous (protein-rich) structure which has two large openings (the anterior and posterior scleral foramina) and a number of smaller apertures that allow for the passage of nerves and blood vessels into the eye. It is through the posterior scleral foramen that three main components sustaining the eye's functions pass: the optic nerve, the central retinal vein, and the central retinal artery.

The eye has three main layers, within which are further specialized divisions. The outer layer consists essentially of the transparent cornea and opaque sclera. The middle layer, called the uvea, is made up of the choroid, which is the outer coating of the layer; the ciliary body, which contains key eye muscles that affect the degree of curvature in the lens; and the iris, which, with the lens located immediately behind it, separates the anterior from the posterior chambers of the eye. This iris itself has two layers, the stroma and the epithelium. The latter is immediately recognizable to the layperson, since its cells are markedly pigmented, giving to each individual a characteristic eye color.

It is the opening in the iris, called the pupil, that allows the passage of light into the inner layer of the eye, which contains the key sensory portion of the organ, the retina. Before light reaches the inner layer and the retina, it passes through the lens of the eye, located immediately behind the iris (which it supports), and through the largest area of open space within the eye, the vitreous cavity. This posterior cavity, like the smaller forward cavity of the eye, is filled with a transparent hydrogel called aqueous humor, made up mainly of water (about 95 percent of its total mass) in a collagenous framework within which the main component is hyaluronic acid. The aqueous humor is very similar to plasma but lacks its protein concentration. The pupil of the eye serves a purpose similar to the diaphragm (or f-stop) on a camera; it opens wider (dilates) or closes (contracts) according to the intensity of light striking the eye. (This reaction explains why, after a few minutes in an apparently totally dark room, the eye adjusts at least in part to the lower intensity of light.) For purposes of examining the internal structures of the eye, ophthalmologists sometimes place special drops in the eye to cause the pupil to dilate.

The lens of the eye, which is held in place behind the pupil by zonular fibers, consists of onionlike lens fibers. These are the product of epithelial cells that "migrate" from their place of origin in a germinative zone next to the edges of the lens to the anterior portion of the concentric structure of the lens. The central or internal layers of lens fibers, called the embryonic nucleus, represent the earliest cell specialization processes before birth. By contrast, the anterior and posterior lens fibers are constantly renewed at the surface.

As light passes through the transparent lens fibers, the phenomenon of refraction results, in the simplest possible explanation, both from the concentric shape of the lens itself and from a differential in the index of refraction occurring in the "younger" outside layers of lens fibers and that of the "older" central layers; the latter have a greater index of refraction than the former. Another phenomenon that increases the refractive power of the lens occurs when the zonular fibers that hold it in place relax under the influence of the ciliary muscle, making the lens more spherical in shape. The resultant increase in refractive power is called accommodation.

It is the retina, located in the last layer of the eye, that receives the light images passing through the lens and transmits them to the brain via the optic nerve. Physiologists consider the nerve-related function of the retina to be comparable in many details with all other sensory phenomena in the body, including touch and smell. The retina itself consists of a very thin outer layer, called the retinal pigment epithelium, and an inner layer, the sensory retina. On the surface of the retina, one finds a layer of photoreceptor cells. Once affected by the absorption of light rays reaching them from the lens, these cells form synapses with an intermediate layer of modulator cells. A synaptic relationship may be defined as an excitatory functional contact between two nerve cells, causing either a chemical or an electrical response. The modulator cells—referred to as neurons when their function is to receive synaptic transmissions from receptor cells—in turn pass the "message" of light to ganglion cells forming the innermost cellular layer of the retina. These cells transmit electrical discharges through the optic nerve to the brain, where they are registered as images.

DIAGNOSTIC AND TREATMENT TECHNIQUES
Ophthalmologists must deal with a wide variety of problems affecting the eyes, ranging from injuries to the diagnosis of vision problems that can be corrected with eyeglasses or contact lenses. Perhaps the most important area of applied ophthalmology, however, involves treating the diseases that may occur in several areas of the eye.

An entire category of diseases can appear in the conjunctiva, the thin mucous membrane that lines the inner portion of the eyelid and covers the exterior of the sclera. Conjunctivitis refers to inflammatory conditions that may attack this membrane. Some conditions cause mere irritation, while others may lead to serious infections. In acute catarrhal, or mucopurulent, conjunctivitis, the conjunctival blood vessels become congested with mucus and then with pus, which accumulates on the margins of the eyelids. If untreated, this form of contagious, easily transmitted infection begins to affect the cornea, by causing prismatic distortions and eventually abrasions that may infect the cornea itself. A more serious form of conjunctivitis is referred to as purulent conjunctivitis; it is sometimes associated with complications of the sexually transmitted disease gonorrhea.

Inflammation of the cornea, or keratitis, usually comes from the passage of virulent organisms from the conjunctival sac, which, although exposed to the external environment, may not itself react to the presence of bacteria. There are many different types of keratitis. Individuals may be vulnerable to infections in the cornea as a result of abrasions (one of the main reasons that all ophthalmologists recommend against rubbing the eye to remove irritating particles) or because of abnormal conditions affecting the surface of the cornea. Among the latter, ophthalmologists list excessive dryness in the eye and the side effects of malnutrition leading to a condition called keratomalacia, which is common in underdeveloped countries.

Bacteria such as pneumococci (the primary contributor to pneumonia in the lungs) may cause infections that result in corneal ulceration, the most common form of keratitis. In such cases, the area affected by the ulceration may increase considerably as epithelial tissue in the cornea attaches itself to the ulcer. Corneal ulcers may be removed by surgery, although the effect of remaining scar tissue may reduce the level of vision. The prospect of success in corneal transplant operations has not eliminated the need for ulcer removal surgery, since transplants depend on the availability of "fresh" cornea donors.

Another form of corneal infection, herpes zoster (a form of skin rash also called shingles), is caused by the virus that causes chickenpox; it is common among aged patients whose cellular immunity systems suffer from decreased efficiency. In herpes zoster ophthalmicus, an infection that begins in the eye spreads via the naso-ciliary branch of the ophthalmic nerves and appears as red blotches on the surface of the skin (usually near the eye orbits on the side of the infection only). Zoster attacks are accompanied by rather severe pain. Ophthalmologists use several key drugs to treat this condition, including Distalgesic, Fortral, or Pethidine. Resultant depression in the patient may be relieved by prescribing amitriptyline.

Inflammation and possible infection of other regions of the eye also occur. Some zones, such as the sclera, tend to be more resistant to invasion because of the density of their fibrous tissues. Superficial inflammation of the sclera, called episcleritis, may be transitory but recurrent. Ophthalmologists will prescribe the anti-inflammatory drug Tandearil in the form of drops. More serious but much less common is the condition called scleritis, which extends much deeper into the tissue of the sclera and may affect the cornea and the uveal tract in the middle layer of the eye. Treatment of scleritis involves the use of steroid therapy, such as the corticosteroid drug prednisolone, often supplemented with Tandearil.

Uveitis is a term that applies to inflammations that occur in the uveal tract. The name suggests that such complications are not limited to one or another of the parts of the uveal zone (the iris or the ciliary body): All are affected and must be treated simultaneously.

The most common vision problem is myopia (near-sightedness). While most people still choose to correct nearsightedness with contact lenses or glasses, laser techniques such as photorefractive keratectomy (PRK) and laser in situ keratomileusis (LASIK) have shown some promise in treating myopia. Early enthusiasm for radial keratotomy has waned because of erratic results.

The most widely known eye disorders are probably glaucoma and cataracts. Glaucoma occurs when pressure caused by an excessive amount of aqueous humor increases inside the eyeball, specifically in the area of the retina. Impairment of vision may be slight, occurring at first in the peripheral area of sight. Further deterioration, however, may lead to blindness in the eye. Regular treatment with drugs that reduce the production of aqueous humor is necessary in patients suffering from chronic glaucoma. Acute glaucoma, which is very sudden, represents only about one-tenth of recorded cases. It must be treated within less than a week to avert permanent blindness.

Cataracts occur when there is a loss of full transparency in the lens of the eye. Cataracts occurring among children are congenital or hereditary in origin. Cataract-like damage to the lens of the eye may also result from exposure to the sun's rays (which is especially dangerous when one views the sun without protection during eclipses), extreme heat, X rays, or nuclear radiation. Most characteristically, however, cataracts (from slight to advanced stages) are associated with the aging process. Formerly, cataract surgery was difficult and the recovery period slow, so patients were advised to wait as long as possible to have cataracts removed. Improvements in surgical techniques and materials mean that patients no longer need to wait until their vision is severely impaired to have this surgery. Most cataract extractions are combined with implantation of an intraocular lens, so that patients do not need to wear specially prescribed contact lenses or thick glasses following surgery.

Ophthalmologists make use of laser surgery for an increasing number of eye disorders. Lasers are used to treat eye problems caused by diabetes and hypertension, to treat or prevent some types of glaucoma, and to treat other, rarer eye conditions. Macular degeneration, an important cause of decreased central vision, may be arrested by laser therapy, but the technique does not repair existing damage.

Microsurgical techniques have further revolutionized eye care and have led to more effective management of conditions (such as retinal detachment) that formerly caused blindness.

Perspective and Prospects

Knowledge of the anatomy and physiology of the eye evolved gradually through history and then spectacularly in the latter half of the twentieth century. The most extraordinary advances in the later period were made in the field of eye surgery. For an understanding of how vision itself worked, it took centuries for surprisingly unscientific views to cede to the first modern theories and then, with the advance of anatomical dissection, the practical possibility of examining both normal and abnormal conditions of the organ in the laboratory.

An early but not widespread theory of how the eye sees, held into the Middle Ages, depended on what now seems to be the fantastic conception of *eidola*, or "skins." Those who believed this theory held (in part correctly) that something must be leaving the objects that one perceives through the eyes. This "something" was thought to be a skinlike picture that, once detached from the object in question, actually entered the eye (after an unexplainable physical contraction) through the pupil, the aperture in the eye that is visible in many different animals. Another widespread theory was a prescientific version not of light rays but of "visual rays" that were thought to leave the interior of the eye, returning to record the colors and shapes of objects encountered.

Historians generally agree that the tenth century Arab scientist Ḥasan ibn al-Haytham, known in the West as Alhazen, was the first to suggest that rays of light entered the eye to stimulate what he called the "sensorium." Although Alhazen's theory predated a scientific explanation of the nature of light itself, he based his views on the phenomenon of the lingering image on the eye's "sensorium" of strong light, particularly that of the sun, even after the eyelids closed out the object emitting light. He even proposed a basic theory of refraction of light inside the eye. According to his theory, the sensorium recorded images according to an exact formula that reconstituted both the "shape" and the "order" in which rays are received by the eye, depending on the angle at which they strike the spherical surface of the cornea. Alhazen even warned that, although the eye's sensorium always duplicated this formula exactly, the observer (actually, the observer's brain) could be "tricked" by the reproduction of certain ray patterns that might resemble something that was not "real"—the optical illusion.

Alhazen's views would be examined and extended during the late sixteenth and mid-seventeenth centuries in the West by the scientific pioneers of optics, specifically the Italian Francesco Maurolico (died 1575) and the famous German astronomer Johannes Kepler (1571-1630). Kepler's best-known work complemented that of his Italian contemporary Galileo Galilei (1564-1642), marking a breakthrough in the science of optics and the use of lenses to make telescopes in order to explore the skies. Only in later generations, however, did the ophthalmological relevance of some of his findings concerning the measurement of light reflected off the objects "seen" by a lens become clear.

As specialized interest in the eye progressed along with the constant advance of science in the eighteenth and nineteenth centuries, exact observation of the internal features of the organ of vision hinged on both the historical progress of anatomical dissection and the development of instruments to look into the living eye. One of the principal figures who contributed to the latter field was the Swedish ophthalmologist Allvar Gullstrand (1862-1930). Gullstrand received the Nobel Prize in Physiology or Medicine in 1911 for his application of physical mathematics to the study of refraction of light in the eye. He gained additional worldwide attention for his research on astigmatism (the failure of rays to be focused by the lens accurately on a single central point) and for devising the so-called slit lamp for viewing the interior of the eye through the use of an intense beam of light.

In the area of eye surgery, a major landmark was achieved in the 1960's when the Spanish ophthalmologist Ramón Castroviejo began to develop a method for surgical transplant of fully transparent corneas from deceased donors to replace damaged corneas in eye patients.

—Byron D. Cannon, Ph.D.;
updated by Rebecca Lovell Scott, Ph.D., PA-C
See also Aging: Extended care; Albinos; Astigmatism; Biophysics; Blindness; Blurred vision; Cataract surgery; Cataracts; Color blindness; Conjunctivitis; Corneal transplantation; Eye infections and disorders; Eye surgery; Eyes; Geriatrics and gerontology; Glaucoma; Keratitis; Laser use in surgery; Macular degeneration; Microscopy, slitlamp; Myopia; Optometry; Sense organs; Trachoma; Vision; Vision disorders.

FOR FURTHER INFORMATION:

Buettner, Helmut, ed. *Mayo Clinic on Vision and Eye Health: Practical Answers on Glaucoma, Cataracts, Macular Degeneration, and Other Conditions.* Rochester, Minn.: Mayo Foundation for Medical Education and Research, 2002. A helpful handbook on all the medical, social, and emotional facets of vision impairment.

Kaufman, Paul L., and Albert Alm. *Adler's Physiology of the Eye: Clinical Application.* 10th ed. St. Louis, Mo.: Mosby, 2003. Provides a technical but generally readable treatment of the photochemical and electrophysiological aspects of vision. Deals in detail with the muscular mechanisms that aid the eye in its work.

Newell, Frank W. *Ophthalmology.* 8th ed. St. Louis, Mo.: Mosby, 1996. Although clearly technical in its treatment of the subject, this textbook, revised over a twenty-year period, is widely cited.

Palay, David A., and Jay H. Krachmer, eds. *Primary Care Ophthalmology.* 2d ed. Philadelphia: Mosby/Elsevier, 2006. While this text is aimed at physicians, it is well illustrated, and much of the material is in an outline format. The sixteen chapters cover the diagnosis and treatment of the eye problems encountered in the primary care setting.

Riordan-Eva, Paul, and John P. Whitcher. *Vaughan and Asbury's General Ophthalmology*. 17th ed. New York: Lange Medical Books/McGraw-Hill, 2007. This well-illustrated textbook is an excellent reference for the serious student who desires detailed information on any aspect of the eye or its diseases.

Ronchi, Vasco. *Optics: The Science of Vision*. Translated and revised by Edward Rosen. Rev. ed. New York: Dover, 1991. Originally published in Italian in 1955, this textbook deals in quite readable detail with the principles of optics as they relate to the eye itself.

Sutton, Amy L., ed. *Eye Care Sourcebook: Basic Consumer Health Information About Eye Care and Eye Disorders*. 3d ed. Detroit, Mich.: Omnigraphics, 2008. A complete guide to eye care that includes such topics as eye anatomy, preventive vision care, refractive disorders and eye diseases, current research and clinical trials, and a list of organizations.

Yanoff, Myron, and Jay S. Duker, eds. *Ophthalmology*. 3d ed. St. Louis, Mo.: Mosby/Elsevier, 2009. Discusses such topics as the anatomy and histology of the eye and ocular physiology and physiopathology. Includes bibliographical references and an index.

OPPORTUNISTIC INFECTIONS
DISEASE/DISORDER

ANATOMY OR SYSTEM AFFECTED: All

SPECIALTIES AND RELATED FIELDS: Bacteriology, immunology, internal medicine, microbiology, virology

DEFINITION: Potentially life-threatening diseases occurring in people with weakened immune systems by microorganisms that typically do not cause severe illnesses in otherwise healthy people.

KEY TERMS:

CD4: a type of white blood cell (specifically a type of T cell) that is affected by the human immunodeficiency virus (HIV)

encephalitis: inflammation of the brain

immunocompromised: the state of having a weakened immune system

lumbar puncture: also known as a spinal tap; a procedure that involves insertion of a needle into the lumbar spinal column

pneumonia: infection of the lung

prophylaxis: a method of preventing a disease

CAUSES AND SYMPTOMS

Opportunistic infections can be caused by various microorganisms, including viruses, bacteria, fungi, and protozoa. While they are capable of infecting healthy persons, the infection is either without symptoms or the disease is mild. It is in those who lack a healthy immune system that these organisms cause disastrous infections. Acquired immunodeficiency syndrome (AIDS), resulting from human immunodeficiency virus (HIV), is a widely known disease that weakens the immune system. There are other situations, however, in which the immune system can be compromised and become susceptible to opportunistic infections, such as being on chronic glucocorticoid therapy, taking immunosuppressive medications after organ transplantation, undergoing chemotherapy for cancer, being malnourished, or having a genetic predisposition.

Pneumocystis jirovecii is a fungus capable of causing life-threatening pneumonia in the immunocompromised. In those with HIV, the majority of *Pneumocystis* pneumonia develops in those with a very low CD4 cell count. Common symptoms include fever, cough, progressive difficulty breathing (especially with exertion), fatigue, chills, chest pain, and weight loss.

Toxoplasmosis is a ubiquitous infection caused by the intracellular protozoan parasite *Toxoplasma gondii*, which makes cats their hosts. Transmission is via ingestion of contaminated soil or undercooked meats that contain the protozoan oocyte. Infection in the healthy person is usually asymptomatic, but the organism can remain dormant in the host indefinitely. In immunocompromised patients such as those with very low CD4 cells, the organism reactivates and causes active infection. The central nervous system is the principal site of involvement. *T. gondii* can cause encephalitis and masses within the brain. Symptoms may include confusion, fever, seizures, and headache. *T. gondii* can also cause pneumonia, with difficulty breathing, fever, and cough. Other organs such as the intestines, liver, bone marrow, bladder, spinal cord, testes, pancreas, eyes, heart, and liver can be infected, although this is less common. Pregnant women who have an active infection can pass it to their offspring, leading to infantile neurological deficits, mental retardation, and eye infections.

Mycobacterium avium complex (MAC) usually causes widespread disease in the immunocompromised and is due to two nontuberculous species, *M. avium* or *M. intracellulare*. These organisms are ubiquitous in the environment such as in soil, with transmission typically through inhalation or ingestion. Acquisition of infection typically takes place when the CD4 count is extreme low. Symptoms include fever, night sweats, abdominal pain, diarrhea, weight loss, weakness, and wasting.

Cytomegalovirus (CMV) is a herpesvirus found worldwide. It is commonly transmitted via feces, saliva, breast milk, urine, and genital secretions. In immunocompetent individuals, the virus remains latent and usually does not cause any severe disease. In the immunocompromised, however, the dormant virus reactivates and infection occurs. Symptoms generally include fever, night sweats, chills, fatigue, and muscle and joint aches. Other symptoms depend on the organ system affected: Gastrointestinal involvement typically produces symptoms of colitis (inflammation of the colon), such as abdominal pain and bloody diarrhea; lung involvement produces a pneumonitis (inflammation of the lung) with cough and difficulty breathing; and eye involvement (retinitis) can lead to blindness. The adrenal gland and the nervous system can also be affected.

Another opportunistic fungus associated with immunocompromised hosts is *Cryptococcus neoformans*, which causes cryptococcosis. The organism is normally found in soil contaminated with pigeon droppings, and transmission is usually through inhalation. The initial site of infection is in the lungs, from where it subsequently spreads to the brain, causing what is known as meningoencephalitis (inflammation of the brain and its surrounding protective tissues). Meningoencephalitis is the most common clinical syndrome in immunocompromised patients, developing slowly over one to two weeks with fever, malaise, headache, stiff neck, photophobia (aversion to bright lights), and vomiting. Disseminated rash is another symptom occurring in those with a weakened immune system.

INFORMATION ON OPPORTUNISTIC INFECTIONS

CAUSES: Viruses, bacteria, fungi, protozoa

SYMPTOMS: Fever, weakness, lack of appetite, rash, cough, difficulty breathing, confusion, headache, blurry vision, chest pain, weight loss, night sweats

DURATION: Acute to chronic

TREATMENTS: Antibiotics, antiviral medications, antifungal medications, antiprotozoan medications

---

There are many other causes of opportunistic infections, including the viruses *Varicella* and herpes simplex; the bacteria *Nocardia*, *Listeria*, and the less common *Mycobacterium* species; the protozoans *Cryptosporidium*, *Isospora*, *Microsporidia*, and *Cyclospora*; and the fungi *Coccidioides*, *Candida*, *Histoplasma*, and *Aspergillus*. While all these organisms are capable of causing disease in the healthy, their impact on the immunocompromised is much more severe.

TREATMENT AND THERAPY

Treatment of specific infections is important in addressing the disease, but what is more important is to correct the underlying deficit, which is the weakened immune system. In some cases, this may not be possible, such as in those who require immunosuppressive therapy after organ transplantation or those undergoing chemotherapy for cancer. However, advances in HIV therapy with the implementation of highly active antiretroviral therapy (HAART) as well as institution of prophylaxis against opportunistic infections have dramatically decreased the mortality rate in these patients.

Treatment of *Pneumocystis* pneumonia requires the demonstration of organisms from respiratory specimens. Treatment is with anti-Pneumocystis regimens typically for twenty-one days, with or without corticosteroids. The latter is used in severe cases when oxygenation becomes problematic. Symptoms typically worsen after two to three days of therapy as a result of increased inflammation in response to dying microorganisms. After initial therapy, prophylactic therapy against future infections is instituted.

Treatment of toxoplasmosis requires antiprotozoan medications for at least six weeks. Prophylaxis against future infection is also required, which is the same medication as that used for *Pneumocystis* prophylaxis. In high-risk persons, as a means of prevention it is important to avoid undercooked meats and cat litter boxes. Treatment of MAC involves combination antibiotics for at least twelve months, with subsequent prophylaxis.

CMV infection is treated with antiviral agents. Immunoglobulin may be used to reduce the risk of infection in certain transplant recipients. If the eye is involved, then a pellet that releases an antiviral agent may be implanted into the eye with surgery. While not curative, this treatment may hinder the progression of the eye disease.

The treatment of cryptococcosis is with antifungal

agents, initially with combination medications for what is known as induction therapy, followed by consolidation therapy, and finally maintenance therapy. Because the disease can also cause an increased pressure surrounding the brain, frequent lumbar punctures are sometimes required to relieve this pressure, or if severe enough, a drain placed in the spinal cord may be necessary to continuously relieve the pressure.

While prophylactic therapy is needed when the CD4 cell count is low, it may be withdrawn when the CD4 cells improve.

PERSPECTIVE AND PROSPECTS

Pneumocystis was originally identified by the Brazilian physician Carlos Chagas in 1909. Chagas was also the discoverer of the protozoan *Trypanosoma cruzi*, the organism that causes trypanosomiasis, or Chagas' disease. Initially, he mistakenly thought that the *Pneumocystis* cysts from the lungs of rats were part of the *Trypanosoma* life cycle. It was in 1910 that the Italian physician Antonio Carini discovered that these cysts were also present in lungs without *T. cruzi* infection, and thus concluded that these cysts were a different type of infection. In 1912, Pierre and Marie Delanoe at the Pasteur Institute also confirmed that these cysts were present in the absence of *T. cruzi* infection, and they subsequently named these cystlike organisms *Pneumocystis carinii*, after Carini. Because these infections appeared to affect only rats, however, the organism did not become a major issue at that time.

It was not until the 1940's that *P. carinii* was found to cause pneumonia in human infants and adults. However, these patients all had some type of immune system compromise, such as malnutrition, genetic immune deficiency, or immunosuppressive medications. Before the AIDS epidemic, there were fewer than one hundred confirmed cases per year in the United States. It was later determined that there were several species of *Pneumocystis*, one of which causes disease in rats and another in humans. It was in 1999 when the term *P. jirovecii* (named after the Czech parasitologist Otto Jiroveci) was officially coined to refer to the disease occurring in humans. *P. carinii* still refers to the disease in rats. It was also in 1999 that *Pneumocystis* was recognized as a fungus rather than a protozoan, as previously thought.

In late 1980 to early 1981, the Centers for Disease Control and Prevention (CDC) described a cluster of five cases of *Pneumocystis* pneumonia in young gay men. Since then, the cases of *Pneumocystis* pneumonia increased, as did the cases of Kaposi's sarcoma (rare HIV-related skin cancer). It was soon realized that both of these illnesses were not exclusive to gay males; they also affected heterosexuals, intravenous drug users, and others who were immunocompromised. In 1982, the CDC officially coined the term "acquired immunodeficiency syndrome," or AIDS, for this syndrome. In 1983, Luc Montagnier and his team from the Pasteur Institute isolated a virus that was thought to be the causative agent of AIDS, which they termed lymphadenopathy-associated virus. In 1984, Robert Gallo and his team from the United States also isolated a virus presumptive to cause AIDS; they named it human T lymphotropic virus type III (HTLV-III). Later, it was recognized that both viruses were the same, and the virus was officially termed human immunodeficiency virus (HIV) in 1986.

In the beginning of the AIDS epidemic, death was certain. Treatment of HIV did not begin until 1986, when the Food and Drug Administration (FDA) approved the first antiviral agent, zidovudine, a nucleoside reverse transcriptase inhibitor (NRTI)—an agent that inhibits viral replication. However, single agent therapy did not prove to be as effective due to drug resistance. In 1995, newer classes of antiviral medications were approved—non-nucleoside reverse transcriptase inhibitor (NNRTI) and protease inhibitors (PI)—and began the trend of combination therapy of what is now known as highly active antiretroviral therapy (HAART). The thought behind combination therapy is that if the virus develops a genetic mutation and becomes resistant to one drug, the other two would still be active against it. However, while successful, even this powerful combination of drugs is still not adequate enough to achieve a complete cure, since the virus is capable of remaining dormant inside cells and become resistant to medications even after a brief episode of missed doses.

In 2007, the FDA approved two new classes of antiretroviral therapy, integrase inhibitors and CCR5 co-receptor antagonists, which are both used for advanced stages of HIV infection.

As of 2010, there are currently no available vaccines against HIV, although there had been trials in the past in its development. A report in 2009 of a study of healthy volunteers with an experimental HIV vaccine in Thailand showed only a modest success rate (about 31 percent) in the prevention of HIV. Nevertheless, the investigation to find a successful vaccine is ongoing.

While there are still obstacles to conquer in the fight

against HIV, the battle against opportunistic infections has largely been successful with the introduction of HAART and prophylactic medications.

—*Andrew Ren, M.D.*

See also Acquired immunodeficiency syndrome (AIDS); Bacterial infections; Fungal infections; Human immunodeficiency virus (HIV); Immune system; Immunodeficiency disorders; Immunology; Kaposi's sarcoma; Protozoan diseases; Terminally ill: Extended care; Viral infections.

FOR FURTHER INFORMATION:

Fauci, Anthony, eds. *Harrison's Principles of Internal Medicine.* 17th ed. New York: McGraw-Hill, 2008. A comprehensive textbook of internal medicine that thoroughly discusses the basic and clinical science on various disease topics, including HIV and infectious diseases. Includes detailed illustrations and detailed reference lists.

Mandell, Gerald, et al., eds. *Mandell, Douglas, and Bennett's Principles and Practice of Infectious Diseases.* 7th ed. Philadelphia: Churchill Livingstone/Elsevier, 2009. A comprehensive textbook covering all aspects of infectious diseases, including epidemiology, the immune system, antimicrobial therapy, and specific disease syndromes and their etiologies.

Rubin, Robert, eds. *Clinical Approach to Infection in the Compromised Host.* 4th ed. New York: Kluwer Academic, 2002. Clinical textbook on opportunistic infections not only in the HIV patient but also in those with cancer and organ transplants.

St. Georgiev, Vassil. *Opportunistic Infections.* Totowa, N.J.: Humana Press, 2003. A detailed discourse on the treatment of various opportunistic infections that, while technical, does provide an introduction to a comprehensive array of organisms.

OPTOMETRY

SPECIALTY

ANATOMY OR SYSTEM AFFECTED: Eyes

SPECIALTIES AND RELATED FIELDS: Ophthalmology

DEFINITION: A field involving the provision of eye exams, the prescription of corrective lenses, and the diagnosis and treatment of eye disease, but not eye surgery.

KEY TERMS:

clinical refraction: the determination of appropriate optical powers and related parameters to promote optimal visual acuity

contact lens: a small, shell-like glass or plastic lens that rests directly on the external surface of the eye to serve as a new anterior surface and thus correct refractive error as an alternative to spectacles, to protect the eye, or to serve as a prosthetic device promoting a more normal appearance of a disfigured eye

ophthalmologist: a physician who specializes in the comprehensive care of the eyes and the visual system; ophthalmologists provide visual, medical, and surgical eye care and diagnose general diseases of the body

prism: an optical element or component that, by virtue of two nonparallel plane faces, deviates the path of a beam of light

spectacles: a pair of ophthalmic lenses held together with a frame or mounting; also called glasses

SCIENCE AND PROFESSION

Optometry has been defined as "the art and science of vision care" by Monroe J. Hirsch and Ralph E. Wick in *The Optometric Profession* (1968). The American Optometric Association has stated that "Doctors of Optometry are independent primary health care providers who specialize in the examination, diagnosis, treatment and management of diseases and disorders of the visual system." Optometrists examine eyes and the visual system. They prescribe spectacles and contact lenses, optimize binocularity (the manner in which the two eyes work together), and improve visual function. Optometrists are trained to detect, treat, and manage disorders and diseases of the eyes and related structures.

Optometry is one of the youngest of the learned professions, which were originally restricted to law, medicine, and theology. Following the earlier lead of organized medicine, optometrists successfully organized and passed the first optometry practice law in 1901. Optometrists today complete a university education and then spend four additional years in a specialized school or college of optometry to receive the O.D. (doctor of optometry) degree. Many optometrists spend an additional year training in special-interest residency programs after graduation. Optometrists practice independently in private offices, although increasing numbers of optometrists also work in groups, the military, public health agencies, and university and hospital environments.

Distinctions are made between optometrists, ophthalmologists, and opticians. Ophthalmologists are physicians who diagnose and treat eye diseases and who perform eye surgery. They complete a premedical university education, four years of medical school, one year of internship, and three or more years of specialized training in ophthalmology. Many ophthalmologists also complete one or more years of fellowship subspecialty training. Opticians are technicians trained in the manufacture and dispensing of optical aids.

DIAGNOSTIC AND TREATMENT TECHNIQUES

A portion of the eye examination performed by optometrists is called clinical refraction. To the physicist, refraction is the bending of light as it passes through an interface separating two differing media (such as water and air). Refraction, however, has also come to mean the clinical evaluation of the human visual system. Clinical refraction generally results in a spectacle prescription; such a prescription will contain the spherical optical power, and the astigmatic optical power and its axis when appropriate, that are necessary to provide optimally focused light on the retina for each eye.

A clinical refraction also includes an assessment of binocularity, which is the way in which both eyes are used simultaneously such that each retinal image contributes to the final visual percept. (The retina is the inner nerve layer of the eye upon which the optics of the eye focuses the image of the outside world.) Much effort is made, during a refraction, to attain maximum visual comfort by optimizing binocularity. Occasionally, it is necessary to utilize a prismatic element in the spectacle prescription as well as optical powers to this end. In other cases, the clinician may suggest a course of eye exercises to assist the patient in achieving improved binocularity without, or in supplement to, spectacles. Some patients may be found to suffer from severe binocular dysfunction and are referred for surgical consideration.

Near vision is tested during a refraction, especially for those people more than forty years of age who might require optical assistance for near work. The cornea is the clear, circular "window" in the front of the eye through which the colored iris is seen. Behind the iris is a crystalline lens. The cornea and the lens act together to focus light on the retina. The cornea provides most of the refractive power of the eye, and the lens serves to fine-tune the image in a process called accommodation. As one ages, however, the ability to accommodate deteriorates. Some form of near correction, either with two pairs of spectacles or with some form of bifocal, is then necessary. Only minimal optical power is needed at first, but as the aging process continues, the need for stronger near correction increases.

For a given patient, an analysis of binocularity, the determination of near vision requirements, and a consideration of additional occupational or avocational tasks (such as sports) make up his or her "functional vision." For some patients, the data gleaned in a standard refraction will provide the optometrist with all the information necessary to recommend comfortable visual correction for all tasks. For other patients, some additional thought and consideration may be required. For example, a very tall,

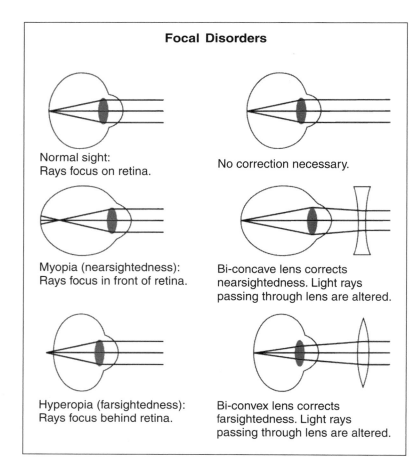

Focal Disorders

Normal sight:
Rays focus on retina.

No correction necessary.

Myopia (nearsightedness):
Rays focus in front of retina.

Bi-concave lens corrects nearsightedness. Light rays passing through lens are altered.

Hyperopia (farsightedness):
Rays focus behind retina.

Bi-convex lens corrects farsightedness. Light rays passing through lens are altered.

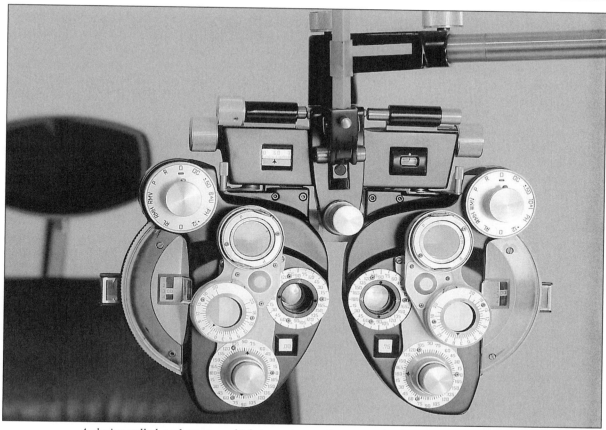

A device called a phoropter, which is used to evaluate a patient's vision. (Digital Stock)

fifty-year-old patient may not require as strong a reading correction as another shorter individual of the same age because the former has longer arms and is more used to holding reading material at a greater distance than the latter. In addition, providing visual care to patients using computers and video display terminals has become a rapidly growing subarea in functional vision.

No clinical refraction would be complete without an assessment of ocular health. This examination consists of observation of the eyes and related structures, as well as a testing of function. Good visual acuity, in and of itself, is fairly good evidence that the function of the eye is normal. Some ocular diseases, however, may occur and—at least initially—leave central vision intact. The structures of the eye are inspected with the assistance of instruments such as a clinical biomicroscope, or slitlamp microscope, to examine the outer ocular structures, and an ophthalmoscope, which allows inspection of the structures of the inner eye. Pupillary dilation with pharmaceutical agents in the form of drops allows inspection of the peripheral retina. The pressure in the

eye should be tested, a process called tonometry, and the field of vision evaluated. Many optometrists also bear the responsibility for the treatment of certain ocular diseases.

As is true for all professionals, when the management of a specific problem is beyond one doctor's training, interest, or licensure, referral is made to another, more appropriate, doctor. For example, a patient with an age-related cataract (clouding of the crystalline lens) may be referred to an ophthalmologist for surgery, and an optometrist who suspects multiple sclerosis will refer the patient to a neurologist.

There are subspecialty areas in optometry, such as the prescription of appropriate visual aids for patients with particularly poor vision, known as low vision rehabilitation. Other subspecialty areas include industrial vision, developmental vision and vision therapy, and ocular disease. Contact lens care has become a large subspecialty in optometry. In fitting contact lenses, the curvature of the cornea, the quality of the patient's tears, and the health of the ocular surface and associated structures (such as eyelids) are all important considerations. Contact lenses are usually intended as devices to provide vision as an alternative to spectacles (although there are occasions when contact lenses may be used as prosthetics, to cover a damaged eye, or as therapy for a specific disease). The clinician must modify the original refractive findings to adjust for the placement of the lens because it will rest directly on the ocular surface instead of being attached to a frame half an inch from the eye. The contact lens must be designed so that the surface of the eye is not compromised by its presence. The proper contact lens care system is vitally important for the initial and continued success of a contact lens fitting. Continuing professional supervision is essential in maintaining optimal vision and safe contact lens wear.

PERSPECTIVE AND PROSPECTS

Evidence suggests that spectacles were first used to assist human vision in Europe at about the end of the thirteenth century. Organizations of spectacle makers were formed in Europe in the fourteenth and fifteenth centuries. These guilds policed the quality of spectacles and the working conditions under which their manufacture occurred. Spectacles were sold to the public in stores and by peddlers. Individuals self-selected the lens or lenses that seemed most appropriate to them for their visual tasks. Retailers selling spectacles eventually began to assist their clientele in making an informed selection. Over time, spectacle vendors evolved into opticians. Some "refracting" opticians tested vision to provide what they believed to be the most appropriate correcting lenses for a particular person. Physicians at that time did not recommend or examine the eyes for spectacles, preferring the use of medication for eye difficulties.

The impetus for optometry's modern development and legal recognition in the United States began with a confrontation between optometry and ophthalmology. A New York refracting optician named Charles Prentice referred a patient to Henry D. Noyes, an ophthalmologist, in 1892. Noyes wrote Prentice a thank-you note for the referral but suggested that Prentice should not have charged a fee (of three dollars) for his services—such being the right reserved to professionals such as physicians. Prentice responded, defending his practice of charging for his services. Noyes sent Prentice's letters to another ophthalmologist, D. B. St. John Roosa, who expressed his opinion that Prentice was in violation of the law by charging a fee for his services. By 1895, Roosa had announced that he would

seek legislation to prevent opticians from practicing, and Prentice responded by organizing the Optical Society of the State of New York. This society eventually introduced a bill to the New York legislature to regulate the "practice of optometry." Optometry was defined as refraction, dispensing (that is, selling) spectacles, and related services.

This bill was quite controversial and never came to a vote. Later, however, another New York optometrist, Andrew J. Cross, while visiting Minnesota to teach a program in optics, scoffed at the notion that Minnesota could pass an optometry practice act before New York. Thus inspired, the Minnesotans passed their law, which included a regulatory board, in 1901. Arguing that optometry was separate and distinct from medicine, optometrists proceeded to obtain practice acts in all the states over the next twenty-three years.

Optometrists sought to be professionals rather than businesspeople and developed an agenda which included the formation of organizations: Both the American Optometric Association (AOA) and the American Academy of Optometry were established early in the twentieth century. Efforts were made both to reduce the commercial aspects of practice and to improve educational standards. A code of ethics and stringent rules of conduct were adopted by the AOA.

The first American optometric schools were extensions of apprenticeships and offered short courses (one to two weeks) in refraction. Eventually, private schools were established to train both physicians and nonphysicians. Academic programs developed from these independent schools, such as the Southern California College of Optometry and the Illinois College of Optometry. A milestone two-year optometry course began at Columbia University in New York in 1910; Cross and Prentice were instrumental in preparing the curriculum. Ohio State University began a four-year program in 1915, and the University of California, Berkeley, established an optometry course in 1923. By the late twentieth century, seventeen schools and colleges of optometry trained optometrists in the United States; many of the university programs also provided academic postgraduate studies. Similar programs were created in England, Australia, Canada, Europe, Asia, Africa, and South America.

Optometrist and lawyer John G. Classe credits the major change in the way optometry developed in the latter half of the twentieth century to contact lenses and modern tonometry. Prior to technical improvements in contact lenses and tonometry, the practice of optometry was limited and nonmedical. The commercial success of contact lenses brought about research in physiology, which in turn expanded biological knowledge and improved contact lenses. The ability to use a tonometer without drops to test for increased intraocular pressure (a condition called glaucoma) gave optometrists additional responsibility in ocular disease management. Unfortunately, the subsequent changes in practice placed optometry in even greater direct conflict with ophthalmology.

In a meeting held in January, 1968, many of the leaders of the schools and colleges of optometry, the chair of the AOA's Council on Optometric Education, and the editor of the *Journal of the American Optometric Association* unofficially discussed the future of the profession. Court decisions had ruled that optometrists had the legal responsibility to detect, diagnose, and refer ocular disease, and many optometrists were frustrated by the limited scope of their practice. This group believed that optometry should discard its original concept of being a drugless profession dedicated solely to ocular function. They argued that optometric education should be expanded in the fields of ocular pharmacology, anatomy, physiology, and pathology so that optometrists would become primary entry points into the health care system for patients. Finally, it was concluded that the state laws which govern the practice of optometry should be updated to allow the optometrist to practice what he or she was taught, including the appropriate use of pharmaceutical agents.

In 1971, Rhode Island became the first state to amend its optometry law to permit the use of diagnostic pharmaceutical drugs. Despite continued opposition from ophthalmology, all fifty states followed over the next twenty years. In 1976, West Virginia became the first state to permit the use of therapeutic drugs, and thirty-two states had enacted similar laws by 1993.

It should be noted, however, that ophthalmologists continue to oppose the expansion of optometry's scope of practice, believing that a physician—medically trained to appreciate both the local and the systemic natures of ocular disease and treatment—is best qualified to treat ocular disease. Optometry is a health care profession providing eye care to a large segment of the public. It remains a field in transition, however, and it is not clear how the dual professions of optometry and ophthalmology, as they become more similar clinically and legally, will work out their future relationship.

—*Barry A. Weissman, O.D., Ph.D.*

See also Aging: Extended care; Astigmatism; Biophysics; Blurred vision; Cataracts; Eye infections and disorders; Eyes; Geriatrics and gerontology; Glaucoma; Myopia; Ophthalmology; Optometry, pediatric; Sense organs; Strabismus; Trachoma; Vision; Vision disorders.

For Further Information:

Buettner, Helmut, ed. *Mayo Clinic on Vision and Eye Health: Practical Answers on Glaucoma, Cataracts, Macular Degeneration, and Other Conditions.* Rochester, Minn.: Mayo Foundation for Medical Education and Research, 2002. A helpful handbook on all the medical, social, and emotional facets of vision impairment.

Classe, John G. "Optometry: A Legal History." *Journal of the American Optometric Association* 59, no. 8 (1988): 641-650. This outstanding paper provides a summary of the history of the profession from a legal standpoint, including much of the more recent history not available elsewhere.

Eger, Milton J. "Now It Can and Should Be Told." *Journal of the American Optometric Association* 60, no. 4 (1989): 323-326. This paper, written by a former editor of the *Journal of the American Optometric Association*, provides insight into the deliberations and conclusions of a very important, although unofficial, meeting which helped to redirect the course of the profession of optometry in the United States.

Gregg, James R. *History of the American Academy of Optometry.* Washington, D.C.: American Academy of Optometry, 1987. This text covers the history of the academic arm of the profession of optometry. It is quite well written and focuses on many of the early proponents of academics and professionalism in the field.

Millodot, Michel. *Dictionary of Optometry and Visual Science.* 7th ed. New York: Butterworth-Heinemann/ Elsevier, 2009. Millodot defines more than four thousand of the most commonly used terms in optometry and visual science, often with clinical advice.

Sutton, Amy L., ed. *Eye Care Sourcebook: Basic Consumer Health Information About Eye Care and Eye Disorders.* 3d ed. Detroit, Mich.: Omnigraphics, 2008. A complete guide to eye care that includes such topics as eye anatomy, preventive vision care, refractive disorders and eye diseases, current research and clinical trials, and a list of organizations.

OPTOMETRY, PEDIATRIC

SPECIALTY

ANATOMY OR SYSTEM AFFECTED: Eyes

SPECIALTIES AND RELATED FIELDS: Neurology, ophthalmology

DEFINITION: The diagnosis and treatment of vision problems and of diseases and injuries to the eye in infants and children.

KEY TERMS:

amblyopia: a problem, related to strabismus but not as severe, in which one eye does not function in conjunction with its partner; also called lazy eye

astigmatism: a vision disorder in which the eyeball is misshapen, causing the resulting image to be distorted

esotropia: a condition in which the eye is turned inward

exotropia: a condition in which the eye is turned outward

hyperopia: a vision disorder, commonly called farsightedness, in which the vocal point of the image falls behind the retina; farsighted people are able to see objects better from a distance than from a short range

myopia: a vision disorder, commonly called nearsightedness, in which the focal point of the image falls in front of the retina; nearsighted people are able to see objects better from a short range than from a distance

nystagmus: jerky eye movements

strabismus: a disorder of vision in which one or both eyes are turned inward or outward

vision: the process by which the brain gives meaning to the images that it receives from the eye through the optic nerve

SCIENCE AND PROFESSION

The pediatric optometrist has received special training in the diagnosis and treatment of vision disorders in children beyond the four years of optometry college that are required for the doctor of optometry (O.D.) degree. Those who choose pediatric optometry as a specialty must, during a one-year residency, develop competency in the diagnosis and treatment of childhood vision disorders as well as develop knowledge about the various aspects of child development. They must learn to prescribe and carry out vision therapy that can help children overcome problems of eye movement, eye coordination, and perception.

The optometrist is concerned with the health and functioning of all parts of the eye: the eyelids, which act as a filter; the cornea, which covers the outer part of the eye, bends light for focusing, allows the light to pass to the retina, and protects the eye from infection; the conjunctiva, which covers the underside of the lid and allows for the proper wetting of the cornea; the lachrymal system, a glandular system that produces and eliminates tears; the orbit, the bony structure that holds the eyeball; the extraocular muscles, which control eye movement; the lens, which provides focus; and the pupil, which regulates the amount of light that enters the eye. Optometry is also concerned with the visual pathway, the route that light takes from an image through the pupil, through the lens, to the optic nerve, and to the brain for interpretation. Optometry also considers problems related to the visual field, which describes the area that can be seen to the left, to the right, up, down, and in front.

In general, children suffer the same range of visual problems that adults suffer, even cataracts and glaucoma. While the vast majority of cataracts are not congenital and occur beyond the age of fifty, a cataract can be present at birth or develop at any time. One of every 10,000 births produces a baby with congenital glaucoma.

Conditions such as amblyopia or strabismus, in which one eye does not function properly with the other eye, are treated by pediatric optometrists. These conditions are characterized by eye turns that may be esotropic (inward) or exotropic (outward). Esotropic turning usually occurs at birth, while exotropic turning generally occurs after six months of age. Whether the eye turns are inward or outward, the pediatric optometrist must work with the patient to establish or restore binocularity, the process of two eyes working together to send an image to the brain; individuals who do not have binocularity have problems with depth perception and distance judgment.

Like adults, children have problems with farsightedness, nearsightedness, and astigmatism, as well as with eye injuries and diseases of the eye such as conjunctivitis, a highly contagious infection of the conjunctiva. Various diseases occurring in childhood, such as rubella and juvenile-onset diabetes, might affect eye functioning and create vision disorders.

Even though children have many of the same eye and vision problems as adults, childhood is a special developmental period. Eye or vision problems can significantly affect the quality of a child's early years as well as the quality of the child's future. A child's ability to read well, to do well in school, to play sports, and to interact effectively with peers may all be hampered by poor eye health or by vision problems. Pediatric optometrists must have knowledge of all aspects of human development and must understand how vision problems can impact development.

DIAGNOSTIC AND TREATMENT TECHNIQUES

Upon the initial examination of a child, the pediatric optometrist first takes the child's health history. A health history is important because many types of diseases, such as diabetes, and many kinds of physical conditions, such as high blood pressure, can create vision problems. The optometrist also obtains a family medical history, since certain visual problems are genetically based.

Next, the pediatric optometrist examines the patient's eyes for disease and injury. Certain tests are performed to determine visual acuity, perception, and reaction. An optometrist may prescribe visual therapy to improve or correct problems related to binocularity, perception, or reaction. Corrective lenses are prescribed to correct problems of acuity. When glasses are needed, the optometrist may work with an optician to make sure that the child receives eyewear that is flattering, as eyewear can affect the child's social life.

In cases of amblyopia and strabismus, surgery may be indicated. If so, the pediatric optometrist refers the patient to a pediatric ophthalmologist. Modern practice generally involves the use of vision therapy to train the eyes to work together. Sometimes, surgery is performed for strabismus, but often such surgery is only cosmetic; vision therapy is still required. Pediatric cases involving glaucoma, cataracts, or tumors also require the optometrist to work closely with an ophthalmologist.

PERSPECTIVE AND PROSPECTS

Research indicates that cultures that rely heavily on work requiring close visual examination, such as reading, have much higher incidences of vision problems than do other cultures. Thus, in the modern world, where there is a high dependence on literacy skills and computer use for recreational purposes, for communica-tion, and for job functions, it is likely that all aspects of pediatric optometry will grow in the foreseeable future.

—*Annita Marie Ward, Ed.D.*

See also Blindness; Blurred vision; Conjunctivitis; Diabetes mellitus; Eye infections and disorders; Eye surgery; Eyes; Myopia; Optometry; Sense organs; Strabismus; Styes; Vision; Vision disorders.

FOR FURTHER INFORMATION:

Behrman, Richard E., Robert M. Kliegman, and Hal B. Jenson, eds. *Nelson Textbook of Pediatrics*. 18th ed. Philadelphia: Saunders/Elsevier, 2007.

Buettner, Helmut, ed. *Mayo Clinic on Vision and Eye Health: Practical Answers on Glaucoma, Cataracts, Macular Degeneration, and Other Conditions*. Rochester, Minn.: Mayo Foundation for Medical Education and Research, 2002.

Clark, Robert. *Does Your Child Really Need Glasses? A Parent's Complete Guide to Eye Care*. New York: Crown, 2003.

D'Alonzo, Thomas L. *Your Eyes! A Comprehensive Look at the Understanding and Treatment of Vision Problems*. Clifton Heights, Pa.: Avanti, 1991.

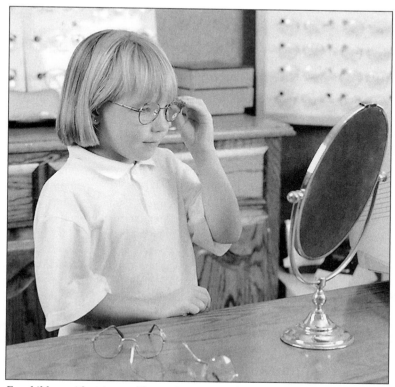

For children with vision problems, glasses provide the safest and easiest means of correction. (Digital Stock)

Jennings, Barbara J., ed. *Pediatric Optometry*. Stamford, Conn.: Appleton & Lange, 1996.

Nathanson, Laura Walther. *The Portable Pediatrician: A Practicing Pediatrician's Guide to Your Child's Growth, Development, Health, and Behavior from Birth to Age Five*. 2d ed. New York: HarperCollins, 2002.

ORAL AND MAXILLOFACIAL SURGERY
SPECIALTY

ANATOMY OR SYSTEM AFFECTED: Gums, head, mouth, teeth

SPECIALTIES AND RELATED FIELDS: Anesthesiology, dentistry, oncology, otorhinolaryngology, plastic surgery

DEFINITION: A specialty of dentistry that deals with the diagnosis and management of diseases or conditions of the mouth, teeth, jaws, and face.

KEY TERMS:

mandible: the lower bone of the jaw

maxilla: two fused bones that make up the upper jaw and the mid-portion of the facial skeleton

nitrous oxide: a chemical compound that at room temperature forms a colorless gas, also known as laughing gas, used to produce anesthesia and analgesia during surgery

obstructive sleep apnea: periods of interrupted breathing during sleep caused by airway obstruction in the nose or throat

orthgnathic surgery: surgical procedures of the jaws to correct structural deformity caused by congenital or growth defects

temporomandibular joint: the hinged joint that attaches the head of the mandible to the skull

SCIENCE AND PROFESSION

The specialist in oral and maxillofacial surgery deals with the anatomical region of the head that includes the oral cavity and the hard and soft tissues that comprise that part of the facial skeleton formed by the mandible and the maxilla. The mandible is the bone that forms the lower jaw and the maxilla is the fusion of the two bones that form the middle part of the face, or the upper jaw.

The maxilla forms the roof of the mouth, the lateral walls and floor of the nose, and the floor of the eye cavities. The maxilla contains the maxillary sinuses and holds the upper teeth. The mandible holds the lower teeth and attaches to the temporal bone of the skull at the temporomandibular joint (TMJ).

The diseases and conditions treated by oral and maxillofacial surgeons are numerous and diverse. They may include extraction of impacted teeth, dental implants, benign and malignant lesions of the oral cavity, TMJ disorders, management of facial pain syndromes, facial fractures, obstructive sleep apnea, and surgical correction of congenital deformities. Oral and maxillofacial surgeons will treat infections of the jaws, oral cavities, and salivary glands and may perform facial cosmetic procedures.

Most oral and maxillofacial surgeons begin their training after dental school. Increasingly, medical doctors are being integrated into the specialty through additional dentistry training and subsequent entry into an oral and maxillofacial training program. The oral and maxillofacial surgical residency includes general surgery, plastic surgery, medicine, and anesthesia. A four-year residency program grants a degree that makes these surgeons board eligible in oral and maxillofacial surgery. About half of American oral and maxillofacial surgeons complete a six-year residency program that grants a medical degree as well. Graduates of the residency program may elect to do additional fellowship training in head and neck cancer, cosmetic facial surgery, pediatric maxillofacial surgery, or maxillofacial trauma.

Oral and maxillofacial surgery is recognized as one of nine dental specialties. The American Board of Oral and Maxillofacial Surgery is responsible for certifying oral and maxillofacial surgeons in the United States. The board is recognized and approved by the Council on Dental Education of the American Dental Association. In order to become board-certified, a typical applicant will have completed four years of undergraduate studies and four years of dental school, followed by an approved training program. Candidates must present letters of recommendation from board-certified oral and maxillofacial surgeons and then pass a written and oral examination. After completion of these qualifications, applicants are granted the title of Diplomat of the American Board of Oral and Maxillofacial Surgery. The board requires that its diplomats be recertified every ten years.

DIAGNOSTIC AND TREATMENT TECHNIQUES

Oral and maxillofacial surgeons take careful and detailed histories of present and past medical conditions, including family history, medication history, and allergy history. Examination of the oral and maxillofacial area includes a complete examination of the oral cavity and the use of radiologic techniques to visualize the soft tissues and bone structure of the jaw and the midface. Many oral and maxillofacial surgeons perform conventional radiographs (X rays) and panoramic radiographs of the upper and lower jaw in their office. The diagnosis of oral and maxillofacial conditions is further aided by the use of diagnostic images from computed tomography (CT) scans and magnetic resonance imaging (MRI).

Oral and maxillofacial surgeons perform surgical procedures both at the hospital and in the office. Because many biopsies and dental procedures are done in the office, these specialists must be proficient in administering oral sedation, local anesthetics, nitrous oxide, intravenous sedation, and general anesthesia. Patients who come to oral and maxillofacial surgeons come from all age groups. They may have multiple medical conditions and require a broad range of medical and surgical care. The oral and maxillofacial surgeon must be part medical doctor, part general surgeon, and part dentist.

Some of the more common treatment techniques in oral and maxillofacial surgery include dental procedures for removal of impacted teeth or teeth that cannot be restored. These surgeons may work along with restorative dentists to reconstruct bone for placement of dental implants. In the event of facial trauma, oral and maxillofacial surgeons may be called upon to repair routine and complex fractures, repair lacerations, and reconstruct damaged nerves and blood vessels. Oral and maxillofacial surgeons may diagnose and treat benign cysts and growths in the oral cavity, including cysts that form in the salivary glands. Head and neck cancer diagnosis and treatment may include malignant lesions of the jaws, lips, or oral cavity.

A major component of the specialty involves reconstructive and orthognathic surgery to correct congenital deformities such as facial asymmetry, bite deformities, and cleft lip or palate. Obstructive sleep apnea is being increasingly recognized and may affect up to 45 percent of the U.S. population. Severe cases may be life threatening and may be an indication for surgical intervention by an oral and maxillofacial specialist. Maxillomandibular advancement surgery may be performed in selected cases. The procedure involves moving the upper and lower jaws forward. The bones are surgically separated and advanced to increase the opening of the airway. The procedure is done in the hospital under general anesthesia and may take three to four hours to complete. In cases of severe obstructive sleep

apnea that do not respond to conservative treatments, this type of orthognatic surgery may be the treatment of choice.

Chronic facial pain disorders that oral and maxillofacial surgeons deal with include TMJ disease and neurogenic pain syndromes. TMJ disorders may cause pain in the ear, headache, or pain when moving the jaw. The oral and maxillofacial surgeon may treat this condition conservatively with medication or splint therapy. In more severe cases, open or arthroscopic joint surgery may be indicated. The most common craniofacial pain syndrome is trigeminal neuralgia. If medications are not effective, then the oral and maxillofacial surgeon may treat this condition with local nerve block, surgical destruction of the nerve, or microvascular decompression of the trigeminal nerve root.

Because of their surgical training, their familiarity with the soft tissue and structural anatomy of the face, and their experience with office-based surgery and anesthesia, oral maxillofacial surgeons are uniquely qualified and positioned to take advantage of recent developments in facial cosmetic surgery. Facial cosmetic surgery may be indicated for birth defects, deformity resulting from injury, or aging process reversal. Facial plastic surgery that may be performed by the oral and maxillofacial surgeon includes cheekbone implants, chin augmentation, facial and neck liposuction, lip enhancement, and face lift surgery. These specialists may also use the surgical laser to remove outer layers of damaged skin, inject collagen to fill wrinkles, and use Botox injections to reduce muscle activity that causes wrinkles.

PERSPECTIVE AND PROSPECTS

Hesy-Re, an Egyptian scribe who lived around 2600 B.C.E., is credited as the first dentist. The Greek physician Hippocrates, who lived between 500 and 300 B.C.E., described treatments of diseased teeth and gums including the use of forceps to extract teeth and wires to stabilize fractured jaws. During the early part of the Middle Ages, most oral surgery was performed by monks; after the popes forbade monks from practicing medicine, barbers became responsible for extracting teeth and draining dental abscesses. In 1723, the French surgeon Pierre Fauchard described the practice of dentistry, including oral anatomy and operative and restorative procedures, and is credited with being the founder of modern dentistry. The American Revolutionary War patriot Paul Revere advertised himself as a dentist, in addition to being a fine silversmith. The first dental school was established in 1840 as the Baltimore College of Dental Surgery, and in 1867 the Harvard Dental School became the first university-affiliated dental school. In 1844, the Connecticut dentist Horace Wells performed the first dental extractions done using nitrous oxide as an anesthetic.

Simon P. Hullihen of Wheeling, West Virginia, both a medical doctor and a dentist, is considered to be the founder of oral surgery. He specialized in operations on defects of the mouth and head and performed hundreds of operations for cleft lip, cleft palate, and other abnormalities of the mouth and jaw.

Another contributing factor to the development of the specialty of oral and maxillofacial surgery was the devastating injuries suffered by soldiers during the great wars of the twentieth century. It became clear to battlefield surgeons that dentists were needed to help align dental occlusion in facial injuries and fractured jaws. Dentists became valued members of the surgical team, and today dentistry is still the field from which most oral and maxillofacial surgeons come.

In 1945, a committee was authorized to establish an American Board of Oral Surgery (ABOS). In 1947, the ABOS was approved by the American Dental Association. The name of the board was changed to the American Board of Oral and Maxillofacial Surgery in 1978 to more accurately reflect the complete scope of the specialty.

Advancements in cosmetic and reconstructive surgery put the oral and maxillofacial surgery specialist at the cutting edge of medical innovation. An example is the French oral and maxillofacial surgeon Bernard Devauchelle, who along with his colleges at the University Hospital Center of Amiens, France, performed the first human face transplant. In November, 2005, Devauchelle and his team transplanted the central and lower face of a thirty-eight-year-old woman whose nose, lips, and chin had been lost as a result of a dog bite. Their success was reported around the world and hailed as a milestone in surgical history. Today, the specialty of oral maxillofacial surgery is a dynamic field that attracts both medical and dental school graduates. Although the residency program is long and arduous, the rewards of the specialty are great.

—Chris Iliades, M.D.

See also Anesthesia; Anesthesiology; Birth defects; Cleft lip and palate; Cleft lip and palate repair; Dental diseases; Dentistry; Dentistry, pediatric; Facial transplantation; Fracture repair; Head and neck disorders; Jaw wiring; Orthodontics; Periodontal surgery; Periodontitis; Plastic surgery; Root canal treatment; Surgery, general; Teeth; Temporomandibular joint (TMJ) syndrome; Tooth extraction; Toothache; Wisdom teeth.

FOR FURTHER INFORMATION:

Ellis, Edward, et al. *Contemporary Oral and Maxillofacial Surgery.* 4th ed. St. Louis: Mosby/Elsevier, 2008. A comprehensive review of the principles of basic oral and maxillofacial problems that may be seen in a general medical practice. The text also details when a patient should be sent to an oral and maxillofacial specialist and how these complex cases are managed in the specialty setting.

Miloro, Michael, et al. *Peterson's Principles of Oral and Maxillofacial Surgery.* 2d ed. Philadelphia: BC Decker, 2004. A detailed but concise and easy-to-read reference text that covers the complete scope or oral and maxillofacial diagnosis and treatment.

Mitchell, David A. *An Introduction to Oral and Maxillofacial Surgery.* New York: Oxford University Press, 2006. An introduction for undergraduates or dental students including core competencies and skills that are required, as well as a comprehensive review of the diagnosis and treatment of oral and maxillofacial problems.

White, R. L. "Oral and Maxillofacial Surgery: Defining Our Present, Shaping Our Future." *Journal of the American College of Dentistry* 76, no. 1. (Spring, 2009): 36-39. A review of the specialty through the eyes of the American Association of Oral and Maxillofacial Surgeons, its guidelines and practice standards, and prospects for future research and development.

ORCHIECTOMY

PROCEDURE

ANATOMY OR SYSTEM AFFECTED: Reproductive system

SPECIALTIES AND RELATED FIELDS: Urology

ALSO KNOWN AS: Testicle removal

DEFINITION: Excision of a testicle, usually performed as part of cancer therapy.

KEY TERMS:

electrocautery: a needle charged with electricity that is heated and placed on the tissue; often used to remove warts and polyps

lymphadenectomy: the removal of lymph nodes, one or more in a group

seminoma: the most common cancer of the testes

INDICATIONS AND PROCEDURES

Orchiectomy is usually performed for benign or malignant conditions. For metastic carcinoma of the prostate, bilateral orchiectomy is often utilized. For primary tumors of the testes that are malignant, radical orchiectomy is performed for the best result.

During simple orchiectomy, the patient is placed in the supine position. Then his genitalia is prepared in a sterile manner. During incision, bilateral orchiectomy is performed either by a transverse incision which would extend across the midline or a single midline incision. The scalpel incises the scrotal skin, and the dartos muscle and immediate underlying tissues are sectioned off by electrocautery. The testis is withdrawn from its sac only after the tunica vaginalis is incised. The spermatic cord is clamped during the procedure, and then it gets divided.

When it comes to radical orchiectomy, the patient is placed in a supine position. The genitalia and the inguinal region are prepared in a sterile manner, and an inguinal skin incision is made. The incision continues on through the subcutaneous tissue whereby the external oblique fascia is identified. The part is incised which opens toward the external ring. Then the spermatic cord is freed and clamped at the same level of the internal ring by tightening the looped one-half-inch Penrose drain. A rubber shod clamp may be used instead. Next, the testis is firmly pulled up from the scrotum. A radical orchiectomy would be necessary if the testis felt and looked grossly abnormal. If there is a question or doubt about the tunica vaginalis being opened, an incisional biopsy of the testis would be performed. Once the tumor is verified, either by gross analysis or by a frozen section, the cord is doubly clamped at the level of the internal ring.

It is important for patients undergoing an orchiectomy to have blood drawn and a urine sample collected and to stop any aspirins that they may be taking a week before the procedure. Also, all nonsteroidal anti-inflammatory drugs (NSAIDs) should be discontinued two days before the procedure.

Orchiectomy can be a part of gender reassignment surgery and is mostly done in clinics that specialize in it. It is considered genital reconstruction. Prior to the genital reconstruction, patients usually undergo hormone therapy for several months or as long as a year before going through the surgery. The patient must be sure that he wants to live life as a woman with real-life experiences as a female with all the social implications.

USES AND COMPLICATIONS

Orchiectomy can be used to treat testicular cancer. Seminoma is a type of testicular cancer that, if the tumors are localized, in 98 percent of the patients is curable with orchiectomy and low doses of adjuvant radiotherapy. Advanced cancer at stage II is curable with orchiectomy and radiation therapy to the involved areas for 85 to 90 percent of patients. In metastatic diseases, stage III or localized advanced disease is primarily curable in 90 percent of the patients if combined with chemotherapy. Nonseminoma germ cell tumors (NSGCTs) seem to resist radiation therapy and are more likely to travel to the lungs, brain, bones, and liver.

Both seminoma and nonseminoma are highly curable if caught early enough, even if the cancer has spread beyond the testes to other body parts and tissues, as compared to other cancers. When it comes to relapse of the disease, the risk is lowered with retroperitoneal lymphadenectomy followed by chemotherapy, but this protocol does not improve survival. It is also possible that removing the lymph nodes may cause infertility.

Patients who have undergone orchiectomy may go to work the next day, if they desire. However, some patients may need a day or two before they feel ready. It is important to drink fluids such as water and to abstain from alcoholic beverages. Sometimes, the patient may feel nauseated if the procedure was performed because of cancer. Some pain and swelling may develop, which is normal, and the physician may prescribe medications to counteract them.

One of the major risks of orchiectomy is a sudden hormone change, and side effects may occur, such as loss of muscle mass, brittle bones, weight gain, fatigue, erection problems, loss of sexual desire, hot flashes, enlargement and tenderness in the breasts, and sterility.

Undergoing orchiectomy for male-to-female genital reconstruction requires a diagnosis from a psychiatrist, as well as letters from mental health counselors in support of this procedure. Such precautions are highly important because the patient's life will completely change.

PERSPECTIVE AND PROSPECTS

In 1941, orchiectomy was first used on a patient suffering from advanced prostate cancer. Indications from this therapy showed no apparent improvement of survival from it. In 1967, the Veterans Administration Cooperative Urological Research Group or (VACURG), presented information on more than two thousand patients who had received different types of therapies, including orchiectomy.

From 1984 through 1993, a study was performed on seventy-two patients with stage C and stage D prostate cancer whereby forty-four out of sixty-one patients had a partial response, and a good response on the tumor markers. Finally, in some states orchiectomy may be used for sex offenders on a case by case basis.

—*Marvin Morris, L.Ac., M.P.A.*

See also Genital disorders, male; Glands; Hydroceles; Men's health; Orchitis; Reproductive system; Surgery, general; Testicles, undescended; Testicular cancer; Testicular surgery; Testicular torsion; Urology; Urology, pediatric; Vascular system.

FOR FURTHER INFORMATION:

Dawson, C. "Testicular Cancer: Seek Advice Early." *Journal of Family Health Care* 12 (2002): 3.

Geldart, T. R., P. D. Simmonds, and G. M. Mead. "Orchiectomy After Chemotherapy for Patients with Metastatic Testicular Germ Cell Cancer." *BJU International* 90 (September, 2002): 451-455.

Incrocci, L., et al. " Treatment Outcome, Body Image, and Sexual Functioning After Orchiectomy and Radiotherapy for Stage I-II Testicular Seminoma." *International Journal of Radiation Oncology, Biology, Physics* 53 (August 1, 2002): 1165-1173.

Khatri, Vijay P., and Juan A. Asensio. *Khatri: Operative Surgery Manual*. Philadelphia: Saunders, 2003.

ORCHITIS

DISEASE/DISORDER

ALSO KNOWN AS: Epididymoorchitis

ANATOMY OR SYSTEM AFFECTED: Genitals, reproductive system

SPECIALTIES AND RELATED FIELDS: Family medicine, virology

DEFINITION: An inflammation of one or both testicles.

CAUSES AND SYMPTOMS

Orchitis is usually a consequence of epididymitis, an inflammation of the tube that connects the vas deferens and the testicles. It can also result from prostate infections. The source of inflammation can be either bacterial or viral organisms. The disease is typically caused by a generalized infection, such as mumps, scarlet fever, or typhoid fever. Chronic cases of orchitis can be produced by syphilis, gonorrhea, chlamydia, tuberculosis, and parasitic infections. In most cases of orchitis, only one testis is infected.

> ## INFORMATION ON ORCHITIS
>
> **CAUSES:** Bacterial or viral infection of epididymis or prostate from mumps, scarlet fever, typhoid fever; chronic cases may result from STDs (syphilis, gonorrhea, chlamydia), tuberculosis, parasitic infections
>
> **SYMPTOMS:** Tenderness and swelling of affected testis; nausea; fever; fatigue; groin pain; pain during urination, intercourse, or ejaculation; penile discharge; blood in semen
>
> **DURATION:** Acute, with possible sterility
>
> **TREATMENTS:** Depends on cause; may include antibiotics, anti-inflammatory drugs, bed rest, elevation and support of testes, pain medications, ice packs

The most frequent cause of orchitis is the mumps, a viral infection. About one-third of males with the mumps develop orchitis at some stage of the illness, usually within four to six days after it begins. In prepubertal boys, about 20 percent develop mumps-induced orchitis. It is much more rare for males who are past puberty.

Symptoms of orchitis include nausea, fever, fatigue, and tenderness and significant swelling of the affected testis. Other effects may include groin pain, pain during urination, discharge from the penis, pain associated with intercourse and ejaculation, and blood in the semen.

TREATMENT AND THERAPY

If orchitis is produced by a bacterial infection, then antibiotics are the most effective treatment. Anti-inflammatory drugs are also commonly prescribed. If the source of infection is viral, then orchitis can be treated only with proper bed rest, elevation and support of the testes, and pain-relieving drugs. The application of ice packs periodically to the infected area helps reduce the pain. If acute pain occurs in the scrotum or testicles, then immediate medical attention is necessary.

When orchitis is properly treated and the cause is bacterial, normal function of the testis is typically preserved. If mumps is the source of orchitis, then shrinking of the testicles often occurs and, in some cases, sterility. Sterility is very rare, however, in cases of unilateral (one-sided) orchitis. Immunization against mumps is the best preventive treatment to avoid these possible complications of orchitis, although there have been a few cases of mumps-induced orchitis developing subsequent to a mumps-measles-rubella (MMR) vaccine. Spread of bacteria associated with sexually transmitted diseases (STDs) that can cause epididymo-orchitis in sexually active men can be minimized through monogamy and the use of condoms.

PERSPECTIVE AND PROSPECTS

The first recorded description of orchitis goes back to Hippocrates in the fifth century B.C.E. Physical examination often reveals a tender, enlarged testicle on the affected side. Tender, enlarged lymph nodes in the groin area may also indicate the presence of orchitis.

Doppler ultrasound of the groin area can be used to confirm a diagnosis of orchitis by showing increased blood flow to the affected region, as well as tissue textures that are associated with infection. This test can also reveal any presence of scrotal abscesses. Nuclear magnetic resonance (NMR) imaging may also be used to help diagnose the presence of orchitis.

—*Alvin K. Benson, Ph.D.*

See also Antibiotics; Bacterial infections; Chlamydia; Gonorrhea; Men's health; Mumps; Parasitic diseases; Prostate gland; Reproductive system; Scarlet fever; Sexually transmitted diseases (STDs); Syphilis; Testicles, undescended; Testicular cancer; Testicular surgery; Testicular torsion; Typhoid fever; Tuberculosis; Viral infections.

FOR FURTHER INFORMATION:

Behrman, Richard E., Robert M. Kliegman, and Hal B. Jenson, eds. *Nelson Textbook of Pediatrics*. 18th ed. Philadelphia: Saunders/Elsevier, 2007.

Rosenfeld, Isadore. *Symptoms*. New York: Bantam Books, 1994.

Standring, Susan, et al., eds. *Gray's Anatomy*. 40th ed. New York: Churchill Livingstone/Elsevier, 2008.

Taguchi, Yosh, and Merrily Weisbord, eds. *Private Parts: An Owner's Guide to the Male Anatomy*. 3d ed. Toronto, Ont.: McClelland & Stewart, 2003.

Van De Graaff, Kent M. *Human Anatomy*. 6th ed. New York: McGraw-Hill, 2002.

ORGANS. *See* SYSTEMS AND ORGANS.

ORTHODONTICS

SPECIALTY

ANATOMY OR SYSTEM AFFECTED: Gums, mouth, teeth
SPECIALTIES AND RELATED FIELDS: Dentistry
DEFINITION: A dental specialty in which the teeth are straightened and moved into positions in the jaws that yield a correct and attractive arrangement.

KEY TERMS:

analgesic: a medication (such as aspirin) that reduces or eliminates pain

dental arch: the arched bony part of the upper and lower jaws, in which the teeth are found

lingual: related to the tongue; in orthodontics, the inner sides or faces of the teeth

malocclusion: an incorrect fit of the upper and lower teeth when they are brought together

mastication: the act of chewing food

occlusion: the fit of the upper and lower teeth when they are brought together

SCIENCE AND PROFESSION

The term "orthodontics" comes from the Greek words meaning "straight teeth." It is practiced by the dental specialist called an orthodontist. Orthodontists graduate from dental school and then specialize in orthodontics. To explore orthodontics as a field, one must first consider teeth and the mouth. Ideally, thirty-two human teeth are arranged in appropriate orientations in the dental arches of each jaw. Four incisors are located in the center of each arch; on either side of them are a cuspid or canine tooth, followed by two bicuspids (premolars) and three molars.

The first molar on the side of each jaw is viewed as particularly important to orthodontics. Appropriate tooth development within the jaw and correct tooth eruption enable proper dental health, which keeps teeth in the mouth for most of an individual's life. They also ensure appropriate mastication of food and good digestive health, as well as self-confidence with an attractive smile.

Teeth are rarely optimally placed in the jaws. One important reason for this is heredity. This facet of orthodontics relates to the teeth and to jaws. The genes that control the size and shape of human teeth and jaws vary considerably. In addition, the genes for teeth and jaws are highly individualized and often poorly related to one another. Hence, it is likely that orthodontic problems caused by tooth-jaw mismatch will occur.

Other aspects of the development of irregular tooth positioning arise from living. In some cases, teeth are damaged by decay, oral diseases, or injury. In others, poor oral habits such as thumb sucking move them out of appropriate positions. In many cases, minor problems may be handled by restorative dentistry, such as filling dental caries or placing crowns. Most treatment of poorly positioned teeth, however, is carried out by orthodontists on nearly 5 million Americans per year.

The majority of these patients are children, but many adults are presently undergoing orthodontic treatment.

There are several main goals of orthodontic treatment involving the bones of the jaws and the teeth. First, occlusion is improved so that all teeth engage one another properly for chewing and swallowing. Speech patterns are also improved, because almost twenty letter sounds involve interactions between tooth, tongue, and jaw movements. Another goal is increased resistance to decay and periodontal disease, which cause havoc in mouths where teeth are too close together or misaligned in other ways. The final orthodontic goal is improved appearance, which is for many individuals the primary reason for undergoing treatment.

Most orthodontic problems are termed malocclusions and are caused by defects of teeth and/or the jaws. Malocclusions are often classified according to the system developed by Edward H. Angle, the originator of orthodontics. Three occlusion classes exist, defined by relationships between the upper and lower first molars.

In normal occlusion (class I), the lower first molars are seen slightly farther forward than their upper counterparts when the mouth is closed. This relationship positions the rest of the teeth for optimum chewing. When the arch length of either jaw is too small for all the teeth to be in appropriate positions, they become crowded. Also, in some individuals bimaxillary protrusion occurs, in which the front teeth of the jaws flare outward. These occurrences are unattractive and lead both to tooth decay and to periodontal disease.

Classes II and III are malocclusions that can be considered together. They are caused by improper positioning in the closed mouth of the lower first molars, either very far back or very far forward. In the first case (class II), the position of the first molars produces buck teeth because of the protrusion of the upper jaw in the closed mouth. The resulting problems are uncosmetic appearance and the ease with which buck teeth can be knocked out. Class II malocclusion is most often attributable to a hereditary size mismatch of the jawbones. Class III malocclusion is often termed crossbite. It causes the lower jaw to be positioned so that the lower front incisors are in front of the upper ones. In some cases, this problem is treated by orthodontics; in others, surgery is required.

The Angle classification system does not include faulty vertical relationships of the jaws, which produce other problems. Examples are overbite, which hides the lower teeth entirely in the closed jaw, and open bite, which leaves a gap between the upper and lower front teeth in the closed mouth. These situations may be asymmetric and make closures lopsided.

Functional malocclusions are also caused by thumb sucking, chewing of the lower lip, or tongue thrusting. With thumb sucking, class II malocclusion may result or be enhanced, or open bite may occur. Chewing the lower lip will cause the upper front teeth to flare outward, and tongue thrusting (often a consequence of mouth breathing because of asthma) may cause open bite, crossbite, or class II malocclusion.

Defects of the teeth themselves occur as well. They are caused by overretention or underretention of the baby teeth and missing or lost permanent teeth. These conditions cause the remaining teeth to drift in the mouth and should be corrected as soon as possible in order to preclude occlusion problems.

DIAGNOSTIC AND TREATMENT TECHNIQUES

The first stage of orthodontic treatment is an extensive diagnostic procedure that requires several office visits. First, the orthodontist compiles a complete dental and medical history. Then, the patient's mouth and teeth are examined thoroughly. This effort, accomplished in one visit, leads to a preliminary treatment plan. During the next visit, complete X rays of the jaws are taken to show their relationship to each other, dental impressions of the teeth and jaws are made, and color photographs of the face and mouth are taken.

On the third visit, the patient is given a comprehensive diagnosis, and a treatment plan is described. At this point, the patient is informed about the problems to be treated, the probable consequences if they are left untreated, the steps to be used and their duration, the results that are expected, and any possible treatment complications. The overall cost of the treatment is also discussed. After agreement is reached, treatment begins and may require up to several years of visits at varied intervals. The process begins with the use of orthodontic appliances worn to move the teeth to new positions. After this, a simpler appliance called a retainer is worn until the bone of the tooth sockets, remodeled by the earlier treatment, is able to maintain the new dental arrangement.

Patient compliance with treatment instructions is crucial. Short-term noncompliance can lengthen the treatment period greatly; extreme noncompliance may completely destroy the endeavor. Most aspects of modern orthodontic treatment are relatively painless. If soreness occurs, it may usually be relieved quickly by combining saltwater gargles, temporary soft diets, and mild analgesics. Soreness caused by the rubbing of metal appliance parts against the inside of the cheeks or lips may be prevented by application of a wax supplied by the orthodontist. Pain that lasts for more than several days should be reported; it can usually be alleviated by an office visit where the orthodontist adjusts the offending portion of the appliance.

Throughout the course of orthodontic treatment, it is recommended that patients keep careful written records of orthodontic instructions and a complete daily record of use of the orthodontic appliance prescribed. The orthodontic appliances also need to be kept clean, stored carefully if removable, and guarded carefully during sports or other physical activities. The teeth must also be kept clean to prevent tooth decay. In addition, hard or sticky foods must be avoided.

The mechanical devices used by orthodontists vary widely. Their purposes are to direct jaw growth, to move selected teeth, to alter the behavior of the jaw muscles, and to maintain the position of the teeth once they have been moved. These appliances operate on two main principles. First, bone growth slows when pressure is applied against it and accelerates when the bone is kept in traction. This is how desired facial bone growth is attained. Second, when pressure is applied to the bone in tooth sockets, bone growth slows on the side to which the pressure is applied. Conversely, the growth of bone is stimulated on the other side of the tooth. This is the principle that generates tooth movement in the mouth. Applied properly, the combination of jaw and tooth treatment achieves results that can be fine-tuned over the treatment period. A lengthy treatment period ensures the minimum amount of pain while this movement occurs.

There are two main categories among the many orthodontic appliances used: fixed and removable appliances. Each category has numerous subcategories, and there are variants within each subcategory. Fixed appliances are firmly affixed in the mouth for the duration of treatment. They are made of metal cylinders shaped to fit snugly around individual teeth and cemented in position. The main fixed appliance types are bracketed appliances, lingual arch wires, habit control appliances, and space retainers.

Bracketed appliances, usually called braces, move teeth and direct growth of bone in the dental arches. Although braces are often disliked by patients on aesthetic grounds, orthodontists view them as an unrivaled means to cause precise tooth movement and directed bone growth. They are made up of several components.

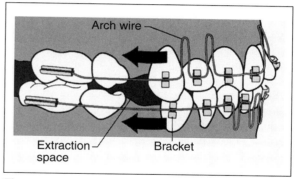

The most common orthodontic appliances are braces, which can be used to realign crooked teeth or correct malocclusion (such as underbite or overbite). In cases of tooth overcrowding, some teeth may be extracted, and the remaining teeth may be repositioned to fill the extraction space (shown here).

First, bands (metal cylinders) are applied around chosen anchor teeth. Then, metal or sturdy synthetic polymer brackets are cemented to each tooth in positions that determine the direction of the force to be applied to it. Next, arch wires are passed across each bracket to the anchor teeth, where they are attached to the bands. Elastic or wire ligatures keep the arch wires in the brackets at all times.

Much of the pressure that engenders tooth movement comes from the shape of the arch wires and their composition. Elastic bands are also used to provide special treatment to a given tooth or tooth group. These bands must be removed before eating and replaced daily. When necessary, external headgear is used to apply pressure to teeth and/or jaws, either pulling them forward or pushing them backward.

Lingual bracketed appliances, a newer device often called "invisible braces," are fixed appliances attached to the teeth on the inside of the dental arch. They are not externally visible except for the bands on the anchor teeth. Thus, they are advantageous aesthetically. They do not function as well as standard braces, however, and often interfere with normal speech. Other fixed appliances include lingual arch wires, habit control devices, and space retainers.

A wide variety of removable appliances may also be used. They are either entirely or partly removable by wearers. Removable appliances are most effective when worn constantly, but they can be removed at meals and on special occasions. Their use gives much less precise results than fixed appliances, however, and requires the continuous, unflagging cooperation of patients. Active, partly removable appliances put pressure on teeth and jaws. Functional appliances, which are completely removable, alter the pressure created by the muscles of the mouth and so act on the teeth and bones (for example, lip bumpers, which keep lips away from teeth).

Removable habit control appliances and space retainers are used, respectively, to prevent activities such as thumb sucking and to maintain desired spaces between teeth until the new dental arrangements have stabilized. They are specially designed bands, acrylic plates, and/or combinations. Space retainers exert enough pressure on teeth to keep them in place but not to move them. Special headgear may also be used as an auxiliary to in-the-mouth appliances. In some cases, diseased or extra teeth must be extracted as part of the treatment regimen.

PERSPECTIVE AND PROSPECTS

Orthodontics has changed markedly since its inception. The changes include efforts at making braces more appealing and a changing clientele, evolving from one in which most patients were children to a population having many adult customers. The new direction in producing more cosmetic bracketed appliances arises from several factors.

First is the development of stronger and better synthetic polymer and ceramic replacements for metals, allowing the creation of materials that are less visible and that still produce the unrivaled therapeutic capabilities of bracketed appliances. A second factor is the interest of adults in orthodontic treatment. This discriminating population wishes to appear as attractive as possible, even in braces, and has both the independence of judgment and the monetary power to drive trends toward the use of such materials.

The adult move toward orthodontics in the United States is founded partly on the funding of orthodontic work by entities as diverse as Medicaid for welfare recipients and third-party group dental insurance plans. In addition, the adult public is being made more aware that it is not necessary to live out life with an unattractive smile simply because orthodontic treatment was not attempted in childhood or adolescence.

Considerable research has been carried out in the treatment of problems associated with orthodontics, including the root tip resorption that often halts such treatment. It is hoped that a combination of these endeavors and factors will continue to improve orthodontics.

—Sanford S. Singer, Ph.D.

See also Bones and the skeleton; Braces, orthodontic; Dentistry; Jaw wiring; Orthodontics; Periodontal surgery; Teeth; Tooth extraction.

FOR FURTHER INFORMATION:

Doundoulakis, James, and Warren Strugatch. *The Perfect Smile: The Complete Guide to Cosmetic Dentistry.* Long Island, N.Y.: Hatherleigh Press, 2003. Covers treatments and products available to today's consumer and explores financial and insurance considerations, effectiveness, duration, and risks of each. Topics include orthodontic braces, bleaching, bonding, implants, and crowns and bridges.

Gluck, George M., and Warren M. Morganstein, eds. *Jong's Community Dental Health.* 5th ed. St. Louis, Mo.: Mosby, 2003. Explores the role of dentistry in public health, examining such topics as dental care delivery, demographic shifts and dental health, distribution of dental disease and prevention, and research in dental public health.

Holt, Robert Lawrence. *Straight Teeth: Orthodontics and Dental Care for Everyone.* New York: William Morrow, 1980. Provides excellent information on teeth; orthodontic principles, procedures, and appliances; and dental health procedures that can help maintain good dentition and cut dental and orthodontic costs. A handy glossary is included.

Houston, W. J. B., C. D. Stephens, and W. J. Tulley. *A Textbook of Orthodontics.* 2d ed. Boston: Wright, 1992. This dental handbook covers all aspects of the field of orthodontics. Includes a bibliography and an index.

Klatell, Jack, Andrew Kaplan, and Gray Williams, Jr., eds. *The Mount Sinai Medical Center Family Guide to Dental Health.* New York: Macmillan, 1991. This excellent family reference work has a fine, well-illustrated chapter on orthodontics. Procedures, appliances, and patient dos and don'ts are included. A wide variety of related dental options is also described.

Mitchell, Laura. *An Introduction to Orthodontics.* 3d ed. New York: Oxford University Press, 2007. This book provides a concise but comprehensive introduction to clinical orthodontics. It is designed to appeal to both undergraduate dental students and the practicing dentist. It is both easy to read and fully illustrated.

Smith, Rebecca W. *The Columbia University School of Dental and Oral Surgery's Guide to Family Dental Care.* New York: W. W. Norton, 1997. This classic text provides easy-to-understand explanations of all common dental problems and procedures and many less common procedures. The text is written for the general reader.

ORTHOPEDIC BRACES. *See* BRACES, ORTHOPEDIC.

ORTHOPEDIC SURGERY
PROCEDURE

ANATOMY OR SYSTEM AFFECTED: Bones, feet, hands, hips, joints, knees, legs, ligaments, muscles, musculoskeletal system, nervous system, spine, tendons

SPECIALTIES AND RELATED FIELDS: General surgery, orthopedics, physical therapy, podiatry, rheumatology, sports medicine

DEFINITION: Surgical procedures involving the bones or joints.

KEY TERMS:

polymethylmethacrylate: a material used in the fixation of bones

valgus: a musculoskeletal deformity in which a limb is twisted outward from the body

varus: a musculoskeletal deformity in which a limb is twisted toward the body

INDICATIONS AND PROCEDURES

Orthopedic surgery encompasses a number of different procedures carried out to repair injuries affecting the skeletal system and joints or to repair tissues associated with these structures. Such surgery may also attempt to correct associated neurological injury. In addition, orthopedic surgery is used to correct musculoskeletal problems that may be congenital in origin.

Among the congenital conditions for which orthopedic surgery may be warranted are bowlegs (valgus knees) and knock-knees (varus knees). In the case of bowlegs caused by a congenital malformation, one or both legs are twisted outward at the knee. In knock-knees caused by congenital conditions, the knees are curved inward, causing the lower legs to twist away from the body.

Treatment begins with a thorough evaluation of the problem. Based on X-ray analysis, an orthopedic surgeon may make a decision as to whether surgery can be used in the correction of the problem. During the surgical procedure itself, the affected limbs are properly aligned; they are splinted upon completion of the surgery. The chances of success are greatest in younger children. In an analogous situation, if a limb is twisted during fetal development, the child may exhibit misalignment of the structure following birth. Since bone at this stage of life is only beginning its growth, maintaining the limb in a splint may correct the problem. If necessary, the surgeon may decide to realign the limb at the joint through orthopedic surgery.

Tumors that originate in bone are uncommon. If they occur, such growths must be removed as quickly as possible because of the speed with which they spread to adjacent and distant structures in the body if the tumor is cancerous. The first signs of bone cancer include pain and swelling in the affected region. Spontaneous fractures may occur. X-ray and biopsy analyses are necessary to confirm the diagnosis of cancer. If the tumor is benign, it may be removed through surgery. Osteomas, which are tumors that arise from connective tissue within the bone, may require radiation or chemotherapy in addition to surgical removal.

Commonly, orthopedic surgery is used to correct fractures or dislocations. As with any procedure, a thorough evaluation is necessary prior to a final decision. This evaluation often includes X-ray and computed tomography (CT) analyses. If the injury involves the spine, treatment must both correct the problem and prevent secondary injury to the spinal cord. Fractures to the vertebral column may produce fragments that pose a threat to the spinal cord. Under these conditions, orthopedic surgery is used to immobilize or straighten the spinal column; this may involve external braces or an internal brace such as a Harrington distraction rod. The patient may be immobilized for weeks to months, depending on the extent of the injury and the course of treatment.

USES AND COMPLICATIONS

One of the most common applications of orthopedic surgery is the repair of trauma or fractures to bones. For example, a blow to the face, either intentional or accidental, may result in fractures to the nose or facial bones. Injuries to other skeletal structures, including the spine, may also result from the incident. This is particularly true if the source of the injury was an automobile accident. Upon clinical examination by a physician, it may be apparent that facial bones have been fractured. X-ray analysis may be used to confirm the initial diagnosis. Proper repair and restoration of features will be the primary concern of the orthopedic surgeon, assuming that the injuries are not life-threatening. In the event of facial injuries, damage to teeth and other periodontal regions will also be a consideration. In many cases, wire fixation may be a sufficient course of treatment. If more severe, the fracture may require screw-plate fixation, particularly in complicated fractures.

If uneventful or uncomplicated, the healing of such injuries usually requires about six weeks of immobilization. The procedure and immobilization, however, are inherently uncomfortable. If a muscle tear is severe or significant, resulting in a pull to the bone or joint, an associated fracture may heal improperly because of the dislocation of tissue. Proper evaluation of surgical options, including the use of metallic plates, can limit any such complications.

Although cancers originating in bone tissue are uncommon, they nevertheless present problems for the orthopedic surgeon. Fractures related to tumor development are generally treated in much the same way as uncomplicated breaks. If damage to the bone, either through the tumor itself or as a result of therapy, is severe, even surgical repair may not be sufficient to heal the structure and allow mobility or normal function. If the fracture is near the joint, the bone may require realignment or resection, resulting in a shortening of the structure. In some cases, internal fixation with polymethylmethacrylate bone cement may be used to augment repair.

PERSPECTIVE AND PROSPECTS

The introduction of CT scanning technology in the 1970's allowed for much more detailed evaluation of bone and joint injuries. Much of the technology is best applicable in a post-traumatic situation, evaluating the result of injury rather than its cause. Magnetic resonance imaging (MRI) is based on different technology but produces results that are similar to CT scans.

The destruction of bone as a function of aging or of disease is not well understood. Degenerative bone disease as a result of arthritis is among the most common of arthritic conditions, affecting nearly half of middle-aged adults in some manner. Such conditions, particularly among the elderly, remain to be fully addressed.

The ability to carry out bone transplants, developed extensively in the latter half of the twentieth century, allowed for at least partial replacement of damaged bone. Replacement structures may come from the patient's own body or from a cadaver. In addition, orthopedic technology has resulted in prostheses for the replacement of most joints in the body.

Joint replacements are dramatic. Individuals with crippling deformities can have nearly normal function restored through replaced joints. The most commonly replaced joints include hips and knees. Other joints can also be replaced. Individuals who have their hips and knees replaced usually start walking on the replaced joint in the first or second postoperative day. Complete rehabilitation requires several months.

—*Richard Adler, Ph.D.; updated by*
L. Fleming Fallon, Jr., M.D., Ph.D., M.P.H.

See also Amputation; Arthroplasty; Arthroscopy; Bone grafting; Bowlegs; Bunions; Casts and splints; Disk removal; Fracture repair; Hammertoe correction; Hammertoes; Heel spur removal; Hip fracture repair; Hip replacement; Jaw wiring; Joints; Kneecap removal; Knock-knees; Laminectomy and spinal fusion; Orthopedics; Orthopedics, pediatric; Physical rehabilitation; Prostheses; Rotator cuff surgery.

FOR FURTHER INFORMATION:

Bentley, George, and Robert B. Greer, eds. *Orthopaedics*. 4th ed. Oxford, England: Linacre House, 1993. A standard textbook of orthopedic surgery. Although the text is quite technical, a nonphysician can easily understand the diagrams.

Brotzman, S. Brent, and Kevin E. Wilk. *Clinical Orthopaedic Rehabilitation*. 2d ed. Philadelphia: Mosby, 2003. Discusses examination techniques, classification systems, differential diagnoses, treatment options, and rehabilitation protocols for common nonoperative and postoperative musculoskeletal problems. This edition includes new chapters on sports injuries and aquatic therapy.

Callaghan, John J., Aaron Rosenberg, and Harry E. Rubash, eds. *The Adult Hip*. 2d ed. Philadelphia: Lippincott Williams & Wilkins, 2007. A standard reference text on surgery of the hip. Complementing the text are more than 1,300 full-color and black-and-white illustrations, including drawings by a noted medical illustrator.

Doherty, Gerard M., and Lawrence W. Way, eds. *Current Surgical Diagnosis and Treatment*. 12th ed. New York: Lange Medical Books/McGraw-Hill, 2006. This book is intended for professionals and provides updated information concerning orthopedic surgical procedures.

Griffith, H. Winter. *Complete Guide to Symptoms, Illness, and Surgery*. Revised and updated by Stephen Moore and Kenneth Yoder. 5th ed. New York: Perigee, 2006. Covers more than five hundred diseases and disorders and includes information about causes and risk factors, preventive techniques, diagnostic tests, and surgical treatment.

Mulholland, Michael W., et al., eds. *Greenfield's Surgery: Scientific Principles and Practice.* 4th ed. Philadelphia: Lippincott Williams & Wilkins, 2006. Covers the scope and practice of surgery and includes reviews of wound biology, immunology, the management of trauma and transplantation, surgical practice according to anatomic region and specialty, and musculoskeletal, neurologic, genitourinary, and reconstructive surgery.

Tapley, Donald F., et al., eds. *The Columbia University College of Physicians and Surgeons Complete Home Medical Guide.* Rev. 3d ed. New York: Crown, 1995. This book is easy for nonmedical readers to understand.

Tierney, Lawrence M., Stephen J. McPhee, and Maxine A. Papadakis, eds. *Current Medical Diagnosis and Treatment 2007.* New York: McGraw-Hill Medical, 2006. This book is revised annually and provides information relating to medical conditions that are associated with orthopedic surgery. It is an excellent and concise text but is written for professionals.

Zollinger, Robert M., Jr., and Robert M. Zollinger, Sr. *Zollinger's Atlas of Surgical Operations.* 8th ed. New York: McGraw-Hill, 2003. A comprehensive examination of surgery. Covers basic surgical anatomy and vascular, gynecologic, musculoskeletal, gastrointestinal, and miscellaneous abdominal procedures.

ORTHOPEDICS

SPECIALTY

ANATOMY OR SYSTEM AFFECTED: Bones, feet, hands, hips, joints, knees, legs, ligaments, muscles, musculoskeletal system, nervous system, spine, tendons

SPECIALTIES AND RELATED FIELDS: Physical therapy, podiatry, rheumatology, sports medicine

DEFINITION: The field of medicine concerned with the prevention and treatment of disorders, either developmental or caused by injury or disease, that are associated with the skeleton, joints, muscles, and connective tissues.

KEY TERMS:

articulation: a joint between two bones of the skeleton; also called an arthrosis

bursa: a connective tissue sac filled with fluid that reduces friction at joints

collagen: a fibrous protein found in skin, bone, ligaments, tendons, and cartilage

inflammation: the reaction of tissue to injury, with its corresponding redness, heat, swelling, and pain

ligament: a structure of tough connective tissue that attaches one bone to another bone

synovial: referring to the lubricating fluid in the joints or the membrane surrounding the joints

tendon: a structure of tough connective tissue that attaches a muscle to a bone

SCIENCE AND PROFESSION

Orthopedics is the branch of medicine primarily concerned with the movement of the human body and its parts, as well as disorders that affect its function. Such activities as maintaining posture, walking, doing manual work, and exercising involve a complex relationship between the nervous system, muscular system, and skeletal system. While orthopedists must be familiar with the nervous system, they focus primarily on the prevention and treatment of disorders of the skeleton and muscles. They also have expertise in the proper development of these systems in childhood and the changes that occur as a result of aging.

When a person decides to make a movement, the brain sends signals to the muscles. The muscles contract and, by pulling on the bones to which they are attached, cause that part of the body to move. The anchor point for the muscle is the origin, and the attachment point to the bone that is being moved is the insertion. Muscles work in groups to perform a movement. The principal muscle involved is the prime mover, or agonist. The muscles that help the prime mover are called synergists. When a prime mover contracts, the muscle on the opposite side of the bone, termed the antagonist, must relax. An illustration of this would be the muscle and bone interaction involved in the flexing of the arm. The biceps muscle, anchored to bone in the shoulder, contracts, pulling on the bone in the lower arm to which it is attached by a tendon. Its synergist, the brachialis, also contracts. On the back of the upper arm, its antagonist, the triceps muscle, relaxes to allow the arm to bend. When the arm is extended, the triceps becomes the prime mover for that action, and the biceps is the antagonist.

The skeletal system is made of bone and cartilage. Bone cells, called osteocytes, take in nutrients from the blood and constantly renew the bony matrix. The chemical composition of bone includes calcium and phosphorus salts, which provide stiffness. The fibrous protein collagen gives bones some flexibility. Cartilage cells, called chondrocytes, manufacture cartilage, which is a mass of collagen and elastic fibers embedded in a gelatin-like substance. The nature of this structure gives cartilage more flexibility than bone, which makes it an ideal substitute for bone in certain areas. The ribs, for example, are attached by cartilage to the sternum, or breastbone. This arrangement allows for the expansion of the chest during breathing.

Tendons, ligaments, and bursas are also part of the skeletal and muscular systems. Tendons attach muscles to bones. They are made of fibrous tissue so strong that, under stress, the muscle will tear or the bone will break before the tendon will be damaged. Ligaments, which are also made of fibrous tissue, attach bones to other bones and provide stability at the joints. Bursas are fluid-filled connective tissue sacs that lie between muscle and bone, tendon and bone, or other areas around joints. They reduce the damage that occurs to the softer tissue as it rubs against bone with each movement. Because of their close interdependence, the skeleton, attached muscles, and other associated structures are often referred to as the musculoskeletal system.

The health of the musculoskeletal system during childhood is of primary importance to an individual in attaining full growth and function as an adult. In the early developmental stages of the embryo and fetus, a skeleton of cartilage is formed. This structure is replaced with bone in a process called ossification that continues for years after birth. Good nutrition is vital to this process. In particular, the body requires adequate amounts of protein, calcium, and vitamin D. The ends of a long bone are separated from the shaft of the bone by cartilage until the child reaches full growth. Care should be taken when participating in sports, since damage to these areas could affect the growth of that limb. Hormonal production influences the development of the skeleton. Adequate amounts of growth hormone are needed to ensure that proper growth is attained. At puberty, sex hormones, especially testosterone, stimulate the final growth spurts and completion of the adult skeleton.

Young adults have attained their full growth, but the skeleton must renew itself continuously to remain strong and maintain its ability to repair injury. A woman of childbearing age must eat a healthy diet since she may need to nourish a fetus that, in turn, is developing its own skeleton. Both men and women must take care to exercise, since the stress of activity not only builds muscle but also sends messages to the bone to maintain its strength. Calcium and vitamin D intake must continue, or the bones may begin to dissolve some of their calcium matrix. Automobile accidents, work injuries, and sports injuries are more likely to occur at this stage of life.

As adults age, metabolic and other cellular processes become less efficient, and care must be taken to maintain functions and prevent further losses. At one time, disorders such as osteoarthritis and osteoporosis were considered an inevitable part of the aging process. While heredity is certainly a risk factor in these conditions, a substantial body of evidence has been accumulated showing that some degenerative processes can be traced to lifestyle and diet. Osteoarthritis is the type of joint tissue degeneration that is associated with wear and tear on the joints. A person who is obese puts excessive pressure on the skeletal system, especially the hips, knees, and ankles. This pressure increases the damage to the joints. A person who fails to exercise begins to lose flexibility in the joints, and muscles become weaker.

Osteoporosis occurs as bones become porous and brittle. As osteocytes age, they become less efficient at calcium absorption and renewal of the bony matrix. At a time in life when more calcium is needed to make up for this inefficiency, most people consume fewer dairy products, either because of lactose intolerance or because of the ingestion of other beverages. Older women are at particular risk because their bones are lighter than are those of men. After the menopause, women lose some of the protection that estrogen provided by stimulating the absorption of calcium and thus bone renewal. If older people lose the ability to move as surely as before and their reflexes slow down, then injuries are more likely to occur as a result of falls. These injuries are much more serious if the bones are brittle. Even if osteoporosis is not a factor, fractures and other injuries in an older individual do not heal as quickly as they would in a younger person.

Because of their knowledge of developmental processes, orthopedists, as well as pediatricians, are able to advise parents concerned about their growing children and the appropriate precautions for sports activities. Recommendations are made by orthopedists with regard to the design and utilization of safety equipment to prevent or reduce injury. Advice on nutrition and exercise for adults may also be given by physicians in an effort to reduce the incidence of problems as a person ages, allowing continuation of an active, independent life.

DIAGNOSTIC AND TREATMENT TECHNIQUES

In nonemergency situations, patients with some pain or disorder of the muscles, bones, or joints are usually referred to an orthopedic surgeon. The first office visit begins with a review of the condition, during which the physician will take a general medical history and obtain a history of the current complaint. This history will include the time frame from onset, any action that may have initiated the condition, and a description of any difficulty in movement that the patient is having. A physician will then perform a physical examination to determine the specific areas affected and observe range-of-motion exercises to determine if function has been lost.

X rays or other imaging methods are ordered to see whether any structural defect can be seen. Blood tests may be ordered if a disease process is expected. Once a diagnosis has been made, a physician may prescribe medication, order physical therapy or home exercises, schedule surgery, or take other therapeutic measures to correct the condition. The types of abnormalities treated by orthopedists generally fall into one of three categories: injuries caused by accidents, repetitive motion disorders, and diseases affecting the skeleton, skeletal muscles, or joints.

The most common situation in which a patient sees an orthopedist is after an accidental injury. If the injury is severe, the patient may be transported to a hospital emergency room, with care taken to keep the injury site immobilized until a physician can see the patient. The type of treatment needed will be determined by the type and severity of the injury. In a closed or simple fracture, the skin is unbroken; the bones are manipulated back in line and then immobilized with a plaster cast or brace. An open or compound fracture occurs when the ends or fragments of the bone protrude through the skin. In this case, or if surgery is needed to align the bones properly, there is a higher risk of infection. In some cases, pins or wires must be used to hold the bone in position. Fractures of the skull or vertebrae are of special concern because of the possibility of permanent damage to the brain or spinal cord; a neurologist (a physician with specialty training in the nervous system) is usually called to assist an orthopedic surgeon.

Because of twisting movements, injuries that affect one or more joints are common. A dislocation occurs when the bones at a joint are separated. An orthopedist must realign the bones as closely as possible to the original positions and immobilize the joint to allow healing to occur. A sprain results from severe twisting of a joint without dislocation. The severity of joint injury and recovery time depend on the extent of the damage to surrounding ligaments, tendons, cartilage, and other tissues. A special procedure called arthroscopy may be scheduled since damage to soft tissue may not be re-

vealed in an X ray. An orthopedic surgeon inserts a flexible tube, called an arthroscope, into the injury site. This tube, combined with lights and a camera, allows the surgeon to view the joint cavity, to see if any abnormality is present, and, if possible, to repair it.

Some damage to the musculoskeletal system is not the result of a single accident but of actions that are repeated over a long period of time as a part of work duties or recreational activities. These are termed repetitive motion disorders. For example, bursitis, or inflammation of the bursas, may arise in a baseball pitcher's shoulder or a tennis player's elbow. Because the same motion is repeated over and over, the rub of the bursa and other soft tissue over bone causes irritation and inflammation, resulting in pain each time the movement is attempted. Treatment consists of reducing the inflammation by using cortisone or other similar drugs, usually by injection at the affected site, coupled with rest. Resumption of the activity may occur following recommendations from an orthopedist or therapist on a change in technique aimed at reducing the trauma. In some cases, the condition becomes chronic, and the patient may have to discontinue the activity altogether.

Many occupations arising in the mid-twentieth century involved relatively small movements of the hands and wrists. A worker on an assembly line who installs a specific part and an employee who uses a computer

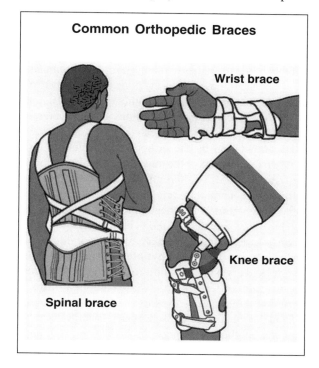

Common Orthopedic Braces

Wrist brace

Knee brace

Spinal brace

keyboard all day are examples of people at high risk for repetitive motion disorders. An understanding of the structure of the wrist leads to better understanding of the problem involved. The median nerve leads from the spinal cord through a tunnel in the carpal bones of the wrist and then branches out to the fingers. It is encircled, together with tendons leading to the fingers, by the transverse carpal ligament. When constant friction causes swelling of the tendons and tissues adjacent to the nerve, the nerve is pinched, resulting in pain, tingling, and weakness in the hand and fingers. This condition is termed carpal tunnel syndrome. Therapy may include changing work positions, wearing a splint to hold the wrist straight, using medications to reduce inflammation, and injecting cortisone at the injury site. If the problem continues, surgery may be needed. In this procedure, the orthopedic surgeon makes an incision in the wrist and cuts the transverse carpal ligament, thus releasing the pressure on the nerve and tendons. If the motion or activity that initially caused carpal tunnel syndrome is not stopped, the condition is likely to recur.

Diseases can affect the bones and joints. Congenital defects and inheritance may result in deformities that can be treated by orthopedic devices or surgery. Hormone therapy may be used by a physician to help a child attain full growth. Nutritional disorders, such as rickets, may cause the softening of the bones, with the corresponding bowed-leg deformity. Caused by a vitamin D deficiency, rickets must be treated not only with vitamin therapy but also with braces to keep the legs straight while the bones harden. Multiple myeloma is a form of cancer that invades the bone and bone marrow and must be treated with chemotherapy as well as surgery to remove the tumor. Infections such as gangrene affect the limbs and, if not treated in time, may necessitate amputation by the orthopedic surgeon.

Of all the diseases of the musculoskeletal system, arthritis and related disorders affect the most people. "Arthritis" is a general term referring to inflammation of a joint. Osteoarthritis is a degenerative disease that results to some extent from the aging process, although it can be exacerbated by obesity, lifestyle, or injury. Arthritis can also be caused by infection or by deposits of uric acid crystals, a condition called gout. The most serious form of joint disease is rheumatoid arthritis, a term that is sometimes used to encompass a group of related disorders. These diseases are classified as autoimmune conditions because the body is making antibodies against itself—in this case, against the tissues associated with the joints. The disease process itself is often treated by a specialist called a rheumatologist, who tries various medications to alleviate the condition. An orthopedic surgeon may be called upon to help correct the deformities resulting from the disease or to replace defective joints with artificial ones. Special care must be taken in cases of juvenile rheumatoid arthritis, since the growth process may also be affected. Systemic lupus erythematosus (SLE), ankylosing spondylitis, and scleroderma are some of the other autoimmune diseases that affect the musculoskeletal system.

PERSPECTIVE AND PROSPECTS

In the study of prehistoric humans, a major source of information is their skeletal remains. Archaeologists have found evidence of broken bones that were set and healed, indicating some rudimentary attempts at the treatment of injuries. Examination of hieroglyphs shows that ancient Egyptians set bones and used wooden splints held in place by the same gum and bandages that were used to wrap mummies. There were no medical specialties, and the treatment of wounds and fractures was part of the duties of any medical practitioner.

The branch of medicine known as orthopedics had its start in the eighteenth century. A physician named Jean André Venel opened an institute in Switzerland with the purpose of correcting skeletal deformities in children. The term "orthopedics" is actually a combination of two Greek words: *orthos*, meaning "straight" or "correct," and *pais*, meaning "child." Treatment of congenital deformities such as clubfoot and defects caused by rickets or injury was the primary function of this type of clinic.

In the nineteenth century, the development of quick-setting plaster for casts aided physicians in the immobilization of broken bones after they were set. The development of anesthesia and antiseptic techniques to prevent infection allowed the practice of orthopedic surgery to expand. Research using the microscope added to the understanding of the structure and function of bone as a living tissue.

In 1895, Wilhelm Conrad Röntgen discovered that radiation from a cathode-ray tube would produce a photographic image of the bones of his hand. By the early twentieth century, the medical X ray came into widespread use, providing an invaluable diagnostic tool for orthopedists. In the 1940's and 1950's, better understanding of radioactive phenomena allowed the development of safer X-ray equipment and techniques. In the 1970's and 1980's, other imaging techniques, such as computed tomography (CT) scanning and magnetic resonance imaging (MRI), increased the ability of orthopedic surgeons to diagnose and treat musculoskeletal disorders.

One of the greatest orthopedic surgical advances has been in the ability to treat badly damaged limbs. At one time, the best the orthopedic surgeon could do for some patients was to amputate the limb to prevent the spread of infection and the development of gangrene, then help the patient cope with the amputations by use of artificial limbs. More sophisticated techniques, incorporating the use of the microscope with computer-directed surgical instruments, allow the reattachment of limbs in many cases by enabling the surgeon to connect even the smallest blood vessels and nerves.

If amputation is necessary, artificial limbs, or prostheses, have also become more sophisticated. Artificial hands have become functional as a result of computer technology that enables the patient to direct the movement of the fingers by contracting and relaxing arm muscles. New plastics and other materials are being developed and used for synthetic joint replacements which increase the mobility of, and decrease the pain for, arthritic patients.

Joints are now routinely replaced. The most common replacements are hip and knee joints, although techniques have been developed to replace other joints in the body. The surgery is performed in a hospital. Recipients are encouraged to begin to use their replaced joints within twenty-four to forty-eight hours after surgery. Complete rehabilitation requires several months of increasingly intense physical activity and exercise. Contemporary materials have an expected useful life of twenty or more years.

A better understanding of the natural healing process at the cellular level has also allowed advances in the treatment of fractures. It has been found that attaching a device that generates a weak electric current can increase the rate of healing in some patients. This current stimulates the multiplication of osteocytes and the growth of new bone in the area.

As the understanding of disease and of degenerative processes increases, better treatments can also be devised. Osteoporosis, for example, is known to be a preventable condition when a correct diet and sufficient physical exercise are obtained throughout life. After the menopause in women, treatment with estrogen replacement therapy gives further protection against osteoporosis. New imaging devices allow osteoporosis to be detected at an earlier stage and more aggressive treatment measures to be applied. The genetic factor in diseases and conditions that trigger autoimmune disorders are other areas of research that are being pursued. While accidents will always occur, orthopedic research into the injury process can help devise methods of prevention, as well as new treatments for the orthopedic problems that do arise.

—Edith K. Wallace, Ph.D.; updated by
L. Fleming Fallon, Jr., M.D., Ph.D., M.P.H.

See also Amputation; Arthritis; Arthroplasty; Arthroscopy; Bone cancer; Bone disorders; Bone grafting; Bones and the skeleton; Bowlegs; Bunions; Bursitis; Cancer; Cartilage; Casts and splints; Chiropractic; Collagen; Craniosynostosis; Disk removal; Dwarfism; Ewing's sarcoma; Feet; Flat feet; Foot disorders; Fracture and dislocation; Fracture repair; Geriatrics and gerontology; Growth; Hammertoe correction; Hammertoes; Heel spur removal; Hip fracture repair; Hip replacement; Jaw wiring; Joints; Kinesiology; Kneecap removal; Knock-knees; Laminectomy and spinal fusion; Ligaments; Lower extremities; Muscle sprains, spasms, and disorders; Muscles; Neurofibromatosis; Orthopedic surgery; Orthopedics, pediatric; Osgood-Schlatter disease; Osteoarthritis; Osteochondritis juvenilis; Osteogenesis imperfecta; Osteomyelitis; Osteonecrosis; Osteopathic medicine; Osteoporosis; Paget's disease; Physical examination; Physical rehabilitation; Pigeon toes; Podiatry; Prostheses; Rheumatoid arthritis; Rheumatology; Rickets; Rotator cuff surgery; Scleroderma; Scoliosis; Slipped disk; Spina bifida; Spinal cord disorders; Spine, vertebrae, and disks; Spondylitis; Sports medicine; Systemic lupus erythematosus (SLE); Tendon disorders; Tendon repair; Upper extremities.

FOR FURTHER INFORMATION:

Cash, Mel. *Pocket Atlas of the Moving Body.* New York: Crown, 2000. An excellent reference guide that covers information about movement and posture of the human body. Full-page anatomical illustrations; tables of muscles, joints, posture, and movement patterns; definitions of technical terms; and a listing of common types of injury are included.

Currey, John D. *Bones: Structures and Mechanics.* 2d ed. Princeton, N.J.: Princeton University Press, 2006. Very accessible overview of a range of information related to whole bones, bone tissue, and dentin and enamel. Topics include stiffness, strength, viscoelasticity, fatigue, fracture mechanics properties, buckling, impact fracture, and properties of cancellous bone.

Delforge, Gary. *Musculoskeletal Trauma: Implications for Sport Injury Management*. Champaign, Ill.: Human Kinetics, 2002. Covers the therapeutic management of sport-related soft tissue injuries, fractures, and proprioceptive/sensorimotor impairments. Reviews the major categories of intervention and presents fifty illustrations to accompany the text.

Marcus, Robert, David Feldman, and Jennifer Kelsey, eds. *Osteoporosis*. 3d ed. Boston: Academic Press/Elsevier, 2008. This book offers a comprehensive, authoritative reference on osteoporosis, covering all aspects of the disease, from basic biology, anatomy, physiology, and pathophysiology to preclinical issues, experimental medicine, management, and therapeutics.

Marieb, Elaine N., and Katja Hoehn. *Human Anatomy and Physiology*. 9th ed. San Francisco: Pearson/Benjamin Cummings, 2010. Nonscientists at the advanced high school level or above will be able to understand this fine textbook. The chapters titled "Bones and Bone Tissue," "The Skeleton," and "Joints" are very well illustrated and include many applications in the fields of physical education and medical science.

Rosen, Clifford J., Julie Glowacki, and John P. Bilezikian. *The Aging Skeleton*. San Diego, Calif.: Academic Press, 1999. Although the target audience of this book is clinicians working in the area of osteoporosis, there is a sound coverage of the underlying biology, including recent developments in bone-cell biology and a useful description of animal models of osteoporosis.

Salter, Robert Bruce. *Textbook of Disorders and Injuries of the Musculoskeletal System*. 3d ed. Baltimore: Williams & Wilkins, 1999. Four sections of the book—"Basic Musculoskeletal Science and Its Applications," "Musculoskeletal Disorders: General and Specific," "Musculoskeletal Injuries," and "Research"—examine the diagnosis and treatment principles of disorders and trauma of the musculoskeletal system.

Tortora, Gerard J., and Bryan Derrickson. *Principles of Anatomy and Physiology*. 12th ed. Hoboken, N.J.: John Wiley & Sons, 2009. This introductory college textbook offers an excellent survey of human anatomy and physiology. Several chapters are devoted to the musculoskeletal system. In addition to normal structure and function, each chapter includes sections on abnormalities (including both injuries and diseases) and their treatment.

ORTHOPEDICS, PEDIATRIC
SPECIALTY

ANATOMY OR SYSTEM AFFECTED: Bones, feet, hands, joints, knees, legs, ligaments, muscles, musculoskeletal system, nerves, nervous system, tendons

SPECIALTIES AND RELATED FIELDS: Exercise physiology, neonatology, orthopedics, pediatrics, physical therapy, rheumatology, sports medicine

DEFINITION: The evaluation and treatment of diseases and injuries of the musculoskeletal system and related nerves in infants and children.

KEY TERMS:

cerebral palsy: a group of nonprogressive disorders of the upper neurologic system resulting in abnormal muscle tone and lack of muscular control

computed tomography (CT) scanning: a computer-assisted method of taking X rays that allows the detailed examination of cross sections of the body

congenital defect: an anatomic deformity present at birth; it is not necessarily hereditary

SCIENCE AND PROFESSION

The pediatric orthopedic surgeon has received additional training in the management of the orthopedic problems of infants and children. Four years of medical school are followed by one year of internship, in either general surgery or primary care. Next come four years of orthopedic residency, then an additional year of fellowship in pediatric orthopedics. After completing training, this specialist usually works in a community with a large referral hospital or in a children's hospital.

The word "orthopedics" comes from two Greek root words, *orthos* ("correct" or "straight") and *pais* ("child"). Childhood musculoskeletal diseases were the original reason for which orthopedic surgery was developed early in the twentieth century. As polio, tuberculosis, and dietary deficiencies came under control, however, the practice of orthopedics grew to encompass adult bone and joint diseases and injuries as well. Nevertheless, a number of orthopedic surgeons continued to work primarily with children.

Infants and children may suffer from a number of congenital musculoskeletal deformities such as clubfoot, hand deformities, congenital dislocation of the hip, and deformities of the spine. Treatment for these disorders may include splints, braces, casts, and surgery. The goal of therapy is to achieve function that is as near normal as possible in the affected part of the skeletal system. Normal appearance, while secondary to function in importance, is also a goal. Some defects require a combination of therapies or repeated operations over a number of years. As the child's musculoskeletal system grows and develops, the mechanics of normal movement change. The pediatric orthopedic surgeon must be aware of these dynamic changes in order to adjust the therapy.

Cerebral palsy, a neuromuscular disorder of infancy and childhood, requires considerable orthopedic evaluation and therapy. As a result of damage to the nerves in the brain that control muscle use, the affected muscles develop abnormal tone (spasticity) and weakness (paralysis). The child cannot control these muscles normally. The asymmetric pull of muscles leads to deformities of the bones and joints and to increasing difficulty in movement as the child grows. Using a combination of splints, braces, and physical and occupational therapy, the pediatric orthopedic surgeon works to keep function as normal as possible in the affected extremities. At times, surgery is necessary to release especially tight muscles. Unfortunately, very little can be done to correct the underlying neurologic defect.

The pediatric orthopedic surgeon also deals with spinal deformities. These conditions may be congenital or may be the result of illness or of some types of surgery, such as removal of a portion of a lung. Scoliosis, the lateral curvature of the spine, may be attributable to factors outside the spine, such as cerebral palsy, or to intrinsic factors in the spine itself. Spinal deformity requires regular observation and the initiation of therapy if the curvature becomes too great. Treatment may involve different types of back braces or, in severe cases, back surgery.

A worry to parents, although often not a significant problem, is the in-toeing and out-toeing that may often be noticed in infants and young children. The pediatric orthopedic surgeon can usually reassure the family that there is no serious problem. Severe toeing problems, however, may require special shoes, splints, or casts.

Childhood fractures must be treated differently from those of adulthood. Children's bones grow at their ends, and growth continues into young adulthood. A fracture at or near the end of a bone may damage the growth area, leading to the loss of normal growth after the injury. Pediatric fractures may be difficult to diagnose, since the growing parts of the bones are cartilage and are not visible on X rays. The pediatric orthopedic surgeon looks for subtle signs of fracture when the growth areas may be involved and follows the patient closely.

DIAGNOSTIC AND TREATMENT TECHNIQUES

The pediatric orthopedic surgeon's practice is divided between the operating room and the clinic. The pediatric specialist spends relatively more time in the clinic than his or her adult practice counterpart because the large percentage of pediatric practice in orthopedics involves chronic deformities.

While taking the patient's history is important, the pediatric orthopedic surgeon relies heavily on a careful and thorough examination of the child's bones, joints, and nervous system. Radiographic studies, especially routine X rays and computed tomography (CT) scans, are often helpful in the evaluation.

Pediatric orthopedic operations must often be carefully planned. It is important for the parents to be involved, so that they can be educated about the child's disorder and can help make appropriate decisions regarding therapy.

PERSPECTIVE AND PROSPECTS

Childhood illnesses and deformities were the original impetus for the development of orthopedic surgery as a specialty early in the twentieth century. Despite the conquest of polio and tuberculosis in the mid-twentieth century, the need for pediatric orthopedic surgeons continues into the twenty-first century. Improved techniques and innovative procedures, such as bone transplantation and metal implants, allow the correction of more musculoskeletal deformities and suggest a bright future for the specialty.

—*Thomas C. Jefferson, M.D.*

See also Amputation; Arthroplasty; Arthroscopy; Bone cancer; Bone disorders; Bone grafting; Bones and the skeleton; Bowlegs; Cancer; Cartilage; Casts and splints; Chiropractic; Collagen; Craniosynostosis; Dwarfism; Ewing's sarcoma; Feet; Flat feet; Foot disorders; Fracture and dislocation; Fracture repair; Growth; Juvenile rheumatoid arthritis; Kinesiology; Knock-knees; Ligaments; Lower extremities; Neurofibromatosis; Orthopedic surgery; Orthopedics; Osgood-Schlatter disease; Osteochondritis juvenilis; Osteogenesis imperfecta; Osteomyelitis; Osteonecrosis; Osteopathic medicine; Paget's disease; Pediatrics; Physical examination; Physical rehabilitation; Pigeon toes; Podiatry; Prostheses; Rickets; Scoliosis; Spina bifida; Spinal cord disorders; Spine, vertebrae, and disks; Sports medicine; Tendon disorders; Tendon repair; Upper extremities.

FOR FURTHER INFORMATION:

Behrman, Richard E., Robert M. Kliegman, and Hal B. Jenson, eds. *Nelson Textbook of Pediatrics*. 18th ed. Philadelphia: Saunders/Elsevier, 2007. Text covering all medical and surgical disorders in children with authoritative information on genetics, endocrinology, etiology, epidemiology, pathology, pathophysiology, clinical manifestations, diagnosis, prevention, treatment, and prognosis.

Kaplan, Deborah. "How to Avoid Orthopedic Pitfalls in Children." *Patient Care* 33, no. 4 (February 28, 1999): 95-116. Missing an orthopedic diagnosis can be hazardous to patients' health. Presents a list of the most common pitfalls in pediatric orthopedic disorders.

Leet, Arabella I., and David L. Skaggs. "Evaluation of the Acutely Limping Child." *American Family Physician* 61, no. 4 (February 15, 2000): 1011-1018. The differential diagnosis of the acutely limping child is explored. The challenge to the family physician is to identify the cause of the limp and determine whether further observation or immediate diagnosis workup is indicated.

Moore, Keith L., and T. V. N. Persaud. *The Developing Human*. 8th ed. Philadelphia: Saunders/Elsevier, 2008. An outstanding textbook on human embryonic development. Includes discussion of the development of the musculoskeletal system.

Patel, Hema, and Victor Bialik. "Hip Dysplasia in Infants." *Pediatrics* 104, no. 6 (December, 1999): 1418. Since the 1960's, it has been recognized that up to 90 percent of infants with developmental dysplasia of the hip, identified at birth by any diagnostic method, require absolutely no intervention.

Rose, Rene, Andy Fuentes, Brenda J. Hamel, and Cynthia J. Dzialo. "Pediatric Leg Length Discrepancy: Causes and Treatments." *Orthopedic Nursing* 18, no. 2 (March/April, 1999): 21-31. Leg length discrepancies have multiple causes with a number of treatment options available to accomplish a goal of equal or near equal leg lengths at skeletal maturity.

Shapiro, Frederic. *Pediatric Orthopedic Deformities: Basic Science, Diagnosis, and Treatment*. San Diego, Calif.: Academic Press, 2001. Reviews major pediatric orthopedic deformities, showing how normal developmental bone biology and abnormal pathobiology relate to their occurrence, diagnosis, and treatments.

Staheli, Lynn. *Fundamentals of Pediatric Orthopedics*. 4th ed. Philadelphia: Wolters Kluwer/Lippincott Williams & Wilkins, 2008. An accessible guide to the diagnosis and management of pediatric orthopedic problems. Treatment plans are reviewed and illustrated, and pitfalls, including normal variations, are discussed. Includes a parent education section, helpful for the layperson.

Wenger, Dennis R., and Mercer Rang. *The Art and Practice of Children's Orthopaedics*. New York: Raven Press, 1993. A thorough look at pediatric orthopedics, which includes bibliographical references and an index.

OSGOOD-SCHLATTER DISEASE

DISEASE/DISORDER

ANATOMY OR SYSTEM AFFECTED: Knees, musculoskeletal system, tendons

SPECIALTIES AND RELATED FIELDS: Orthopedics, pediatrics

DEFINITION: Pain caused by the patellar (kneecap) tendon pulling away from the tibia (shin bone).

CAUSES AND SYMPTOMS

Osgood-Schlatter disease is most frequently found in young athletes during their years of rapid growth. It is more common in boys, who are typically affected between the ages of thirteen and fourteen. Girls usually are affected at younger ages, ten to eleven. However, children are at risk between the ages of ten and eighteen, especially during their rapid skeletal growth years. Children who play sports that involve running or repetitive jumping have the highest risk.

The most common symptom of Osgood-Schlatter disease is pain below the kneecap. There is usually a swollen, bony bump in that area. Pain is often felt when the bump is touched or when the knee is bent or fully extended in activities such as running, jumping, kneeling, squatting, or lifting weights. As the child matures, Osgood-Schlatter disease will usually go away. When children stop growing, the patellar tendon is stronger and the pain and swelling disappear. Very seldom does the disease continue after rapid growth stops.

If the pain persists, then the child should see a pediatrician or orthopedist. The physician will examine the knee area and the location of pain in order to make a diagnosis. If the source of the pain is unclear, then an X ray will be taken of the knee to verify Osgood-Schlatter disease.

TREATMENT AND THERAPY

The best treatment for Osgood-Schlatter disease is simply rest. Depending on the severity of the condition, the child may have to decrease activity levels or stop playing sports for several months. Deep knee bending and jumping should be minimized, and running may need to be limited. To treat the pain, the knee should get more rest, and ice should be applied for twenty minutes three times per day. Elastic bandages should be used to compress the knee area, and the leg should be elevated when possible. Over-the-counter pain relievers can be taken. In extreme cases, a brace or cast may be used.

After recovery from the pain, the child can slowly return to previous activity levels. Additionally, a physical therapist can prescribe exercises that will help strengthen the leg muscles around the knee to minimize the chances of a recurrence.

There is no surgical procedure for Osgood-Schlatter disease unless the patellar tendon is fully torn from the tibia. This should not happen if the patient gets proper rest, in which case Osgood-Schlatter disease will resolve itself.

—*Bradley R. A. Wilson, Ph.D.*

See also Bone disorders; Bones and the skeleton; Growth; Orthopedic surgery; Orthopedics; Orthopedics, pediatric; Physical rehabilitation; Sports medicine; Tendon disorders; Tendon repair.

FOR FURTHER INFORMATION:

Dunn, J. F., Jr. "Osgood-Schlatter Disease." *American Family Physician* 41, no. 4 (1990): 173.

Globus, S. "Osgood-Schlatter: More than Growing Pains." *Current Health* 2 28, no. 4 (2002): 20.

Lackey, E., and R. Sutton. "Rest Is Best for Common Knee Swelling." *GP: General Practitioner* 1c (2003): 75.

Parker, James N., and Philip M. Parker, eds. *The Official Patient's Sourcebook on Osgood-Schlatter Disease.* San Diego, Calif.: Icon Health, 2002.

Woodward, A. H. "Osgood-Schlatter Disease." *Pediatrics for Parents* 11, no. 1 (1990): 11.

OSTEOARTHRITIS
DISEASE/DISORDER

ANATOMY OR SYSTEM AFFECTED: Joints, musculoskeletal system

SPECIALTIES AND RELATED FIELDS: Exercise physiology, orthopedics

DEFINITION: A degenerative joint disease that results from the wearing away of the cartilage of bones, causing inflammation, swelling, and pain in affected joints and eventually causing joint stiffness and limitation of movement, misalignment, and knoblike bone growths in the hands.

KEY TERMS:

Bouchard's nodes: osteophytes or bony spurs that develop as a result of destruction of joint cartilage in proximal interphalangeal joints

cartilage: a smooth material covering the ends of bone joints that cushions the bone, allowing the joint to move easily

collagen: a fibrous protein substance in connective tissue, bone, tendons, and cartilage

crepitus: the scraping or grinding sound heard or felt when bone rubs over bone in joint spaces

degenerative: marked by progression to a state below what is considered normal or desirable

distal: away from the point of origin

distal interphalangeal joints: the distal joints of the fingers

Herberden's nodes: osteophytes or bony spurs that develop as a result of destruction of joint cartilage in distal interphalangeal joints

inflammatory: irritation that causes swelling, heat, and discomfort

joints: the junctions at the ends of bones that allow for movement

proximal: toward the point of origin

proximal interphalangeal joints: the proximal joints in the fingers

synovial fluid: fluid contained in the synovium of joint margins that reduces friction during movement of the joints

synovium: fluid-filled sacs in joint margins

CAUSES AND SYMPTOMS

There are several causes of osteoarthritis (OA), including traumatic injuries, joint overuse or repetitive movement of a joint, obesity, and genetic or metabolic diseases. The most commonly affected joints are in the hands, hips, knees, and spine. An inherited genetic defect in the production of collagen leads to defective cartilage and to more rapid joint deterioration. OA in the hands or hips may be hereditary. OA in the knees is linked to excess weight. X rays of more than half the population over sixty-five would show evidence of osteoarthritis in at least one joint.

Cartilage containing synovial fluid and elastic tissue reduces friction as joints move. Osteoarthritis develops when the cartilage wears away and bone rubs against bone. The most prominent symptom of osteoarthritis is joint pain. Other symptoms include morning stiffness or stiffness after long periods of immobility. Early in the disease, individuals may experience joint pain after strenuous exercise. As the disease progresses, joints stiffen and diminished joint mobility is experienced even with slight activity. As joint mobility decreases, the muscles surrounding the joint weaken, thereby increasing the likelihood of further injury to the joint. As the cartilage wears away, crepitus can often be heard as bone moves against bone. The development of Herberden's nodes on the distal interphalangeal joints and Bouchard's nodes on the proximal interphalangeal joints of the hands is not uncommon.

Confirmation of osteoarthritis is based on a history of joint pain and physical findings that indicate arthritic changes in the joints. An X ray shows a loss of joint space, osteophytes, bone cysts, and sclerosis of subchondrial bone. Sometimes, a computed tomography

INFORMATION ON OSTEOARTHRITIS

CAUSES: Traumatic injuries, joint overuse, obesity, genetic or metabolic diseases

SYMPTOMS: Joint pain (commonly in hands, hips, knees, spine); stiffness in morning or after long periods of immobility; development of nodes

DURATION: Chronic and progressive

TREATMENTS: Occupational therapy; physical therapy; moderate exercise; heat therapy (warm soaks, paraffin, mud treatments); pain medications such as topical analgesic ointments, acetaminophen, NSAIDs (ibuprofen, naproxyn); COX-2 inhibitors; glucosamine; chondroitin; injections of cortisone or hyaluronic acid; surgery in severe cases

(CT) scan or magnetic resonance imaging (MRI) may be helpful in confirming the presence of osteoarthritis.

TREATMENT AND THERAPY

The goal of treatment for OA is to preserve physical function and reduce pain. Education, physical therapy, and occupational therapy are instrumental in maintaining independence and improving muscle strength around affected joints. Pacing activities to avoid overexertion of the affected joints is an effective means to prevent further pain and injury. Heat therapies such as warm soaks, paraffin, and mud treatments may help to lessen the discomfort in tender joints. Moderate exercise such as walking, swimming, strength training, and stretching all may help to maintain mobility in arthritic joints and to improve posture and balance. Relaxation techniques, stress reduction activities, and biofeedback may also be helpful.

Topical analgesic ointments may help to reduce joint swelling and pain. Acetaminophen is very effective for controlling OA pain. However, persons who take blood-thinning medicines, have liver disease, or consume large amounts of alcohol should use acetaminophen with caution. Nonsteroidal anti-inflammatory drugs (NSAIDs) such as ibuprofen and naproxen are also effective for pain relief, but they may cause gastrointestinal bleeding. COX-2 selective inhibitors are the most recently introduced NSAIDs. This class of drugs selectively blocks the enzyme COX-2, thus controlling the production of prostaglandins, natural chemicals that contribute to body inflammation and cause the pain

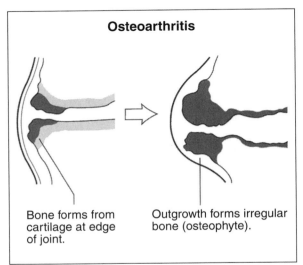

Osteoarthritis

Bone forms from cartilage at edge of joint.

Outgrowth forms irregular bone (osteophyte).

Osteoarthritis results when irregular bone growth occurs at the edge of a joint, causing impaired movement of the joint and pressure on nerves in the area.

and swelling of arthritis. Since they do not block the COX-1 enzyme cyclooxygenase-1, which is present in the stomach and inflammation sites, the natural mucous linings of the stomach and intestine are protected, thereby reducing the incidence of upset, ulceration, or bleeding. This feature of blocking COX-2 but not COX-1 makes these drugs unique among traditional NSAIDs. COX-2 selective inhibitors include Celebrex (celecoxib), Vioxx (rofecoxib), and Bextra (valdecoxib); the latter two are no longer on the market, however. Other COX-2 inhibitors sold outside the United States include Prexige (lumiracoxib) and Arcoxia (etoricoxib). Any medication used to treat OA should be taken under the direction of a health care provider.

Glucosamine and chondroitin naturally occur in the body. Both have been promoted for the treatment of OA. Glucosamine may promote the formation and repair of cartilage, while chondroitin may promote water retention and elasticity in cartilage and prevent cartilage breakdown.

When interventions to relieve symptoms of OA no longer work, an orthopedic surgeon may inject cortisone or hyaluronic acid into joint spaces such as the knee. Hyaluronic acid is used to replace the synovial fluid that a joint has lost in order to maintain knee movement without pain. Cortisone may be injected into affected joint spaces to provide temporary relief of joint pain. Surgical intervention to trim torn and damaged cartilage from joint spaces, to partially or totally replace severely damaged joints in the knees and hips, or to fuse bones together are effective treatments in the most severe, debilitating stages of OA. Realignment of a joint (osteotomy) is another possible procedure.

PERSPECTIVE AND PROSPECTS

Arthritis comprises more than one hundred diseases and conditions and is the major cause of disability in the United States. The incidence of OA increases with age, but it can affect individuals as young as eighteen. More than sixteen million people in the United States have OA, and it is the most common form of arthritis. OA is three times more common among women, although before forty-five years of age, it is more common in men. Costs for treatment of arthritis in the United States exceed $65 billion annually. There is no cure for OA, but a healthy diet, regular exercise, and weight control are measures that can slow its progress.

—*Sharon W. Stark, R.N., A.P.R.N., D.N.Sc.;*
updated by Victoria Price, Ph.D.

See also Arthritis; Bursitis; Cartilage; Collagen; Gout; Joints; Juvenile rheumatoid arthritis; Obesity; Rheumatoid arthritis; Rheumatology.

FOR FURTHER INFORMATION:

Foltz-Gray, Dorothy. *The Arthritis Foundation's Guide to Good Living with Osteoarthritis.* 2d ed. Atlanta: Arthritis Foundation, 2004. Discussion of the effects of osteoarthritis on the body, diagnosis and treatment, genetic links, and implications for pain and depression.

Lane, Nancy E., and Daniel J. Wallace. *All About Osteoarthritis: The Definitive Resource for Arthritis Patients and Their Families.* New York: Oxford University Press, 2002. Discussion and diagrams of causes, signs, symptoms, treatment with exercise, medications, and surgery.

Nelson, Miriam E., et al. *Strong Women and Men Beat Arthritis.* New York: G. P. Putnam's Sons, 2002. Discusses strategies for dealing with arthritis, including nutrition and exercise, medication, surgery, and complementary approaches.

Sayce, Valerie, and Ian Fraser. *Exercise Beats Arthritis: An Easy to Follow Program of Exercises.* Palo Alto, Calif.: Bull, 1998. Offers discussion, illustrations, and pictorial review of daily exercises for joint mobility, increased muscle strength, strong bones and ligaments, and improved overall quality of life.

Sutton, Amy L., ed. *Arthritis Sourcebook: Basic Consumer Health Information About Osteoarthritis, Rheumatoid Arthritis, Other Rheumatic Disorders, Infectious Forms of Arthritis, and Diseases with Symptoms Linked to Arthritis.* 2d ed. Detroit, Mich.: Omnigraphics, 2004. A comprehensive guide.

Yelin, E. "The Economics of Osteoarthritis." In *Osteoarthritis*, edited by K. Brandt, M. Doherty, and L. Lohmander. New York: Oxford University Press, 1998. Provides a comprehensive overview of risk factors, clinical aspects, differential diagnosis, and medical and surgical treatments for OA.

OSTEOCHONDRITIS JUVENILIS
DISEASE/DISORDER

ALSO KNOWN AS: Legg-Calvé-Perthes disease, coxa plana, pseudocoxalgia

ANATOMY OR SYSTEM AFFECTED: Bones, circulatory system, hips, joints, musculoskeletal system

SPECIALTIES AND RELATED FIELDS: Orthopedics, vascular medicine

DEFINITION: The disturbance of the blood supply to the tops of the thigh bones, resulting in their destruction.

CAUSES AND SYMPTOMS

Osteochondritis juvenilis is believed to be the result of trauma and damage to the blood vessels that serve the thigh bone. The patient, who in 80 percent of cases is male, usually experiences tenderness in the hip joint area during the early stages of the disease, accompanied by limping, pain in the thigh or knee, and limited movement of the leg. Usually it is difficult to rotate the leg or move it sideways. In 90 percent of cases, only one leg is affected. In such cases, one leg is shorter than the other, and the child favors the affected leg. If the disease is not treated, atrophy of the thigh results.

TREATMENT AND THERAPY

Most cases of osteochondritis juvenilis do not require treatment beyond observation, particularly with children under the age of six who have a small amount of damage. For children over six with most of the joint affected, a more aggressive therapy is needed.

Physical therapy, coupled with braces and crutches or bed rest with traction, is used only in the most severe cases. For most children, a Scottish Rite brace is used. Such a brace is belted around the waist and wrapped around the thighs, with a bar holding the knees apart so that the legs are held at a slight angle away from the body. The child wears the brace until the bone begins to form again, usually in six months.

If the child is more than eight years old, if the brace is too restrictive for an active child, or if the brace must be worn more than six months, surgical correction is recommended. In these cases, the affected bone is cut away and the tip of the thigh bone placed back into its socket. Occasionally, the hip bone must be cut away instead.

—*Rose Secrest*

See also Blood vessels; Bone disorders; Bones and the skeleton; Braces; Circulation; Joints; Lower extremities; Orthopedics; Orthopedics, pediatric; Osteonecrosis; Vascular system.

FOR FURTHER INFORMATION:

Behrman, Richard E., Robert M. Kliegman, and Hal B. Jenson, eds. *Nelson Textbook of Pediatrics.* 18th ed. Philadelphia: Saunders/Elsevier, 2007.

Currey, John D. *Bones: Structures and Mechanics.* 2d ed. Princeton, N.J.: Princeton University Press, 2006.

Goldberg, Kathy E. *The Skeleton: Fantastic Framework.* Washington, D.C.: U.S. News Books, 1982.

Shapiro, Frederic. *Pediatric Orthopedic Deformities: Basic Science, Diagnosis, and Treatment.* San Diego, Calif.: Academic Press, 2001.

Staheli, Lynn T. *Fundamentals of Pediatric Orthopedics.* 4th ed. Philadelphia: Wolters Kluwer/Lippincott Williams & Wilkins, 2008.

Wenger, Dennis R., and Mercer Rang. *The Art and Practice of Children's Orthopaedics.* New York: Raven Press, 1993.

OSTEOGENESIS IMPERFECTA
DISEASE/DISORDER

ANATOMY OR SYSTEM AFFECTED: Bones, ears, ligaments, musculoskeletal system, spine, teeth

SPECIALTIES AND RELATED FIELDS: Biochemistry, dentistry, genetics, orthopedics, pediatrics

DEFINITION: A genetic disorder of variable severity that results in frequent bone breaks.

KEY TERMS:

chondrocytes: cartilage cells

collagen: organic material that provides a matrix for bone formation

osteoblasts: bone-forming cells

osteogenesis: new bone formation and repair during development and after trauma

osteogenesis imperfecta congenita: a genetic disorder of collagen formation that begins to show signs during gestation

osteogenesis imperfecta tarda: a genetic disorder of collagen formation that begins to show signs after infancy

CAUSES AND SYMPTOMS

Osteogenesis imperfecta, a rare genetic disorder occurring in 1 in 20,000 people, affects the formation of collagen, which in turn alters bone formation, as collagen provides the foundation for mineralization of developing and healing bone. As the name implies, patients

---

INFORMATION ON OSTEOCHONDRITIS JUVENILIS

CAUSES: Trauma and damage to blood vessels that serve thigh bone

SYMPTOMS: In early stages, tenderness in hip joint, limping, pain in thigh or knee, limited leg movement

DURATION: Chronic

TREATMENTS: Physical therapy, braces and crutches, bed rest with traction

with this disorder have imperfect bone formation, resulting in multiple, recurrent fractures.

Bones are composed of a complex matrix including strands of cross-linked collagen. Collagen is produced by chondrocytes in newly forming bone. Osteoblasts then add the mineral matrix (calcium salts), which forms a complex with collagen to create bone. Children with osteogenesis imperfecta do not produce collagen molecules that allow for a well-organized, strong, stable structure. Fractures can take place without outside stresses such as those occurring in a fall. Normal muscle contractions can produce enough force in some children to induce a bone break.

The long-term outcome of the disease is variable. Most severely affected infants die from complications of lung disease. Patients with less severe disease usually survive but have fractures of their long bones. Most breaks occur between the ages of two and three and again during puberty, between ten and fifteen. From late adolescence through the adult years, the fracture incidence drops unless the patient becomes pregnant, is nursing, or becomes inactive.

> ### INFORMATION ON
> ### OSTEOGENESIS IMPERFECTA
>
> **CAUSES:** Genetic disorder
> **SYMPTOMS:** Imperfect bone formation, multiple and recurrent fractures, bluish sclera of eyes, thin skin that bleeds easily, frequent nosebleeds, elevated body temperatures
> **DURATION:** Chronic
> **TREATMENTS:** Hormonal therapy, exercise

There are two main types of osteogenesis imperfecta. The more severe form, osteogenesis imperfecta congenita, affects bone development during gestation and results in bone fractures before birth. These children continue to have fractures without adequate bone repair. Because of the malformation of bony tissues and frequent fractures, they do not grow normally and have numerous bone deformities.

Other tissues with abundant collagen are also affected in osteogenesis imperfecta congenita. Because

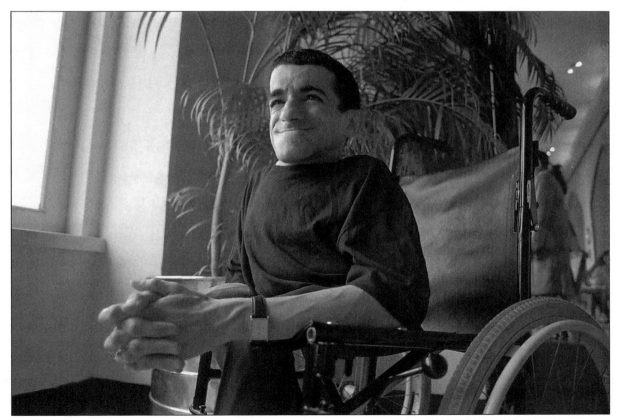

Writer Firdaus Kanga of Bombay was born with osteogenesis imperfecta. (AP/Wide World Photos)

these tissues include tendons and ligaments, joints become more mobile and less stable. The small bones in the middle ear are similarly affected, resulting in otosclerosis, in which the ossicles stiffen and do not allow the normal transition of sound from the eardrum to the inner ear. Thus, patients have hearing difficulties and subsequent language delays. Because the white parts of the eyes (the sclera) are composed mainly of collagen, these patients tend to have bluish sclera. They also have thinner skin that bleeds easily. Epistaxis (nosebleeding) is likewise common and difficult to control. Patients have deformed teeth, as tooth development is also affected. They tend to have elevated body temperatures, causing them to sweat excessively; because this can become dangerous during surgery under general anesthesia, the anesthesiologist should be made aware of such a possibility. It is important to note that the nervous system, and thus the intelligence, of children with osteogenesis imperfecta congenita is not affected.

The second type of osteogenesis imperfecta is known as osteogenesis imperfecta tarda. Patients with this type have a slower onset and milder course of disease. Fractures begin after birth, do not occur as frequently, and tend to heal better, causing less deformity.

Treatment and Therapy

Unfortunately, there is no effective way to control osteogenesis imperfecta with medication. Drug therapies include the hormones calcitonin, estrogen, and testosterone and supplements of fluoride, calcium, and magnesium. Hormonal therapy seems to stabilize the bone matrix by stimulating bone-forming cells (osteoblasts) and inhibiting the cells which break down bone tissue (osteoclasts). This is likely why patients tend to improve during and after puberty, since levels of these hormones naturally rise.

Activity is encouraged, as exercise strengthens bones. Activities with a high potential for fractures, however, should be avoided. If fractures occur, pediatric orthopedic specialists often place metal rods in the long bones when repairing a fracture to help prevent deformities.

Perspective and Prospects

Unfortunately, the prognosis for some children with osteogenesis imperfecta is poor, and most are confined to wheelchairs as adults. Others are more fortunate and have relatively few fractures after adolescence.

Some advancements in the understanding of osteogenesis imperfecta have occurred using molecular biology techniques to help identify the errors in collagen formation. It is hoped that these data will result in future gene therapy techniques.

—*Matthew Berria, Ph.D.*

See also Bone disorders; Bones and the skeleton; Cartilage; Collagen; Congenital disorders; Ear infections and disorders; Ears; Fracture and dislocation; Genetic diseases; Hearing loss; Hip fracture repair; Ligaments; Nosebleeds; Orthopedics; Orthopedics, pediatric.

For Further Information:

Behrman, Richard E., Robert M. Kliegman, and Hal B. Jenson, eds. *Nelson Textbook of Pediatrics.* 18th ed. Philadelphia: Saunders/Elsevier, 2007. Offers detailed information intended mainly for pediatricians.

Green, Morris. *Pediatric Diagnosis: Interpretation of Symptoms and Signs in Infants, Children, and Adolescents.* 6th ed. Philadelphia: W. B. Saunders, 1998. An excellent text providing information on physical diagnosis.

Hay, William W., Jr., et al., eds. *Current Diagnosis and Treatment in Pediatrics.* 19th ed. New York: Lange Medical Books/McGraw-Hill, 2009. A basic pediatric text detailing general pediatric diseases.

Jones, Kenneth Lyons. *Smith's Recognizable Patterns of Human Malformation.* 6th ed. Philadelphia: Saunders/Elsevier, 2006. This classic text discusses pediatric malformations.

Kimball, Chad T. *Childhood Diseases and Disorders Sourcebook: Basic Consumer Health Information About Medical Problems Often Encountered in Preadolescent Children.* Detroit, Mich.: Omnigraphics, 2003. Offers basic facts about cancer, sickle cell disease, diabetes, and other chronic conditions in children and discusses frequently used diagnostic tests, surgeries, and medications. Long-term care for seriously ill children is also presented.

Parker, James N., and Philip M. Parker, eds. *The Official Patient's Sourcebook on Osteogenesis Imperfecta.* San Diego, Calif.: Icon Health, 2002. Draws from public, academic, government, and peer-reviewed research to provide a wide-ranging handbook for adult patients with osteogenesis imperfecta.

Van De Graaff, Kent M., and Stuart I. Fox. *Concepts of Human Anatomy and Physiology.* 5th ed. Dubuque, Iowa: Wm. C. Brown, 2000. A basic anatomy and physiology textbook. See especially chapters 8, 9, and 10.

OSTEOMYELITIS

DISEASE/DISORDER

ANATOMY OR SYSTEM AFFECTED: Bones, joints, musculoskeletal system

SPECIALTIES AND RELATED FIELDS: Bacteriology, orthopedics

DEFINITION: A secondary bacterial infection of the bone and bone marrow.

CAUSES AND SYMPTOMS

After a cut, open bone fracture, or puncture wound to the heel becomes infected, a secondary infection, caused 80 percent of the time by the bacterium *Staphylococcus aureus*, can take place. In children, the bacterium usually enters the body via an infection of the mucous membranes in the throat or an infected sore on the body. In the case of a heel puncture, a bacterium that breeds in old athletic shoes, called *Pseudomonas aeruginosa*, can be the culprit. In children, osteomyelitis tends to be located at the growing ends of the long bones.

Osteomyelitis is generally accompanied by fever, drowsiness, dehydration, bone pain, and swelling and redness in the affected region. When a joint near the infected area is flexed, severe pain and tenderness can result. With a heel puncture, the heel tends to hurt and swell, but there is often no fever. Over time, the bacteria form pus.

TREATMENT AND THERAPY

If osteomyelitis is discovered within seven to ten days from the onset of the infection, large doses of antibiotics can be administered with success. In children, oral antibiotics are not recommended because compliance is hard to achieve. Patients must ingest two to four times the recommended daily dose of the antibiotic over four to six weeks, which can cause severe side effects. Usually, children are hospitalized and given intravenous antibiotics. During this time, the affected bones should not be exposed to undue stress until easy,

---

INFORMATION ON OSTEOMYELITIS

CAUSES: Bacterial infection
SYMPTOMS: Fever, drowsiness, dehydration, bone pain, localized swelling and redness
DURATION: Several days to weeks
TREATMENTS: Hospitalization, intravenous antibiotics, surgery

---

pain-free movement is achieved. Risks during the time of treatment include broken bones and the onset of severe osteoporosis.

In severe cases or in cases in which the infection was not discovered early, surgery that removes the infected bone or bone marrow is necessary. If the osteomyelitis is not treated, the infection enters the bloodstream and the disease becomes chronic. Extensive bone damage, arthritis, and extrusion of pus will follow. Treatment may involve occasional removal of pus and pieces of dead bone or, in extreme cases, amputation.

—*Rose Secrest*

See also Antibiotics; Arthritis; Bacterial infections; Bone disorders; Bone marrow transplantation; Bones and the skeleton; Joints; Orthopedics; Orthopedics, pediatric; Osteonecrosis.

FOR FURTHER INFORMATION:

Biddle, Wayne. *A Field Guide to Germs*. 2d ed. New York: Anchor Books, 2002.

Currey, John D. *Bones: Structures and Mechanics*. 2d ed. Princeton, N.J.: Princeton University Press, 2006.

Icon Health. *Osteomyelitis: A Medical Dictionary, Bibliography, and Annotated Research Guide to Internet References*. San Diego, Calif.: Author, 2004.

National Institute of Arthritis and Musculoskeletal and Skin Diseases. Osteoporosis and Related Bone Diseases, National Resource Center. http://www.niams.nih.gov/health_info/bone.

Norden, Carl W., ed. *Osteomyelitis*. Philadelphia: W. B. Saunders, 1990.

Wilson, Michael, Brian Henderson, and Rod McNab. *Bacterial Disease Mechanisms: An Introduction to Cellular Microbiology*. New York: Cambridge University Press, 2002.

OSTEONECROSIS

DISEASE/DISORDER

ALSO KNOWN AS: Aseptic necrosis, avascular necrosis, ischemic necrosis

ANATOMY OR SYSTEM AFFECTED: Bones, hips, joints, knees, musculoskeletal system

SPECIALTIES AND RELATED FIELDS: Orthopedics, rheumatology

DEFINITION: A disorder that occurs when the blood supply to bone is cut off, causing the death of bone tissue and leading to the collapse of joints in the affected areas.

CAUSES AND SYMPTOMS

Osteonecrosis—from *osteo*, meaning "bone," and *necro*, meaning "death"—may be either post-traumatic or nontraumatic, in some cases with risk factors identified and in others with no known cause (idiopathic). Approximately twenty thousand new cases are diagnosed each year in the United States, most commonly between the ages of twenty and fifty, with the average age of onset at thirty-eight. Osteonecrosis is of equal prevalence in men and women.

Some risk factors seem to predispose people to osteonecrosis, including the use of corticosteroids (to treat inflammatory conditions) as well as excessive alcohol ingestion. Both steroid and alcohol use may lead to a buildup of lipids in the blood vessels, decreasing blood flow to bones. Injury to a bone or joint (such as a fracture) may damage the blood vessels, decreasing the blood supply and causing bone death. Medical conditions which affect the bone (gout, osteoarthritis, osteoporosis) may predispose someone to osteonecrosis. Cancer treatments (radiation and chemotherapy) and organ transplantation also increase the risk of osteonecrosis, as do other medical conditions including sickle cell disease and acquired immunodeficiency syndrome (AIDS). Recently, the medication Fosamax, a bisphosphenate used to treat osteoporosis, has been linked to osteonecrosis of the jaw.

Often, few symptoms occur in early stages of the disease. Preliminary symptoms include pain in the affected joint, followed by collapse of joint surfaces and increased pain. Pain occurs initially only when the joint is in use and later even at rest. The bones most commonly affected are the ends of the femur, the upper arm bone, and the knees, shoulders, and ankles. Within months to two years from the onset of symptoms, individuals may lose range of motion and suffer severe disability. Appropriate treatment must be undertaken to prevent the breakdown of joints, Therefore, immediate diagnosis is important. X rays, magnetic resonance imaging (MRI), computed tomography (CT) scan, and bone scans serve as diagnostic tools when an individual is symptomatic.

TREATMENT AND THERAPY

Once the condition has been diagnosed, treatment should begin immediately. To decide on most effective treatments, physicians consider the age of the patient, the progression of the disease, the location of the bones involved, and the underlying cause. Treatment can be either medical or surgical. Medical treatments include the

---

INFORMATION ON OSTEONECROSIS

CAUSES: Interruption of blood supply to bone; may result from trauma, corticosteroid use, excessive alcohol consumption, bone disorders, cancer treatment

SYMPTOMS: Joint pain and loss, death of bone tissue

DURATION: Chronic and progressive

TREATMENTS: Nonsteroidal anti-inflammatory drugs (NSAIDs), anticoagulants, statins, exercises, electrical stimulation, surgery (core decompression, bone grafting, osteotomy, joint replacement)

---

use of nonsteroidal anti-inflammatory drugs (NSAIDs) to decrease pain, anticoagulants (blood thinners) to improve blood supply to bone, and statins (cholesterol-lowering medications) to decrease lipid buildup in blood vessels, allowing improved blood flow to bone. Other medical treatments involve range of motion exercises, electrical stimulation to induce bone growth, and decreased weight-bearing on affected joints.

Surgical techniques used to treat osteonecrosis include core decompression, bone grafting, osteotomy, and joint replacement. In core decompression, the inner core of the bone is removed, thus reducing pressure within the bone. Core decompression is often followed by bone grafting to the decompressed area to support the joint. Osteotomy is a surgical reshaping of the bone to decrease stress on affected areas. Joint replacement is the surgical treatment of choice in advanced cases. Treatment may be an ongoing process that continues for years, as the disease progresses. Adequate treatment allows afflicted individuals to continue to live reasonably normal lives.

—*Robin Kamienny Montvilo, R.N., Ph.D.*

See also Alcoholism; Arthritis; Bone disorders; Bones and the skeleton; Circulation; Corticosteroids; Gout; Grafts and grafting; Joints; Necrosis; Orthopedics; Osteoarthritis, Osteoporosis; Steroids; Vascular medicine; Vascular system.

FOR FURTHER INFORMATION:

Icon Health. *Osteonecrosis: A Medical Dictionary, Bibliography, and Annotated Research Guide to Internet References*. San Diego, Calif.: Author, 2004.

National Osteonecrosis Foundation. http://www.nonf .org.

Soucacos, Panayotis N., and James R. Urbaniak, eds. *Osteonecrosis of the Human Skeleton*. Philadelphia: W. B. Saunders, 2004.

Urbaniak, James R., and John Paul Jones, eds. *Osteonecrosis: Etiology, Diagnosis, and Treatment*. Rosemont, Ill.: American Academy of Orthopaedic Surgeons, 1997.

Osteopathic medicine

Specialty

Anatomy or system affected: Bones, muscles, musculoskeletal system

Specialties and related fields: Critical care, emergency medicine, family medicine, geriatrics and gerontology, internal medicine, physical therapy, preventive medicine, public health

Definition: The practice of medicine as dictated by the philosophy of treating the individual instead of merely the disease, by the belief that the musculoskeletal system is crucial to the health of the entire body, and by an emphasis on the interrelatedness of all bodily systems.

Key terms:

allopathic medicine: the traditional course of study leading to a doctorate in medicine; most practicing physicians are allopathic physicians

family medicine: the practice of medicine in which the physician cares for the basic needs of the family and emphasizes preventive health care, as well as the importance of the patient's environment

immune system: the system of the body that is responsible for the maintenance of health; includes the spleen, the thymus, bone marrow, and the lymphatic system

Medical College Admission Test (MCAT): a test of problem-solving skills taken by all candidates for medical school in the United States; used to predict which students will be successful

musculoskeletal system: the system of the body consisting of the muscles and skeleton particularly in relation to their role in the maintenance of health

obstetrics/gynecology: the practice of medicine which deals with the health of the female reproductive system; includes care of the pregnant woman and delivery of her baby, as well as care for infertile couples who need assistance in becoming pregnant

osteopathy: philosophy of medicine which emphasizes the treatment of the whole person, rather than only the disease; from the Greek *osteo*, meaning bone, and *pathos*, meaning to suffer or be in sympathy with

The History of Osteopathy

Osteopathy is a medical philosophy which treats disease in the context of the whole person, taking into consideration the functions and interrelationships of all body systems as well as such factors as nutrition, environment, and psychology. The first college of osteopathic medicine was founded in Kirksville, Missouri, in 1892, by Andrew Taylor Still, a frontier physician and Civil War surgeon. A hundred years later, there were fifteen colleges of osteopathic medicine located in various parts of the United States.

Still was the son of the Reverend Abraham Still, a doctor as well as a minister. As a youth, Andrew often accompanied his father on house calls, where he helped with basic medical procedures. His study of medicine led to a doctorate of medicine (M.D.), and he was licensed in the state of Missouri.

During the Civil War and in his practice as a frontier doctor, Still became frustrated by his inability to cure patients using the available techniques. The suffering of his patients was difficult for him to tolerate. The lack of knowledge about diseases and their treatment drove him to reconsider ways to improve the lot of the ill and injured. He also suffered a great personal loss when an epidemic of spinal meningitis spread through Kansas. Three of his children died of the disease, and three others died shortly after they were born. These tragedies nearly caused Still to abandon his career, but, in spite of the fact that the practice of modern medicine was in its infancy, he was determined to find the answers that would help him conquer disease and improve the health of his patients.

After the war ended, Still spent his life studying, observing, comparing, and experimenting in the treatment of disease. His observations closely paralleled the theories that the Greek physician Hippocrates proposed two thousand years earlier. Both Still and Hippocrates encouraged the physician to concentrate on the patient, not the disease.

Still wanted to establish the first school of osteopathy at Baker University in Baldwin, Kansas. He was refused permission to do so, however, because his philosophy of medicine did not conform to the accepted medical practice of the day. He was ostracized in Kansas, and in 1874, he moved to Missouri, where he was still licensed as a doctor and was legally able to practice medicine. As an itinerant doctor, he gained fame throughout the area and was affectionately known as the "bonesetter." It was during this time that he perfected his practice of osteopathy. Still's reputation and popularity spread, and he soon required assistance in treating the patients who sought him out. He established the first school of osteopathic medicine in Kirksville, Missouri, as the American School of Osteopathy under the law governing scientific institutions in 1892.

In 1894, he received a new charter from the state of Missouri for an educational institution. By the authority of the charter, the school could have awarded an M.D. degree, but Still wanted his degree to be different and chose to award a doctor of osteopathy (D.O.) degree instead. During the next few years, osteopathic colleges became a fad, and at one time, thirty-seven of them existed, many of which were correspondence or diploma schools.

The American School of Osteopathy taught the art of manipulative therapy. Still and his followers believed that if they could regulate and correct malfunctions of musculoskeletal function, they could return the body to a healthful state. When possible, they also eliminated the use of drugs to treat disease. Although this approach now sounds extreme, at that time few, if any, drugs were on the market, and most had severe side effects.

At the time that Still was establishing the roots of osteopathy, many significant advances were made in medical knowledge and techniques, including germ theory, the development of antiseptic surgery, the development of anesthesia, and the reorganization of medical education. The emphasis of Still on the treatment of the entire person has taken on more importance in modern times with the development of the fields of holistic medicine and preventive care.

SCIENCE AND PROFESSION

The philosophy of osteopathic medicine suggests that a human being is an ecologically and biologically unified whole. Among its tenets are that the various body systems are joined through the nervous, endocrine, and circulatory systems and that if one region of the body is diseased, the entire body is diseased.

There are five basic premises of osteopathy. First, the unity of all body parts is a benefit which assists in the maintenance of health and the resistance to disease. Second, when the body is properly nourished and structural relationships are normal, the body is able to adapt to physiologic changes that might otherwise put the body out of balance. Third, a healthy body depends on a healthy circulatory system and a nervous system that is able to conduct information to all areas of the body. Fourth, the musculoskeletal system does more than simply provide a framework for the body, and its normal function is critical to a healthy body. Fifth, it is not in the patient's best interest for the physician to treat only one aspect of the disease; the physician must treat the entire body and mind if the patient is to be cured. In modern times, the osteopathic physician uses manipulative therapy—in which rhythmic stretching and thrusting movements are used to realign joints and muscles properly—as one of many tools to cure the patient.

Osteopathic physicians and allopathic physicians have much in common. Both are members of the health care community who are fully trained physicians, who have taken a prescribed amount of undergraduate work, and who received four years of training in a medical school. After completing medical school, osteopathic physicians take a one-year rotating internship in hospitals with approved intern training programs. They may then enter a medical specialty program which may require a three- to four-year residency program.

Both allopathic and osteopathic medical programs use scientifically accepted methods of diagnosis and treatment. In the United States, the graduates of these programs are licensed by the same state medical boards and can practice in all phases of medicine in all states.

Admission to a college of osteopathic medicine in the United States requires a minimum of three years of preprofessional education in an accredited college or university. Virtually all students in osteopathic school, however, have been awarded undergraduate degrees. Many osteopathic students were science majors in undergraduate school, but all areas of study are represented. Most schools require a minimum of two semesters of study in biology, physics, and inorganic and organic chemistry. Students are also required to take the Medical College Admission Test (MCAT), submit letters of recommendation, and demonstrate an understanding of osteopathic medicine.

During the first two years in a college of osteopathic medicine, students receive basic science and preclinical instruction in a classroom or laboratory environment. Students are required to take courses in anatomy, biochemistry, physiology, pharmacology, pathology, and microbiology.

Schools are organized along one of two lines. They teach either by discipline or by system. In a discipline curriculum, the student concentrates on one subject at a time, such as biochemistry or physiology. In those programs with a curriculum that is organized by system, the student will study one organ system from the perspective of various basic science disciplines. For example, when studying the circulatory system, the student would concentrate on the anatomy, biochemistry, physiology, and pathology of the blood vessels and heart before moving on to another system.

Most students of osteopathy are required to take the first part of an examination prepared by the National Board of Examiners in Osteopathic Medicine and Surgery near the end of their second year. At the end of the second year or in the third year, the student concentrates on clinical instruction. Students of osteopathy may do clinical rotations in teaching hospitals, community hospitals, or physicians' offices in both urban and rural areas. Clinical instruction is designed to give the student experience in the diagnosis and treatment of a patient's symptoms. Students also attend seminars and conferences which are more specialized and which emphasize the disease process and the healing process.

The second part of the national boards is taken during the last year, and the third part is taken after the student has received the D.O. degree. After completion of the degree, the student participates in a one-year rotating internship in an approved hospital prior to selection of a residency program. Approximately 70 percent of all doctors of osteopathy enter one of the primary care specialties, including general practice, general internal medicine, obstetrics/gynecology, and pediatrics.

DIAGNOSTIC AND TREATMENT TECHNIQUES

Osteopathic medicine stresses the interdependence of structure and function. The application of manipulative therapy, and in particular joint mobilization, has been a hallmark of osteopathic medicine since its inception. Osteopathic physicians recognize human beings as complex biomechanical, biophysical, and biochemical organisms. They believe that structural disturbances can have wide-ranging effects that may spread to interconnecting systems. The biologic foundations of osteopathic medicine are based in the concepts of holism, homeostasis, unity of the body, environmental influences, and health-versus-disease.

Holism suggests that humans are whole beings that are not resolvable into component parts and that each "whole" is more than the sum of its parts. This premise can also be extended to mean that people are not isolated units—they are a part of their surroundings and thus are a part of their environment and the universe. The increased tendency toward specialization in health

care would seem to be in conflict with this principle. Osteopathic medicine suggests a need to increase the number of generalists or primary care physicians to ensure adequate care of the whole person. It further requires time to know and understand the patient as a person in his or her own environment.

The concept of body unity suggests that the normal healthy body contains all the elements necessary to maintain optimum function. Osteopathic physicians would argue that when disease alters body function, there is adequate flexibility within the system to compensate for change and to return the body to a state of wellness. This concept is similar to the principle of general physiology known as homeostasis.

Homeostasis recognizes the fact that essential body functions such as acidity of the blood, body temperature, and blood pressure are maintained within relatively narrow limits. It is not unusual for these parameters to drift slightly from the norm, but they must be quickly and efficiently returned to normal if the body is to survive. Deviations that cannot be readjusted quickly lead to poor body function and even death. Therefore, the body expends much time and energy in maintaining homeostasis, which prevents changes in the environment from having a significant effect on body function.

The philosophy of osteopathic medicine presents the position that musculoskeletal function is important in the maintenance of homeostasis. If this system is "out of line" or in any way unhealthy, the body will have a more difficult time maintaining homeostasis. It further argues that a healthy musculoskeletal system is necessary for a healthy immune system and that an unhealthy immune system can interfere with homeostasis.

The role of the environment in health is emphasized by the osteopathic physician. There is general agreement that a healthy environment contributes to a healthy body. A healthy environment here refers not only to the working and living environment of the patient but also to all associates and family members who are directly involved with the patient.

The concept of health-versus-disease is central to the philosophy of osteopathic medicine. The osteopathic physician is not as concerned with the treatment of the disease as with the cause of the disease and the methods that can be used to prevent its continuation or recurrence. The concept of health implies that all components of the body are functioning as a unit and that all are contributing to the maintenance of homeostasis.

Consequently, properly functioning circulatory, nervous, and endocrine systems are required. Disease, on the other hand, is present when cells do not receive appropriate circulation and/or nervous or endocrine regulation, causing a breakdown in the immune system or impairment of the adaptive mechanisms.

Although there are many similarities between allopathic and osteopathic physicians, some distinctions can be made. While the allopathic physician's philosophy emphasizes the value of the type of intervention used, the osteopathic physician stresses the importance of the body's ability to heal itself. Osteopathic medicine recognizes the musculoskeletal system as an important factor in the body's efforts to resist and overcome illness and disease. The major factor that separates osteopathic medicine from allopathic medicine is manipulative treatment, which is often called biomechanics. Osteopathic manipulative treatment is used in conjunction with other practices to provide the body with the means to cure itself.

PERSPECTIVE AND PROSPECTS

In 1894, when Andrew Taylor Still opened the first osteopathic medical school in Kirksville, Missouri, the medical community was skeptical of the methods of the osteopathic physician. Although Missouri was the first state to recognize an osteopathic medical school, there was resistance to licensing the graduates. In 1896, Vermont was the first state to enact legislation legalizing the licensing of osteopathy. Licensing in Missouri followed in 1897. By 1924, thirty-eight states had legally recognized osteopathy. In 1897, the American Osteopathic Association was formed to establish professional standards of practice. Its objectives were to promote the public health and to maintain high standards of medical education in osteopathic colleges.

Members of the American Medical Association (AMA) were not as accepting of osteopathic physicians as was the general public. When World War I broke out, some allopathic physicians claimed that the osteopaths were insufficiently trained for military service. Although there was widespread disagreement across the country, these allopathic physicians were successful, and the osteopathic physicians were kept at home. This situation ultimately proved to be to the benefit of osteopathy: While allopaths were serving in foreign countries, health care in the United States was left to osteopaths.

In 1923, the AMA continued its efforts to limit the practice of osteopathic physicians by declaring that it was unethical for M.D.'s to consult with D.O.'s. In 1938, M.D.'s were forbidden to engage in any professional relationship with D.O.'s.

Acceptance of osteopathic physicians finally came in 1967, when the AMA voted to negotiate for the merger of the two professions. The American Osteopathic Association was not interested in such a merger, but allopaths and osteopaths were allowed to work side by side in hospitals, community health clinics, and offices throughout the United States.

In the United States in the late twentieth century, there were approximately 32,000 osteopathic physicians across the nation, constituting 10 percent of practicing physicians and delivering 15 percent of American health care. The education of osteopathic physicians is expected to have an increasingly important role in the United States as people continue to emphasize preventive and family medicine. In efforts to cut costs and to improve the availability of health care, the government and health care insurance providers have stressed the need for primary care—an area that has always been important to the osteopathic physician.

Two monthly journals are available in libraries throughout the United States: the *Journal of the American Osteopathic Association* and *The D.O.* These journals contain research studies from osteopathic physicians as well as articles regarding the profession and the education of its students.

—Annette O'Connor, Ph.D.

See also Alternative medicine; Bones and the skeleton; Exercise physiology; Family medicine; Holistic medicine; Massage; Muscle sprains, spasms, and disorders; Muscles; Nutrition; Physical rehabilitation; Preventive medicine.

FOR FURTHER INFORMATION:

American Association of Colleges of Osteopathic Medicine. *The Education of the Osteopathic Physician.* Rev. ed. Rockville, Md.: Author, 1990. In addition to a thorough discussion of the educational requirements for entrance into an osteopathic medical school, this book outlines the courses required for the osteopathic physician.

Lederman, Eyal. *Fundamentals of Manual Therapy: Physiology, Neurology, and Psychology.* New York: Churchill Livingstone, 1997. This text discusses orthopedic manipulation as a means of therapy. Includes a bibliography and an index.

McKone, Walter Llewellyn. *Osteopathic Medicine: Philosophy, Principles and Practice.* Malden, Mass.:

Blackwell Scientific, 2001. Discusses the philosophy of osteopathic medicine and the way in which anatomy, physiology, signs, and symptoms all merge at the point of treatment.

Siegel, Irwin M. *All About Bone: An Owner's Manual.* New York: Demos Medical, 1998. Includes chapters on osteoporosis, arthritis, fractures, scoliosis, and low back pain.

Ward, Robert C., et al., eds. *Foundations for Osteopathic Medicine.* 2d ed. Philadelphia: Lippincott Williams & Wilkins, 2003. An introductory text that covers osteopathic principles and techniques as they relate to basic science and clinical medicine. Topics include osteopathic philosophy and history, clinical problem solving, clinical specialties, palpatory diagnosis and manipulative treatment, and health restoration.

OSTEOPOROSIS
DISEASE/DISORDER

ANATOMY OR SYSTEM AFFECTED: Back, bones, hips, legs, spine

SPECIALTIES AND RELATED FIELDS: Geriatrics and gerontology, nutrition, orthopedics, physical therapy

DEFINITION: A condition resulting from reduced bone mass; fractures are the major complications and are associated with significantly increased risks of morbidity and mortality, especially in older women.

KEY TERMS:

biochemical diagnostic procedures: a series of blood tests to evaluate the presence or absence of diseases, such as those aggravating osteoporosis

bone densitometry: a technique of bone scanning to measure mineral content, calcium content, and density

bone mineral density: the amount of mineralized bone, reported in grams per square centimeter of bone tissue, as measured by densitometry

cancellous bone: also called spongy or trabecular bone; bone that makes up 20 percent of the bone mass, is present in the ends of the long bones and throughout the vertebrae, provides the microstructure that gives bone its strength, and is the site for osteoporotic fractures

dual energy X-ray absorptiometry (DEXA): a method used to evaluate the regional and total bone mineral content considered the standard or criterion measure for bone mineral density

fracture risk: an estimate of the likelihood that a fracture will occur in an individual

CAUSES AND SYMPTOMS

Bone is constantly being remodeled by cells: Old bone is reabsorbed by the osteoclasts, and new bone is formed by the osteoblasts. Several factors control these processes of bone formation and resorption, which are about equal in adults. In children, formation exceeds resorption, and the bone mass increases. In old age, however, bone resorption exceeds bone formation and bone mass is lost. When bone mass is reduced, the bone becomes mechanically weak and vulnerable to fractures. This condition of reduced bone mass is known as osteoporosis and is part of the aging process. At this time, there is no known cure for osteoporosis. Prevention is the only strategy for combating bone mineral loss and the development of osteoporosis.

Type I osteoporosis is related to aging alone. It has two forms: postmenopausal (occurring in women between the ages of fifty-one and sixty-five, with fractures of the vertebrae and wrist) and senile (occurring in both men and women past the age of seventy, with fractures of the hip and vertebrae). Type II osteoporosis is associated with an underlying disease such as hyperparathyroidism or multiple myeloma and may occur in younger as well as older individuals. A third type has been found in young women who are amenorrheic (having no menstrual cycles) in association with eating disorders. Osteoporotic fractures are occurring in women in their twenties and thirties who have been amenorrheic for several years. Because it was found in athletic women, the link between eating disorders, amenorrhea, and osteoporosis was named the Female Athlete Triad. No matter the type of osteoporosis, it remains a clinically silent disease until a fracture occurs. In the United States, one to three million fractures related to osteoporosis occur yearly. The frequency of osteoporosis and related fractures is expected to increase in parallel with the increase in the older population. Women are more vulnerable to this condition, especially after the menopause. As the life span for men increases, however, so will their risk for osteoporosis.

In the early postmenopausal period, the distal end of the radius and ulna are particularly susceptible to fractures; a few years later, the patient is likely to sustain vertebral fractures. The most common presentation of such a fracture is a sudden onset of very severe, localized back pain, often occurring spontaneously. The pain is so severe that it incapacitates the patient and may require the administration of narcotics for relief. Unlike the pain caused by a disk rupture, this pain does not radiate to the legs, although some radiation anteriorly may be present. The pain usually lasts about four weeks and is then spontaneously relieved unless nerve compression or secondary arthritic changes complicate the condition.

When multiple vertebrae have collapsed, the body height is reduced and the patient's arms appear to be disproportionately long. Normally, both measurements—body height and arm span—are equal. In osteoporosis complicated by several vertebral fractures, body height is reduced, but the arm span is unchanged. When multiple thoracic vertebrae collapse, kyphosis (an increased spinal curvature) develops, a condition sometimes referred to as dowager's hump. The space between the ribs and the pelvic cavity is also reduced. When lumbar vertebrae are collapsed, the lower end of the ribs may lie over the pelvic cavity. At this stage, the patient's lung functions may be compromised because the chest movements are limited. Pneumonia is a common, fatal complication.

Progressive and long-standing osteoporosis may be complicated by fractures of the femoral neck. Although most of these fractures are preceded by a fall, it is probable that in some cases the bones are so weakened and fragile that they fracture spontaneously and cause the patient to fall. Fractures of the femoral neck are associated with significant mortality and morbidity risks, with 12 to 20 percent of the patients dying within six months of the fracture and about half losing the ability to live independently.

A number of factors predisposing an individual to osteoporosis have been identified. Some of these factors cannot be changed. For example, the older patients are, the more likely they are to develop osteoporosis. Furthermore, although both sexes are affected by osteoporosis, women tend to be more vulnerable because, in addition to the accelerated rate of bone loss which oc-

curs at the menopause, women tend to have smaller skeletons than men do and, therefore, are likely to reach the threshold at which bone fragility is increased well before men do. Caucasians in Europe and North America are more susceptible to osteoporosis than are African Americans or Latinos, in whom this condition is relatively rare. The reasons for these racial differences are not well known. It is possible, however, that African Americans statistically have larger skeletons, and weight may be a factor in both African Americans and Latinos. Asians have about the same bone densities as Caucasians. Because a difference in stature means that their hip axis length is shorter and therefore less likely to fracture, however, they have about half the number of hip fractures. Finally, people with large body frames are less likely to develop osteoporosis than those with small body frames, probably because their bone reserve allows them to lose bone for a longer period before reaching the threshold at which the bone fragility is significantly increased. Genetic research has also determined that variations in the gene for the vitamin D receptor (VDR) may contribute to 7 to 10 percent of the difference in bone mass density because of its influence on calcium intake. For those with a family history of osteoporosis, this factor could lead to identification of an individual's risk factor and enable early intervention.

A number of risk factors that can be reversed have also been identified. A low dietary calcium intake is associated with a reduced bone mass and an increased fracture rate. Conversely, an elevated calcium intake, particularly before puberty, is associated with an increased mass. In 1994, the National Institutes of Health consensus statement recommended an increase in daily calcium, and in 1997 the National Academy of Sciences' dietary reference intake (DRI), formerly the recommended dietary allowance (RDA), increased from 800 milligrams per day to 1,300 milligrams at age nine up to age eighteen. Some researchers are recommending a daily intake of 1,300 to 1,500 milligrams for all young people during puberty and up to at least age thirty to obtain optimal peak bone mass. Women during pregnancy and lactation also need a higher amount, up to 1,300 milligrams. Men from age thirty to sixty-four should take in 1,000 milligrams, increasing to 1,200 milligrams at age sixty-five. Women from age nineteen to the menopause should take in 1,000 milligrams, increasing to 1,200 milligrams when they are no longer producing estrogen. Amenorrheic women should be taking in 1,300 to 1,500 milligrams. The maximum allowable intake has been increased from 2,000 to 2,500

INFORMATION ON OSTEOPOROSIS

CAUSES: Aging, disease (e.g., hyperparathyroidism, multiple myeloma), amenorrhea, anorexia nervosa, physical inactivity

SYMPTOMS: Increased bone fractures, severe and localized back pain, reduced height

DURATION: Chronic

TREATMENTS: Hormonal therapy (estrogens, calcitonin); drug therapy (bisphosphonates, teriparatide, slow-release sodium fluoride, calcitriol, raloxifene), calcium supplements

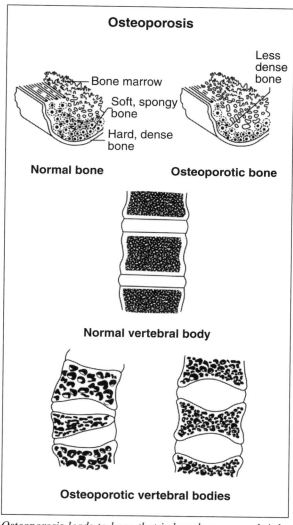

Osteoporosis

Bone marrow

Soft, spongy bone

Hard, dense bone

Less dense bone

Normal bone

Osteoporotic bone

Normal vertebral body

Osteoporotic vertebral bodies

Osteoporosis leads to bone that is less dense, more brittle, more easily broken, and degenerative.

During the formative years, exercise is imperative to develop the highest bone density possible. Then throughout the rest of life, exercise is essential to slow the rate of bone loss. Research on amenorrheic and eumenorrheic young female athletes has contributed much to the body of knowledge of the relationship of exercise to bone density. It is not only the exercise that is important but also the presence of estrogen (or testosterone in males) that enhances the process of bone formation. Several factors modulate the response of the skeleton to exercise. These include the subject's age and gender; the intensity, frequency, and type of exercise; and the subject's endocrinal status. The current recommendation for exercise in relationship to osteoporosis is preventive: a variety of exercise, both weight-bearing and vigorous, to be done regularly (thirty to sixty minutes per day, three to five days per week) throughout life. Variety is essential because no single exercise stresses all bones equally. The stimulus to build bone comes from the muscle that is attached to the bone pulling on the attachment site, which makes the bone remodel itself to resist the stress.

In the elderly, exercise may have a secondary benefit. Often, a fracture is precipitated by a fall, and the cause of the fall may be a loss of balance or coordination. Maintaining an active lifestyle helps with balance and coordination as well as confidence, all of which may help in the prevention of a fall. Studies in the elderly have demonstrated that a general exercise such as walking is not enough to maintain gains in bone density for very long. Exercise studies of one or two years' duration show a decline begins after about one year. To combat that loss, a regular strength training regimen, targeting the most common fracture sites, done two or three times a week for twenty minutes to stimulate specific bones, should be added to any other activities that are done.

Cigarette smoking is associated with osteoporosis; however, the underlying mechanism is not clearly understood. It is possible that cigarette smokers are more likely to lead a sedentary life and have a reduced dietary calcium intake compared to nonsmokers. Cigarette smoking may have a direct effect on the bone cells, or it may have an indirect effect by modulating the release of substances that may affect the activity of these cells, such as the parathyroid hormone or calcitonin secretion.

At one time, caffeine ingestion was thought to have a significantly adverse effect on calcium absorption. The craze of drinking lattes (espresso coffee mixed with hot

milligrams. Higher doses may be detrimental, as they may cause the formation of kidney stones, so the benefit must be weighed against the risk in each case. Getting the greatest percentage of the calcium from the diet is preferred, but, if it is to be taken as a supplement, no more than 500 milligrams should be taken at one time and always with meals. Calcium is not absorbed well, so having stomach acid present, as well as vitamin D and protein, enhances the absorption.

Physical inactivity is associated with a reduced bone mass and therefore an increased predisposition to developing osteoporosis. There is also evidence that people who have a sedentary lifestyle are more susceptible to osteoporosis than those who are physically active.

milk) stimulated more research, and the findings suggested that the advantage of drinking about 14 ounces of milk in a latte resulted in an increased calcium intake of about 400 milligrams. The amount of calcium lost as a result of the caffeine amounted to only about one teaspoon of milk, which is insignificant. Since many American women surveyed have been drinking little or no milk, the popularity of lattes may have a beneficial effect on the members of the thirty- to fifty-year-old population.

A number of drugs may induce osteoporosis. Among them, cortisone preparations are particularly notorious. Therefore, the long-term administration of these drugs should be avoided. If cortisone must be administered, then the lowest effective dose should be chosen. Studies are underway on a drug, etidronate (Didronel), which, when given along with corticosteroid drugs, may act as a bone-sparing therapy and lower the chance of fractures in people who must take the corticosteroids. The long-term administration of potent diuretics also should be avoided, as they induce a negative calcium balance by increasing renal urinary calcium excretion. (Milder diuretics, on the other hand, may actually induce a positive calcium balance by reducing renal calcium excretion.) Other drugs that have been added to the list include anticonvulsive drugs, antacids that contain aluminum, some forms of cancer chemotherapy, and heparin, which is used to prevent blood clots. For a person at risk for osteoporosis, anytime that medications are prescribed, calcium interaction should be considered.

TREATMENT AND THERAPY

Several tests are available to confirm the diagnosis of osteoporosis, quantify its degree, and identify underlying diseases that might cause or aggravate the osteoporosis.

Plain X rays used to be the only way to evaluate patients with osteoporosis. Although they are helpful in assessing bone involvement from other diseases, they are not useful for the detection of early osteoporosis because the characteristic appearances are seen only when at least 40 percent of the bone mass has been lost. In the 1990's, a new analysis technique was developed using a simple X ray of the hand and then computer analysis. It is able to reveal as little as 1 percent bone loss.

The most accurate technique now available to measure bone density uses a technique called dual energy X-ray absorptiometry (DEXA). DEXA is based on the principle that if a beam of radiation is directed at a bone, the amount of radiation trapped by the bone is proportional to the amount of mineral and calcium inside. By knowing the amount of radiation aimed at the bone and the amount reaching a detector crystal across the bone, the amount of mineral can be calculated. To differentiate the radiation trapped by the surrounding muscles and fat from the radiation trapped by the bone itself, radiation with two different peaks (which are absorbed to a different extent by bone and soft tissue) is used. The exposure to radiation is minimal, one-fiftieth the radiation as in a chest X ray. The same densitometry machine can do whole-body or single-site readings, making it even more useful for diagnosis. The only problem is that the number of DEXA machines available for diagnosis does not allow everyone to be assessed. Therefore, the criteria for who should be screened is determined by perceived risk. The physician must assess a patient's known risks to determine when and how often densitometry should be done. Bone density determination is also useful in monitoring the bone mass of patients requiring long-term cortisone therapy in order to determine whether bone loss is occurring and therefore whether some other medication needs to be prescribed.

Osteoporosis therapy includes several options. Several drugs are currently being used or investigated for use. For decades, the most commonly prescribed regimen for women was hormone therapy, the use of estrogen, usually in combination with progesterone. Despite findings in 2002 by the long-term study called the Women's Health Initiative that the overall risks of hormone therapy outweighed its benefits, this therapy is effective in arresting the bone loss that occurs after the menopause and even increasing the bone mass, particularly if started within the first five years and combined with calcium and exercise. With increased concerns about the safety of estrogens, however, other drugs are increasingly used to prevent or treat osteoporosis.

Calcitonin, a hormone produced by the thyroid gland, specifically inhibits the osteoclasts, which are the bone resorbing cells. As a result, there is a relative increase in the rate of bone formation, and the bone mass increases. After the initial increase, however, the bone mass tends to stabilize, and the continued administration of calcitonin beyond this point may be associated with an actual decline in bone mass. Many physicians, therefore, administer calcitonin in cycles of six to twelve months. One of the main advantages of calcitonin is that, unlike hormone therapy, it is effective in both sexes and in patients of all ages, including the very old. Calcitonin also appears to have an analgesic effect, which may be quite useful following a vertebral collapse. The main disadvantages of calcitonin are cost and form of administration. A synthetic form that is administered as a nasal spray has received Food and Drug Administration (FDA) approval. This is a relief to patients who have had to give themselves a daily injection. The only disadvantage of this drug is that it does not appear to be as effective in thickening bones as other drugs being studied.

A more effective class of drugs used to treat osteoporosis are the bisphosphonates, which include etidronate (Didronel), pamidronate (Aredia), alendronate (Fosamax), risedronate (Actonel), and zolendronate (Zometa). Fosamax was the first nonhormonal osteoporosis drug. In very large studies, dramatic increases in bone density have been seen, along with fewer fractures. The cost is about the same as calcitonin, but considerably more than hormone therapy. The cost, coupled with the lack of long-term use studies to determine side effects, suggests that alendronate should be the drug of choice for the elderly with severe bone loss rather than a preventive measure for a newly postmenopausal woman, unless her risk is very high.

In 2002, the FDA announced the approval of the drug teriparatide, sold as Forteo, which works by increasing the action of osteoblasts and causes bones to become denser and more resistant to fractures. It is especially effective for osteoporosis in postmenopausal women. Forteo differs from Fosamax by stimulating the body to build new bone, rather than by helping bones retain their density. The drug is given by daily injection and can be used in combination with the older approved drugs because the drugs work by different mechanisms in the body.

Several other drugs are showing promise in controlled studies, including slow-release sodium fluoride, calcitriol, and raloxifene (Evista). Sodium fluoride causes significant increases in bone densities, as much as 5 percent a year for four years. The side effects, however, include peptic ulcers, and, unfortunately, the bone that is built is sometimes brittle. Also, fluoride can be toxic, so the levels must be monitored carefully. The slow-release form seems to avoid some of the side effects, but larger studies need to be completed before the drug can be approved. Calcitriol, or synthetic vitamin D, is used in many countries as a treatment for osteoporosis. Currently, it is used in the United States only to treat a bone disorder that can result from kidney dialysis. Calcitriol helps in the absorption of calcium and stimulates osteoblasts. Evista be-

IN THE NEWS: NEW OSTEOPOROSIS DRUG PROLIA

A new investigational medication that works unlike others currently on the market offers a promising alternative for the treatment of osteoporosis in both men and women. Prolia (denosumab) blocks the ability of bone cells to break down bone. Prolia is injected subcutaneously (into the skin) every six months in men or women to prevent osteoporosis and bone loss. If approved by the Food and Drug Administration (FDA), this first-in-its-class biologic therapy would be used in breast cancer patients or prostate cancer patients undergoing therapy to decrease natural hormone levels or in postmenopausal women.

In August, 2009, two Prolia studies were published in *The New England Journal of Medicine*. Patients included men with prostate cancer (about 1,500) and postmenopausal women (about 7,800) with osteoporosis who were enrolled and followed for three years. At the conclusion of the study, treatment with Prolia reduced radiographic spine fractures significantly. Thus, the results of these randomized, placebo-controlled trials indicated that the drug was similarly effective in treating osteoporosis as a bisphosphonate medication.

In another study, Prolia was found to slow the time to a skeletal-related event (such as a bone fracture) in patients with breast cancer. Patients received either Prolia or Zometa every four weeks for bone metastases. At the conclusion of the study, patients taking Prolia experienced both a delay to time to first skeletal-related event and delay to subsequent skeletal-related events.

While the efficacy results from the registration trials and the comparative trials are impressive, further research is warranted to address safety concerns with the medication, including whether the medication increases cancer recurrence. Also, concerns have been raised that Prolia may block immune cells and liver cells from functioning properly. According the manufacturer, clinical trials are underway.

—*Jesse Fishman, Pharm.D.*

longs to the class of drugs known as selective estrogen receptor modulators (SERMs), or so-called designer estrogens. This compound attaches to estrogen receptors in the body to mimic the effect of estrogen on the bones. It appears to work without increasing the risk of breast or uterine cancer.

Calcium supplements are useful if the patient's dietary calcium intake is less than required. There is no evidence to support any beneficial effect of supplements if the daily dietary intake of calcium exceeds the DRI. Unfortunately, only 14 percent of girls and 35 percent of boys aged twelve to nineteen are achieving the DRI. According to the FDA, either supplementation or education needs to occur in this population in order to avoid an epidemic of osteoporosis in the future. Similarly, if the daily vitamin D intake is below the recommended level of 400 milligrams in the elderly population, supplementation is recommended. Vitamin D supplements may also be necessary in patients who are taking a medication that interferes with vitamin D metabolism, such as anticonvulsant drugs which increase the rate of vitamin D breakdown in the liver. The determination of proper dosage is based on some vitamin D formation from sunlight. If a person is not exposed to a minimum of twenty minutes of sunlight a day, the requirement increases by 200 milligrams. An excessive vitamin D and calcium intake, however, may lead to the development of kidney stones. Furthermore, excessive vitamin D (greater than 1,000 milligrams a day) may increase the rate of bone resorption and, because vitamin D is lipid soluble and it is stored in the body-fat tissue, its toxicity may last for months.

Although fluorides are sometimes used in the treatment of osteoporosis, they are associated with a high incidence of adverse effects, such as gastritis, kidney damage, and joint pain. In addition, investigators are trying to identify the optimum fluoride dose that will encourage the deposition of calcium in the bone and yet keep the side effects to a minimum.

Considerable research has been conducted on the use of different preparations, such as growth hormone, testosterone, and anabolic steroids, in the treatment of osteoporosis, particularly in men. Some experts are recommending that in men with low testosterone, a biweekly injection or the daily application of a testosterone patch may be needed. More research is needed on men with the new drugs that have been approved for use for women. Also, studies of heart disease risk or prostate problems in men using testosterone need to be conducted.

PERSPECTIVE AND PROSPECTS

Osteoporosis is a major public health problem, affecting at least 25 million Americans, with about 1.5 million fractures occurring each year. It is often silent until a fracture occurs. Up to one of every five older patients sustaining a hip fracture dies within six months of the fracture. One-half of the survivors need some help with their daily living activities, and as many as 25 percent of these patients need care in a nursing home. The 1995 estimated cost for treating osteoporotic fractures was nearly $14 billion.

The early diagnosis of osteoporosis and the ability to quantify its degree have represented major strides in the diagnosis, management, and prevention of this disease. It is now recommended that all women approaching the menopause be checked to determine a baseline density reading and to help with prevention and possible treatment options. Indeed, physicians can now identify patients with early osteoporosis and assess their response to treatment accurately. Additionally, modifiable risk factors increasing the likelihood of developing osteoporosis have been identified; these include a low dietary calcium intake, cigarette smoking, excessive alcohol use, amenorrhea, anorexia nervosa or bulimia nervosa, and a sedentary lifestyle. Education of the public, therefore, has an important part to play in the prevention and management of osteoporosis. Working with young people may be the best way to combat osteoporosis. For many people, making the right choices early in life may have great influence in preventing this debilitating disease later in life. For the older adult, attempts are being made to develop "risk profiles" that can be used to estimate the individual patient's fracture risk. This in turn will allow physicians to identify those in the population who are particularly likely to benefit from specific therapy. Moreover, the increased understanding of bone formation, bone resorption, and bone metabolism has led to a considerable amount of research work on the development of effective treatment programs. Drugs that can build strong bones, or ones that can prevent further bone loss, will need to be continually studied in both men and women, and everything that can be done to reduce side effects from these or other drugs that affect calcium stores in the bones must be a top priority of research dollars spent.

—*Ronald C. Hamdy, M.D., Larry Hudgins, M.D., and Sharon Moore, M.D.; updated by Wendy E. S. Repovich, Ph.D.*

See also Aging; Aging: Extended care; Amenorrhea; Anorexia nervosa; Bone disorders; Bones and the skeleton; Eating disorders; Exercise physiology; Fracture and dislocation; Fracture repair; Hip fracture repair; Hormone therapy; Hormones; Malnutrition; Menopause; Nutrition; Orthopedic surgery; Orthopedics; Preventive medicine; Spinal cord disorders; Spine, vertebrae, and disks; Sports medicine; Supplements; Vitamins and minerals.

FOR FURTHER INFORMATION:

Bilger, Burkhard. "Bone Medicine." *Health* 10, no. 3 (1996). This article summarizes the new drugs approved by the FDA for the treatment of osteoporosis in women, as well as other drugs that are being researched for approval.

Bohme, Karine, and Frances Buddin. *The Silent Thief: Osteoporosis, Exercises and Strategies for Prevention and Treatment*. Toronto, Ont.: Firefly Books, 2001. A thorough exploration of osteoporosis, discussing hereditary and lifestyle factors that contribute to its onset, outlining dietary and supplementary options, and illustrating detailed exercise programs for prevention and treatment at any age.

Heaney, Robert P. "Osteoporosis." In *Nutrition in Women's Health*, edited by Debra A. Krummel and Penny M. Kris-Etherton. Gaithersburg, Md.: Aspen, 1996. This chapter highlights the role of nutrition in the prevention and treatment of osteoporosis in the postmenopausal woman.

Hodgson, Stephen F., ed. *Mayo Clinic on Osteoporosis: Keeping Bones Healthy and Strong and Reducing the Risk of Fractures*. Rochester, Minn.: Mayo Clinic, 2003. A comprehensive overview of the disorder.

Meredith, C. M. "Exercise in the Prevention of Osteoporosis." In *Nutrition of the Elderly*, edited by Hamish Munro and Gunter Schlierf. Nestle's Nutrition Workshop Series 29. New York: Raven Press, 1992. This report emphasizes the positive effect of sustained exercise programs on bone mineral stabilization.

National Osteoporosis Foundation. http://www.nof .org. A leading resource for people seeking updated, medically sound information on the causes, prevention, detection, and treatment of osteoporosis.

Nelson, Miriam E., and Sarah Wernick. *Strong Women, Strong Bones: Everything You Need to Know to Prevent, Treat, and Beat Osteoporosis*. Rev. ed. New York: Berkley Books, 2006. Basics of osteoporosis, adopting a therapeutic lifestyle, treatment and prevention, and research resources are covered.

Rosen, Clifford J., Julie Glowacki, and John P. Bilezikian. *The Aging Skeleton*. San Diego, Calif.: Academic Press, 1999. This book is a substantial addition to the texts available in the area of osteoporosis. Its large-format pages are divided into forty-nine chapters that range widely across such topics as the biology of aging, determinants of peak bone mass, the biology of age-related bone loss, assessment of bone loss, the epidemiology of osteoporotic fractures, and the therapeutics of osteoporosis.

Van Horn, Linda, and Annie O. Wong. "Preventive Nutrition in Adolescent Girls." In *Nutrition in Women's Health*, edited by Debra A. Krummel and Penny M. Kris-Etherton. Gaithersburg, Md.: Aspen, 1996. Discusses the role that nutrition in adolescents may play in the prevention of osteoporosis later in life.

OTOPLASTY

PROCEDURE

ANATOMY OR SYSTEM AFFECTED: Ears, skin

SPECIALTIES AND RELATED FIELDS: Audiology, family medicine, general surgery, pediatrics, plastic surgery

DEFINITION: Cosmetic or reconstructive surgery performed on the outer ear.

INDICATIONS AND PROCEDURES

Otoplasty is performed to improve the appearance of the outer ear, typically to flatten protruding ears or to repair or reconstruct a missing or badly damaged ear. Since the ears have reached 90 percent of their adult size by the time a child reaches age five, the surgery can be performed either at this early age or later.

The first step in flattening protruding ears is to remove a flap of skin from the back of each ear. The underlying cartilage is then remolded, and the two edges of the wound are stitched together, bringing the ear closer to the head. Dressings are applied to the ears and left for a few days, when they are replaced by a headband that is worn for several weeks. The stitches are removed approximately one week after the surgery.

The reconstruction of a missing or badly damaged ear is a complex procedure that typically involves more than one operation, and long healing intervals are necessary between operations. The first step is to remove a piece of cartilage from a rib and sculpt it to resemble a normal ear. The cartilage is then transferred to a fold of skin where the ear will be located. A skin graft may be necessary. Dressings are applied to the ear for up to two weeks, and the stitches are then removed. In many cases, hearing in the reconstructed ear may not be normal. As long as hearing is normal in the other ear, however, no attempt is usually made to improve hearing in the reconstructed ear.

USES AND COMPLICATIONS

Possible complications associated with otoplasty operations include sensitivity of the ear to cold weather, especially during the first year after surgery, and skin graft failure. On rare occasions, excessive bleeding or infection of the surgical wounds may arise. For minor pain, the patient can take acetaminophen or ibuprofen. As the ear heals, a hard ridge usually forms along the incision, but it will gradually recede. The scar will be hidden in the crease between the scalp and the ear.

—Alvin K. Benson, Ph.D.

See also Ear infections and disorders; Ears; Hearing loss; Plastic surgery; Surgery, pediatric.

FOR FURTHER INFORMATION:

Converse, J. M. *Reconstructive Plastic Surgery.* 2d ed. Philadelphia: W. B. Saunders, 1977.

Davis, Jack. *Otoplasty: Aesthetic and Reconstructive Techniques.* 2d ed. New York: Springer, 1997.

Stedman, Thomas Lathrop. *Stedman's Plastic Surgery/ENT/Dentistry Words.* 4th ed. Baltimore: Lippincott Williams & Wilkins, 2005.

Townsend, Courtney M., Jr., et al., eds. *Sabiston Textbook of Surgery.* 18th ed. Philadelphia: Saunders/Elsevier, 2008.

OTORHINOLARYNGOLOGY

SPECIALTY

ANATOMY OR SYSTEM AFFECTED: Ears, nose, respiratory system, throat

SPECIALTIES AND RELATED FIELDS: Audiology, neurology, pediatrics, plastic surgery

DEFINITION: The study of the diseases and disorders of the ears, nose, and throat.

KEY TERMS:

audiometer: an electronic device, often used in combination with a computer, that measures a patient's range of hearing

fenestration: the surgical opening of a passage in a closed or narrowing ear canal through which sound can pass

mastoidectomy: the surgical removal of the temporal or mastoid bone, which is located behind the ear

maxillofacial surgery: surgery of the face and neck, a form of cosmetic and reconstructive surgery

otologist: a medical doctor who specializes in diseases and disorders of the ear

stapedectomy: the surgical removal of all or part of the stapes or innermost ossicle of the ear

tomography: an X ray used in combination with sophisticated computers to create an image of a specific organ, blotting out everything in front or behind

SCIENCE AND PROFESSION

Otorhinolaryngology—whose practitioners are often referred to simply as otolaryngologists or ear, nose, and throat (ENT) doctors—is a medical specialty that requires a doctor of medicine degree followed by a hospital or medical center residency ranging from four to five years, depending on the institution in which it is served. Many physicians in this field develop subspecialties, for which additional training is requisite. Among the most common subspecialties are oncology of the head and neck, ear surgery, pediatric otolaryngology, and maxillofacial surgery.

The scope of the otorhinolaryngologist's job is broad and overlaps several other medical specialties, notably general surgery, neurosurgery, plastic surgery, pediatrics, ophthalmology, and oncology. The otorhinolaryngologist treats all diseases and lesions that occur above the clavicle or collarbone except for those belonging to two categories: diseases and disorders of the eyes, which fall into the province of ophthalmology, and brain lesions, which are usually treated by neurosurgeons.

Otorhinolaryngology has existed as a specialty since the late nineteenth century. The need for it was great because ear, nose, and throat problems had, through the centuries, been among the most persistent killers of human beings. The areas affected have much to do with the ability to take in food and air. They also are directly connected with speech, smell, taste, hearing, and balance. Dysfunction of the ears, nose, or throat can profoundly affect a person's well-being physically, emotionally, and socially.

Among the medical conditions and diseases that most frequently come under the purview of otorhinolaryngology are the following: cleft lip and palate deformities (which are often treated as well by plastic surgeons); thyroid tumors (which are also treated by oncological surgeons); skin cancers (which also fall within the practices of plastic surgeons and oncological surgeons); face lifts, the treatment of facial lacerations, and other reconstructive surgery (which plastic surgeons also handle); lumps on the salivary glands (which

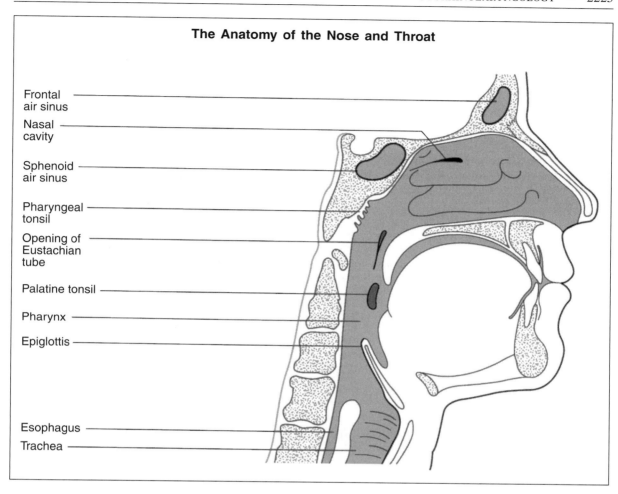

The Anatomy of the Nose and Throat

Frontal air sinus
Nasal cavity
Sphenoid air sinus
Pharyngeal tonsil
Opening of Eustachian tube
Palatine tonsil
Pharynx
Epiglottis
Esophagus
Trachea

are sometimes treated by oncological surgeons); and jaw injuries, including fractures (which are treated by maxillofacial surgeons, many of them board-certified in otorhinolaryngology).

Some of the surgery once done by otorhinolaryngologists is now virtually unnecessary because of the development of antibiotics. For example, drugs can combat effectively the kinds of infections that used to result in mastoiditis (inflammation of the mastoid bone), which frequently required a mastoidectomy. The flexible fiber-optic endoscope permits doctors to look into areas that previously could be exposed only through surgery. Advances in research have revealed that nasal polyps, which had a high rate of recurrence and were removed on a continuous basis, can usually be treated effectively with antibiotics, making such surgery unnecessary.

Until the mid-twentieth century, the most serious operation performed by otorhinolaryngologists was the laryngectomy (removal of the larynx, or voice box). By the end of the century, however, many practitioners in this specialty were routinely performing surgeries on tongue cancers and thyroid tumors because otorhinolaryngologists are often the ones who initially discover these conditions during head and neck examinations.

Because otorhinolaryngologists have long dealt with the grafting of bone and skin and the surgical management of skin flaps, much reconstructive and cosmetic surgery now falls into their specialty. Removal of tumors from the base of the skull, the interior ear canal, or the posterior cranial depression by means of modified craniotomies can be done by otorhinolaryngologists, who sometimes work in tandem with neurosurgeons in such cases.

DIAGNOSTIC AND TREATMENT TECHNIQUES
The illnesses treated by otorhinolaryngologists have plagued the human race throughout history but could

not be treated effectively until technology was developed that enabled physicians to look into the crowded crevices deep inside the body that were the source of many illnesses. In 1854, Manuel Garcia invented a concave mirror with a hole in its center through which doctors, attaching the implement to their heads, could peer as light from the mirror illuminated a patient's ears, nose, and throat. Doctors discovered that, using the reflecting head mirror in combination with an angled mirror held as far back as possible in the throat, they could illuminate the laryngeal area and the pharynx as well as the area behind the nose, all previously unavailable for visual inspection. Eventually, rather than examining affected areas with the bare eye, physicians had available to them, imbedded in the eyepiece of a hollow instrument with a light at the end, a magnifying telescope through which they could examine remote cavities with considerable ease and in great detail.

Modern otorhinolaryngologists can also examine patients under mild local anesthetic with sophisticated endoscopes, flexible devices that can easily be inserted into the nose, mouth, or ear of the patient. Such procedures are usually carried out in the doctor's office or in a hospital on an outpatient basis. These endoscopes, originally lighted with bulbs that heated up and burned out quickly, now carry light through light-bearing fiberoptic strands. In combination with small magnifying devices and cameras designed for this purpose, physicians can examine almost any area of the ears, nose, and throat and create color images, which can be invaluable in determining the presence of disease and in making an accurate diagnosis.

Modern technology has also made available to otorhinolaryngologists laser scalpels that permit extremely intricate surgery and accurate electronic audiometers. Audiometers eliminate the subjectivity of past tests of hearing acuity: In the nineteenth century, doctors either whispered into patients' ears, increasing the volume until their whispers could be heard, or used tuning forks to determine how much their patients could hear.

Treatment of disorders and diseases of the ear, nose, and throat have changed rapidly with the introduction of increasingly sophisticated surgical equipment and with the development of new drugs to control many conditions that once could be managed only by surgery. Computers have also been a valuable tool in diagnosing many of the problems that fall within this specialty.

All the anatomical areas with which otorhinolaryngologists must deal are interconnected; therefore a disease that begins in the ears can affect the nose and the throat, and vice versa. The most common diseases of the ears include deafness and Ménière's disease, an illness caused by an accumulation of fluid in the ear's labyrinth that results in loss of balance. Both of these disorders are most common among people over fifty, although they can afflict people at any age. One out of every ten thousand babies born in the United States has some hearing deficit, and many—particularly those whose mothers contracted rubella (German measles) during pregnancy—are almost totally deaf.

Otologists (physicians who treat diseases and disorders of the ear) have made considerable headway in treating some forms of deafness, particularly conductive deafness, which results from a narrowing of the ear canal to the point of closure. Shortly before 1920, it was discovered that considerable hearing can be restored through fenestration—that is, through making a small surgical opening in the eardrum through which sound can pass. The complications associated with this procedure have been largely overcome with stapedectomy (the removal of all or part of the stapes, one of the bones of the middle ear) and the insertion of a prosthetic device, which is made of wire or Teflon and used in combination with a gelatin sponge or the patient's own veins, connective tissue, and fat. Although fenestration is highly successful in cases in which deafness is conductive, it does not alleviate deafness whose cause is sensorineural, so-called nerve deafness, which is often treated palliatively with hearing aids. These devices are constantly improving, however, as they are decreasing in size and increasing in effectiveness.

Tumors of the inner ear can now be successfully removed through a translabyrinthine approach. The ear canal is entered with tiny, well-illuminated laser instruments to which magnifying devices are attached. Such surgery is often performed by otologists, although many undertake it collaboratively with a neurologist. Pituitary tumors, once the responsibility almost solely of neurosurgeons who performed craniotomies to reach the diseased area of the brain, are often treated by otorhinolaryngologists, who approach the tumor through the nose. Thus the tumor can be removed without the need for debilitating surgery.

From the earliest beginnings of otorhinolaryngology, the larynx has been among the parts of the anatomy most often treated by its practitioners. The laryngectomy, with its radical side effect of rendering the patient unable to speak, was once the treatment of choice for malignant laryngeal tumors. Such tumors can now be treated successfully with radiation, obviating the need for more drastic treatment. Teflon injections have been used to treat patients whose vocal cords have been compromised by surgery or by radiation. Because the larynx is in the area of the thyroid glands, otorhinolaryngologists also possess expert knowledge of thyroid disorders and may perform a thyroidectomy (removal of the thyroid), a procedure that is now emphasized in their residencies.

Two of the most frequent surgical procedures of the field in the mid-twentieth century were the removal of the tonsils (tonsillectomy) and of the adenoids, the masses of lymphoid tissue in the lining at the back of the tongue that produce white blood cells, which fight disease. Tonsils and adenoids were once removed routinely if children suffered from frequent colds. Now this surgery is discouraged because it has been discovered that the tonsils and adenoids help children develop a resistance to infection. When these tissues become inflamed, they can be treated conservatively and successfully through medication.

Otorhinolaryngologists regularly work in concert with physicians in other specialties, particularly neurosurgery. An internist treating a patient who suffers from loss of balance usually refers that patient to an otologist, who orders diagnostic tests to check for fluid in the inner ear, which would suggest Ménière's disease. If such tests fail to reveal a buildup of fluid in the inner ear, the otologist usually refers the patient to a neurologist or neurosurgeon to check for other causes, including a tumor or a disorder in the central nervous system.

Otologists sometimes perform plastic surgery on ears that are abnormally protrusive. This reduction is a form of cosmetic surgery. By the end of the twentieth century in the United States, it was common for otorhinolaryngologists to perform most cosmetic and reconstructive surgeries related to these areas of the body. Consequently, residencies in this specialty offer considerable training in plastic surgery, especially in the procedures that otorhinolaryngologists have come to perform routinely in connection with thyroid, nasal, and other surgeries. They are often the physicians of choice in cases of cleft lip and cleft palate, the treatment of which normally falls largely within the province of reconstructive surgery. Because much cosmetic and reconstructive surgery involves the face, maxillofacial surgeons are often otorhinolaryngologists.

The common cold, although usually treated by an internist or family doctor if it is referred to a physician at all, sometimes involves complications such as bronchitis, pneumonia, or ancillary infections of the ears and sinuses. In such cases, an otorhinolaryngologist may be consulted for treatment. Dealing with the common cold is merely a waiting game: Colds generally go away after a week or ten days. Colds afflict the average adult about four times a year and the average child twice that often (because young children have not yet built up the immunity that prevents infection).

PERSPECTIVE AND PROSPECTS

Many of the illnesses that fall within the purview of otorhinolaryngology became more threatening and more frequent when the Industrial Revolution of the eighteenth century caused the relocation of large numbers of people from rural to urban settings. Cities grew as factories opened. Living conditions were often deplorable and, at best, overcrowded. Added to this situation was the pollution of the air by the waste products expelled by smokestack industries. Wherever pollution is prevalent, diseases of the upper respiratory tract are endemic.

The eighteenth century spawned conditions that compromised the environment and severely affected humans, but until physicians had a way of examining the body's more remote crevices, the diagnosis and treatment of ear, nose, and throat problems were difficult. Such treatments as bleeding frequently killed rather than cured patients. Surgery was a treatment of last resort because the major anesthetic was whiskey. Patients sometimes died of shock from the unbearable pain that they suffered during surgical procedures.

Once physicians had reliable means of seeing into the body by using such equipment as reflective mirrors, endoscopes, X rays, tomography, and ultrasonography, they could treat many illnesses nonsurgically. It is hoped that in the future even less invasive surgery will be done in all fields of medicine, including otorhinolaryngology.

Even when surgery is indicated, in the field of otorhinolaryngology it can often be performed without an incision by entering the body through the ear canal, nose, or throat. Advanced technology has produced surgical instruments that, in combination with computer imaging, work precisely and with less trauma. In cases where incisions are necessary, the opening is often so small that it is almost undetectable a year after the procedure.

—R. Baird Shuman, Ph.D.

See also Antihistamines; Aromatherapy; Audiology; Cleft lip and palate; Cleft lip and palate repair; Common cold; Deafness; Decongestants; Ear infections and disorders; Ear surgery; Ears; Earwax; Esophagus; Epiglottitis; Halitosis; Hearing; Hearing loss; Hearing tests; Laryngectomy; Laryngitis; Ménière's disease; Motion sickness; Mouth and throat cancer; Myringotomy; Nasal polyp removal; Nasopharyngeal disorders; Nosebleeds; Otoplasty; Pharyngitis; Pharynx; Plastic surgery; Quinsy; Rhinoplasty and submucous resection; Sense organs; Sinusitis; Sjögren's syndrome; Smell; Sneezing; Sore throat; Strep throat; Taste; Tonsillectomy and adenoid removal; Tonsillitis; Tonsils; Voice and vocal cord disorders.

FOR FURTHER INFORMATION:

Benjamin, Bruce, et al. *A Color Atlas of Otorhinolaryngology.* Edited by Michael Hawke. Philadelphia: J. B. Lippincott, 1995. This atlas explores the diseases that can affect the ears, nose, and throat. Includes a bibliography.

Chasnoff, Ira J., Jeffrey W. Ellis, and Zachary S. Fainman, eds. Rev. ed. *The New Illustrated Family Medical and Health Guide.* Lincolnwood, Ill.: Publications International, 1994. The fourteen-page chapter on disorders of the ear, nose, and throat is distinctly directed toward a nonspecialized audience. The text is enhanced by useful illustrations.

Crumley, Roger L. "Otolaryngology—Head and Neck Surgery." In *Planning Your Medical Career: Traditional and Alternative Opportunities*, edited by T. Donald Rucker and Martin D. Keller et al. Garrett Park, Md.: Garrett Park Press, 1986. Presents a comprehensive overview of the field in language that, although occasionally specialized, is, on the whole, not difficult for readers who lack a medical background.

Ferrari, Mario. *PDxMD Ear, Nose, and Throat Disorders.* Philadelphia: PDxMD, 2003. A clinical yet accessible reference text that provides a comprehensive list of disorders, with a summary of the condition, background, diagnosis, treatment, outcomes, prevention, and resources.

Gulya, Aina J., and William R. Wilson. *An Atlas of Ear, Nose, and Throat Diagnosis and Treatment.* New York: Parthenon, 1999. Authoritative, updated color atlas and textbook on diagnosing and treating ear, nose, and throat disorders. Published expressly for otorhinolaryngology physicians, it contains more than ninety distinctive color photographs along with many other figures and tables.

Kennedy, David W., and Marilyn Olsen. *Living with Chronic Sinusitis: A Patient's Guide to Sinusitis, Nasal Allergies, Polyps, and Their Treatment Options.* Long Island, N.Y.: Hatherleigh Press, 2007. Provides a wealth of general information on sinusitis, including causes, new drug options and surgical procedures, and information about related respiratory allergies.

Woodson, Gayle E. *Ear, Nose, and Throat Disorders in Primary Care.* Philadelphia: W. B. Saunders, 2001. Discusses such topics as the examination of the head and neck; hearing loss, tinnitus, and otalgia; dizziness and vertigo; facial paralysis; the nose and sinus disease; and the oral cavity and throat.

OVARIAN CANCER. *See* CERVICAL, OVARIAN, AND UTERINE CANCERS.

OVARIAN CYSTS

DISEASE/DISORDER

ANATOMY OR SYSTEM AFFECTED: Reproductive system

SPECIALTIES AND RELATED FIELDS: Gynecology

DEFINITION: Benign growths that develop in the ovaries.

CAUSES AND SYMPTOMS

Ovarian cysts may occur at any age, individually or in numbers, on one or both ovaries. The cyst consists of a thin, transparent outer wall enclosing one or more chambers filled with clear fluids, aged blood that presents as thick brownish, or jellylike, material; in some cases tissue material may be present as well. Such cysts range in size from that of a raisin to that of a large orange. The normal ovary measures 3 centimeters by 2 centimeters; the cystic ovary requiring investigation is one which is enlarged to more than twice its normal size. Large cysts may cause a feeling of fullness in the abdominal area, cramping pain with various levels of severity, or pain during vaginal intercourse. Often, however, there are no apparent symptoms, and the cyst is discovered only during a routine gynecologic examination when the clinician, on bimanual examination, discovers that one ovary is considerably enlarged. At this point, it is important to rule out malignancy, because ovarian cancers in their early stages also have no warning symptoms and can occur at any age.

Polycystic ovaries (ovaries containing multiple cysts) causing significant enlargement occur in a variety of conditions. For example, polycystic ovaries can result from an enzyme deficiency in the ovaries which interferes with the normal biosynthesis of hormones, resulting in the release of an abnormal amount of androgen (a substance producing or stimulating the development of male characteristics).

More than half of all ovarian cysts are functional; that is, they arise out of the normal functions of the ovary during the menstrual cycle. These cysts are relatively common. A cyst can form when a follicle (a small, spherical, secretory structure in the ovary) has grown in preparation for ovulation but fails to rupture and release an egg; this type is called a follicular cyst. Sometimes the structure formed from the follicle after ovulation, the corpus luteum, fails to shrink and forms a cyst; this is called a corpus luteum cyst.

Another type of ovarian cyst, most often found in younger women, is the dermoid cyst, which contains particles of teeth, hair, or calcium-containing tissue that are thought to be an embryologic (developmental) remnant; such cysts usually do not cause menstrual irregularity and are very common. Dermoids are bilateral in 25 percent of cases, making careful examination of both ovaries mandatory. The cyst has a thickened, white, opaque wall and is more buoyant than other types of cysts.

Ovarian cysts cause problems when they become very large, when they rupture and cause severe internal bleeding, or when a cyst's pedicle (a tail-like appendage) suddenly twists and cuts off its blood supply, creating severe pain and possibly gangrene. Rupture of a cyst is followed by the acute onset of severe lower abdominal pain radiating to the vagina and lower back. The most severe symptoms of pain and collapse are associated with rupture of a dermoid cyst, as the cyst contents are extremely irritating.

Torsion (twisting) of a cyst may occur at any age but most often in the twenties; it may be associated with pregnancy. A twisted dermoid cyst is the most common, probably because of its increased weight. The onset of pain often occurs in the umbilical region and radiates to one or the other side of the pelvis. Pain on the right is frequently confused with appendicitis. Hemorrhage may sometimes occur from a vessel in the wall of the cyst or within the capsule.

TREATMENT AND THERAPY

The diagnosis of an ovarian cyst is made with consideration of the patient's age, medical and family history, symptoms, and the size of the enlarged ovary. In women under age thirty, clinicians, after a manual examination, will usually wait to see if the ovary will return to its normal size. If it does not, and pregnancy has been ruled out, a pelvic X ray or a sonogram (the use of sound to produce an image or photograph of an organ or tissue), or both, can determine the exact size of the ovaries and distinguish between a cyst and a solid tumor. In women age forty and older, X rays and sonograms may be done sooner. If uncertainty still exists, the physician may recommend laparoscopy, the visual examination of the abdominal cavity using a de-

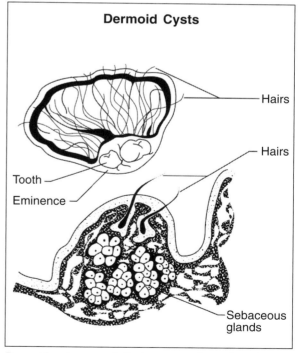

Dermoid Cysts

Hairs

Hairs

Tooth

Eminence

Sebaceous glands

Dermoid cysts are a relatively common form of ovarian cyst often found in younger women.

vice consisting of a tube and optical system inserted through a small incision. The physician may also suggest the option of a larger incision and a biopsy.

In the case of the functional ovarian cyst, if no severe pain or swelling is present, the clinician may adopt "watchful waiting" for one or two more menstrual cycles, during the course of which this type of cyst frequently disappears on its own accord. Sometimes this process is hastened by administering oral contraceptives for several months, which establishes a very regular menstrual cycle. Women already taking oral contraceptives rarely develop ovarian cysts.

In the case of torsion or rupture, surgical treatment is indicated, preferably the removal of the cyst only and preservation of as much of the normal ovarian tissue as possible. Sometimes, with a very large cyst, the ovary cannot be saved and must be removed, a procedure called oophorectomy or ovariectomy.

—*Genevieve Slomski, Ph.D.*

See also Biopsy; Cyst removal; Cysts; Genital disorders, female; Infertility, female; Laparoscopy; Ovaries; Polycystic ovary syndrome; Women's health.

FOR FURTHER INFORMATION:

Altcheck, Albert, Liane Deligdisch, and Nathan Kase, eds. *Diagnosis and Management of Ovarian Disorders.* 2d ed. San Diego, Calif.: Academic Press, 2003. A text that blends the perspectives of clinicians, surgeons, pathologists, basic scientists, and related medical researchers to discuss reproductive technology, early diagnosis of ovarian cancer, cysts, and management of the menopause, among other topics.

Ammer, Christine. *The New A to Z of Women's Health: A Concise Encyclopedia.* 6th ed. New York: Checkmark Books, 2009. A respected classic that covers the full spectrum of women's health issues, including reproduction, the aging process, methods of contraception, childbearing, herbal medicines, mammography, and advances in infertility research and hormone therapy. Includes helpful charts and illustrations.

Berek, Jonathan S., ed. *Berek and Novak's Gynecology.* 14th ed. Philadelphia: Lippincott Williams & Wilkins, 2007. A standard text covering all aspects of gynecology with an emphasis on diagnosis and treatment. Topics include biology and physiology, family planning, sexuality, evaluation of pelvic infections, early pregnancy loss, benign breast disease and benign gynecologic conditions, malignant diseases of the reproductive tract, and breast cancer.

Kovacs, Gabor T., ed. *Polycystic Ovary Syndrome.* New York: Cambridge University Press, 2000. This publication provides an essential guide to the diagnosis of polycystic ovary syndrome and its etiology, pathology, and effective medical management. This comprehensive account summarizes advances in the molecular basis of the syndrome, its genetic basis, and long-term health effects.

Leung, Peter C. K., and Eli Y. Adashi, eds. *The Ovary.* 2d ed. San Diego, Calif.: Academic Press, 2004. Contributed by leading investigators, the material presented in this volume links molecular and cellular physiology with traditional physiology. Moving from follicular and oocyte maturation to ovulation and corpus luteum formation, it addresses all phases of the ovarian life cycle.

Mahajan, Damodar K., ed. *Polycystic Ovarian Disease.* Philadelphia: W. B. Saunders, 1988. In addition to polycystic ovary syndrome, this text discusses Stein-Leventhal syndrome. Includes bibliographical references and an index.

OVARIES

ANATOMY

ANATOMY OR SYSTEM AFFECTED: All

SPECIALTIES AND RELATED FIELDS: Biochemistry, embryology, endocrinology, genetics, gynecology, obstetrics

DEFINITION: The ovaries produce eggs and sex hormones in females.

KEY TERMS:

atresia: the programmed process of cell death

corpus luteum: the structure that develops from an emptied ovarian follicle after ovulation

Fallopian tubes or oviducts: tubular structures attached at their lower ends to the uterus; the passageways for ova following ovulation

follicle: a structure composed of an oocyte and surrounding granulosa cells

hormone: a chemical messenger secreted by one cell type and acting on another to cause a predictable response

oocyte: a female germ cell that differentiates to become a mature ova

ovum (pl. *ova):* an egg cell

STRUCTURE AND FUNCTIONS

Ovaries develop from undifferentiated gonadal tissue in the absence of a Y chromosome. They are ductless glands located in the female pelvis, attached on either side of the uterus by the ovarian ligaments. Each is a flattened lumpy oval about 5 centimeters (cm) in length, 2.5 cm wide, and less than 1 cm in thickness. They are often described as being about the size and shape of an almond. There are three regions to each ovary: An outer cortex contains the developing oocytes, an inner medulla produces steroid hormones, and the hilum serves as the point of attachment and entry of blood vessels and nerves.

A principal function of the ovaries is gametogenesis, the production of ova through meiosis. This process actually begins during fetal life, and about 1 to 2 million immature oocytes are present in the cortex of the ovaries at birth. By puberty, this number has been reduced to about 300,000 through the process of atresia. Within the mature ovarian cortex are many follicles, each containing an oocyte. At any given time, there are oocytes in all stages of development, and only a small percentage of available oocytes ever undergo ovulation; the rest undergo atresia and are recycled by the body.

Starting at puberty, eggs mature successively, and one breaks through the ovarian wall each cycle in the process of ovulation. This continues until menopause, or cessation of reproductive functioning in the female. After release from the ovary, the ovum passes through the Fallopian tube and into the uterus. If the ovum is fertilized, then pregnancy ensues and the ovum (now a blastocyst) implants in the uterine lining.

Following ovulation, the empty follicle becomes the corpus luteum. It appears as a yellow body (because of lipid droplets in the cells) on the surface of the ovary and secretes progesterone to prepare the uterine lining for implantation. The corpus luteum deteriorates after ten to twelve days if conception does not occur.

The ovarian medulla is also responsible for hormonogenesis. The primary steroids produced here are estradiol (estrogen) and progesterone. Androgens (particularly androstenedione and testosterone) are also secreted, but most of them are converted to estradiol within the ovary. Estrogens are essential for the development of ova and female body characteristics (including breasts, body shape, fat deposition, and body hair distribution) and for implantation and pregnancy maintenance. They also initiate mammary gland maturation and contribute to bone mineralization. Progesterone prepares the uterine lining for implantation and pregnancy, regulates the release of luteinizing hormone (LH) from the pituitary, and contributes to the maturation of mammary gland alveoli.

In addition to the steroid hormones, peptide hormones are produced by the ovaries. Relaxin is secreted from the corpus luteum and induces relaxation of the pelvic bones and ligaments, inhibits myometrial motility, softens the cervix, and induces uterine growth. Activins stimulate the release of follicle-stimulating hormone (FSH) from the pituitary, and inhibin causes decreasing FSH output, although the mechanism is not yet understood. The ovary has been found to produce a variety of neuropeptides such as β-endorphin, adrenocorticotropin, α-melanocyte-stimulating hormone, vasopressin, and oxytocin. The physiologic roles that these peptides may play in the ovary are uncertain.

Human ovaries display a regular cycle in reproductively mature females. This cycle, known as menstruation, includes a follicular phase, during which FSH promotes growth and maturation of the granulosa cells, partial maturation of oocytes, synthesis of proteins, and estrogen secretion. Next is the ovulatory phase, during which one mature oocyte and the surrounding cells are discharged. Lastly is the luteal phase, in which progesterone is secreted. The average ovarian cycle is twenty-eight days, with a normal range between twenty-four and thirty-two days in length.

DISORDERS AND DISEASES

Polycystic ovary syndrome (PCOS), or Stein-Leventhal syndrome, is the most common ovarian disorder, affecting 6 to 10 percent of all women. The ovarian stroma becomes enlarged and produces excessive amounts of androgens. Atretic follicles accumulate and large numbers of cysts (fluid-filled sacs) may form; most are harmless and require no treatment. Ovarian follicle development is incomplete, and menstrual cycles are usually irregular. Symptoms can be alleviated with combination contraceptives and anti-androgens. Ovulation can sometimes be induced by clomiphene.

Ovulatory dysfunction is one of the causes of infertility. Most often this is hormonal in nature, and many cases of infertility can be overcome by hormone treatments.

Ovarian cancer is a major cause of death in females and comes in a variety of forms. The lifetime risk is about 1.6 percent, but it increases with age and in women with relatives who have had reproductive cancers. In women with an altered *BRCA1* or *BRCA2* gene, the risk is 25 to 60 percent, depending on the specific mutation. Pregnancy decreases the overall risk, as do oral contraceptives. Surgery is the treatment of choice, often followed by chemotherapy. Prognosis is poor overall, mostly due to the lack of clear symptoms that would lead to early diagnosis.

PERSPECTIVE AND PROSPECTS

The human ovary was first described by Renier De Graaf in 1672. In 1701, the first surgery to remove an ovarian tumor was performed by Robert Houston, and in 1809 the first known ovary removal (ovariectomy or oophorectomy) was performed by Ephraim McDowell. Throughout the nineteenth and early twentieth centuries, study of the ovaries centered on their anatomy and physiology, while during the later part of the twentieth century studies turned to their endocrine functions.

Many postulated ovarian hormones are still being searched and studied for their effects. They include transforming growth factor beta (TGF-β), anti-Mullerian hormone (AMH), folliculostatins, and many other peptides involved in the control of growth and differentiation. Gonadotropin surge attenuating factor (GnSAF) has also been hypothesized to be physiologically involved in the control of LH secretion during the menstrual cycle.

—Kerry L. Cheesman, Ph.D.

See also Amenorrhea; Assisted reproductive technologies; Cervical, ovarian, and uterine cancers; Contraception; Endometrial biopsy; Endometriosis; Gamete intrafallopian transfer (GIFT); Genital disorders, female; Gynecology; Hormone therapy; Hormones; Hot flashes; Hysterectomy; In vitro fertilization; Infertility, female; Menopause; Menorrhagia; Menstruation; Obstetrics; Ovarian cysts; Pap test; Pelvic inflammatory disease (PID); Polycystic ovary syndrome; Pregnancy and gestation; Premenstrual syndrome (PMS); Puberty and adolescence; Reproductive system; Sterilization; Tubal ligation; Uterus; Women's health.

FOR FURTHER INFORMATION:

Futterweit, Walter, and George Ryan. *A Patient's Guide to PCOS: Understanding—and Reversing—Polycystic Ovary Syndrome.* New York: Holt, 2006.

Kaipia, Antti, and Aaron Hsueh. "Regulation of Ovarian Follicle Atresia." *Annual Review of Physiology* 59 (1997): 349-363.

Plourde, Elizabeth. *Your Guide to Hysterectomy, Ovary Removal, and Hormone Replacement: What All Women Need to Know.* Ashland, Ohio: New Voice/Atlas Books, 2002.

OVER-THE-COUNTER MEDICATIONS

TREATMENT

ANATOMY OR SYSTEM AFFECTED: All

SPECIALTIES AND RELATED FIELDS: Family medicine, pharmacology, preventive medicine

DEFINITION: Pills, capsules, tablets, or syrups that can be purchased without prescription for the self-treatment of common illnesses, such as colds, fever, and headache.

KEY TERMS:

brand name: the name under which a drug is marketed by a pharmaceutical company

excipients: fillers, coloring, or coatings added to pills, tablets, capsules, or syrups

generic name: the unique name of a drug, typically the active chemical ingredient; a drug may be marketed under the generic name or the brand name

self-diagnosis: a determination of medical condition or illness without the benefit of a physician's input

self-prescription: the selection of over-the-counter medications without consulting a physician

self-treatment: the self-administration of one or more over-the-counter medications

INDICATIONS AND PROCEDURES

Drugs or medications that can be purchased directly, without a prescription, are called over-the-counter (OTC) medications or drugs. These medications may be suggested by physicians or simply purchased for consumption as a result of self-diagnosis and self-prescription. Most of the common OTC medications are used to treat common ailments such as cold and fever symptoms, headache, coughs, and similar complaints. Such self-treatment may be initiated at will and discontinued at any time.

Dozens of pharmaceutical companies produce and market hundreds of drugs for sale as over-the-counter medications, but they fall into only a few categories. The basic types of OTC medications, along with some brand examples, include analgesics (Advil, Tylenol), antacids (Milk of Magnesia), antidiarrheal medications (Imodium), antifungal agents (Tinactin), antihistamines (Benadryl), antiacne treatments (Clearasil), anti-inflammatory drugs (Motrin), decongestants (Sudafed), motion sickness (Meclizine), laxatives (Metamucil, Dulcolax), dandruff treatments (Selsun Blue), expectorants (Robitussin), hair growth formulas (Rogaine), and sleep aids (L-Tryptophan).

The most frequently used category of OTC medications is analgesics, which are more popularly known as painkillers. Analgesics include a diverse group of drugs that are used to relieve soreness, general body pain, and headaches. Probably the most common analgesic is aspirin, which is part of a group of medications termed nonsteroidal anti-inflammatory drugs (NSAIDs) that chemically affect the central and possibly the peripheral nervous system by leading to a decrease in prostaglandin production. Many analgesics are used in combination with other drugs such as vasoconstriction drugs that contain pseudoephedrine, which is especially important for the relief of sinus congestion, and in combination with antihistamine drugs, which relieve the worst symptoms of allergy.

Decongestants must certainly rank as the second most common category of OTC medications. Generally, decongestants are taken to relieve nasal congestion and allied symptoms of colds and flu by acting to reduce swelling of the mucous membranes of the nasal passageways. A recurring problem with most nasal decongestants is that they increase hypertension, but this effect is lessened by including one or more antihistamines in the preparation. The brand name drug Dimetapp, for example, is both an antihistamine and a decongestant, while various Tylenol products may contain drugs that collectively work to soothe sore throat, relieve nasal congestion, or suppress coughing.

Despite the fact that over-the-counter drugs are available to everyone, their marketing and use is restricted by the Food and Drug Administration (FDA) in the United States and similar agencies with regulatory powers in many other countries. The FDA mandates ingredients and labeling of OTC drugs and specifies rigid testing and safety standards that must be met prior to marketing. Pharmaceutical companies must apply to the New Drug Agency (NDA) for the approval of drugs. The NDA specifies testing requirements prior to issuing a license for the sales and marketing of the proposed new drug. Following approval, the FDA regularly reviews and maintains the right to remove or restrict marketing and sales of OTC drugs that create adverse side affects or are potentially addictive.

Following discovery, testing, and FDA approval of a new drug, it is given a unique trade name or brand name. The pharmaceutical company is awarded an exclusive patent to manufacture and market the drug for a specified period of time, usually seventeen years in the United States but of variable length in other countries. At the end of this time, the company no longer has proprietary rights to the drug, which may then be manufactured and marketed by other pharmaceutical compa-

nies. These drug companies may choose to market the drug under a new brand name of their choosing but not under the original label, which may still be manufactured by the original pharmaceutical company that designed and patented the drug. Spin-off products of these companies must still pass rigid FDA quality control standards which demonstrate that their product contains sufficient amounts of the active ingredients to promote bioequivalency before it can be marketed as an OTC medication—that is, the new drug has to be the therapeutic equal of the original drug.

Drugs manufactured by other pharmaceutical companies following patent expiration are typically called generic drugs and are strictly regulated by the U.S. Drug Price Competition and Patent Term Restoration Act (also known as the Hatch-Waxman Act), which was enacted in 1984. Tylenol, for example, is the exclusive brand name of an analgesic over-the-counter medication that contains the active chemical ingredient acetaminophen. Following the release of its patent, many other pharmaceutical companies started marketing pain relief drugs containing products for pain relief under the their own trade name or brand name. These copies are considered generic drugs and provide the consumer with a wide choice of the most popular drugs, usually at greatly reduced cost.

Manufacture and marketing of a generic drug by new companies usually means that their product costs considerably less, partly because of competition but mostly because the new drug companies did not bear the initial costs of development, marketing, and promotion that were part of the original financial investment of the parent company. Furthermore, manufacturers of generic drugs enjoy all the benefits of prior marketing, public acceptance, and possibly dependence on the most popular OTC medications. Generally, however, the parent company enjoys a certain competitive advantage of brand name recognition that promotes continued use of their marketed product, thereby reducing the impact of cheaper competition.

Over-the-counter medications may take the form of packets, tablets, capsules, pills, drops or droplets, ointments, inhalants, lotions, creams, suppositories, or syrups. Except for creams and topical ointments, OTC medications are administered orally, in contrast to drugs that are taken by injection. This mode of delivery places natural limits on their therapeutic effectiveness in several ways.

After being swallowed, OTC medications pass down the esophagus, through the stomach, and into the small intestine, where they are digested and absorbed. This mode of delivery requires a certain time interval between oral intake of the drug and its arrival in the bloodstream that transports it to target cells, tissues, and organs, thus delaying the effects of the drug. Tablets or capsules sometimes get stuck in the back of the mouth or on the lining of the esophagus, where they start to dissolve. When this happens, the ingredients may cause irritation, nausea, and sometimes vomiting, and the therapeutic value is lost. Furthermore, a certain amount of each key ingredient will be destroyed by the digestive enzymes of the gastrointestinal system, may be metabolized by cells of the intestinal epithelia, or may simply pass through the gut without being absorbed. Even following absorption into the blood, a certain amount of the drug may be lost because liver and other body cells set about removing foreign substances in the blood almost as soon as they are detected, generally by metabolizing the ingredient into a harmless chemical that will be excreted into the bile or be removed by the kidneys. This process explains why all drugs, including OTC medications, must be taken in repeated doses at regularly prescribed intervals in order to obtain maximum therapeutic value.

A final factor complicating delivery efficiency and thus the therapeutic value of OTC medications involves their packaging. Capsules, tablets, and pills in particular all contain substances in addition to the chemical ingredient, such as coatings, fillers, stabilizers, and often color additives. These substances, called excipients, do not contribute to the actual working of the drug itself, but they often modify both the rate and the extent of dissolution of the drug as it travels the gastrointestinal tract. While most excipients ultimately reduce the overall degree of delivery, some have important functions of permitting them to transit through the stomach, which has limited absorption ability, and into the small intestine, where chemical dissolution and absorption occurs at an optimum rate. For some drugs, the natural limits placed on delivery efficiency by gastrointestinal processes and excipient components can be sharply reduced by placing the capsule or tablet directly under the tongue, thus entirely bypassing the alimentary tract.

USES AND COMPLICATIONS

Primarily because of liability issues, all OTC medications include labels that are sometimes extensive. Label components typically consist of a list of one or more symptoms addressed by the medication, active ingredients contained in the drug, warnings, directions for use, and the date after which the medication should be dis-

carded. For example, the label on a common OTC medication used to treat severe colds notes that it is to be used to relieve symptoms of nasal congestion, cough, sore throat, runny nose, headache and body ache, and fever. Directions for use are specific as to number of times a day, hours between use, and factors involving taking the medication, such as with or without glasses of water prior to or following administration and limits regarding food intake.

Most labels also carry prominent warnings regarding use with respect to age, alcohol consumption, sedatives or tranquilizers, and combinations of medications. Most over-the-counter medications also state that use should be continued only for a specified time and that, if symptoms persist, the user should stop taking the medication and consult a physician. Finally, the user is usually cautioned to stop taking the OTC medication immediately if headache, rash, nausea, or similar symptoms appear. Despite these warnings, even commonly used OTC medications pose certain health hazards, and the user is advised to take these medications with full recognition of potential problems.

In the United States, while the FDA periodically issues warnings regarding OTC medications, their actual use by consumers normally is not regulated, documented, or monitored. This has led to a number of concerns regarding real and potential overuse of OTC drugs, particularly for reasons unrelated to their medicinal intent. It has also led directly to the modification of certain OTC medications to engineer drugs that are highly addictive.

Because their use is unregulated—or, more correctly, cannot be regulated—over-the-counter medications can be deliberately abused. Overdosing with certain types of painkillers, for example, has become a frequent method of suicide attempt. The use of Tylenol in suicide attempts is increasing. Tylenol overdosing causes the destruction of liver cells that synthesize blood coagulants. Loss of these blood coagulants results in uncontrolled bleeding, most evidently through the eyes, nose, and mouth but also internally. Internal bleeding continues until death occurs, usually within a few days following onset.

Perhaps the most egregious misuse of OTC medications is to induce or achieve temporary "highs" that parallel those obtained by use of street or hard drugs. Cough suppressants that contain the drug dextromethorphan, for example, affect the central nervous system and can be used as mood-altering drugs that cause brain damage and even death at high doses. An even more serious abuse is the cooking of common drugs to obtain the highly addictive drug methamphetamine, popularly called meth. Also known as ice or speed, meth is a highly addictive drug that is often devastating and sometimes deadly. In some regions of the United States, it ranks with heroin and cocaine as the popular drug of choice. Record growth in use and the ability to cook meth from readily obtained OTC drugs has led to the creation of National Methamphetamine Awareness Day to draw attention at all levels to this problem.

This cooking process involves the conversion of certain OTC medications into meth. Some other sources for cooking meth include diet aids, tincture of iodine or other iodine solutions, and household cleaning solutions. In response to the widespread home manufacture of meth, a national federal law was enacted to require pharmacies to check photo identification and keep records of over-the-counter sales of cold medications that contain pseudoephedrine and ephedrine, which are the two popular ingredients in many cold medications. By-products of in-home meth cooking labs are garbage cans filled with Sudafed packages and a distinct odor of cat urine. The cooking process itself releases potentially harmful toxic chemicals that can pose serious health hazards to lungs and the respiratory system and also poses the risk of fire.

PERSPECTIVE AND PROSPECTS

Originally, OTC medications were available for purchase only at pharmacies, along with physician-prescribed drugs. Today, a varied selection of OTC medications is available at many retail outlets, including supermarkets, food stores, and even convenience stores, although pharmacies still continue to offer the greatest selection. This can lead to a confusion of terms, as such medications or drugs are often no longer sold "over the counter" but instead can be found on shelves alongside other items for sale.

To complicate matters, certain drugs are offered as OTC medications at low dosages but must be obtained by prescription at higher dosages. For example, the popular analgesic ibuprofen (Advil, Motrin) can be purchased as an OTC medication at dosages of less than 200 milligrams, but higher dosages can be obtained only via prescription. Similarly, the antidiarrheal medication Imodium, an opiate, is available as an OTC medication in liquid form, while tablets of Imodium are available only by prescription.

The status of over-the-counter medications may change over time, depending on effectiveness and safety issues. While some OTC drugs are removed from the general market following various concerns regarding safety, other drugs are transferred from prescription drugs to OTC medications. Examples include the antihistamine drug Benadryl, which is used to relieve symptoms of allergy and guard against allergic reactions, and the painkiller ibuprofen, both of which were, until recently, sold as prescription drugs only but are now available as OTC medications.

While the distribution and sale of over-the-counter medications is strictly regulated by state and federal laws in the United States, certain drugs that are deemed harmless may be offered for sale as medical cures for many ailments and thereby compete with OTC medications. These so-called miracle drugs have become increasingly popular because of the Web, which opens the door to purchases without prescription. Media promotions also sometimes offer these medications, complete with testimonials that dramatically describe their success as a cure-all for ailments. These types of medications are often labeled "quack" drugs. They pose a threat to users of prescription and OTC medications in several ways. First, they are generally useless, offering a nonexistent cure for health problems. Second, they are manufactured without regard to quality control measures that legitimate drug manufacturers must follow. Third, time may be lost in using the quack drug, especially if the condition is chronic and the symptoms need to be treated immediately. Finally, while some may be harmless, other quack drugs contain chemical ingredients that are potentially dangerous when used in combination with genuine over-the-counter medications.

—*Dwight G. Smith, Ph.D.*

See also Aging: Extended care; Antihistamines; Anti-inflammatory drugs; Aphrodisiacs; Clinical trials; Decongestants; Digestion; Food and Drug Administration (FDA); Herbal medicine; Homeopathy; Metabolism; Pain management; Pharmacology; Pharmacy; Polypharmacy; Sports medicine; Veterinary medicine.

FOR FURTHER INFORMATION:

Griffith, H. Winter, and Stephen Moore. *Complete Guide to Prescription and Non-Prescription Drugs.* Rev. ed. New York: Penguin Group, 2010. This book provides easy-to-read descriptions of common drugs, covering both drugs prescribed by doctors and drugs available over the counter.

Litin, Scott C., ed. *Mayo Clinic Family Health Book.* 4th ed. New York: HarperResource, 2009. This clear and comprehensive volume details all aspects of family health. Includes good overview sections on categories, issues, concerns, and treatments with OTC medications.

Prescription and Over-the-Counter Drugs. Rev. ed. Pleasant View, N.Y.: Reader's Digest, 2001. This nine-hundred-page introduction to OTC drugs is as clearly and comprehensively written as a *Reader's Digest* issue.

Sanberg, Paul, and Richard M. T. Krema. *Over-the-Counter Drugs: Harmless or Hazardous?* New York: Chelsea House, 1986. From the series the Encyclopedia of Psychoactive Drugs. The subtitle defines the thrust of this slim book aimed at cautioning the need for intelligent use of OTC medications.

OVERTRAINING SYNDROME
DISEASE/DISORDER

ANATOMY OR SYSTEM AFFECTED: Endocrine system, lymphatic system, muscles, nervous system, psychic-emotional system

SPECIALTIES AND RELATED FIELDS: Exercise physiology, psychology, sports medicine

DEFINITION: Perceptible and lasting decrease in athletic performance, often coupled with mood changes, which does not quickly resolve following a normal period of rest.

CAUSES AND SYMPTOMS

To achieve peak athletic performance, increased effort in training, sometimes to the point of overexertion, is required. Initial periods of overexertion followed by a brief decrease in performance are often referred to as overreaching, which is distinguishable from overtraining syndrome by the desired increase in performance following a brief period of rest. Overtraining syndrome appears to develop from an overload of training, psychosocial stressors, and performance without adequate recovery or rest periods.

Diagnosing this syndrome can be complicated because a single diagnostic test or tool has yet to be developed. Symptoms may vary depending on the individual athlete or the sport so other possible causes for a long-term decrease in performance, such as diet or disease, should be ruled out first. More than eighty-four symptoms or markers have been attributed to overtraining syndrome. Most often noted in diagnosis are impaired performance, variations in heart rate, variations in blood pressure, loss of coordination, elevated basal metabolic rate, decreased body fat, weight loss, chronic fatigue, sleep disturbances, increased thirst, headaches, nausea, elevated C-reactive protein (CRP), hormone

---

INFORMATION ON OVERTRAINING SYNDROME

CAUSES: Training overload, stress, inadequate recovery or rest periods

SYMPTOMS: Impaired performance, loss of coordination, elevated metabolism, body fat loss, chronic fatigue, sleep disturbances, increased thirst, headaches, nausea, depression, muscle soreness

DURATION: Chronic

TREATMENTS: None; prevention through rest periods, stress management

---

changes, excessive production of cytokines, mood changes, depression, increased susceptibility to colds, difficulty concentrating, restlessness, increased aches and pains, and muscle soreness. Sport-specific stress tests conducted to the point of exhaustion may aid in the diagnosis.

TREATMENT AND THERAPY

Rest from training, performance, and/or competition is needed. The recovery period may take anywhere from several weeks to years. As the rest period needed to fully recover from overtraining syndrome may vary greatly from one athlete to the next, prevention is seen as the better option. To reduce the risk of developing this condition, a training schedule that alternates high and low training intensities with at least one day of rest is suggested. Other possible preventive measures include managing stress and maintaining a log to track training intensities, diet, and sleep.

PERSPECTIVE AND PROSPECTS

Research on the characteristics of overtraining syndrome, such as how it affects men and women differently, or athletes from various sports, continues to offer new insight. More research, especially longitudinal research, is needed to better understand the condition—its diagnosis, prevention, and treatment. A number of physiological tests to aid in detecting overtraining syndrome, including hormone levels, enzyme levels, and blood plasma changes, have been tested, but none thus far have proved to be a valid measure for diagnosing this condition.

—*Susan E. Thomas, M.L.S.*

See also Ergogenic aids; Exercise physiology; Fatigue; Kinesiology; Metabolism; Muscle sprains, spasms, and disorders; Muscles; Nutrition; Physical rehabilitation; Physiology; Preventive medicine; Sports medicine; Stress; Stress reduction.

FOR FURTHER INFORMATION:

Kreider, Richard B., Andrew C. Fry, and Mary L. O'Toole, eds. *Overtraining in Sport*. Champaign, Ill.: Human Kinetics, 1998.

Romain, Meeusen, et al. "Prevention, Diagnosis, and Treatment of the Overtraining Syndrome." *European Journal of Sport Science* 6, no. 1 (2006): 1-14.

Urhausen, Axel, and Wilfried Kindermann. "Diagnosis of Overtraining: What Tools Do We Have?" *Sports Medicine* 32, no. 2 (2002): 95-102.

OXYGEN THERAPY

TREATMENT

ANATOMY OR SYSTEM AFFECTED: Chest, circulatory system, heart, lungs, respiratory system

SPECIALTIES AND RELATED FIELDS: Anesthesiology, cardiology, critical care, emergency medicine, preventive medicine, pulmonary medicine

DEFINITION: Giving air enhanced by added oxygen to persons suffering from hypoxia, lack of sufficient oxygen in the tissues.

INDICATIONS AND PROCEDURES

The major indication for oxygen therapy is cyanosis, in which the skin assumes a bluish tint as a result of hypoxia, a reduced arterial saturation of oxygen to the tissues. In cases of extreme breathlessness, which may be caused by extreme physical exertion, hypoxia may occur, but the condition in most cases reverses itself within minutes if the affected person rests.

In older people whose circulatory systems have been compromised by such conditions as arteriosclerosis (narrowing of the arteries), hypoxia may be chronic. Asthmatics often require immediate oxygen therapy during severe attacks. People suffering from influenza or pneumonia may have accumulated secretions in their airways that limit the amount of oxygen that can reach their tissues. Such people are usually given oxygen administered through either a nasal catheter or a face mask.

In instances where respiratory difficulties persist, as in emphysema or chronic bronchitis, patients often receive prescriptions for oxygen cylinders for home use. They may also benefit from the home installation of an oxygen concentrator, a machine that removes oxygen from the atmosphere and remixes it in high concentrations with air. Such machines can supply oxygen-enhanced air to various rooms within a house so that ambulatory patients can breathe it for prolonged periods without being confined to one location. Some patients must breathe oxygen-enhanced air for up to fifteen hours a day.

USES AND COMPLICATIONS

Oxygen therapy is routinely used by anesthesiologists during many surgical procedures, but very high oxygen concentrations are usually avoided. Warm, humidified oxygen is preferred in surgical situations to prevent condensation and inordinate cooling, which can lead to complications. Such therapy is often administered through a catheter and used postoperatively for up to five days to prevent hypoxemia (reduced oxygen in the blood). In emergency rooms, pure oxygen is frequently given to patients in acute distress.

In some situations, physicians must use medications such as naftidrofuryl to reduce the brain's requirement for oxygen where hypoxemia is present, and brain damage may result if this complication is not addressed immediately. A thrombus (blood clot) may reduce blood flow substantially and reduce to dangerous levels the supply of oxygen to the brain and tissues. In such situations, anticoagulants such as heparin or warfarin often reduce or eliminate the thrombus and restore the body's circulation of oxygen.

—*R. Baird Shuman, Ph.D.*

See also Alternative medicine; Altitude sickness; Asbestos exposure; Asthma; Brain damage; Bronchitis; Chronic obstructive pulmonary disease (COPD); Circulation; Drowning; Ergogenic aids; Exercise physiology; Hyperbaric oxygen therapy; Hypoxia; Influenza; Lungs; Pneumonia; Pulmonary diseases; Pulmonary hypertension; Pulmonary medicine; Pulmonary medicine, pediatric; Respiration; Sports medicine; Thrombosis and thrombus; Vascular medicine; Vascular system; Wheezing.

FOR FURTHER INFORMATION:

Perry, Anne Griffin, and Patricia A. Potter, eds. *Clinical Nursing Skills and Techniques*. 6th ed. St. Louis, Mo.: Mosby/Elsevier, 2006.

Rosdahl, Caroline Bunker, and Mary Kowalski, eds. *Textbook of Basic Nursing*. 9th ed. Philadelphia: Lippincott Williams & Wilkins, 2008.

Sheldon, Lisa Kennedy. *Oxygenation*. 2d ed. Sudbury, Mass.: Jones and Bartlett, 2008.

Tallis, Raymond C., and Howard M. Fillit, eds. *Brocklehurst's Textbook of Geriatric Medicine and Gerontology*. 7th ed. Philadelphia: Saunders/Elsevier, 2010.

PACEMAKER IMPLANTATION

PROCEDURE

ANATOMY OR SYSTEM AFFECTED: Chest, circulatory system, heart

SPECIALTIES AND RELATED FIELDS: Biotechnology, cardiology

DEFINITION: The introduction into the heart of a permanent instrument that uses electrical pulses to regulate its rhythm.

KEY TERMS:

atrium: one of the two upper chambers of the heart; the right atrium receives blood returning through the veins; the left atrium receives oxygenated blood from the lungs

catheter: a thin tube that can be inserted into blood vessels, such as a vein leading into the heart, to carry electrical wires or optical fibers

circus movement: electrical impulses in the heart that continue firing instead of reaching a normal resting phase, causing heart flutter and fibrillation

electrocardiogram (ECG or EKG): a recording of electrical signals generated by the heart that are detected by electrodes placed on the chest, arms, and legs; used to diagnose heart abnormalities

fibrillations: rapid and chaotic contractions of the heart muscle that are usually fatal when they occur in the ventricles because of insufficient blood flow

heart block: a delay or blockage of the electrical signal traveling through the heart muscle, which upsets the synchronization between contractions of the upper and lower chambers

sinoatrial (S-A) node: a cluster of cells above the right atrium that emit electrical signals which initiate contractions of the heart; also called natural pacemaker cells

ventricles: the two lower chambers of the heart; the right ventricle pumps blood to the lungs, and the left ventricle pumps oxygenated blood to the body

INDICATIONS AND PROCEDURES

The first human-made pacemaker, which used electronic pulses to stimulate a regular heart rhythm, was built in the 1950's. Since then, the device has evolved into a sophisticated and reliable instrument. It was miniaturized so that it could be implanted under the skin of the patient. Tiny batteries that would last from five to fifteen years were developed. A microprocessor that can sense the need for different heart rates during sleep or strenuous exercise has become a standard component. Most recently, a small automatic defibrillator was incorporated into the pacemaker to supply several large jolts of electrical energy in case of heart stoppage or other emergencies.

The normal rhythm of a healthy heart is regulated by natural pacemaker cells. These unique cells are located at the sinoatrial (S-A) node near the top interior of the heart, where blood empties from the veins into the right atrium. Electrical impulses originating at the S-A node travel to the atrioventricular (A-V) node, which is located where the four chambers of the heart come together. From there, the signal is relayed to the ventricles, causing the muscle fibers to contract. This pumping action forces blood to flow from the two ventricles to the lungs and the body arteries.

If the natural pacemaker cells or the nerve pathways do not function properly, the heart may beat too rapidly, too slowly, irregularly, or not at all. For example, the condition called heart block interrupts or delays the electrical signal at the A-V node. It can happen that only every second or third pacemaker signal triggers a contraction. Sometimes, the ventricles will start a contraction on their own, but it will not be synchronized with the blood flow from the atrium. An artificial electronic pacemaker can be used to overcome heart block.

The electrical activity of the heart is observed in an electrocardiogram (ECG or EKG). Metal electrodes are placed in contact with a patient's left arm, right arm, left leg, and sometimes the chest. After suitable amplification, the signal can be displayed on a video screen or recorded by an ink pen on moving paper.

For a healthy heart, the normal ECG pattern starts with a small pulse (the P wave), which is followed by a group of three closely spaced pulses (the QRS complex) and a final small pulse (the T wave). This pattern is repeated approximately seventy-two times per minute for a person sitting at rest.

In brief, the P wave indicates contraction of the atrium, the QRS complex shows contraction of the ventricles, and the T wave represents the muscles' return to the resting state. If the heart "skips a beat" because of a heart block at the A-V node, the ECG will show a missing or delayed pulsation in the otherwise regular pattern. If this happens in a sustained fashion, electronic stimulation is needed.

Two other serious malfunctions of the heart's electrical system are flutter and fibrillation. Flutter is a very rapid but still constant rhythm that may produce 200 to 300 beats per minute. Fibrillations are much more serious, causing chaotic, random contractions that can occur as often as 500 times per minute. There is insuffi-

Locations of Internal Pacemakers

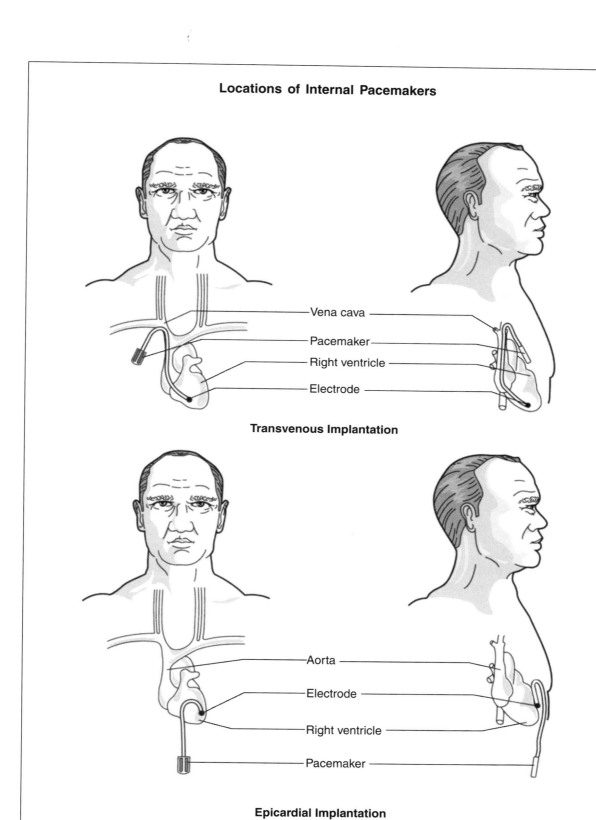

Vena cava

Pacemaker

Right ventricle

Electrode

Transvenous Implantation

Aorta

Electrode

Right ventricle

Pacemaker

Epicardial Implantation

cient time between contractions for blood to fill the ventricles. Pumping action becomes very inefficient, and death is likely to occur if the fibrillations continue.

To restore normal heart rhythm, a defibrillator is used to send a strong electric shock through the ventricular muscle fibers, which inactivates the heart's electrical system for several seconds. An electronic pacemaker may then replace the natural pacemaker cells to prevent the recurrence of fibrillations.

The cause of flutter and fibrillation is a process called "circus movement." Suppose the electrical impulses are diverted from their normal pathway by thickened or dead heart tissue. In such a case, the timing may be thrown off so that the ventricles are restimulated to contract again without waiting for the pacemaker's signal. Therefore, the heart is unable to reach its resting state.

In the ECG pattern, flutter shows up as a rapid pulsation with an indistinct QRS complex. Fibrillation is indicated by irregularly spaced pulses of random size that have no pattern at all. It is something like electrical noise coming from the heart, with no synchronization. Heart cells at many locations fire at random, producing ripples similar to those made by a handful of pebbles thrown into a lake.

The first artificial pacemaker was developed by Paul Zoll in 1952. When a patient suffering from heart block went into heart failure during surgery, Zoll inserted a needle electrode into the man's chest and applied regular voltage pulses from an external circuit. After two days, the man's heart resumed beating on its own, and the circuit was disconnected.

A portable artificial pacemaker was developed in 1957 by C. W. Lillehei and Earl Bakken. The electrode was inserted directly against the outer surface of the heart, and a battery pack and timer circuit were worn around the patient's waist. Three years later, the pacemaker was miniaturized sufficiently to be implanted under the skin of the patient's chest. This had the advantage of reducing the risk of infection.

The next major improvement was to redesign the fixed-rate pacemaker so that it could respond to variable demand during exercise or sleep. The demand pacemaker has a built-in sensor that monitors the heart's electrical system. An electronic microprocessor is programmed to recognize abnormal ECG pulses. Generally, the demand pacemaker is set to deliver a trigger pulse only when the heart rate falls below a certain point.

For people with a potential for unpredictable heart stoppage or fibrillation, an automatic implantable defibrillator has been developed. The unit, which is comparable to the external defibrillators used by emergency medical technicians, can deliver several large jolts directly to the heart. Since implanted batteries are quite small, the circuit requires some time to recharge between shocks. The circuit is quite similar to the flash attachment of a camera, with its "slow charge, fast discharge" process.

USES AND COMPLICATIONS

The implantation of a pacemaker may become necessary as a result of a coronary artery disease, in which a buildup of plaque leads to irregularities in the heart's rhythm. Coronary artery disease is the leading cause of death in the United States. It claims more than one-half million American lives per year and disables another 2 million. It is primarily a disease of modern, industrial society and is less frequently found in more rural, underdeveloped countries. In the United States, the death rate from heart attacks increased sharply after 1920, reached a peak in the mid-1960's, and has declined substantially since then.

A heart attack is usually caused by an oxygen deficiency in the heart muscle. The attack may come suddenly and without warning, but most often there is previous tissue damage that has weakened the heart over a period of time. A buildup of plaque in the coronary artery, called atherosclerosis, can reduce the flow rate to a dangerously low level. The heart muscle tries to compensate for its reduced pumping power and may develop rhythmic irregularities. Eventually, heart block or ventricular fibrillations can ensue, leading to heart failure and death.

The famous Framingham study, initiated in 1948, has been following the medical histories of approximately 5,000 men and women in order to identify the most important risk factors for heart disease. For example, the rate of heart disease among male smokers in this study was three times as high as that among nonsmokers. (This result is in addition to the much higher rate of lung cancer among smokers.) Other risk factors are excessive alcohol consumption, lack of exercise, high blood cholesterol, emotional or physical stress, and excess weight. Some unalterable risk factors are age, sex, and a family history of heart disease. The decline in heart attack deaths in recent years has been attributed to widespread changes of lifestyle to reduce the risk factors, as well as to improvements in medical diagnosis and treatment.

Modern pacemakers are remarkably reliable and safe. One of the few precautions for pacemaker wearers is to avoid standing near high-level microwave sources (although household microwave ovens are harmless). The problem is that the metal wire going into the heart acts like an antenna; it can pick up stray microwave radiation, which can disrupt the electronics in the sensitive pacemaker circuit. Also, the battery in a pacemaker must be changed at five- to ten-year intervals to ensure proper operation.

Thousands of people receive implanted pacemakers each year. The procedure has become so routine that even small community hospitals are equipped to handle it. Many patients with heart block and irregular rhythm, especially elderly patients, have benefited greatly from this technological development.

The creation of effective electronic pacemakers depends on an understanding of the structure and function of the human heart. Also, instruments such as X-ray machines and electrocardiographs are indispensable for monitoring an individual patient's response. This section will review the progress of the medical ideas and the instruments that were the essential prerequisites for modern pacemakers. Good starting points are the pioneering studies of human anatomy made by Leonardo da Vinci (1452-1519) and Andreas Vesalius (1514-1564).

Leonardo dissected and studied the human body and made anatomical sketches in his notebooks. He recognized that the heart had four chambers, and he also drew the heart valves in detail. His interest in anatomy was that of an artist rather than that of a physician.

Vesalius was a professor of medicine at the University of Padua, in Italy. He taught anatomy and wrote a famous seven-volume treatise on the structure of the human body that had many excellent illustrations. His knowledge of anatomy came from the dissection of animals and of human cadavers obtained at night from paupers' graves. Some of his anatomical investigations contradicted traditional medical doctrine and brought him into conflict with the Church. Like Galileo, he believed that experimental information was superior to ancient textbooks.

William Harvey, a British physician, received his medical degree from the University of Padua in 1602. He is known for formulating the first accurate description of the circulation of the blood through the body. He showed that the volume of blood is fairly constant, so the function of the heart is to act as a recirculating pump. He had a clear understanding of the way in which the right ventricle pushes blood through the lungs and the left one circulates it to the rest of the body. There was, however, one missing link in Harvey's theory: How did the blood get from the arteries to the veins for its return flow? The invention of the microscope in the 1670's made it possible to see the tiny, previously invisible capillaries, thus providing final confirmation of the circulation process.

The scientific investigation of electricity began in the eighteenth century. Benjamin Franklin studied lightning rods, and scientists learned how to build a friction machine that produced electricity in the laboratory. Taking an electric shock became an amusing, although somewhat dangerous, entertainment at parties.

About 1790, the Italian anatomist Luigi Galvani made an important, though accidental, discovery. A metal scalpel lying near an electrostatic machine came into contact with the leg of a recently dissected frog, causing a sudden twitching of the muscle. Evidently, there was a connection between the electric shock and the muscle contraction.

The modern pacemaker that stimulates the heart muscle works in the same way that Galvani's scalpel worked; however, a major evolution in physiological knowledge and medical practice had to take place before the pacemaker could be developed.

Mary Wollstonecraft Shelley picked up the idea of animal electricity and popularized it in her famous science-fiction story *Frankenstein*, which was published in 1809. If electricity could make a dead muscle twitch, perhaps enough electricity could make a dead body come to life. Shelley's story was a frightening exaggeration. Nevertheless, present-day emergency medical technicians use electric shocks to revive a stopped heart—an accepted procedure for a person at the borderline between life and death.

The nineteenth century was a fertile period for new inventions and discoveries in electrical technology. Among these were the telephone, the electric lightbulb, and radio waves. The most basic diagnostic tool for checking the heart is the stethoscope. Its invention is attributed to a French physician in the early nineteenth century who first used a kind of ear trumpet with a flexible hollow tube. Measuring blood pressure is done routinely today to indicate possible heart problems. The method of using a tourniquet on the arm together with a mercury column pressure gauge was not invented until 1896.

Wilhelm Conrad Röntgen was experimenting with high voltages in his laboratory in 1896 when he observed a mysterious new type of radiation, which he called X rays. Unlike light, X rays were able to pass through black paper, wood, and even thin metal sheets. They could cause certain paints to glow in the dark and could expose photographic film that was still in its light-tight box. For the medical profession, the discovery of X rays was a major breakthrough.

The immediate usefulness of X rays was to show broken bones, objects that had been swallowed, bullets or shrapnel embedded in tissue, and large tumors. The heart and lungs, however, showed up only as faint outlines. Physicians learned to inject opaque dye into the blood vessels to increase the contrast. A new technique of inserting a catheter through a vein directly into the heart chambers was developed after experimentation was performed with animals. Combining catheters and X rays, doctors could obtain diagnostic information about the interior of the heart.

X-ray technology has been improved in recent years. Electronic image intensifiers were developed in the 1950's in order to brighten the dim pictures on a fluorescent screen. A major breakthrough in the 1970's was the invention of computed tomography (CT) scanning. Instead of using film or a fluoroscope, a computer generates images of the heart and other internal organs on a video screen. For pacemaker implantation, X-ray apparatus is indispensable in order to observe the electrode's precise placement into the interior of the heart.

The heart is a mechanical pump, but its rhythm is controlled by electrical impulses. The instrument that provides essential electrical information about the heart to the physician is the electrocardiograph. It was invented in 1903 by the Dutch physician Willem Einthoven. The voltage fluctuations produced by the heart are typically only one-thousandth of a volt at the peak, so a very sensitive meter is necessary to observe them.

IN THE NEWS: IMPLANTABLE CARDIOVERTER DEFIBRILLATOR

A device that acts much like a pacemaker, called an implantable cardioverter defibrillator (ICD), has become very popular in recent years because of important technological advances. The ICD is indicated for patients who have experienced one or more episodes of spontaneous sustained ventricular tachycardia (VT) or ventricular fibrillation (VF) unrelated to a myocardial infarction or other causes amenable to correction.

The ICD can offer high-energy defibrillation therapy, low-energy cardioversion therapy, tachycardia pacing, and posttherapy bradycardia pacing. It is predominantly used, however, to monitor a patient's heartbeat continuously and to jolt the heart automatically to restore its rhythm in the case of cardiac arrest. The jolt changes ventricular fibrillation to an organized ventricular rhythm or changes a very rapid and ineffective cardiac rhythm to a slower, more effective rhythm.

In July, 2002, the Food and Drug Administration (FDA) approved a broadened indication for ICDs that included patients with a history of a heart attack and depressed heart function. The ICDs were previously approved for patients who had survived cardiac arrests and for patients who had undergone invasive electrical testing (done through a catheter from the groin to the heart) to determine if they were suitable candidates for an ICD. The expanded approval enabled three to four million Americans to receive the devices. The FDA made the change after Guidant Corporation, the manufacturer, demonstrated in clinical trials of twelve hundred heart attack survivors that the device reduced patients' chances of dying by one-third. Innovations in technology will only improve the capability of ICDs: The next generation of the devices will include telemetry and Holter capabilities that store and recall effective and ineffective therapies. Tomorrow's ICDs will also be much smaller in size and have longer life spans.

—*Janet Mahoney, R.N., Ph.D., A.P.R.N.*

A typical electric meter has a coil of wire mounted between the poles of a magnet. When current flows through the coil, the coil rotates. A pointer is attached to the coil, indicating the amount of current by its deflection. Einthoven's ingenious adaptation was to hang the coil from a very thin fiber that allowed it to rotate with almost no resistance. Attached to the fiber was a small mirror. A beam of light shining on the mirror would be deflected to different angles as the mirror rotated. This so-called "string galvanometer" worked very well and won for Einthoven the 1924 Nobel Prize in Physiology or Medicine.

The electrodes of most pacemakers are installed with a catheter that is inserted through a vein, through the right atrium, through the valve, and finally touches the inside of the right ventricle. The first human heart catheterization is credited to Werner Forssmann in 1929, when he was a young intern at a hospital in Berlin, Germany. He requested permission to try the procedure on a patient, but his supervisor refused. Forssmann then decided to try it on himself. He anesthetized his left elbow, opened a vein, and inserted the catheter tube. As he pushed it up the arm, he watched its progress on an X-ray fluoroscope, which he had to view by reflection in a mirror held by a nurse. When the catheter had gone in 65 centimeters, Forssmann asked an X-ray technician to record it on film to prove that it had entered his heart. During the next two years, he repeated the procedure several times, but criticism by his medical colleagues forced him to discontinue it. He became a small-town doctor and was amazed to learn in 1956 that he had been awarded the Nobel Prize for Medicine.

Accumulated knowledge about the structure of the heart, improvements in surgery, the development of new drugs, and the availability of modern instrumentation have all contributed to a substantial improvement in the medical treatment of heart ailments in modern times.

The development of artificial heart valves, the heart-lung machine, the success of heart bypass surgery, the use of laser beams for surgery, and the use of drugs to control high blood pressure are recent developments.

An important contribution from the field of electronics was the development of the transistor in the early 1950's. It made possible the whole technology of miniaturized electronics, replacing the bulky vacuum tubes that were used in old radio circuits. Implantable pacemakers and microprocessor sensors would not have been possible without transistors.

Human ingenuity no doubt will continue to develop new instruments for cardiac diagnosis and rehabilitation, building on the accomplishments of the innovators of the past.

—*Hans G. Graetzer, Ph.D.*

See also Arrhythmias; Cardiac arrest; Cardiac rehabilitation; Cardiac surgery; Cardiology; Cardiology, pediatric; Cardiopulmonary resuscitation (CPR); Circulation; Echocardiography; Electrocardiography (ECG or EKG); Exercise physiology; Heart; Heart attack; Heart disease; Heart valve replacement; Vascular medicine; Vascular system.

FOR FURTHER INFORMATION:

Corona, Gyl Garren. "Pacemakers: Keeping the Beat Today." *RN* 62, no. 12 (December, 1999): 50-52. To-day's permanent pacemakers not only send electrical impulses to the right atrium and ventricle but also can be programmed to respond to a variety of metabolic cues, bringing medicine ever closer to duplicating the heart's own pacing system.

Crawford, Michael, ed. *Current Diagnosis and Treatment—Cardiology.* 3d ed. New York: McGraw-Hill Medical, 2009. Discusses advances in cardiac diagnostics, treatments, and prognostic indicators and includes information on pacemakers.

Davis, Goode P., Jr., and Edwards Park. *The Heart: The Living Pump.* Washington, D.C.: U.S. News Books, 1981. An excellent book about the structure and functioning of the heart, with many full-color photographs and diagrams, intended for a general audience of nonspecialists. Good explanations of the electrocardiogram, rheumatic fever, coronary bypass surgery, and new diagnostic technology. Highly recommended.

Eagle, Kim A., and Ragavendra R. Baliga, eds. *Practical Cardiology: Evaluation and Treatment of Common Cardiovascular Disorders.* 2d ed. Philadelphia: Lippincott Williams & Wilkins, 2008. Details advances in cardiac medicine.

Gersh, Bernard J., ed. *The Mayo Clinic Heart Book.* 2d ed. New York: William Morrow, 2000. One of the most respected texts for laypeople on heart disease. Covers all aspects of anatomy, physiology, diagnosis, treatment, and prevention.

Jeffrey, Kirk. *Machines in Our Hearts: The Cardiac Pacemaker, the Implantable Defibrillator, and American Health Care.* Baltimore: Johns Hopkins University Press, 2001. Traces the way in which pacemakers and defibrillators became a multibillion-dollar manufacturing and service industry in the United States, examines the development of knowledge about the human heartbeat, and follows surgeons, cardiologists, and engineers as they invent and test a variety of electronic devices.

Sonnenberg, David, Michael Birnbaum, and Emil A. Naclerio. *Understanding Pacemakers.* New York: Michael Kesend, 1982. The authors discuss the way in which the normal heart works, rhythm disorders that may occur, the way in which a pacemaker is surgically implanted, and new developments in pacemaker technology and technique.

Urone, Paul Peter. *Physics with Health Science Applications.* New York: John Wiley & Sons, 1986. An introductory work describing how the principles of physics apply to human physiology. A chapter on basic electric circuits is followed by a discussion of the electrical hazards of medical instruments. Contains a thorough description of bioelectricity, including electrocardiograms and the artificial pacemaker.

PAGET'S DISEASE
DISEASE/DISORDER
ALSO KNOWN AS: Osteitis deformans, Paget's disease of bone
ANATOMY OR SYSTEM AFFECTED: Bones, head, hips, legs, musculoskeletal system, spine
SPECIALTIES AND RELATED FIELDS: Genetics, orthopedics, rheumatology, virology
DEFINITION: A chronic disorder resulting in enlarged and deformed bones.

CAUSES AND SYMPTOMS
Paget's disease of bone is a disorder characterized by excessive and abnormal formation of bone, most commonly in the spine, skull, pelvis, thighs, and lower legs. (Paget's disease of the nipple is a different disorder re-lated to breast cancer.) The cause of this disease is under investigation. Genetic factors are a major component. Between 15 and 40 percent of all patients with Paget's disease have a positive family history of the disease, and the risk of developing Paget's disease is seven to ten times higher in relatives of those who have Paget's disease compared with relatives of those who do not have this disease. Several genes are known to regulate the cells that remodel bone, and mutations in some of these genes seem to be the main cause of Paget's disease in some patients.

In adult, nongrowing bone, the structure of bone is the result of the interplay between two types of cells— one that deposits bone, the osteoblast, and another that resorbs bone, a multinucleate cell called the osteoclast. A signaling system called the RANK-RANKL-OPG system regulates osteoclast recruitment. RANK is a receptor on the surface of osteoclast precursor cells. RANKL is the ligand, or molecule that binds to RANK to activate it. RANKL is secreted by bone marrow cells; when RANKL binds to the RANK molecules on the

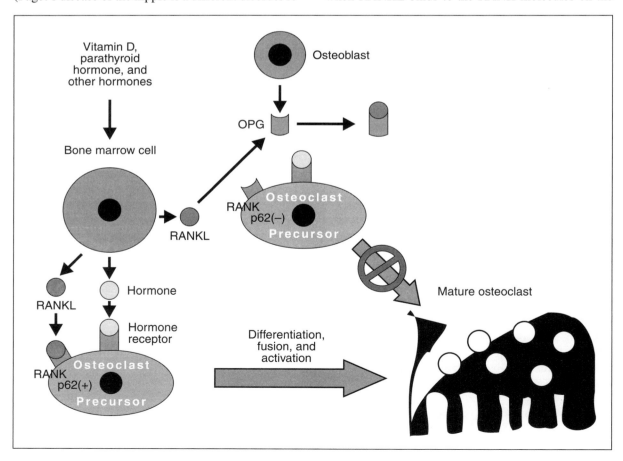

INFORMATION ON PAGET'S DISEASE

CAUSES: Unknown; possibly viral infection and genetic factors
SYMPTOMS: Excessive and abnormal formation of bone (commonly in spine, skull, pelvis, thighs, lower legs); increased risk of fractures; curving of spine or legs; bone and joint pain
DURATION: Chronic and progressive
TREATMENTS: Bisphosphonates (pamidronate, alendronate, risedronate, tiludronate); pain medications (acetaminophen, NSAIDs); exercise; adequate intake of calcium and vitamin D; surgery

surface of osteoclast precursor cells, it activates an internal protein called p62. The activation of p62 pushes osteoclast precursor cells toward becoming mature, bone-resorbing osteoclasts. Osteoblasts, however, also secrete OPG, a soluble receptor that competitively binds RANKL and prevents osteoclast recruitment (see figure on page 2244). Mutations in the genes that encode RANK, OPG, or p62 cause various inherited forms of Paget's disease with varying severities and times when the disease manifests itself. Not all individuals who harbor these mutations, however, suffer from full-blown Paget's disease.

Paget's disease might also result from viral infections. Experimental infection of mouse osteoblasts with measles virus can cause Paget's disease in mice. Furthermore, osteoblasts from human patients with Paget's disease sometimes harbor measles virus or other closely related viruses. It is possible that the presence of mutations in genes that increase osteoclast activity in combination with chronic infection of osteoclasts by measles virus or similar viruses create an environment that nurtures the development of clinical Paget's disease.

Paget's disease is more common in people over the age of forty. The disease usually starts without any symptoms. It is often diagnosed when a person has radiographs taken for other reasons or has a higher-than-normal level of alkaline phosphatase in the blood. As the disease progresses, the patient may develop an enlarging skull, sometimes accompanied by headaches; increased risk of fractures; curving of the spine or legs; and bone and joint pain. Rarely, Paget's disease may lead to kidney stones, loose teeth when bones of the face are involved, and loss of hearing and vision when the enlarging skull compresses nerves to the eye and

ear. People with severe Paget's disease may have heart problems such as congestive heart failure or abnormal heart rhythms. Less than 1 percent of people with Paget's disease will develop bone cancer.

TREATMENT AND THERAPY

Bisphosphonates (such as etidronate, pamidronate, alendronate, risedronate, or tiludronate) are the main treatment for Paget's disease. Subcutaneous injections of salmon calcitonin successfully reverse the symptoms of Paget's disease, but 50 percent of all patients who receive this treatment develop an immune response against calcitonin and 10 to 20 percent of all patients become resistant to it. In patients with severe symptoms who do not respond to these more typical treatments, the antibiotic mithramycin has been used successfully, but the toxicity of this drug militates against its use for anything but worst-case scenarios.

Treatment is given when patients experience pain, deformities, nerve compression, or other symptoms or to prevent the risk of future complications when the skull, spine, legs, and/or pelvis are involved. Therapy is given until the levels of alkaline phosphatase in the blood return to normal, and it may need to be repeated if that level increases again. Acetaminophen or nonsteroidal anti-inflammatory drugs (NSAIDs) may be used to treat pain. Exercise and adequate intake of calcium and vitamin D are also recommended. Surgery may be needed to stabilize fractures, replace joints affected with severe pain from arthritis, or decompress nerves.

PERSPECTIVE AND PROSPECTS

Paget's disease likely has been around for many centuries, as it has been observed in a grossly thickened Egyptian skull dating from about 1000 B.C.E. The disorder is named after a British surgeon, Sir James Paget, who was the first to describe this condition in 1876. He noted five patients with thickened bones that were prone to fracture and deformity. Paget thought that the disorder resulted from chronic inflammation and named it osteitis deformans. Subsequently, researchers have shown that Paget's disease of bone arises from the overproduction of poor-quality bone, rather than from chronic inflammation.

Identification of mutations in candidate genes in patients who have active Paget's disease, coupled with the expression of these mutant genes in transgenic mice in which the endogenous copy of the same gene has been eliminated (so-called knockout mice), represents one of the most powerful techniques for studying the cause and pathology of Paget's disease. Combining Paget's disease-specific mutations in transgenic mice whose osteoblasts have been chronically infected with measles virus or respiratory syncytial virus has also greatly elucidated the nongenetic causes of this disease.

—*Meika A. Fang, M.D.;*
updated by Michael A. Buratovich, Ph.D.
See also Bone disorders; Bones and the skeleton; Fracture and dislocation; Orthopedic surgery; Orthopedics; Orthopedics, pediatric.

FOR FURTHER INFORMATION:

Daroszewska, Anna, and Stuart H. Ralston. "Genetics of Paget's Disease of Bone." *Clinical Science* 109, no. 3 (September, 2005): 257-263.

Delmas, Pierre D., and P. J. Meunier. "Drug Therapy: The Management of Paget's Disease of Bone." *New England Journal of Medicine* 336, no. 8 (February 20, 1997): 558-566.

Kanis, John A. *Pathophysiology and Treatment of Paget's Disease of Bone.* 2d ed. London: Martin Dunitz, 1998.

Klippel, John H., ed. *Primer on the Rheumatic Diseases.* 13th ed. New York: Springer, 2008.

Litin, Scott C., ed. *Mayo Clinic Family Health Book.* 4th ed. New York: HarperResource, 2009.

Roodman, David G., and Jolene J. Windle. "Paget Disease of Bone." *Journal of Clinical Investigation* 115, no. 2 (February, 2005): 200-208.

PAIN

DISEASE/DISORDER

ANATOMY OR SYSTEM AFFECTED: All

SPECIALTIES AND RELATED FIELDS: Most, especially anesthesiology, general surgery, genetics, internal medicine, neurology, oncology, physical therapy, psychiatry, rheumatology, sports medicine

DEFINITION: An unpleasant, subjective experience of physical or mental suffering, a symptom of a real or potential underlying cause, condition, or injury.

KEY TERMS:

acute pain: sudden, extreme pain that is short-term; serves as a warning of damage or disease

analgesic: a drug or medication that alleviates pain by blocking pain receptors

chronic pain: a deeper, aching pain that comes on slowly and lasts longer than the normal course for a specific injury or condition; may be constant or intermittent

cutaneous pain: caused by injuries to the skin or superficial tissues; brief and localized

endorphins: brain chemicals released by the body that act as natural painkillers

nociception: the process of transmitting pain messages to the brain through the spinal cord by sensitive nerve endings in skin and tissues

referred pain: pain experienced at a site other than the site of origin

substance P: a peptide found in nerve cells in the body, which serves as a chemical messenger (neurotransmitter) that carries pain messages along pathways to the brain

visceral pain: throbbing or aching pain that originates in the deeper body tissues and organs; of longer duration than cutaneous pain

CAUSES AND SYMPTOMS

Not all causes of pain are known or understood, but some basic causes of the most commonly reported pain include inflammation, as in arthritis, rheumatism, and infection; work-related and sports-related injuries; stress and tension; nerve pain, as from shingles, diabetic neuropathy, and sciatica; and pain related to such diseases as osteoporosis and cancer.

People have similar pain thresholds but different levels of pain tolerance, or how much pain they can bear. One congenital anomaly actually inhibits or eliminates the perception of pain. Pain tolerance is therefore subjective and can be influenced by socioeconomic status, cultural background, and socialization, with disparities noted in who suffers pain, what type of pain a person suffers, and how pain is perceived by the individual.

The most commonly reported types of pain are associated with the lower back, with severe or migraine headache, and with joint pain, particularly in the knees. Physiological pain is a response of the body associated with tissue damage or inflammation, or as a warning system to alert the body to potential physical harm. Al-

---

INFORMATION ON PAIN

CAUSES: Infection, trauma, disease

SYMPTOMS: Sensation may range from mild to severe

DURATION: Acute to chronic

TREATMENTS: Wide ranging; may include drug therapy, surgery, physical therapy, alternative medicine

though pain may be produced without a defined stimulus, such as with emotional or psychological pain, physiological pain is transmitted through stimulation of nerve pathways, a process called nociception. Nociceptors are free, sensitive nerve endings located outside the spinal column; they are found in skin and on internal surfaces, such as on the joints. Nociceptors, when stimulated, send signals through sensory neurons to the posterior horn of the spinal cord that are then transmitted to other nerve fibers, which travel upward through the brain stem to the thalamus, the gateway to conscious action in the brain. There, information is coordinated and localized and then sent to the cerebral cortex, where a conscious reaction to the stimulus is produced.

Pain is said to be referred when it is experienced at a location other than its site of origin. This occurs when nerve fibers carrying pain messages enter the spinal cord at the same place as other nerve fibers from other parts of the body using the same pathways. The other nerve fibers may become stimulated and result in painful perceptions in healthy areas of the body, such as referred pain from the heart to the neck, arm, and stomach.

Among theories of pain transmission, the gate control theory of Ronald Malzack and Patrick Wall helps to explain the differing degrees of pain that people may suffer. It is related to the amount of substance P, a peptide found in nerve cells throughout the body, that actually reaches the brain. The transmission of neurons is generally very rapid, as when touching a hot stove produces immediate action to protect the body from damage. Messages carried by substance P, however, travel more slowly, since they must pass through a special gateway in the spinal cord. At the same time, pain signals are also prompting the brain to release chemical endorphins, the body's natural painkillers, which must also pass downward through the same gate. Thus, there is some competition for passage, and the fewer receptors for substance P that actually arrive in the brain and attach to nerve cells there, the lower the pain perception. With healing, the gate closes, but when chronic

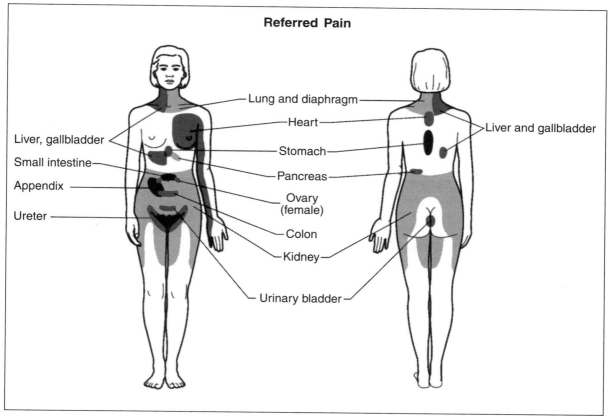

Referred Pain

Lung and diaphragm

Heart

Liver, gallbladder

Small intestine

Appendix

Ureter

Stomach

Pancreas

Ovary (female)

Colon

Kidney

Liver and gallbladder

Urinary bladder

Internal organs do not have the same type of neural sensors found in surface tissues; as a result, damage to internal organs may manifest itself in areas of the body away from the organ's location.

pain occurs, it remains open even after healing or without an identified underlying cause.

The two basic types of pain are chronic and acute. Acute pain comes on suddenly and, although extreme, is generally brief in duration. Acute pain is a warning to the body about damage or disease, is localized, and is more easily treated. Chronic pain, however, occurs daily and lasts longer than would be common for a specific injury. It no longer serves to warn, and it is much more difficult to treat, although most sufferers can be helped. Chronic pain may last beyond resolution of an underlying cause, or it may grow out of an acute condition. In this case, it may become a learned response that no longer has a purpose but continues to hurt. Chronic pain may also occur without any apparent cause, creating disability, depression, and suffering.

Pain may be medically classified as either superficial or deep. Superficial pain, also called fast or cutaneous pain, is carried by nerve fibers on the skin and outer linings of the organs. These nerve fibers are plentiful in the intestines, cornea, and nose, for example, and pain messages are quickly delivered to the brain, such as when one is cut or burned. Also termed somatic pain, it is experienced as intense, or burning. Kidney stones or acid reflux from the stomach may create waves of this burning pain. Deep pain, on the other hand, also referred to as slow or visceral pain, comes from nerve fibers located in muscles, bones, and tissues of the internal organs, and it travels more slowly, taking longer to reach the brain. It may be experienced as dull aching or throbbing pain. The two types of pain may also occur at the same time.

TREATMENT AND THERAPY

The major treatment for pain in the United States has been analgesic medications, or drug therapy, with sufferers spending over an estimated $18 billion a year for relief, both prescription and over-the-counter medications. There are no standard guidelines for the use of analgesics, since the degree of relief varies from one patient to another. These medications are classified as narcotic, such as morphine or opium-based addictive drugs, and non-narcotic, such as aspirin, ibuprofen, and acetaminophen. Since patients respond differently, and many of the analgesics can carry significant side effects with cardiovascular, renal, and gastrointestinal toxicity, the lowest dose of the preferred medication is usually recommended to start. Painkillers must also often be administered with other medications directed to the underlying cause of the pain, and must therefore be compatible.

One subcategory of non-narcotic analgesics is made up of nonsteroidal anti-inflammatory drugs (NSAIDs). Another alternative, acetaminophen, addresses pain but has no effect on inflammation. Another non-narcotic class of drugs, known as COX-2 inhibitors, suppress the COX-2 enzyme, which triggers inflammation. Although these drugs are seemingly well-tolerated and effective, it was found that many of them endanger the heart, and several were withdrawn from the market.

Narcotic analgesics are the most effective, but long-term use can create dependency, and these drugs are stringently protected in the United States by state and federal laws. Doctors have therefore been hesitant to use them for severe chronic pain, even in patients dying from cancer or other painful diseases, when other medications are not working. This situation appears to be changing.

Nondrug therapies include such techniques as transcutaneous electrical nerve stimulation (TENS), massage therapy, neurosurgery, physical therapy and exercise, and mind-body therapies such as guided imagery, meditation, relaxation, and hypnosis. These therapies attempt to alleviate chronic pain in various ways by stimulating blood circulation, blocking nerve pain messengers, and enlisting the help of the brain, where pain messages are processed.

A combination of biomedical and nonbiomedical therapies also utilizes a number of alternative therapies for pain. Acupuncture and acupressure, the foundation of Chinese medicine, are thought to stimulate blood circulation and possibly the autonomic nervous system through insertion of very fine needles at crucial points in the body. Herbal medicine uses substances that are derived from plants with therapeutic or pharmacologic properties and benefits. Many of today's medicines have ingredients that originated in plants and can be synthesized in the laboratory. Guided imagery, aromatherapy, creative arts therapy, magnet therapy, and therapeutic touch are often used as adjuncts to dealing with pain, but most have not been proven. Like analgesics, these therapies address the control and management of pain, rather than offering a cure.

Although many of these complementary therapies are not biomedically sanctioned or recognized, it is estimated that almost all sufferers of chronic pain try some form of complementary medicine. Little or no research has been done on many of these therapies, but their popularity relates to the fact that chronic pain is closely connected with the brain, affecting emotions, attitudes, and psychological stability, which are not addressed by conventional medicine and treatment. Some of these therapies may work through the placebo effect—meaning that if one expects the therapy to alleviate pain, then it will. Some approaches are backed by positive evidence, while others may have been shown to have no effect. Very little evidence exists about how or why many of these therapies are successful, but combination therapies are vital in alleviating pain, however they may work.

PERSPECTIVE AND PROSPECTS

The development of pain medicine and pain clinics, devoted solely to the study and alleviation of pain, are of fairly recent occurrence. Since pain was traditionally seen as a symptom rather than as a disease or condition in itself, the medical profession has generally focused on treating the cause, considering pain to be purely a diagnostic tool. The discovery and development of anesthetics for surgical procedures in the latter nineteenth century, however, was a huge advance in medical care and treatment and was a precondition for the later development of pain medicine. Anesthesiologists not only had to address traumatic and postoperative pain but also worked to refine techniques and developed expertise in management relating to other types of pain.

Anesthesiology progressed rapidly during World War II, with improved use of nerve blocking and analgesics. Anesthesiologist John Bonica contributed significantly to this development of pain medicine. He was faced with extreme, intractable, complex, and phantom limb pain (the sensation of pain felt in a limb no longer there) in the injured during wartime and lacked knowledge or methods to treat them. As pain persisted and when physiological causes could not be identified, it became necessary to look elsewhere for the source of the pain. It became obvious that numerous specialists, including psychologists and psychiatrists, needed to consult and discuss their varied findings and opinions.

Practitioners of pain medicine mostly come from other medical fields most closely related to pain, such as neurology, anesthesiology, and rehabilitation. As defined by the American Academy of Pain Medicine, the specialty is concerned with the study, prevention, evaluation, treatment, and rehabilitation of people in pain. Many are certified as pain specialists through the American Board of Anesthesiology. While some pain clinics focus on specific types of pain, such as bone and joint, others address a broader spectrum of suffering and tend to use a variety of methods and treatments, including alternative therapies, to find whatever works.

Some pain cannot be eliminated but can be minimized or controlled to allow the patient to function.

The need to study and understand the causes and alleviation of pain have become more urgent. According to the National Center for Health Statistics, one in four adults in the United States reported suffering pain lasting for at least twenty-four hours during the previous month, and one in ten reported pain lasting a year or more. Pain is usually seen as a result of another physical condition, but considering the costs that accompany pain and resulting disability in terms of dollars and loss of individual function reflected in absenteeism in the workplace, pain places an increasing burden on the American health care system. The general cost of pain and pain-related items is estimated to top $100 billion each year.

Research is being conducted into the origins and mechanics of pain in an attempt to identify new and more effective therapies. A study funded by the National Institutes of Health found that the perception of pain (the extent to which one feels pain) is inherited through a gene with a specific variant. This gene variant affects sensitivity to acute pain as well as the risk of developing chronic pain. Other genes may also play a role. This study opens up pathways for developing new treatments and approaches to pain.

Such professional organizations as the American Academy of Pain Medicine, the American Pain Foundation, the American Pain Society, and the International Association for the Study of Pain represent only a few of the growing number of resources for the study of pain and pain management. Alternative approaches are represented through organizations for specific therapies and the National Center for Complementary and Alternative Medicine.

—*Martha Oehmke Loustaunau, Ph.D.*

See also Acupressure; Acupuncture; Alternative medicine; Amputation; Anesthesia; Anesthesiology; Arthritis; Back pain; Bruises; Burns and scalds; Cancer; Fibromyalgia; Headaches; Healing; Hypnosis; Local anesthesia; Massage; Meditation; Narcotics; Nervous system; Neuralgia, neuritis, and neuropathy; Neurology; Over-the-counter medications; Pain management; Physical rehabilitation; Prescription drug abuse; Self-medication; Skin; Stress; Stress reduction; Substance abuse; Toothache; Touch; Wounds.

FOR FURTHER INFORMATION:

American Pain Foundation. http://www.painfounda tion.org. Web site of one of the major advocacy and support organizations for persons in pain and for health professionals and caregivers. Includes links to helpful resources, including academic journals, and links to information on "pain law and ethics" and finding care.

Baszanger, Isabelle. *Inventing Pain Medicine: From the Laboratory to the Clinic.* New Brunswick, N.J.: Rutgers University Press, 1998. Explores the progressive development of approaches to and perceptions of pain and suffering, using science, history, and sociology. Shows how patients and physicians are redefining pain. Documents the need for medical recognition of pain as a medical problem and medical interventions for pain management. Includes explanations of major pain theories, extensive notes, and references.

Bellenir, Karen, ed. *Pain Sourcebook: Basic Consumer Health Information About Specific Forms of Acute and Chronic Pain.* 2d ed. Detroit, Mich.: Omnigraphics, 2002. Describes the management of various types of pain, including head, back, nerve, cancer, and surgery. Includes resources for pain management.

Coakley, Sarah, and Kay Kaufman Shelemay, eds. *Pain and Its Transformations: The Interface of Biology and Culture.* Cambridge, Mass.: Harvard University Press, 2008. An interdisciplinary collection of essays exploring the human experience of pain, especially chronic pain, and how the world's cultures make sense of pain and ascribe meaning to it.

Fishman, Scott, with Lisa Berger. *The War on Pain: How Breakthroughs in the New Field of Pain Medicine Are Turning the Tide Against Suffering.* New York: HarperCollins, 2001. Discusses the field of pain medicine, including holistic approaches, analgesia, alternative treatments, and mind-body therapies. Includes appendixes listing pain clinics by state, Web sites, associations, and organizations and a glossary.

Vertosick, Frank T., Jr. *Why We Hurt: The Natural History of Pain.* New York: Harcourt, 2000. A popular history of how pain has been perceived, its place in life, its biological nature, and human efforts to deal with it through knowledge and understanding.

PAIN MANAGEMENT

TREATMENT

ANATOMY OR SYSTEM AFFECTED: All

SPECIALTIES AND RELATED FIELDS: Alternative medicine, anesthesiology, critical care, emergency medicine, geriatrics and gerontology, oncology, pharmacology, physical therapy, psychiatry, psychology

DEFINITION: Any treatment or management technique to lessen or eliminate pain or make it more tolerable.

INDICATIONS AND PROCEDURES

Pain is experienced as an unpleasant reaction to either an external stimulus (such as a burn) or an internal process (such as a disease). The initial evaluation of pain is aimed at determining the cause. A good description by the patient aids diagnosis. The person experiencing the pain must be able to communicate the intensity, location, pattern (such as throbbing, steady, intermittent) and type (crushing, burning, sharp, or dull). In addition, factors that make the pain better or worse must be known and communicated. Duration is important; recent onset is termed "acute" pain while long-standing pain or pain that returns periodically is termed "chronic."

Generally, the best way to treat pain is to prevent its occurrence. Failing that, a number of different interventions should be used together. Whatever treatment is used, the therapy must be tailored both to the patient and to the nature and severity of the pain. When medications are used, review of some important principles is essential, such as the pharmacology, duration of effectiveness, and optimal dose of a certain medication. Even the route of administration must be considered in every case.

Treatment may include combinations of simple analgesics, narcotics, and other treatments. Combinations take advantage of the additive pain relief while sparing the patient potential side effects. When choosing pain medications, a stepwise approach is often used. It starts with the simple analgesics: aspirin, acetaminophen, and nonsteroidal anti-inflammatory drugs (NSAIDs). These medications are generally well tolerated, although aspirin and NSAIDs can produce gastrointestinal distress ranging from mild heartburn to bleeding ulcers. Additionally, adjuncts to these types of medications might be icing or heat, depending on the nature of the problem.

For more severe pain, the second step often includes a narcotic analgesic with or without the simple analgesics. Narcotics are very potent and have a potential for addiction. Furthermore, they may produce problems such as confusion, nausea and vomiting, constipation, and drowsiness. If the pain has a significant inflammation component that does not resolve easily with milder analgesic approaches or with narcotics, then corticosteroids may be used to alleviate the pain. This approach does not lend itself well to longer-term pain management, however, because of side effects such as fluid retention, stomach irritation, thrush, muscle weakness, weight gain, bone loss, suppressed adrenal function, and increased risk of infections, among others.

The third step in pain control involves alternative methods of pain control. Treatments here include phys-

IN THE NEWS: FDA PANEL RECOMMENDS PERCOCET, VICODIN BAN

In June, 2009, a Food and Drug Administration (FDA) advisory committee convened to discuss the use of acetaminophen (Tylenol) in combination drugs, the risk of acetaminophen-associated liver damage, and possible interventions to reduce the incidence of liver injury. The issue with the combination drugs Percocet (oxycodone/acetaminophen) and Vicodin (hydrocodone/acetaminophen) is their potential for severe liver damage as a result of an overdose of acetaminophen. Acetaminophen is a key drug in the treatment of pain and fever. When it is used according to directions, the risk of developing liver injury is very low. However, many people are unaware that acetaminophen overdose can cause serious liver damage. Between 1998 and 2003, acetaminophen-related liver damage was the leading cause of acute liver failure in the United States, with 48 percent of cases associated with accidental overdose. It is noteworthy that there is only a small difference between the maximum recommended daily dose and a potentially damaging dose of acetaminophen, and some people may be more susceptible to liver damage than others, such as those who use alcohol. Additionally, a multitude of over-the-counter and prescription acetaminophen products are available with a range of doses indicated for a variety of different conditions, and it may not be obvious that acetaminophen is an ingredient in some prescription drugs—for example, the label on pharmacy-dispensed containers are often identified as containing APAP.

The FDA panel voted twenty to seventeen in favor of banning Percocet and Vicodin, as well as seven other drugs that combine a narcotic with acetaminophen. Though the FDA is not required to follow the recommendations of its advisory committees, it frequently does. However, if prescription acetaminophen combination products continue to be marketed, the panel recommends implementing additional safety measures by requiring "unit-of-use" packaging and/or requiring an additional boxed warning for prescription acetaminophen combination products. "Unit-of-use" would require packaging by the manufacturer for sale in a pharmacy, with no need for repackaging at the pharmacy. Standardized information would be displayed on the prescription package (for example, prominent display of "ACETAMINOPHEN" as an active ingredient and a warning about potential liver damage). Regardless of a ban on these combination drugs, acetaminophen would continue to be available as an over-the-counter medication and opioids would be available as single-ingredient painkillers.

—*Anita P. Kuan, Ph.D.*

---

ical therapy, nerve-blocking injections, transcutaneous electrical nerve stimulation (TENS), and behavioral approaches. The latter method seeks to identify the causes of preventable pain (physical or mental) and takes steps to minimize pain.

Recent medical research is leading to interesting discoveries about the management of pain. In 2002, researchers announced that they had identified a key protein that controls severe pain, a discovery that might lead to better pain management for patients who suffer from chronic pain or pain associated with terminal cancer. The protein, known by the acronym DREAM, protects the neural reflex critical to survival, allowing individuals to feel pain and quickly pull away from its source, but over time, DREAM seems to help sharp pain fade as the protein becomes disabled. Moreover, while there are many types of pain, disabling the DREAM protein appears to reduce the severity of all of them. The next step in research will be to examine ways to disable the protein, a task that scientists deem difficult because of its location deep within individual cells. Additional research in this area recognizes that pain has different causes and that it may be more productive to examine mechanisms of pain rather than taking a disease-based approach.

—*Charles C. Marsh, Pharm.D.;*
updated by Nancy A. Piotrowski, Ph.D.

See also Acupressure; Acupuncture; Alternative medicine; Anesthesia; Anesthesiology; Biofeedback; Chiropractic; Hypnosis; Local anesthesia; Marijuana; Meditation; Narcotics; Over-the-counter medications; Pain; Palliative medicine; Pharmacology; Prescription drug abuse; Self-medication; Substance abuse.

FOR FURTHER INFORMATION:

Cousins, Michael J., and P. O. Bridenbaugh, eds. *Cousins and Bridenbaugh's Neural Blockade in Clinical Anesthesia and Management of Pain.* 4th ed. Philadelphia: Lippincott Williams & Wilkins, 2009.

Dillard, James M. *The Chronic Pain Solution: The Comprehensive, Step-by-Step Guide to Choosing the Best of Alternative and Conventional Medicine.* New York: Bantam Books, 2002.

Ferrari, Lynne R., ed. *Anesthesia and Pain Management for the Pediatrician.* Baltimore: Johns Hopkins University Press, 1999.

Ferrer-Brechner, Theresa. *Common Problems in Pain Management.* Chicago: Year Book Medical, 1990.

Fishman, Scott, with Lisa Berger. *The War on Pain: How Breakthroughs in the New Field of Pain Medicine Are Turning the Tide Against Suffering.* New York: HarperCollins, 2001.

Loeser, John D., ed. *Bonica's Management of Pain.* 4th ed. Philadelphia: Lippincott Williams & Wilkins, 2010.

Raj, Prithvi, and Lee Ann Paradise, eds. *Pain Medicine: A Comprehensive Review.* 2d ed. St. Louis, Mo.: Mosby, 2003.

Rosenfeld, Arthur. *The Truth About Chronic Pain: Patients and Professionals on How to Face It, Understand It, Overcome It.* Rev. ed. New York: Basic Books, 2005.

PALLIATIVE MEDICINE

SPECIALTY

ANATOMY OR SYSTEM AFFECTED: All

SPECIALTIES AND RELATED FIELDS: Cardiology, critical care, ethics, geriatrics and gerontology, hematology, immunology, internal medicine, nephrology, neurology, nursing, oncology, osteopathic medicine, proctology, psychiatry, psychology, pulmonary medicine, radiology, rheumatology, urology

DEFINITION: The practice of relieving or reducing the symptoms of life-threatening conditions, providing comfort—but not cure—to patients suffering from serious or terminal illnesses to improve their quality of life and improve their strength to enable them to better tolerate treatments. Palliative medicine addresses the physical, emotional, and spiritual needs of patients and their families.

KEY TERMS:

multidisciplinary: involving several medical specialties, requiring health care practitioners from various perspectives to work closely together to meet the needs of the patient

opioid medications: pain medications derived from opiates, such as morphine, oxycodone, codeine, and fentanyl; intended to control severe pain

SCIENCE AND PROFESSION

Palliative medicine is a specialty that spans disciplines. The goal is to comfort and support patients as they face life-threatening illnesses, not only relieving their suffering but also addressing their emotional and spiritual needs. Although palliative medicine is typically associated with the final stages of life-threatening conditions, patients may also benefit from the care while they are still undergoing active treatment. In that case, symptom relief and other interventions to improve their quality of life helps improve their strength and stamina to endure additional cycles of therapy.

Palliative care may be provided in a long-term care facility, a hospital, or the patient's home. Care is provided by a team consisting of general practice physicians, specialists in the patient's condition (for example, oncologists, cardiologists, or pulmonologists), nurses, social workers, mental health specialists (psychologists, psychiatrists, or counselors), nutritionists, and clergy. The level and type of care provided are guided by the wishes and needs of the patient. Pain management is often the greatest need, but the patient may also require relief of other symptoms associated with the condition or its treatment, such as nausea, constipation or diarrhea, fatigue, depression, or inability to eat.

Palliative medicine is recognized as a basic human right in the International Bill of Human Rights of the United Nations. The document declares that all people have the right to adequate health and medical care, and further states that patients with chronic and terminal illnesses have the right to avoid pain and die with dignity. Following these principles, Canada decreed that every citizen has the right to palliative care. The European Committee of Ministers and the South African Department of Health declared that palliative care is a right of all citizens. Palliative medicine is formally recognized as a specialty in the United States, the United Kingdom, Ireland, and Australia.

Palliative medicine is an essential component of care for patients suffering from any chronic, life-threatening illness, but the specialty has taken on an added significance in the field of oncology. In the United States, the Institute of Medicine stated in 1997 that any comprehensive cancer care plan should include palliative care. A 2005 resolution of the 58th World Health Assembly to improve cancer care placed palliative medicine on equal footing with surgery, radiation, and medical oncology.

Although recognized as a medical specialty, palliative medicine relies on the unique contributions of numerous disciplines. Education in palliative techniques begins at the undergraduate level and is incorporated into the training of a number of medical specialties, such as oncology and gerontology. Continuing education programs focus on educating health care professionals in quality palliative care techniques. Other projects build on these efforts, using trained health care professionals to develop quality palliative medicine programs in their institutions.

The American Society for Clinical Oncology (ASCO) actively promotes continuing education in palliative medicine. Palliative care is incorporated into educational materials and programs developed by ASCO. The society published an educational curriculum for continuing medical education on palliative medicine, and it has a study program devoted to supportive care. Palliative medicine is included in the training for internists, as adopted by the American Board of Internal Medicine.

The National Consensus Project for Quality Palliative Care issued guidelines for palliative care to establish continuity of care across institutions. The clinical practice guidelines have been incorporated into the hospital accreditation standards of The Joint Commission (formerly the Joint Commission for the Accreditation of Hospitals). Institutions are assessed on the eight domains of palliative care: structure and process, physical aspects, psychological and psychiatric aspects, spiritual and religious aspects, cultural aspects, care of the imminently dying patient, the ethical aspects of care, and the legal aspects of care. Additionally, the Center for the Advancement of Palliative Care developed the State-by-State Report Card on Access to Palliative Care in Our Nation's Hospitals. The report card measures patient access to palliative care and to palliative medicine specialists, access of medical students to training in palliative care, and access of physicians to specialty training in palliative care. The report card emphasizes the importance of a multidisciplinary approach to palliative medicine.

DIAGNOSTIC AND TREATMENT TECHNIQUES

Patient care is traditionally disease-oriented. Specialists in particular tend to focus narrowly on a specific organ or body system. Palliative care, however, takes a holistic, patient-centered approach. The emphasis is on communicating with the patient and family to assess the patient's specific needs and desires.

Palliative care can be divided into primary and secondary teams. The primary team is responsible for assessing and managing symptoms, communicating with the patient and family, and providing expertise regarding psychosocial services. This team consists of generalists trained in palliative care. If, however, the patient's condition worsens and the primary team can no longer manage the symptoms, a specialist in the patient's condition is called. The disease specialist may consult on specific issues as needed or become a core member until the patient's death.

The whole-patient assessment begins with the patient's description of symptoms and level of function. Diagnostic tests may be used to evaluate symptom severity, but diagnosis is not the purpose. The emphasis is always on symptom relief.

Pain is a significant issue that must be managed properly. Inadequately controlled pain may reduce the effectiveness of treatment and wear the patient down psychologically. Proper pain management involves communication with and education of the patient and family members as well as continuous assessment of the effectiveness of pain medications. A stepwise approach is recommended, beginning with nonsteroidal anti-inflammatory drugs (NSAIDs), such as ibuprofen, and progressing through acetaminophen combined with an opioid medication, such as acetaminophen with codeine, and lastly to opioid medications such as morphine or oxycodone. The goal is to relieve pain while keeping the patient alert and in control.

The effect of the condition on the emotions and cognitive functioning of the patient is an important aspect of the palliative medicine assessment. Patients are facing serious issues while they battle their illnesses. They must cope with imminent death and the grief of their loved ones along with the fear of loss of control and dignity. Patients must be evaluated for depression and anxiety. Practical needs, such as relationship issues, legal affairs, and financial management, also need attention. The patient's spiritual needs should also be addressed. Spiritual counseling can be traditional religious advisement from a clergyperson or an informal discussion of personal beliefs, according to the desires of the patient.

Depression and anxiety are common among patients coping with life-threatening conditions. Feelings of sadness and depression are to be expected, but they are not expected to be permanent. The members of the primary team who are in closest contact with the patient need to be alert for symptoms of depression that surpass the normal grieving process. Signs of major depression include persistent feelings of worthlessness, hopelessness, helplessness, and loss of self-esteem. Physical symptoms may include weight loss or changes in sleep habits, although these symptoms may also be attributed to the patient's underlying condition. Thoughts of suicide or requests by the patient to hasten death are not part of the coping process and are a sign of major depression. If the signs of depression fail to resolve after a few weeks, then the mental health specialists on the team are consulted and the depression should be treated.

Similarly, anxiety is an understandable and natural emotion as patients juggle financial concerns, family issues, medical concerns, and preparations for their own death. Anxiety may be managed through counseling or, if it is severe, with antianxiety medications.

The role of the palliative care team is not limited to the patient. The team assists family members in accepting the patient's condition, managing financial and insurance matters, and coping with grief. The health care team can advise family members on what to expect as the patient's condition deteriorates. Breathing difficulties, delirium or dementia, wasting, and incontinence can be upsetting for family members to experience if they are not properly prepared. After the patient's death, the palliative care team assists family members through the grieving process. The team follows up with the family through phone calls and visits, providing grief counseling or referral to support groups or other mental health professionals when needed. Bereavement services often last for several months to a year after the patient's death.

PERSPECTIVE AND PROSPECTS

In the span of two decades, palliative medicine progressed from haphazard training through chance experiences to a recognized specialty. A 1998 member survey by ASCO revealed 90 percent of the oncologists who responded had no formal training in palliative medicine. Rather, they indicated they learned through "trial and error." Alarmingly, more than one-third claimed that their education in palliative medicine was from a "traumatic experience" with a patient. Most had little training in how to discuss a poor prognosis with patients and their families, and only 10 percent had completed clinical training in palliative care.

Since that survey, ASCO and other professional societies have incorporated palliative medicine into their continuing education curricula. More important, national and international groups have formally recognized the importance of palliative medicine in preserving the dignity and well-being of patients nearing the end of their lives. Within the next decade, palliative medicine is expected to be incorporated as a routine part of comprehensive cancer care plans in the United States.

Despite these advances, much work remains. The need for palliative medicine is increasing. The population is growing older while the prevalence of cancer is rising. Cancer treatments are becoming more effective. Although cancer death rates are declining, more people are living longer with the disease, resulting in growing numbers of people who will benefit from palliative medicine.

To meet the growing need, health care practitioners must be educated in palliative medicine. Fellowships in palliative medicine, continuing education, and readily available educational resources are necessary. Guidelines must be adopted to ensure consistency in the quality of palliative medicine across states and individual institutions. The concept of palliative medicine must be incorporated into care plans across medical disciplines.

Improving end-of-life care requires more than educational and quality control initiatives; it also requires political will. Unless palliative medicine is viewed as a priority by administrators and policy makers, quality care cannot be ensured. Policies establishing comprehensive education and consistent care standards need to be adopted.

Pain management is an integral piece of palliative medicine. Unfortunately, misconceptions remain among health care practitioners as well as the general public regarding the use of opioid medications. The fear of addiction frequently results in less than optimal pain control. The need for higher doses of pain medications does not indicate addiction; it is more likely a sign the pain is inadequately controlled or the condition is progressing. The United Nations elevated effective pain control to a fundamental right. In a formal statement, the U.N. equated inadequate pain control with "cruel, inhuman, and degrading treatment" and called for nations to supply adequate pain medications to patients.

Collectively, the United Nations, individual countries, and medical societies are striving to ensure that all patients suffering from terminal illnesses receive compassionate and comprehensive care. The strength of palliative medicine is in considering the patient as a whole rather than focusing exclusively on a particular diagnosis. Palliative medicine breaks from traditional medical practice and creates a multidisciplinary team to care for the patient. The direction of care is dictated by the wishes of the patient and encompasses physical, emotional, and spiritual needs.

—*Cheryl Pokalo Jones*

See also Aging; Cancer; Death and dying; Depression; Ethics; Euthanasia; Grief and guilt; Hospice; Narcotics; Pain; Pain management; Phobias; Psychiatry; Psychiatry, child and adolescent; Psychiatry, geriatric; Stress; Suicide; Terminally ill: Extended care.

FOR FURTHER INFORMATION:

Chochinov, Harvey M., and William Breitbart. *Handbook of Psychiatry in Palliative Medicine.* New York: Oxford University Press, 2000. Discussion of the role of psychiatry in palliative medicine.

Doyle, Derek, et al., eds. *Oxford Textbook of Palliative Medicine.* New York: Oxford University Press, 2005. Comprehensive text on palliative medicine, including the role of different medical specialties in patient care.

Field, M. J., and C. K. Cassel, eds. *Approaching Death: Improving Care at the End of Life.* Washington, D.C.: National Academies Press, 1997. The documents from the Institute of Medicine establishing the role of palliative medicine in comprehensive cancer care.

Woodruff, Roger. *Palliative Medicine: Evidence-Based Symptomatic and Supportive Care for Patients with Advanced Cancer.* 4th ed. New York: Oxford University Press, 2004. Review of recent research in the principles of palliative medicine and related ethical issues.

PALPITATIONS

DISEASE/DISORDER

ALSO KNOWN AS: Skipping beats, irregular heartbeat

ANATOMY OR SYSTEM AFFECTED: Chest, circulatory system, heart, muscles

SPECIALTIES AND RELATED FIELDS: Cardiology

DEFINITION: A perceived irregularity of the normal heartbeat.

CAUSES AND SYMPTOMS

Individuals experiencing palpitations often describe a slight discomfort and uneasiness accompanied by a flutter or sudden change in heart rate. Palpitations are often a symptom of an abnormal heart rhythm known as an arrhythmia. Arrhythmias involve a change in the electrical activity of the heart resulting in a chaotic or

---

> **INFORMATION ON PALPITATIONS**
>
> **CAUSES:** Abnormal heart rhythm, high caffeine intake, alcohol or tobacco use, fatigue, extreme physical exertion, stress and anxiety, poor diet
>
> **SYMPTOMS:** Flutter or sudden change in heart rate, slight discomfort and uneasiness; in severe cases, decreased blood flow leading to dizziness, loss of consciousness, chest pain, shortness of breath
>
> **DURATION:** Brief, sometimes recurrent
>
> **TREATMENTS:** Removal of underlying cause; in severe cases, medications (beta-blockers, calcium-channel blockers), surgery (implantable defibrillator)

---

irregular contraction of the heart muscle. The location of these arrhythmias within the heart muscle determines the type, duration, and intensity of the palpitations.

Palpitations are common among many people, regardless of age or gender. They are often diagnosed by cardiologists using several techniques aimed at measuring the electrical activity of the heart. Such tests include electrocardiograms (ECGs), Holter monitoring, and stress tests. Most palpitations do not indicate the presence of a serious cardiac problem. Instead, they are often the result of one cause or a combination of several causes. Several underlying causes of heart palpitations include a high caffeine intake, alcohol and tobacco use, fatigue, extreme physical exertion, stress and anxiety, and a poor diet.

Palpitations have not been shown to cause any damage to the heart muscle. Extended palpitations, however, may lead to decreased blood flow to areas of the brain, heart, or other parts of the body. This decreased blood flow can create oxygen deficits in these areas, leading to dizziness, loss of consciousness, chest pain, or shortness of breath. Palpitations accompanied by such symptoms may be a sign of other structural problems of the heart muscle or surrounding blood vessels and may be diagnosed with the use of an echocardiogram (an ultrasound technique) or invasive catheterization.

TREATMENT AND THERAPY

Most palpitations are treated by removing the underlying causes. Decreasing intake of caffeine, alcohol, and tobacco products often succeeds in lowering the frequency and severity of palpitations. Reducing levels of physical and emotional stress while maintaining proper diet and sleep patterns has also been successful in treating palpitations. Medications such as beta-blockers or calcium-channel blockers or other methods such as surgery or implantable defibrillators may be used to treat palpitations in more severe cases.

PERSPECTIVE AND PROSPECTS

Advances in medical technology have shown heart palpitations to be much more common than once thought. Today, heartbeat irregularities perceived as palpitations are rarely considered to be a sign of serious disease and are often easily treated or prevented.

—Paul J. Frisch

See also Addiction; Alcoholism; Anxiety; Arrhythmias; Caffeine; Cardiology; Cardiology, pediatric; Echocardiography; Electrocardiography (ECG or EKG); Exercise physiology; Heart; Nicotine; Panic attacks; Smoking; Stress; Stress reduction.

FOR FURTHER INFORMATION:

American Medical Association. *American Medical Association Family Medical Guide.* 4th rev. ed. Hoboken, N.J.: John Wiley & Sons, 2004.

Berne, Robert M., and Matthew N. Levy. *Cardiovascular Physiology.* 8th ed. St. Louis, Mo.: Mosby, 2001.

Icon Health. *Heart Palpitations: A Medical Dictionary, Bibliography, and Annotated Research Guide to Internet References.* San Diego, Calif.: Author, 2004.

Litin, Scott C., ed. *Mayo Clinic Family Health Book.* 4th ed. New York: HarperResource, 2009.

Zaret, Barry L., Marvin Moser, and Lawrence S. Cohen, eds. *Yale University School of Medicine Heart Book.* New York: William Morrow, 1992.

PALSY

DISEASE/DISORDER

ANATOMY OR SYSTEM AFFECTED: Muscles, musculoskeletal system, nerves, nervous system

SPECIALTIES AND RELATED FIELDS: Neurology, physical therapy

DEFINITION: A paralysis or partial paralysis that is usually accompanied or followed by muscle weakness and muscle wasting over the affected area; in some cases, there may be residual electrical activity present, but the amount is usually small and the activity cannot be controlled.

KEY TERMS:

Bell's palsy: paralysis of the seventh cranial nerve (facial nerve)

cerebral palsy: a palsy arising prenatally, at birth, or early in life within the central nervous system, affecting large portions of the cerebral hemispheres, with extensive paralysis of many major muscles

hemiplegia: paralysis involving an arm and a leg on the same side of the body

palsy: a paralysis or partial paralysis involving loss of motor control, usually accompanied or followed by muscle weakness and muscle wasting over the affected area

Parkinson's disease: also called shaking palsy; a degenerative paralysis resulting from destruction of certain cells in the substantia nigra, a structure near the base of the cerebral hemispheres

quadriplegia: paralysis involving all four extremities more or less equally

spastic: characterized by uncontrollable spasms

substantia nigra: a clump of cells located near the base of the cerebral hemispheres that secrete the neurotransmitter dopamine

CAUSES AND SYMPTOMS

In general, the term "palsy" describes any type of dysfunction of the motor nerves that impairs or reduces the conscious control of muscles. The paralysis or loss of motor control is usually accompanied or followed by weakness and wasting of the muscles in the affected area.

The most common type of palsy is Bell's palsy, a paralysis of the seventh cranial nerve, or facial nerve, often accompanied by pain over part or all of the affected area. The number of muscles involved varies. The paralysis usually occurs on one side of the face at a time, with the result that the undamaged muscles of the opposite side pull the facial skin to that side. Typically, the eye on the affected side remains open all the time because the muscles that close it have been affected; attempts by the patient to close the eye merely result in the eyeball rotating upward. The rest of the face on the affected side generally droops but remains flat; the brow fails to wrinkle, and the cheeks never thicken. Smiles and other facial expressions are asymmetrically contorted.

Thorough neurological testing is needed to assess how much damage has been done and which branches of the facial nerve have been affected. If the damage affects either hearing or taste, this finding indicates that the damage is closer to the root of the facial nerve, and the patient's chances for recovery are correspondingly much lower. If only a few muscles are involved, it indicates that the damage is farther from the root of the nerve, which usually forecasts a better chance of recovery. In most cases, Bell's palsy is thought to arise from a reduced blood supply to the affected nerves. Viral infection by herpes simplex or herpes zoster (shingles) is also a frequent cause; the viral infections are believed to cause demyelination (deterioration of the myelin sheath that insulates nerves) of the affected parts of the facial nerve. Other causes include injuries to the area just below or in front of the external ear, resulting from blows to the head, surgery in this region, or other types of trauma.

Another common type of palsy is cerebral palsy, an impairment of movement and posture caused in most cases by injury, malformation, or other damage to the immature brain. Cerebral palsy is actually a group of paralytic disorders that begin during intrauterine development, at birth, or in early infancy. The extent of the paralysis may vary, often involving large groups of muscles while sparing others. Those muscles that are not totally paralyzed are often uncoordinated in their movements or poorly controlled; this is especially true of large muscle movements such as those of the limbs. In many cases, the patient exhibits a "scissors gait" in which the lower limbs are crossed and the one behind must be swung sideways before it is placed in front of the other limb. In addition to the lack of muscular control of the limbs, other symptoms variously include spasms, athetoid (slow, rhythmic, and wormlike) movements, or muscular rigidity. Speech is in many cases difficult or unclear if the muscles used in speaking are affected.

Mental deterioration may occur in some cases but not in others: Some patients with cerebral palsy are retarded, while others have managed to display brilliant artistic or literary talents with the use of whatever muscles still function in their bodies. Some cerebral palsy patients also suffer from seizure disorders such as epilepsy. Almost all cases of cerebral palsy are accompanied by some other type of neurological impairment, the nature of which varies greatly. In general, cerebral palsy is a nonprogressive type of disease; that is, it does not continually worsen. Afflicted individuals generally experience a normal life span, though with impaired motor functions.

The most common types of cerebral palsy are those that occur in infancy or earlier. Of this group, injuries received at birth (during forceps delivery, for example) form one of the largest and most well defined groups. Cerebral hemorrhage, a cause of many cerebral palsies, may occur either during intrauterine life or at birth. Cerebral palsy may also result from embryonic malformations, from injuries received during intrauterine life, or from injuries or other damage during the first two years of life. In addition to birth trauma, many other factors may contribute to a risk of cerebral palsy: premature delivery, breech delivery, toxemia of pregnancy, impairment of the baby's oxygen supply, maternal infection (especially rubella, also called German measles), premature detachment of the placenta during the birth process, and incompatibility between the Rh blood types of mother and child. Brain injuries caused by low oxygen levels (anoxia or hypoxia) can arise before, during, or after birth and can result from damage to the blood vessels, birth trauma, or infectious diseases such as meningitis or encephalitis.

Cerebral palsies are classified into two general types: pyramidal (or spastic) and extrapyramidal (or nonspastic). The pyramidal or spastic types show muscular spasms and other symptoms that persist with age and hardly vary with changes in emotion, tension, movement, or sleep. The pyramidal tracts of the brain stem are damaged in these forms of cerebral palsy. The extrapyramidal or nonspastic types are more variable and are subdivided into several subtypes according to the types of movement exhibited: none (rigid type), weak (dystonic type), rhythmic and wormlike (athetoid type), or uncoordinated shaking (ataxic type). The extrapyramidal tracts of the brain stem are damaged in

---

INFORMATION ON PALSY

CAUSES: May include genetic and environmental factors, birth defects, trauma during childbirth, reduced blood flow to affected nerves, viral infection, injury in front of ear (trauma, surgery)

SYMPTOMS: May include paralysis (partial or complete); muscle weakness, wasting, or rigidity; awkward gait; impaired facial movement; impaired speech; mental impairment; seizure disorders

DURATION: Acute to chronic

TREATMENTS: Drug therapy (vasodilators drugs such as cortisone, antiviral drugs such as acyclovir); surgery; application of warmth and avoidance of cold drafts

all these forms of the disease. Most forms of cerebral palsy can also be described as hemiplegia (involving both extremities on one side of the body only), diplegia (involving both legs more than the arms), bilateral hemiplegia (involving the arms more than the legs), or quadriplegia (involving all four extremities more or less equally). Attempts to group the various forms of cerebral palsy by their causes have generally resulted in a lack of agreement among experts. One scheme divides the causes into subependymal hemorrhage among premature infants, damage from oxygen deprivation to the growing brain (the vast majority of cases), and developmental abnormalities of the nervous system.

The most common form of cerebral palsy is infantile spastic hemiplegia, which accounts for about one-third of all cerebral palsies. Most cases of spastic hemiplegia (about 65 percent) are thought to result from birth trauma, either from forceps delivery or from the difficult passage of a very large head through the mother's pelvic girdle. Another 30 percent arise after birth, during the first year of life, either from head injury or from infections such as meningitis and encephalitis. Only 5 percent of spastic hemiplegias arise before birth from embryonic malformations or from toxemia of pregnancy. The rate at which cerebral palsy occurs is higher for babies born prematurely than for those born at term. It is also higher for large babies that may suffer injury during a difficult passage through the birth canal. In the United States, there is a somewhat higher incidence rate among Caucasians than among African Americans.

Parkinson's disease (also called paralysis agitans or shaking palsy) is a progressive or degenerative type of palsy. The disease usually produces a tremor which includes a distinctive "pill-rolling" movement of the thumb and forefinger; this tremor usually stops if a voluntary movement of some other kind is begun. Muscle weakness, stiffness, and muscular rigidity are common but intermittent symptoms that come and go; movements generally become slow and difficult. The muscles involved in chewing and swallowing are often affected in Parkinson's disease, so patients are often advised to eat high-calorie, semisoft foods that require no chewing and are more easily swallowed than liquids. Involvement of the muscles of facial expression results in a masklike expression that does not alter with changes in emotion. Patients suffering from Parkinson's disease often have difficulty in initiating voluntary movements; this difficulty is often described by patients as a feeling of "being frozen in place."

The walking gait of Parkinson's disease patients is also very characteristic: The body above the waist leans forward, the head and shoulders droop, the feet shuffle slowly (and are barely lifted from the ground), and the arms are generally held slightly flexed and motionless rather than swinging. Many patients break into a trot or a run when they attempt to walk; as a result, patients often fall, most often forward. To prevent such falls, they frequently shuffle forward in very small steps. The shuffling gait is believed to result from a partial paralysis of the extrapyramidal motor system of neurons, which is generally responsible for controlling posture and coordinating motor activities.

Parkinson's disease is known to result from a disorder in the production of dopamine, a neurotransmitter chemical normally secreted by certain parts of the brain. The affected parts of the brain are the basal ganglia deep within the cerebral hemispheres, and especially the substantia nigra, a deeper structure that sends dopamine-secreting nerve fibers to the basal ganglia. In patients with Parkinson's disease, cells of the substantia nigra are often degenerate and pale from the loss of normal pigments, but this may be a result, rather than a cause, of the primary defect: an impairment of the brain's ability to convert dopa (dihydroxyphenylalanine) into the neurotransmitter dopamine.

The chemical n-methyyl-4-phenyl-1,2,3,4-tetrahydropyridine has been found to produce in experimental animals a disease very similar to Parkinson's disease. For this reason, many researchers suspect that the disease has an environmental cause that leads to the production of a related toxic chemical, one that presumably interferes with the production of dopamine.

Parkinson's disease is uncommon before the age of forty, but it becomes so common in people over sixty that it is the leading neurological disorder in this age group. In the United States, the incidence rate is about 130 per 100,000 in the general population and is roughly the same in all races and ethnic groups. About 10 to 15 percent of patients show mental deterioration (dementia) as the disease progresses. Patients often experience depression, social withdrawal, and generalized apathy.

Other, less common palsies include brachial birth palsy, Erb's palsy, Klumpke's palsy, true or progressive bulbar palsy, pseudobulbar palsy, Féréol-Graux palsy, posticus palsy, lead palsy, scrivener's palsy, pressure palsy, compression palsy, and creeping or wasting palsy.

Brachial birth palsy is a paralysis of the infant's arm resulting from an injury received at birth, involving the whole arm, the upper arm only (Erb's palsy), or the lower arm only (Klumpke's palsy). Erb's palsy, a brachial birth palsy of the upper arm, is caused by an injury at birth to the brachial plexus or the posterior roots of the fifth and sixth cervical nerves; the muscles involved generally include the deltoideus, biceps brachii, and brachialis, impairing the raising of the upper arm, flexion of the elbow, or supination movements involving the forearm. In Klumpke's palsy, which results from an injury at birth, the muscles of the forearm and the small muscles of the hand undergo atrophy; this form is often accompanied by paralysis of the cervical sympathetic nerves.

True or progressive bulbar palsy, a palsy and progressive atrophy of the muscles of the tongue, lips, palate, pharynx, and larynx, often occurs late in life and is caused by degeneration of the motor neurons leading to these muscles. Twitching or atrophy of the tongue and other affected muscles causes drooling, difficulties in swallowing, and ultimately a respiratory paralysis that results in death. Many experts consider true bulbar palsy to be a manifestation of the same disease that causes amyotrophic lateral sclerosis (ALS), which is popularly known as Lou Gehrig's disease.

Pseudobulbar palsy ("laughing sickness") is a paralysis of the lips and tongue that mimics true or progressive bulbar palsy, but it arises in the brain itself and is accompanied by difficulties in swallowing and by spasmodic laughter at inappropriate times. Féréol-Graux palsy, a one-sided (unilateral) paralysis of the motor nucleus of the lateral rectus muscle of one eye and the medial rectus muscle of the other eye, results from damage to the medial longitudinal fasciculus and impairs the ability to direct either eye toward the affected side. Posticus palsy is a paralysis of the posterior cricoarytenoideus muscle (cricoarytenoideus posticus), resulting in the vocal cords being held close to the midline.

Lead palsy is a paralysis of the extensor muscles of the wrist resulting from lead poisoning, while scrivener's palsy ("writer's cramp") is a repetitive motion disorder resulting in damage to the nerve controlling the small muscles of the hand. Pressure palsy is a paralysis caused by repeated or persistent compression of a nerve or nerve trunk. Compression palsy results from nerve compression, especially of the arm, caused by pressure from the use of a crutch (crutch palsy) or from compression of a nerve during sleep. Creeping palsy and wasting palsy are general terms for progressive muscle atrophy, such as that associated with ALS.

TREATMENT AND THERAPY

Bell's palsy is treated by various methods, including the application of warmth, the avoidance of cold drafts, or the administration of vasodilating drugs such as cortisone or antiviral drugs such as acyclovir. In unusual cases, surgery is performed to enlarge the passages through which the facial nerve passes, thus relieving compression on the nerve. In past generations, physicians often recommended treating eyes that could not be closed by taping them shut, especially in sleep. This treatment is no longer recommended. Instead, physicians usually advise patients who cannot close an affected eye to wear dark glasses during the day.

Many patients with Bell's palsy recover spontaneously on their own. The chances that a particular individual will spontaneously recover depend on the location of the damage and the extent of muscle involvement; the cases with the most favorable outcomes are those in which the damage is more peripheral and fewer muscles are involved. Frequent, repeated testing of each small group of facial muscles is needed to assess the extent of damage and the extent of any recovery.

Diagnosis of cerebral palsy is best made by a trained neurologist through observation of the patient's spontaneous motor movements and reflex actions. Infants who exhibit any reflex that persists beyond its appropriate age range, or any voluntary motor pattern that fails to develop at the appropriate age, should be examined more carefully for signs of nerve damage. For example, most babies can lift their heads by one month of age and their chests by two months. By three months of age, most babies can raise themselves up on their elbows, and by four months on their wrists. Newborn babies exhibit reflexes such as the Moro reflex, a flexion and "embracing" reflex in reaction to a sudden noise or other sudden stimulus or "startle"; however, the persistence of this reflex beyond six months of age (or its asymmetrical performance) may be indicative of some form of cerebral palsy. Another reflex often used in diagnosis is the "fencer" reflex, or asymmetric tonic neck reflex: Turning the baby's head toward one side usually causes extension movements in both the arm and leg on the side toward which the chin faces, while flexion movements usually take place on the opposite side of the body. This reflex is present at birth and disappears in a few months; its persistence after six months of age should be considered suspicious.

There is no cure for cerebral palsy. Treatment generally consists of physical rehabilitation and training the patient to use whatever muscles are still capable of being consciously controlled. This is a difficult form of therapy that must be tailored to the needs of each patient because individuals experience unique combinations of motor abilities and disabilities. Few patients with cerebral palsy are capable of walking on their own. Depending on the extent of impairment of muscle movements, some patients may require crutches or braces, while others use motorized wheelchairs. In cases in which there is speech impairment, speech therapy may also be needed to teach the patient to speak more clearly. Most types of cerebral palsy are already present during infancy; therapy for these types is always rather difficult because the patient is learning the necessary motor skills (such as walking or speaking) for the first time. Palsies that arise during adolescence or adulthood respond differently to therapy because the patient is relearning skills that had already been mastered.

Treatment for Parkinson's disease includes the administration of a number of drugs that are chemically related to dopamine, the missing neurotransmitter. The drug most often used is levodopa, or L-dopa, a derivative of a naturally occurring amino acid in the brain. The drug carbidopa is also given to help deliver most of the levodopa into the brain. Dopamine agonists (enhancers) such as bromocriptine and pergolide are frequently given. The antiviral drug amantadine has also been shown to have effects that counter the disease.

PERSPECTIVE AND PROSPECTS

The various palsies were identified in the nineteenth century. Bell's palsy was first described by Sir Charles Bell (1774-1842), a renowned Scottish anatomist. Parkinsonism was first described by James Parkinson (1755-1824), who called it "shaking palsy"; the understanding of the neurotransmitter dopamine and the use of L-dopa in the treatment of Parkinson's disease were development of the late twentieth century. Cerebral palsy was first described in 1861 by a London physician, William J. Little; the famous psychoanalyst Sigmund Freud (1856-1939) published an account of this disease in 1883. The most thorough early work on this disease was published in 1889 by the distinguished Canadian physician Sir William Osler (1849-1919), who coined the term "cerebral palsies" to describe the several types of the disease.

Several types of cerebral palsy that were more common in the early twentieth century, such as those caused by the use of obstetrical forceps during delivery,

have decreased in incidence as a result of improved medical procedures. For larger babies that formerly faced a greater risk of cerebral hemorrhage and other brain injury from passage through the mother's pelvic girdle at birth, the increased frequency of cesarean sections has greatly reduced the rates of cerebral palsy arising at birth.

—*Eli C. Minkoff, Ph.D.*

See also Amyotrophic lateral sclerosis; Bell's palsy; Cerebral palsy; Hemiplegia; Herpes; Motor neuron diseases; Nervous system; Neuralgia, neuritis, and neuropathy; Neurology; Neurology, pediatric; Paralysis; Paraplegia; Parkinson's disease; Physical rehabilitation; Quadriplegia; Shingles; Tremors.

FOR FURTHER INFORMATION:

Behrman, Richard E., Robert M. Kliegman, and Hal B. Jenson, eds. *Nelson Textbook of Pediatrics.* 18th ed. Philadelphia: Saunders/Elsevier, 2007. The treatment of cerebral palsy is brief and to the point, including advice for diagnosis and treatment.

Bloom, Floyd E., M. Flint Beal, and David J. Kupfer, eds. *The Dana Guide to Brain Health.* New York: Dana Press, 2006. An easy-to-understand health guide to the brain from neuroscience, neurology, and psychiatry perspectives. More than seventy psychiatric and neurological disorders, their diagnoses, and their treatments are covered.

Chipps, Esther, Norma J. Clanin, and Victor G. Campbell. *Neurologic Disorders.* St. Louis, Mo.: Mosby Year Book, 1992. Written for nurses, this reference work uses nontechnical language and an easy-to-read style. Includes sections on Bell's palsy and Parkinson's disease but does not cover cerebral palsy. Illustrations are provided.

Daube, Jasper R., ed. *Clinical Neurophysiology.* 3d ed. New York: Oxford University Press, 2009. Covers the basics of clinical neurophysiology, considers the assessment of disease by anatomical system, and explains how clinical neurophysiologic techniques are used in the clinical assessment of diseases of the nervous system.

Parker, James N., and Philip M. Parker, eds. *The Official Patient's Sourcebook on Bell's Palsy.* San Diego, Calif.: Icon Health, 2002. Guides patients in using the Web to educate themselves about Bell's palsy and draws from public, academic, government, and peer-reviewed research to provide comprehensive information on a range of topics related to Bell's palsy.

_____. *The Official Patient's Sourcebook on Peripheral Neuropathy.* San Diego, Calif.: Icon Health, 2002. Guides patients in using the Web to educate themselves about neuropathies and draws from public, academic, government, and peer-reviewed research to provide information on virtually all topics related to neuropathic diseases, from the essentials to the most advanced areas of research.

Stanley, Fiona J., Eva Alberman, and Eva Blair. *Cerebral Palsies: Epidemiology and Causal Pathways.* New York: Cambridge University Press, 2000. Covers the advances in the understanding of cerebral palsies and their epidemiology and causation.

Stanton, Marion. *The Cerebral Palsy Handbook.* London: Vermilion, 2002. A guide for caregivers of cerebral palsy patients. Covers the early stages, routine care, types of treatment available, support networks, school and legal rights, and benefits.

United Cerebral Palsy. http://www.ucp.org. A leading source of information on cerebral palsy, acting as a pivotal advocate for the rights of persons with any disability. One of the largest health charities in the United States, UCP helps advance the independence, productivity, and full citizenship of people with cerebral palsy and other disabilities.

Victor, Maurice, and Allan H. Ropper. *Adams and Victor's Principles of Neurology.* 9th ed. New York: McGraw-Hill, 2009. A good if somewhat technical text. Contains a nonstandard (and incomplete) classification of types of cerebral palsy according to their causes.

Waxman, Stephen G. *Correlative Neuroanatomy.* 25th ed. New York: Lange Medical Books/McGraw-Hill, 2002. Balances basic information about functioning of nerves with clinical discussions. A readable treatment for college students.

PANCREAS

ANATOMY

ANATOMY OR SYSTEM AFFECTED: Abdomen, endocrine system, gastrointestinal system, glands, immune system

SPECIALTIES AND RELATED FIELDS: Endocrinology, gastroenterology, immunology, internal medicine

DEFINITION: A vital organ that produces enzymes used in the digestive process and hormones such as insulin, which regulates blood sugar levels.

KEY TERMS:

autoimmunity: a disorder in which the immune system starts to attack the body's cells as foreign matter

autosomal recessive disease: a disease caused by a gene (other than the X or Y chromosome) that must be on both chromosomes to be expressed

concordance: the inheritance of the same trait by both twins

duodenum: the initial part of the small intestine, where most of the digestion of food occurs

endocrine glands: ductless glands that secrete hormones directly into the bloodstream; these glands help to maintain homeostasis

exocrine glands: glands that excrete their products into tubes or ducts

STRUCTURE AND FUNCTIONS

The pancreas is an organ about 15 to 18 centimeters long and weighing 100 grams that is located in the abdominal cavity. The head of the organ is situated in the loop of the small intestine that forms at the site where the small intestine joins the stomach. The pancreas is enclosed in a thin connective tissue capsule. As an accessory gland of the digestive system, the pancreas is an exocrine gland. Scattered within the tissue of this exocrine gland, however, are small distinct regions known as the islets of Langerhans, which are a part of the endocrine system. The exocrine portion composes by far the greatest mass of tissue. For example, in the guinea pig about 82 percent of pancreatic cells are exocrine cells, while the endocrine portion is about 2 percent. The remaining cells are associated with the duct system and the blood vessels.

The exocrine pancreas is an arrangement of tubules that continue to branch until they form very fine ducts called the intercalated ducts. Along the edges of the intercalated ducts are the acinar cells. These cells produce the pancreatic juices that aid in the digestion of food in the small intestine and help neutralize the contents of the small intestine. The products drain from the ducts into the main collecting duct, which joins the common bile duct and empties into the duodenum.

The islets of Langerhans, as is the case with all endocrine glands, have a well-developed blood supply. The hormones produced by these endocrine cells are emptied into the surrounding capillaries. The hormones flow into the general circulation, where they are distributed to target cells throughout the body. Since the two portions of the pancreas are anatomically as well as functionally different, they will be considered independently.

The exocrine portion of the pancreas produces about 1 liter of aqueous fluid per day that is delivered directly to the duodenum. The two major components of the pancreatic juices are ions, which are used to neutralize the stomach contents as they enter the small intestine, and enzymes, which metabolize intestinal contents for absorption.

The various ions that are secreted include sodium, potassium, chloride, and bicarbonate ions. The sodium, potassium, and chloride are present in concentrations similar to their concentrations in the bloodstream. The bicarbonate ions act as the major buffer of the body. With only a few exceptions, the bloodstream and the contents of the body must be maintained at a pH of 7.4. Bicarbonate ions ensure that there is no change in pH.

The stomach is one of the areas of the body in which the pH varies. It may be as low as pH 1, which is highly acidic. The contents of the stomach empty directly into the duodenum, and while the cells of the stomach are capable of withstanding an acid environment, the cells of the small intestine are not. The acid must be rapidly neutralized in order to protect these cells. In addition,

the enzymes that help to digest the food reaching the small intestine work optimally at about pH 7. If the pH varies significantly, the food will not be properly digested and vital nutrients will not be absorbed by the intestinal cells.

The production of bicarbonate by the duct cells is controlled by a hormone called secretin. The contents of the small intestine become acidic as food moves into the area from the stomach. When the pH is lowered, the cells of the small intestine release secretin, which in turn stimulates the pancreas to produce more bicarbonate. As bicarbonate enters the small intestine, it neutralizes the acid, and the stimulus to produce secretin is removed.

The pancreas also produces a variety of enzymes that digest proteins, sugars, lipids, and nucleic acids. In order for protein to be absorbed by the cells of the small intestine, it must be broken down into its building blocks, amino acids. This breakdown is an enzymatic process that occurs only when the appropriate enzymes are present and at a pH near neutrality. The enzymes that digest proteins include trypsin, chymotrypsin, and carboxypeptidase. Like protein, sugars, nucleic acids, and lipids must be digested to their subunits if they are to be absorbed. Sugars are metabolized by amylase, nucleic acids by either ribonuclease or deoxyribonuclease, and fats by lipase, phospholipase, or cholesterol esterase.

The secretion of enzymes by the pancreas is controlled by the hormone cholecystokinin. As the content of protein and fat increases in the lumen of the duodenum, the duodenal cells release cholecystokinin, which acts on the acinar cells of the pancreas to release the enzymes. As the food is digested, the level of cholecystokinin decreases and the release of enzymes from the pancreas also decreases.

The islets of Langerhans have four different cell types and produce four different hormones. The alpha and beta cells produce glucagon and insulin, respectively. The delta cells produce somatostatin, which inhibits the secretion of hormones by the

The Pancreas

Liver

Gallbladder

Duodenum

Head of pancreas

Stomach

Tail of pancreas

Pancreatic duct

The pancreas is an unusual gland that contains both endocrine tissue and exocrine tissue; the inset shows the location of the pancreas within the gastrointestinal system.

alpha and beta cells. The F cells produce pancreatic polypeptide, the function of which is not yet understood.

Insulin secretion is stimulated or inhibited by a large number of factors. Blood glucose levels are the most important factor in the release of insulin from the beta cells. If blood glucose increases, insulin is released until glucose levels return to normal. When insulin is released into the bloodstream, it stimulates the uptake of glucose by target cells. Although insulin is best known for its action on glucose, it also stimulates the uptake of amino acids and fatty acids from the bloodstream during periods of adequate nutrition. Glucagon is an antagonist of insulin. It is released in response to low levels of glucose and acts on cells to release glucose, amino acids, and fatty acids into the circulatory system.

DISORDERS AND DISEASES

Diseases of the pancreas can be divided into two basic categories: diseases of the exocrine cells of the organ and those diseases that effect the function of the endocrine portion, the islets of Langerhans. The exocrine cells of the pancreas can be affected by various conditions, including acute pancreatitis, chronic pancreatitis, cystic fibrosis, and carcinoma of the pancreas. Also, because the pancreas is a gland and glandular organs typically have a large blood supply, it is at risk of injury any time that circulation is impaired. The islets of Langerhans may be affected by diabetes mellitus.

Inflammation of the pancreas (pancreatitis) can be either acute or chronic. While some cases are mild, it is considered a serious disease and has a high mortality rate. Although the acute form is more serious, patients with chronic pancreatitis may suffer from acute episodes.

Acute pancreatitis may result from obstruction of the pancreatic duct (possibly by gallstones from the gallbladder or by mucous plugs, as in cystic fibrosis), bile reflux, acute intoxication by alcohol, shock, infection by the mumps virus, hypothermia, or trauma. The diagnosis, pathology, and prognosis are the same regardless of the cause.

The onset of the disease is usually quite sudden, with severe pain in the abdomen, nausea, and vomiting. Diagnosis is made by the presence of amylase in the blood serum. Amylase is an enzyme produced by the pancreas that is used to digest carbohydrates in the small intestine. The presence of elevated levels of the enzyme is an indication that it is not reaching the small intestine and is spilling over into the bloodstream.

The powerful enzymes produced by the pancreas are used to digest proteins, carbohydrates, and fats. If for any reason these substances are not released from the pancreas, they will digest the cells of the pancreas and destroy them. As pancreatitis progresses, it will cause tissue inflammation and will lead to swelling of the organ. In addition, the enzymes may start to digest the cells of the blood vessels in the immediate area, causing bleeding into the tissue. The inflammation, combined with the bleeding, may lead to greater swelling and further inflammation.

Acute pancreatitis can lead to complications in other tissue as well, such as fat necrosis leading to the release of fatty acids from adipose tissue. The fatty acids bind to circulating calcium and may cause tetanus of the skeletal muscle as a result of calcium deficiency. If the enzymes released from the exocrine cells destroy the endocrine cells, the resulting loss of hormone production will lead to hyperglycemia and the complications that stem from it. Cysts or abscesses may also result from acute pancreatitis. Although this disease is usually self-limiting, in many cases it will lead to death.

Chronic pancreatitis is a recurring disease that may also demonstrate acute episodes. It has generally been associated with chronic alcoholism, which seems to be the major cause. Chronic pancreatitis is primarily a disease of middle age and occurs more frequently in men than in women. The patient generally complains of abdominal or back pain, often after a large meal or excessive alcohol consumption. Because of the lack of enzymes for lipid digestion, patients often excrete large quantities of undigested lipids. Without fat absorption, many fat-soluble substances such as vitamins A, D, E, and K will not be absorbed.

Because the patient with chronic pancreatitis is often malnourished from inadequate digestion and absorption of food and from vitamin deficiencies, there is associated weight loss and muscular wasting. The exocrine portion of the pancreas is gradually replaced by scar tissue, but the endocrine cells remain unaffected.

Disease of the pancreas can also be caused by cystic fibrosis. Cystic fibrosis, also known as mucoviscidosis, is an autosomal recessive disease of the exocrine glands. It occurs in about 1 in 2,500 live births of Caucasians but rarely occurs in blacks or Asians. Cystic fibrosis affects the mucus-secreting glands in the body and leads to the production of abnormally thick mucus. About 80 percent of these patients have involvement of the pancreas. The onset and severity of the disease vary widely, but most infants born with cystic fibrosis have a pancreas that appears to be normal. As the abnormal mucus is produced, however, it may block the ducts of the exocrine glands and lead to the destruction of the exocrine tissue. The glandular tissue is progressively replaced by fibrous or adipose tissue or by cysts. The loss of pancreatic activity may lead to malabsorption of nutrients and vitamins. Although the islets of Langerhans are not affected by the disease in its early stages, eventually they also may be destroyed.

Tumors of the pancreas are primary tumors; there is almost no incidence of tumors metastasizing to the pancreas from other locations in the body. The exocrine tumors are generally adenocarcinomas, a type of cancer which is increasing in frequency throughout the world. An association with cigarette smoking and diabetes mellitus has been established. The tumors most commonly occur in the area of the gland where the major ducts leave the pancreas. As the tumors enlarge, they may put excessive pressure on the common bile duct, which is located in the same region. This pressure leads to the backup of bile in the liver known as obstructive jaundice; this is one of the earliest signs of pathology. Tumors located at other sites will not be detected until much later because they do not produce symptoms. Metastases of these tumors may be to the liver or surrounding lymph nodes. Because diagnosis is usually after the disease has progressed, the prognosis is poor even in operable cases.

The most common disease of the endocrine portion of the pancreas is diabetes mellitus. Each year, about 35,000 patients die of diabetes in the United States. Diabetes is a chronic disorder affecting carbohydrate, fat, and protein metabolism. It may be further classified as insulin-dependent or juvenile diabetes (type 1), non-insulin-dependent or adult-onset diabetes (type 2), or secondary diabetes. All forms of diabetes have a common pattern in which insulin is present in insufficient quantities, is absent, or does not function normally— all of which lead to hyperglycemia. Both type 1 and type 2 diabetes are inherited. In identical twins, there is a 50 percent concordance rate for type 1 and a 90 percent concordance for type 2. The latter figure indicates that heredity plays a more important role in type 2 diabetes.

Patients with type 1 diabetes are insulin-dependent. The disease starts at an early age and is sometimes referred to as juvenile diabetes. The decrease in insulin supply is caused by a decrease in functional beta cells in the islets of Langerhans. Evidence indicates that the beta cells are damaged or destroyed by an autoimmune reaction, which may follow a viral infection. Type 1 diabetics often have other endocrine disorders that are a result of autoimmunity. Type 2 diabetics produce some insulin, but not sufficient quantities. It appears that the tissues of these patients are resistant to insulin. The symptoms are less severe than those associated with type 1. Secondary diabetes is a result of some other disease that causes injury or destruction of beta cells. Diseases such as chronic pancreatitis or carcinoma of the pancreas can interfere with insulin production. The severity of the three forms of the disease varies widely, as does the treatment. The type 1 diabetic requires insulin for survival, while in many type 2 diabetics the disease may be controlled by diet and exercise.

Although the presence of insulin has several effects on the body, the lack of insulin has the most pronounced effect on serum glucose levels. If insulin supply is diminished or if the cells do not respond to the insulin produced, there is a rise in blood glucose levels exceeding the amount that the kidney can retain. As a result, glucose is excreted in the urine along with large quantities of water. The loss of glucose and water may lead to hypoglycemia and dehydration. The problem is further complicated by the fact that if there is inadequate glucose available, the cells will metabolize fats. One of the by-products of fat metabolism is the production of chemicals known as ketones, which are acids. Thus the dehydration may be accompanied by a more acidic serum.

The symptoms described above are acute and demand immediate attention. In addition to these symptoms, many abnormalities may appear in patients who have diabetes for ten or more years. The cardiovascular system is highly vulnerable to the disease, and the cause of death in about 80 percent of diabetics is a cardiovascular abnormality.

PERSPECTIVE AND PROSPECTS

Since the pancreas is a vital organ, any disease or injury to it will have serious consequences. Problems with the pancreas may be magnified because the diseases associated with the exocrine portion of the gland are not easily detected. In acute cases of pancreatitis, the onset is sudden and requires immediate treatment to control the extent of the disease. Even when the disease is treated early, many patients die. Surgery is complicated by the inflammation and hemorrhaging that may have previously occurred.

Chronic pancreatitis and cancer of the pancreas are even more difficult to diagnose since many of the symptoms are common to other ailments and may not even be present until the disease has progressed to an acute stage. The chronic condition is complicated because the body cannot absorb nutrients and vitamins. By the time that the diagnosis has occurred, the patient is weakened by the loss of weight and muscular wasting from malnutrition.

Diabetes presents its own unique set of problems. In type 1 diabetes, the patient is often unable to follow the prescribed diet and must continually monitor his or her glucose levels to ensure that the insulin doses are appropriate. Assuming that the patient is able to follow the diet and takes the medication as prescribed, there will still be complications—particularly of the cardiovascular system—that may include renal damage.

Many advances have occurred which provide hope for the sufferers of diseases of the pancreas. Physicians are able to provide pancreatic transplants to patients who have no other recourse. The success rate is improving, and techniques are available that should continue to improve the prognosis for the patient. The limitations are the competition for the available organs and the expense of an organ transplant.

New techniques have been employed that are particularly promising for the type 1 diabetic. Instead of complete organ transplants, techniques are being perfected that will allow the transplantation of only the beta cells of the islets of Langerhans. As scientists become more adept at genetically altering cells, it may be possible to replace the defective genes with healthy ones.

There is also hope in the fact that scientists have become more successful in the treatment of autoimmune disease. With early diagnosis, it may be possible to treat children with type 1 diabetes with immunosuppressive drugs before the disease does any damage. It is likely that there will be significant progress with the treatment of diabetes as more becomes known about somatic gene therapy, cell transplants, immunosuppression, and the control of insulin receptors.

—Annette O'Connor, Ph.D.

See also Abdomen; Abscess drainage; Abscesses; Diabetes mellitus; Digestion; Endocrine glands; Endocrinology; Endocrinology, pediatric; Enzymes; Fetal tissue transplantation; Food biochemistry; Gastroenterology; Gastroenterology, pediatric; Gastrointestinal disorders; Gastrointestinal system; Glands; Hormones; Internal medicine; Metabolic syndrome; Metabolism; Pancreatitis; Stomach, intestinal, and pancreatic cancers; Systems and organs; Transplantation.

For Further Information:

Goodman, H. Maurice. *Basic Medical Endocrinology.* 4th ed. Boston: Academic Press/Elsevier, 2009. Contains good background information regarding endocrinology. Covers the endocrine activity of the pancreas and gives a thorough discussion of the physiological role of insulin and the other pancreatic hormones.

Howard, John M., and Walter Hess. *History of the Pancreas: Mysteries of a Hidden Organ.* New York: Kluwer Academic, 2002. A unique examination of the pancreas and its historical role in the science of medicine. Gives anecdotal vignettes of the researchers who have worked on this organ and details such events as the discovery of the islets of Langerhans and of insulin, gastrin, and their tumors.

Marieb, Elaine N. *Essentials of Human Anatomy and Physiology.* 9th ed. San Francisco: Pearson/Benjamin Cummings, 2009. This introductory anatomy and physiology textbook, easily accessible to those with little science background, is richly illustrated with diagrams and photographs that help to illuminate body systems and processes.

O'Reilly, Eileen, and Joanne Frankel Kelvin. *One Hundred Questions and Answers About Pancreatic Cancer.* 2d ed. Sudbury, Mass.: Jones and Bartlett, 2010. Gives both a doctor's and patient's points of view and covers treatment options, post-treatment quality of life, and sources of support.

Pizer, H. F. *Organ Transplants: A Patient's Guide.* Cambridge, Mass.: Harvard University Press, 1991. An excellent treatment of organ transplants, with a chapter on pancreatic transplants. There is a wealth of general knowledge about such operations, including information on how candidates are chosen, the transplant team, antirejection drugs and side effects, and surgical procedures.

Valenzuela, Jorge E., Howard A. Reber, and André Ribet, eds. *Medical and Surgical Diseases of the Pancreas.* New York: Igaku-Shoin Medical, 1991. A well-written book that describes the diseases of the pancreas, with a clear description of the causes and treatment. Although written for the medical community, it is not too technical and should be clear to most readers.

PANCREATIC CANCER. *See* STOMACH, INTESTINAL, AND PANCREATIC CANCERS.

PANCREATITIS

DISEASE/DISORDER

ANATOMY OR SYSTEM AFFECTED: Abdomen, endocrine system, gastrointestinal system, pancreas

SPECIALTIES AND RELATED FIELDS: Endocrinology, gastroenterology, internal medicine

DEFINITION: Inflammation of the pancreas, which may be acute or chronic.

CAUSES AND SYMPTOMS

Linked to the small intestines by the pancreatic duct, the pancreas contributes the enzymes necessary to digestion. When the pancreas is damaged or its duct is blocked, the enzymes may begin to digest the pancreatic tissue itself, a process called autodigestion. Inflammation ensues, resulting in acute pancreatitis. Although there may be complications, most cases are self-correcting once the damaging agent is eliminated, and the pancreatitis does not recur. With continuing damage to the pancreas, however, the disease may become self-perpetuating and either break out periodically in attacks that mimic the acute form or cause few symptoms until much of the pancreas has been destroyed, a chronic form of pancreatitis that is difficult to treat. Either form can be fatal. Acute pancreatitis causes death in less than 5 percent of cases and generally does so because of complications, such as extensive tissue destruction and hemorrhage or infection. Complications from chronic pancreatitis can be fatal in as many as 50 percent of cases.

Medical science has not yet uncovered the exact biochemical processes responsible for pancreatitis. Although a variety of damaging agents are known to lead to the disease, in as many as 30 percent of cases no clear cause is detectable; doctors call these cases idiopathic pancreatitis. Of detectable causes, alcoholism and biliary tract disease account for about 80 percent of both acute and chronic cases in the United States and Europe (the percentages vary widely in other parts of the world). Alcohol is the most common toxic agent causing pancreatitis, although susceptibility varies and only a minority of heavy drinkers develop acute pancreatitis; however, a long history of steady drinking is by far the most common cause of chronic pancreatitis. Gallstones in the common bile duct, or any other

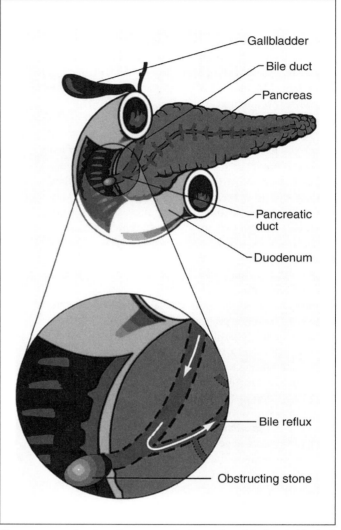

The pancreas, showing the pancreatic duct; when this duct is blocked, bile may reflux, leading to "autodigestion" of the pancreas.

stricture or obstruction that backs up bile into the pancreatic duct, can trigger pancreatitis. Because surgeons can correct this problem by removing the obstruction, it seldom leads to chronic pancreatitis. Other, rarer causes include traumatic injury (especially the damage done by the steering wheel or seat belt during an automobile accident), damage incurred during abdominal surgery or endoscopic procedures in the small intestine, reactions to some medicines, viral infections, very high levels of fats in the blood (hyperlipidemia), structural abnormalities in the pancreas, or hereditary disease.

Despite the variety in causes, patients present a fairly limited set of symptoms, at least during an acute episode. Usually (but not always), they initially complain of steady pain in the upper abdomen that in severe cases seems to bore into them and radiate to the back. They may also have an enlarged abdomen, run a fever, experience nausea, and vomit. The physician is likely to find the abdomen distended, while the patient feels tenderness when it is touched. In severe cases, the patient may develop signs of shock, unstoppable hiccuping, jaundice, discoloration around the navel, fluid buildup in the peritoneal cavity, and impaired bowel function. While abdominal pain is a prominent feature of chronic pancreatitis as well, the most common associated symptoms are diarrhea, fatty stool, weight loss from poor digestion, and the development of diabetes mellitus.

Because none of these symptoms belongs exclusively to pancreatitis, physicians must conduct tests to establish the diagnosis; however, no single test is conclusive. Only by carefully showing that other possible diseases, such as pancreatic cancer, are not responsible for the symptoms can doctors be sure that pancreatitis is the culprit. Blood tests that detect elevated levels of amylase and lipase (pancreatic digestive enzymes) support the diagnosis. X rays, ultrasonography, computed tomography (CT) scanning, and endoscopic inspection of the pancreas and common bile duct can identify both causes and complications of pancreatitis.

TREATMENT AND THERAPY

The treatment for pancreatitis depends on its cause. If the problem is abuse of alcohol or other drugs, physicians usually let an attack of acute pancreatitis run its course while the patient abstains from the offending substance. Nevertheless, even mild attacks frequently require hospitalization because painkillers and intravenous hydration therapy are needed. If gallstones are thought to be the problem, plans are made to remove them by surgery. Patients with severe acute pancreatitis

---

INFORMATION ON PANCREATITIS

CAUSES: Sometimes unknown; often alcoholism and biliary tract disease; possibly trauma, certain medications, viral infections, hyperlipidemia, structural abnormalities in pancreas, hereditary disease
SYMPTOMS: Pain, inflammation
DURATION: Acute or chronic
TREATMENTS: Pain medications, intravenous hydration, antibiotics, surgery, intensive care

---

are sent to the hospital's intensive care unit, since they urgently need supportive treatment to stay alive. There doctors insert a tube through the patient's nose and into the stomach to suck out excess gastric fluids and relieve pressure on the pancreas. They may give antibiotics if there is evidence of infection. Extra oxygen or mechanical assistance may be needed to support breathing. Surgery may rarely be called for even in pancreatitis not caused by gallstones in order to cut away dead, infected tissue or drain fluid accumulations known as pseudocysts. Following an attack and treatment, a patient may require intravenous nourishment for weeks before the pancreas is ready to resume its full function.

Continued alcohol abuse will generally spur recurrent bouts of pancreatitis. Sometimes, however, the alcohol (or, rarely, slowly developing biliary tract disease) causes more subtle, gradual impairment of pancreatic function with few symptoms; in fact, some patients do not go to the doctor until the damage has become extensive and permanently disabling. Others have intense, continual upper abdominal pain that painkillers cannot reduce easily. (In fact, drug addiction from high dosages of painkillers often becomes a problem.) The doctor's first step is to stop the patient's alcohol intake. If gallstones or other obstructions are present, clearing the bile duct with surgery or an endoscopic procedure will decrease pain. Sometimes, high doses of pancreatic enzymes may be helpful in relieving pain.

In cases of uncontrollable pain, however, surgery may be needed to block the sympathetic nerves or even to remove all or part of the pancreas. The chance of surviving some forms of pancreatic surgery is not high—as low as 50 percent—and the procedure often causes further complications. Because pancreatic function is destroyed, most chronic pancreatitis patients digest food poorly and require enzyme supplements to avoid continued weight loss. Since insulin is made in the pancreas, most such patients will also need treatment for diabetes, which may be difficult to manage.

—*Roger Smith, Ph.D.*

See also Alcoholism; Diabetes mellitus; Endocrine disorders; Endocrinology; Endocrinology, pediatric; Enzymes; Gallbladders; Gallbladder diseases; Hypoglycemia; Obstruction; Pancreas; Stomach, intestinal, and pancreatic cancers; Stone removal; Stones.

FOR FURTHER INFORMATION:

Büchler, M. W., et al., eds. *Acute Pancreatitis: Novel Concepts in Biology and Therapy.* Boston: Blackwell Science, 1999. Covers the pathophysiology and repair mechanisms, diagnosis, and treatment options of pancreatitis.

Feldman, Mark, Lawrence S. Friedman, and Lawrence J. Brandt, eds. *Sleisenger and Fordtran's Gastrointestinal and Liver Disease: Pathophysiology, Diagnosis, Management.* 2 vols. Philadelphia: Saunders/Elsevier, 2010. A comprehensive textbook of gastrointestinal diseases and physiology. Contains information on pancreatic disorders.

Kronenberg, Henry M., et al., eds. *Williams Textbook of Endocrinology.* 11th ed. Philadelphia: Saunders/Elsevier, 2008. Text that covers the spectrum of information related to the endocrine system, including diabetes, endocrinology and aging, kidney stones, and endocrine hypertension.

Levine, Joel S., ed. *Decision Making in Gastroenterology.* 2d ed. Philadelphia: B. C. Decker, 1992. This text for physicians contains detailed information about the symptoms and development of cancers. Accompanying charts explain the sequence of examination, testing, and treatment, and dedicated laypersons can glean much of value from them.

Munoz, Abilio, and David A. Katerndahl. "Diagnosis and Management of Acute Pancreatitis." *American Family Physician* 62, no. 1 (July 1, 2000): 164-174. Acute pancreatitis usually occurs as a result of alcohol abuse or bile duct obstruction. A careful review of the patient's history and appropriate laboratory studies can help the physician identify the etiology of the condition and guide management.

Pancreatitis Supporters' Network. http://www.pancreatitis.org.uk. A group based in the United Kingdom that provides medical information and support. Although physician referrals and insurance information are specific to the United Kingdom, readers can still obtain valuable information on drugs, advances in medical research, and book and Web resources.

Parker, James N., and Philip M. Parker, eds. *The Official Patient's Sourcebook on Pancreatitis.* San Diego, Calif.: Icon Health, 2002. Draws from public, academic, government, and peer-reviewed research to provide a wide-ranging handbook for patients with pancreatitis.

Sachar, David B., Jerome D. Waye, and Blair S. Lewis, eds. *Pocket Guide to Gastroenterology.* Baltimore: Williams & Wilkins, 1991. Discusses such topics as gastroenterology, the digestive organs, and digestive system diseases. Includes bibliographical references and an index.

PANIC ATTACKS
DISEASE/DISORDER

ANATOMY OR SYSTEM AFFECTED: Psychic-emotional system

SPECIALTIES AND RELATED FIELDS: Psychiatry, psychology

DEFINITION: Sudden attacks of intense apprehension, fear, doom, and/or terror.

CAUSES AND SYMPTOMS

The physical symptoms of panic attacks include shortness of breath, palpitations, chest pain, smothering sensations, tingling sensations, chills, nausea, sweating, and light-headedness. During attacks, individuals frequently report fears of "going crazy," losing control, or dying. A panic attack is a time-limited experience: Symptoms appear suddenly, build to a peak, and end in a period of time often briefer than ten minutes.

Panic attacks can be related to specific situations in which there is an almost invariable likelihood for a person to have an attack. They may also be partially related to situations, such that they occur in specific situations but not invariably or immediately. Finally, panic attacks may occur spontaneously, unrelated to specific cues or situations.

Agoraphobia, or anxiety about and active avoidance of specific panic-related situations, is often a complicating problem. The situations typically avoided are those from which escape or the attainment of assistance might be difficult. As a result, an individual's range of activities can become quite limited. The unpredictability of symptoms, and the patient's lack of ability to control them, can create a sense of helplessness. Additionally, agoraphobia often results in depression because of decreases in the number of pleasurable activities attempted.

The physical condition mitral valve prolapse (or mitral insufficiency) is also often associated with panic attacks. It occurs when blood leaks back into the heart because the mitral valve did not close properly. For some individuals, it may be noticed as something as mild as a flutter in the chest; for others, it may be characterized by chest pain, palpitations, headache, giddiness, and/or a systolic murmur of the heartbeat. It most cases, it is not a life-threatening condition; however, its presence in individuals who experience panic attacks is often associated with psychological distress because the symptoms of mitral valve prolapse are often misinterpreted as signs of cardiac arrest, leading to feelings of worry, distress, and sometimes panic. At the same time, be-

INFORMATION ON PANIC ATTACKS

CAUSES: Psychological disorder
SYMPTOMS: Shortness of breath, palpitations, chest pain, smothering sensation, tingling, chills, nausea, sweating, light-headedness
DURATION: About ten minutes, with recurrent episodes
TREATMENTS: Psychotherapy, drug therapy, behavioral and cognitive therapies

cause other conditions can also mimic panic attacks, the presence of such attacks requires medical evaluation. These conditions include hypoglycemia, temporal lobe epilepsy, pheochromocytoma (in which an adrenal tumor of the medulla produces excess adrenaline), hyperthyroidism or hypothyroidism, and Cushing's syndrome. If these conditions have been ruled out and mitral valve prolapse is the resulting diagnosis, then patients can be assured that a serious problem does not exist. They may, however, be advised by a physician to monitor the symptoms and take certain preventive actions so that the mitral valve prolapse does not worsen into a more pressing problem.

Both biological and psychological theories attempt to explain the etiology of panic attacks. They are best understood, however, as being determined by a combination of these factors. Physically, panic attacks may result from normal "fight or flight" responses to dangerous situations or either constitutional or state-related hypersensitivity to physical and environmental stimuli. Hyperventilation has also been implicated as a cause of panic attacks. When individuals experiencing panic do not breathe properly, they may be come light-headed and actually create more paniclike symptoms from breathing too quickly and hyperventilating. Similarly, drug withdrawal, drug effects, and drug intoxication can set the stage for panic attacks because many drugs cause similar effects to panic when the person is intoxicated and/or sometimes withdrawing from the drugs. Finally, physical conditions such as mitral valve prolapse that simulate the symptoms of serious heart trouble and of panic can trigger panic attacks.

Panic attacks also may result from thought-related and behavioral processes. It is important to remember, however, that anxiety and panic may be experienced differently depending on a person's culture of origin. For instance, in one culture anxiety may be thought of a medical problem, yet in another it may be seen as a spir-

itual problem. Therefore, culture may have a hand in determining the best type of treatment approach. More generally, from a strictly behavioral perspective, panic attacks may arise from conditioning, in which a person learns via association to experience panic in certain situations. In terms of thought processes, panic attacks may result from learned, maladaptive ways of interpreting and responding to physical and environmental cues. For example, a person might experience a tickling sensation in his or her chest, misinterpret it as a heart attack, and then begin to hyperventilate in response to this misinterpretation, setting the stage for a panic attack. In general, these types of cognitive distortions, combined with biological factors, seem to play a critical role in the development and maintenance of panic-related problems.

TREATMENT AND THERAPY

Four therapies are available to treat panic: bibliotherapies, pharmacotherapies, behavioral therapies, and cognitive therapies. Bibliotherapies involve dispensing information. Books are used at treatment initiation to provide corrective or background information. Bibliotherapy is also useful for individuals with mild panic disorders who are not in need of intensive therapy, as well as for the family members of individuals experiencing panic.

Pharmacotherapies are drug treatments. Historically, sedatives were used to treat panic-related problems. Once problems with dependence on such drugs were discovered, however, their use for this purpose was reduced. Instead, use of other antianxiety agents and certain antidepressant medications have become popular for treatment. Relatedly, the use of stimulating drugs (such as caffeine, diet pills, amphetamine, or cocaine) and hallucinogenic drugs is often discouraged in individuals complaining of panic attacks. The managed detoxification of drugs, where use or withdrawal is related to panic (such as alcohol or Valium use), is also a treatment strategy. It is important to remember that side effects from drugs may differ depending on the individual's ethnic and racial background, in part as the result of biological differences in how individuals respond to different drugs. While side effects may be more mild or minimal for one person, for persons of different ethnic or racial backgrounds they may be more pronounced. Consequently, careful monitoring of side effects is needed to ensure maximum therapeutic benefits and good compliance with prescribed drug regimens.

Other behavioral strategies include social and life skills training, relaxation, and desensitization. Desensitization helps individuals learn to relax in situations that would cause them to panic inappropriately. Behavioral therapies may also integrate family therapy to enlist support and/or to correct for the family-related aspects of a panic problem.

Cognitive therapies focus on identifying irrational beliefs contributing to panic. Individuals work with therapists to identify maladaptive thinking styles. Such styles typically serve to heighten anxiety by magnifying patients' fears and/or minimizing their beliefs that they can cope with feared situations. Through therapy, individuals learn to identify and correct maladaptive thinking patterns, substituting more adaptive thinking where necessary.

Finally, it also important to remember that panic attacks may not occur in isolation. They may be part of a formal panic disorder, they may occur within the context of other psychiatric disorders, or they may occur with other psychiatric disorders, such as depression. It is important that treatment providers monitor the occurrence of panic attacks in conjunction with other psychiatric disorders, such as mood disorders or substance use disorders, to insure proper treatment.

PERSPECTIVE AND PROSPECTS

Panic attacks are experienced by both males and females in every culture, affecting 3.0 to 5.6 percent in a lifetime. Similarly, the formal condition of panic disorder affects approximately 1.5 to 5.0 percent of the population in a lifetime. Women are disproportionately affected. Understanding the origins and relevance of this apparent gender difference will be important to treatment advances. Similarly, understanding why panic disorders are more prevalent in some families than in others will be key in creating better behavioral and pharmacological therapies. Finally, though the incidence of panic attacks is higher in individuals between late adolescence and middle adulthood, both the very young and the very old endure problems related to panic attacks. Though the available therapies have promise for these groups, challenges are evident. Tailoring treatments to the dynamic physical, social, and cognitive developmental needs of children and the elderly will be critical. This is particularly important for individuals who are not able to remain on drug regimens as a result of other health conditions. Similarly, increasing knowledge regarding how ethnic and cultural background may interact with different types of therapies, including drug therapies, is likely to increase the specificity of treatments in this area of work.

—*Nancy A. Piotrowski, Ph.D.*

See also Antianxiety drugs; Anxiety; Factitious disorders; Hyperventilation; Hypochondriasis; Mitral valve prolapse; Neurosis; Palpitations; Phobias; Psychiatric disorders; Psychiatry; Psychiatry, child and adolescent; Psychiatry, geriatric; Psychoanalysis; Stress.

FOR FURTHER INFORMATION:

Barlow, David H., ed. *Clinical Handbook of Psychological Disorders*. 4th ed. New York: Guilford Press, 2008. This collection defines and describes psychological disorders and uses case histories as illustrations for treatment.

Bloom, Floyd E., M. Flint Beal, and David J. Kupfer, eds. *The Dana Guide to Brain Health*. New York: Dana Press, 2006. An easy-to-understand health guide to the brain from neuroscience, neurology, and psychiatry perspectives. More than seventy psychiatric and neurological disorders, their diagnoses, and their treatments are covered.

Davidson, Jonathan, and Henry Dreher. *The Anxiety Book*. New York: Penguin, 2003. The director of the Anxiety and Traumatic Stress Program at Duke University Medical Center provides an informed overview of each category of chronic anxiety, including its symptoms and manifestations. Self-assessment tests are included to help readers identify which type of anxiety is troubling them.

Friedman, Steven, ed. *Cultural Issues in the Treatment of Anxiety Disorders*. New York: Guilford Press, 1997. Provides an overview of anxiety disorders, including panic, and how these disorders may present themselves in individuals of different backgrounds. Attention to interactions between pharmacotherapy and ethnicity are also discussed.

Rachman, Stanley, and Padmal de Silva. *Panic Disorder: The Facts*. 3d ed. New York: Oxford University Press, 2010. This concise volume covers many aspects of panic disorder. Includes bibliographical references and an index.

Root, Benjamin A. *Understanding Panic and Other Anxiety Disorders*. Jackson: University Press of Mississippi, 2000. Root explains physical and mental problems that can mimic panic disorders and that the differentiating diagnosis in an emergency room or clinic is often a major hurdle. Describes those likely to suffer from panic attacks and discusses drug and psychotherapy treatments.

PAP TEST

PROCEDURE

ALSO KNOWN AS: Pap sampling, Pap smear

ANATOMY OR SYSTEM AFFECTED: Genitals, reproductive system, uterus

SPECIALTIES AND RELATED FIELDS: Gynecology, oncology

DEFINITION: A sampling of cells from the cervix or vagina used to screen for dysplasia (precancer) and cancer.

INDICATIONS AND PROCEDURES

Pap testing guidelines have recently changed. Formerly, the procedure was recommended for all women over the age of eighteen or for women who are sexually active. New guidelines have been issued by three authoritative groups: the American Cancer Society, the American College of Obstetricians and Gynecologists, and the Preventive Services Task Force, part of the U.S. Department of Health and Human Services. While there are minor differences among these new guidelines, they are similar in stipulating that there is no need for Pap tests to begin in women younger than age twenty-one unless a woman has been sexually active for three years. New guidelines have been issued as well for testing for human papillomavirus (HPV), which frequently accompanies the procedure; it is now recommended that HPV testing be done in women age twenty-one and older because HPV is usually a transient infection that will clear without need for intervention.

The guidelines also recommend less frequent Pap testing for women who have had three consecutive negative tests; the guidelines also call for a cutoff to Pap testing in older women without abnormalities. Pap testing guidelines for women who have had a hysterectomy (with sampling of the vaginal cuff) vary depending on whether the hysterectomy was done for benign or malignant causes. The guidelines recommend that only women who have had malignant disease continue Pap testing.

A Pap test is performed easily in an office visit. Generally the patient lies on her back with legs flexed and knees apart, although alternative positions can be utilized for women with limited mobility or with disabilities. A speculum is then carefully inserted into the vagina, and the cervix is visualized. A wooden or plastic spatula is used to gently scrape off cells from the transition zone of the cervix. A cytobrush samples cells from the cervical canal. These cells are then placed in a preservative and sent to a pathology laboratory for analysis. The term "Pap smear" derives from the fact that before the recent advent of liquid preservative methods of collecting samples, samples were "smeared" on a glass slide and then sent to a laboratory for analysis.

USES AND COMPLICATIONS

The main use of Pap testing is to identify asymptomatic cases of dysplasia (abnormal growth) of the cervix and vagina. With early treatment of dysplasia, the incidence of and number of deaths from cervical cancer have decreased dramatically. Although cancer screening is the primary purpose and use of Pap testing, incidental findings may include vaginal infections of bacteria, fungi, or parasites. In rare cases, Pap tests may also detect abnormal cells shed from the endometrium.

There are no serious risks from the procedure. Women may see a small amount of spotting after the procedure as a result of abrasions from the spatula or cytobrush.

PERSPECTIVE AND PROSPECTS

The Pap test was introduced in 1943 by George N. Papanicolaou and Herbert F. Traut. Since then, the incidence of invasive cervical cancer has decreased by 50 percent. A screening test analogous to cervical Pap sampling, called the anal Pap test, has been developed to screen for anal dysplasia and cancer. It has been used primarily on high-risk patients, such as those with HIV and HPV.

—Clair Kaplan, A.P.R.N./M.S.N.;
additional material by Anne Lynn S. Chang, M.D.

See also Biopsy; Cervical, ovarian, and uterine cancers; Cervical procedures; Genital disorders, female; Gynecology; Reproductive system; Screening; Women's health.

FOR FURTHER INFORMATION:

Kumar, Vinay, et al., eds. *Robbins Basic Pathology.* 8th ed. Philadelphia: Saunders/Elsevier, 2007.

Stenchever, Morton A., et al. *Comprehensive Gynecology.* 4th ed. St. Louis, Mo.: Mosby/Elsevier, 2006.

Wright, Thomas C., Jr., et al. "2001 Consensus Guidelines for the Management of Women with Cervical Cytological Abnormalities." *Journal of the American Medical Association* 287, no. 16 (April, 2002): 2120-2129.

PARALYSIS

DISEASE/DISORDER

ANATOMY OR SYSTEM AFFECTED: Legs, muscles, musculoskeletal system, neck, nerves, nervous system, spine

SPECIALTIES AND RELATED FIELDS: Neurology, physical therapy

DEFINITION: Pronounced weakness or the inability to produce movement in a part of the body resulting from a variety of causes.

KEY TERMS:

brain cortex: the outer layer of the brain, or gray matter; divided into many areas, each with a different function, such as motion (the motor cortex) or sensation (the sensory cortex)

central nervous system: a system consisting of the brain, the brain stem, the cerebellum, and the spinal cord

hemiplegia: paralysis of one side of the body

motor: referring to parts of the nervous system having to do with movement production

nerve cell: the type of cells that make up the brain, spinal cord, and all the nerves; some initiate nerve impulses, some transmit impulses from one nerve cell to another, some transmit impulses from nerve cells to muscle cells, and some function to regulate other impulses

nerve impulse: a weak, localized electrical current generated by the movement of charged particles across and along a nerve cell membrane

nerves: bands of nervous tissue that carry both motor and sensory nerve impulses between the central nervous system and the rest of the body

neurotransmitters: chemical substances, such as acetylcholine, that are released by nerve cells into synapses when the nerve is stimulated; they stimulate the next nerve cell to fire in turn, thus passing the impulse from cell to cell

paraplegia: paralysis of the legs and lower trunk

peripheral nervous system: a system consisting of the nerves not located in the central nervous system; these nerves carry impulses from the central nervous system to the target muscles and relay sensory impulses from the rest of the body to the central nervous system

quadriplegia: paralysis of all four limbs

spinal cord: a large collection of nerve cells that relay impulses between the brain and the rest of the body; sometimes the spinal cord initiates nerve impulses of its own, such as reflexes

NERVOUS SYSTEM FUNCTIONS

To understand the causes of paralysis—weakness or the inability to move a part of the body—it is necessary to review briefly the motor nervous system and muscles. Following an action from initiation to completion through the motor nervous system may clarify this process. One may begin, for example, with a voluntary movement. An alarm clock rings early one morning. A sleeper hears the noise and decides to hit the "snooze" button. This decision is made in the cerebral cortex, which sends impulses to the nerves in the arm via the spinal cord.

The actual microscopic actions that result in a nerve impulse traveling from the motor cortex all the way to individual muscles will be briefly reviewed. An individual nerve cell, or neuron, comprises three parts: The dendrites, the cell body, and the axon. The cell body conducts the metabolism for the cell and otherwise keeps things in running order, but it has little direct involvement with the transmission of nerve impulses.

Dendrites are similar in appearance to the roots of plants. They are numerous and relatively short. Their function is to pick up impulses received either from sensory organs or from other cells. They do this when the receptors on their surface become activated by certain chemical signals released by neighboring nerve cells. Once these receptors are activated, they initiate a process known as depolarization.

In the most basic description, depolarization refers to the generation of a minute electrical charge on nerve cell membranes. It occurs through the motion of charged molecules, or ions, across the cell membrane. The specific ions involved include potassium, sodium, and calcium. Depolarization progresses down the length of the nerve cell. It passes through the dendrite to the cell body of the nerve cell and then to the axon. The axon is long and thin, some axons reaching lengths of three or more feet. Depending on its type and function, the axon may split into small filaments that go to several nerve or muscle cells, or it may remain single.

The sending axons do not touch the receiving cells when passing an impulse. Instead, they come close to the receiving cell's dendrites but leave a small gap (the synapse). Once a nerve impulse reaches the end of an axon, the axon releases chemical compounds called neurotransmitters.

Synthesized by the nerve cell, the neurotransmitter is collected and stored in small packets resting at the end of the axon. In response to depolarization, the small packets of neurotransmitter are released into the synapse, and the original electrical nerve impulse is converted into a chemical impulse. When the neurotransmitter is released, it diffuses across the gap and contacts specific receptors on the dendrite of the receiving nerve cell. The receiving nerve cell's receptors then depolarize the receiving nerve cell, converting the chemical impulse back into an electrical one.

The receiving nerve cell is forced to continue depolarizing until the neurotransmitter is no longer in contact with the receptor, or until the nerve cell itself becomes exhausted and cannot depolarize again. To allow the receiving nerve cell to stop firing and to prepare itself for another signal, the neurotransmitter must be removed rather quickly from the receptor. This can be done by the axon of the sending cell, which takes it back in, or by enzymes located within the synapse that actually destroy the neurotransmitter. The most common neurotransmitter is acetylcholine, and the most frequently encountered form of enzyme that destroys neurotransmitters is called acetylcholinesterase.

The transmission of the nerve impulses signaling the hand to press the alarm clock's snooze button involves passing the impulses through several nerves. The impulses form synapses on nerve cells in the spinal cord before those cells pass the impulse down the spinal cord toward the arm to cause the desired action.

The spinal cord is protected inside the vertebral column, a hollow column of bone. This column is made up of a stack of vertebrae supported by solid bone in the front and a hollow ring of thinner bone in the back through which the spinal cord runs. The vertebrae are anchored to one another by bony connections; the facets and vertebral spines; fibrous ligaments to the front,

---

INFORMATION ON PARALYSIS

CAUSES: May include injury; infection, exposure to toxins, stroke, central nervous system disorders

SYMPTOMS: Range from muscle weakness to complete immobility

DURATION: Acute or chronic, depending on cause

TREATMENTS: Depend on cause; may include surgery, physical therapy, spinal alignment and stabilization, drug therapy, toxin removal, hormonal therapy

---

back, and side; and the intervertebral disks. Disks are made up of soft, gelatinous material surrounded by fibrous tissue. The disks and joints in the vertebral column allow the spine to flex and turn, while the bony column surrounding the spinal cord provides protection.

When the nerve leaves the spinal cord, it travels in what is called the motor ramus, or "root." The ramus passes through an opening in the vertebral column called a foramen. While passing through the foramen, the ramus passes near the intervertebral disk. The motor nerve fibers (and consequently the nerve impulses sent out to turn off the alarm clock) in the motor ramus join with the sensory nerve fibers in the sensory ramus just outside the vertebral column, and together they form the spinal nerves. These spinal nerves regroup to form peripheral nerves.

A peripheral nerve is the part of the nervous system that finally contacts the muscles that turn off the alarm clock. Peripheral nerves carry both sensory and motor information in the same nerve. They are the only locations in which sensory and motor nerve fibers are so completely joined. Peripheral nerves must sometimes pass through relatively tight or exposed locations. An example of an exposed nerve is the "funny bone," the ulnar nerve, which causes an unpleasant sensation when struck. Nerves that pass through tight spaces may suffer entrapment syndromes. A common nerve entrapment syndrome is carpal tunnel syndrome, in which the median nerve is squeezed in the fibrous band around the wrist.

Finally, the arm muscles themselves become involved in the process of turning off the alarm. The muscles are made up of numerous muscle fibers, and each muscle fiber is made up of numerous muscle cells. Inside each muscle cell are two active protein filaments, actin and myosin, which pull together when activated, causing the muscle cell to shorten. When the majority of muscle cells "fire" at once, the whole muscle contracts. The signal from nerve to muscle cell is transmitted across a synapse. The snooze button is pushed, and the alarm ends. Finally, the signals to the arm end, and the filaments slide back to their initial positions, relaxing the muscle cells.

For actin and myosin to move well, there must be adequate blood flow and adequate concentrations of substances such as oxygen, glucose, potassium, sodium, and calcium. Many other substances are needed indirectly to keep muscle cells functioning optimally, including thyroid hormone and cortisone.

TYPES OF PARALYSIS

True paralysis is the inability to produce movement of a part of the body. Paralysis may result from problems at many locations in the body, such as the motor cortex of the brain, the spinal cord, the nerves in the arms or legs, the blood, or the muscle cells themselves. Doctors must determine the specific cause of paralysis or weakness since the treatment of each disease is different. The first task is to determine whether the weakness or paralysis is caused by a disease of the nervous system, the muscle cells, or one of the substances that interferes with nerve conduction or muscular contraction. Some characteristics of specific problems are helpful in this diagnosis.

Disease of the nervous system is most often associated with complete paralysis. Diseases affecting the muscle cells or the factors controlling them are usually associated with a partial rather than complete paralysis—there is weakness rather than a lack of movement. When weakness is severe, however, it may be mistaken for complete paralysis. The fact that diseases of the nervous system cause paralysis of one side of the body (hemiplegia) or one part of the body is helpful in diagnosis. Paralyzing conditions that affect muscle cells tend to result in whole-body weakness, although some muscles may be more severely affected than others. Another aid in differentiation is that neurologic diseases are almost always associated with some degree of impairment in sensation, while muscular causes are never associated with sensory loss.

Damage to the central nervous system and to the peripheral nervous system can be differentiated by features of the dysfunction. Central nervous system problems affect either half of the body or one region of the body, while peripheral damage affects only the muscles controlled by the damaged nerve or nerves. Central nervous system damage leaves pronounced reflexes, while damage to peripheral nerves results in an affected area without any reflexes. There is some muscle wasting with either type of paralysis, but the wasting seen after a peripheral nerve disease appears more quickly and more severely. When central nervous system damage occurs, the muscles involved are generally tight (spastic paralysis). Conversely, in patients with peripheral nervous system damage, muscles are usually loose. Through attention to these differentiating features, the source of paralysis can usually be discovered.

In adults, the most common cause of paralysis is stroke. A stroke results from interruption of the blood supply to a part of the brain. After being cut off from blood flow, the affected area dies. Brain tumors may also cause paralysis. Unlike strokes, however, which cause most of their damage as soon as the blood supply is interrupted, the damage produced by tumors tends to increase slowly as the tumor grows. An interesting feature of brain tumors is that they are surrounded by an area of swelling called edema. The edema, not the tumor itself, causes most of the neurologic changes. This distinction is important because edema is usually responsive to medical treatment.

Subdural hematomas are collections of blood that are outside the brain but inside the skull. They are seen most frequently in older people and alcoholics. To form a subdural hematoma, a small blood vessel becomes injured in such a way that blood slowly oozes from it, accumulates, and clots. Interestingly, the trauma may be so slight as to not be remembered by the patient. This clot may cause pressure on the motor cortex that results in paralysis. Generally, subdural hematomas are slow in onset.

Multiple sclerosis, a disease affecting the nervous system, causes scattered, multiple small areas of destruction virtually anywhere in the brain or spinal cord. The extent of paralysis depends on the sites and extent of the damaged areas. Patients often have impairments in vision, speaking, sensation, and coordination.

If the spinal cord is the cause, the extent and location of the paralysis and numbness depend on the size, location, and level of the lesion. Spinal cord paralysis may result from trauma, tumors, interruption of blood flow, blood clots, or infections such as abscesses. These disorders are similar, except for location, in most respects to the previously described conditions in the brain. One of the conditions, however—trauma of the spinal cord—is very different from trauma of the brain.

Significant trauma may result in fracture of the vertebral column. Spinal fractures may be classified as stable or unstable. Unstable fractures, unlike stable ones, are often associated with paralysis because unstable fractures allow subluxation to occur. Subluxation is a dislocation of the vertebral column that compresses the spinal cord. If it occurs in the neck, quadriplegia (paralysis of all four limbs) results. If it occurs lower down the spine, paraplegia (paralysis of both lower limbs) is seen. On occasion, through inadvertent or excessive movement, overenthusiastic rescuers cause permanent paralysis by converting a nonsubluxated fracture to a subluxated one during rescue attempts.

Another unique type of spinal cord trauma is the rupture of an intervertebral disk, which allows the gelatinous material to press on the spinal cord or on the rami leaving the spinal cord. In addition to causing severe pain, an intervertebral disk rupture may cause weakness or paralysis. It usually affects only one or two rami and spares the spinal cord itself. Trauma to the spinal cord is particularly dangerous to individuals with conditions that weaken the bony spine. These conditions include osteoporosis of all types and rheumatoid arthritis.

Peripheral nerve damage can occur through a number of conditions that may result in nerve degeneration, including diabetes mellitus, vitamin deficiencies, use or abuse of certain medications, and poisoning by toxins such as alcohol and lead. Sometimes, a temporary nerve degeneration called Guillain-Barré syndrome follows upper respiratory tract infections and may be quite serious if the respiratory muscles are affected. A peripheral nerves may also be damaged by direct trauma, or by pressure as it passes through a narrow compartment, as happens in carpal tunnel syndrome. Peripheral nerve conditions are accompanied by numbness, tingling, and weakness or paralysis of only the area served by the affected nerve.

Paralysis may complicate diseases affecting muscles, although in these cases the patients usually demonstrate weakness rather than paralysis. In muscular diseases, the paralysis (or weakness) tends to affect all the muscles of the body, although some may be more affected than others. The most frequent causes of paralysis in children are inherited diseases such as muscular dystrophy. In adults, muscular diseases are mainly attributable to hormonal imbalances caused by problems such as an underactive thyroid gland or an overactive adrenal gland.

Paralysis may result if the concentration of certain substances in the body is significantly altered, although weakness is a much more common occurrence. The concentration of potassium, sodium, calcium, glucose, and specific hormones may dramatically affect muscle strength. A specific, though uncommon, disease of this Type is periodic hypokalemic paralysis, a condition that runs in families. In this disorder, the amount of potassium in the blood can be dramatically reduced for short periods of time, resulting in brief periods of severe weakness or paralysis. These episodes rarely have serious consequences.

Weakness or paralysis may result if the body is unable to produce adequate amounts of acetylcholine, or if this neurotransmitter is destroyed in the synapse before it can pass on its message. Myasthenia gravis is the most common example of this type of disorder. Affected patients initially have adequate strength, but they develop weakness and paralysis in muscles during periods of use because acetylcholine stores become depleted. The weakness in this condition tends to become more prominent as the day wears on. The most frequently used muscles are the most affected. This type of paralysis temporarily improves after rest or medication.

Another unique type of paralysis, called Todd's paralysis, may follow a generalized epileptic seizure. It happens only when the seizure has been so extensive and prolonged that the nerve cells in the brain are literally exhausted and no longer able to initiate the nerve impulses needed to generate movements. This paralysis is temporary.

Paralysis may be caused by a variety of psychiatric disorders, including hysteria, catatonic psychosis, conversion disorder, factitious disorder, and somatization disorder. In psychological paralysis, the patient's inability to move parts of the body is psychological. This paralysis is particularly common during periods of high stress such as combat. Psychological paralysis should be differentiated from malingering. In a psychological paralysis, the patients genuinely believe that they are paralyzed, whereas malingerers, though they deny it, know that they are not paralyzed. Malingering is usually seen when some benefit resulting from the paralysis is anticipated.

PERSPECTIVE AND PROSPECTS

Once a nerve cell has been destroyed, it cannot be repaired. This is the main reason that the outlook is quite poor when most types of paralysis occur. The only thing that doctors can do is to try to limit the extent of the paralysis. Improvements can be made only by training the neighboring cells to take over the functions of the lost cells.

After suffering a paralyzing event, a patient begins rehabilitation using a number of exercises. These activities are usually carried out with the help of physical therapists, occupational therapists, or kinesiotherapists. Unfortunately, progress is rather limited, and most patients are not able to resume their old lifestyle after suffering extensive paralysis.

It is very important to take seriously paralysis or weakness that is localized to a single muscle or single group of muscles. Doctors need to find out the cause of this weakness as soon as possible and take steps to minimize or reverse the damage prior to complete destruction of the nerve cells. Initial and subsequent stroke prevention, tumor treatments, hematoma evacuation, spinal alignment and stabilization, intervertebral disk surgery, toxin removal, hormonal manipulation, and ion correction are all currently available methods of dealing with paralysis.

Because of the poor prognosis for overcoming paralysis, research has focused on understanding how nerve cells grow. Some lower animals possess an ability to regenerate nerve cells when they are damaged. It is well known that a lobster which has lost one of its claws can regenerate that claw, as well as the nerves that control the claw's functioning. A lower animal nerve growth factor has been identified and is being examined by a number of researchers. It is likely that drugs which could aid regeneration of damaged nerve cells in higher animals will be discovered. Once available, these drugs will improve the outlook for recovery of patients with paralysis. These medications may also help with other conditions associated with nerve cell damage, such as Alzheimer's disease and Parkinson's disease.

Progress in medical treatment and an increased health awareness by the public will reduce the incidence of diseases such as diabetes mellitus and the intake of toxins, such as alcohol, that may cause paralysis. Seat belt laws and motorcycle helmet laws may reduce the incidence of paralysis by reducing the severity of injuries in motor vehicle accidents.

Progress in neurosurgery should also improve a patient's hope for recovery in trauma cases. Although dead nerve cells cannot regenerate, cut nerve filaments may be able to regenerate and reattach, which is why surgeons have been able to reattach severed limbs. With progressively finer techniques and equipment, the success rate should improve further. Future progress in neurosurgery may also benefit patients whose paralysis is attributable to causes other than trauma. Progress in genetic research may allow scientists to isolate the genes responsible for diseases causing paralysis. Diseases such as myasthenia gravis and muscular dystrophy could respond to treatment if genetic therapies are found.

—*Ronald C. Hamdy, M.D., Mark R. Doman, M.D., and Katherine Hoffman Doman*

See also Amyotrophic lateral sclerosis; Ataxia; Bell's palsy; Botox; Brain; Brain damage; Brain disorders; Brain tumors; Cerebral palsy; Epilepsy; Fracture and dislocation; Guillain-Barré syndrome; Hemiplegia; Motor neuron diseases; Multiple sclerosis; Muscular dystrophy; Nervous system; Neuralgia, neuritis, and neuropathy; Neuroimaging; Neurology; Neurology, pediatric; Neurosurgery; Numbness and tingling; Palsy; Paraplegia; Parkinson's disease; Quadriplegia; Seizures; Spinal cord disorders; Spine, vertebrae, and disks; Strokes.

FOR FURTHER INFORMATION:

Bear, Mark F., Barry W. Connors, and Michael A. Paradiso. *Neuroscience: Exploring the Brain*. 3d ed. Philadelphia: Lippincott Williams & Wilkins, 2007. Undergraduate text that introduces the topics of neuroscience, neurobiology, neurodiseases, and physiological psychology.

Christopher and Dana Reeve Foundation, Paralysis Resource Center. http://www.christopherreeve.org. Site describes this advocacy organization that supports research into spinal cord injuries and nervous system disorders that cause paralysis.

Cure Paralysis Now. http://www.cureparalysisnow .org. Site offers information for professionals and patients on aims to advance progress toward a cure for spinal cord paralysis.

Goroll, Allan H., and Albert G. Mulley, eds. *Primary Care Medicine*. 5th ed. Philadelphia: Lippincott Williams & Wilkins, 2006. One of the best resources for problem-oriented medical diagnosis and management. Can be used by physicians and laypersons alike.

Kandel, Eric R., James H. Schwartz, and Thomas M. Jessell. *Principles of Neural Science*. 5th ed. Norwalk, Conn.: Appleton and Lange, 2006. Although this book is used in many college graduate courses, the discussion involving peripheral neuropathies should be understandable to the general reader. Provides examples of neuropathies as well as their syndromes, causes, diagnosis, and history.

Nicholls, John G., A. Robert Martin, and Bruce G. Wallace. *From Neuron to Brain*. 4th ed. Sunderland, Mass.: Sinauer, 2007. In this comprehensive work, which includes the text *Neurons in Action 2*, three leading neurophysiologists describe contemporary knowledge of the neuron: its structure, its function, and its roles in the central and peripheral nervous systems.

Tortora, Gerard J., and Bryan Derrickson. *Principles of Anatomy and Physiology*. 12th ed. Hoboken, N.J.: John Wiley & Sons, 2009. This text clearly explains the functions of many individual muscles. Furthermore, it provides many examples of clinical applications involving muscles, including diseases and the use of medical tests for the diagnosis of muscle disease.

Paramedics

Specialty

Anatomy or system affected: All

Specialties and related fields: Cardiology, critical care, emergency medicine, geriatrics and gerontology, pulmonary medicine

Definition: Trained professional emergency medical technicians (EMTs) who provide sophisticated advanced life support in the field, especially intravenous therapy, cardiac monitoring, drug administration, cardiac defibrillation, and advanced airway management.

Key terms:

advanced life support (ALS): procedures such as intravenous therapy, pharmacology, cardiac monitoring, and defibrillation

basic life support (BLS): simple emergency lifesaving procedures that can aid a person in respiratory or circulatory failure

cardiopulmonary resuscitation (CPR): the artificial establishment of circulation of the blood and movement of air into and out of the lungs in a pulseless, nonbreathing patient

certification: the formal notice of certain privileges and abilities after completion of specified training and testing

defibrillation: the termination of atrial or ventricular fibrillation (irregular heart muscle contractions), with restoration of the normal rhythm

emergency medical services (EMS): the combined efforts of several professionals and agencies to provide prehospital emergency care to the sick and injured

intravenous therapy: the introduction of medication into a vein with a special needle

intubation: the introduction of a tube into a body cavity, as into the larynx

Science and Profession

Emergency medical technician-paramedics (EMT-Ps) provide hospital emergency care in the field under medical command authority to acutely ill and/or injured patients and then transport those patients to the hospital by ambulance or other appropriate vehicle. The clinical knowledge possessed by the EMT-P includes the following systems and areas: the cardiovascular system, including the recognition of arrhythmias, myocardial ischemia, and congestive heart failure; the respiratory system, including acute airway obstruction, pneumothorax, chronic obstructive pulmonary disease (COPD), and respiratory distress; trauma to the head, neck, chest, spine, abdomen, pelvis, and extremities; medical emergencies, including acute abdominal infections, diabetes mellitus, and allergic reactions; the central nervous system, including strokes, seizures, and alterations in levels of consciousness; obstetrical emergencies such as eclampsia; pediatric cases, including croup, epiglottitis, dehydration, child abuse, and care of the newborn; psychiatric emergencies, including problems with individuals who are suicidal, assaultive, destructive, resistant, anxious, confused, amnesiac, or paranoid; drug-related problems, including alcoholism, drug addiction, or overdoses; sexual assault and abuse; and various special situations, such as carbon monoxide and other noxious inhalations, poisoning, near drownings, overexposure to heat and cold, electrocution, burns, and exposure to hazardous materials.

The EMT-P must be able to fulfill many roles. First, paramedics must recognize a medical emergency, assess the situation, manage emergency care, and, if needed, extricate the patient. They must also coordinate their efforts with those of other agencies that may be involved in the care and transport of the patient. Paramedics should establish a good rapport with patients and their significant others in order to decrease their state of anxiety.

The next step is to assign priorities to emergency treatment data for the designated medical control authority. Emergency treatment priorities must be assigned in cases where the medical direction is interrupted by communication failure or in cases of immediate, life-threatening conditions. Paramedics must record and communicate pertinent information to the designated medical command authority.

Meanwhile, they must initiate and continue emergency medical care under medical control, including the recognition of presenting conditions and the initiation of appropriate treatments. Such conditions include traumatic and medical emergencies, airway and ventilation problems, cardiac arrhythmias or standstill, and psychological crises. Paramedics must also assess the response of patients to treatment, modifying the medical therapy as directed by the medical control authority. EMT-Ps exercise personal judgment; provide such emergency medical care as has been specifically authorized in advance; direct and coordinate the transport of the patient by selecting the best available methods in concert with the medical command authority; record, in writing, the details related to the patient's emergency care and the incident; and direct the maintenance and preparation of emergency care equipment and supplies.

EMT-Ps must have a good working knowledge of human anatomy and must be familiar with its topographical language. Even though paramedics are not expected to diagnose every injury or illness, they can aid emergency department personnel by conveying correct information using medical terminology. Such information is gathered after examination of a patient at the scene of an accident or sudden illness.

The most important functions of the paramedic are to identify and treat any life-threatening conditions first and then to assess the patient carefully for other complaints or findings that may require emergency treatment or transportation to a hospital setting. Paramedics must distinguish between signs (measured information such as pulse, respiration, and temperature) and symptoms (patient complaints). They must be able to take complete patient histories, document all medications, and transfer this information to medical control.

The vital role of the respiratory system is stressed in all paramedical training courses. The function of the respiratory system is to provide the body with oxygen and to eliminate carbon dioxide. Paramedics must fully understand the breathing process, including gas exchange and the role and anatomic position of the air passages and lungs. They must understand the mechanics of breathing—how the diaphragm and intercostal muscles contract and relax during inspiration and expiration—and must realize that breathing is controlled by the brain's response to levels of carbon dioxide and oxygen present in the arterial blood. Of special concern to the paramedic is the patient with COPD, who needs specialized oxygen support and careful watching.

Basic life support (BLS), formerly called cardiopulmonary resuscitation (CPR), is a series of emergency lifesaving procedures that are carried out in order to treat respiratory arrest, cardiac arrest, or both. CPR is a method of providing artificial ventilation and circulation. Its effectiveness depends on the prompt recognition of respiratory and/or cardiac arrest and the immediate start of treatment. Very often, the paramedic is able to defibrillate the patient immediately after cardiac arrest and restart the heart. Knowledge of how to provide BLS to the laryngectomy patient is part of

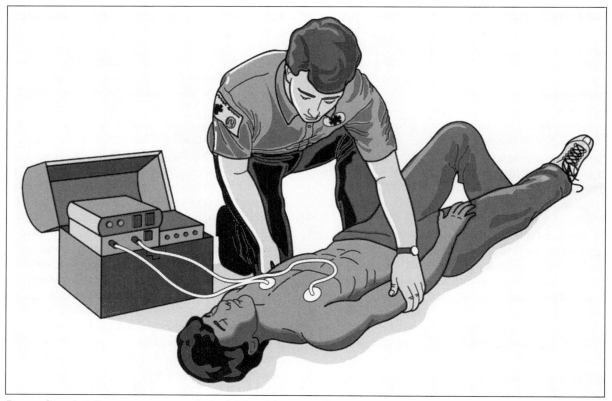

Paramedics administer emergency care in the field to sick or injured patients; among their primary tools are portable monitoring devices, such as an electrocardiograph (ECG or EKG) machine to check the electrical activity of the heart.

paramedic education; in such cases, ventilation is often given via a stoma (opening) in the neck of the patient. Basic life support procedures must be modified for infants and children, since their respiration and pulse rates are higher than those of adults and require more rapid delivery of ventilatory and cardiac assistance.

Although breathing and heart rate are the primary interests of the paramedic, serious bleeding can also be life-threatening. Hence, paramedics must be well versed in blood circulation routes, control of bleeding, and the pressure points that can help in the control of serious hemorrhage. Serious bleeding often brings on a type of shock that is termed hypovolemic (meaning low blood volume). Paramedics must be alert to signs of impending shock and deal with this condition as soon as possible. Medical antishock trousers (MAST) are often used by paramedics to autotransfuse volumes of blood from the patient's lower extremities to the heart, lungs, and brain. These trousers are also used to control severe hemorrhage or the complications of pelvic fractures. The paramedic must be aware of the contraindications to the use of these devices as well; for example, persons with head injuries should not have the MAST device applied to them.

Paramedics need to identify the many types of shock. Anaphylactic shock is caused by an unusual or exaggerated allergic reaction of a person to a foreign protein. Psychogenic shock (fainting) is often self-correcting. Septic shock is caused by severe bacterial infections, while metabolic shock may arise from severe, untreated illnesses. Cardiogenic shock arises from an underlying cardiac condition and inefficient blood flow. In each case, the paramedic must be alert to the signs of each type of shock and be prepared to treat it, either with drugs delivered under medical control or with equipment present on the paramedic ambulance.

The more common types of injuries encountered by the paramedic are soft tissue injuries, caused by falls or accidents. The skin is the largest single organ of the body. It protects the body from the environment, regulates the body temperature, and transmits information from the environment to the brain. Soft tissue injuries can cause breaks in the skin, leaving the body vulnerable to infection and bleeding. Paramedic training includes treatment for massive traumatic wounds, such as gunshot or knife wounds.

Dealing with fractures is another part of paramedic training. While most fractures are not life-threatening, they can be painful and bring on patient shock; hence, paramedics need to deal with them quickly. Knowledge of the body's musculoskeletal system is vital to the performance of a paramedic.

Head injuries are a very challenging part of paramedic treatment, since the scalp contains many blood vessels and bleeding from head injuries is often profuse. The more serious head injury is often bloodless externally, but internal bleeding brings on pressure buildup in the skull and sudden coma. Such injuries are life-threatening and often require rapid treatment and transport.

Other medical emergencies include strokes (cerebrovascular accidents), diabetic coma or insulin shock, acute abdominal infections, and seizures. Prompt recognition and treatment by the paramedic are essential. Finally, treating the pediatric patient can be one of the most difficult emergencies, but saving a child's life or rescuing a child from permanent, disabling injury is very rewarding. The broad range of knowledge required of paramedics makes them a very special part of the health care team.

DIAGNOSTIC AND TREATMENT TECHNIQUES

Three technologies that distinguish the paramedic from the basic EMT are intravenous therapy, advanced airway management, and defibrillation.

Intravenous (IV) therapy may be an important procedure during the resuscitation of a patient who is suffering from hypovolemia, burn injury, blood loss, heatstroke, shock, electrolyte imbalance, or many other medical and surgical conditions. IV therapy is also important in providing an avenue of medication delivery in many medical situations, such as cardiac arrest, seizures, and asthma attacks. IV therapy is an invasive procedure that requires extensive training in its use in order for the paramedic to maintain the necessary skill level. In addition, paramedics must be aware of the indication for the use of IV therapy, the maintenance of such therapy, and possible complications.

Infusion is the introduction of fluid other than blood or blood products into the vascular system. This technique is used to establish and maintain direct access to the circulation or to provide fluids in order to maintain an adequate circulating blood volume. Fluids used for IVs are often referred to as electrolyte solutions because the chemical compounds that they contain are electrolytes. The most common electrolyte solutions used are sodium chloride solutions; for example, NS is a normal saline solution containing 0.9 percent sodium chloride. Occasionally, paramedics use plasma expanders or colloids, including Dextran. A common intravenous fluid is D5W, which is a 5 percent dextrose solution. The procedure for starting an IV includes preparing the solution, selecting the proper catheter size, selecting and preparing the site, and performing the venipuncture. Local complications to IV therapy may include some pain from the needlestick, hematoma formation at failed IV sites, infection, accidental arterial puncture, nerve damage, and thrombophlebitis. Environmental complications include cold climates, which cause IV solutions to freeze, and the danger of a needlestick to medical personnel during disposal. Proper precautions and periodic retraining keep paramedics up to date in their skills.

Advanced airway management means placing a cylindrical tube into the patient's airway to maintain an open passage, to prevent aspiration of foreign bodies and stomach contents, and to allow the delivery of oxygen-enriched air. Three types of devices are employed in advanced airway management to achieve these objectives: the endotracheal tube (ENT), the esophageal obturator airway (EOA), and the pharyngeotracheal airway. The use of any of these devices by paramedics requires the consent of a medical director and adherence to written protocols. These devices require skill and instruction for proper insertion and use.

The ENT is placed through a patient's mouth or nose and directly through the larynx between the vocal cords. The tube may be placed blindly through the vocal cords using sounds of labored respirations as a guide, or it may be placed by feel through the cords. After placement, a soft balloon cuff near the end of the tube is then inflated with approximately 10 cubic centimeters of air to seal the trachea and anchor the tube, so that air can be blown directly into the lungs. The ENT prevents aspiration and gastric distension. It facilitates airway suctioning and enables the delivery of high volumes of oxygen at higher-than-normal pressures. In addition, certain medications may be given down the tube. ENT placement and use are difficult skills to master, requiring considerable practice and expert initial instruction. Direct visualization of the vocal cords is an important skill to have in order to prevent tracheal damage. If intubation takes too long, the resulting delay in oxygenation may lead to brain damage. Constant monitoring of lung sounds is needed to ensure that the tube stays in place.

The EOA has been in use since 1973 to facilitate airway management in cardiopulmonary resuscitation. The EOA is a plastic, semirigid tube 34 centimeters long and 13 millimeters in diameter. The lower end of the tube is smooth, rounded, and closed. The upper one-third of the EOA is designed to function as an airway. It has sixteen holes in its wall at the junction of the middle and upper sections; when properly inserted, these holes will lie at the level of the pharynx and provide free passage of oxygen-enriched air to the lungs. The lower two-thirds of the EOA should lie in the esophagus. The balloon surrounding the end of the tube is normally inflated to block the esophagus and prevent the regurgitation of stomach contents backward into the airway. The face mask that comes with the EOA is designed to fit snugly about the patient's nose and mouth and must provide a tight seal. The EOA is used only for short-term airway management. It should be removed when the unconscious patient awakens and is able to protect the airway or when ENT placement has been performed over the EOA. At the time that the balloon is deflated and the EOA is removed, there is a high risk of vomiting and/or regurgitation of gastric contents. The EOA is not to be used on patients who are awake, on small children, or on patients with known esophageal disease.

The pharyngeotracheal airway is designed to provide lung ventilation when placed in either the trachea or the esophagus. This device is designed to be inserted blindly into the oropharynx and esophagus by paramedics who have received training and are authorized to use it. A pharyngeotracheal airway is contraindicated in conscious or semiconscious patients with a gag reflex. It should not be used with children under the age of fourteen or with adults under five feet tall.

With the use of any of these airway devices, the patient may regain consciousness while intubated. Such patients will usually gag, choke, and grasp at the device in an attempt to remove it, often resulting in injury to the airway. The patient's hands must be immediately restrained while the airway device is removed.

Defibrillation is the delivery of an electric current through a person's chest wall and heart for the purpose of ending ventricular fibrillation. The device used for this procedure is called a defibrillator; it is typically a portable, battery-powered instrument that is used to record cardiac rhythm and to generate and deliver an electrical charge. Defibrillation can be a lifesaving measure in the treatment of sudden cardiac arrest in which the heart is in an arrhythmia known as ventricular fibrillation or ventricular tachycardia (VT). These two conditions occur when cardiac muscle becomes oxygen deficient or is injured or dies, causing the electrical system of the heart to be disturbed. Sometimes, the injured area of the heart begins to fire off uncoordinated electrical impulses. These irregular impulses can initiate abnormal beats called premature ventricular contractions (PVCs). If several of the PVCs occur close together, they produce the rhythm called ventricular tachycardia. If VT does not spontaneously convert back to a normal heart rhythm, it rapidly degenerates into ventricular fibrillation. The heart in VT beats faster and faster until its oxygen supply is depleted, at which point tissue injury begins and electrical impulses become completely uncoordinated and are fired at random.

If a defibrillator is applied to the patient and an electrical shock is given to the heart during the time of ventricular fibrillation, there is a good chance of restoring more normal electrical activity. This electrical countershock is thought to depolarize the cardiac muscle and conducting tissues instantaneously, thus resetting the electrical energies to the depolarized state. The patient's heart can then begin its normal conduction and contractions without having to contend with randomly generated electrical impulses. The electrical current delivered by defibrillators is measured in units called joules. In most protocols, the first shock is 200 joules, the second is between 200 and 300 joules, and the third and subsequent shocks are at the full 360-joule level. Paramedics using defibrillators need frequent continuing education in order to emphasize the practical skills of proper attachment of the electrodes, proper device operation, and recognition of cardiac arrhythmias.

PERSPECTIVE AND PROSPECTS

Emergency medical services (EMS) in the United States had its beginnings in 1966. In that year, the Committees on Trauma and Shock of the National Academy of Sciences National Research Council jointly published *Accidental Death and Disability: The Neglected Disease of Modern Society.* This joint report brought public attention to the inadequate emergency medical care being provided to the injured and sick in many parts of the United States. Two federal agencies initiated reform measures: The Department of Transportation (DOT) initiated the Highway Safety Act in 1966, and the Department of Health, Education, and Welfare enacted the Emergency Medical Services Act in 1973. Both created funding sources to develop prehospital emergency care in an effort to eliminate the majority of prehospital deaths. Local EMS systems were established in the early 1970's. In the 1980's, practitioners took a hard look at what had been done in the past, and

the focus changed from establishing EMS systems to developing educational programs to provide consistent levels of quality care to the sick and injured.

The EMS system is made up of various components that work together to provide the sick and injured with the best possible emergency care in the shortest possible time. The EMS system represents the combined efforts of the first responder, the EMT with basic life support skills, the EMT-paramedic with advanced life support skills, emergency department personnel, physicians, allied health personnel, hospital administrators, EMS system administrators, and the overseeing governmental agencies.

Emergency medical technology is an exciting field of study. Few areas offer more direct application of theory and skills. All the information received in an EMT class will be important when it comes to saving lives and lessening human suffering. Emergency medical technology combines theoretical information, practical skills, and common sense. Above all, the EMS person dealing with a patient must possess great compassion and understanding.

The certification of an EMT-paramedic is formal notice of certain privileges and abilities after the completion of specific training and testing. The possession of a certificate obligates the individual to conform to the standard of care of other certified emergency medical care personnel. Nearly every state exempts emergency medical care from the licensure requirements of the Medical Practices Act for nonmedical personnel. (Because many emergency medical care procedures may be construed by the public to be the performance of a medical act, the EMT must be protected legally in those situations.) The need for prehospital care providers is ongoing, and recruiting people to enter this field continues to be a challenge to the agencies that oversee this work.

—*Jane A. Slezak, Ph.D.*

See also Accidents; Arrhythmias; Burns and scalds; Cardiac arrest; Cardiopulmonary resuscitation (CPR); Choking; Critical care; Critical care, pediatric; Drowning; Electrocardiography (ECG or EKG); Emergency medicine; First aid; Fracture and dislocation; Heart attack; Heat exhaustion and heatstroke; Intravenous (IV) therapy; Respiration; Resuscitation; Shock; Strokes; Tracheostomy; Wounds.

FOR FURTHER INFORMATION:

American Academy of Orthopaedic Surgeons. *Emergency Care and Transportation of the Sick and In-*

jured. Edited by Benjamin Gulli, Les Chatelain, and Chris Stratford. 9th ed. Sudbury, Mass.: Jones and Bartlett, 2005. A text covering both basic and advanced life support procedures for the EMT and the EMT-paramedic. Contains many illustrative diagrams.

Copass, Michael K., Mickey S. Eisenberg, and Steven C. Macdonald. *The Paramedic Manual*. 2d ed. Philadelphia: W. B. Saunders, 1987. This volume in the Saunders Blue Books series examines the function of the emergency medical technician and the paramedic, addressing the skills and knowledge that are required of these individuals. Includes an index.

Hamilton, Glenn C., et al. *Emergency Medicine: An Approach to Clinical Problem-Solving*. 2d ed. New York: W. B. Saunders, 2003. Addressed to students of medicine, this text provides a detailed, well-written script for the clinical setting. Facilitates the reader's understanding of the emergency scene. Actual medical cases are integrated into the chapters in order to reinforce concepts.

Limmer, Daniel, et al. *Emergency Care*. 11th ed. Upper Saddle River, N.J.: Pearson/Prentice Hall Health, 2009. This simple text has been acclaimed for its comprehensive, accurate, and up-to-the-minute treatment of emergency care. Easy to read, this book provides the contemporary standards on CPR from the American Heart Association and a full treatment on many emergency medical protocols for prehospital treatment.

Markovchick, Vincent J., and Peter T. Pons, eds. *Emergency Medicine Secrets*. 4th ed. Philadelphia: Mosby/Elsevier, 2006. Details all aspects of emergency medicine in a question-and-answer format. Topics include nontraumatic illness, hematology/oncology, infectious disease, environmental emergencies, neonatal and childhood disorders, toxicologic emergencies, emergency medicine administration and risk management, and disaster management.

Rella, Francis J. *Manhattan Medics: The Gripping Story of the Men and Women of Emergency Medical Services Who Make the Streets of the City Their Career*. Hightstown, N.J.: Princeton Book Company, 2003. The author, a registered EMT-P serving in New York City, gives a firsthand account of the emergency response to the terrorist attacks on the World Trade Center in 2001 and, in the process, sheds light on the "turf wars" between the city's paramedics and fire department personnel.

Sanders, Mick J. *Mosby's Paramedic Textbook*. Rev. ed. St. Louis, Mo.: Mosby/Elsevier, 2007. Designed to help students pass their exams, this text nonetheless offers valuable information for the layperson on the paramedic's role, characteristics of prehospital care, patient assessment and emergency care for acutely ill and traumatically injured patients, and the principles and practice of emergency cardiac care, emergency pharmacology, care of infectious diseases, and pediatric and geriatric emergencies.

Shapiro, Paul D., and Mary B. Shapiro. *Paramedic: The True Story of a New York Paramedic's Battles with Life and Death*. New York: Bantam Books, 1991. Paul Shapiro recounts his experiences in the field as a paramedic. A valuable firsthand account of the profession.

Tangherlini, Timothy R. *Talking Trauma: Paramedics and Their Stories*. Jackson: University Press of Mississippi, 1998. Tangherlini, a folklorist, reports the stories told by Alameda County, California, paramedics and explores what roles the stories play in their self-conceptions and their relations with colleagues and supervisors.

PARANOIA

DISEASE/DISORDER

ANATOMY OR SYSTEM AFFECTED: Psychic-emotional system

SPECIALTIES AND RELATED FIELDS: Psychiatry, psychology

DEFINITION: Pervasive distrust and suspiciousness of others and a tendency to interpret others' motives as malevolent.

CAUSES AND SYMPTOMS

Paranoia is characterized by suspiciousness, heightened self-awareness, self-reference, projection of one's ideas onto others, expectations of persecution, and blaming of others for one's difficulties. Conversely, though paranoia can be problematic, it can also be adaptive. In threatening or dangerous situations, paranoia might instigate proactive protective behavior, allowing an individual to negotiate a situation without harm. Thus, paranoia must be assessed in context for it to be understood fully.

Paranoia can be experienced at varying levels of intensity in both normal and highly disordered individuals. As a medical problem, paranoia may take the face of a symptom, personality problem, or chronic mental disorder. As a symptom, it may be evidenced as a fleeting problem; an individual might have paranoid feelings that dissipate in a relatively brief period of time once an acute medical or situational problem is rectified.

As a personality problem, paranoia creates significant impairment and distress as a result of inflexible, maladaptive, and persistent use of paranoid coping strategies. Paranoid individuals often have preoccupations about loyalties, overinterpret situations, maintain expectations of exploitation or deceit, rarely confide in others, bear grudges, perceive attacks that are not apparent to others, and maintain unjustified suspicions about their relationship partner's potential for betrayal. They are prone to angry outbursts, aloof, and controlling, and they may demonstrate a tendency toward vengeful fantasies or actual revenge.

Finally, paranoia may be evidenced as a chronic mental disorder, most notably as the paranoid type of schizophrenia. In paranoid schizophrenia, there is a tendency toward delusions (faulty beliefs involving misinterpretations of events) and auditory hallucinations. Additionally, everyday behavior, speech, and emotional responsiveness are not as disturbed as in other variants of schizophrenia. Typically, individuals suffering from paranoia are seen by others as anxious, angry, and aloof. Their delusions usually reflect fears of persecution or hopes for greatness, resulting in jealousies, odd religious beliefs (such as persecution by God, thinking they are Jesus Christ), or preoccupations with their own health (such as the fear of being poisoned or of having a medical disorder of mysterious origin).

Paranoia may best be understood as being determined by a combination of biological, psychological,

and environmental factors. It is likely, for example, that certain basic psychological tendencies must be present for an individual to display paranoid feelings and behavior when under stress, as opposed to other feelings such as depression. Additionally, it is likely that certain physical predispositions must be present for stressors to provoke a psychophysiological response.

Biologically, there are myriad physical and mental health conditions that may trigger acute and more chronic paranoid reactions. High levels of situational stress, drug intoxication (such as with amphetamines or marijuana), drug withdrawal, depression, head injuries, organic brain syndromes, pernicious anemia, B vitamin deficiencies, and Klinefelter syndrome may be related to acute paranoia. Similarly, certain cancers, insidious organic brain syndromes, and hyperparathyroidism have been related to recurrent or chronic episodes of paranoia.

In terms of the etiology of chronic paranoid conditions, such as paranoid schizophrenia and paranoid personality disorder, no clear causes have been identified. Some evidence points to a genetic component; the results of studies on twins and the greater prevalence of these disorders in some families support this view. More psychological theories highlight the family environment and emotional expression, childhood abuse, and stress. In general, these theories point to conditions contributing toward making a person feel insecure, tense, hungry for recognition, and hypervigilant. Additionally, the impact of social, cultural, and economic conditions contributing to the expression of paranoia is important. Paranoia cannot be interpreted out of context. Biological, psychological, and environmental factors must be considered in the development and maintenance of paranoia.

TREATMENT AND THERAPY

Three major types of therapies are available to treat paranoia: pharmacotherapies, community-based therapies, and cognitive-behavioral therapies. For acute paranoia problems and the management of more chronic, schizophrenia-related paranoia, pharmacotherapy (the use of drugs) is the treatment of choice. Drugs that serve to tranquilize the individual and reduce disorganized thinking, such as phenothiazines and other neuroleptics, are commonly used. With elderly people who cannot tolerate such drugs, electroconvulsive therapy (ECT) has been used for treatment.

Community-based treatment, such as day treatment or inpatient treatment, is also useful for treating chronic

---

INFORMATION ON PARANOIA

CAUSES: May include psychological disorder (depression, schizophrenia), situational stress, drug intoxication or withdrawal, head injury, organic brain syndromes, pernicious anemia, B vitamin deficiencies, Klinefelter syndrome

SYMPTOMS: Pervasive distrust and suspiciousness of others, tendency to interpret others' motives as malevolent, aloofness, heightened self-awareness, self-reference, blaming of others for one's difficulties, angry outbursts, controlling behavior

DURATION: Acute to chronic

TREATMENTS: Drug therapy, community-based therapy, cognitive and behavioral therapies

paranoid conditions. Developing corrective and instructional social experiences, decreasing situational stress, and helping individuals to feel safe in a treatment environment are primary goals.

Finally, cognitive-behavioral therapies focused on identifying irrational beliefs contributing to paranoia-related problems have demonstrated some utility. Skillful therapists help to identify maladaptive thinking while unearthing concerns but not agreeing with the individual's delusional ideas.

PERSPECTIVE AND PROSPECTS

Certain life phases and social and cultural contexts influence behaviors that could be labeled as paranoid. Membership in certain minority or ethnic groups, immigrant or political refugee status, and, more generally, language and other cultural barriers may account for behavior that appears to be guarded or paranoid. As such, one can make few assumptions about paranoia without a thorough assessment.

Clinically significant paranoia is notable across cultures, with prevalence rates at any point in time ranging from 0.5 to 2.5 percent of the population. It is a problem manifested by diverse etiological courses requiring equally diverse treatments. Increased knowledge about the relationship among paranoia, depression and other mood disorders, schizophrenia, and the increased prevalence of paranoid disorders in some families will be critical. As the general population ages, a better understanding of more acute paranoid disorders related to medical problems will also be necessary. Better understanding will facilitate the development of more effective pharmacological and nonpharmacological treatments that can be tolerated by the elderly and others suffering from compromising medical problems.

—*Nancy A. Piotrowski, Ph.D.*

See also Antianxiety drugs; Anxiety; Delusions; Hallucinations; Post-traumatic stress disorder; Psychiatric disorders; Psychiatry; Psychiatry, child and adolescent; Psychiatry, geriatric; Psychoanalysis; Schizophrenia; Shock therapy; Stress.

FOR FURTHER INFORMATION:

Barlow, David H., ed. *Clinical Handbook of Psychological Disorders*. 4th ed. New York: Guilford Press, 2008. This collection defines and describes psychological disorders and uses case histories as illustrations for treatment.

Bloom, Floyd E., M. Flint Beal, and David J. Kupfer, eds. *The Dana Guide to Brain Health*. New York: Dana Press, 2006. An easy-to-understand health guide to the brain from neuroscience, neurology, and psychiatry perspectives. More than seventy psychiatric and neurological disorders, their diagnoses, and their treatments are covered.

Kring, Ann M., et al. *Abnormal Psychology*. 11th ed. Hoboken, N.J.: John Wiley & Sons, 2010. This college text addresses the causes of psychopathology and treatments commonly used to treat various disorders. The book is well organized, readable, and interesting. An extensive reference list and a glossary are included.

Munro, Alistair. *Delusional Disorder: Paranoia and Related Illnesses*. New York: Cambridge University Press, 1999. Discusses the various subtypes of delusional disorders, such as the somatic, jealous, erotomanic, persecutory/litigious, and grandiose subtypes. Also discusses treatments.

Robbins, Michael. *Experiences of Schizophrenia: An Integration of the Personal, Scientific, and Therapeutic*. New York: Guilford Press, 1993. Discusses such topics as the psychological system, the family system, society and culture, and the treatment of schizophrenia and includes a number of case studies.

Siegel, Ronald K. *Whispers: The Voices of Paranoia*. New York: Simon & Schuster, 1996. In a mesmerizing journey into mental illness, the author captures the suspicion, terror, and rage that possess the minds of paranoids.

PARAPLEGIA

DISEASE/DISORDER

ANATOMY OR SYSTEM AFFECTED: Legs, nervous system, spine

SPECIALTIES AND RELATED FIELDS: Neurology

DEFINITION: A motor or sensory loss in the lower extremities, with or without involvement of the abdominal and back muscles.

CAUSES AND SYMPTOMS

Paraplegia, the loss of motor and sensory function in the lower body, results in paralysis that may be complete or incomplete, spastic or flaccid, symmetric or asymmetric, and permanent or temporary. Almost half of the 10,000 to 12,000 spinal cord injuries reported each year result in paraplegia. This condition occurs twice as often in men as in women, and the incidence is highest between ages sixteen and thirty-five. Most spinal cord injuries result from trauma, especially automobile, motorcycle, and sporting accidents; gunshot wounds and falls also contribute. Less common causes are nontraumatic lesions, such as spina bifida, scoliosis, and chordoma.

In many patients, the onset of total or partial paralysis is immediate, resulting in loss of motion, sensation, and reflexes below the level of the lesion, with urinary retention and absence of perspiration in the paralyzed parts. In some patients, careful questioning and gentle examination are necessary to determine the extent of motor or sensory loss. Spinal cord injuries with motor and sensory loss may result in bowel, bladder, and sexual dysfunctions, depending on the level of the lesion and whether damage to the cord is complete or incomplete. In an incomplete spinal cord injury, perianal sensation, voluntary toe flexion, or sphincter control is still present. In a complete spinal cord injury, lack of sensation or voluntary muscle control is apparent and persists for twenty-four hours. Any return of functional muscle power distal to the injury is unlikely.

Diagnosis requires a clinical history, neurologic examination, and computed tomography (CT) scans. A lumbar puncture may rule out blocked cerebrospinal fluid circulation. Laboratory studies include a complete blood count (CBC), prothrombin time, electrolytes, twenty-four-hour urine for creatinine clearance, serum creatinine, and urinalysis. Weekly urine samples for culture and sensitivity are advisable during the entire rehabilitation period.

TREATMENT AND THERAPY

The four goals of treatment for any spinal cord injury are restoration of normal alignment for the spine, early insurance of complete stability of the injured spinal area, decompression of compressed neurologic structures, and early rehabilitation to an active and productive life.

Treatment begins at the scene of the accident by not moving the patient until the spine and head have been stabilized through strapping the patient to a board. Even after reaching the hospital, the patient is not removed from the board but placed on a stretcher while still strapped to it. Such stabilization helps prevent reversible damage from becoming permanent through additional injury to the neuraxis. Supportive treatment corrects systemic shock and controls local hemorrhage. Insertion of a Foley catheter insures uninterrupted urine drainage.

Whenever possible, the care of spinal cord injuries emphasizes conservative treatment, such as closed reduction of fractures. However, unstable fractures and

---

INFORMATION ON PARAPLEGIA

CAUSES: Spinal cord injuries, usually resulting from vehicle or sporting accidents, gunshot wounds, falls

SYMPTOMS: Total or partial paralysis with loss of motion, sensation, and reflexes below lesion; urinary retention; absence of perspiration in paralyzed parts

DURATION: Permanent or temporary

TREATMENTS: Spinal alignment and stabilization, laminectomy, drug therapy (nitrofurantoin, vitamin C, analgesics and narcotics)

---

fracture dislocations require fusion following reduction, combined with recumbent immobilization until healing occurs. Bone fragments pressing on the spinal cord may require laminectomy (surgical removal of the vertebral arch). Drug therapy may include nitrofurantoin to prevent bladder infection; large doses of vitamin C to enhance utilization of protein and help minimize infection by acidifying the urine; diazepam, baclofen, or dantrolene sodium to relieve skeletal muscle spasms from upper motor neuron disorders; and, sparingly, analgesics and narcotics to relieve pain. The extent of paralysis cannot be accurately assessed until a year after the spinal cord injury.

—*Jane C. Norman, Ph.D., R.N., C.N.E.*

See also Accidents; Emergency medicine; Hemiplegia; Laminectomy and spinal fusion; Nervous system; Neuralgia, neuritis, and neuropathy; Neuroimaging; Neurology; Neurology, pediatric; Paralysis; Physical rehabilitation; Quadriplegia; Spinal cord disorders; Spine, vertebrae, and disks.

FOR FURTHER INFORMATION:

Asbury, Arthur K., et al., eds. *Diseases of the Nervous System: Clinical Neuroscience and Therapeutic Principles.* 3d ed. New York: Cambridge University Press, 2002.

Bromley, Ida. *Tetraplegia and Paraplegia: A Guide for Physiotherapists.* 6th ed. New York: Churchill Livingstone/Elsevier, 2006.

Rowland, Lewis P., ed. *Merritt's Textbook of Neurology.* 12th ed. Philadelphia: Lippincott Williams & Wilkins, 2010.

Victor, Maurice, and Allan H. Ropper. *Adams and Victor's Principles of Neurology.* 9th ed. New York: McGraw-Hill, 2009.

Parasitic diseases
Disease/disorder

Anatomy or system affected: All

Specialties and related fields: Environmental health, epidemiology, family medicine, internal medicine, public health, virology

Definition: Diseases borne by parasites, or organisms that live within "host" organisms; parasites travel to their hosts via vectors that may include fleas, mosquitoes, rats, and other animals.

Key terms:

commensalism: a relationship in which one symbiont, the commensal, benefits from a host symbiont, but the host neither benefits nor is harmed by the commensal

host: a living plant or animal harboring or affording subsistence to a parasite

hyperparasitism: a relationship in which parasites act as hosts to other parasites

mutualism: a relationship between symbionts in which both members benefit from the association

parasitism: a relationship in which one symbiont, a parasite, harms its host symbiont or in some way lives at the expense of the host

phoresis: when two symbionts "travel together" but neither is physiologically dependent on the other

symbiont: any organism involved in a symbiotic relationship with another organism

symbiosis: a relationship in which two symbionts live in close association with each other; commonly, one symbiont lives in or on the body of the other

TYPES OF PARASITES

Parasites are organisms that take up residence, temporarily or permanently, on or within other living organisms for the purpose of procuring food. They include plants such as bacteria and fungi; animals such as protozoa, helminths (worms), and arthropods; and forms such as spirochetes and microscopic viruses.

The study of parasitism is a study of symbiosis. Symbiosis occurs when two organisms, known as symbionts, live in close association with each other, usually with one organism living in or on the body of the other. Such a living arrangement is called a symbiotic relationship. In a symbiotic relationship, the symbionts are usually, but not always, of different species, and the relationship need not be beneficial or damaging to either organism.

Often, two symbionts will exist together merely as traveling companions. Such a symbiotic relationship is called phoresis. In such cases, neither partner is physio-

logically dependent on the other, but the smaller of the two organisms has simply attached itself for the ride. Examples of phoresis are bacteria carried on the legs of a cockroach and fungus spores on the feet of ants and beetles.

If a situation exists in which both symbionts benefit from an association, the partnership is referred to as a mutual relationship. In most cases, mutualism is obligatory because both symbionts have evolved to a point at which they are physiologically dependent on each other and the survival of both symbionts requires a continuous interrelationship. Such a relationship exists between termites and the protozoan fauna that live in their guts. Termites are unable to digest cellulose fibers, because their bodies cannot produce the proper enzyme, but protozoa that live in a termite's gut synthesize the ingested cellulose fibers and excrete a fermented product that nourishes the host termite. The protozoa benefit by living in a stable, secure environment, with a constant supply of food, and the termite is supplied with sustenance.

Another form of mutualism that is not obligatory is called cleaning symbiosis. In this instance, certain animals, called cleaners, remove other parasites, injured tissues, fungi, or invading organisms from a cooperating host. Examples of cleaning relationships include birds that groom the skins of rhinoceroses and the mouths of crocodiles, and tiny shrimp that remove parasites from the body surfaces of fish.

When one symbiont benefits from its relationship with its host but the host neither benefits nor is harmed, the condition is called commensalism. Examples of commensals are pilot fish and remoras, which attach themselves to turtles or other fish, using their hosts as transportation and scavenging food left over when the hosts eat; in no way, however, do they harm their hosts or rob them of food. Another example of commensalism exists between humans and the amoeba

---

INFORMATION ON PARASITIC DISEASES

Causes: Infection with parasites, often through vectors

Symptoms: Wide ranging; may include fever, malaise, vomiting, inflammation, joint pain, muscle aches, diarrhea

Duration: Acute to chronic

Treatments: Drug therapy, supportive care

Entamoeba gingivalis. This amoeba lives in the human mouth, feeding on bacteria, food particles, and dead epithelial cells, but it never harms its human host. The amoeba is transmitted from person to person by direct contact and cannot exist outside the human mouth.

When one member of a symbiotic relationship actually harms its host or in some way lives at the expense of the host, it is then a parasite. The word "parasite" is derived from the Greek *parasitos,* which means "one who eats at another's table" or "one who lives at another's expense." A parasite may harm its host by causing a mechanical injury, such as boring a hole into it; by eating, digesting, or absorbing portions of the host's tissue; by poisoning the host with toxic metabolic products; or by robbing the host of nutrition. It has been found that most parasites inflict a combination of these conditions.

The majority of parasites are obligate parasites—that is, they must spend at least a portion of their lives as parasites to survive and complete their life cycles. Most of these obligate parasites have free-living stages outside their hosts in which they exist in protective cysts or eggs. Certain symbionts are referred to as facultative parasites, which means that the organism is not normally parasitic, but if the proper situation arises, it becomes a parasite. The most common facultative parasites are those that are accidentally eaten or enter a host through a wound or body orifice. One facultative parasite whose infection of humans is almost always fatal is the amoeba *Naegleria,* which is responsible for amebic meningitis. Many obligate parasites are also hyperparasites. Hyperparasitism exists when parasites play host to other parasites; for example, the malaria-causing parasite *Plasmodia* is carried in mosquitoes, and juvenile tapeworms live in fleas.

Parasites that live their entire adult lives within or on their hosts are called permanent parasites. Other parasites, such as mosquitoes and ticks, are called temporary parasites because they feed on their hosts and then leave. Temporary parasites are actually micropredators that prey on different hosts, or on the same host at different times, as the need for nourishment arises. There are many parallels between parasitism and predation in that both parasites and predators live at the expense of their hosts or prey. Parasites, however, do not normally kill their hosts, because to do so results in their own death. It is the mark of a well-adapted parasite to produce as few pathological conditions in the host as possible.

Despite the knowledge that parasites are a major cause of disease, it is wrong to assume that an animal hosting a parasite must ultimately be in danger. The healthiest human or wild animal is probably harboring some type of parasite, and while the host and parasite may live for years without interfering in each other's existence, at any given time, the healthy host can fall victim to a disease brought on by the parasite, or some change in the host may destroy the parasite.

Whether the host reacts to its symbiotic partner with indifference, annoyance, or illness is the result of many factors. The most important is how many parasites are being hosted. A single hookworm takes approximately 0.5 milliliter of blood per day from its host. This is about the same amount of blood lost when one pricks oneself with a needle. This amount of blood loss is so low that the host will never miss it and, in most instances, will not even know that the parasite is there. If a host harbors five hundred hookworms, however, the blood loss per day becomes 250 milliliters, approximately one half pint, and the result is physically devastating to the host.

CAUSES AND SYMPTOMS

Medical parasitology is the study of human diseases caused by parasitic infection. It is commonly limited to the study of parasitic worms (helminths) and protozoa. The science places nonprotozoan parasites in separate disciplines, such as virology, rickettsiology, and bacteriology. The branches of parasitology known as medical entomology and medical arthropodology deal with insects and noninsect arthropods that serve as hosts and transport agents for parasites, as well as with the noxious effects of these pests. The study of fungi (molds and yeasts), including those that cause human disease, is called mycology.

Throughout history, human welfare has suffered greatly because of parasites. Fleas and bacteria killed one-third of the human population of Europe during the seventeenth century, and malaria, schistosomiasis, and African sleeping sickness have killed additional countless millions. Despite successful medical campaigns against yellow fever, malaria, and hookworm infections worldwide, parasitic diseases in combination with nutritional deficiencies are the primary killers of humans. Medical research suggests that parasitic infections are so widespread that if all the known varieties were evenly distributed among the human population, each living person would have at least one.

Most serious parasitic infections occur in tropical, less modernized regions of the world, and because most of the planet's industrially developed and affluent populations live in temperate regions, many people are unaware of the magnitude of the problem. On an annual ba-

Common Human Parasites

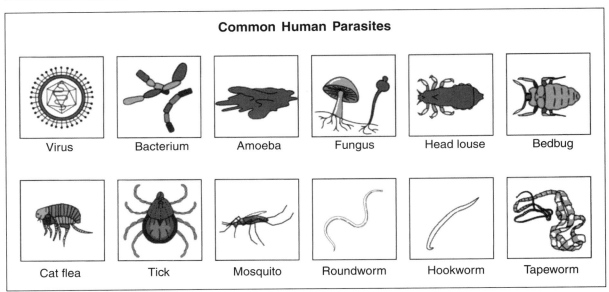

Virus	Bacterium	Amoeba	Fungus	Head louse	Bedbug
Cat flea	Tick	Mosquito	Roundworm	Hookworm	Tapeworm

Any organism that, temporarily or permanently, lives on or in another organism for the purpose of procuring food is considered a parasite; these parasites may cause infection in their human hosts.

sis, 60 million deaths occur worldwide from all causes; of these deaths, half are children under five years of age. Fifty percent of these, 15 million child deaths per year, are directly attributable to a combination of malnutrition and intestinal parasitic infection. It must be noted that less than 15 percent of the world's present population is served by adequate clean water supplies and sewage disposal programs, and that almost all intestinal parasitic infections are the result of ingesting food or water contaminated with human feces.

The transmission of parasitic diseases involves three factors: the source of the infection, the mode of transmission, and the presence of a susceptible host. The combined effect of these factors determines the dispersibility and prevalence of a parasite at a given time and place, thus regulating the incidence of a parasitic disease in a population. Because of host specificity, other humans are the chief source of most human parasitic diseases. The various manifestations of any human parasitic disease are a result of the particular species of parasite involved, its mode of transport, the immunological status of the host, the presence or absence of hosts, and the pattern of exposure.

Humans transmit parasitic diseases to one another through the intestinal tract, nose and mouth, skin and tissue, genitourinary tract, and blood. It is fecal discharge, however, that offers the most convenient and common means for a parasite or its ova and larvae to leave its host, since the majority of parasites inhabit the gastrointesti-

nal tract. For this reason, the proper disposal of fecal material is the most important method of preventing the spread of parasitic disease. Since most parasites inhabit the intestinal tract, food and water are also important means of transmitting parasitic infections. The infective organism may be present in contaminated drinking water, in animal and fish flesh used as food, in human feces used as fertilizer, or on the hands of food handlers.

Arthropods are one of the main sources of parasitic diseases in humans. Arthropods act as both mechanical carriers of and intermediate hosts to many diseases—bacterial, viral, rickettsial, and parasitic—which they transmit to humans. In most tropical countries, basic preventive medicine for many devastating parasitic diseases depends on the control or eradication of insects and arachnids.

There are four major groups of parasites that most often invade human hosts: nematodes, trematodes, cestodes, and protozoa. Most nematodes, or roundworms, are free-living, and nematodes are found in almost every terrestrial and aquatic environment. Most are harmless to humans, but some parasitic nematodes invade the human intestinal tract and cause widespread debilitating diseases. The most prevalent intestinal nematodes are *Ascaris lumbricoides*, which infect the small intestine and affects more than a billion people; the whipworm *Trichuris trichiura*, which infects the colon and is carried by an estimated 500 million individuals; the human hookworms *Necator americanus* and *An-*

cylostoma duodenale, which suck blood from the human small intestine and cause major debilitation among undernourished people; and *Enterobius vermicularis*, the human pinworm, which infects the large intestine and is common among millions of urban dwellers because it is easily transmitted from perianal tissue to hand to mouth.

Nonintestinal, tissue-infecting nematodes are spread most often by hyperparasitic bloodsucking insects such as mosquitoes, biting flies, and midges. The most common tissue-infecting nematode is *Trichinella spiralis*, the pork or trichina worm, which is the agent of trichinosis. Other important parasitic nematodes include *Onchocerca volvulus*, which is transmitted by blackflies in tropical regions and causes blindness, and the mosquito-transmitted filarial worms that are responsible for elephantiasis.

Trematodes, or flatworms, are commonly called flukes. Flukes vary greatly in size, form, and host living location, but all of them initially develop in freshwater snails. The human intestinal fluke, the oriental liver fluke, and the human lung fluke are all transmitted to humans by the ingestion of raw or undercooked aquatic vegetables, fish, or crustaceans. An important group of trematodes consists of the blood flukes of the genus *Schistosoma*, which enter the body through skin/water contact and are responsible for schistosomiasis.

Cestodes, commonly called tapeworms, are parasitic flatworms that parasitize almost all vertebrates, and as many as eight species are found in humans. The two most common cestodes—*Taenia saginata*, the beef tapeworm, and *Taenia solium*, the pork tapeworm—are transmitted to humans by infected beef or pork products obtained from livestock that grazed in fields contaminated by human feces, or by contaminated water. The resulting disease, cysticercosis, which is potentially lethal, develops mostly in the brain, eye, and muscle tissue. Another animal-transmitted cestode is the dog tapeworm, *Echinococcus granulosus*, which dogs ingest by eating contaminated sheep viscera and then pass on to humans, who ingest the parasite's eggs after petting or handling an infected dog. The human infestation of *E. granulosus* results in hydatid disease. Probably the most dramatic of the cestode parasites is the gigantic tapeworm *Diphyllobothrium latum*, which may reach a length of 10 meters and a width of 2 centimeters. This tapeworm is transmitted to humans by the ingestion of raw or undercooked fish. This tapeworm, like most cestodes, can be effectively treated and killed by drugs, but if the worm merely breaks, leaving the head and anterior segments attached, it can regenerate its original body length in less than four months.

Protozoa that can infect human hosts are found in the intestinal tract, various tissues and organs, and the bloodstream. Of the many varieties of protozoa that can live in the human intestinal tract, only *Entamoeba histolytica* causes serious disease. This parasite, which is ingested in water contaminated by human feces, is responsible for the disease amebiasis, also known as amebic dysentery. A less serious, though common, waterborne intestinal protozoan is *Giardia lamblia*, which causes giardiasis, a common diarrheal infection among campers who ingest water fouled by animal waste.

Another group of protozoa parasites specializes in infecting the human skin, bloodstream, brain, and viscera. *Trypanosoma brucei*, carried by the African tsetse fly, causes the blood disease trypanosomiasis (African sleeping sickness). In Latin America, infection by the protozoa *Trypanosoma cruzi* results when the liquid feces of the reduviid bug is rubbed or scratched into the skin; it causes Chagas' disease, which produces often fatal lesions of the heart and brain. Members of the protozoan genus *Leishmania* are transmitted by midges and sandflies, and their parasitic infestation manifests in long-lasting dermal lesions and ulcers; the destruction of nasal mucous, cartilage, and pharyngeal tissues; or in the disease kala-azar, resulting in the destruction of bone marrow, lymph nodes, and liver and spleen tissue.

Two other types of protozoa are parasitic to humans. The first is the ciliate protozoa, which are mostly free-living, and of which only a single species, *Balantidium coli*, is parasitic in humans. This species is responsible for balantidiasis, an ulcerative disease. The second is the sporozoans, all of which are parasitic. Many species of sporozoans are harmful to humans, the most important being *Plasmodium*, the agent of malaria. The sporozoan parasite *Toxoplasma gondii*, the agent of toxoplasmosis, is responsible for encephalomyelitis and chorioretinitis in infants and children and is thought to infect as much as 20 percent of the world's population. *Pneumocystis* pneumonia, a major cause of death among persons with acquired immunodeficiency syndrome (AIDS), was formerly considered a result of sporozoan infection but is now thought to be fungal.

PERSPECTIVE AND PROSPECTS

Because of their size, the large parasitic worms were among the first parasites to be noted and studied as possible causes of disease. The Ebers papyrus, written about 1600 B.C.E., contains some of the earliest records of the presence of parasitic worms in humans. In early Egypt, trichinosis, cysticercosis, and salmonellosis were all likely to be acquired from pigs. This knowledge is reflected in the law of Moses, later reinforced in the Qur'ān, which forbids the eating of "unclean swine" or the touching of their dead carcasses—a clear indication that people knew of the relationship between parasitic worms and human disease. Persian, Greek, and Roman physicians were also familiar with various parasitic worms, and many of their early medical writings describe the removal of worm-induced cysts. The Arabic physician and philosopher Avicenna (979-1037 C.E.) was the first to separate parasitic worms into classifications: long, small, flat, and round.

The modern study of parasites began in 1379 with the discovery of the liver fluke, *Fasciola hepatica*, in sheep. During the eighteenth century, many parasitic worms and arthropods were described, but progress was slow prior to the invention and widespread use of the microscope. The microscope made possible the study of small protozoan parasites and allowed for detailed anatomic and lifecycle studies of larger parasites.

In 1835, *Trichinella spiralis*, the parasite responsible for the disease trichinosis, was described, and quickly thereafter knowledge concerning the parasitic worms of humans began to accumulate. Many new species were discovered, prominent among which were the hookworm and the blood fluke.

Between 1836 and 1901, the first protozoan parasites of humans were recognized and described; among the most important of these were the parasites responsible for giardiasis, gingivitis, vaginitis, trichomoniasis, kala-azar, and Gambian trypanosomiasis (sleeping sickness).

Although arthropods had been recognized as parasites since early times, their role in transporting other parasites and in spreading disease was not noted until 1869, when the larval stages of the dog tapeworm were found in the dog louse. Further investigations led to the identification in 1893 of ticks as the transmitting agents of Texas fever in cattle. By 1909, parasitologists had observed the development of the malarial parasite in mosquitoes, had proved the transmission of yellow fever by the mosquito *Aedes aegypti*, and had linked the tsetse fly to African sleeping sickness, the tick to African relapsing fever, the reduviid bug to Chagas' disease, and the body louse to the transmission of typhoid fever.

—*Randall L. Milstein, Ph.D.*

See also Amebiasis; Babesiosis; Bacterial infections; Bacteriology; Biological and chemical weapons;

Bites and stings; Chagas' disease; Coccidiodomycosis; Dengue fever; Ehrlichiosis; Diarrhea and dysentery; Elephantiasis; Encephalitis; Fungal infections; Giardiasis; Insect-borne diseases; Leishmaniasis; Lice, mites, and ticks; Lyme disease; Malaria; Microbiology; Pinworms; Protozoan diseases; Rocky Mountain spotted fever; Roundworms; Schistosomiasis; Shigellosis; Sleeping sickness; Tapeworms; Toxoplasmosis; Trichinosis; Tropical medicine; Typhoid fever; Viral infections; Worms; Yellow fever.

FOR FURTHER INFORMATION:

Despommier, Dickson D., et al. *Parasitic Diseases*. 5th ed. New York: Apple Tree, 2006. This source provides a list of parasitic diseases of current concern to public health professionals. It also describes the assessment of and treatment options for a variety of these diseases.

Frank, Steven A. *Immunology and Evolution of Infectious Disease*. Princeton, N.J.: Princeton University Press, 2002. Blends research from molecular biology, immunology, pathogen biology, and population dynamics to discuss how and why parasites vary to escape recognition by the immune system, vaccine design, and the control of epidemics.

Gittleman, Ann Louise. *Guess What Came to Dinner? Parasites and Your Health*. Rev. ed. New York: Putnam, 2001. Discusses the role of parasites in many ailments, from allergies to chronic fatigue syndrome and bowel disorders, and explains methods of detection, antiparasitic treatments, and herbal cures.

Klein, Aaron E. *The Parasites We Humans Harbor*. New York: Nelson Books/Elsevier, 1981. An overview of common human-infecting parasites written for the general reader. The text is nontechnical, is easy to follow, and presents numerous examples.

Roberts, Larry S., and John Janovy, Jr., eds. *Gerald D. Schmidt and Larry S. Roberts' Foundations of Parasitology*. 7th ed. Boston: McGraw-Hill Higher Education, 2005. A graduate-level textbook covering all aspects of parasitology. The text is highly technical and intended for the informed reader. The book is well illustrated, but sensitive readers may be disturbed by many of the case study photographs.

Salyers, Abigail A., and Dixie D. Whitt. *Bacterial Pathogenesis: A Molecular Approach*. 2d ed. Washington, D.C.: ASM Press, 2002. Examines the molecular mechanism involved in bacterial-host interactions that can produce infectious disease. Introductory chapters discuss host-parasite relationships.

SALEM HEALTH

MAGILL'S
MEDICAL
GUIDE

ENTRIES BY ANATOMY OR SYSTEM AFFECTED

Hearing tests
Histiocytosis
Leukodystrophy
Ménière's disease
Motion sickness
Myringotomy
Nervous system
Neurology
Neurology, pediatric
Osteogenesis imperfecta
Otoplasty
Otorhinolaryngology
Pharynx
Plastic surgery
Quinsy
Rubinstein-Taybi syndrome
Sense organs
Speech disorders
Tinnitus
Vasculitis
Vertigo
Wiskott-Aldrich syndrome

ENDOCRINE SYSTEM
Addison's disease
Adrenal glands
Adrenalectomy
Adrenoleukodystrophy
Assisted reproductive technologies
Bariatric surgery
Biofeedback
Breasts, female
Carbohydrates
Congenital adrenal hyperplasia
Congenital hypothyroidism
Contraception
Corticosteroids
Diabetes mellitus
Dwarfism
Eating disorders
Emotions: Biomedical causes and effects
End-stage renal disease
Endocrine disorders
Endocrine glands
Endocrinology
Endocrinology, pediatric
Ergogenic aids
Failure to thrive
Fibrocystic breast condition
Gender reassignment surgery
Gestational diabetes
Gigantism
Glands

Goiter
Hashimoto's thyroiditis
Hormone therapy
Hormones
Hot flashes
Hyperhidrosis
Hyperparathyroidism and hypoparathyroidism
Hypoglycemia
Hypothalamus
Klinefelter syndrome
Liver
Melatonin
Nonalcoholic steatohepatitis (NASH)
Obesity
Obesity, childhood
Overtraining syndrome
Pancreas
Pancreatitis
Parathyroidectomy
Pituitary gland
Placenta
Plasma
Polycystic ovary syndrome
Postpartum depression
Prader-Willi syndrome
Prostate enlargement
Prostate gland
Prostate gland removal
Sexual differentiation
Small intestine
Steroid abuse
Steroids
Sweating
Systems and organs
Testicular cancer
Testicular surgery
Thymus gland
Thyroid disorders
Thyroid gland
Thyroidectomy
Turner syndrome
Weight loss medications

EYES
Adenoviruses
Adrenoleukodystrophy
Agnosia
Albinos
Antihistamines
Astigmatism
Auras
Batten's disease
Behçet's disease

Blindness
Blurred vision
Botox
Cataract surgery
Cataracts
Chlamydia
Color blindness
Conjunctivitis
Corneal transplantation
Cornelia de Lange syndrome
Cytomegalovirus (CMV)
Dengue fever
Diabetes mellitus
Dyslexia
Enteroviruses
Eye infections and disorders
Eye surgery
Eyes
Face lift and blepharoplasty
Galactosemia
Glaucoma
Gonorrhea
Gulf War syndrome
Jaundice
Juvenile rheumatoid arthritis
Keratitis
Kluver-Bucy syndrome
Laser use in surgery
Leukodystrophy
Macular degeneration
Marfan syndrome
Marijuana
Microscopy, slitlamp
Motor skill development
Multiple chemical sensitivity syndrome
Myopia
Ophthalmology
Optometry
Optometry, pediatric
Pigmentation
Ptosis
Refractive eye surgery
Reiter's syndrome
Rubinstein-Taybi syndrome
Sarcoidosis
Sense organs
Sjögren's syndrome
Strabismus
Sturge-Weber syndrome
Styes
Tears and tear ducts
Toxoplasmosis
Trachoma

Dyskinesia
Electroencephalography (EEG)
Embolism
Epilepsy
Esophagus
Facial transplantation
Fetal tissue transplantation
Fibromyalgia
Hair loss and baldness
Hair transplantation
Head and neck disorders
Headaches
Hydrocephalus
Lice, mites, and ticks
Meningitis
Migraine headaches
Nasal polyp removal
Nasopharyngeal disorders
Neuroimaging
Neurology
Neurology, pediatric
Neurosurgery
Oral and maxillofacial surgery
Pharynx
Polyps
Rhinoplasty and submucous
 resection
Rubinstein-Taybi syndrome
Seizures
Shunts
Sports medicine
Strokes
Sturge-Weber syndrome
Subdural hematoma
Tears and tear ducts
Temporomandibular joint (TMJ)
 syndrome
Thrombosis and thrombus
Tinnitus
Unconsciousness
Whiplash

HEART
Acidosis
Aneurysmectomy
Aneurysms
Angina
Angiography
Angioplasty
Anxiety
Apgar score
Arrhythmias
Arteriosclerosis
Atrial fibrillation

Biofeedback
Bites and stings
Blood pressure
Blood vessels
Blue baby syndrome
Bypass surgery
Caffeine
Cardiac arrest
Cardiac rehabilitation
Cardiac surgery
Cardiology
Cardiology, pediatric
Cardiopulmonary resuscitation
 (CPR)
Carotid arteries
Catheterization
Circulation
Congenital heart disease
Cornelia de Lange syndrome
Coronary artery bypass graft
Defibrillation
DiGeorge syndrome
Diuretics
Echocardiography
Electrical shock
Electrocardiography (ECG or EKG)
Embolism
End-stage renal disease
Endocarditis
Enteroviruses
Exercise physiology
Fatty acid oxidation disorders
Glycogen storage diseases
Heart
Heart attack
Heart disease
Heart failure
Heart transplantation
Heart valve replacement
Hemochromatosis
Hypertension
Hypotension
Infarction
Internal medicine
Intravenous (IV) therapy
Juvenile rheumatoid arthritis
Kinesiology
Lyme disease
Marfan syndrome
Marijuana
Methicillin-resistant *Staphylococcus
 aureus* (MRSA) infections
Mitral valve prolapse
Nicotine

Obesity
Obesity, childhood
Pacemaker implantation
Palpitations
Plaque, arterial
Plasma
Prader-Willi syndrome
Pulmonary edema
Pulse rate
Respiratory distress syndrome
Resuscitation
Reye's syndrome
Rheumatic fever
Rubinstein-Taybi syndrome
Sarcoidosis
Scleroderma
Shock
Sports medicine
Stenosis
Stents
Steroid abuse
Strokes
Thoracic surgery
Thrombolytic therapy and TPA
Thrombosis and thrombus
Toxoplasmosis
Transplantation
Ultrasonography
Uremia
Yellow fever

HIPS
Aging
Arthritis
Arthroplasty
Arthroscopy
Bone disorders
Bones and the skeleton
Chiropractic
Dwarfism
Fracture and dislocation
Fracture repair
Hip fracture repair
Hip replacement
Liposuction
Lower extremities
Orthopedic surgery
Orthopedics
Orthopedics, pediatric
Osteoarthritis
Osteochondritis juvenilis
Osteonecrosis
Osteoporosis
Physical rehabilitation

Colorectal surgery
Constipation
Crohn's disease
Diarrhea and dysentery
Digestion
Diverticulitis and diverticulosis
E. coli infection
Eating disorders
Endoscopy
Enemas
Enterocolitis
Fiber
Fistula repair
Food poisoning
Gastroenteritis
Gastroenterology
Gastroenterology, pediatric
Gastrointestinal disorders
Gastrointestinal system
Gluten intolerance
Hemorrhoid banding and removal
Hemorrhoids
Hernia
Hernia repair
Hirschsprung's disease
Ileostomy and colostomy
Indigestion
Infarction
Internal medicine
Intestinal disorders
Intestines
Irritable bowel syndrome (IBS)
Kaposi's sarcoma
Kwashiorkor
Lactose intolerance
Laparoscopy
Malabsorption
Malnutrition
Metabolism
Nutrition
Obesity
Obesity, childhood
Obstruction
Peristalsis
Pinworm
Polyps
Proctology
Rectum
Rotavirus
Roundworm
Salmonella infection
Small intestine
Soiling
Sphincterectomy

Stomach, intestinal, and pancreatic
  cancers
Tapeworm
Toilet training
Trichinosis
Tumor removal
Tumors
Typhoid fever
Ulcer surgery
Ulcers
Vasculitis
Worms

JOINTS
Amputation
Arthritis
Arthroplasty
Arthroscopy
Braces, orthopedic
Bursitis
Carpal tunnel syndrome
Cartilage
Casts and splints
Chlamydia
Collagen
Corticosteroids
Cyst removal
Cysts
Endoscopy
Exercise physiology
Fracture and dislocation
Fragile X syndrome
Gout
Gulf War syndrome
Hammertoe correction
Hammertoes
Hip fracture repair
Juvenile rheumatoid arthritis
Klippel-Trenaunay syndrome
Kneecap removal
Ligaments
Lyme disease
Methicillin-resistant *Staphylococcus
  aureus* (MRSA) infections
Motor skill development
Orthopedic surgery
Orthopedics
Orthopedics, pediatric
Osteoarthritis
Osteochondritis juvenilis
Osteomyelitis
Osteonecrosis
Physical rehabilitation
Reiter's syndrome

Rheumatoid arthritis
Rheumatology
Rotator cuff surgery
Sarcoidosis
Scleroderma
Spondylitis
Sports medicine
Systemic lupus erythematosus
  (SLE)
Temporomandibular joint (TMJ)
  syndrome
Tendinitis
Tendon disorders
Tendon repair
Von Willebrand's disease

KIDNEYS
Abdomen
Abscess drainage
Abscesses
Adrenal glands
Adrenalectomy
Babesiosis
Carbohydrates
Corticosteroids
Cysts
Dialysis
Diuretics
End-stage renal disease
Galactosemia
Hantavirus
Hematuria
Hemolytic uremic syndrome
Hypertension
Hypotension
Infarction
Internal medicine
Intravenous (IV) therapy
Kidney cancer
Kidney disorders
Kidney transplantation
Kidneys
Laparoscopy
Lithotripsy
Metabolism
Methicillin-resistant *Staphylococcus
  aureus* (MRSA) infections
Nephrectomy
Nephritis
Nephrology
Nephrology, pediatric
Nuclear medicine
Nuclear radiology
Polycystic kidney disease

Glycogen storage diseases
Hematology
Hematology, pediatric
Hemochromatosis
Hemolytic disease of the newborn
Hepatitis
Histiocytosis
Internal medicine
Jaundice
Jaundice, neonatal
Kaposi's sarcoma
Liver
Liver cancer
Liver disorders
Liver transplantation
Malabsorption
Malaria
Metabolism
Methicillin-resistant *Staphylococcus aureus* (MRSA) infections
Niemann-Pick disease
Nonalcoholic steatohepatitis (NASH)
Polycystic kidney disease
Reye's syndrome
Schistosomiasis
Shunts
Thrombocytopenia
Transplantation
Wilson's disease
Yellow fever

LUNGS
Abscess drainage
Abscesses
Acute respiratory distress syndrome (ARDS)
Adenoviruses
Allergies
Altitude sickness
Anthrax
Antihistamines
Apgar score
Apnea
Asbestos exposure
Aspergillosis
Asphyxiation
Asthma
Bacterial infections
Bronchi
Bronchiolitis
Bronchitis
Cardiopulmonary resuscitation (CPR)

Chest
Childhood infectious diseases
Choking
Chronic obstructive pulmonary disease (COPD)
Coccidioidomycosis
Common cold
Coronaviruses
Corticosteroids
Coughing
Croup
Cystic fibrosis
Cytomegalovirus (CMV)
Diaphragm
Diphtheria
Drowning
Edema
Embolism
Emphysema
Endoscopy
Exercise physiology
Fetal surgery
Hantavirus
Heart transplantation
Heimlich maneuver
Hiccups
Histiocytosis
H1N1 influenza
Hyperbaric oxygen therapy
Hyperventilation
Hypoxia
Infarction
Influenza
Internal medicine
Interstitial pulmonary fibrosis (IPF)
Intravenous (IV) therapy
Kaposi's sarcoma
Kinesiology
Legionnaires' disease
Lung cancer
Lung surgery
Lungs
Marijuana
Measles
Mesothelioma
Multiple chemical sensitivity syndrome
Nicotine
Niemann-Pick disease
Oxygen therapy
Plague
Pleurisy
Pneumonia

Pneumothorax
Pulmonary diseases
Pulmonary edema
Pulmonary hypertension
Pulmonary medicine
Pulmonary medicine, pediatric
Respiration
Respiratory distress syndrome
Resuscitation
Rhinoviruses
Sarcoidosis
Scleroderma
Severe acute respiratory syndrome (SARS)
Smoking
Sneezing
Thoracic surgery
Thrombolytic therapy and TPA
Thrombosis and thrombus
Toxoplasmosis
Transplantation
Tuberculosis
Tularemia
Tumor removal
Tumors
Vasculitis
Wheezing
Whooping cough
Wiskott-Aldrich syndrome

LYMPHATIC SYSTEM
Adenoids
Angiography
Antibodies
Bacillus Calmette-Guérin (BCG)
Bacterial infections
Biological therapies
Blood and blood disorders
Blood vessels
Breast cancer
Breast disorders
Breasts, female
Bruises
Burkitt's lymphoma
Cancer
Cervical, ovarian, and uterine cancers
Chemotherapy
Circulation
Colon cancer
Coronaviruses
Corticosteroids
DiGeorge syndrome
Edema

Palsy
Paralysis
Paraplegia
Parkinson's disease
Periodontitis
Physical rehabilitation
Pigeon toes
Poisoning
Poliomyelitis
Prader-Willi syndrome
Precocious puberty
Quadriplegia
Rabies
Radiculopathy
Respiration
Restless legs syndrome
Rheumatoid arthritis
Rheumatology
Rickets
Sarcoma
Scoliosis
Seizures
Sleepwalking
Slipped disk
Speech disorders
Sphincterectomy
Spinal cord disorders
Spine, vertebrae, and disks
Sports medicine
Systemic lupus erythematosus
   (SLE)
Systems and organs
Teeth
Tendinitis
Tendon disorders
Tendon repair
Tetanus
Tics
Tourette's syndrome
Trembling and shaking
Trichinosis
Upper extremities
Weight loss and gain
Yellow fever

NAILS
Anemia
Dermatology
Fungal infections
Malnutrition
Nail removal
Nails
Nutrition
Podiatry

NECK
Asphyxiation
Back pain
Botox
Braces, orthopedic
Carotid arteries
Casts and splints
Chiari malformations
Choking
Congenital hypothyroidism
Dyskinesia
Endarterectomy
Esophagus
Goiter
Hashimoto's thyroiditis
Head and neck disorders
Heimlich maneuver
Hyperparathyroidism and
   hypoparathyroidism
Laryngectomy
Laryngitis
Mouth and throat cancer
Otorhinolaryngology
Paralysis
Parathyroidectomy
Pharynx
Quadriplegia
Spine, vertebrae, and disks
Sympathectomy
Thyroid disorders
Thyroid gland
Thyroidectomy
Tonsillectomy and adenoid removal
Tonsillitis
Torticollis
Trachea
Tracheostomy
Vagus nerve
Whiplash

NERVES
Agnosia
Anesthesia
Anesthesiology
Back pain
Bell's palsy
Biofeedback
Brain
Carpal tunnel syndrome
Cells
Creutzfeldt-Jakob disease (CJD)
Cysts
Dyskinesia
Electromyography

Emotions: Biomedical causes and
   effects
Epilepsy
Facial transplantation
Fibromyalgia
Guillain-Barré syndrome
Hearing
Hemiplegia
Huntington's disease
Leprosy
Leukodystrophy
Listeria infections
Local anesthesia
Lower extremities
Marijuana
Motor neuron diseases
Motor skill development
Multiple chemical sensitivity
   syndrome
Multiple sclerosis
Nervous system
Neuralgia, neuritis, and neuropathy
Neuroimaging
Neurology
Neurology, pediatric
Neurosurgery
Numbness and tingling
Palsy
Paralysis
Paraplegia
Parkinson's disease
Physical rehabilitation
Poliomyelitis
Ptosis
Quadriplegia
Radiculopathy
Sarcoidosis
Sciatica
Seizures
Sense organs
Shock therapy
Skin
Spina bifida
Spinal cord disorders
Spine, vertebrae, and disks
Sturge-Weber syndrome
Sympathectomy
Tics
Tinnitus
Touch
Tourette's syndrome
Upper extremities
Vagotomy
Vasculitis

NERVOUS SYSTEM

Abscess drainage
Abscesses
Acupressure
Addiction
Adenoviruses
Adrenoleukodystrophy
Agnosia
Alcoholism
Altitude sickness
Alzheimer's disease
Amnesia
Amputation
Amyotrophic lateral sclerosis
Anesthesia
Anesthesiology
Aneurysmectomy
Aneurysms
Anosmia
Antidepressants
Anxiety
Apgar score
Aphasia and dysphasia
Apnea
Aromatherapy
Ataxia
Atrophy
Attention-deficit disorder (ADD)
Auras
Autism
Back pain
Balance disorders
Batten's disease
Behçet's disease
Bell's palsy
Beriberi
Biofeedback
Botulism
Brain
Brain damage
Brain disorders
Brain tumors
Caffeine
Carpal tunnel syndrome
Cells
Cerebral palsy
Chagas' disease
Chiari malformations
Chiropractic
Chronic wasting disease (CWD)
Claudication
Cluster headaches
Cognitive development
Coma

Computed tomography (CT)
  scanning
Concussion
Congenital hypothyroidism
Craniotomy
Creutzfeldt-Jakob disease (CJD)
Cysts
Deafness
Defibrillation
Dementias
Developmental disorders
Developmental stages
Diabetes mellitus
Diphtheria
Disk removal
Dizziness and fainting
Down syndrome
Dwarfism
Dyskinesia
Dyslexia
E. coli infection
Ear surgery
Ears
Ehrlichiosis
Electrical shock
Electroencephalography (EEG)
Electromyography
Emotions: Biomedical causes and
  effects
Encephalitis
Endocrinology
Endocrinology, pediatric
Enteroviruses
Epilepsy
Eye infections and disorders
Eyes
Facial transplantation
Fetal alcohol syndrome
Fetal tissue transplantation
Fibromyalgia
Frontotemporal dementia (FTD)
Gigantism
Glands
Guillain-Barré syndrome
Hallucinations
Hammertoe correction
Head and neck disorders
Headaches
Hearing aids
Hearing loss
Hearing tests
Heart transplantation
Hemiplegia
Histiocytosis

Huntington's disease
Hydrocephalus
Hypnosis
Hypothalamus
Insect-borne diseases
Intraventricular hemorrhage
Irritable bowel syndrome (IBS)
Kinesiology
Lead poisoning
Learning disabilities
Leprosy
Light therapy
Listeria infections
Local anesthesia
Lower extremities
Lyme disease
Malaria
Maple syrup urine disease
  (MSUD)
Marijuana
Memory loss
Meningitis
Mental retardation
Mercury poisoning
Migraine headaches
Motor neuron diseases
Motor skill development
Multiple chemical sensitivity
  syndrome
Multiple sclerosis
Myasthenia gravis
Narcolepsy
Narcotics
Nausea and vomiting
Nervous system
Neuralgia, neuritis, and neuropathy
Neurofibromatosis
Neuroimaging
Neurology
Neurology, pediatric
Neurosurgery
Niemann-Pick disease
Nuclear radiology
Numbness and tingling
Orthopedic surgery
Orthopedics
Orthopedics, pediatric
Overtraining syndrome
Paget's disease
Palsy
Paralysis
Paraplegia
Parkinson's disease
Pharmacology

Appetite loss
Aromatherapy
Asperger's syndrome
Attention-deficit disorder (ADD)
Auras
Autism
Bariatric surgery
Biofeedback
Bipolar disorders
Body dysmorphic disorder
Bonding
Brain
Brain disorders
Bulimia
Chronic fatigue syndrome
Club drugs
Cluster headaches
Cognitive development
Colic
Coma
Concussion
Corticosteroids
Death and dying
Delusions
Dementias
Depression
Developmental disorders
Developmental stages
Dizziness and fainting
Domestic violence
Down syndrome
Dyskinesia
Dyslexia
Eating disorders
Electroencephalography (EEG)
Emotions: Biomedical causes and effects
Endocrinology
Endocrinology, pediatric
Facial transplantation
Factitious disorders
Failure to thrive
Fibromyalgia
Frontotemporal dementia (FTD)
Gender identity disorder
Grief and guilt
Gulf War syndrome
Hallucinations
Headaches
Hormone therapy
Hormones
Hydrocephalus
Hypnosis
Hypochondriasis

Hypothalamus
Kinesiology
Klinefelter syndrome
Learning disabilities
Light therapy
Marijuana
Memory loss
Menopause
Mental retardation
Midlife crisis
Migraine headaches
Miscarriage
Morgellons disease
Motor skill development
Narcolepsy
Narcotics
Neurology
Neurology, pediatric
Neurosis
Neurosurgery
Nicotine
Nightmares
Obesity
Obesity, childhood
Obsessive-compulsive disorder
Overtraining syndrome
Palpitations
Panic attacks
Paranoia
Pharmacology
Pharmacy
Phobias
Pick's disease
Postpartum depression
Post-traumatic stress disorder
Prader-Willi syndrome
Precocious puberty
Prescription drug abuse
Psychiatric disorders
Psychiatry
Psychiatry, child and adolescent
Psychiatry, geriatric
Psychoanalysis
Psychosis
Psychosomatic disorders
Puberty and adolescence
Rabies
Rape and sexual assault
Restless legs syndrome
Schizophrenia
Seasonal affective disorder
Separation anxiety
Sexual dysfunction
Sexuality

Shock therapy
Sibling rivalry
Sleep
Sleep disorders
Sleepwalking
Soiling
Speech disorders
Sperm banks
Stammering
Steroid abuse
Stillbirth
Stress
Strokes
Stuttering
Substance abuse
Suicide
Synesthesia
Tics
Tinnitus
Toilet training
Tourette's syndrome
Weight loss and gain
Wilson's disease

REPRODUCTIVE SYSTEM
Abdomen
Abdominal disorders
Abortion
Acquired immunodeficiency syndrome (AIDS)
Adrenoleukodystrophy
Amenorrhea
Amniocentesis
Anatomy
Anorexia nervosa
Assisted reproductive technologies
Breast-feeding
Breasts, female
Candidiasis
Catheterization
Cervical, ovarian, and uterine cancers
Cervical procedures
Cesarean section
Childbirth
Childbirth complications
Chlamydia
Chorionic villus sampling
Circumcision, female, and genital mutilation
Circumcision, male
Conception
Congenital adrenal hyperplasia
Contraception

STOMACH
Abdomen
Abdominal disorders
Abscess drainage
Abscesses
Acid reflux disease
Adenoviruses
Allergies
Bariatric surgery
Botulism
Bulimia
Burping
Bypass surgery
Campylobacter infections
Chyme
Clostridium difficile infection
Coccidioidomycosis
Colitis
Crohn's disease
Digestion
Eating disorders
Endoscopic retrograde
    cholangiopancreatography (ERCP)
Endoscopy
Esophagus
Food biochemistry
Food poisoning
Gastrectomy
Gastroenteritis
Gastroenterology
Gastroenterology, pediatric
Gastrointestinal disorders
Gastrointestinal system
Gastrostomy
Gluten intolerance
Halitosis
Heartburn
Hernia
Hernia repair
Indigestion
Influenza
Internal medicine
Kwashiorkor
Lactose intolerance
Malabsorption
Malnutrition
Metabolism
Motion sickness
Nausea and vomiting
Nutrition
Obesity
Obesity, childhood
Peristalsis
Poisoning

Poisonous plants
Pyloric stenosis
Radiation sickness
Rotavirus
Roundworm
Salmonella infection
Small intestine
Stomach, intestinal, and pancreatic
    cancers
Ulcer surgery
Ulcers
Vagotomy
Vitamins and minerals
Weaning
Weight loss and gain

TEETH
Braces, orthodontic
Cavities
Cornelia de Lange syndrome
Crowns and bridges
Dental diseases
Dentistry
Dentistry, pediatric
Dentures
Endodontic disease
Fluoride treatments
Forensic pathology
Fracture repair
Gastrointestinal system
Gingivitis
Gum disease
Jaw wiring
Lisping
Nicotine
Nutrition
Oral and maxillofacial surgery
Orthodontics
Osteogenesis imperfecta
Periodontal surgery
Periodontitis
Plaque, dental
Prader-Willi syndrome
Root canal treatment
Rubinstein-Taybi syndrome
Teeth
Teething
Temporomandibular joint (TMJ)
    syndrome
Thumb sucking
Tooth extraction
Toothache
Veterinary medicine
Wisdom teeth

TENDONS
Carpal tunnel syndrome
Casts and splints
Collagen
Connective tissue
Cysts
Exercise physiology
Ganglion removal
Hammertoe correction
Joints
Kneecap removal
Orthopedic surgery
Orthopedics
Orthopedics, pediatric
Osgood-Schlatter disease
Physical rehabilitation
Sports medicine
Tendinitis
Tendon disorders
Tendon repair

THROAT
Acid reflux disease
Adenoids
Antihistamines
Asbestos exposure
Auras
Bulimia
Catheterization
Choking
Croup
Decongestants
Drowning
Epiglottitis
Epstein-Barr virus
Esophagus
Fifth disease
Gastroenterology
Gastroenterology, pediatric
Gastrointestinal disorders
Gastrointestinal system
Goiter
Head and neck disorders
Heimlich maneuver
Hiccups
Histiocytosis
H1N1 influenza
Laryngectomy
Laryngitis
Mouth and throat cancer
Nasopharyngeal disorders
Nicotine
Nosebleeds
Otorhinolaryngology

Entries by Specialties and Related Fields

ALL
Accidents
African American health
American Indian health
Anatomy
Asian American health
Biostatistics
Clinical trials
Diagnosis
Disease
Emergency rooms
First aid
Geriatrics and gerontology
Health maintenance organizations
  (HMOs)
Iatrogenic disorders
Imaging and radiology
Internet medicine
Invasive tests
Laboratory tests
Men's health
Neuroimaging
Noninvasive tests
Pediatrics
Physical examination
Physiology
Polypharmacy
Preventive medicine
Prognosis
Proteomics
Screening
Self-medication
Signs and symptoms
Syndrome
Systems and organs
Telemedicine
Terminally ill: Extended care
Veterinary medicine
Women's health

ALTERNATIVE MEDICINE
Acidosis
Acupressure
Acupuncture
Allied health
Alternative medicine
Antioxidants
Aphrodisiacs
Aromatherapy
Biofeedback

Biological therapies
Chronobiology
Club drugs
Colon therapy
Enzyme therapy
Fiber
Healing
Herbal medicine
Holistic medicine
Hydrotherapy
Hypnosis
Magnetic field therapy
Marijuana
Massage
Meditation
Melatonin
Nutrition
Oxygen therapy
Pain management
Stress reduction
Supplements
Yoga

ANESTHESIOLOGY
Acidosis
Acupuncture
Anesthesia
Anesthesiology
Catheterization
Cesarean section
Critical care
Critical care, pediatric
Defibrillation
Dentistry
Hyperbaric oxygen therapy
Hyperthermia and hypothermia
Hypnosis
Hypoxia
Intravenous (IV) therapy
Local anesthesia
Oral and maxillofacial surgery
Pain management
Pharmacology
Pharmacy
Pulse rate
Surgery, general
Surgery, pediatric
Surgical procedures
Surgical technologists
Toxicology

AUDIOLOGY
Adrenoleukodystrophy
Aging
Aging: Extended care
Audiology
Biophysics
Deafness
Dyslexia
Ear infections and disorders
Ear surgery
Ears
Earwax
Hearing
Hearing aids
Hearing loss
Hearing tests
Ménière's disease
Motion sickness
Neurology
Neurology, pediatric
Otoplasty
Otorhinolaryngology
Sense organs
Speech disorders
Tinnitus
Vertigo

BACTERIOLOGY
Amebiasis
Anthrax
Antibiotics
Antibodies
Bacillus Calmette-Guérin (BCG)
Bacterial infections
Bacteriology
Biological and chemical weapons
Blisters
Boils
Botulism
Campylobacter infections
Cells
Childhood infectious diseases
Cholecystitis
Cholera
Clostridium difficile infection
Cystitis
Cytology
Cytopathology
Diphtheria
Drug resistance

Thrombolytic therapy and TPA
Toxic shock syndrome
Tracheostomy
Transfusion
Tropical medicine
Wounds

CYTOLOGY

Acid-base chemistry
Bionics and biotechnology
Biopsy
Blood testing
Cancer
Carcinoma
Cells
Cholesterol
Cytology
Cytopathology
Dermatology
Dermatopathology
E. coli infection
Enzymes
Fluids and electrolytes
Food biochemistry
Gaucher's disease
Genetic counseling
Genetic engineering
Genomics
Glycolysis
Gram staining
Healing
Hematology
Hematology, pediatric
Histology
Hyperplasia
Immune system
Immunology
Karyotyping
Laboratory tests
Lipids
Melanoma
Metabolism
Microscopy
Mutation
Oncology
Pathology
Pharmacology
Pharmacy
Plasma
Pus
Rhinoviruses
Sarcoma
Serology
Side effects

Stem cells
Toxicology

DENTISTRY

Abscess drainage
Abscesses
Aging: Extended care
Anesthesia
Anesthesiology
Braces, orthodontic
Canker sores
Cavities
Crowns and bridges
Dental diseases
Dentistry
Dentistry, pediatric
Dentures
Endodontic disease
Fluoride treatments
Forensic pathology
Fracture and dislocation
Fracture repair
Gastrointestinal system
Gingivitis
Gum disease
Halitosis
Head and neck disorders
Jaw wiring
Lisping
Local anesthesia
Mouth and throat cancer
Nicotine
Oral and maxillofacial surgery
Orthodontics
Osteogenesis imperfecta
Periodontal surgery
Periodontitis
Plaque, dental
Plastic surgery
Prader-Willi syndrome
Prostheses
Root canal treatment
Rubinstein-Taybi syndrome
Sense organs
Sjögren's syndrome
Teeth
Teething
Temporomandibular joint (TMJ)
    syndrome
Thumb sucking
Tooth extraction
Toothache
Von Willebrand's disease
Wisdom teeth

DERMATOLOGY

Abscess drainage
Abscesses
Acne
Adrenoleukodystrophy
Age spots
Albinos
Anthrax
Anti-inflammatory drugs
Athlete's foot
Bedsores
Bile
Biopsy
Birthmarks
Blisters
Body dysmorphic disorder
Boils
Burns and scalds
Carcinoma
Chickenpox
Coccidioidomycosis
Corns and calluses
Corticosteroids
Cryotherapy and cryosurgery
Cyst removal
Cysts
Dermatitis
Dermatology
Dermatology, pediatric
Dermatopathology
Eczema
Electrocauterization
Enteroviruses
Facial transplantation
Fungal infections
Ganglion removal
Glands
Gluten intolerance
Grafts and grafting
Gray hair
Hair
Hair loss and baldness
Hair transplantation
Hand-foot-and-mouth disease
Healing
Histology
Hives
Hyperhidrosis
Impetigo
Itching
Laser use in surgery
Lesions
Lice, mites, and ticks
Light therapy

ETHICS

Abortion
Animal rights vs. research
Assisted reproductive technologies
Circumcision, female, and genital
  mutilation
Circumcision, male
Cloning
Defibrillation
Ergogenic aids
Ethics
Euthanasia
Fetal surgery
Fetal tissue transplantation
Gender identity disorder
Gene therapy
Genetic engineering
Genomics
Gulf War syndrome
Health Canada
Health care reform
Hippocratic oath
Law and medicine
Living will
Malpractice
Marijuana
Münchausen syndrome by proxy
Palliative medicine
Sperm banks
Stem cells
Xenotransplantation

EXERCISE PHYSIOLOGY

Acidosis
Back pain
Biofeedback
Blood pressure
Bone disorders
Bones and the skeleton
Cardiac rehabilitation
Cardiology
Carotid arteries
Circulation
Defibrillation
Dehydration
Echocardiography
Electrocardiography (ECG or EKG)
Ergogenic aids
Exercise physiology
Fascia
Glycolysis
Heart
Heat exhaustion and heatstroke
Hypoxia

Kinesiology
Ligaments
Lungs
Massage
Metabolism
Motor skill development
Muscle sprains, spasms, and
  disorders
Muscles
Nutrition
Orthopedic surgery
Orthopedics
Orthopedics, pediatric
Overtraining syndrome
Oxygen therapy
Physical rehabilitation
Physiology
Pulmonary diseases
Pulmonary medicine
Pulmonary medicine, pediatric
Pulse rate
Respiration
Sports medicine
Stenosis
Steroid abuse
Sweating
Tendinitis
Vascular system

FAMILY MEDICINE

Abdominal disorders
Abscess drainage
Abscesses
Acne
Acquired immunodeficiency
  syndrome (AIDS)
Alcoholism
Allergies
Alzheimer's disease
Amyotrophic lateral sclerosis
Anemia
Angina
Anosmia
Antianxiety drugs
Antidepressants
Antihistamines
Anti-inflammatory drugs
Antioxidants
Arthritis
Athlete's foot
Atrophy
Attention-deficit disorder (ADD)
Bacterial infections
Bed-wetting

Bell's palsy
Beriberi
Biofeedback
Birthmarks
Bleeding
Blisters
Blood pressure
Blurred vision
Body dysmorphic disorder
Boils
Bronchiolitis
Bronchitis
Bunions
Burkitt's lymphoma
Burping
Caffeine
Candidiasis
Canker sores
Carotid arteries
Casts and splints
Chagas' disease
Chickenpox
Childhood infectious diseases
Chlamydia
Cholecystitis
Cholesterol
Chronic fatigue syndrome
Cirrhosis
Clinics
Clostridium difficile infection
Cluster headaches
Coccidioidomycosis
Cold sores
Common cold
Constipation
Contraception
Corticosteroids
Coughing
Cryotherapy and cryosurgery
Cytomegalovirus (CMV)
Death and dying
Decongestants
Deep vein thrombosis
Defibrillation
Dehydration
Dengue fever
Depression
Diabetes mellitus
Diaper rash
Diarrhea and dysentery
Digestion
Dizziness and fainting
Domestic violence
Earwax

FORENSIC MEDICINE
Autopsy
Blood and blood disorders
Blood testing
Bones and the skeleton
Cytopathology
Dermatopathology
DNA and RNA
Forensic pathology
Genetics and inheritance
Genomics
Hematology
Histology
Immunopathology
Laboratory tests
Law and medicine
Pathology

GASTROENTEROLOGY
Abdomen
Abdominal disorders
Acid reflux disease
Acidosis
Adenoviruses
Amebiasis
Amyotrophic lateral sclerosis
Anal cancer
Anthrax
Anus
Appendectomy
Appendicitis
Bariatric surgery
Bile
Bulimia
Bypass surgery
Campylobacter infections
Celiac sprue
Cholecystectomy
Cholecystitis
Cholera
Chyme
Clostridium difficile infection
Colic
Colitis
Colon
Colonoscopy and sigmoidoscopy
Colorectal cancer
Colorectal polyp removal
Colorectal surgery
Computed tomography (CT)
    scanning
Constipation
Critical care
Critical care, pediatric

Crohn's disease
Cytomegalovirus (CMV)
Diarrhea and dysentery
Digestion
Diverticulitis and diverticulosis
E. coli infection
Emergency medicine
Endoscopic retrograde
    cholangiopancreatography (ERCP)
Endoscopy
Enemas
Enterocolitis
Enzymes
Epidemics and pandemics
Esophagus
Failure to thrive
Fiber
Fistula repair
Food allergies
Food biochemistry
Food poisoning
Gallbladder
Gallbladder cancer
Gallbladder diseases
Gastrectomy
Gastroenteritis
Gastroenterology
Gastroenterology, pediatric
Gastrointestinal disorders
Gastrointestinal system
Gastrostomy
Giardiasis
Glands
Gluten intolerance
Heartburn
Hemochromatosis
Hemolytic uremic syndrome
Hemorrhoid banding and removal
Hemorrhoids
Hernia
Hernia repair
Hirschsprung's disease
Ileostomy and colostomy
Indigestion
Infarction
Internal medicine
Intestinal disorders
Intestines
Irritable bowel syndrome (IBS)
Lactose intolerance
Laparoscopy
Lesions
Liver
Liver cancer

Liver disorders
Liver transplantation
Malabsorption
Malnutrition
Metabolism
Nausea and vomiting
Nonalcoholic steatohepatitis (NASH)
Noroviruses
Nutrition
Obstruction
Pancreas
Pancreatitis
Peristalsis
Poisonous plants
Polycystic kidney disease
Polyps
Proctology
Pyloric stenosis
Rectum
Rotavirus
Roundworm
Salmonella infection
Scleroderma
Shigellosis
Small intestine
Soiling
Stenosis
Stevens-Johnson syndrome
Stomach, intestinal, and pancreatic
    cancers
Stone removal
Stones
Tapeworm
Taste
Toilet training
Trichinosis
Ulcer surgery
Ulcers
Vagotomy
Vagus nerve
Vasculitis
Von Willebrand's disease
Weight loss and gain
Wilson's disease
Worms

GENERAL SURGERY
Abscess drainage
Adenoids
Adrenalectomy
Amputation
Anesthesia
Anesthesiology
Aneurysmectomy

GENETICS

Fetal surgery
Fragile X syndrome
Fructosemia
Galactosemia
Gaucher's disease
Gender identity disorder
Gene therapy
Genetic counseling
Genetic diseases
Genetic engineering
Genetics and inheritance
Genomics
Grafts and grafting
Hematology
Hematology, pediatric
Hemophilia
Hermaphroditism and
    pseudohermaphroditism
Huntington's disease
Hyperadiposis
Immunodeficiency disorders
In vitro fertilization
Karyotyping
Klinefelter syndrome
Klippel-Trenaunay syndrome
Laboratory tests
Leptin
Leukodystrophy
Malabsorption
Maple syrup urine disease (MSUD)
Marfan syndrome
Mental retardation
Metabolic disorders
Motor skill development
Mucopolysaccharidosis (MPS)
Muscular dystrophy
Mutation
Neonatology
Nephrology
Nephrology, pediatric
Neurofibromatosis
Neurology
Neurology, pediatric
Niemann-Pick disease
Obstetrics
Oncology
Osteogenesis imperfecta
Ovaries
Pediatrics
Phenylketonuria (PKU)
Polycystic kidney disease
Polydactyly and syndactyly
Polyps
Porphyria

Prader-Willi syndrome
Precocious puberty
Reproductive system
Retroviruses
Rh factor
Rhinoviruses
Rubinstein-Taybi syndrome
Sarcoidosis
Screening
Severe combined immunodeficiency
    syndrome (SCID)
Sexual differentiation
Sexuality
Sperm banks
Stem cells
Synesthesia
Tay-Sachs disease
Tourette's syndrome
Transplantation
Turner syndrome
Wiskott-Aldrich syndrome

GERIATRICS AND GERONTOLOGY

Age spots
Aging
Aging: Extended care
Alzheimer's disease
Arthritis
Assisted living facilities
Atrophy
Bed-wetting
Blindness
Blood pressure
Blurred vision
Bone disorders
Bones and the skeleton
Brain
Brain disorders
Cartilage
Cataract surgery
Cataracts
Chronic obstructive pulmonary
    disease (COPD)
Corns and calluses
Critical care
Crowns and bridges
Deafness
Death and dying
Dementias
Dentures
Depression
Domestic violence
Dyskinesia

Emergency medicine
End-stage renal disease
Endocrinology
Euthanasia
Family medicine
Fatigue
Fiber
Fracture and dislocation
Fracture repair
Gray hair
Hearing aids
Hearing loss
Hip fracture repair
Hip replacement
Hormone therapy
Hormones
Hospitals
Incontinence
Joints
Memory loss
Nursing
Nutrition
Ophthalmology
Orthopedics
Osteoporosis
Pain management
Palliative medicine
Paramedics
Parkinson's disease
Pharmacology
Pick's disease
Psychiatry
Psychiatry, geriatric
Radiculopathy
Rheumatology
Safety issues for the elderly
Sleep disorders
Spinal cord disorders
Spine, vertebrae, and disks
Suicide
Vision disorders
Wrinkles

GYNECOLOGY

Abortion
Amenorrhea
Amniocentesis
Assisted reproductive technologies
Biopsy
Bladder removal
Breast biopsy
Breast cancer
Breast disorders
Breast-feeding

Thrombocytopenia
Thrombolytic therapy and TPA
Thrombosis and thrombus
Transfusion
Uremia
Vascular medicine
Vascular system
Von Willebrand's disease

HISTOLOGY
Autopsy
Biopsy
Cancer
Carcinoma
Cells
Cytology
Cytopathology
Dermatology
Dermatopathology
Fluids and electrolytes
Forensic pathology
Healing
Histology
Laboratory tests
Microscopy
Nails
Necrotizing fasciitis
Pathology
Tumor removal
Tumors

IMMUNOLOGY
Acquired immunodeficiency
  syndrome (AIDS)
Adenoids
Adenoviruses
Allergies
Antibiotics
Antibodies
Antihistamines
Arthritis
Aspergillosis
Asthma
Autoimmune disorders
Bacillus Calmette-Guérin (BCG)
Bacterial infections
Biological and chemical weapons
Biological therapies
Bionics and biotechnology
Bites and stings
Blood and blood disorders
Boils
Bone cancer
Bone grafting

Bone marrow transplantation
Breast cancer
Cancer
Candidiasis
Carcinoma
Cervical, ovarian, and uterine
  cancers
Childhood infectious diseases
Chronic fatigue syndrome
Colorectal cancer
Coronaviruses
Corticosteroids
Cytology
Cytomegalovirus (CMV)
Dermatology
Dermatopathology
DiGeorge syndrome
Emerging infectious diseases
Endocrinology
Endocrinology, pediatric
Epidemics and pandemics
Epstein-Barr virus
Facial transplantation
Food allergies
Fungal infections
Gluten intolerance
Grafts and grafting
Healing
Hematology
Hematology, pediatric
Histiocytosis
Hives
Homeopathy
Host-defense mechanisms
Human immunodeficiency virus
  (HIV)
Hypnosis
Immune system
Immunization and vaccination
Immunodeficiency disorders
Immunology
Immunopathology
Impetigo
Juvenile rheumatoid arthritis
Kawasaki disease
Laboratory tests
Leprosy
Liver cancer
Lung cancer
Lymph
Lymphatic system
Microbiology
Multiple chemical sensitivity
  syndrome

Myasthenia gravis
Nicotine
Noroviruses
Oncology
Opportunistic infections
Oxygen therapy
Palliative medicine
Pancreas
Prostate cancer
Pulmonary diseases
Pulmonary medicine
Pulmonary medicine, pediatric
Rheumatology
Rhinitis
Rhinoviruses
Sarcoidosis
Sarcoma
Scleroderma
Serology
Severe combined immunodeficiency
  syndrome (SCID)
Side effects
Skin cancer
Small intestine
Stem cells
Stevens-Johnson syndrome
Stomach, intestinal, and pancreatic
  cancers
Stress
Stress reduction
Systemic lupus erythematosus (SLE)
Thalidomide
Thymus gland
Transfusion
Transplantation
Tropical medicine
Wiskott-Aldrich syndrome
Xenotransplantation

INTERNAL MEDICINE
Abdomen
Abdominal disorders
Acidosis
Adenoids
Adrenal glands
Amebiasis
Anatomy
Anemia
Angina
Antianxiety drugs
Antibodies
Anti-inflammatory drugs
Antioxidants
Anus

Occupational health
Opportunistic infections
Osteopathic medicine
Paget's disease
Pain
Palliative medicine
Palpitations
Pancreas
Pancreatitis
Parasitic diseases
Parkinson's disease
Peristalsis
Peritonitis
Pharyngitis
Pharynx
Phlebitis
Physical examination
Physician assistants
Physiology
Plaque, arterial
Plasma
Pneumonia
Polyps
Proctology
Psoriasis
Puberty and adolescence
Pulmonary edema
Pulmonary medicine
Pulmonary medicine, pediatric
Pulse rate
Pyelonephritis
Radiopharmaceuticals
Rashes
Rectum
Renal failure
Reye's syndrome
Rheumatic fever
Rheumatoid arthritis
Roundworm
Rubella
Sarcoidosis
Scarlet fever
Schistosomiasis
Sciatica
Scurvy
Septicemia
Severe acute respiratory syndrome
  (SARS)
Sexuality
Sexually transmitted diseases
  (STDs)
Shingles
Shock
Sickle cell disease

Small intestine
Sneezing
Sports medicine
Staphylococcal infections
Stevens-Johnson syndrome
Stone removal
Stones
Streptococcal infections
Stress
Supplements
Systemic lupus erythematosus
  (SLE)
Tapeworm
Tetanus
Thrombosis and thrombus
Toxic shock syndrome
Tumor removal
Tumors
Ulcer surgery
Ulcers
Ultrasonography
Viral infections
Vitamins and minerals
Weight loss medications
Whooping cough
Wilson's disease
Worms
Wounds

MICROBIOLOGY
Abscesses
Amebiasis
Anthrax
Antibiotics
Antibodies
Aspergillosis
Autopsy
Bacillus Calmette-Guérin (BCG)
Bacterial infections
Bacteriology
Bionics and biotechnology
Campylobacter infections
Clostridium difficile infection
Coccidioidomycosis
Dengue fever
Drug resistance
E. coli infection
Enteroviruses
Epidemics and pandemics
Epidemiology
Fluoride treatments
Fungal infections
Gangrene
Gastroenteritis

Gastroenterology
Gastroenterology, pediatric
Gastrointestinal disorders
Gastrointestinal system
Genetic engineering
Genomics
Gram staining
Hematuria
Immune system
Immunization and vaccination
Immunology
Impetigo
Laboratory tests
Listeria infections
Methicillin-resistant *Staphylococcus*
  aureus (MRSA) infections
Microbiology
Microscopy
Opportunistic infections
Pathology
Pharmacology
Pharmacy
Plasma
Protozoan diseases
Pus
Serology
Severe acute respiratory syndrome
  (SARS)
Smallpox
Toxic shock syndrome
Toxicology
Tropical medicine
Tuberculosis
Urinalysis
Urology
Urology, pediatric
Viral infections

NEONATOLOGY
Apgar score
Birth defects
Blue baby syndrome
Bonding
Cardiology, pediatric
Cesarean section
Childbirth
Childbirth complications
Chlamydia
Cleft lip and palate
Cleft lip and palate repair
Congenital disorders
Congenital heart disease
Critical care, pediatric
Cystic fibrosis

Asphyxiation
Bacillus Calmette-Guérin (BCG)
Back pain
Biofeedback
Blurred vision
Carcinogens
Cardiac rehabilitation
Carpal tunnel syndrome
Defibrillation
Environmental diseases
Environmental health
Gulf War syndrome
Hearing aids
Hearing loss
Home care
Interstitial pulmonary fibrosis
   (IPF)
Lead poisoning
Leukodystrophy
Lung cancer
Lungs
Mercury poisoning
Mesothelioma
Multiple chemical sensitivity
   syndrome
Nasopharyngeal disorders
Occupational health
Pneumonia
Prostheses
Pulmonary diseases
Pulmonary medicine
Pulmonary medicine, pediatric
Radiation sickness
Skin cancer
Skin disorders
Stress
Stress reduction
Tendinitis
Tendon disorders
Tendon repair
Toxicology

ONCOLOGY
Aging
Aging: Extended care
Amputation
Anal cancer
Antibodies
Antioxidants
Anus
Asbestos exposure
Biological therapies
Biopsy
Bladder cancer

Bladder removal
Blood testing
Bone cancer
Bone disorders
Bone grafting
Bone marrow transplantation
Bones and the skeleton
Brain tumors
Breast biopsy
Breast cancer
Breasts, female
Burkitt's lymphoma
Cancer
Carcinogens
Carcinoma
Cells
Cervical, ovarian, and uterine
   cancers
Chemotherapy
Colon
Colorectal cancer
Colorectal polyp removal
Cryotherapy and cryosurgery
Cytology
Cytopathology
Dermatology
Dermatopathology
Disseminated intravascular
   coagulation (DIC)
Embolization
Endometrial biopsy
Epstein-Barr virus
Ewing's sarcoma
Fibrocystic breast condition
Gallbladder cancer
Gastrectomy
Gastroenterology
Gastrointestinal disorders
Gastrointestinal system
Gastrostomy
Gene therapy
Genital disorders, female
Genital disorders, male
Gynecology
Hematology
Histology
Hodgkin's disease
Human papillomavirus (HPV)
Hysterectomy
Imaging and radiology
Immunology
Immunopathology
Intravenous (IV) therapy
Kaposi's sarcoma

Karyotyping
Kidney cancer
Laboratory tests
Laryngectomy
Laser use in surgery
Lesions
Liver cancer
Lung cancer
Lung surgery
Lungs
Lymph
Lymphadenopathy and lymphoma
Malignancy and metastasis
Mammography
Massage
Mastectomy and lumpectomy
Melanoma
Mesothelioma
Mouth and throat cancer
Necrosis
Nephrectomy
Nicotine
Oncology
Oral and maxillofacial surgery
Pain management
Palliative medicine
Pap test
Pathology
Pharmacology
Pharmacy
Plastic surgery
Proctology
Prostate cancer
Prostate gland
Prostate gland removal
Prostheses
Pulmonary diseases
Pulmonary medicine
Radiation sickness
Radiation therapy
Radiopharmaceuticals
Rectum
Retroviruses
Sarcoma
Serology
Skin
Skin cancer
Skin lesion removal
Small intestine
Smoking
Stem cells
Stenosis
Stomach, intestinal, and pancreatic
   cancers

Poliomyelitis
Polydactyly and syndactyly
Porphyria
Prader-Willi syndrome
Precocious puberty
Premature birth
Progeria
Psychiatry, child and adolescent
Puberty and adolescence
Pulmonary medicine, pediatric
Pulse rate
Pyloric stenosis
Rashes
Reflexes, primitive
Respiratory distress syndrome
Reye's syndrome
Rheumatic fever
Rhinitis
Rickets
Roseola
Rotavirus
Roundworm
Rubella
Rubinstein-Taybi syndrome
Safety issues for children
Scarlet fever
Seizures
Severe combined immunodeficiency
    syndrome (SCID)
Sexuality
Sibling rivalry
Soiling
Sore throat
Steroids
Stevens-Johnson syndrome
Strep throat
Streptococcal infections
Sturge-Weber syndrome
Styes
Sudden infant death syndrome
    (SIDS)
Surgery, pediatric
Tapeworm
Tay-Sachs disease
Teething
Testicles, undescended
Testicular torsion
Thumb sucking
Toilet training
Tonsillectomy and adenoid removal
Tonsillitis
Tonsils
Trachoma
Tropical medicine

Urology, pediatric
Weaning
Well-baby examinations
Whooping cough
Wiskott-Aldrich syndrome
Worms

PERINATOLOGY
Amniocentesis
Assisted reproductive technologies
Birth defects
Breast-feeding
Cesarean section
Childbirth
Childbirth complications
Chorionic villus sampling
Congenital hypothyroidism
Critical care, pediatric
Embryology
Fatty acid oxidation disorders
Fetal alcohol syndrome
Glycogen storage diseases
Hematology, pediatric
Hydrocephalus
Karyotyping
Metabolic disorders
Motor skill development
Neonatology
Neurology, pediatric
Nursing
Obstetrics
Pediatrics
Perinatology
Pregnancy and gestation
Premature birth
Reflexes, primitive
Shunts
Stillbirth
Sudden infant death syndrome
    (SIDS)
Trichomoniasis
Umbilical cord
Uterus
Well-baby examinations

PHARMACOLOGY
Acid-base chemistry
Acidosis
Aging: Extended care
Anesthesia
Anesthesiology
Antianxiety drugs
Antibiotics
Antibodies

Antidepressants
Antihistamines
Anti-inflammatory drugs
Bacteriology
Blurred vision
Chemotherapy
Club drugs
Corticosteroids
Critical care
Critical care, pediatric
Decongestants
Digestion
Diuretics
Drug resistance
Dyskinesia
Emergency medicine
Emergency medicine, pediatric
Enzymes
Epidemics and pandemics
Ergogenic aids
Fluids and electrolytes
Food biochemistry
Genetic engineering
Genomics
Geriatrics and gerontology
Glycolysis
Herbal medicine
Homeopathy
Hormones
Laboratory tests
Marijuana
Melatonin
Mesothelioma
Metabolism
Narcotics
Nicotine
Oncology
Over-the-counter medications
Pain management
Pharmacology
Pharmacy
Poisoning
Polycystic ovary syndrome
Prader-Willi syndrome
Prescription drug abuse
Psychiatry
Psychiatry, child and adolescent
Psychiatry, geriatric
Rheumatology
Self-medication
Side effects
Sports medicine
Steroid abuse
Steroids

Substance abuse
Thrombolytic therapy and TPA
Toxicology
Tropical medicine

PHYSICAL THERAPY
Aging: Extended care
Amputation
Amyotrophic lateral sclerosis
Arthritis
Atrophy
Back pain
Bell's palsy
Biofeedback
Bowlegs
Burns and scalds
Cardiac rehabilitation
Casts and splints
Cerebral palsy
Cornelia de Lange syndrome
Disk removal
Dyskinesia
Electromyography
Exercise physiology
Fascia
Grafts and grafting
Hemiplegia
Hip fracture repair
Hip replacement
Home care
Hydrotherapy
Kinesiology
Knock-knees
Leukodystrophy
Ligaments
Lower extremities
Massage
Motor skill development
Muscle sprains, spasms, and
   disorders
Muscles
Muscular dystrophy
Neurology
Neurology, pediatric
Numbness and tingling
Orthopedic surgery
Orthopedics
Orthopedics, pediatric
Osteopathic medicine
Osteoporosis
Pain management
Palsy
Paralysis
Paraplegia

Parkinson's disease
Physical examination
Physical rehabilitation
Plastic surgery
Prostheses
Pulse rate
Quadriplegia
Radiculopathy
Rickets
Scoliosis
Slipped disk
Spina bifida
Spinal cord disorders
Spine, vertebrae, and disks
Sports medicine
Tendinitis
Tendon disorders
Torticollis
Upper extremities
Whiplash

PLASTIC SURGERY
Aging
Amputation
Bariatric surgery
Birthmarks
Body dysmorphic disorder
Botox
Breast cancer
Breast disorders
Breast surgery
Breasts, female
Burns and scalds
Cancer
Carcinoma
Circumcision, female, and genital
   mutilation
Circumcision, male
Cleft lip and palate
Cleft lip and palate repair
Craniosynostosis
Cyst removal
Cysts
Dermatology
Dermatology, pediatric
DiGeorge syndrome
Face lift and blepharoplasty
Facial transplantation
Gender reassignment surgery
Grafts and grafting
Hair loss and baldness
Hair transplantation
Healing
Jaw wiring

Laceration repair
Liposuction
Malignancy and metastasis
Moles
Necrotizing fasciitis
Neurofibromatosis
Obesity
Obesity, childhood
Oral and maxillofacial surgery
Otoplasty
Otorhinolaryngology
Plastic surgery
Prostheses
Ptosis
Rhinoplasty and submucous
   resection
Skin
Skin lesion removal
Sturge-Weber syndrome
Surgical procedures
Tattoo removal
Tattoos and body piercing
Varicose vein removal
Varicose veins
Vision
Wrinkles

PODIATRY
Athlete's foot
Bone disorders
Bones and the skeleton
Bunions
Cartilage
Corns and calluses
Feet
Flat feet
Foot disorders
Fungal infections
Hammertoe correction
Hammertoes
Heel spur removal
Joints
Lesions
Lower extremities
Nail removal
Orthopedic surgery
Orthopedics
Physical examination
Pigeon toes
Podiatry
Polydactyly and syndactyly
Tendon disorders
Tendon repair
Warts

PREVENTIVE MEDICINE

Acidosis
Acupressure
Acupuncture
Aging: Extended care
Alternative medicine
Antibodies
Aromatherapy
Assisted living facilities
Bacillus Calmette-Guérin (BCG)
Biofeedback
Braces, orthopedic
Caffeine
Cardiac surgery
Cardiology
Chiropractic
Cholesterol
Chronobiology
Disease
Echocardiography
Electrocardiography (ECG or EKG)
Environmental health
Exercise physiology
Family medicine
Fiber
Genetic counseling
Geriatrics and gerontology
Holistic medicine
Host-defense mechanisms
Hypercholesterolemia
Immune system
Immunization and vaccination
Immunology
Mammography
Massage
Meditation
Melatonin
Mesothelioma
Noninvasive tests
Nursing
Nutrition
Occupational health
Osteopathic medicine
Over-the-counter medications
Pharmacology
Pharmacy
Physical examination
Phytochemicals
Polycystic ovary syndrome
Preventive medicine
Psychiatry
Psychiatry, child and adolescent
Psychiatry, geriatric
Rhinoviruses

Screening
Serology
Spine, vertebrae, and disks
Sports medicine
Stress
Stress reduction
Tendinitis
Tropical medicine
Yoga

PROCTOLOGY

Anal cancer
Anus
Bladder removal
Colon
Colonoscopy and sigmoidoscopy
Colorectal cancer
Colorectal polyp removal
Colorectal surgery
Crohn's disease
Diverticulitis and diverticulosis
Endoscopy
Fistula repair
Gastroenterology
Gastrointestinal disorders
Gastrointestinal system
Genital disorders, male
Geriatrics and gerontology
Hemorrhoid banding and removal
Hemorrhoids
Hirschsprung's disease
Internal medicine
Intestinal disorders
Intestines
Irritable bowel syndrome (IBS)
Palliative medicine
Physical examination
Proctology
Prostate cancer
Prostate gland
Prostate gland removal
Rectum
Reproductive system
Urology
Polyps

PSYCHIATRY

Addiction
Adrenoleukodystrophy
Aging
Aging: Extended care
Alcoholism
Alzheimer's disease
Amnesia

Amyotrophic lateral sclerosis
Anorexia nervosa
Antianxiety drugs
Antidepressants
Anxiety
Appetite loss
Asperger's syndrome
Attention-deficit disorder (ADD)
Auras
Autism
Bariatric surgery
Bipolar disorders
Body dysmorphic disorder
Bonding
Brain
Brain damage
Brain disorders
Breast surgery
Bulimia
Chronic fatigue syndrome
Circumcision, female, and genital
  mutilation
Club drugs
Corticosteroids
Delusions
Dementias
Depression
Developmental disorders
Developmental stages
Domestic violence
Dyskinesia
Eating disorders
Electroencephalography (EEG)
Emergency medicine
Emotions: Biomedical causes
  and effects
Factitious disorders
Failure to thrive
Family medicine
Fatigue
Frontotemporal dementia
  (FTD)
Gender identity disorder
Gender reassignment surgery
Grief and guilt
Gynecology
Hallucinations
Huntington's disease
Hypnosis
Hypochondriasis
Hypothalamus
Incontinence
Intoxication
Kluver-Bucy syndrome

Light therapy
Marijuana
Masturbation
Memory loss
Mental retardation
Midlife crisis
Morgellons disease
Münchausen syndrome by proxy
Neurosis
Neurosurgery
Nicotine
Nightmares
Obesity
Obesity, childhood
Obsessive-compulsive disorder
Pain
Pain management
Palliative medicine
Panic attacks
Paranoia
Penile implant surgery
Phobias
Pick's disease
Postpartum depression
Post-traumatic stress disorder
Prader-Willi syndrome
Prescription drug abuse
Psychiatric disorders
Psychiatry
Psychiatry, child and adolescent
Psychiatry, geriatric
Psychoanalysis
Psychosis
Psychosomatic disorders
Rape and sexual assault
Restless legs syndrome
Schizophrenia
Seasonal affective disorder
Separation anxiety
Sexual dysfunction
Sexuality
Shock therapy
Single photon emission computed
    tomography (SPECT)
Sleep
Sleep disorders
Speech disorders
Steroid abuse
Stress
Stress reduction
Substance abuse
Sudden infant death syndrome
    (SIDS)
Suicide

Synesthesia
Tinnitus
Toilet training
Tourette's syndrome

PSYCHOLOGY
Addiction
Aging
Aging: Extended care
Alcoholism
Amnesia
Amyotrophic lateral sclerosis
Anorexia nervosa
Anxiety
Appetite loss
Aromatherapy
Asperger's syndrome
Attention-deficit disorder (ADD)
Auras
Bariatric surgery
Bed-wetting
Biofeedback
Bipolar disorders
Bonding
Brain
Brain damage
Brain disorders
Bulimia
Cardiac rehabilitation
Cirrhosis
Club drugs
Cognitive development
Death and dying
Delusions
Depression
Developmental disorders
Developmental stages
Domestic violence
Dyslexia
Eating disorders
Electroencephalography (EEG)
Emotions: Biomedical causes
    and effects
Environmental health
Factitious disorders
Failure to thrive
Family medicine
Forensic pathology
Gender identity disorder
Gender reassignment surgery
Genetic counseling
Grief and guilt
Gulf War syndrome
Gynecology

Hallucinations
Holistic medicine
Hormone therapy
Huntington's disease
Hypnosis
Hypochondriasis
Hypothalamus
Juvenile rheumatoid arthritis
Kinesiology
Klinefelter syndrome
Kluver-Bucy syndrome
Learning disabilities
Light therapy
Marijuana
Meditation
Memory loss
Mental retardation
Midlife crisis
Motor skill development
Münchausen syndrome by proxy
Neurosis
Nightmares
Nutrition
Obesity
Obesity, childhood
Obsessive-compulsive disorder
Occupational health
Overtraining syndrome
Pain management
Palliative medicine
Panic attacks
Paranoia
Phobias
Pick's disease
Plastic surgery
Polycystic ovary syndrome
Postpartum depression
Post-traumatic stress disorder
Prescription drug abuse
Psychosomatic disorders
Puberty and adolescence
Restless legs syndrome
Separation anxiety
Sexual dysfunction
Sexuality
Sibling rivalry
Sleep
Sleep disorders
Sleepwalking
Speech disorders
Sports medicine
Steroid abuse
Stillbirth
Stress

Stress reduction
Sturge-Weber syndrome
Stuttering
Substance abuse
Sudden infant death syndrome (SIDS)
Suicide
Synesthesia
Temporomandibular joint (TMJ) syndrome
Tics
Toilet training
Tourette's syndrome
Weight loss and gain
Yoga

PUBLIC HEALTH
Acquired immunodeficiency syndrome (AIDS)
Acute respiratory distress syndrome (ARDS)
Adenoviruses
Aging: Extended care
Allied health
Alternative medicine
Amebiasis
Anthrax
Antibodies
Asbestos exposure
Assisted living facilities
Babesiosis
Bacillus Calmette-Guérin (BCG)
Bacteriology
Beriberi
Biological and chemical weapons
Biostatistics
Blood banks
Blood testing
Botulism
Carcinogens
Chagas' disease
Chickenpox
Childhood infectious diseases
Chlamydia
Cholera
Chronic obstructive pulmonary disease (COPD)
Clinics
Club drugs
Common cold
Coronaviruses
Corticosteroids
Creutzfeldt-Jakob disease (CJD)
Dengue fever

Department of Health and Human Services
Dermatology
Diarrhea and dysentery
Diphtheria
Domestic violence
Drug resistance
E. coli infection
Ebola virus
Elephantiasis
Emergency medicine
Environmental diseases
Epidemics and pandemics
Epidemiology
Fetal alcohol syndrome
Food poisoning
Forensic pathology
Gonorrhea
Gulf War syndrome
Hantavirus
Health Canada
Health care reform
Hepatitis
H1N1 influenza
Hospitals
Human immunodeficiency virus (HIV)
Immunization and vaccination
Influenza
Insect-borne diseases
Kwashiorkor
Lead poisoning
Legionnaires' disease
Leishmaniasis
Leprosy
Lice, mites, and ticks
Lyme disease
Macronutrients
Malaria
Malnutrition
Managed care
Marburg virus
Marijuana
Measles
Medicare
Meningitis
Methicillin-resistant Staphylococcus aureus (MRSA) infections
Microbiology
Monkeypox
Multiple chemical sensitivity syndrome
Mumps
Necrotizing fasciitis

Nicotine
Niemann-Pick disease
Nursing
Nutrition
Occupational health
Osteopathic medicine
Parasitic diseases
Pharmacology
Pharmacy
Physical examination
Physician assistants
Pinworm
Plague
Pneumonia
Poliomyelitis
Polycystic ovary syndrome
Prion diseases
Protozoan diseases
Psychiatry
Psychiatry, child and adolescent
Psychiatry, geriatric
Rabies
Radiation sickness
Rape and sexual assault
Retroviruses
Rhinoviruses
Roundworm
Rubella
Salmonella infection
Schistosomiasis
Screening
Serology
Severe acute respiratory syndrome (SARS)
Sexually transmitted diseases (STDs)
Shigellosis
Sleeping sickness
Smallpox
Syphilis
Tapeworm
Tattoos and body piercing
Tetanus
Toxicology
Toxoplasmosis
Trichinosis
Trichomoniasis
Tropical medicine
Tuberculosis
Tularemia
Typhoid fever
Typhus
Whooping cough
World Health Organization

TOXICOLOGY

Acidosis
Biological and chemical weapons
Bites and stings
Blood testing
Botulism
Club drugs
Critical care
Critical care, pediatric
Cyanosis
Defibrillation
Dermatitis
Eczema
Emergency medicine
Environmental diseases
Environmental health
Food poisoning
Forensic pathology
Gaucher's disease
Hepatitis
Herbal medicine
Homeopathy
Intoxication
Itching
Laboratory tests
Lead poisoning
Liver
Mold and mildew
Multiple chemical sensitivity
    syndrome
Nicotine
Occupational health
Pathology
Pharmacology
Pharmacy
Poisoning
Poisonous plants
Rashes
Sarcoidosis
Side effects
Snakebites
Toxicology
Toxoplasmosis
Urinalysis

UROLOGY

Abdomen
Abdominal disorders
Adenoviruses
Bed-wetting
Bladder cancer
Bladder removal
Catheterization
Chlamydia

Circumcision, male
Congenital adrenal hyperplasia
Cystitis
Cystoscopy
Dialysis
Diuretics
E. coli infection
Endoscopy
Erectile dysfunction
Fetal surgery
Fluids and electrolytes
Gender reassignment surgery
Genital disorders, female
Genital disorders, male
Geriatrics and gerontology
Gonorrhea
Hemolytic uremic syndrome
Hermaphroditism and
    pseudohermaphroditism
Hydroceles
Hyperplasia
Hypospadias repair and
    urethroplasty
Incontinence
Infertility, male
Kidney cancer
Kidney disorders
Kidney transplantation
Kidneys
Lesions
Lithotripsy
Nephrectomy
Nephritis
Nephrology
Nephrology, pediatric
Orchiectomy
Palliative medicine
Pediatrics
Pelvic inflammatory disease (PID)
Penile implant surgery
Polycystic kidney disease
Polyps
Prostate cancer
Prostate enlargement
Prostate gland
Prostate gland removal
Proteinuria
Pyelonephritis
Reiter's syndrome
Reproductive system
Schistosomiasis
Semen
Sexual differentiation
Sexual dysfunction

Sexually transmitted diseases
    (STDs)
Sterilization
Stevens-Johnson syndrome
Stone removal
Stones
Syphilis
Testicles, undescended
Testicular cancer
Testicular surgery
Testicular torsion
Toilet training
Transplantation
Trichomoniasis
Ultrasonography
Uremia
Urethritis
Urinalysis
Urinary disorders
Urinary system
Urology
Urology, pediatric
Vas deferens
Vasectomy

VASCULAR MEDICINE

Acidosis
Amputation
Aneurysmectomy
Aneurysms
Angiography
Angioplasty
Anti-inflammatory drugs
Arteriosclerosis
Biofeedback
Bleeding
Blood and blood disorders
Blood pressure
Blood vessels
Bruises
Bypass surgery
Cardiac surgery
Carotid arteries
Catheterization
Cholesterol
Circulation
Claudication
Defibrillation
Dehydration
Diabetes mellitus
Dialysis
Embolism
Embolization
End-stage renal disease

Endarterectomy
Exercise physiology
Glands
Healing
Hematology
Hematology, pediatric
Hemorrhoid banding and removal
Hemorrhoids
Histology
Hypercholesterolemia
Hyperlipidemia
Infarction
Ischemia
Klippel-Trenaunay syndrome
Lesions
Lipids
Lymphatic system
Mitral valve prolapse
Necrotizing fasciitis
Nicotine
Osteochondritis juvenilis
Phlebitis
Plaque, arterial
Plasma
Podiatry
Preeclampsia and eclampsia
Progeria
Pulse rate
Shunts
Smoking
Stents
Strokes
Sturge-Weber syndrome
Thrombolytic therapy and TPA
Thrombosis and thrombus
Toxemia
Transfusion
Transient ischemic attacks (TIAs)

Varicose vein removal
Varicose veins
Vascular medicine
Vascular system
Venous insufficiency
Von Willebrand's disease

VIROLOGY
Acquired immunodeficiency
  syndrome (AIDS)
Biological and chemical weapons
Chickenpox
Childhood infectious diseases
Chlamydia
Chronic fatigue syndrome
Common cold
Coronaviruses
Creutzfeldt-Jakob disease (CJD)
Croup
Cytomegalovirus (CMV)
Dengue fever
Drug resistance
Ebola virus
Encephalitis
Enteroviruses
Epidemics and pandemics
Epstein-Barr virus
Fever
Gastroenteritis
Hantavirus
Hepatitis
Herpes
H1N1 influenza
Human immunodeficiency virus
  (HIV)
Human papillomavirus (HPV)
Infection
Influenza

Laboratory tests
Marburg virus
Measles
Microbiology
Microscopy
Monkeypox
Mononucleosis
Mumps
Noroviruses
Opportunistic infections
Parasitic diseases
Pelvic inflammatory disease (PID)
Poliomyelitis
Pulmonary diseases
Rabies
Retroviruses
Rheumatic fever
Rhinitis
Rhinoviruses
Roseola
Rotavirus
Rubella
Sarcoidosis
Serology
Severe acute respiratory syndrome
  (SARS)
Sexually transmitted diseases
  (STDs)
Shingles
Smallpox
Tonsillitis
Tropical medicine
Viral hemorrhagic fevers
Viral infections
Warts
Yellow fever
Zoonoses